1 MONTH OF
FREE
READING

at

www.ForgottenBooks.com

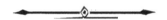

By purchasing this book you are
eligible for one month membership to
ForgottenBooks.com, giving you
unlimited access to our entire
collection of over 1,000,000 titles via
our web site and mobile apps.

To claim your free month visit:

www.forgottenbooks.com/free870141

ISBN 978-0-266-58034-8
PIBN 10870141

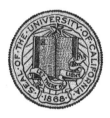

ELEMENTS

OF

GENERAL AND PATHOLOGICAL

ANATOMY.

OF

GENERAL AND PATHOLOGICAL ANATOMY,

PRESENTING A

VIEW OF THE PRESENT STATE OF KNOWLEDGE IN THESE BRANCHES OF SCIENCE.

BY

DAVID CRAIGIE, M.D., F.R.S.E.

FELLOW OF THE ROYAL COLLEGE OF PHYSICIANS, EDINBURGH,
AND HONORARY CONSULTING PHYSICIAN
TO THE ROYAL INFIRMARY.

SECOND EDITION,
ENLARGED, REVISED, AND IMPROVED.

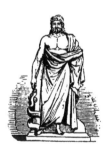

PHILADELPHIA:
LINDSAY AND BLAKISTON.
1851.

PREFACE

TO THE FIRST EDITION.

THE value of Morbid Anatomy as the basis of rational Pathology was early recognized by physicians; and the works of Wepfer, Gerard Blasius, Schenke, Pechlin, Harder, Plater, Van der Wiel, and Fantoni, demonstrate the diligence with which the pathologists of the 17th century laboured to investigate the nature and effects of morbid action. The elaborate, but somewhat confused, collection of Bonetus was the first attempt to classify the facts observed by these and previous authors. To Morgagni, however, was reserved the merit of publishing a work, distinguished equally by critical knowledge of the labours of his predecessors and contemporaries, and by accurate personal observation. From the days, indeed, of Fantoni, Valsalva, and Morgagni, to those of Sandifort, Baillie, Meckel, and Laennec, the study of Morbid Anatomy has been assiduously cultivated by all who were interested in the progress of accurate knowledge.

At no period, however, has this department of science been pursued with greater zeal than during the last twenty years, in the course of which the observation and collection of pathological facts has engrossed the attention of numerous observers, both in this country and in France and Germany. Of this the result has been, more accurate distinction of diseases formerly confounded, fuller and more precise information regarding those which were imperfectly known, and an extraordinary accumulation of matter on all topics. In some instances the boundaries of the science have been extended; in others, departments already known have been more

diligently explored; and if the result has not at all times been absolute discovery, some advantage has accrued from the correction
or the modification of former statements.

The advantage to the science at large has nevertheless been accompanied with great and increasing inconvenience to the student.
The recorded information is scattered through so many volumes,
that the usual period allotted to the acquisition of knowledge is
quite inadequate to consult them in the most cursory manner.
Many of the most valuable papers also are contained in periodical
works, in which it is not always easy to peruse them. In short, so
great is the accumulation of materials, yet so dispersed and multiplied, that the most intrepid diligence is disconcerted, and the
most indefatigable perseverance is exhausted.

To alleviate, if not to remove, some of these difficulties, the most
obvious plan is to classify the principal facts, which it is important
for the student to know; to reduce to general heads the numerous,
isolated, and not unfrequently unarranged facts, recorded by different observers; to reconcile what is discordant; to explain what is
anomalous; to distinguish the essential from the accidental,—the
important from the trivial; and to exhibit in a connected and systematic shape those deductions and inferences, which are justified
by accurate analytic comparison of the best authenticated facts.
Though these are the objects which have been held in view in the
composition of the present volume, it can only be determined by
others, with what success they have been attained.

In the arrangement of the materials of which it consists, I found
it impossible to adopt the methods in ordinary use. Without pre-
tending to determine the comparative merits of the methods of
Baillie, Conradi, Meckel, and Cruveilhier, each of which has peculiar advantages, I may be permitted to observe, that the first object in tracing the progress and effects of pathological processes is
to fix the boundary between what is sound and what is morbid, and
that every morbid process always bears some relation to the proper
characters of the texture in a sound state. For these reasons, I
have chosen as the basis of arrangement, the distinctions of the com-

ponent tissues of the animal body, as derived from the similitude and difference of their anatomical characters; and, though the advantages of .this method have been recognized by John Hunter, Carmichael Smyth, Bichat, Dr Thomson, and Beclard, I am not aware that any complete system of pathological anatomy has been hitherto constructed according to its principles. The present attempt is, I believe, the first instance, in which it has been carried to the length of a full though elementary treatise.

It is almost superfluous to enter into any detailed account of the principles on which this work is composed. In describing both the sound and morbid states of the different organic tissues, I have in general indicated the sources of my information. On the subject of the normal or healthy states, without neglecting the labours of previous authors, it has been my study to give accurate descriptions of the objects from frequent and careful personal dissection. Whatever I have stated on my own authority has been from repeated and rather elaborate examination; and if I have erred or misrepresented, it is not from carelessness or indifference in the endeavour to insure accuracy.

In describing the pathological changes incident to each tissue, it has been my study not so much to speak from personal observation, as to generalize with fidelity the results of the researches of others. In a subject so extensive and so complicated as Morbid Anatomy, individual observation and research are of little avail, unless as they tend to confirm, to correct, or to modify the results obtained by other inquirers. The duty of the author of an elementary treatise in such circumstances is chiefly to compare and generalize these results. For these reasons, I have seldom spoken of what I have seen myself, unless where that tended either to confirm some uncertain inference; to settle some controverted or ambiguous point; or to verify views, in favour of which information was either scanty, deficient, or contradictory. I must, however, say, that, in adducing the testimony of other observers, I have in no instance spoken on subjects which I have not taken care to verify myself. Of every morbid change described, the description is derived in some instan-

ces from repeated inspection,—in all from more or less personal
examination of its physical and anatomical characters.   Of my own
observation, however, I say nothing, but leave the reader to judge
both of its extent and its accuracy.

  Though I have been thus studious to avoid intentional errors, it
is possible that many have been committed in the course of the volume, both from ignorance and from oversight.   These I will not
extenuate by any apology derived either from the difficulty and complicated nature of the subject, or from the calls of other professional
engagements.   When such apology is admissible, its first interpretation is,—that the author should have left the undertaking to some
one better qualified by opportunities and attainments to execute it
creditably.   On some points I have gone less into detail than the
nature of the subject may seem to require; on others unnecessary
diffuseness may be perceived; and in some, perhaps, omissions may
be detected.

  In the section on the Diseases of the Nerves, though I refer to
the cases of Mojon and Covercelli, I confess that I had at the time
some doubts regarding the connection between existence of the tumour and the epileptic motions.   Since that sheet was printed I
met with the remarkable case of Dr Short,* which has tended to
remove these doubts; and I have elsewhere offered a conjecture on
the connection between these tumours and the sensation called
epileptic aura.   This it was unnecessary to notice, had not my
friend, Mr William Wood, attaching to the conjecture more value
than it really merited, resumed with his usual acuteness the investigation of a subject, on which he was the first to communicate exact information.   The monograph of Mr Wood, published in the
third volume of the Edinburgh Medico-Chirurgical Transactions,
is now not only the fullest, but the best account of the neuromatic
tubercle; and had it been composed previous to the sheet in which
the account in the present volume is contained, would have enabled
me to give a much better description of that disease.

  To the peculiar disease of the intestinal mucous membrane in

---

        * * Medical Essays and Observations, Vol. iv. p. 416.

children described by Dr Crampton, I have not assigned a separate place in the text, from difficulty of understanding its exact nature. In some of the cases recorded by that physician, the *villi* seemed converted into tubercles. In others the presence of pustular ulcers not unlike small-pox seems to indicate the usual follicular disease of that membrane. And in others the granular appearance of the villous membrane appears to correspond with the usual effects of dysenteric inflammation. These appearances the ingenious author of the account ascribes to inflammation operating on the strumous habit.*

The work of Dr Abercrombie on the Pathology of the Intestinal Canal, I did not receive till the sheets on the diseases of the Mucous and Serous Membranes were printed. It was therefore impossible for me to avail myself of the researches of that acute observer.

On one department of Pathological Anatomy the reader will find little or no information in the present volume. I allude to local diseases, and to those varieties of malformation which consist in misapplications of the component parts of organs. These, it is almost superfluous to remark, cannot, without violation of the principles of arrangement, be introduced in a work on General Anatomy; and I have therefore, however reluctantly, excluded them almost entirely, unless so far as their general characters could be stated.

Farther, it was my intention to conclude the work with an account of the healthy structure and the morbid changes of the glandular system. I found it, however, difficult to give such a general sketch of the healthy anatomy of these organs as would be applicable to all without being untrue of any,—and by no means easy, without swelling a volume already too large, to exhibit such a view of the anormal deviations as would be either just or useful. This, therefore, I am obliged to defer for the present.

Lastly, The limits within which it is requisite to confine this work, principally intended for the student of pathology, have com-

* Dublin Reports, Vol. ii. p. 286.

pelled me to touch very cursorily on many points, which, from
their importance, would have required fuller details. Though I
have throughout been solicitous to present the unbroken chain of
evidence, on which the inferences and deductions are made to rest,
I have often been obliged to state the latter only, and in a form
perhaps too dogmatic, with the view of saving the time of the
reader. In no instance, however, has this been done without
deliberate examination of the authorities for every fact, and of the
evidences for each conclusion. On ordinary points, on which
pathological opinion is unanimous, I have been sparing of reference,
or omitted it entirely. On subjects, on the contrary, on which
information is doubtful and scanty, or on which there is room for
diversity of sentiment, I have, by referring the reader to the best
sources, enabled him to appreciate the validity of the conclusions
stated. Without attempting, however, to refer to all the authorities extant, which must have uselessly enlarged the work, I have
directed him chiefly to those which are at once most useful and
most accessible.

EDINBURGH, 4th November 1828.

ADVERTISEMENT.

In preparing the present Edition all the materials of the first have been employed. But they have been greatly increased by the introduction of new matter under the proper heads, in order to carry forward to the present time the information acquired since the appearance of the first edition. Numerous rectifications, both in healthy and morbid anatomy, have also been made.

Besides the changes now mentioned, two new books have been added; one on the Structure and Morbid States of the Glands; the other on the Structure and Morbid States of the Lungs and Heart.

The object of the author throughout the volume has been to communicate precise and useful information in a perspicuous and methodical manner. Of the difficulties attending the undertaking he is fully aware; and it is possible, that, after all endeavours to render the work perfect, it may still present defects. In a subject so extensive and complicated as morbid anatomy, and which is cultivated by so many assiduous inquirers, the difficulty of presenting the most recent views must always be great. This, however, the author has studied to do, so far as the limits of the work permit.

Novelty, however, is not the only object which the author of a work on pathological anatomy should keep in view. His great object must be to furnish correct statements and useful information on the nature and distinctive characters of diseases. On this account the author has adhered, as formerly, to the principle of judicious selection.

By some it may be expected that this work should have been illustrated with delineations, more especially in reference to micrscopical anatomy. These, however, would have added so much to the expense of the work, without otherwise increasing its value, that it was thought best for the present to dispense with their assistance. The most effectual way to obtain information in microscopical anatomy is for the student to take frequent opportunities of examining, by the microscope, the textures in their healthy and diseased states. In this, as in all other branches of knowledge, nothing can be compared to practice and experience; and no information is equal to that which is obtained by frequent personal observation.

In conclusion, the author trusts, that while the work in its present form may be useful to students and practitioners, it is still more worthy of that degree of favour, with which it was received by those distinguished members of the profession, whose approbation it must always be an honour to obtain.

20, QUEEN STREET,
4th November 1847.

CONTENTS.

BOOK I.

SIMPLE ELEMENTARY TISSUES.

BOOK II.

NERVOUS SYSTEM.

BOOK III.

KINETIC TEXTURES.—STEREOMORPHIC
TEXTURES.

4

BOOK IV.

MEMBRANOUS OR INVESTING TEXTURES.

BOOK V.

THE GLANDS.

BOOK VI.

THE LUNGS AND HEART.

CHAPTER I.

CHAPTER II.

ELEMENTS

OF

GENERAL AND PATHOLOGICAL ANATOMY.

BOOK I.

CHAPTER I.

DIVISION OF THE TEXTURES.

THE Human Body has been said to consist of solid and fluid parts, the former of which are organized, and determine the shape of the body and its parts. In the same manner the solid parts were distinguished into simple and vital; the first of which were believed to possess only the general properties of matter, as weight, cohesion, elasticity, flexibility, &c. but to be destitute of sensibility and mobility, the great characteristics of the vital solids. Under the head of vital solids it is evident that the brain, *cerebellum*, spinal chord, and nervous branches on the one hand, and the whole of the muscles on the other, were comprehended. Of the simple solids, on the contrary, bone, tooth, cartilage, tendon, and ligament were conceived to be examples. This division, which was made at a time when the attention of physicians was more attracted by physical and mathematical, than by physiological and vital properties, may now be safely set aside, while we adopt another which, though less scholastic, is more suited to the nature of living bodies.

In the living body, it may be observed, there is no solid which is not alive, and which does not possess vital properties; and there is no vital solid which does not possess all the properties ascribed to the simple solid, or the usual attributes of inanimate matter. The great characteristic of living or organic bodies is, that every substance which enters into their composition possesses not only the usual properties of matter, as weight, cohesion, flexibility, elasticity, &c., but also peculiar properties not found in inorganic bo-

A

dies, and which have therefore been termed indiscriminately *animal
or living properties.*

Every animal body consists of several kinds of organic substance, which differ from each other in various modes, and each
of which is characterized by peculiar properties. In the human
body, and in those of all mammiferous animals, these various kinds
of organic substances are believed to be presented in their most
perfect state; and it is to these more especially that the attention
of the pathologist is directed, and from their examination that his
knowledge is derived.

At an early period of the study of anatomy, the human body
was distinguished into various kinds of animal substance; and we
find even in the writings of JACOPO BERENGER of Carpi, (1521),
but more distinctly in the great work of VESALIUS, an enumeration and general description of the different kinds of substance
found to constitute the human body. The example given by these
founders of the science was imitated to a greater or less extent,
and in different degrees of perfection by succeeding systematists;
and we find in the works of RIOLAN,* ADRIAN SPIGEL,† CASPAR
and THOMAS BARTHOLIN,‡ DIONIS,§ MARCHETTIS,|| WILLIS,¶ and
WINSLOW,** but especially in the bulky compilation of SAMUEL
COLLINS,†† various attempts to communicate a just idea of the in-

* Joannis Riolani Ambiani Medici Parisiensis Opera Omnia. Parisiis, 1610. Folio.
† Adriani Spigelii de Corporis Humani Fabricâ, libri x. 4to, 1632.
‡ Thomæ Bartholini, Anatomia Reformata, ex [Casparis Bartholini Parentis Insti-
tutionibus omniumque Recentiorum et propriis observationibus. 8vo, Hagæ Comi-
tum, 1660.
§ The Anatomy of Human Bodies improved, &c., publicly demonstrated in the
Royal Garden at Paris, by Monsieur Dionis, Chief Surgeon to the late Dauphiness,
and to the present Duchess of Burgundy. Translated from the third edition. Lon-
don, 1703.
|| Dominici de Marchettis Anatomia. Batav. 1652, 4to.
¶ Thomæ Willis, M. D. Opera Omnia. Amstelædami, 1682. 4to. Pharmaceutice
Rationalis. This treatise contains much information on the anatomical structure of
the textures and organs.
** Exposition Anatomique de la Structure du Corps Humain. Par Jacques-Benigne
Winslow, de l'Academie Royale, &c. &c. A Paris, 1732. 4to.
†† A System of Anatomy treating of the Body of Man, Beasts, Birds, Fish, Insects,
and Plants, illustrated with many Schemes, consisting of a variety of elegant Figures
drawn from the Life, and engraven in twenty-four folio Copperplates. By Samuel
Collins, Doctor of Physic, Physician-in-Ordinary to his late Majesty of blessed memory,
and Fellow of the King's most famous College of Physicians in London, and formerly
a Fellow of the Royal Foundation of Trinity College, in the most flourishing University of Cambridge. In the Savoy, printed by Thomas Newcomb, 1685. Two volumes folio.

timate structure and properties of the several animal textures. In general, however, these notices are meagre and scanty. Sometimes they are too generalizing, and hastily refer every variety of texture to one or two hypothetical elements; too often they consist of fanciful conjectures substituted for accurate observation; and they are never so clear and satisfactory as to afford useful instruction to the pathological inquirer.

MARCELLO MALPIGHI, born in 1628, professor of medicine successively in the universities of Bologna, of Pisa, and of Messina, and finally invited to Rome as physician to Innocent XII., was the first anatomist in whose hands the knowledge of intimate structure became a science of accurate observation. In this manner (1660) he investigated assiduously the minute structure of the lungs and the disposition of their vessels; he examined the omentum, (1661), and inquired into the manner in which fat and marrow are secreted; he studiously endeavoured (1665) to unfold by dissection and microscopical observation the minute structure of the brain; he demonstrated the organization of the skin, and considered its constituents as the organ of touch; he studied the structure of bone, and exposed the errors of Gagliardi; he traced the formation and explained the structure of the teeth; and he finally carried his researches into the substance of the liver, the spleen, the kidneys, and the conglobate glands, (1666.) In these delicate and difficult inquiries, the observations of Malpighi are in general faithful to nature, and his descriptions accurate. The information which he collected was new and curious, and it is communicated in perspicuous language, and in an interesting manner. He may be justly regarded as the founder of that part of anatomical science which treats of structure and organization; and even in the present day his writings on this subject are by no means destitute either of interest or instruction.

About the same time (1641) the researches of DE GRAAF and RUYSCH tended to throw some light on the intimate structure of several organs. De Graaf, who was young, while Malpighi was declining in years, (1664), studied particularly the structure of the pancreas, and of the organs of generation in both sexes, (1668), and at once removed many popular errors, and communicated a large proportion of accurate information. Had he not been cut off at the early age of thirty-two, (1673), it cannot be doubted that his zeal in prosecuting the true knowledge of minute structure would have greatly advanced this department of anatomy.

FREDERIC RUYSCH, (1638), professor of anatomy and surgery at Amsterdam, was more fortunate. Assiduously devoted during a long life to the cultivation of anatomy, and eminent for the perfection to which he carried the art of injecting, he was enabled to obtain more correct views than his predecessors of the arrangement of minute vessels in the interior of organs, and to demonstrate peculiarities of organization, which had escaped the scrutiny of previous anatomists. Scarcely a part or texture of the human body eluded the penetration of his syringe; and his discoveries were proportionally great, (1665). His researches on the lungs, on the vascular structure of the skin, of the bones and their epiphyses, of the spleen, of the glans penis, the clitoris, (1691), and the womb, impregnated and unimpregnated, were sufficient to give him the reputation. of a most able and accurate anatomist, (1701). These, however, were but a limited part of his anatomical labours. He studied the minute structure of the brain, (1715); he demonstrated the organization of the choroid plexus; he described the state of the hair when affected with Polish plait; he proved the vascular structure of the teeth; he injected the dura mater, the pleura, the pericardium, and peritoneum; he investigated the structure of the synovial apparatus placed in the interior of the joints, and he discovered many curious particulars relating to the lacteals, the lymphatics, and the lymphatic glands. So assiduously, indeed, did Ruysch study by injection the tissues and organs of the animal body, that it is less easy to say what he did than what be neglected. We are indebted to him for many of the facts of which anatomy at the present day consists, (1731.)

The labours of these ingenious and indefatigable inquirers added considerably to the stock of accurate knowledge, and tended to diffuse a taste for correct observation in the study of the minute structure of the parts of the animal body. Not much, however, had been done for the arrangement of the materials thus collected. Though many isolated facts had been established, and several curious discoveries had been made, they were not yet digested in that systematic order which renders them useful to the purposes of pathology.

It is in the great work of HALLER (1757), that we recognise the first tráces of a better spirit and more philosophical views. This accomplished scholar and indefatigable observer was the first who attempted to present, in a collected form, the most correct information on the intimate structure of the animal tissues. Assiduous in his cultivation of anatomy, and deeply impressed with the necessity of accuracy in research, Haller scrutinized with the eye of rigorous observation every point in anatomical structure advanced by his predecessors and contemporaries. In his description of the cellular web, of the adipose membrane, of arterial texture of the veins, of the structure of the heart, of that of the brain and nerves, of the lungs, of the minute structure of the muscles, of the membranes, and of the organs in general, the reader perceives, that, while Haller did not disdain to avail himself of the results of previous and coeval inquiry, he scrupulously avoided adopting what he had not verified by personal observation. The work which he modestly styled Elements of Physiology shows, that, in extent of information and soundness of judgment, he had no rival in the day in which he lived; and though something has been added to science since his death, it is more by the combined efforts of many than by the labours of any individual.

Amidst so much excellence it was unfortunate that the vain search after an elementary fibre or rudiment, into which every variety of animal substance was supposed to be resolved, led him to indulge in some fanciful conjecture and gratuitous generalization.*

The distinction of the animal body into separate kinds of texture (1757), thus introduced and recognised, was confined principally to anatomy and physiology. The merit of applying them to pathology is divided between William Hunter, William Cullen, and John Hunter. The first, in a paper on Emphysema, in the second volume of the Medical Observations and Inquiries (1762,) gave in 1757 an ingenious account of the difference between the cellular tex-

---

* It will scarcely be credited that Haller could speak of this hypothetical fibre in the following terms. "*Fibra* quo communi nomine multiplex genus elementorum comprehendimus, et cujus discrimina continuo exponemus, communis toti humano corpori materies est, etiam, ut alibi ostendemus, cerebro et medullæ spinali. Fragilis aut mollis, elastica, aut penitus pultacea, longa absque fere latitudine, vel lata ut longitudini par fere latitudo sit, ossa, cartilagines, membranas, vasa, ligamenta, tendines, musculos, nervos, cellulosum textum, viscerum parenchymata, pilos et ungues sola constituit." Here it is represented as constituting the most opposite animal substances, and entering into the composition of every texture. The composition of this ideal fibre is not less wonderful. "Invisibilis ea fibra, quam sola mentis acie attingimus, ex solis elementis terreis et glutine, non ex minoribus fibris composita, cum sui similibus abit in duo conspicua elementa solida corporis animalis."

ture and the adipose membrane, with some observations on the serous membranes, and showed in what manner the respective properties of each tend to modify their different morbid states. In the Nosology, Physiology, and First Lines of Dr Cullen, (1765, 1769), we find the author making frequent allusion to the organic properties of the various substances which enter into the composition of the animal body, (1777), and employing these distinctions as the foundation of his Pathology. In the hands of John Hunter this system was carried to still greater perfection; and his work on Inflammation contains the rudiment of many of the improvements which Pathology has derived from this source.

General anatomy was thus beginning to attain insensibly the form of a science, and to be cultivated with assiduity as the surest basis of pathological knowledge. I must not omit to mention, that in the time of the elder Hunter and Cullen it underwent a valuable improvement in the hands of an ingenious foreigner. This consisted in the systematic and connected view which ANDREW BONN of Amsterdam delineated of the mutual connections of the membranes of the human body. In his Inaugural Dissertation, *De Continuationibus Membranarum*, published at Leyden in 1763, this author, after some preliminary observations on membranes in general, and on their structure and organization, unfolds the structure of the skin and its component parts, as ascertained by the best anatomists. He then proceeds to trace its continuation or transition into the mucous membranes, which he regards as productions of the skin; 1*st*, By the eyelids into the lacrymal passages; 2*d*, Into the external ear-hole; 3*d*, Into the nasal passages in the form of the Schneiderian, or pituitary membrane; 4*th*, Into the mouth, throat, and Eustachian tube and tympanal cavity; 5*th*, By the larynx and windpipe into the bronchial tubes and lungs; 6*th*, By the pharynx and œsophagus into the stomach and bowels, where, at the lower extremity of the rectum, its continuity with the skin may again be traced. He concludes this part of his essay with a short view of the transition of the skin into the mucous membrane of the urinary and genital organs, or what has since been named the genito-urinary surface. This may be regarded as the first division of his subject.

In the second, in which he treats of the membranes beneath the skin, he considers, 1*st*, Those of the muscles, as the cellular membrane and aponeurotic expansions; 2*d*, The periosteum and perichondrium, with their modifications and uses; and shows that one or other of these membranes invests and connects every bone of the skeleton.

In the third division he places the internal membranes of cavities, or those which are now denominated serous and fibro-serous membranes. He first traces at great length the course and divisions of the *dura mater* and *pia mater*, and contends that they accompany each nerve and nervous branch; then examines the course of the pleura and pericardium, and the relations of the mediastinum; and, lastly, he describes the extent of the peritoneum and its several divisions in connection with the organs contained in the abdominal cavity.*

The quantity of accurate information which Bonn has here collected, and the new and interesting views which he communicates are truly wonderful. This essay is one of the best specimens of correct and useful generalization which can be imagined; and it is an example of the capricious nature of scientific reputation, that, while the work of Bichat, which was published forty years after, though little more than the thesis of Bonn expanded, has given its author an imperishable name, the small treatise of Bonn is equally unknown and unregarded, and has scarcely served to rescue his name from utter oblivion.

I have already alluded to the application of the distinctions of general anatomy to pathology in the writings of Cullen and John Hunter (1790). A more complete specimen of this was given in 1790 by Dr Carmichael Smith. In a paper published in the second volume of the Medical Communications of London,† this physician took a view of the phenomena and peculiarities of inflammation as they are observed in the different sorts of organic substance found in the animal body. This may be regarded as the first systematic attempt in this country to trace the influence which different peculiarities of structure exercise on the phenomena and progress of morbid action.

After this time various attempts were made to enumerate and

* Specimen Anatomico-Medicum Inaugurale de Continuationibus Membranarum, quod publicæ ac solemni disquisitioni submisit, Andreas Bonn, Amstelædamo-Batavus ad diem 14 Octobris 1763. Extat in Thesauro Dissertationum, Programmatum, alio. rumque Opusculorum Selectorum, Eduardi Sandifort, M. D., &c. Vol. II. Rotterodami, 1769, xii. p. 265.

† Transactions of a Society for Promoting Medical Knowledge, Vol. II. London, 1790.

classify the several animal substances of which the human body consists, and to describe, in general terms, their obvious and distinctive characters and properties. M. Pinel, in his *Nosographie Philosophique*, first published in 1798, made the distinctions of the membranes and other animal tissues the foundation of his arrangement and pathology.

Soon after Xavier Bichat, (1800), in his Treatise on the Membranes, gave a neat and comprehensive view of the general structure of these tissues, and of their connection with the vital and morbid processes carried on at their respective surfaces. This, however, was merely the introduction to a work still more extensive and elaborate. In his Treatise on the Membranes he confined himself to the examination of the structure and properties of the mucous, serous, and fibrous membranes, and a short view of the fibro-mucous and fibro-serous tissues. In his General Anatomy, which appeared in 1801, he delineated the first, and perhaps the most perfect arrangement of the different organic textures of the human body that has yet appeared.

This author considers the human body as an assemblage of many different organs (1801), each of which consists of a greater or smaller number of animal substances, which, though thus combined in the formation, or entering into the composition of the same part or organ, are very different in structure and properties from each other. Each of these distinct forms of animal matter he calls a *tissue* or texture, (*textus, tela ;*) and he refers the whole of those which anatomists have enumerated, or which accurate discrimination can distinguish in the human body, to twenty-one general heads.

1. CELLULAR. Subdivided into
  - Subcutaneous, connecting the skin to the subjacent parts.
  - Subserous, connecting the serous or transparent membranes to the contiguous parts.
  - Submucous, connecting the mucous membranes to the subjacent parts.
  - Arterial, surrounding and enclosing arteries.
  - Venous, ...   veins.
  - Excretory, ...   excretory ducts.
  - Enveloping, surrounding and enclosing organs.
  - Penetrating, entering into the substance of organs.

2 and 3. NERVOUS. { *a* Animal life. { *b* Organic life.

4. ARTERIAL.
5. VENOUS.
6. EXHALANT.
7. ABSORBENT. { Absorbent vessels. { Absorbent glands.
8. OSSEOUS. { Bones proper, long, flat, and short. { Teeth.
9. MEDULLARY. { Marrow of short and flat bones, or the ends of long bones. { Marrow of the shafts, or bodies of long bones.

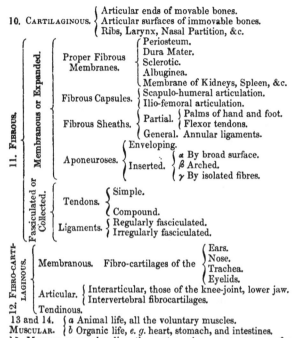

10. CARTILAGINOUS.
- Articular ends of movable bones.
- Articular surfaces of immovable bones.
- Ribs, Larynx, Nasal Partition, &c.

11. FIBROUS.

Membranous or Expanded.

Proper Fibrous Membranes.
- Periosteum.
- Dura Mater.
- Sclerotic.
- Albuginea.
- Membrane of Kidneys, Spleen, &c.

Fibrous Capsules.
- Scapulo-humeral articulation.
- Ilio-femoral articulation.

Fibrous Sheaths.
- Partial. { Palms of hand and foot. / Flexor tendons.
- General. Annular ligaments.

Aponeuroses.
- Enveloping.
- Inserted. { α By broad surface. / β Arched. / γ By isolated fibres.

Fasciculated or Collected.

Tendons. { Simple. / Compound.

Ligaments. { Regularly fasciculated. / Irregularly fasciculated.

12. FIBRO-CARTILAGINOUS.

Membranous. Fibro-cartilages of the { Ears. / Nose. / Trachea. / Eyelids.

Articular. { Interarticular, those of the knee-joint, lower jaw. / Intervertebral fibrocartilages.

Tendinous.

13 and 14. MUSCULAR. { a Animal life, all the voluntary muscles. / b Organic life, e. g. heart, stomach, and intestines.

15. MUCOUS, comprehending the gastro-pulmonary mucous surface, and genito-urinary mucous surface.

16. SEROUS, comprehending the arachnoid membrane, pleura, pericardium, peritonæum, and vaginal coat.

17. SYNOVIAL.

18. GLANDULAR, comprehending the secreting glands only.

19. DERMOID or CUTANEOUS.

20. EPIDERMOID or CUTICULAR.

21. PILOUS or HAIRY.

These different forms of animal substance he considers as the organic elements, or proximate principles, to use the language of chemistry, into which animal bodies may be resolved. These elementary tissues he again refers to two great orders,—one generally distributed and everywhere present, so as to form an integrant part of every other animal substance. To this order, which he termed *general or generating systems,* he referred cellular membrane, arterial and venous tissue, the nerves, and the exhalants and absorbents. The substances of the second kind, which are placed in determinate situations, and confined to particular regions, consist of the bones, cartilages, fibrous substances, muscles, and muscular parts, the mucous, serous, and synovial membranes, glandular organs, the skin and its appendages, the nails, hair, &c.

All the substances of this latter order consist of a peculiar matter, by which they are distinguished, and more or fewer of the general tissues.

As the structure and properties of the same elementary tissue are nearly the same in whatever region of the body it is found, or undergo only such modifications as its peculiar use or local connections render requisite, a just idea of the structure of the human body suggests the propriety of considering the extent, disposition, structure, and most obvious properties, mechanical and vital, of each tissue by itself. The examination of these circumstances constitutes the subject of his General Anatomy, a work which, in originality of plan, and general excellence of performance, notwithstanding occasional defects and errors, has not yet been surpassed.

The arrangement, however, of Bichat has been found incorrect or inconvenient; and various alterations or modifications of it have been proposed by subsequent authors. The first which we shall notice is that proposed by Dupuytren and Richerand, which has been generally esteemed in France as more correct and comprehensive. It may be exhibited in the following tabular form :—

1. CELLULAR.		
2. VASCULAR,	. .	{ Arterial. { Venous. { Lymphatic.
3. NERVOUS,	. .	{ Cerebral. { Gangliar.
4. OSSEOUS.		
5. FIBROUS,	. .	{ Fibrous. { Fibro-cartilaginous. { Dermoid.
6. MUSCULAR,	. .	{ Voluntary. { Involuntary.
7. ERECTILE.		
8. MUCOUS.		
9. SEROUS.		
10. HORNY OR EPIDERMAL,		{ Pilous. { Epidermal.
11. PARENCHYMATOUS,	.	{ Parenchymatous. { Glandular.

In this enumeration several important differences from that of Bichat will be recognized. It presents altogether nineteen separate tissues, of which five are so decidedly peculiar, that they do not admit of being associated with any similar, and consequently form distinct systems by themselves; while the other fourteen are referred to the general heads of vascular, nervous, fibrous, muscular, horny, or parenchymatous systems. The result of this arrangement is to diminish the number of organic systems from twenty-one to eleven, one of which, the *erectile*, comprehending the peculiar structure of the cavernous body, the clitoris, the nipple, and the spleen, is not found in the original arrangement of Bichat, but has been added by MM. Dupuytren and Richerand.

A less neat and elegant arrangement is that given by Hippolytus Cloquet, who admits in the human body the following fifteen tissues: 1. The cellular; 2. The membranous; 3. The vascular, including blood-vessels, and lymphatics; 4. Bone; 5. Cartilage; 6. Fibro-cartilage; 7. Ligament; 8. Muscle; 9. Tendon; 10. Aponeurosis, or fascia; 11. Nerve; 12. Glandular structure; 13. Follicle; 14. Lymphatic ganglion, or gland; 15. The *Viscera*. It is evident that the last mentioned term is greatly too vague, and that the structure which it is intended to denote may be either united with several of those already noticed, or is so different or opposite in different situations, that admitting it as a separate tissue becomes of no use whatever in a correct classification.

Not unlike to the arrangement of MM. Richerand and Dupuytren is that proposed by John Frederic Meckel, who looked on the arrangement of Bichat as too detailed, and embarrassed with too many and minute distinctions. According to this anatomist, the medullary system should be united with the cellular; the synovial should be viewed as a modification of the serous system; the pilous and epidermal systems ought not to be separated from the cutaneous or dermal; and even this last, along with the glandular and mucous, ought to be referred to the same general head. According to these principles all the organized substances composing the human body are referred by Meckel to the following ten heads:—

1. Mucous, or cellular.	6. Fibro-cartilaginous.
2. Vascular.	7. Fibrous.
3. Nervous.	8. Muscular.
4. Osseous.	9. Serous.
5. Cartilaginous.	10. Cutaneous.

Against this arrangement Mayer, professor of anatomy at Bonn, has urged the following objections:—That it is impossible to consider the scarf-skin, or cuticle, and the hairs, as of the same or similar structure with the cutaneous tissue in general: that glandular structure cannot be regarded as pertaining to the same order with the mucous membranes; that the fibro-cartilages ought neither in this arrangement nor in that of Bichat to be considered as distinct from cartilage; and that in both several parts of the ani-

mal body are omitted, or can have no convenient place of reference.   Mayer therefore reduces the twenty-one tissues of Bichat to
seven, and adds an eighth, comprehending the crystalline lens, the
cornea, epidermis, hair, nails, &c. to which he gives the general
name of *lamellar* tissue.   The classification of organic tissues given
by this anatomist would stand in the following order :—*

I. LAMELLAR.
- Crystalline lens,   Cornea.
- Cuticle.
- Hair, nails in whatever form, as claws, bill, hoof.
- Horns, scales, &c.
- Teeth.

II. FILAMENTOUS. CELLULAR.
1. Cellular system,   S. Cellulosum.
2. Adipose system,   S. Adiposum.
3. Medullary system,   Medullare.
4. Serous system,   Serosum.
5. Synovial,   Synoviale.
6. Vascular,   Vasculosum.
7. Dermoid,   Dermodeum.
8. Mucous,   Mucosum.
9. Structure of the womb and reservoirs of secreted
   fluids,   Uterus.

III. FIBROUS.
1. Hard membrane,   Dura meninx, Dura mater.
2. Periosteum.
3. Cartilage.
4. Proper membrane of intestinal tube,   T. Nervosa.
5. Membrane of synovial capsules.
6. Ligaments.
7. Sheaths,   Vaginæ tendinum.
8. Aponeurosis,   Fascia.
9. Tendon.
10. Neurilema.
11. Soft membrane,   Meninx tenuis, Pia mater.

To these may be added a series of parts pertaining at once to the fibrous and the
filamentous cellular system, since their structure presents a predomination of fibrous
filaments.   These are,
1. The Sclerotic.
2. The Tunica albuginea of the testicle.
3. The Proper tunic of the spleen and kidneys.
4. The Cellulo-fibrous sheath of conglomerate and conglobate
   glands.
5. The Corpus cavernosum and C. spongiosum.

IV. CARTILAGINOUS.
V. OSSEOUS.
VI. GLANDULAR.
1. Lymphatic ganglion or glands.
2. α Granular glands, or those provided with excreting duct, the
   lacrymal gland, the salivary glands, the pancreas, liver,
   kidneys.
   β Glandular organs without excreting duct, as the spleen, thymus, renal capsules.

These three forms of glandular organs are considered by Professor Mayer as combi-
nations of minute lymphatics, or blood-vessels, or both united.
VII. MUSCULAR.   1. Animal or voluntary.
2. Organic or involuntary.
VIII. NERVOUS.

* Sur l'Histologie, avec une division nouvelle des tissus du corps humain.   Par le
Docteur Mayer, Prof. d'Anatomie et de Physiologie.   Bonn, 1819.—Journal de Medecine, &c.   Vol. XII. 193, XII. 99.

This arrangement, which is undoubtedly very elaborate, and perhaps more comprehensive than either that of Bichat or any other author, is not, however, quite faultless. It may be doubted whether the lens is an organic body at all, and it is certainly much less an organic substance than the cornea, with which it is arranged. Cellular and cutaneous tissue are certainly not so similar as to admit of being referred to the same rank ; and the organs destined to contain secreted fluids are so opposite and different in structure, that it appears rather violent to connect them in one group. The proper membrane of the intestinal tube is, according to the result of my observations, nothing but the corion of the villous membrane ; at least I cannot conceive any other part to which the description will apply; and surely the soft cerebral membrane (*pia mater*) cannot justly be associated with such substances as ligaments, tendons, or aponeurotic sheaths.

The system termed glandular by Professor Mayer is still more awkwardly situate. For not only is it doubtful with what justice the lymphatic glands are associated with the proper secreting glands, but the latter are themselves much varied in structure and anatomical characters ; and as to the old notion of glandular structure being merely an expansion of vessels arranged in a peculiar manner, I fear that is not only too general to be true, but that there is no tissue in the human body which might not be defined in the same manner.

In the formation of any arrangement of the organic tissues of which the human body consists, two extremes must be sedulously avoided. First, care should be taken not to diminish too much the number of individual or distinct tissues, and to avoid the useless and unnatural system of referring the several substances employed in the construction of the human body to a small number of general heads. This was the error of the ancient physiologists, who, from a wish to simplify more than nature admitted, referred the various animal substances to an elementary fibre or fibres, which they imagined formed the basis or ground-work of the whole animal organization.

The second extreme which ought to be avoided in this matter is the practice of dividing the substances of the animal body into a greater number of distinct kinds and species than is convenient or necessary. Very superficial inspection, indeed, shows that they are not the same either in anatomical or physical characters, or in chemical composition, and that the idea of considering one tissue as a modification of another, or one animal substance as forming or generating another, is, if not unnatural and impossible, at least much more remote from the truth, than to consider them as actually differing in kind, and possessing the properties of a separate form of organized matter. This, therefore, though an evil in its way, is one of much less injurious consequence than the former, which, by its generalizing spirit, has a tendency to supersede investigation, and to consider the nature of the animal tissues as sufficiently established. This perhaps was the error of Bichat, if his arrangement is chargeable with fault. But with still greater justice it may be said, that the recent attempts at classification, like the imperfect ones of the ancient physiologists, are to be blamed in diminishing too much the number of separate tissues, and in delivering arrangements, the principles of which are more general and comprehensive than nature warrants.

It may indeed be assumed as a safe principle, that all the substances employed in the construction of the animal body, which are not very obviously alike, may be considered as separate or distinct proximate principles, till careful examination shall show that they ought to be associated with others. This indeed defeats the purpose of classification, which is useful in proportion as it discovers genuine analogies and general resemblances for the purpose of communicating knowledge with facility; but it also prevents the approach or insinuation of error, by the caution with which it examines, and the discrimination with which it adopts.

In the short view which I propose here to take of the organic tissues, I shall not adhere scrupulously to either of those arrangements which I have already noticed, but attempt to modify that of Bichat, which is perhaps the least objectionable, by adopting as many of the suggestions of his commentators and followers as the nature of the subject and personal observation may seem to authorize. In the course of this exposition I shall have frequent occasion to refer to the best and most complete commentary that has yet appeared,—that by Professor Beclard, who has availed himself of the researches of J. F. Meckel, and Dr J. Gordon of Edinburgh, the Prodromo of Mascagni, the Histologie of Mayer, and the View of Bock.

The human body consists of solid and fluid substances, the former of which are organized, and determine the shape of the body and its parts. These organized solids are not in a strict physical sense solid and impenetrable. Most of them are soft, compressible, and elastic, by reason of the fluid matter contained in their interstices; and when deprived of this by desiccation, they shrink in various degrees, and lose both bulk and weight. The general ratio of the fluid to the solid parts varies from 7 to 1, to 9 to 1. An adult carcass weighing perhaps from 9 to 10 stones, has been reduced by desiccation to $7\frac{1}{2}$ lbs. A human body may be reduced to nearly the weight of its skeleton, which varies from 150 ounces $= 9\frac{3}{8}$ lbs. to 200 ounces $= 12\frac{1}{2}$ lbs.

These organized solids agree in the possession of certain general characters. Their internal structure consists of a union of solid and liquid matter, which is observed to exude in drops more or less abundant from the surface of sections. The solid parts are generally arranged in the form of collateral lines, sometimes oblique, sometimes perfectly parallel, sometimes mutually intersecting. Such lines are denominated *fibres*, and occasionally *filaments*. In other instances the solids are observed to consist of minute globular or spheroidal particles, which are shown by the microscope to be cells or membranous cavities with a central nucleus, connected generally by delicate filaments. Most of these solids anatomists and microscopical observers have attempted to resolve into what they conceive to be an ultimate fibre or last element; but this inquiry leads beyond the bounds of strict observation.

Most of the solids may be demonstrated to be penetrated by minute ramifying tubes or blood-vessels, which traverse their substance in every direction, and in which is contained the greater part, perhaps the whole, of the fluid matter found in the solids. In a few, in which ramifying vessels cannot be positively demonstrated, their existence is inferred by analogy from those in which they can. The filamentous, fibrous, or globular or cellular arrangement, with the distribution of arborescent vessels, constitutes organization. The substances so constructed are named *organized tissues* (*telæ, textus,*) or *textures*, or simply *tissues*.

The organized solids also resemble each other in chemical constitution. They may be resolved into proximate principles, either the same or very closely allied. The proximate principles most generally found are albumen, fibrin, and gelatine, one or other of which, sometimes more, form the basis of every tissue of the human body. Next to these are mucus, and oily or adipose matter. Osmazome or extractive matter is found in certain tissues.

And lastly, several saline substances, as phosphate of lime, carbonate of lime, soda, hydrochlorate of soda, are found in variable proportions in most of them. Of these principles albumen and fibrin, which are closely allied and pass into each other, are the most common and abundant. Osmazome, which is probably a modification of fibrin, is less frequent. These also are contained in the blood, and are derived from that fluid. Gelatine, though not found in the blood, is nevertheless a principle of extensive distribution, being found in skin, cellular tissue, tendon, cartilage, and bone. These proximate principles are resolved, in ultimate analysis, into carbon, oxygen, hydrogen, azote, phosphorus, and sulphur. From the saline substances, calcium, potassium, sodium, chlorine, iron, and manganese may be obtained.

Mulder maintains the existence of another element named proteine, obtained by a particular process from albumen. Its character is that it is a common element to albumen, fibrin, and various of the elements of the tissues.

The different organized solids which enter into the composition of the human body may be referred to the following seventeen simple tissues. Filamentous or cellular tissue, including the ordinary cellular membrane and adipose membrane; artery, vein, with their minute communications, termed capillary vessels, and the erectile vessels; lymphatic vessel and gland; nerve, plexus, and ganglion; brain; muscle; white fibrous system, including ligament, periosteum, and fascia; yellow fibrous system, including the yellow ligaments, &c.; bone and tooth; gristle or cartilage; fibro-cartilage; skin; mucous membrane; serous membrane; synovial membrane; compound membranes, for instance the fibro-mucous, and fibro-serous; and lastly, the peculiar matter which forms the liver, the kidneys, the female breast, the testicle, and other organs termed glands.   To these may be added the compound textures or organs; in which two or more simple textures are united; as the heart and lungs; the larynx; the stomach, *duodenum*, and alimentary canal; the bladder, prostate gland, and penis; and the female organs of generation, as the uterus, ovaries, Fallopian tubes, and vagina with appendages.

These tissues may be distinguished into orders, according to the mode of their distribution in the animal frame. Several, for instance filamentous tissue, artery and vein, lymphatic vessel, and nerve, are most extensively distributed, and enter into the composition of all the other simple tissues. To these, therefore, which are named by Bichat general or generating systems, the character of *textures of distribution* may be applied. A second order, consisting of substances confined to particular regions and organs, and placed in determinate situations, viz. brain, muscle, white fibrous system, yellow fibrous system, bone, cartilage, fibro-cartilage, and gland, may be denominated *particular tissues.* To a third order, consisting of substances which assume the form of a thin membrane, expanded over many different tissues and organs, may be referred skin, mucous membrane, serous membrane, and synovial membrane, under the denomination of *enveloping tissues.* It may indeed be objected, that the circumstance of mechanical disposition is insufficient to communicate a distinctive or appropriate character, and several of the tissues referred to the second head, *e. g. fascia*, must, on this principle, be referred to the third. The objection is not unreasonable. But it may be answered, that it is almost vain to expect an arrangement entirely faultless; and the present is convenient in being on the whole more natural, and therefore more easily remembered, than any other. A distinct idea of it may be formed from the following tabular view.

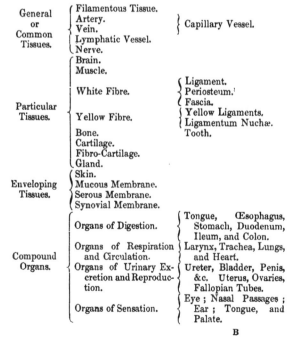

General or Common Tissues.
- Filamentous Tissue.
- Artery.
- Vein.
- Lymphatic Vessel.
- Nerve.
  - Capillary Vessel.

Particular Tissues.
- Brain.
- Muscle.
- White Fibre.
  - Ligament.
  - Periosteum.
  - Fascia.
- Yellow Fibre.
  - Yellow Ligaments.
  - Ligamentum Nuchæ.
- Bone.
  - Tooth.
- Cartilage.
- Fibro-Cartilage.
- Gland.

Enveloping Tissues.
- Skin.
- Mucous Membrane.
- Serous Membrane.
- Synovial Membrane.

Compound Organs.
- Organs of Digestion.
  - Tongue, Œsophagus, Stomach, Duodenum, Ileum, and Colon.
- Organs of Respiration and Circulation.
  - Larynx, Trachea, Lungs, and Heart.
- Organs of Urinary Excretion and Reproduction.
  - Ureter, Bladder, Penis, &c. Uterus, Ovaries, Fallopian Tubes.
- Organs of Sensation.
  - Eye; Nasal Passages; Ear; Tongue, and Palate.

B

CHAPTER II.

THE FLUIDS OF THE HUMAN BODY.

SECTION I.

THE solid or organized textures contain fluids, some for purposes within the system, others destined to be expelled from it. I shall give a short account of the characters and properties of the principal fluids of the body, preparatory to a view of their morbid states.

The fluids of the animal body are various, but may be distinguished into three sorts; the circulating nutritious fluid named the blood, the fluids which are incessantly mixed with the blood for its renewal, and those which are separated from it by secretion.

The blood is well known to be a viscid liquid, of red colour, peculiar odour, and saline, something nauseous taste. Its temperature in the living body is about 97°; its specific gravity is about 105 to water as 100. Its quantity is in the adult considerable, varying from 8 or 10 to 80 or 100 pounds; the average is about 30 pounds.

According to the results of microscopic observation, it consists of red particles suspended in a serous or sero-albuminous fluid. On the shape of these red particles various opinions have been maintained. Generally represented as globular, Hewson describes them as flattened spheroids, or lenticular bodies, a view which is confirmed by the observations of Prevost and Dumas, Beclard, of Hodgkin and Lister, and Mr Wharton Jones. The opinion of Home and Young, that the flattening of these globules is a process posterior to the discharge of the fluid, is not improbable. These particles have since the time of Hewson been almost universally represented as consisting of a central transparent whitish globule, inclosed in a red translucent vesicle, which gives them the shape of an oblate spheroid. In man and the mammalia they are circular discs, often with a depression on the sides. The diameter of these particles is estimated, by the subdivided scale of Kater, the micrometer of Wollaston, and the eriometer of Young, at $\frac{1}{3000}$, and by the common micrometer, at $\frac{1}{1700}$ of an inch. (*Phil. Trans.*) Mr Gulliver estimates the average thickness of the human blood-corpuscle at $\frac{1}{1200}$th part of an English inch, and the diameter at $\frac{1}{3200}$. This description applies to the blood circulating in the vessels.

The flattening of the corpuscles is greatest in reptiles, amphibia, and fishes; and it is most remarkable in the salamander. In birds the red globules are flattened, but in less degree than in the amphibia.

The red particles are largest in the amphibia. In birds, reptiles, and fishes they are smaller. In mammalia they are smallest. (Gulliver apud Hewson, p. 236.)

Discharged from the vessels, it exhales, during the process of cooling, a thin watery vapour, consisting of water suspending animal matter capable of impressing the sense of smell, and undergoing decomposition. During the same space it is observed to be converted into a firm mass, which, though still soft and elastic, is entirely void of fluidity. As this process advances, a thin watery fluid, straw-coloured, not perfectly transparent, is observed to exude from every part of the solid mass, which also diminishes in size, till at length it is found floating like a tolerably thick cake in the thin watery fluid. The thick solid mass is named the clot or *coagulum ;* the watery fluid is denominated *serum ;* and the process of the separation, which is spontaneous, is termed *coagulation.* The blood at the same time is said to discharge carbonic acid.

The clot, if divided and washed in water often changed, or in alcohol or *aqua potassæ,* may be deprived of its red colour, and made to assume a gray or bluish-white tint. This gray mass, which is tough, coherent, opaque, and more or less dense, homogeneous, but void of traces of organic structure, consists chiefly of albumen or fibrin, or a substance partaking of several of the characters of both. To this substance the blood owes its viscidity and its property of spontaneous coagulation ; and from the circumstance of its resemblance to the lymph or albuminous fluid which is effused from wounds and inflamed surfaces, and to the fibrin of muscle, and the albumen of many of the tissues, it may be regarded as the most vital and nutritious part of that fluid. It is a mistake, nevertheless, to assert, as is done by Beclard and others, that this substance presents to the microscope the aspect and structure of muscular fibre. Its aspect is by no means so regular as this, nor can its particles be said to present traces of organic structure or arrangement.

The red matter removed by washing is a mixture of serum, of globules, and of a peculiar colouring matter. Modern chemistry shows that the latter is a particular substance, insoluble in water, but susceptible of suspension in it to an extreme extent, and consisting of animal matter combined with peroxide of iron. It is distinguished by the name of *zoohematine*. Deprived of this, the globules are estimated by Bauer at $\frac{1}{2000}$ of an inch in diameter.

The serum, with the taste and odour of the blood, rather alkaline, coagulates at 162° F. or on the addition of acids, nitrate of silver, or corrosive sublimate, and then resembles boiled white of egg. The coagulated matter is albumen; and a little water containing soda and salts of soda may be separated. It is a remarkable difference between this albumen, which is suspended in the serum, and that which constitutes the clot, that while the former requires heat as a re-agent, the latter assumes the solid form spontaneously.

The proportion of serum to clot varies in different animals, in different individuals, and in different states of the system, healthy and morbid.

In the human body a quantity of five ounces of blood usually furnishes about one ounce and two drachms, or one ounce and four drachms of serum. In inflammatory diseases the amount of the serum is usually increased. Thus in acute rheumatism and in pneumonia, if the buffy coat be thick and strong, the serum afforded by five ounces amounts to one ounce and six drachms, or two ounces. In fever, again, the proportion of serum is diminished. Thus five ounces of blood will afford not more than one ounce, or only six drachms of serum. At advanced periods of the disease, for instance after the first eight days or towards the close of the first septenary period, the serum afforded by five ounces is not more than six or four drachms; and in some instances it is about three drachms or two drachms, or not more than one and a half.

In these circumstances the clot is less firm than usual, and is loose and flabby.

In purpura most commonly no serum is separated; and the clot appears alone as a mass of gelatinised blood imperfectly coagulated.

These phenomena depend on the degree of the coagulating power; and they may be taken to measure its force. Thus in the healthy state, and in certain inflammatory diseases, the coagulating power is greatest. In fever the coagulating power is weakened in proportion as the disease advances. And in purpura and at the close of fever the coagulating power is very nearly null.

. This, however, is merely the relation of the serum to the clot, when under spontaneous coagulation. After this is completed, the clot still retains so much serum, that it must be subjected to repeated pressure, or to evaporation, or both, before the clot can be obtained in a solid and dry state, quite free from serum. When this has been done, it is found that the spontaneously coagulable part of the blood is always much less than the fluid part; in other words, that it is in the ratio of minority to the serum, or numerically in the ratio of 13 to 87 in 100 parts of blood.

Liquid fibrin, or the spontaneously coagulable part of the blood, is most abundant in warm-blooded animals; and among these it is more abundant in the blood of birds than in that of the mammalia. In fishes it is very scanty; and it is sparing also in the blood of the reptile family. In fishes and reptiles it is more in the form of a liquid gore, viscid and semifluid, but scarcely coagulating, than in that of blood.

It is a well-known fact that in frogs the blood does not coagulate on exposure of the vessels to air, as it does in the mammalia. This must be owing either to the blood of these animals containing a much smaller proportion of fibrin than that of the mammalia, or the fibrin having much less coagulating power. In either case it comes to the same result.

This has been supposed by De Saissy and others to bear some relation to the state of respiration in these several classes; and the idea seems accordant with the facts. In birds the function of respiration is most fully developed. In reptiles and fishes it is very imperfectly developed.

When blood drawn from the veins of a person labouring under acute rheumatism and other inflammatory diseases is undergoing coagulation in a glass vessel, a colourless fluid may be perceived round the edge of the surface; and after an interval of four or five minutes, a bluish appearance is observed, forming an upper layer of the blood, in consequence of the subsidence of the red particles to a certain distance below the surface, and the clear liquor being left between the place of the red particles and the edge of the vessel. This liquid may be collected by a spoon and placed in another vessel, where it is first clear, though opalescent, viscid, and homogeneous. After some time, however, it undergoes separation into two parts; one coagulated, the other fluid. The coagulated part is the fibrin of the blood or that which is spontaneously coagulable; the fluid part the serum. The opalescent liquor has been named *liquor sanguinis*, (Babington.)

Gmelin, Chevreul, and Lecanu obtained from the blood stearine and elaine.

The colour of the blood varies in different parts of the system. In the left auricle, ventricle, and arterial trunks generally, its colour is bright scarlet, a tint which it loses in the capillary vessels. In the veins, venous trunks, right auricle, right ventricle, and pulmonary artery, its colour is a dark or purple-red, or modena. As it moves from the trunk and branches through the minute divisions of the pulmonary artery, it gradually parts with this tint; and in the branches of the pulmonary veins it is found to have acquired the bright scarlet colour which it has in the left auricle, ventricle, and aorta. Hence the modena or dark-coloured blood is distinguished as venous, or proper to the veins; and the bright red or scarlet-coloured as proper to the arteries.

In the fœtus, the blood contains little coagulable matter; and this principle is entirely wanting in the blood of the menstrual discharge.

The fluids received by the blood are chyle and lymph. Chyle is derived from chyme, a gray pulpy substance, formed from the alimentary mass in the stomach and duodenum. Detached from this substance, and received by the chyliferous tubes, it is whitish and scarcely coagulable. In the mesenteric glands it becomes more coagulable, and assumes a rose colour. Lastly, in the thoracic duct, and before joining the mass of blood, it is distinctly rose-coloured, coagulable, and globular in its particles. In the branches of the pulmonary artery it appears to become perfect blood. Lymph is a colourless, viscid, albuminous fluid, imperfectly known.

Of the fluids separated from the blood, all cannot be said to belong to the animal body. Several, for instance the perspired fluid of the skin and lungs, the fluid of the cutaneous and mucous follicles, and the urine, become, after secretion, foreign to the body, and require to be removed. Those belonging to the body are such as are prepared for some purpose within it, and after this are either re-absorbed, or, being decomposed, are expelled. Of the former kind, fat, serum of serous membranes, and synovia, afford examples. To the latter description belong tears, saliva, pancreatic fluid, bile, the seminal fluid of the male, and the milk of the female, all of which are the result of a distinct glandular secretion for a specific purpose, after which they are expelled from the economy.

The urine, though also the result of glandular secretion, is nevertheless exempt from this rule, and though separated from arterial blood, is forthwith eliminated. Its chief purpose seems to be to afford a convenient vehicle for ridding the system of superfluous azote, and to maintain the due proportion between this and the other ultimate principles, carbon, hydrogen, and oxygen. The fluids which fulfil a purpose in the economy are regarded as secretory, and are remarkable for a predominance of alkali; those which do not, are excrementitial, and are generally acid.

Bile, the secreted product of the liver, may be regarded as a choleate of soda with taurine; both containing sulphur.

Urine may be regarded as urea suspended or dissolved in water. Urea is the peculiar and characteristic element of the secretion. It contains also a little uric acid, which is probably produced from the urea, as it can scarcely be said to be a constituent of healthy urine. The other ingredients are saline matters common to the blood and the urine, or complementary between these fluids.

The density of healthy urine varies from 1015 to 1033, water being as 1000; and the average, as determined from the examination of the urine in fifty instances of persons in good health, is at the highest 1.026, and at the lowest 1017. The general average, therefore, amounts to 1022. If it be stated between 1022 and 1026 it cannot be far wrong. This is understood while the quantity discharged daily is from 45 to 53 ounces, which is about the general average in healthy individuals who consume liquids at the ordinary rate.

This density above that of water urine owes to the presence of urea and saline matters. If the urea and saline matters be increased, the density of the urine is increased; and if they be diminished, the density of the urine is also diminished.

It may be here observed that urea is the form which the elements of the fibro-albuminous parts of the blood assume after these fibro-albuminous have been employed in repairing the waste of the tissues. If we compare the proximate chemical principles of albumen with those of urea, we shall see that the latter are the complement of the former. Thus

	Hydrogen.	Carbon.	Oxygen.	Azote.
Albumen consists of	7.77	50.00	26.66	15.55
Urea consists of .	6.66	20.00	26.66	46.66

Thus while albumen and urea contain the same proportion of oxygen, the former contains one-seventh more hydrogen, three-fifths more carbon, and one-third less azote. It is known that the former proportions are employed in repairing the waste of the albuminous tissues, especially the muscular system, and while carbon and oxygen are discharged by the lungs, and carbon, oxygen, and hydro-gen by the liver, the large superfluous portion of nitrogen not required is left in the form of urea, to pass through the blood, and by means of the kidneys to be expelled from the system.

In the healthy state urine is always acid when discharged. It is prone, however, to undergo the putrefactive decomposition; and then its acid reaction disappears, and it becomes alkaline. This change is much favoured if not wholly occasioned by the presence of mucus, purulent matter, or other azotized substances; for if the urine be filtered so as to remove these substances, and placed in a close vessel, secluded from the air, it may be preserved for a long time without undergoing change or presenting any odour indicating the presence of decomposition.

Section II.

A. The morbid states of the blood are mostly, if not all, connected with morbid states of the system at large, of the organs of respiration, or the organs of secretion. The most important are the following.

1. In diseases of plethora it has been supposed that the blood is more abundant than usual in quantity, and that its fibrine is increased in proportion. The first point it is not easy to determine. The fibrine, however, is not increased. The red globules are stated by Andral to be the only element in which an increase actually takes place. In 31 blood-lettings he found for the medium the cypher 141 in 1000, 127 in 1000 being the average of health; for the minimum, 131; and for the maximum, 154. There is, in short, in the blood of the plethoric an increased amount of red globules, and a great deal less water than the average.

2. In chlorosis, dyspeptic and other diseases in which the leading character is *anæmia*, the red globules are diminished in proportion. Andral found, as the medium of the cypher for the globules in fifteen cases of incipient anæmia, the number 109, and in twenty-four cases of confirmed anæmia, the number 65. In spontaneous anæmia, mild or violent, the globules alone are diminished; the fibrine and the albumen of the serum preserving their normal proportion. In hemorrhagic anæmia, at first the globules only are diminished. But if the morbid condition continue, the fibrine and the albumen of the serum are also diminished. There is a form of anæmia which may be called *toxic*, as it depends on the influence of the mineral poisons. In that from lead, Andral finds that the

red globules are as much diminished as in spontaneous anæmia, while the fibrine and albumen preserve their normal proportions.

In chlorosis it is a curious fact that the blood is occasionally buffy. This Andral ascribes to the circumstance, that in these patients, while the blood loses its colouring matter, it preserves all its fibrine. It must be observed, nevertheless, that in many chlorotic patients, processes are present which give the blood the tendeney to the buffy coat.

It is also to be observed that in renal dropsy ofttimes, while the blood is deteriorated by diminution of red particles, and while the patient is pale and dropsical, yet blood if drawn presents the buffy coat. This merely shows that the blood is altogether in an unnatural and probably diseased condition. The textures are unable to take from it the fibrine which they do in the healthy state, and hence this fibrine remains ready to be separated in the form of buffy coat.

3. *State of the blood in inflammatory diseases.*—In inflammation the blood assumes the property of forming what is called the buffy coat, (*tunica coriacea*). This consists in the clot presenting at its surface a covering variable in thickness, whitish-grey in colour, and of considerable toughness. In the slightest degree it is very thin, and a mere pellicle. In more considerable degrees of inflammation, it is thicker, as thick as a shilling or a half-crown piece, and firm and tenacious. In the most intense degree, it is as thick as a crown piece or a penny piece; extremely firm, hollow on the top and elevated at the edges; and being contracted from the circumference to the centre, it is much cupped. This condition of the blood is most common in acute rheumatism, pneumonia, pleurisy, *peritonitis*, *hepatitis*, disease of the kidney, the early stage of pulmonary consumption, and similar disorders. It is also observed during pregnancy.

The cause of the buffy coat has been a subject of great inquiry; but regarding it little is ascertained. It may often be observed in the act of formation, by the surface of the blood drawn, as it is coagulating, assuming a peculiar bluish colour, which is evidently dependent on the *liquor sanguinis* undergoing spontaneous coagulation, while the red part of the blood subsides from it. In general the blood coagulates more slowly in inflammatory diseases than in the healthy state. But the rate of the diminution does not correspond to the amount of the buffy coat. If, however, we bear this fact in remembrance, that when it takes place as in inflammatory diseases and in pregnancy, there is in the vessels of some part of the body a process of separating fibrin or fluid fibrin in the shape of lymph, which afterwards undergoes spontaneous coagulation, it may be regarded as most probable, that, while the process of normal nutrition, that is, deposition of fluid fibrin in the different textures and organs, is suspended or diminished, the albuminous matter which ought to be employed in this process is left free in the blood, and therefore is found in that fluid.

Buffy blood is less thick than healthy blood; but its *liquor sanguinis* contains more fibrin. The red globules are very numerous, and they are aggregated rapidly and closely. (W. Jones, Ed. Med. and Surg. Journal, lx.)

In fever, and especially in typhous fever, the blood loses part of its spontaneously coagulating property. The serum is diminished in quantity, or rather is not separated from the clot, which is loose, flaccid, and commonly dark-coloured, and as it were semifluid.

4. *Oil in the blood.*—In certain states of the system the serum is observed to be turbid, opalescent in colour, and not unlike milk. The clot is then in general of a peculiar pink colour, whether from some intrinsic change, or the optical effect of the milky serum. This state of the serum is owing to its being mixed with fatty matter, or rather oil. If serum of this kind be agitated in a phial with a quantity of sulphuric ether, the latter dissolves the oil, which is after some time found floating in the form of a clear yellow oil on the surface of the serum, which is then clear and of its usual characters. The oil may be then withdrawn by the pipette or poured off, and is found to leave on paper an oleaginous stain.

This state of the blood, which was originally observed by Tulpius, Schenke, Morgagni, and Hewson and several of his friends,* and afterwards by Dr Traill, Dr Ziegler, and Dr Christison, takes place in various wasting diseases, and is often observed in granular degeneration of the kidney. The oil appears to be mixed with the serum in the form of an emulsion. It is most usual in corpulent persons; and appears especially, or has been noticed mostly, when they are attacked by disease. It is connected also with an imperfect state of digestion.

5. In jaundice and various diseases of the liver, even in inflammation of the liver affecting the lower surface of the organ and the

* Experimental Inquiries, Part the First, containing an Inquiry into the Properties of the Blood, with Remarks on some of its Morbid Appearances. 3d Edition. By William Hewson, F. R. S. London, 1780. Pp. 191.

vicinity of the capsule of Glisson, the serum occasionally presents a considerable proportion of bile. It is then of a pale green colour; and on the addition of hydrochloric acid, it undergoes immediate coagulation, with the formation of a bright grass-green precipitate.

6. Urea is found in the blood in instances of granular disease of the kidney, and those cerebral and urinary affections in which the secretion of the kidneys is suspended or suppressed. It may be detached from the serum by treating the latter with nitric acid, when crystals of nitrate of urea are found.

7. Purulent matter is found in the blood in certain diseases in which suppuration is going on at the internal surface of a membrane or in the interior of an organ. The most usual preceding state, however, is inflammation and suppuration of a vein or veins, and the secondary effects thence resulting, especially suppuration within one of the joints. If the blood in cases of this kind be inspected under the microscrope, it is observed to present globules of purulent matter. In certain forms of disease of the spleen, purulent matter is found mixed with the blood in the veins after death, to which this state leads.

B. Of chyle and lymph the morbid states are too little known to speak of them with certainty.

C. Of the morbid changes of bile also very little is known. During the process of digestion it is decomposed; at least in the healthy state it is never seen pure in the intestinal discharges.

The bile is liable to be formed into concretions or gall-stones, varying in size. When small these are numerous; when large there may be only one or at most two. A large sized gall-stone is one that is one inch or more in diameter. These bodies consist of inspissated bile, cholesterine, and colouring matter.

D. The morbid states of the urine are manifold. They may be referred to the following heads. 1. Increase in the proportion of nitrogenous matter, e. g. urea increased in quantity generally with formation of uric acid; 2. Diminished cohesion of elements of urea; 3. Increase in saline matter; and 4. By the presence of new substances, as albumen, purulent matter, sugar, &c.

1. The first and most usual is excess of urea, generally with uric acid. The urine, if allowed to evaporate in a watch-glass, one or two drops of nitric acid having been previously poured on it, presents in no long time crystals of nitrate of urea. At the same time uric acid is usually deposited from the urine.

2. Another form of disorder consists in the formation of urate of

ammonia. The uric acid being formed in the urine as in the last case, it is probable that part of the urea itself is decomposed, the nitrogen and hydrogen combining to form ammonia. This takes place in birds and serpents at all times, and carnivorous animals and the human body when living mostly on animal food.

3. A form more intense still is denoted by the formation of carbonate of ammonia. There can be little doubt that when this product appears, it is the result of the spontaneous decomposition of the urea; the carbon and oxygen forming carbonic acid, and the nitrogen and hydrogen ammonia.

4. A form still different is indicated by the formation of phosphate of ammonia and magnesia. The causes and the mechanism of this production are not well known. It is only known that it takes place most readily under a state of the system of impaired strength; that the urine is either not acid or speedily becomes alcaline; and that the urine is most prone to the putrefactive decomposition. As the addition of ammonia to urine causes a precipitate of phosphate of lime, there is strong reason to believe that the urea is first decomposed and its hydrogen and azote made to furnish ammonia, and that this latter substance causes the precipitate either of phosphate of lime or phosphate of magnesia according to circumstances.

5. Other morbid products are purpuric acid, purpurate of ammonia, oxalate of lime.

6. Blood may be contained in the urine either in consequence of wounds and injuries of the kidneys, ureters, bladder, or prostate gland, or in consequence of calculi in any of these parts, or inflammatory and hemorrhagic diseases. The urine is either like blood, containing a considerable proportion of that liquid, or it is only of a dark brown colour, coagulable by heat or acids, and presenting to the microscope blood-globules. The physician has most frequent occasion to see it in the latter state; and sometimes the urine is clear, but depositing the colouring matter of the blood at the bottom of the vessel. This I have observed during scarlet fever, at its close, and especially during the dropsical affection which often succeeds that disorder.

7. Albumen is contained in urine in the form of serum or serous urine. It is known by the urine being paler than usual, by its specific gravity being lowered, that is, being below 1015, generally about 1009, 1010, or 1011, and by being coagulable on the application of heat between 160° and 212° F. The proportion of serum varies from one-tenth to one-fifth, in which case it forms a

3

dense firm jelly adhering to the tube.* The presence of albumen always denotes more or less disease of the kidney, particularly the granular degeneration described by Dr Bright; and, with certain exceptions, the greater the amount of the coagulum, the more intense and decided is the degree of degeneration. In scarlet fever it occasionally indicates merely a state of the kidney allied to acute inflammation.

8. Purulent matter is contained in the urine in various purulent or puriform affections of the kidneys and bladder. Its presence is known by being observed at the bottom of the vessel after the urine has been allowed to rest for some time. When the urine is first voided it is turbid and opaque with numerous *flocculi*, and the colour is generally pale straw with an opalescent tint. After standing some time the upper portion becomes clear, and a layer more or less thick of yellow or whitish grey purulent matter is observed at the bottom of the tube or glass jar. The supernatant urine is often coagulable by the application of heat or the addition of acids. The lower deposit may be recognised by the eye to be purulent matter with shreds of lymph; but it is more easily seen by a good glass; and the microscope exhibits distinctly the purulent globules.

In this state of the urine, as in the last, the patient feels frequent and urgent calls to empty the bladder, in which accordingly the urine seldom accumulates beyond two or three ounces.

9. *Melituria.*—Sugar is the most important foreign or new substance which may be found in the urine. The secretion has in that state, when voided, a smell of whey, or milk, or new hay, less agreeable, however, and somewhat nauseous. Its colour is generally a pale honey yellow, but in some instances it is as deep as that of porter. Its density is always increased, being generally above 1020, and rising from that to 1030, or 1035, or 1050. This is caused by the considerable increase of the solid matters; for not only is there a new substance in the sugar contained, but the urea is increased in quantity and is rarely diminished. It is supposed, however, that in saccharine urine the urea is diminished as the disease advances.

The presence of saccharine matter in urine constitutes the pathological character of the disease named diabetes. With the increase in the amount of urea and the presence of this new element, the quantity of the whole secretion is greatly increased, so that within

* Elements of Practice of Medicine, Vol. II. p. 1122.

24 hours the amount of urine voided is about six or seven times greater than in the state of health.

The presence of saccharine matter in the urine enables it, by the addition of yeast, to undergo fermentation and furnish alcohol.

In this state of the urine, saccharine matter is found also in the gastric juice, and in the blood; and may be obtained from the fluids by chemical analysis. There is, therefore, the best reason to believe, that sugar, when it appears in the urine, is previously formed in the stomach by some great perversion in the digestive and assimilative power.

CHAPTER III.

FILAMENTOUS OR CELLULAR TISSUE. (*Tela cellulosa,—Tissu cellulaire,—Tissu muqueux* of Bordeu,—*Corpus Cribrosum*, Hippocratis,—*Corps Cribleux* of Fouquet,—Reticular membrane of William Hunter.)

SECTION I.

THE general distribution of the filamentous or cellular tissue was first maintained by Haller, and Charles Augustus de Bergen, and afterwards made the subject of more elaborate discussion by William Hunter and Bordeu. It may be described as a substance consisting of very minute thready lines, which follow no uniform or invariable direction, but which, when gently raised by the forceps, present the appearance of a confused and irregular net-work. As these minute lines cross each other, they form between them spaces of a figure not easily determined, and perhaps not uniform. By some authors these spaces or intervals have been named cells; but, accurately speaking, the term is not fortunately applied. The component lines, which do not exceed the size of the silk-worm threads, are so slender, that they do not form those distinct partitions which the term *cell* implies; and though by forcible distension, such as takes place in insufflation or separation by forceps, cavities appear to be formed, these, it will be found, are artificial, and result from the separation of an infinity of the slender filaments of which the part is composed. These interlineal spaces necessarily communicate on every side with each other; and indeed the most distinct way of forming a true idea of the structure of the cellular tissue is to suppose a certain space of the animal body

which is divided and intersected into an infinite multitude of minute spaces, (*areolæ*,) by slender thready lines crossing each other.

This description, originally derived from personal observation,
led me to apply to this tissue the name of *filamentous* as more appropriate than that of *cellular*, by which it is generally known.   I
find, however, that in this I am anticipated by Charles Augustus
de Bergen, the most accurate observer who has treated of its anatomical structure.   His description is so faithful, that it should be
known to the student of general anatomy.   " Alteram vero non
adeo distincté saltem paucissimis, ut mihi videtur, observatam."
He alludes here to the filamentous as distinct from the adipose
tissue.   " Ubi sic dicta cellulosa ex innumerâ atque intricatissimâ
congerie *staminum aut filamentorum*, nullatenus cellulas pingue-
dinem continentes efformantium, componitur ; quæ tenerrima mi-
rificé obliqué disposita, inexplicabili adeo contentu viscerum om-
nium et musculorum substantiam internam perreptant, ut nihil
certi, vel microcospiis adjutus, hic effari queas ; quam proin *substantiam filamentosam* vocabo."[*]

The interstitial spaces resulting from the interlacement of these
filaments do not exist as distinct cavities in the healthy state, so that
they cannot be said to contain any substance solid or fluid.   But
when an incision is made into this tissue in the living body, it is
found, that, if we except those fluids which issue from divided vessels, nothing is observed to escape, but a thin exhalation or vapour,
which is evidently of an aqueous nature.   This is what some authors have termed, from its resemblance to the serous part of the
blood, the *cellular* serosity, (Bichat,) and the quantity of which has
been greatly exaggerated.   In the living body it appears not to
exist as a distinct fluid, but merely as a thin vapour, which communicates to the tissue the moist appearance which it possesses.

This fluid is understood to be derived from the minute colourless
capillaries named *exhalants ;* and it is supposed to be no sooner poured forth in an insensible manner, than it is removed by the absorbing power either of lymphatics, according to the followers of the
Hunterian hypothesis, or of minute veins, according to Magendie.
It is of no great moment whether this process of absorption be ascribed to lymphatics or to veins, or be understood, as is probably the
truth, to be effected by both.   It is sufficient to remark, that, whatever serous fluid is secreted into the insterstitial spaces or cells of

---

[*] Caroli Augusti a Bergen, Programma de Membrana Cellulosa.   Francofurti ad
Viadrum, de 21 Aug. 1732.   Apud Haller, Disputat. Anatomic. Select., Vol. III. p.
82.

the filamentous tissue, makes no long abode in that situation, but in the healthy state is speedily removed; so that if we suppose exhalation, absorption must be also admitted; and the filamentous tissue is therefore represented as the seat of an incessant exhalation and absorption.

The serous fluid of the filamentous tissue varies in quantity in different regions. In the cellular tissue of those parts which are free from fat, as in the eyelids, the prepuce, the *nymphæ* and *labia*, and the scrotum, it is said to be somewhat more abundant than in others. The peculiar structure of those parts, which is cellular, may render any excess of serous fluid more conspicuous; for it is matter of observation, that in many persons otherwise healthy these parts are not unfrequently distended with serous fluid. On the other hand, it must be remarked that the submucous cellular tissue, and that which surrounds arteries, veins, and excreting ducts, which is delicate in substance and compact in structure, contains but a small proportion of serous fluid, and does not readily admit its presence.

This fluid has been generally said to be of an albuminous nature; and if it be identical with the serum of the blood, from which it is believed to be secreted, this character is not unjustly given it. Bichat, who maintained this opinion, injected alcohol into the filamentous tissue of an animal previously rendered emphysematous, and found in various parts *whitish flocculi*, which he regarded as coagulated albumen. He also obtained the same result by immersing a portion of the scrotum in weak nitric acid; and when a considerable quantity of this tissue was boiled, it furnished much whitish foam, which Bichat regarded as albuminous.* These experiments, however, are liable to this objection, that the effects in question may have arisen from coagulation of part of the filamentous tissue itself, which contains a considerable proportion of albuminous matter. The best mode of determining the point is to obtain the fluid apart, and to try the effects of the usual tests on it when isolated from the tissue in which it is lodged.

The description here given applies to the proper filamentous tissue. This substance was shown by Ruysch, and afterwards by William Hunter and Mascagni, to be penetrated by arteries and veins. Exhalants, absorbents, and nerves, it is also said to receive. The arteries certainly belong in the healthy state to the order of colourless capillaries, which is nearly the same with exhalants. It

* Anatomie General, Tome i. p. 50.

does not appear that the nervous twigs observed to pass through this tissue are lost in it, for in general they have been traced to some contiguous part.

Such are the general properties of this tissue considered as an elementary organic substance extensively diffused through the body. In particular regions it undergoes some modifications, which may be referred to the following heads. 1. Beneath the skin, or rather under the adipose membrane ; the subcutaneous and intermuscular cellular tissue; 2. Beneath the villous or mucous membranes; the submucous cellular tissue; 3. Beneath the serous membranes; the subserous cellular tissue; 4. Round blood-vessels, excreting ducts, or other organs; the enclosing tissue, vascular sheaths, &c.; 5. In the substance of organs; the penetrating cellular tissue.

The situation of the subcutaneous filamentous tissue deserves particular notice.   Though generally represented as below the skin, it is not immediately under this membranous covering.   The skin rests on the adipose membrane, beneath which again is placed the filamentous tissue, extending like a web over the muscles and blood-vessels, penetrating between the fibres and bundles of the former, surrounding the tendons and ligaments, and connected by these productions with a deep-seated layer, on which the muscles move, where they do not adhere to the periosteum and to bones.

The extensive distribution of the subcutaneous filamentous tissue, the mutual connection of its parts, and its ready communication with the filamentous tissue of the mucous and serous membranes, were demonstrated by Haller, William Hunter, and Borden, and have been clearly explained by Portal and Bichat.   The principal points worthy of attention may be stated in the following manner.

The filamentous tissue of the head and face communicate freely with each other, and with that of the brain by the cranial openings, and with the submucous tissue of the eyelids, nostrils, lips, and the inner surface of the mouth and cheeks.   It communicates also with the subcutaneous tissue of the neck all round ; and at the angle of the jaw in the vicinity of the parotid gland is the common point of re-union.   To this anatomical fact is referred the frequency of swellings and purulent collections in the region of the parotid in the course of various diseases of the head, face, and neck.

The filamentous tissue of the neck may be viewed as the connecting medium between that of the head and trunk.   From the former region it may be traced downwards along the back, loins, breasts sides, flanks, and belly. ` At the cervical region, and between the shoulders, it is dense and abundant; and, surrounding the dorsal part of the vertebral column it is connected with the mediastinal tissue, the submucous tissue of the lungs, and the subserous tissue of the costal pleura. At the fore part of the neck it is in like manner connected with the abundant tissue of the pectoral region, and by means of that surrounding the larynx and trachea, 1*st*, with the submucous tissue of the bronchi; and, 2*d*, with the anterior mediastinum. Passing downwards, the same communication may be traced with the intermuscular tissue of the loins and belly, the tissue surrounding the lumbar and sacral portion of the vertebral column, that connecting the mesentery and large vessels to the vertebræ, and extending all round under the muscular peritonæum, and into the pelvis, where, by means of the tissue at the posterior surface of the abdominal muscles, at the anterior surface of the *iliacus internus,* and through the obturator hole and ischiatic notch, it communicates with the filamentous tissue of the lower extremities. From the rectum and branches of the ischium it is continued along the perinæum by the urethra, and into the scrotum.

In the whole of this course it is abundant in the space before the vertebræ round the *psoæ* and *iliacus internus* muscles, and round the bladder, rectum, prostate gland, and womb. The tissue surrounding the vertebral column communicates with that in the interior of the column by the intervertebral holes.

The arm-pit may be considered as the point of union between the filamentous tissue of the trunk and that of the upper extremities, while the groin is the corresponding spot for the lower extremities. These facts should be kept in mind in observing the phenomena of diseases of this tissue.

Notwithstanding this general connection, however, certain parts of the tissue are so dense and close as to diminish greatly the facility of communication. Thus along the median line it is so firm, that air injected invariably stops, unless impelled by a force adequate to tear open its filaments, and water is rarely found effused in this situation. In the neighbourhood of some parts of the skeleton also, as at the crest of the ilium, over the great trochanter, and on the shin, the filamentous tissue is very dense and coherent.

In chemical composition it consists principally of gelatin, but contains some albuminous matter.

Section II.

The filamentous tissue is liable to inflammation, acute and ebro-nic, circumscribed, and with exudation of lymph, or diffusive and spreading, generally without this exudation, and with the production of purulent matter; to induration; to hemorrhage; to serous infiltration; to aerial distension; and to new growths.

1. Inflammation of the subcutaneous tissue when circumscribed constitutes phlegmon, a name applied rather in reference to our observation of it near the surface of the body, than with a view to the natural relation between an organized texture and its pathological processes.

In other situations, as it is seldom recognized before it has passed to the stage of suppuration, inflammation of cellular tissue is generally implied in those abscesses or collections of purulent matter, (*apostemata, abscessus*), acute or chronic, which frequently form in the human body.

Various facts, nevertheless, show that inflammation of the filamentons tissue is a process consisting of several stages. At first the vessels become distended with blood, which moves rather slowly and is accompanied with a throbbing or beating sensation. This is attended with more or less swelling of the part, heat, and pain; and if it be near the surface, with redness. In the second place, the distended and overloaded state of the vessels never continues long without giving rise to more or less change in the blood in the part. Serum is poured out into the cells, often sero-albuminous fluid; sometimes blood even is extravasated. The sero-albuminous fluid is separated into lymph and serum. The former gives rise to the hardness usually observed. Thirdly, if the process continue, the secretion of sero-albuminous fluid is followed by that of purulent matter; and sometimes the serum first effused appears to be afterwards converted into purulent matter.

This purulent matter is usually contained within a body of lymph more or less regular; and which forms a sort of boundary between it and the sound or uninflamed part of the tissue. If this boundary be complete so as to surround and inclose the purulent matter, it is denominated a cyst. This may take place either in acute or in chronic inflammation.

After the matter has been deposited in the manner now described, it evinces a tendency to proceed towards the nearest surface. This may be either the skin or any of the mucous membranes. At first it may be seated at so great a depth that it is impossible to recognize its presence. In a short time, however, it may be felt by the practised finger. In most cases, even where there is much hardness, it is generally possible to predicate the presence of purulent· matter. The tendency to advance to the surface is connected with a tendency in other parts of the purulent tumour to contract; and as the former process advances, the latter keeps pace with it, so that in general, when the tumour bursts or is opened, the extent of the bottom of the abscess has sensibly and considerably been diminished.

If inflammation of cellular tissue do not terminate in suppuration, nor is resolved, it terminates in effusion of lymph, with concretion or agglutination of its filaments through a space more or less extensive. This is known by slight swelling, hardness, and immobility of the part. The phenomena of inflammation in this tissue are best observed in deep wounds, which divide a considerable extent of it. If the wound be what is called *simply incised,·* the constitution good, and the inflammation moderate, lymph is effused, and the cut edges are united by what was anciently named the *first intention.* This mode of union was termed by John Hunter adhesive inflammation, (p. 226,) and union by adhesion.

It is not always, however, that the process is so simple. When the wound is extensive or complicated, and involves the cellular web of several different tissues, the lymph effused is inadequate to effect reunion at once: and another process termed granulation! takes place. The basis of this indeed consists in exudation of lymph, which is effused in minute masses of no definite form, and which are soon penetrated by blood-vessels, and thereby become organized, (Hunter, p. 477.) Their surface becomes covered with more or less lymph, which, as they increase in size, causes them mutually to cohere; and by the successive production, growth and union of these granular bodies, the divided surfaces are made eventually to unite. The process of granulation in the filamentous tissue is accompanied with more or less suppuration; but as the granulations coalesce, this is gradually diminished.

2. The second form of inflammation occurring in filamentous tissue is when it spreads, or is diffused along the membrane, or through its substance. John Hunter was aware of the tendency which the inflammatory process in certain circumstances manifests to spread; and referring it to a sympathetic disposition in the surrounding parts, suggests an illustration in the opposite qualities of

dry and damp paper. " If dry," says he, " then it will not spread; it will be confined to its point; but if damp, it will spread, being attracted by the surrounding damp to which it has an affinity," (p. 262.) Though this is a mere illustration, and is a statement of a physical, not a physiological phenomenon, it affords no imperfect idea of the distinction between the limited or circumscribed, and the spreading or diffused inflammation.

Two circumstances, however, appear to have perplexed the principles both of this author and of his successors. The first of these was the sense in which the terms *erysipelas* and *erysipelatous* inflammation were to be understood; the second the constant search for final causes, or ultimate intentions. By most physicians and surgeons, previous to the time of Carmichael Smyth and Willan, and even later, every spreading inflammation was termed *erysipelatous*, whether it existed in skin, mucous membrane, serous membrane, or cellular tissue; and the character of nomenclature was derived, not from the texture, but from the supposed nature of the morbid process. This practice, if not positively wrong, was attended with confusion in arrangement and description; and it is well that the general usage of correct pathologists has now restricted the term to inflammation of a particular tissue. The second source of confusion in the views of Hunter consisted in his regarding the exudation of lymph as an invariable barrier against the diffusion of the morbid process. This exudation doubtless constitutes the character of the limited form of inflammation; but Hunter appears to have forgotten that, in certain circumstances, as in the sort of inflammation now considered, this barrier does not exist, and the morbid process therefore spreads, or is diffused over the membrane. It is further evident from what he says, (p. 271, 272, and 367,) that he regarded the spreading inflammation of the cellular membrane as erysipelas attacking that tissue, and that he considered its pathological peculiarity to consist in the absence of lymphy effusion, and the consequent want of limitation. Though it may be disputing about a name only, to question this, it is perhaps better to regard this form of inflammation as entirely different from erysipelas, which must be referred to the outer surface of the corion; and to represent it as a process tending to spread without adequate effusion of coagulable lymph.

Another point in the pathology of this disorder may be here noticed. Certain facts favour the notion, that it consists in affec-

tion of the adipose membrane, as distinct from the filamentous tissue.   Thus, diffuse inflammation occurs mostly in those parts in
which the adipose membrane is abundant, *e. g.* in the neck, on the
chest between the two pectoral muscles, in the arm-pits, in the extremities immediately beneath the skin, and on the buttock at the
verge of the anus.   In the following passage Hunter seems to have
this in view.   " The cellular membrane, free from the adipose, appears to be more susceptible of the adhesive inflammation than the
adipose membrane, and much more readily passes into the suppurative.   Thus we see that the cellular membrane connecting parts
together as muscles, and the cellular membrane connecting the
adipose to muscles, easily inflames, and runs readily into suppuration, and, as it were, separates the muscles from their lateral connections, and even separates the adipose from the muscles, while
the skin and adipose membrane shall only be highly inflamed," (p.
234.)   •

Diffuse inflammation of the filamentous tissue has been described
by Kirkland, (p. 282, Vol. II.) Willan, Thomson, and Copland
Hutchinson, under the name of *phlegmonoid erysipelas,* noticed by
various authors as inflammation of the *fascia,* (Abernethy, Kirkland, 268,) and was fully investigated by Dr Duncan Junior in
1823, under its proper denomination.

Its general characters are diffuse swelling spreading over the
limb or affected region, compressible, but not elastic, often doughy ;
deep-seated pain, with an oppressive sensation of weight ; and tension of the skin, sometimes with a dull red tinge, not unfrequently
without change of colour.   At a period, varying from the fifth to
the tenth day, the swelling presents in sundry parts a peculiar,
compressible, but not very elastic character, as if the subjacent tissues were floating in a fluid or semi-fluid matter.

If the affected part or limb be examined after death, the whole
cellular tissue, subcutaneous and intermuscular, is found enlarged,
gray, or ash-coloured, and distended with blood-coloured fluid or
serum, sero-purulent or purulent matter.   It is detached extensively from the several tissues which it connects in the healthy
state.   Between the muscles are long sinuous caverns filled with
dirty ash-coloured fluid ; sloughs or mortified shreds are seen
here and there hanging from aponeurotic sheaths, tendons, or even
blood-vessels ; and, while in most cases shreds or filaments of the
subcutaneous or subfascial cellular tissue are the only traces of its

existence, in not a few instances the muscles are detached from the periosteum, and the periosteum from the bone. These shreds are mortified pieces of sloughs or filamentous tissue; and correspond to the pieces of wet tow mentioned by Hunter and Sir E. Home, and the wads of wet chamois leather noticed by Mr James. This process is attended with much disturbance in the circulation, loss of appetite, heat, thirst, dry skin, and more or less derangement of the intellectual functions. Towards the close of the disease, the pulse becomes quick, small, and sometimes intermitting; the strength of the muscular system is greatly impaired; the raving is accompanied with muttering, and starting of the tendons, and alternates with stupor; and the breathing becomes quick, panting, and laborious, or slow, languid and interrupted, and terminates in death.

This may be regarded as the most severe form of the disease. In such circumstances its duration varies. It appears from the result of Dr Duncan's observations, that death does not take place before the sixth day, but may occur on any subsequent one to the twelfth or fifteenth. Perhaps in the average number of cases, the seventh, eighth, or ninth may be stated as the day on which the termination occurs. In milder cases it may terminate in resolution or in abscess. When the latter result takes place, the inflammatory action changes its character, and instead of spreading, shows a tendency to stop. Lymph is effused; healthy purulent matter is formed; and adhesion taking place in one or more points, the disease terminates in phlegmonic suppuration and granulation.

When recovery takes place after suppuration and sloughing of the cellular tissue, it is effected partly by direct adhesion taking place between the muscles, or their cellular substance, partly by the formation of new cellular tissue, similar to the new membranes formed on the serous surfaces. The former is the cause of the stiffness, immobility, and condensation of parts after this inflammation has taken place.

In some instances the circumscribed, or limited, and the spreading forms of inflammation may be combined. The latter proceeds at one part of the affected tissue; while the limited, with lymphy exudation and adhesion, takes place at another. This appears to be the variety of those tedious cases in which the disease is prolonged for weeks, and the patient either recovers, or ultimately dies hectic.

Diffuse inflammation may occur in any part of the filamentous tissue of the whole body, and may affect either the subcutaneous and superficial, or the intermuscular and deep-seated layer. But the regions in which it is most commonly observed may be enumerated in the following order :—

 a. The neck and throat. (Case by Wells in Transactions of a Society, Vol. III. p. 360, and by Wilson, p. 367. *Angina interna* of Kirkland, Vol. II. p. 158, and James, p. 187, &c.)
In persons, generally females, of full gross habit and bloated appearance, swelling diffuse, deep-seated, on the side of the neck towards the angle of the jaw, causing much pain in the side of the head ; attended with much fever, general disorder, loss of appetite, raving, stupor, or coma. It terminates in sloughs of the tissue, foul, ill-conditioned purulent matter ; does not point, but may burst internally, and cause suffocation. In some cases death takes place from the constitutional disorder with the affection of the brain.

 b. The breast, or outer surface of the chest and arm-pit and the side ; *abscess in the axilla* of Kirkland. Several cases in Dr Duncan's Essay. Diffuse painful swelling of the side occurring in middle-aged subjects, male or female, terminating in suppuration all over the side, or between the pectoral muscles, or in the arm-pit.

 c. An upper extremity, and passing to the arm-pit and side of the chest. This is the form which takes place after venesection, after punctured wounds in dissecting, or the application of animal matter or fluid to a wounded surface.

 d. An inferior extremity. The swelled leg of puerperal women is to be referred to this head, (see Hunter, p. 204.) Certain injuries of the foot and toes, more especially when the fibrous tissues have been much lacerated, appear also to be of the same kind. The phlegmonoid erysipelas of the lower extremities of seamen, as described by Mr Copland Hutchinson, comes under this head.

 e. The buttock and the perinæum. (*Proctia, phyma* of the ancients. *Proctitis, Proctalgia* and *Clunesia* of the nosologists. *Suppuration gangreneuse* of the French. Described by Pott in his 2d section on *Fistula ani*, p. 49. Case given by Hunter in his 3d chapter, section xiv., on the use of the adhesive inflammation. Abscess *juxta anum* of Mr James, p. 189.) In persons of gross habit, either naturally or rendered so by intemperance, hard diffuse swelling of the verge of the anus on each side, skin doughy and unresisting, sometimes colourless, generally of a dusky red or pur-

3

plish colour, with shivering, sickness, vomiting, great restlessness, heat, and thirst; pulse at first hard, quick, full and jarring, afterwards weak, fluttering, and irregular; brown tongue and mental disorder. After three, four, or five days, a small quantity of ill-conditioned matter, and sloughs of the cellular and adipose membrane are formed. This inflammation may spread along the urethral and scrotal filamentous tissue, and form the urethral abscess (*abscessus juxta urethram*) of Mr James. Of this an instructive example is related by John Hunter at the passage above referred to. The disease is distinguished according to him by the combination of the suppurative with the erysipelatous spreading inflammation. " It is not so circumscribed as the former; nor does it spread along the skin like the latter. But the skin is shining and œdematous; and the inflammation goes deep into the filamentous tissue, and forms dusky, fetid, purulent fluid, sometimes with air in a bag or abscess, without previous adhesion." The inflammation may pass downward and forward into the scrotum and beside the urethra, and upwards by the dense filamentous tissue of the belly and loins; and when openings are made, either artificially or by the process of ulceration, matter is discharged, and the mortified membrane hangs out like wet dirty tow. (Hunter, p. 368.) Yet, notwithstanding this extensive destruction both of filamentous tissue and even of skin, it is remarkable that the rectum generally escapes.

f. When this disease appears in other parts of the body after wounds with foul instruments, bites of poisonous animals, as the rattlesnake or the cobra di capello, morbid animal secretions, or the juice of the acrid plants, applied in any manner to the exposed corion, its characters and phenomena may be easily understood from the description already given.

g. I am uncertain whether to this head should be referred the peculiar fatal inflammation which succeeds punctured and lacerated wounds of the extremities, compound fractures with much contusion, compound luxations and severe gun-shot wounds. This is commonly regarded as gangrene, and is familiarly termed traumatic gangrene. It consists, however, in a peculiar form of inflammation, spreading rapidly along the subcutaneous and intermuscular cellular tissue, accompanied with emphysematous distension, and causing great constitutional disturbance, in which disorder of the brain and its functions are conspicuous characters. Death generally takes place before any of the tissues are mortified, in consequence of the violence of the constitutional symptoms, chiefly the affection of the brain.

3. *Inflammation of a chronic nature* is not uncommon in the filamentous tissue. In the ordinary acute form, the process is attended with more or less pain and swelling, and proceeds quickly to suppuration.   In other circumstances, however, little or no pain is felt; swelling is not perceived till late; and the first intimation of the existence of the disease is a collection of purulent matter, which, when discharged, is not homogeneous, but consists of flaky or curd-like shreds floating in a thinnish watery fluid.   This constitutes the cold abscess (*apostema frigidum*) of the surgeons of the Saracen school, and is the chronic abscess of modern surgeons. (Boyer.)

The cold abscess may be formed in any part of filamentous tissue; but it is most frequent where this tissue is loose and abundant.   Seldom seen in the head, it is frequent in the neck, in the chest, in the back, especially in the lumbar region, and in the extremities.   I have seen this tumour most generally in the loins, where it is liable to be confounded with lumbar abscess; in the cellular tissue of the *glutæi* muscles; and in the thigh and leg, especially the posterior and internal region.   In these situations it is not unfrequently the cause of sinuous cavities, which are difficult to be healed.   Several of the forms of lumbar abscess, in which there is no affection of the vertebræ or of their ligaments, are examples of this abscess occurring in the abundant loose filamentous tissue, which connects the mesentery, the large vessels, and the psoæ muscles to the spine.   Boyer also states that they are sometimes seen in the filamentous tissue which connects the serous membranes of the chest and belly to the walls of these cavities.   Of the latter I have seen one instance simulating hernia, and by the destruction which it caused of the fibres of the *recti* muscles, actually leaving a space through which the intestines were protruded.

Ileo-cæcal Abscess. (*Apostema Ileo-cæcale.*)—The filamentous tissue connecting the posterior surface of the cæcum to the lumbar muscles is occasionally the seat of inflammation and suppuration, apparently of a chronic character.   Swelling and fulness take place slowly in the space round the cæcum.   At length pain is felt; and when the part is examined a doughy solid tumour is recognized in the right iliac region, while dulness on percussion is observed.   The pulse is at this time a little quicker than natural, (86–90); the skin is dry; the tongue is furred; the abdomen is a little full; and the bowels are slow or obstinately bound. These symptoms increase until fever is established, with more considerable pain of the right iliac region and abdomen in general, and the sense of a hard firm resisting mass in the right iliac region. The swelling may terminate fatally at this time ; or it may end in suppuration, either into the interior of the cæcum, or round the cæcum, and into the iliac fossa, or with an outlet in the region on the surface of the belly. The disease shall be considered more fully under affections of the cæcum, to which it belongs.

4. *Hemorrhage.* Effusion of blood into the filamentous tissue independent of external violence is not common. Of spontaneous and idiopathic hemorrhage no authentic example has been recorded. It occurs, however, in a secondary manner in land and sea scurvy, (*Purpura* and *Scorbutus*). In the former disease it is rarely to any great extent, save when the complaint has terminated fatally with large and repeated hemorrhage from the mucous membranes. In sea scurvy it is at once frequent and considerable. Scarcely a case of this disorder attains any height, without much effusion of blood into the subcutaneous and intermuscular filamentous tissue. On this effusion in general depend the hard, livid tumours, deep in the limbs, with which sea scurvy is attended. The cause of this hemorrhage, or rather the state of the vessels which gives rise to it, is not well known. That the blood is probably altered, may be inferred from the fact, that it is dark-coloured, imperfectly coagulated and grumous, and does not separate into clot and serum ; but the capillaries of the tissue are much affected, certainly overloaded, probably disorganized.

Similar effusion is occasionally found in the filamentous tissue in malignant agues, remittents, especially those of tropical countries, and sometimes in the fever of temperate regions. Extravasation of blood, dark-coloured and semi-coagulated, are observed in cases of typhous fever during bad epidemics, and in broken and impaired constitutions. The patches vary from the size of a pea, or a sixpenny piece, to large irregular shaped masses one or two inches square, and sometimes larger. These effusions take place in the cellular tissue beneath the skin, in the intermuscular, and sometimes apparently among the muscles themselves. These it is important to distinguish from the effects of blows and falls. They are common in bad cases of typhous fever. But it is possible that they may be aggravated by pressure.

5. *Induration.* *L'Endurcissement du Tissu Cellulaire* of Andry,

Auvity, &c. *Engelure.* *Scleroma* of Chaussier, (σκληρωμα; σκληρος.) Skin-bound of Underwood and Burns. Compact œdema of M. Leger and other French authors. First observed by John Andrew Uzembezius in 1718, this affection was not accurately described till 1780, when Denman and Underwood in England, and Doublet in France, published the result of their observations. In 1787 it was fully investigated by Andry, in a memoir crowned by the prize of the Royal Society of Medicine of Paris; and afterwards, in 1789, in those of Auvity and Hulme. Since this it has undergone the successive researches of Naudeau and Bard in France, Went, Henke, Golis, &c. in Germany, Liberali and Palletta in Italy, and again of Trocon, Leger, Denis, and Breschet in France. Notwithstanding the research of these several inquirers, however, the nature of this change in the filamentous tissue is still imperfectly understood.

It has hitherto been observed only in infants, and very often immediately after birth. According to Leger, it appears most frequently eight, twelve, or twenty-four hours after, and very seldom takes place later than the seventh day. Generally in the legs, not so often in the arms; the soft parts become unusually firm, dense, and diffusely swelled either continuously or in patches. The skin over these parts is hard, rough, and does not move easily; and it assumes a red, purple, or violet colour, which when pressed gives place to a yellow tint, with more or less depression. The same change is very generally remarked in the cheeks, the skin of which becomes quite immovable; and it appears successively in the belly and chest, the integuments of which feel as stiff as a board. At the same time the surface, especially the extremities, are unusually cold; the pulse is quick and very small; the breathing is much constrained and panting; the infant ceases to cry, becomes blue in the face, and seems to expire suffocated.

The duration of the disease varies. The greatest number of infants die on the first, second, or third day from the date of attack. In less rapid cases death takes place about the tenth or twelfth day, and in some so late as the twenty-first day.

After death the surface of the body appears in general hard, firm, and leathery, and presents a violet or brownish colour, interspersed with yellow patches. The cheeks, the extremities, and other parts affected during life are firm, rigid, and immovable. The subjacent filamentous tissue is very dense and granular, and when cut communicates the sensation as if it were like collared brawn. From the sections slowly oozes a reddish serous fluid, which coagulates quickly; and in the tissue itself may be observed grayish or yellowish granules, which give the brawny aspect and sensation already mentioned. (Leger.) The greatest firmness and induration are generally remarked in the outer region of the legs, and in the dorsal region of the foot and hand; and this gives the members the air of a peculiar twist or distortion. The adipose membrane appears to be not much less the seat of this disease than the filamentous tissue.

The bodies of infants cut off by this disease are small, being of the medium height of seventeen inches; and all the organs are imperfectly developed. Thus the lungs are hard, marbled, uncrepitating, and sink in water; the windpipe is small, and the alimentary canal is shorter than usual in healthy infants of the same age. The heart, however, is large, and generally contains blood in clots. The *foramen ovale* is often open, and the arterial duct is never closed. The pericardium, and frequently the cavities of the serous membranes, contain more or less serous fluid.

The nature of this morbid change is unknown. The old notion of Uzembezius revived by Andry and Auvity, that it was occasioned by coagulation of the fluids frozen by extreme cold, is completely contradicted by the fact recorded by Leger, that among forty-four infants dead during the month of June 1823 in the Foundling Hospital of Paris, twenty-one were cut off by induration of the cellular tissue. The notion of Alard, that it is allied with the glandular disease of Barbadoes, scarcely deserves mention. On the contrary, its early occurrence after birth, the imperfect developement of the several organs, especially of the lungs, its occasional appearance previous to birth, and its frequency among infants born before the full time, (Palletta,) show that it bears some relation to the fœtal mode of existence. The peculiar nature of the filamentons tissue in the fœtus and in the new-born infant may have some influence in the production of this malady.

6. Serous infiltration, (*œdema, anasarca.*) Under the operation of various causes, as exposure to cold, the use of mercury, inflammation, or injury, the quantity of serous fluid in the filamentous tissue may be considerably increased; and this increase gives rise to a pale, white, or wan-coloured and cold swelling of the skin, which is distinguished by receiving the impression of the finger or any other sub-

stance forcibly applied.　The swelling may be local, or confined to⸰ one arm, to one leg, to a hand, to part of a limb, to the scrotum, to the face, or so forth; or it may extend in different degrees to the greater part or the whole of the person.　In the former case it is termed *Œdema*, (οιδημα) or swelling; in the latter it receives the name of *Anasarca*, (ὑδρωψ ανα σαρκα, dropsy in the flesh,) and is the *aqua intercus* of the Romans.　It was the white or pale and blanched colour of this sort of swelling which procured for it the name of *Leucophlegmatia* (Λευκοφλεγματια), or white inflammation among the ancient physicians.

The fluid of the filamentous tissue may coagulate spontaneously, (Blackall, 263;) but it always undergoes coagulation on the application of heat or the addition of re-agents.

The preternatural increase of the cellular serosity now mentioned is supposed to arise either from diminished absorption or increased exhalation.　This point will be considered afterwards when speaking of the exhalants.

7. *Emphysema.　Pneumatosis spontanea et traumatica*, Cullen. The filamentous tissue may be distended with air, which causes a uniform swelling, crepitating or emitting a crackling sound when pressed.　The situations in which this aerial swelling may take place vary according to the cause by which it is produced.　It may take place spontaneously (Baillie,) when it is commonly general, and is supposed to depend on a process of secretion from the blood-vessels.　It may arise from rupture or laceration of the mucous membrane of the larynx or windpipe, (De Villars, Cheselden, Holyoke, O'Brien,) when the swelling appears chiefly over the face, neck, and upper part of the chest.　It may succeed a broken rib, or any injury of the lungs, (Littre, Berger, William Hunter, Cheston, Leake, Gooch, Halliday,) when it appears sometimes over the neck, face, and chest, sometimes over the chest and side only.　It may arise from rupture of the bronchial membrane during violent efforts, (Blagden, Hicks, Simmons;) and in this manner emphysema happens in puerperal women.　Lastly, it may appear as an effect of gangrenous inflammation and mortification, when it is confined solely to the affected limb.　In the latter case the air is produced by the decomposition of the serum of the blood in the morbid parts.

8. *Vascular Sarcoma*, Abernethy.　The tumour known under this name is, of all the new growths incident to the animal tissues, the most simple in structure.　I refer it to this head for two

reasons. 1st, It appears to occur chiefly where filamentous or cellular tissue is found; and when it occurs among muscles, or in the substance of organs, it appears still to be referable to the filamentous tissue, which enters into the composition of the texture, in which it appears. 2d, The structure of this tumour is principally filamentous tissue condensed or modified by the local morbid action. Every instance of vascular sarcoma may be viewed as a new developement and hypertrophic augmentation of its proper substance in a particular point of the filamentous tissue. The tumour is always liberally supplied with blood from vessels which, if not more numerous, are greatly larger and more capacious than in the natural state; and if this be not the cause of the unusual deposition of substance, it must be regarded as the channel by which the additional matter is conveyed. It is also possible that the irritation resulting from the first effusion of blood, or other coagulable matter, which, according to Mr Abernethy, is the usual cause of tumours, may excite the vessels of the neighbouring parts so much as to cause their capacity to be enlarged, and to convey a more copious supply of blood. This cause of the great vascularity, and its influence in increasing the size of the tumour, are particularly insisted on by Mr John Bell, and afterwards by Mr Abernethy.

The vascular sarcoma is enclosed in a thin capsule, which is formed of filamentous tissue much condensed by the pressure of the enclosed tumour. It may occur in any part or organ of the human body where filamentous tissue penetrates; but it is also found in the female breast, in the testicle of the male, and in the absorbent glands of both sexes. When it occurs in the testicle the vessels are said to be numerous and small. When it affects the female breast the vessels seem to be rather large than numerous, and the organization appears less complete. (Abernethy.)

9. *Melanosis.* The black deposite named *Melanosis* is often found in this tissue; and perhaps when it is said to occur in the interior of muscles, glands, and other tissues, it is in their filamentous substance that it is deposited. As it is, however, still more frequent in the adipose membrane, the points of its history deserving notice shall be introduced under that head.

10. *Tubercle.* I am uncertain whether to this tissue should be referred every variety of the small painful bodies situate beneath the skin, so well described by Mr Wood.* Though situate, as de-

* Edinburgh Medical and Surgical Journal, Vol. VIII. p. 83 and 429.

scribed by Mr Wood, in the subcutaneous cellular tissue, some
facts tend to confirm the notion originally entertained by Camper,*
that it is a morbid growth seated in one of the subcutaneous nerves,
or probably in its neurilema.†

11. *Cysts.* Bichat has taken considerable pains to show the influence of this tissue on the formation of cysts. These, it is well
known, are shut sacs containing fluids of different sorts. But however these fluids may differ, the containing cyst, which is a secreting membrane, has been regarded as formed of condensed and modified filamentous tissue. Against this doctrine Bichat urges the
following objections. 1. Cysts are analogous in all respects to
serous membranes, and should therefore have the same origin. 2.
This mechanical hypothesis of their origin, in which all the vessels,
ought to be obliterated, does not accord with the exhaling and absorbing function of cysts, nor with their mode of inflammation. 3.
If these sacs are formed by the mutual application and agglutination or adhesion of cells, (that is, of the filaments,) the contiguous
tissue ought to be diminished, or to disappear when they are bulky,
which is not observed to take place. 4. If cysts are formed by
condensation of the filamentous tissue, and if their fluid is effused
by exhalation, this fluid ought to exist in the organ which separates
them from the blood.

For these reasons he infers that cysts begin at first to be developed, and to grow in the midst of the filamentous tissue, according
to laws analogous to those of the growth of parts in general, and
which appear to be unknown aberrations, or unnatural applications of these laws. When the cyst is once formed, the process of
exhalation commences, and though scanty at first, it increases as
the cyst enlarges. In short, the formation and growth of the organ precedes the accumulation of the fluid.

12. *Degeneration.* This term is obviously vague and indefinite.
Under it, however, Sandifort has described in the body of a female
infant a preternatural state of the cellular tissue of the breast, back,
and axillary regions.‡ In some respects this change resembles the
disease described above as induration. In others, however, it was
different.

---

* Demonstrationum Anatomico-Pathologicarum, Lib. i. p. 11.

† Ed. Journal, Vol. XI. p. 468.

‡ Observationes Anatomico-Pathologicæ Eduardi Sandifort, Lib. iv. cap. ii. p. 24.
Lugduni Batavorum, 1777. 4to

CHAPTER IV.

ADIPOSE TISSUE, (*Tela adiposa,— Tissu adipeux,— Tissu graisseux.*)

SECTION I.

THE separate existence of an adipose membrane was suspected by Malpighi, distinctly taught by De Bergen and Morgagni, and demonstrated by William Hunter. It was, however, confounded with the filamentous tissue, under the general name of cellular membrane, adipose membrane, and cellular fat, by Winslow, by Portal, by Bichat, and most of the continental anatomists, till distinguished and positively described by M. Beclard himself.

According to the dissections of De Bergen and Morgagni, the demonstrations of Hunter, and the observations of M. Beclard, its structure consists of rounded packets or parcels separated from each other by furrows of various depth, of a figure irregularly oval, or rather spheroidal, varying in diameter from a line to half an inch, according to the degree of corpulence and the part submitted to examination. Each packet is composed of small spheroidal particles, which may be easily separated by dissection, and which are said to consist again of an assemblage of vesicles still more minute, and agglomerated together by very fine and delicate cellular tissue. The appearance of these ultimate vesicles is minutely described by Wolff in the subcutaneous fat, and by Clopton Havers* and Monro in the marrow of bones, in which the two last authors compared them to strings of minute pearls. If the fat with which these vesicles are generally distended should disappear, as happens in dropsy, the vesicles collapse, their cavity is obliterated, and they are confounded with the contiguous cellular tissue, without leaving any trace of their existence.

Hunter, however, asserts, that in such circumstances the cellular tissue differs from the tissue of adipose vesicles, in containing no similar cavities; and justly remarks that the latter is much more fleshy and ligamentous than the filamentous tissue, and contends, that though the adipose receptacles are empty and collapsed, they still exist. When the skin is dissected from the adipose membrane

---

* *Osteologia Nova ;* or some New Observations on the Bones and the Parts belonging to them. By Clopton Havers, M. D., F. R. S. London, 1691. 8vo. P. 167.

D

it is always possible to distinguish the latter from the filamentous tissue, even if it contain no fat, by the toughness of its fibres, and the coarseness of the web which they make.

The distinguishing characters between the cellular or filamentous and the adipose tissue may be stated in the following manner. 1st, The vesicles of the adipose membrane are closed all round, and, unlike the cellular tissue, they cannot be generally penetrated by fluids which are made to enter them. If the temperature of a portion of adipose membrane be raised by means of warm water to the liquefying point of the contents, they will remain unmoved so long as the structure of the vesicles is not injured by the heat. If, again, an adipose packet be exposed to a solar heat of + 40 centigr. though the fat be completely liquefied, not a drop will escape, until the vesicles are divided or otherwise opened, when it appears in abundance. The adipose matter, therefore, though fluid or semi-fluid in the living body, does not, like dropsical infiltration, obey the impulse of gravity. 2d, The adipose vesicles do not form, like cellular tissue, a continuous whole, but are simply in mutual contiguity. This arrangement is demonstrated by actual inspection, but becomes more conspicuous in the case of dropsical effusions, when the filamentous tissue interposed between the adipose molecules is completely infiltrated, while the latter are entirely unaffected. 3d. The anatomical situation of the adipose tissue is different from that of the filamentous tissue. The former is found, 1st, In a considerable layer immediately beneath the skin ; 2d, Between the peritoneal folds which form the omentum and mesentery ; 3d, Between the serous and muscular tissues of the heart ; and 4th, Round each kidney.

In each of these situations it varies in quantity and in physical properties. In the least corpulent persons a portion of fat is deposited in the adipose membrane of the cheeks, orbits, palms of the hand, soles of the feet, pulp of the fingers and toes, flexures of the joints, round the kidney, beneath the cardiac serous membrane, and between the layers of the mesentery and omentum. In the more corpulent, and chiefly in females, it is found not merely in these situations, but extended in a layer of some thickness almost uniformly over the whole person ; but is very abundant in the neck, breasts, belly, *mons veneris*, and flexures of the joints.

Besides the delicate cellular tissue by which the packets and vesicles are united, the adipose tissue receives arterial and venous branches, the arrangement of which has been described by various authors from Malpighi, who gave the first accurate account,* to Mascagni, to whom we are indebted for the most recent. According to the latter, who has also delineated these vessels, the furrow or space between each packet contains an artery and vein, which being subdivided penetrates between the minute grains or particles of which the packet is composed, and furnishes each with a small artery and vein. The effect of this arrangement is, that each individual grain or adipose particle is supported by its artery and vein as by a foot-stalk or peduncle, and that those of the same packet are kept together not only by contact, but by the community of ramifications from the same vessel. These grains are so closely attached, that Mascagni, who examined them with a good lens, compares them to a cluster of fish-spawn, (un aggruppimento di uova). Grutzmacher found much the same arrangement in the grains and vesicles of the marrow of bones.†

It has been supposed that the adipose tissue receives nervous filaments, and Mascagni conceives he has demonstrated its lymphatics. Both points, however, are so problematical, that of neither of these tissues is the distribution known.

The substance contained in these vesicles is entirely inorganic. Always solid in the dead body, it has been represented as fluid during life by Winslow,‡ Haller,§ Portal,‖ Bichat,¶ and most au-

---

* Malpighi's description is not much less accurate than that of Mascagni. " Vasa sanguinea expandunter in ramos arborum adinstar, quorum extremitatibus appenduntur membranosi sacculi, seu lobuli, pinguedinosis globulis referti, qui veluti folia ramis adnata arboris exactam figuram complent."—" Per has membranas excurrunt minima vasa in modum retis expansa, quæ tenue omentum representant. Hæc a venis et arteriis, ut videre potui, ortum ducunt, et non tantum levitur exterius piguedinis lobulos, sed etiam intime penetrant, et pinguedinosis globulis nectuntur."—" Quandoque autem co-operiuntur levi superextensa membrana, ita ut in conspectum non erumpant ; emergunt autem, quotiescunque vetustate et carie membranosæ portiones corrumpuntur. Per hanc eandem membranam diramificantur adiposa vasa in omento reperta, quæ pinguedine turgent, si præcipue in de recenti mactato animali inspiciantur."—De Omento, Pinguedine et Adiposis Ductibus, p. 41.

† De Ossium Medulla, 1748. Extat in Haller, Vol. VI. p. 390.

‡ " La graisse ou matiere graisseuse est plus coulante dans les vivans que dans les morts."—Winslow, Traité des Tegumens, sec. 73.

§ Elementa Physiologiæ, Lib. i. sect. 4.

‖ " La chaleur de la vie maintient la graisse dans une espece de fluidité ; elle se fige par le froid de la mort ; ce qui fait qu'elle est compacte dans les cadavres."—Portal, Tome ii. p. 17.

¶ " La graisse est presque toujours solide et figée dans les cadavres, mais sur le vivant elle s'approche plus de l'etat liquide, au moins dans certaines parties, comme aux

thors on anatomy. The last writer indeed states, that under the skin it is more consistent, and that in various living animals he never found it so fluid as is represented. The truth is, that in the human body, and in most mammiferous animals during life, the fat is neither fluid nor semifluid. It is simply soft, yielding, and compressible, with a slight degree of transparency or rather translucence. This is easily established by observing it during incisions through the adipose membrane, either in the human body or in the lower animals.

The properties and composition of fat form a subject for chemical rather than anatomical inquiry; and in this respect its nature has been particularly investigated by M. Chevreul. According to the researches of this chemist, fat consists essentially of two proximate principles, *stearine* (ςεαρ, *sebum*, *supo*), and *elaine*, (ελαιον, *oleum*.) The former is a solid substance, colourless, tasteless, and almost inodorous, soluble in alcohol, and preserving its solidity at a temperature of 138° centigrade. Elaine, on the contrary, though colourless, or at most of a yellow tint, and lighter than water, is fluid at a temperature of from 17° to 18° centigrade, and is greatly more soluble in alcohol. Of this substance marrow appears to be merely a modification; and the membranous cavities or medullary membrane in which it is contained may be viewed as an intraosseous adipose tissue.

Little doubt can be entertained that animal fat is the result of a process of secretion. But it is no easy matter to determine the mode in which this is effected. Malpighi, departing, however, from strict observation, imagined a set of ducts issuing from glands, in which he conceived the fat to be elaborated and prepared. To this he appears to have been led by his study of the lymphatic glands, and inability to comprehend how the process of secretion could be performed by arteries only. This doctrine, however, was overthrown by the strong arguments which Ruysch derived from his injections; and Malpighi himself afterwards acknowledged its weakness and renounced it. In short, neither the glands nor the ducts of the adipose membrane have ever been seen.

Winslow, though willing to adopt the notion of Malpighi, admits, however, that the particular organ by which the fat is separated from the blood was unknown. Haller, on the contrary, aware

environs du cœur, des gros vaisseaux, &c. Sous la peau elle est constamment plus consistante."—Anatomie General, Tome I. p. 59.

of the permeability of the arteries, and their direct communication with the cells of the adipose tissue, and trusting to the testimony of Malpighi, Ruysch, Glisson, and Morgagni, that it existed in the arterial blood, saw no difficulty in the notion of secretion, or rather of a process of separation; and upon much the same grounds the opinion is adopted by Portal and others. Bichat, again, contends, that no fat can be recognized in the arterial blood, and adduces the fact, that none can be distinguished in blood drawn from the temporal artery. It may be doubted, nevertheless, whether adequate means to ascertain this point were adopted. Gmelin obtained from blood cholesterine, stearine, elaine, and stearic acid. Chevreul obtained from fibrin, by means of ether, a fatty matter. Leeanu found in large quantities of blood small proportions of crystallizable fatty and oily matter; and lastly, Dr R. D. Thomson and others have since that shown, that after meals of certain kinds of food the blood contains adipose and oily matter. From these facts it may be inferred, that adipose matter is conveyed in minute quantities into the blood, and is rapidly deposited from the vessels in various parts of the adipose tissue, where it is afterwards found. From the phenomena of various diseases also, and those of the hybernating animals, which retire in the beginning of winter fat and heavy, and come out in spring meagre and extenuated, there is reason to believe that fat is absorbed by the veins and lymphatics.

It must be observed, nevertheless, that fat or oily matter is found in the free state, and in appreciable quantity, only in certain conditions of the system; and as arteries are not habitually opened for blood-letting, the circumstance of fat or oil not being observed in certain cases of arteriotomy, forms only a degree of negative evidence. This result is not at variance with the facts observed, as already stated, by Hewson[*] and Dr Traill,[†] who found oily matter in venous blood in two instances, or with those observed by Mr Anderson,[‡] Dr Ziegler, Dr Christison,[§] and myself, all of whom have

[*] Hewson's Experimental Inquiries, p. 191, *loco citato.*

[†] On the presence of Oil in Human Blood. By Thomas Stewart Traill, M. D. Edin. Med. and Surgical Journal, XVII., 236, 637, and XIX. 319.

[‡] On White or Milk-like Serum. Edin. Med. and Surgical Journal, Vol. XXXIII. p. 215.

[§] On the Causes of the Milky and Whey-like Appearance sometimes observed in the Blood. By R. Christison, M. D. &c. Edin. Med. and Surg. Journal, Vol. XXXIII. p. 274.

found the blood in certain morbid states to contain oil.   In wounds in the human body during life, and in living animals, oily particles may be seen floating on the surface of the blood; but these proceed from division of the adipose vesicles.

That fat does not exist in the arterial blood in health, or is in very minute quantity, may be therefore admitted as an established point. The idea that it is separated, or strained from this fluid, therefore, must also be gratuitous; and as such it is viewed by Bichat, who considers the deposition of fat as the effect of exhalation.   This, it must be confessed, is little more than a different name for the process termed by Haller *secretion*.   Lastly, an opinion has been delivered by Mascagni, that, while the arteries deposit or pour forth an imperfect or crude oily fluid, the lymphatics absorb the thin parts, and leave the residue in a more solid and perfect form.

In conclusion, all that can be affirmed regarding the formation of this substance is, that it is deposited by the blood-vessels, but by what particular process, or in what form, is entirely unknown.   The process by which the arteries of the adipose membrane secrete fat appears to be equally mysterious as that by which the vessels of muscle deposit fibrine, those of bone deposit osseous matter, and those of cartilage form that animal substance.

It appears, therefore, that the adipose tissue may be distinguished into two elements, one organic and secreting; the other, inorganic and secreted.

The adipose membrane is one of the most extensively distributed tissues in the animal body; and this circumstance, with its peculiar organic and physiological properties, exercises remarkable influence on its inflammatory and other morbid states.

In distribution it may be distinguished in the following manner. 1. The subcutaneous adipose tissue, extended in a uniform layer, variable in thickness, beneath the skin all over the body, excepting at certain parts where the skin communicates with the mucous membrane, as the eyelids, the lips, the penis of the male, the *labia* in the female, where there is no adipose tissue, and beneath the hairy scalp, where the adipose tissue is extremely thin ; 2. the periangial adipose tissue, surrounding and enclosing the large bloodvessels and nerves in the trunk and extremities, forming a sort of sheath to these organs, and sustaining their nutrient vessels, (*vasa vasorum*) ; 3. the subserous adipose tissue, deposited, more or less abundantly, beneath the different serous membranes, and between their folds, often round blood-vessels, for instance between the pericardium and muscular substance of the heart, between the peritoneal folds, forming the *omentum* and the mesentery; 4. round each kidney; 5. between the folds of the synovial membranes; and, 6. the endosteal, or intra-osseous, or the medullary membrane within the canals of the longitudinal bones and the cells of the flat and short bones.

SECTION II.

The pathological relations of the adipose tissue have not been distinctly indicated.

1. *Pimelitis.* Is it subject to inflammation? I have already said that certain facts lead to the inference, that the peculiar phenomena of diffuse inflammation may depend on the influence of the adipose membrane. This may be regarded as established by many facts. But it must be observed, at the same time, that the physical properties and the physiological relations of the adipose tissue, combined with its anatomical position, exert a peculiar influence over its morbid states.

In the *first* place, as the adipose membrane consists of two parts, organic or vital tissue, and an inorganic secreted substance, and as the former bears a small proportion to the latter, the vital properties of the tissue are accordingly much less prominent than the mere physical properties. The component *sacculi*, or vesicles of the adipose membrane, are not possessed of highly or strongly marked vital powers; and the vessels distributed to them, which are neither large nor numerous, seem to be merely adequate to their nutrition in ordinary circumstances, but quite unable to maintain the energies of the tissue when subjected to disease or injury. Pressure or stretching the adipose tissue bears very imperfectly; and when it is subjected to violence or injury of this kind along with other tissues, as skin, muscle, cellular membrane, or artery, its vitality is destroyed first, and long before these tissues are much affected. In continued fever (*synochus ; typhus,*) the adipose membrane of the sacral region is often killed to a large extent long before the skin is affected; and its death involves necessarily ulceration of the incumbent skin, in order to allow the escape of the dead adipose membrane in the form of a large flat slough. It is perhaps of no great moment whether this imperfect and feeble vital energy depends on the want of nerves, or on the smaller number and size of its nutrient vessels. The fact of feeble vitality is well established by many circumstances of daily occurrence, and is further illustrated, as shall be seen, by the different appearance and effects of the phenomena of inflammation in tissues more completely organized, and endowed also with more active vital properties.

In the *second* place, as to anatomical position, the adipose tissue is in many situations of the human body so closely confined, that when inflamed, and consequently distended, it cannot easily expand. This is particularly the case, not only with the subcutaneous fat which is compressed by the skin, but with the dense adipose cushion surrounding the blood-vessels and nerves, which, in the extremities at least, and in the neck, is closely packed and compressed, as it were, by all the incumbent and surrounding tissues,—muscles, fascia, and skin. When we examine the adipose cushion surrounding the carotid artery in the neck, that accompanying the axillary and brachial artery in the arm-pit and arm, and that enclosing the femoral and popliteal arteries in the leg, it must appear obvious, that little or no space is left in either of these regions for the casual expansion of the adipose membrane, from whatever cause proceeding. Not only is the adipose cushion there closely confined by condensed filamentous tissue, but it is further inclosed and compressed by the incumbent *fasciæ*, muscles, subcutaneous adipose membrane, and skin ; and the degree of tightness may be estimated from the fact, that even when cut into in the healthy state, it is forthwith protruded, and is with difficulty replaced. This tightness is one great cause of the readiness and celerity with which the adipose tissue in this situation passes so readily into mortification. As it is distended by the inflammatory vascular congestion, and as the surrounding parts do not yield with proportional facility, it is as if inclosed within a long tight ligature, and is in a manner strangled by its own enlargement. This result is clearly illustrated by the effects of inflammation of the periangial adipose membrane.

In the *third* place, the inflammatory states of the adipose membrane are not only in themselves of the highest importance, from the anatomical and physiological properties of the tissue itself, but in consequence of the uses to which this tissue is applied in enclosing and supporting others, and especially the nutrient vessels of blood-vessels, nerves, tendons, and bones, these states may exercise on the economy a most important influence, which I believe has not hitherto been fully understood.

Inflammation attacking the subcutaneous adipose tissue is liable to produce death, not only in that membrane but in the skin, inflammation and death in the muscles, inflammation in the subcutaneous veins, and inflammation and death in the tendons.

Inflammation attacking the periangial adipose tissue is liable to be followed not only by death in that tissue itself, but by inflammation, death, and ulceration of the arterial tunics, and consequent hemorrhage, inflammation of the veins, with obliteration of their canal, and denudation of the nerves.

Inflammation attacking the medullary or endosteal adipose tissue produces suppuration and causes death in the bone, (*Necrosis*,) and in the cancellated tissue the phenomena of the disease named *Spina ventosa*.

When inflammation affects the adipose membrane it may assume either the limited or the diffuse form, but is most frequently perhaps seen in the latter state.

It appears to have been an opinion entertained by Boerhaave and several of his pupils, that phlegmon, or common acute circumscribed inflammation, is seated in the adipose membrane ; and one of these writers, Hulsebusch, announces this proposition formally in a dissertation.   The same doctrine was afterwards taught in this country by Bromfield, who allowed that the adipose membrane is quite distinct from the filamentous tissue,* and further believed, that extravasated fluid would sooner be converted into purulent

---

* " I may be singular in what I am going to advance, viz. that in general the *adipose* membrane is the seat of abscesses, especially those that are circumscribed.

" I hope I am understood, that I suppose what is generally defined a *phlegmon* or critical abscess, in which a large quantity of matter is collected, to be formed in the *membrana adiposa*."   In the following passage he gives the first description of diffuse inflammation.   " Nevertheless, I am extremely sensible, that the cellular or connecting membrane is frequently the seat of mischief, as the receptacle of some extravasated humour, where the fluids in general have a tendency to sphacelation ; and under such circumstances it is well known, that the humour, instead of being collected and forming an abscess, will be diffused proportionate to the quantity extravasated, and form sloughs, throughout a whole limb, and where probably, the external appearance of sphacelation shall not exceed the size of a crown-piece, the mortification will then discover itself soon after, at a small distance ; and we shall find in the end, that it has not only crept under the skin, but has burrowed deep between the muscles, and through some of these sphacelated parts, sloughs of an immense length are frequently drawn out, which prove to be the cellular membrane ; in which case, if the patient does not sink under the discharge, the neighbouring parts must, in healing, unavoidably unite, and consequently the limb be abridged of its motion, as far as the free motion of the muscles, one over the other, is hardened by this union."—Chirurgical Observations, Vol. I. chapter iii. p. 94 and 95.

matter when lodged in the adipose than in the cellular membrane. It is further remarkable that, while he gives the earliest good description of the phenomena and effects of diffuse or disjunctive inflammation, he refers the seat of circumscribed inflammation to the adipose membrane, and that of disjunctive inflammation to the cellular membrane. The converse of this notion was maintained by J. Hunter, who represents the cellular membrane free from the adipose, to be more susceptible of the adhesive inflammation than the adipose membrane, and much more readily to pass into the suppurative.* This, however, he afterwards in some manner controverts by giving the same view of the effects of cellular inflammation, as that previously furnished by Bromfield.

All that it appears to me can be concluded at present on this subject is, that, though inflammation with tendency to circumscription may attack the adipose tissue, yet that tissue is much more liable to assume the diffuse, spreading, and disjunctive form of the disease.

Among the proofs adduced in favour of this view may be mentioned the following. In cases of diffuse inflammation affecting the arm, the inflammation spreads along the adipose membrane, producing sero-purulent secretion and sloughs of the adipose tissue. In cases of inflammation at the verge of the anus, the disease spreads in the same manner, and affects almost exclusively the adipose tissue round the anus and rectum, and along the *glutaei* muscles. It is in the same manner that the adipose cushion with which the blood-vessels are surrounded is occasionally the seat of a species of bad inflammatory action, terminating in fetid and sloughing suppuration.

I have in a considerable number of instances observed inflamma-

* "The cellular membrane, free from the adipose, appears to be more susceptible of the adhesive inflammation than the adipose membrane, and much more readily passes into the suppurative. Whether this arises from surfaces inflaming more readily than other parts, I will not pretend to say. Thus we see that the cellular membrane connecting parts together as muscles, and the cellular membrane connecting the adipose to muscles, easily inflames, and runs readily into suppuration, and as it were separates the muscles from their lateral connection, and even separates the adipose from the muscles, while the skin and adipose membrane shall only be highly inflamed ; and the matter so formed must produce ulceration through all this adipose membrane to get to the skin, and then through the skin, in which last-mentioned parts it is much more tedious." (P. 234, iii. 282, P. ii. Ch. ii. § 3.) Hunter appears in this place to have confounded the two kinds of inflammation, the adhesive or limited, and diffuse or suppurating.

tion of the adipose tissue, presenting the external signs described by my late friend, Dr Duncan, Junior, as those of diffuse inflammation of the cellular membrane. The process then produced all the effects now specified, and, by the peculiar manner in which the inflammatory process spreads along the meshes of the tissue, detached extensively the skin from the muscles, and the muscles and *fasciæ* from each other, and, in consequence of the intricate manner in which it insinuates itself between the muscles and their *fasciculi*, it produced extensive disjunctive destruction of the different parts which it affected. Thus, on the side of the chest, I have seen it first disjoin, and then kill the fibres of the intercostal muscles, and, affecting the *pleura costalis* at its muscular surface, pass to the free surface, and give rise to pleurisy and *empyema*. In the buttock, at the margin of the anus, I have seen it detach the skin completely from the subjacent muscles, dissect round the *sphincter* and *levator ani* as completely as if done by the knife, and produce such disjunction and separation as to render the whole of the muscles completely useless as organs of motion.

In the course of these destructive processes, this disease, which though first confined with extreme accuracy to the adipose tissue, eventually affects muscles, tendons, blood-vessels, and nerves, by killing and detaching that texture which supports and encloses them, and conveys their nutrient blood-vessels, is ever attended with febrile symptoms, remarkable for their character in deranging all the functions, and impairing more or less, sometimes very considerably, the muscular strength. The pulse is rapid, but generally much oppressed, and though sometimes at the commencement sharp, is generally contracted, wiry, and even vermicular. The skin is pungently hot and dry; the tongue more or less furred, with much thirst; and in severe cases, where the disease assumes a violent character, the patient raves or mutters, and sometimes passes into a state of *typhomania* (*coma vigil*,) or even afterwards coma. The complexion is often of a dingy colour, as it is in typhous fever, or in cases of traumatic gangrene, or in cases of death by animal poisoning; and the eyes, though they may be free from injection, are generally suffused, watery, and turbid. At the same time, almost all the great secretions are more or less completely suspended, or as it were locked up, by the perverted and diminished action of the capillary vessels. The skin is dry and imperspirable, and only at the termination of the disorder betrays the

existence of clammy moisture.   The urine is scanty and clear till
the close, when it becomes sedimentous.   No cathartic medicines,
however powerful, can produce feculent discharges from the intestines, and all that escapes is a watery secretion with minute black
specks, grains, and patches of undecomposed bile, without the characteristic feculent odour or aspect.

The peculiar characters of this form of fever have procured for
it, from Dr Butter* the name of Irritative, and from Mr Travers,†
that of Constitutional Irritation; denominations which may be perfectly correct, if they either denoted a new form of general disorder, or established as a new principle in pathology, the circumstance,
that when any individual texture is in a morbid state, it gives rise
to derangement, perversion, and irregularity, in the motions of the
sanguiferous system and the dependent secretions.   It appears to
me that there is in this nothing new nor even singular, when we
know, that it is an established principle in physiology and pathology, that all the textures of the animal body are so allied, that one
cannot be long in an unhealthy state without inducing general disorder, and that all the properties and actions of these textures are
so intimately associated, that those of one organ are almost never
impaired or perverted, without betraying the existence of this impairment or perversion, by disorder in the motions and actions of
the sanguiferous system, and, its great dependent, the secreting apparatus of the different organs.

The disease, however, is not in all cases a simple and exclusive
affection of one tissue; and the singular feature of this inflammation is, that, either simultaneously or successively, it affects a considerable number of different tissues.   It hence results that the concomitant symptoms are by no means uniform, and assume various
types according to the tissues affected.

Thus, in inflammation of the adipose tissue, the disease is very
liable to attack the filamentous tissue, which it disjoins and destroys
in the manner already described.   It also very commonly attacks
the veins; and the symptoms are then complicated with those of
venous inflammation; and may eventually give rise to the secondary suppurations observed to ensue on that disorder.   The venous

---

* Remarks on Irritative Fever.   By John Butter, M.D., F. R. S., &c.   Devonport,
1825, 8vo. pp. 302.

† An Inquiry concerning Constitutional Irritation.   By Benjamin Travers, F. R. S.
London, 1826, 8vo, pp. 556.

tunics are then observed to be thickened, and sometimes adhering, with obliteration of the canal; and in several instances matter, or lymph, or both, are found within the veins. Lastly, it may produce denudation of the arteries exactly as a broad ligature, or any foreign substance in the neighbourhood of, or around the arterial tubes, and in this manner induce erosion, and rupture of the artery with fatal hemorrhage.

In ordinary circumstances, the course of phenomena appears to be nearly the following. Sometimes without previous warning, in other instances after slight. sensations of chilness and languor, or even after distinct shivering, heavy dull pain is felt in one part particularly, as the neck, the breast, or an extremity, according to the situation which the disease affects. This painful sensation spreads or extends, amounting to stiff soreness of the whole region, with more or less tenderness of the integuments. If the part is examined, it is found affected with diffuse or extensive swelling, compressible, but not very elastic, considerable tension of the skin, great heat, and in some instances a dull red tinge. In some instances the skin retains its natural colour,—a circumstance which is to be ascribed to the depth of the inflammatory action, and perhaps the early period of the disease. In some it is of a faint red, inclining to yellow or orange, which becomes more distinct when pressure is applied; and in some the disease passes through every stage without even producing redness of the skin. In others long red patches, of no determinate shape, may be remarked; but this appearance is more common when the superficial adipose tissue is affected, and when the disease is verging to suppuration. These symptoms, which may be considered as indicating the first or inflammatory stage, last from thirty hours to three or four days,— seventy-two, eighty, or ninety-six hours.

As they proceed, the swelling increases and may become more prominent at one part than another, but still retains its diffuse and shapeless character. The pain, which is continual, becomes occasionally more acute, and is attended with an insufferable sensation of oppressive weight. If the disease affect an extremity, the patient feels as much difficulty in raising it as if it were a dead mass, or unconnected with his person. At length, about the fifth, sixth, or seventh day, according to the rapidity of the disease, the swelling presents in sundry parts a peculiar compressible, but not very elastic character, as if the subjacent tissues were floating in some fluid or semifluid matter.

At this period the constitutional symptoms, which consist in quick sharp pulse, great heat, thirst, loss of appetite, languor, and sometimes delirium, assume the appearance of extreme oppression and mortal weakness.   The pulse becomes much quicker, small and fluttering, sometimes intermittent ; the tongue, which had previously been covered with a thick, gray, or yellow, moist, viscid fur, or was red and glossy, is covered with a rough fur, dry, brown, and hard, yet the patient is insensible of thirst.   The skin is dry, or partially moistened with cold unctuous sweats; the urine is scanty and high-coloured, sometimes entirely suppressed, or passes with the stools involuntarily ; low mutturing alternates with stupor ; the breathing becomes quick, panting, and laborious, or slow, languid, and interrupted, and terminates in death.

If the affected part or limb be examined after death, the whole subcutaneous adipose tissue, and the intermuscular cellular tissue, are found enlarged, gray, or ash-coloured, and distended with blood-coloured fluid, oily serum, or sero-purulent, or purulent matter.   It is detached, in general, extensively from the several organs which it connects in the healthy state.   Between the muscles, which are dark-coloured, softened, lacerable, and emit a fetid odour, are found long sinuous caverns filled with dirty ash-coloured purulent fluid ; sloughs or mortified shreds are seen here and there hanging from aponeurotic sheaths, tendons, or even blood-vessels ; and while in most cases shreds or filaments of the subcutaneous adipose and the cellular tissue are the only traces of its existence, in not a few instances the muscles are detached from the periosteum, and the *periosteum* from the bone.   These shreds or filaments are mortified pieces or sloughs of adipose membrane and cellular tissue, and correspond to the pieces of wet tow mentioned by Hunter and Sir E. Home, and the wads of wet shamoy leather noticed by Mr James.

This may be regarded as the most exquisite and severe form of the disease.   Its duration in such circumstances varies.   It appears from the result of Dr Duncan's observations, that death does not take place before the sixth day, but may occur in any subsequent one to the twelfth or fifteenth.   Perhaps in the average number of cases, the seventh, eighth, or ninth may be stated as the day on which the termination occurs.

In milder cases it may terminate in resolution.   The general swelling subsides slowly, the pain disappears, the skin becomes cool; and the constitutional symptoms decline upon the eruption of a copious sweat, a cutaneous disease or other critical action.

It may terminate in abscess. The inflammatory action changes its character, and, instead of spreading, shows a disposition to stop. Lymph is effused, healthy purulent matter is formed, and adhesion taking place in one or more points, the disease terminates in phlegmonic suppuration.

In some instances the spreading and limited may be combined. The spreading or diffuse inflammation proceeds at one part of the affected tissue, while the limited with lymphy effusion and adhesion appears at another. This appears to be the fact in those tedious cases in which the disease is prolonged for weeks, and the patient either recovers, or ultimately dies hectic.

When recovery takes place after suppuration and sloughing of the adipose and cellular tissue, it is effected partly by direct adhesion taking place between the muscles or their cellular substance, and the skin, partly by the formation of new cellular tissue similar to those new membranes which are formed in the serous surfaces. The former is the cause of the stiffness, immobility, and condensation of parts after this inflammation has taken place.

The causes of this disease are not well known. There is reason to believe that it requires for its production a peculiar state of the constitution; for it more readily attacks the bloated and those of broken constitutions than the spare and the vigorous; it is more common and more severe in the corpulent and plethoric than in those of healthy and active habits; it is more common in those liable to mental inquietude and peevishness than to those of equable or indifferent temperament; and the same exciting cause which produces in a young and healthy subject a common phlegmonic abscess, will be followed in a sallow or middle-aged person, of dry or unctuous skin, with a fatal inflammation of the diffuse character. Something also appears to be attributable to epidemic influence; for several cases are generally remarked to occur much about the same time; and it has been further remarked, that when rose, scarlet fever, and bad sore throat prevail, instances of diffuse inflammation are not unfrequent.

With regard to agents which appear to possess exciting power, it may occur spontaneously : but has been observed to succeed the following circumstances; venesection and punctured wounds in general, application of a ligature to a vein, puncture by a cutting instrument during dissection, inoculation by morbid secretions from living animals, the bite of a venomous serpent, acrid or poisonous substances of the acrid family applied directly to the skin or adipose membrane, sprains or injuries of the fibrous tissues, and contused or lacerated wounds.

Though this disease may arise both spontaneously, and also in consequence of lacerated or punctured wounds, or even mere scratches or abrasions, and in consequence of various poisonous substances applied to the skin or the adipose membrane, it appears further, in certain circumstances, to ensue on the application to the skin of various acrid and irritant poisons. Thus, in the experiments of Orfila upon the mode of operation of these poisons, it was a frequent occurrence, to observe diffuse inflammation in the adipose tissue ensue on the application of such substances as bryony-root, elaterium, colocynth, gamboge, spurge-flax, euphorbium, &c. to the skin or the adipose membrane exposed by wound. Dr Duncan relates a case communicated by Dr Spens, in which it followed the application of an ammoniacal plaster for the removal of rheumatic pains. It has been observed to follow or attend malignant pustule. (Practice of Medicine, Vol. i. p. 656.)

The account of the necroscopic appearances, however, above given, is applicable principally to the disease as it takes place in the subcutaneous adipose tissue ; and perhaps, as it spreads to the intermuscular filamentous tissue. These appearances, though in all general characters similar in other tissues, are varied according to the portion of adipose membrane attacked.

The disease may either, when originally commencing in the subcutaneous adipose tissue, spread to the periangial, or it may commence in the latter at once, and produce destructive ravages in the periangial sheath, and most pernicious effects on the blood-vessels. Thus, I have elsewhere recorded the principal circumstances of a case in which the disease attacked the periangial adipose tissue of the right carotid artery and jugular vein, destroyed the sheath for the space of eight inches, denuded and exposed both vessels, produced gangrene and erosion of the artery and inflammation of the jugular vein, with obliteration of its canal, and denudation of the trunk of the pneumogastric nerve. (Edin. Med. and Surgical Journal, Vol. xlviii. p. 396.)

The adipose tissue connected with the internal organs is also liable to be attacked by inflammation. That enclosing the kidneys in particular has been found affected with, and destroyed by, the true disjunctive inflammation. One of the most characteristic examples of this disease on record is given by Dr Thomas Turner, in the fourth volume of the Medical Transactions of the Royal College of Physicians. In this case the disease commenced with sickness, vomiting, and pain in the bowels, followed by pain in the back and loins; and at the end of about thirty-eight hours with great restlessness, anxiety, laborious, panting respiration, and loss of pulse at the wrist. Death took place at the end of forty-eight hours. The whole adipose tissue enclosing the kidneys was in a gangrenous state, exhibiting a large mass of black pulpy matter. The capsules of both kidneys were inflamed, that of the right kidney mortified, and slight traces of inflammation were observed in the internal structure of both kidneys. In the winter of 1816–17, I examined the body of a man in whom I found the whole of the adipose cushion surrounding the left kidney, converted into an ash-coloured fetid, semifluid pulp, similar to a mixture of train oil and jelly, mingled with shreddy filaments, and in which this suppurative sloughing process had opened a passage from the fat of the left kidney into the interior of the transverse arch of the colon. In this case, though the patient did not complain of much pain, and presented chiefly the general languor, oppression, and stupor observed in typhoid fever, the pulse was quick and small, the tongue brown and dry, the thirst intense, afterwards not felt, the countenance dingy and lurid, and the eyes heavy, the bowels difficult to be affected by medicine, the urine scanty and high-coloured, and at length suppressed; and the patient, after muttering delirium and *typhomania* on the second day of the attack, with *subsultus tendinum*, passed into a comatose state, which terminated on the fourth day in death.

The endosteal or intra-osseous adipose tissue, in other words, the medullary membrane, is liable in like manner to both forms of inflammation, but especially the suppurative and disjunctive; and the invariable effect of this is to kill the compact tissue of the bone, and produce atomical death or caries of the cancellated tissue. *Necrosis* is the result of the former, and *spina ventosa* and caries of the latter. The full consideration of this variety of the disease, however, belongs to another subject.

I have now described the usual characters of this disease in its

E

most acute, intense, and rapid form.   But it sometimes happens that it is slower in progress and less intense in severity ; and in this case it may be said to be subacute or chronic.   Thus I have seen an instance in which the disease attacked the adipose tissue of the arm, and though attended with well-marked fever, yet without the overpowering symptoms of prostration so often observed,— and advancing so slowly as to admit of the employment of local depletion by leeches, and the effect of antimonials and purgatives, so as eventually to terminate in resolution.

The foregoing account may communicate some idea of the seat of this disease, of its effects, and of its dangerous tendency.   I have yet to offer a few remarks on its nature, its pathological peculiarities, and the causes on which its developement may seem to depend. Some of these points I have indeed anticipated.   But others are entitled to more systematic examination.

The most remarkable circumstance in the pathological history of *Pimelitis,* is the extreme rapidity with which it generally proceeds to sero-purulent infiltration and disjunctive destruction.   In several cases this has been known to take place within thirty-six hours from the appearance of the first symptoms of uneasiness.   In others it occurs in the course of about seventy-two hours; and in very few cases is this event protracted beyond the fourth day.

Very nearly at the same rate may be estimated the fatality of the disease.   Wherever the inflammation is very extensive, and especially if it occur in middle-aged or elderly corpulent persons, death is very likely to ensue in the course of the third, or at most, the fourth day.   In young and robust persons, on the contrary, and in whom the adipose tissue is not much loaded, the disease is slower in progress, and less frequently fatal in termination.   The most rapidly fatal case which I think I have yet witnessed occurred in a male patient in the Royal Infirmary this season.   He had been under treatment for slight diarrhœa, which disappeared under the use of chalk mixture and opiates, alternated with gentle eccoprotics, and the use of nutritious diet, and for several days expressed himself well.   He was in his usual health at the visit preceding the last day of his life; but in the afternoon, about four, he was attacked with pain of the left thigh and iliac region, which speedily became swelled, hot, red, and livid, and presented a large detachment of the cuticle, containing livid serum (*phlyctæna.*)   Next day the features were decomposed, the face pale, the countenance Hippocratic; and death took place the same evening, within twenty-six hours from the first appearance of symptoms. Upon inspection, the whole adipose membrane was found extensively infiltrated with dirty oily-like serum. The arteries were not diseased.

ANATOMICO-PATHOLOGICAL CAUSES OF DISJUNCTIVE INFLAMMATION.—Though I do not deny that this disease is occasionally to be seen in the filamentous tissue, yet I think. this is a much rarer occurrence than in the adipose membrane; and several circumstances appear to prove, that it is, if not the only, at least by far the most common, form of inflammation in that tissue. This conclusion is founded not only on the anatomical fact of the adipose membrane being found most usually the seat of the disease, and of its affecting parts where this texture is most abundant, as already stated, but also in another circumstance, viz. that the disease is most frequent in corpulent persons, in whom the adipose tissue is abundant. This circumstance again seems to be referable to the low vital energy of that tissue, as already in some degree explained.

In the corpulent, either by habit or age, in whom this disease assumes its most exquisite, intense, and unmanageable forms,—who are generally not only plethoric, but bloated, and liable to imperfect circulation, and disorders of the circulation and secretion generally,—and in whom slight causes are often followed by serious disorders, the adipose tissue appears to lose a great proportion of the small degree of vital energy which it possesses, and the more abundant the secreted product is, the less active are its vessels and the inherent properties of the membrane. In consequence of this greatly impaired energy, slight causes, as cold, scratches, or abrasions, punctures, contusions, &c. are suddenly followed by a more or less complete loss of circulation and action in the tissue; for the disease consists not in increased, but diminished action; and this impaired energy continues, until the natural functions of the tissue become extinct. In these circumstances, with few and inert blood-vessels, the secreted or inorganic matter of the adipose tissue becomes, as it were, a cause of strangulation of the tissue itself, or at least tends so directly to suppress the energies of its organic part, that it is incapable of resisting the influence of morbific agents of ordinary power; and hence, the organic portion either may be smitten with immediate death, or is easily made to assume a very low, languid, and imperfect form of morbid action, which speedily terminates in death.

This low degree of vital energy seems the principal if not the sole cause of the disjunctive, and, as it may be termed, the disorganizing character of the inflammation, of which the adipose membrane becomes the seat. If we compare the different elementary tissues of the animal body, we find that the nature of the inflammatory process, of which each becomes the seat, bears a relation more or less intimate and direct to the nature of its organization. All parts well provided with blood-vessels, and, therefore, highly organized, seem to have high vital energies, and great powers of resisting disorganization. Parts, on the other hand, less highly organized, and which have few or small-sized blood-vessels, may be said to have inferior degrees of organization, and to be less capable of resisting the vascular perversion in which inflammation consists. Thus the skin, the serous membranes, and the mucous membranes, all of which are highly vascular, possess also great powers of resisting the disorganizing effects of inflammation ; and, when these take place, either counteract this by some supplementary process, which inflicts no serious injury on the structure of the inflamed membrane, and does not permanently injure its functions, or, if actual destruction ensue, it is not by direct death of the part, but by the minute atomical absorption named ulceration ; and at the same time the vessels make attempts, though sometimes abortive, to repair this species of destruction.

My limits do not allow me to consider at length the apparent exceptions to this principle, otherwise it would appear distinctly that these were only confirmations of the fact now stated,—that the protecting faculty of any tissue against the ravages of inflammation depends very much upon, if it be not directly proportioned to, its organization, or the size and number of its nutrient vessels. This principle is also very clearly illustrated in the inflammation of the adipose membrane, in which an imperfect, and, indeed, an inferior degree of organization seems to be the main cause of the destructive effects of that process. In that tissue inflammation is no sooner established than it proceeds rapidly to death, chiefly because the texture has not powerful vital energies, and is less capable than others of resisting the tendency to destruction. It possesses less of the independent form of vitality which the vascular system communicates to all the elementary tissues of the frame, and hence sinks more easily and promptly under the influence of the perverted or impaired vascular disorder in which inflammation, consists.

It is not unlikely that this is also one of the principal causes of the peculiar irritative characters of the febrile disorder with which the inflammation of the adipose tissue is attended. We know that in the case of inflammation of highly organized tissues, as the serous membranes, the character of the concomitant fever is often distinct and acutely inflammatory,—much perverted action of the vascular system, but little of the nervous system, and much less of the overpowering prostration and oppression of all the vital powers which attend inflammation of the adipose membrane. In the one case, the actions of life seem to be simply increased, and are certainly perverted, and in one respect augmented in intensity. In the other, they are oppressed and overpowered; and the full vigour of reaction, as it has been named in the mechanical language of the iatro-mathematical schools, is not permitted to develope itself.

But it is not only in its constitutional effects that inflammation of the adipose tissue is a malady so important. From its intimate union with the parts which it incloses, its destruction entails their destruction; and, if it do not prove fatal by the severity of the febrile disorder which it induces, it may do so by the ravages which it causes among muscles, nerves, and blood-vessels. I mentioned its tendency to expose and denude the blood-vessels; because in almost all the dissections which I have seen and performed of this disease, I have found the vascular sheath more or less diseased, sometimes destroyed, and the vessels exposed, the veins thickened and inflamed, and the arteries brittle, softened, and sloughy. In all these cases, however, the disease proves fatal, either by the intensity of the febrile disorder, or by causing inflammation of the veins, or passing to some internal organ, as for instance when it affects the adipose membrane of the chest, and thence passes, as I have seen it, to the *pleura* and lungs. It cannot be doubted, however, that, were life not terminated in either of these modes now mentioned, the destruction of the adipose tissue, forming the sheath of the vessels, would have the effect of producing death in the arterial tunics, and rupture of these vessels. We know, that when the sheath is by any means detached from the arterial tunics, either by disease, or accident, or in consequence of operation, a result almost inevitable is death of these tunics, chiefly in consequence of the destruction, which the nutrient vessels, the *vasa vasorum*, necessarily sustain by the inflammation of the adipose sheath, by which these vessels are supported. That this has not been more frequently observed in cases of spontaneous inflammation of the adipose cushion, is to be ascribed to the fact, that the disease in general proves fatal by the severity of the constitutional disorder, or by the induction of inflammation of the veins, passing from their external to their internal coat.

It is proper to remark, that in an abstract of the case of inflammation of the periangial adipose tissue above referred to, in the *Archives Generales*, (iii. New Series, Dec. 1837,) M. Godin, the author of that notice, has attempted to oppose the view that the disease consists in inflammation of the adipose membrane, by representing it to be diffuse phlegmon. I have only to remark, that this is a contradiction in terms, which, instead of conveying a correct view of the disease, tends to confuse still more than formerly. The view given by me rests on the accuracy of the anatomical observations; and unless these are shown to be erroneous, I see no mode of denying the fact, that in most of the cases of diffuse inflammation the adipose membrane is the chief seat of the disease.

2. *Hemorrhage.* Effusion of blood into the adipose tissue is not very common. It is observed in the same circumstances nearly in which it occurs in the filamentous tissue. Thus it has been seen in land and sea scurvy. Huxham observed it in fevers with petechial eruptions. And Cleghorn states that one of the appearances after death in the continuous and malignant tertians of Minorca was extravasation of blood in the form of black patches in the adipose layer of the mesentery, omentum, and colon.

3. *Excessive Deposition.* In certain subjects, and in peculiar circumstances, the quantity deposited is enormous. The average weight of the human subject at a medium size is about 160 pounds, or between eleven and twelve stones. Yet instances are on record of its attaining by deposition of fat in the adipose membrane the extraordinary weight of 510, and 600 pounds, or from thirty-five to forty stones. Cheyne mentions a case in which the weight was 448 pounds, equal to thirty-two stones. In the Philosophical Transactions are recorded two cases of persons so corpulent, that

one weighed 480 pounds, and another 500 pounds. And the Breslau Collections contain cases in which the human body weighed 580 and 600 pounds.

In females and in eunuchs it is more abundant than in males; in females deprived of the ovaries it is more abundant than in those possessed of these organs; and it is well known that sterility is frequent among the corpulent of both sexes. In some circumstances this accumulation may be so great as to constitute disease, (*Polysarcia adiposa*, Cyrilli, Sauvages, Cullen, and Good;) and in other circumstances the deposition of fat is a means which the secreting system seems to employ to relieve fulness and tension of the vessels, and if not to cure, at least to obviate morbid states of the circulation. (Parry.) Accumulations of fat are said to take place in some animals in a few hours in certain states of the atmosphere. During a fog of twenty-four hours' continuance, thrushes, wheatears, ortolans, and red-breasts are reported to become so fat that they are unable to fly from the sportsman. (Bichat.)

4. *Local Hypertrophy.* The adipose membrane is liable to a form of hypertrophy, local in situation, and of a peculiar character. The surface of the person and extremities presents many small tumours, varying in size from a garden pea to that of a filbert, soft, compressible, movable under the skin, and indolent. In some the surface acquires a bluish tint, apparently from compression of the vessels of the skin. In the most marked case of this which I have seen, the number was very considerable, probably not less than eighty or ninety of different sizes. On inspection after death, which was the consequence of another disease, these bodies were found to consist of globular or spheroidal masses of fat, not different from that of the ordinary fat, contained within membranous capsules, with walls a little firm. The individual was corpulent; but the presence of these bodies seemed, from the account of his medical attendants, to exert no appreciable influence on the state of his health.

These bodies appear to be merely the result of hypertrophy affecting many separate points of the adipose membrane.

5. *Extreme Diminution.* The diminution or disappearance of fat is much more frequent than its extraordinary abundance. This diminution is said to depend on one or other of the following causes. 1st, Long abstinence, as in fasting, and the periodical sleep of dormant and hybernating animals; 2d, Organic diseases,

as consumption, cancer, disease of the liver, especially cirrhosis,⸱ disease of the heart, granular degeneration of the kidneys, ulceration of the intestines, &c. ; 3*d*, Purulent collections or secretions ; 4*th*, Leucophlegmatic and dropsical states; 5*th*, Gloomy and melancholy thoughts or passions ; 6*th*, Long and uninterrupted effort of the intellectual powers ; 7*th*, Preternatural increase of the natural evacuations, as in cholera, diarrhœa, diabetes, &c. mucous discharges, especially from the pulmonary and intestinal membranes, as in chronic catarrh, inflammation of the intestines and dysentery ; 8*th*, Long and intense heat, whether natural, as during hot summers, or artificial, as in furnaces, hot-houses, &c. ; 9*th*, Running, riding, and every species of fatiguing exercise long continued, as is exemplified in the case of grooms at Newmarket, Doncaster, &c. ; 10*th*, States of long disease not organic; 11*th*, Night-watching and want of sleep in general ; 12*th*, Immoderate use of spirituous liquors ; 13*th*, Habit of eating bitter and spiced or acid aliments.

Yet even in these states the fat of the animal body is seldom entirely wasted. In several organic diseases, in which great emaciation takes place, a considerable quantity of fat is always found in the orbits behind the eyeball, round the substance of the heart, around the kidneys, in the colon, and in the mesentery and omentum.* According to the observation of William Hunter, anasarcous dropsy is the only disease in which the fat of the adipose membrane is entirely consumed. " This disorder, when inveterate, has that effect in such a degree, that we find the heart or mesentery of such subjects as free from fat as in the youngest children." This, however, is in some degree denied by Bichat, who contends that it is not uncommon to find much subcutaneous fat in subjects greatly infiltrated, (Vol. I. p. 57.) It is obvious that much will depend on the stage of the disease. It cannot be expected, that the moment serous infiltration appears in the filamentous tissue, all the fat should be at once removed from the adipose. The process of ab-

---

* An instance of this, which occurred within the last few days, may be now mentioned. I had occasion to examine the body of a young gentleman, (3d October 1827,) who had laboured under symptoms of pulmonary disease during the three months previous to his death. Though the left lung was completely occupied with small whitish amorphous masses of tubercular matter of different degrees of consistence, and the right lung in addition to this was in the second stage of pulmonic inflammation, yet a considerable layer of fat was found between the skin and muscles on the chest and belly.

sorption is gradual as that of deposition; and the inference of Hunter may be regarded as nearly exact in reference to long continued, or what he terms inveterate dropsy. It is certain, that, while it is, very difficult to deprive the bones of ordinary subjects of oil, those of dropscal subjects are the only ones which it is possible to obtain free from this substance.

Lastly, I have to observe, that the remark of Dr Hunter is applicable chiefly to granular disease of the kidney, which, whether accompanied with anasarca or not, has a remarkable effect in removing the fat and various other animal substances.

The removal of the fat from its containing membrane is effected by the process of absorption, the agents of which are supposed by William Hunter, Portal, Bichat, and Mascagni, to be the lymphatics. According to the results of the experiments of Magendie, Mayer, Tiedemann and Gmelin, Segalas, &c. it must, in some measure at least, be ascribed to the influence of minute veins. It is a point of some interest to know in what form it is absorbed, whether as oily matter, or after undergoing a process of decomposition. The observation of Hewson, of Dr Traill, and Dr Christison, above quoted, would lead to the former view; but it is not easy to conceive that this should be uniform. We want, in short, correct facts on the point at issue.

5. *Adipose Sarcoma.* This consists in an unusual deposition of firm fatty matter in cells, the component fibres of which are sufficiently firm to give its consistence. The tumour, which is generally globular, is always surrounded by a thin capsule formed by the condensation of the contiguous filamentous tissue. The tumour is supplied by a few blood-vessels, which proceed from the capsule, but which form so slender an attachment that they are readily broken, and the tumour is easily scooped from its seat. This sort of tumour occurs almost invariably in the adipose membrane, and seems to consist in a local hypertrophy of the part in which it is found. It may have a broad basis, but is often pendulous, or attached by a narrow neck or stalk. It is the most common form of sarcomatous tumour, and may occur in any part of the body in which there is adipose membrane, but is chiefly found on the front and back of the trunk, and not unfrequently on two places at the same time.

6. *Steatoma.* In adipose sarcoma the adipose matter is deposited in cells, and the tumour derives a degree of firmness from the

fibres with which it is thus traversed in every direction. In other instances, however, the adipose matter is deposited in a mass in the cavity of a spherical or spheroidal cyst, formed in the filamentous or the adipose tissue; and the tumour is soft and compressible, and seems to contain fluid or semifluid matter. When cut open it is found to contain a soft semifluid matter of the consistence of honey, but of oily or adipose properties. In such circumstances the inner surface of the cyst, or at least the vessels of this surface, are the agents which secrete the fatty matter. This tumour may occur either in the filamentous or the adipose tissue; but is to be regarded as an example of local deposition of adipose matter. It may appear in any region of the filamentous tissue, but is most frequent about that of the head and face. Small steatoms are not unfrequent in the eyelids and in the scalp. Larger ones are more frequent about the neck.

The other forms of encysted tumours, distinguished by the names of *atheroma*, (*αθηρωμα pulticula* ab *αθαρα pultis genus*), and *meliceris* (*μελιχηρις mel* and *cera*, honey; wax), are to be viewed rather as varieties of the steatom than as generically different. The substance contained may differ in consistence, but is nearly the same in essential qualities.

7. *Melanosis.* I have already spoken of the melanotic deposition taking place in the filamentous tissue. The adipose membrane is also a frequent seat of this singular change. The black or melanose matter is found in the subcutaneous adipose membrane and the subjacent cellular tissue of the chest and belly; it is not uncommon in the fat of the orbit; it is very commonly seen in the adipose cushion on the fore-part of the vertebral column, that surrounding the kidneys, and in the fat of the anus and rectum; it is found in the anterior and posterior mediastinum; and it is found between the folds of the mesentery, of the mesocolon, and of the omentum. It is also found in the substance of the marrow of bones; and perhaps in most cases in which the osseous system appears to be stained with the melanose deposite, the dark matter may be traced to the medullary particles, the situation of which it is found accurately to occupy.

In all these situations it appears in various degrees of perfection, and in different forms. It may be disseminated in black or inky spots through the adipose membrane; it may be accumulated in spherical or spheroidal masses of various size and shape; or it may be found in the form of brown or ebon-coloured fluid or semifluid, enclosed in a cyst formed of the contiguous tissue more or less condensed.

The melanose matter is entirely destitute of organization, and is' to be regarded as the result of a peculiar secretion. No vessels have been traced into it; and when bodies affected with this deposite are minutely injected, the vessels can be traced no farther than the enveloping cyst. (Breschet.) It is also to be noticed that it is never deposited exactly in the site of organic fibres, but always between them, and very generally in the precise situation of the adipose particles. These several circumstances show that the melanose disease consists not in a degeneration or conversion into another substance, but in the deposition of a new form of matter in the manner of a secretion.

In what form the melanose substance is first deposited we have few accurate facts to enable us to form a judgment. Laennec is of opinion that it is first deposited in a solid form, and afterwards becomes fluid. The former he considers the stage of crudity, the latter that of softening, (ramollissement.) Several facts, however, would lead to the conclusion, that when first deposited it was fluid, and afterwards acquired consistency. Thus, in several dissections performed by Dr Cullen and Mr Carsewell, the matter of the small tumours, which are supposed to be of short duration, were found to be softest, and sometimes as fluid as cream.* In like manner, in a case recorded by M. Chomel, in which the disease was found in the liver in the shape of large cysts, the melanose matter was more fluid in the centre than in the circumference of the cysts.† Upon the whole, if the melanose deposite be, as is supposed, an inorganic secretion, the idea of its being poured forth from the vessels at first in a fluid or semifluid state is most probable, and most consistent with the usual phenomena and laws of animal processes.

8. *Acephalo-cysts.* This form of hydatid is occasionally found situate beneath the skin, partly in the adipose tissue, partly in the cellular membrane. When present in numbers, they form an extensive superficial tumour over the person, most commonly the back, and in rare cases in the extremities. They present the usual characters of acephalo-cysts in other regions; that is, they are glo-

* Transactions of the Medico-Chirurgical Society of Edinburgh, Vol. I. p. 264.
† Nouveau Journal de Medecine, Tome III. p. 41.

bular cysts, sometimes solitary, more frequently associated or con-
gregated with membranous coverings, thin, opaque, and almost
translucent. In some instances they give rise to suppuration, and
by this means come to the surface. If they do not, they seem to
cause inconvenience by their size, number, and situation. One
incision made through the skin often allows the escape of a great
number, leaving an extensive cavity in the adipose and cellular
membrane.

9. *Induration.* I think it probable that the peculiar affection which
takes place in the bodies of infants described at p. 43 in chapter iii.
should be referred to this tissue. But after this mention of the subject, I think it unnecessary to alter the arrangement.

CHAPTER V.

ARTERY, ARTERIAL TISSUE, (*Arteria,—Tissu arteriel.*)

SECTION I.

THE structure of the arteries has been so much the subject of
examination at all periods of the history of anatomy, that to mention the authors by whom it has been described would be much the
same as to enumerate all the anatomists who have ever written.
To omit Galen, and some of those who wrote shortly after the revival of literature, descriptions of the structure of arteries have
been given with different degrees of minuteness and accuracy by
Willis, Vieussens, Verheyen, Lancisi, Bidloo, the first Monro,
Morgagni, Ludwig, Haller, De La Sône, Bichat, Gordon, Magendie, and by Mondini. Yet the descriptions given by these observers are so discordant, that Ludwig complains of the difficulty of re-
conciling them, and Haller evidently felt it; and with the exception of those given by the four last authors, they do not accord with
the characters which this substance actually presents.

The following account is derived principally from repeated examination of the arteries of the human subject, occasionally compared with those of the more familiar domestic animals.

Every arterial tube greater than one line in diameter is visibly
composed of one adventitious and two essential substances. The

.first, the sheath, reputed to consist of condensed filamentous tissue: the two last, the proper arterial and internal tissues. (*Tunica propria et membrana intima.*)

1. The inner surface of the arterial tube is formed by a very' thin semitransparent polished membrane, which is said to extend not only in the one direction over the inner surface of the left ventricle, auricle, and pulmonary veins, but in the other to form the minute vascular terminations which are distributed through the substance of the different organs. This membrane is particularly described by Bichat under the name of *common membrane of the system of red blood,* because he believed it to exist wherever red blood was moving,—in the pulmonary veins, in the left side of the heart, and over the entire arterial system.

The inner membrane may be demonstrated by cutting open or inverting any artery of moderate size, when it may be peeled off in the form of thin slips by the forceps. Or, if the tube be fitted on a glass rod, by removing the layers of the proper membrane in successive portions, the inner one at length comes into view in the form of a thin translucent pellicle, of uniform, homogeneous aspect, without fibres or other obvious traces of organization. This membrane is supposed to be prolonged to form those minute vessels in which the proper coat cannot be traced. It is very brittle, and is distinguished during life by a remarkable activity in forming the morbid states to ,which arteries are liable. In other respects it is deemed by Bichat peculiar, and, though similar to the proper membrane, is to be considered as unlike any other tissue. Its chemical composition is not known.

2. Exterior to this *common or inner* membrane is placed a dense strong tissue of considerable thickness, of a dun yellowish colour, which is found to consist of fibres disposed in concentric circles placed contiguous to each other round the axis of the artery. If this substance be examined either from without or in the opposite direction, it will be found that, by proper use of forceps, its fibres can be separated to an indefinite degree of minuteness, even to that of a hair, and that they uniformly separate in the same direction. Longitudinal fibres are visible neither in this nor in any other tissue of the arterial tube. This is the proper arterial tissue, (*tunica propria.*) Its uniform dun yellow colour is perceived through the semitransparent inner membrane, and is most conspicuous either when this is removed, or when the outer cellular envelope is de-

tached and the component threads separated from each other; and if it be less distinct in the smaller branches, it is because the tissue on which the colour depends is here considerably thinner. In this respect it varies in different regions. Though in general less dense and abundant as the arteries recede from the heart, it is thicker, *cæteris paribus*, in those of the lower than in those of the upper extremities. In the vertebral and internal carotid arteries, and in those distributed in the substance of the liver, spleen, &c. it is thinner than in vessels of the same size in the muscular interstices.

The nature of this tissue has been the subject of much controversy. It was long believed to be muscular, and to possess the properties of muscular fibre. Bichat showed that the arguments by which this opinion was supported are inconclusive, and that the arterial tissue has very few qualities in common with the muscular. The circumstances from which he derived his proofs were its physical and physiological properties.

The arguments derived from the physical properties of this tissue are chiefly the following. The arterial tissue is close, elastic, fragile, and easily divided by ligature; muscular fibre is more loose in structure, by no means elastic, and, instead of being divided or cut by ligature as artery is, undergoes a sort of strangulation. The action of alcohol, diluted acids, and caloric, by means of hot fluids, which are not corrosive, affords a proof of the chemical difference of these animal substances. All of them produce, in the arterial tunic, a species of shrivelling or crispation, which seems to depend on more complete coagulation of one of the chemical principles; but no similar effect takes place in muscular fibres. According to Berzelius the proper arterial tunic contains no fibrine.* Beclard, however, asserts, that he has ascertained that it contains a portion of this principle; but nevertheless hesitates to consider it as a muscular or fibrinous tissue, and expresses his opinion, that it would be with greater propriety referred to that order of substances which he has named yellow or tawny fibrous system.

The consideration of the physiological or organic properties leads to similar results. Neither mechanical or chemical agents applied as stimulants produce any change or motion in the living arterial membrane. 1. The arteries of an amputated limb, exposed the moment after amputation, while the muscles are in active motion,

* A View of the Progress of Animal Chemistry. By J. J. Berzelius, M. D. &c. &c. London, 1813. Pp. 24, 25.

do not contract or move when punctured by the scalpel.   2. The experiments of Bikker and Van-den-Bos with the electric spark, and those of Vassalli-Eandi, Giulio, and Rossi with the galvanic , pile, may be considered as disproved by the experiments of Nysten,* who found no contraction in the human aorta after violent death, while the heart and other muscles could still be excited.   In performing the same experiment with the artery of the living dog this physiologist was equally disappointed.   3. The circular contraction of the calibre of an artery, either partially or wholly divided, depends not on irritability, but either on its elasticity, or on that property which it possesses of contracting strongly, the instant the distending agent is removed.   This power, which was rather happily named by Bichat *contractilité par defaut d'extension*, is quite different from muscular contraction or irritability, and must not be confounded with them ; but it depends in a degree not much less on the living state of the body and the individual arterial tube.   4. The contraction said to take place in living arteries after the application of alcohol, acids, or alkalis, is to be ascribed to the chemical *crispation*, and not to stimulant power.   It does not relax.   5. These inferences are not inconsistent with the experiments of Thomson, Philips, Hastings, and Kaltenbrunner, on minute arterial tubes, which may be admitted to possess something like irritability, or rather susceptibility of contraction, without the necessity of supposing the same property in the large branches and trunks.   6. This is so much more probable, as in these minute arteries the proper arterial tunic is either wanting, or is so much thinner and so modified, that it is impossible to conceive its presence capable of affecting the result of experiments made to determime the degree or kind of arterial contraction.

3. The outer surface of the proper arterial tissue is enveloped, as above noticed, in a layer of dense filamentous or cellular membrane, which is very firmly attached to it, and which was formerly considered as part of the arterial tissue.   It is adventitious; a modification of filamentous or cellular texture which establishes a communication between the artery and the contiguous parts, and is necessary to the nutrition and healthy state of the vessel.   It incloses and transmits the minute vessels anciently denominated *vasa vasorum*, (*arteriolæ arteriarum*, Haller ;) and if detached even through

* Nouvelles Experiences Galvaniques, &c.   Par P. H. Nysten, &c.   A Paris, An. XI. pp. 235 and 236.

a trifling extent, the arterial portion thus isolated is sure to become
dead; to be affected with inflammatory and sloughing action; and
ultimately to give way and discharge the contents of the vessel. M.
Beclard considers it a fibro-cellular membrane, which may in the
larger arteries be divided into two layers, one exterior, similar to
the general filamentous tissue; the other inside between the outer
layer and the proper tissue, yellowish and firm, but still sufficiently
distinct from the proper tunic. In the cerebral arteries it is wanting, and in most parts of the chest and belly its absence is supplied
by a portion of pericardium, pleura, or peritonæum. Yet even
there a thin layer of fine cellular tissue appears to connect these
membranes to the proper tunic. In the extremities the cellular
sheath is removed in dissecting arterial preparations.

At different periods several anatomists have maintained the existence of longitudinal fibres in arterial tissue; and even at the present day this notion is not entirely abandoned. Morgagni was the
first who, trusting to mere observation, the only sure guide in anatomical science, doubted the existence of these fibres, and was not
ashamed to say he was unable to perceive them.[*] Upon the same
ground Haller would not admit their existence;[†] and Bichat and
Meckel positively deny them. I have repeatedly examined almost
every considerable artery of the human body, and I have never
been able to recognize any longitudinal fibres either in the middle
or proper coat, or in the thin internal membrane, as taught by
Willis, Douglas, and De La Sône.

Though arterial tissue does not appear to be very vascular, it is
furnished with arteries and veins (*vasa vasorum*; *arteriolæ arteriarum,*) which do not come from the artery or vein itself, but from the
neighbouring vessels.[‡] Thus the aorta at its origin is supplied with
minute arteries from the right and left coronary, and in some instances with a proper vessel adjoining to the orifice of the right coronary artery, which Haller regards as a third coronary. The rest
of the thoracic aorta derives its vessels from the upper bronchials,
from twigs of the internal mammary arteries, from the bronchials,
from the œsophageals, and from the phrenics. The abdominal por-

---

* Adversaria Anatomica, II. p. 78.

† " Verum anatome et microscopium omnino fibros longitudinem sequentes num-
quam demonstravit, aut mihi, aut aliis, ante me, scriptoribus, quorum auctoritate
meam tueor."—Elementa, Lib. ii. sect. 1, sect. 7.

‡ Hunter, IV. p. 131.

tion is supplied from the spermatics, the lumbar, and in some instances the mesocolic artery. The same arrangement nearly is observed with regard to the veins.

Few textures are more liberally supplied with nerves than arteries are. Almost every considerable trunk or vessel is surrounded with numerous plexiform filaments of nerves, many of which may be traced into the tissue of the artery. The anterior part of the arch of the aorta is abundantly supplied with branches from the superficial cardiac nerves, which Haller was unable to trace beyond the artery. The cœliac, the mesenteric, and the mesocolic arteries are invested with numerous plexiform nervous filaments derived from the large semilunar ganglion of the splanchnic nerve. The renal arteries in like manner are surrounded with numerous twigs of the renal plexus. And each of the intercostal arteries at its origin receives nervous threads from the intercostal nerves. In the face the branches of the fifth pair may often be traced enveloping the arteries. This arrangement, which is observed chiefly in the blood-vessels going to the internal organs, led Bichat to announce it as a general fact, that the arteries derived their nerves almost exclusively from the ganglions, and the gangliar nerves.* The inference does not rest upon strict observation, and evidently owes its birth to the hypothetical opinions of this ingenious physiologist. All the arteries going to the extremities, the axillary, and iliac, and their branches, receive nerves from the neighbouring nervous trunks, which are formed chiefly from cerebral or spinal nerves, and have no immediate connection with the system of the ganglions. In the internal carotid and the vertebral arteries, and their branches, nerves cannot be distinctly traced.†

Organized in the manner now described, it is requisite to take a short view of the anatomical connections of the arterial system, or to consider it in its origin, its course, and its termination.

The arterial system of the animal body may be viewed as one large trunk divided into several branches, which again are subdivided and ramified to a degree of minuteness which exceeds all calculation. It is requisite, therefore, to consider the origin, 1st, Of the aorta, the large trunk ; 2d, Of the branches which arise from it ; and, 3dly, Of the small vessels into which these are divided.

---

* " Le grand arbre à sang rouge ou l'arteriel, est presque exclusivement embrassé par la premiere classe des nerves."—Anatomie General, Tom. I. p. 302.

† H. A. Wrisberg De Nervis Arterias Venasque comitantibus, Tome III.

Every one knows that the aorta is connected at its origin with the upper and anterior part of the left ventricle. The manner of this connection has been well examined by Lancisi, by Ludwig, and particularly by Bichat. It may be demonstrated by dissection, but is much more distinctly shown by boiling the heart with the blood-vessels attached. In a heart so treated the thin internal membrane may be traced passing from the interior of the ventricle along the margin of its orifice to the inside of the arterial tube. Exactly at the point of union it is doubled into three semicircular folds, forming semilunar valves, and thence is continued along the whole course of the artery. This membrane is entirely distinct from the proper or fibrous coat. Of the latter, the cardiac extremity or beginning is notched into three semicircular sections, each of which corresponds to the base or attached margin of a semilunar valve. These sections are attached to the aortic orifice of the ventricle by delicate filamentous tissue, but are not connected with the fleshy fibres of the heart; and at the angle or point of attachment, the thin inner membrane is folded in so as to fill up a space or interval which is left between the margin of the orifice and the circumference of the proper arterial tissue, where it is notched or trisected.

The aorta is soon divided into branches, which again are subdivided into small vessels. With the mathematical physiologists, it was a favourite problem to ascertain the number of branches into which any vessel might be subdivided. Keill made them from forty to fifty. Haller states, that, counting the minutest ramifications, he has found scarcely twenty. The inquiry is vain and useless, and cannot be subjected to accurate calculation. In no two subjects is the same artery found to be subdivided the same number of times, and in no two subjects are the very same branches found to arise from the same trunk.

A branch issuing from a trunk generally forms with it a particular angle. Most generally, perhaps, these angles are acute; but in particular situations they approach nearly to a right angle. Thus the *innominata*, left carotid, and left subclavian, issue from the arch of the aorta nearly at a right angle, at least to the tangent of the arch. The intercostals form a right angle with the thoracic aorta; the renal and lumbar arteries form a large acute angle, approaching to right with the abdominal; and the coeliac comes off nearly in the same manner from the anterior part of the vessel. The internal and external carotids, again, the external and internal iliacs, the branches of the humeral, and those of the femoral, form angles more or less acute with each other. The angle which the spermatics make is, generally speaking, the most acute in the arterial system.

It is convenient to distinguish the branches and divisions of the arterial system into different classes or orders, according to their size and their proximity to, or distance from, the heart. Though the arterial system may be considered as one single artery divided and subdivided into a multiplicity of branches and twigs, yet in reference to the communications between the latter, they may be distinguished into the following orders.

First order, the aorta and *innominata*; the second order, the common carotid arteries, the subclavian arteries, and the common iliac arteries; the third order, the external and internal carotid arteries, the axillary arteries, the external and internal iliac arteries; the fourth order, the brachial arteries, the femoral arteries, and the sacromedian arteries; the branches of the subclavian and axillary trunks, as the vertebrals, transverse cervicals, scapular arteries, the pelvic and other branches of the posterior and anterior iliac arteries; the fifth order, the superficial and deep brachial arteries, the radial and ulnar, the superficial and deep femoral arteries, the popliteal, the anterior tibial, and posterior tibial, and the peroneal arteries; and the sixth order, all other small vessels beneath the size and capacity of those already specified.

This division is useful in reference to the phenomena of obstruction of arteries, and the means and channels by which the inconveniences of obstruction are compensated. It will be seen afterwards that obliteration or contraction of vessels of the fourth, fifth, and sixth orders, and obstruction of their canals, are evils much less serious and important than contraction or obliteration of vessels of the first, second, and third orders. In short, the functions of arteries in the first, second, and third orders of vessels are in this respect more necessary and indispensable than in the three last orders of vessels. Hemorrhage, also, from the first two or three orders of vessels is much more dangerous than from the fourth, and from the fourth than from the fifth or sixth.

I have already alluded to the structure of the arterial tissue at the divarications. These changes relate both to the inner and to the proper membrane. In the inside of the vessel, the inner membrane is folded somewhat so as to form a prominent or elevated point, the disposition of which varies according to the angle of divarication.   1st, When this is rectangular, the prominence of the inner membrane is circular, and is equally distinct all round.   2d, When the angle is obtuse, as in the mesenteric artery, the prominence is distinct, and resembles a semicircular ridge, between the continuation of the trunk and the branch given off, but indistinct on the opposite side where the angle is obtuse.   3d, If the angle is acute, and that formed by the branch with the continuation of the trunk is obtuse, the beginning of the artery presents an oblique circle, the elevated half of which is near the heart, the other more remote.

The arrangement of the fibres of the proper tissue is described by Ludwig from the divarication of the iliac arteries, and may be seen in any part of the arterial system where the vessels are large. The circular fibres separating form on each side a half ring, from which is produced a complete ring which incloses the smaller rings formed by the circular fibres of the vessel given off.   These circular fibres proceed to the prominence of the internal membrane already described, and are arranged round it much in the same manner, in which those of the large vessels surround its inner membrane.   In this, however, no continuity between the rings of the large vessel and those of the small one can be recognized.   The latter are inserted as it were into the former, and they are connected by the continuity of the inner membrane only.

. In observing the course or transit of arterial tubes, the principal point deserving notice is the sheltered situation which they generally occupy, their tortuous course, and their mutual communications.   In the extremities they are always found towards the interior or least exposed part of the limb, generally deep between muscles, and sometimes lying along bones.   When they are minutely subdivided, they enter into the interior of organs, without, however, sinking at once into their intimate substance.   In the muscles, they are lodged between the fibres; in the brain, in the convolutions; in glands, between their component lobes.   In such situations they are generally observed to be more or less tortuous in the course which they follow.   On the reasons of this, much difference of opinion still prevails.   (Bichat and Magendie.)

In the course of the arteries, no circumstance is of greater mo_ ment than their mutual communications or inosculations, (*anastvmoses.*) Of this there may be two forms; the first when two equal trunks unite, the second when a large vessel unites with a smaller one. Of the first, three varieties have been mentioned. 1*st*, Two equal trunks may unite at an acute angle to form one vessel. Thus, in the fœtus, the *ductus arteriosus* and the aorta are conjoined; and the two vertebral arteries unite to form the basilar trunk. 2*d*, Two trunks may communicate by a transverse branch, as the two anterior cerebral arteries do in forming the anterior segment of the circle of Willis. 3*d*, Two trunks may, by mutual union, form an arch, from the convexity of which the minute vessels arise, as is seen in the branches of the mesenteric arteries.

The second mode of inosculation is frequent in the extremities, especially round the joints. The multiplied communications of the arterial system in these regions, though well known to anatomists, and enumerated by Haller, were first clearly and systematically explained by Scarpa, and afterwards by Cooper and Hodgson. The importance of this arrangement in facilitating the motions of the circulation, in obviating the effects of local impediment in any vessel or set of vessels, and in enabling the surgeon to tie an arterial trunk when wounded, affected with aneurism or any other disease, has been clearly established by these authors. Their researches have shown that there is not a single vessel which may not be tied with full confidence in the powers of the collateral circulation. Even the aorta has been found contracted or obliterated, and its channel obstructed in the human subject in twelve instances, (Paris,*) (Graham,†)(Winstone,‡)(Otto,§)(Meckel,‖)(Reynaud,¶)

* Retrecissement considerable de l'Aorte Pectorale, observé a l'Hotel Dieu de Paris. Journal de Chirurgie. Par Desault. Tome II. p. 107. Paris, 1791.

† Case of Obstructed Aorta. By Robert Graham, M. D., Medico-Chirurgical Transactions, Vol. V. p. 287. London, 1814.

‡ Surgical Essays. By Astley Cooper, F. R. S., and Benjamin Travers, F. R. S. Part I. p. 115. Third Edition. London, 1818.

§ Neue Seltene Beobachtungen zur Anatomie, Physiologie und Pathologie gehorig. Von Adolph Wilhelm Otto. Berlin, 1824. 4to. Dritter Abshnitt, C. XXIX. Seite 66.

‖ Verschliessung der Aorta am Viertel Brustwirbel. Von A. Meckel zu Bern. Archiv für Anatomie und Physiologie. Herausgegeben Von Johan Friederich Meckel, 1827. Leipzig. Seite 345.

¶ Observation d'une Obliteration presque complete de l'Aorte, &c. Par M. Reynaud. Journal Hebdomadaire de Medecine, Tome Premier, 1828. P. 161. Paris, 1828.

(Jordan,*) (Le Grand,†) (Nixon,‡) (Craigie,§) (Eichler and Romer,‖) (Tiedemann,¶) ; and a ligature has been put on its abdominal
portion, (Cooper.)

To ascertain the several modes in which arteries terminate has
been a problem of much interest to the physiologist, and of no
small difficulty to the anatomist.　The alleged terminations as believed to be established, are minutely and elaborately enumerated
by Haller, who, however, multiplied them too much according to
the modern acceptation of the term.

1. The first undoubted termination of arteries is immediately in
veins.　It is unnecessary to adduce in support of this fact the long
list of observers enumerated by Haller.　It is sufficient to say that
it was clearly established by the microscopical observations of Leu-
wenhoeck, Cowper, and Baker, by Haller himself, and by Spallanzani in his beautiful experiments on the circulation of the blood.

2. The second termination which may be mentioned here is that
into the colourless artery, (*arteria non rubra*.)　This is sufficiently
well established by the phenomena of injections.

3. A third termination which is supposed to exist, but of which
no sensible proofs can be given, is that into colourless vessels supposed to open by minute orifices on various membranous surfaces,
and therefore termed exhalants.　The nature of these vessels shall
be considered afterwards.

Haller admits a termination in, or communication with lymphatic vessels, but allows that it is highly problematical.　Partial communications have been traced between arteries and lymphatics by
several anatomists; but the point requires to be again submitted
to accurate researches.

* A Case of Obliteration of the Aorta.　By Joseph Jordan, Esq., Surgeon to the
Lock Hospital, Manchester.　The North of England Medical and Surgical Journal,
Vol. I.　London, 1830-31.　P. 101.

† Du Retrecissement de l'Aorta : Du Diagnostic et du Traitement de cette Maladie, &c.　Par le Docteur a Le Grand.　Paris, 1832.　8vo. Pp. 58.

‡ Case of Constriction of the Aorta, with Disease of its Valves, &c.　By R. L.
Nixon, Surgeon.　Dublin Medical Journal, Vol. V. p. 386.　Dublin, 1834.

§ Instance of Obliteration of the Aorta beyond the Arch, illustrated by similar
Cases and Observations.　By David Craigie, M. D., Physician to the Royal Infirmary.
Edinburgh Medical and Surgical Journal, Vol. LVI. p. 427.

‖ Eichler und Romer in Medicinische Iahrbucher des Osterreichischen Staats, 1830.
B. XXIX. N. 2, S. 200.

¶ Friedrich Tiedemann, Von der Verengung und Schliessung der Pulsadern in
Krankheiten, Heidelberg, und Leipzig, 1843.　Fall 9.

3

Another mode of termination, that, namely, into excreting ducts, admitted by Haller, scarcely requires particular mention. So far as an artery can be said to terminate in such a manner, it would come under the head of that into exhalant vessels. Many of the proofs mentioned by Haller, however, may be shown to be examples of a morbid state of the mucous membranes of these ducts, in which their capillary vessels are disorganized.

In considering the several terminations of arteries, it is not unimportant to advert to the distribution of these vessels. Injections show that they penetrate into every texture and organ of the animal body, excepting one or two substances in which they have never yet been traced. But in different textures they are found in different degrees; and they may vary in extent even in the same texture in two different conditions. The parts which receive the largest and most numerous vascular ramifications are the brain and spinal chord, the glandular organs, the muscles, voluntary and involuntary, the mucous membranes, and the skin. In the fibrous membranes, and their modifications, tendons, and ligaments, and in the serous membranes few arteries are seen to penetrate; and these are generally minute, sometimes only colourless capillaries. Bones hold in this respect an intermediate position, being well supplied with blood-vessels, especially in early life, though to less extent than the muscles, and in greater proportion than the fibrous tissues. In some textures arteries cannot be traced, though their properties indicate that they must receive vessels of some kind. Such are cartilage and the arachnoid membrane. (Ruysch and Haller.) Lastly, arteries are not found in the scarf-skin, in nails, the enamel of the teeth, the hair, nor in the membranes of the umbilical chord. In early life bones are much more vascular than in adult age; and in the bones of young subjects arteries may be traced going out through the epiphyses into the cartilages, in which they cannot at a later period of life be demonstrated.*

SECTION II.

The morbid states of arteries belong either to the inner membrane, or to the proper arterial tissue, or to both.

1. *Adhesive Inflammation. Arteritis.* Acute, limited. The inner membrane is liable to inflammation, terminating generally in effusion of lymph, adhesion of the sides, and obliteration of the

* Hunter in Philosophical Transactions, No. 470.

canal of the tube. This process takes place in all circumstances in which the corresponding surfaces of the vessel are mutually applied, while the current of blood through the vessel is interrupted. The pressure of a tourniquet, or any mechanical object moderately firm; the pressure of a tumour, or of an aneurism in some instances; the application of a ligature not so tight as to divide the coats; and in the case of small vessels, the spontaneous retraction and collapse of its sides after complete division by a cutting instrument, are conditions which have been followed by adhesion and obliteration of the canal. On the knowledge of this property depends the practice of tying arterial tubes in wounds, and in the cure of aneurism.

Inflammation of the internal arterial membrane may also take place spontaneously, or independent of mechanical causes. Thus the inner membrane of the aorta may be inflamed in persons labouring under general or severe inflammation of the thoracic viscera. (Portal, Hodgson.) The anatomical characters are deep red colour of the membrane, and more or less effusion of lymph within the cavity of the vessel.

If the individual survives such a disease, the lymph thus effused becomes penetrated with blood-vessels, and forms a new body adhering to the inner surface of the vessel. This is the origin of several of the granulated bodies, fungous growths, or vegetations, which have been described by Senac, Morgagni, Portal, Baillie, Corvisart, Burns, and Bertin, as often found at the origin of the aorta, attached to the semilunar valves, or even on the mitral valve, the structure of which is not dissimilar.

A red or crimson staining of the inner membrane, especially in the aorta, has been mentioned by Corvisart, Frank, Hodgson, and Laennec, and may be often seen in persons who have died without symptoms of pectoral or arterial disorder. Its nature is not well known. It seems to be the effect of a dyeing or tinging property of the blood, either during the last moments of life, or after the heart has ceased to beat. It must not be confounded with inflammation or its effects.

2. *Arteritis Diffusa.* It has been believed that an extended or diffuse attack of inflammation might take place over several divisions of the arterial system simultaneously and successively; and the existence of such a disease has been maintained by Reil, and the two Franks. The only unequivocal facts in proof of such a disease, however, have been given by Thomson and Meli. In the case ob-

served by the former, the inflammatory attack which appeared successively in the femoral and humeral arteries appears to have been the consequence of previous chronic inflammation of these vessels; and consequently the case is not a pure example of idiopathic acute *arteritis.* In the case given by Meli, there is no reason to believe that the acute attack was preceded by chronic disease of the arteries; and that probably is the least objectionable example of the disease. The symptoms during life were pain along the course of the large vessels; violent throbbing and beating in all the arteries of the extremities which were felt like tense chords; much heat; great and intense fever, thirst, restlessness; and finally delirium and death. The arteries were found covered with lymph outside, thickened, and containing internally clots of blood and lymph; and the tunics were roughened.*

Inflammation less extensive but not less intense takes place in arteries about to be, or already affected with aneurism. In almost all cases of aneurism the arterial tunics are previously in a state of inflammation. The tunics are reddened and softened, though lacerable; sometimes ulceration takes place in various points; clots of blood and lymph are deposited; and pain is felt in the site and along the course of the artery. When aneurismal enlargement has actually taken place, it is attended with manifest tokens of the presence of inflammation. Pain, generally severe and lasting, is felt along the course of the vessel and on the seat of the aneurismal dilatation. In cases of aneurism of the aorta or innominata, pain is felt proceeding upwards to the neck and head on the left side; and though much of this is caused by pressure of the tumour on nerves, yet much also is caused by inflammation in the aneurismal tumour, and in the vessel or vessels proceeding from. They are found red, softened, thickened, lined with lymph and clots of blood, and presenting points of ulceration and steatomatous and osseous deposit, the effects of the chronic inflammation.

3. *Chronic Inflammation.* In persons who have long laboured under the constitutional effects of the syphilitic poison, or who have been repeatedly and permanently under the influence of mercury, especially in cold and variable climates, the arterial tissue is not unfrequently affected by a slow insidious process of inflammation. It is not easy to determine to what extent this may affect the inner membrane exclusively; for probably both suffer at the same time, and from the same causes; but the effects of the process differ in

* On Acute Aortitis. By Norman Chevers, M. D. Guy's Hospital Reports, Vol. VI. p. 304.

the two tissues. In the inner membrane chronic inflammation may cause partial effusion of lymph, which becoming organized gives rise, as already mentioned, to the production of fungous growths and vegetations. It may render the membrane opaque and thick, and give it a shrivelled puckered appearance. It may cause a tubercular thickening either of the membrane or of the semilunar valves. It may induce gristly induration especially in these and in the mitral valve. Or, lastly, there is reason to believe it is often the agent of the processes next to be considered,—calcareous deposition, steatomatous deposition, and atheromatous deposition.

When it causes tubercular thickening, the inner surface of the aorta from the semilunar valves upwards along the whole course of the arch is covered with small irregular-shaped orbicular eminences, placed at irregular intervals along the course of the cylinder of the artery. From this they extend into the *innominata*, the left carotid and left subclavian, and often they are found beyond the arch at the origin of the intercostal arteries.

These bodies, for which their shape and appearance has procured the name of tubercles and warts, I think are merely lymph of a particular kind deposited either by the inner coat, or, as sometimes seems to be the case, by the middle coat, in a state of chronic inflammation, and assuming the tubercular or verrucose shape, appearance, and disposition.

The opinion that cartilaginous and osseous induration of the semilunar and mitral valves depends on chronic inflammation, derives great probability from several circumstances observed in the origin and progress of these changes. In the first place, in the serous membranes the formation of cartilaginous and osseous patches is often preceded by distinct marks of inflammation. Though we cannot prove absolute identity between these textures and the inner cardiac and arterial membrane, yet, as in many of their properties they are very similar, there is reason to believe that in this also they resemble each other. In the second place, after or along with rheumatic attacks, it is not uncommon to observe symptoms of a morbid state in one or both sets of valves; symptoms of rigidity and immobility; and symptoms of more or less contraction of the orifices which they form. Thirdly, the presence of more or less disease in the semilunar aortic valves is usually associated with indications of the effects of chronic inflammation of the aortic lining membrane; roughness of its interior caused by tubercular, steatomatous, or atheromatous growths.

It is doubtless true that these changes in the valves may be regarded as effects and examples of misnutrition, (*paratrophia*.) This, however, would not alter much the essential merits of the question ; for most instances of misnutrition are accompanied with marks of chronic inflammation, and one of the leading characters of chronic inflammation may be said to be the derangement in the nutrition of the parts which it attacks. It must be allowed also that often the changes take place insidiously and in an imperceptible manner. The most decided evidence, however, as to the cause of these changes being inflammation or not is found in the examination of the changes themselves.

In the semilunar aortic valves they are as follow.

1. The valves may be mutually adherent by their edges; that is, two valves may adhere; or the whole three may be mutually adherent. In other instances two valves only may adhere; and the coalescence may be so perfect that there shall appear to be only two semilunar valves instead of three. When all the three adhere they produce very great occlusion of the orifice of the aorta. In one case which I knew well, the aperture scarcely admitted a silver catheter of calibre No. 10.

2. The semilunar valves may be, without mutual accretion, rigid, firm, and immovable, or at least not readily movable. This state is manifestly caused partly by deposition on their upper and under surface, partly by thickening of their substance. In general this deposit and thickening is greatest at the attached margin of the valves. They are at the same time shrivelled or drawn irregularly from the free margin to the attached. In this state the blood regurgitates from the aorta into the left ventricle.

3. The whole surface and margins of the valves may be covered by small tubercular bodies, varying in size, like pin-heads, or split vetches, and sometimes irregular on the *apices* like warts. The valves are thickened and rendered rigid and shrivelled. If these be not the effects of chronic inflammation, they are products of misnutrition. They are deposited at first as lymph.

4. I have seen the following state of the semilunar valves. The whole three valves were thickened, stiffened, and indurated ; and their surfaces were covered with a series or crop of hair-like or bristly processes, growing from the attached margin and both surfaces of the valves, and projecting into the area of the artery, not unlike a hair-like fringe. It seems difficult to understand the for-

mation of these bodies unless they were from chronic inflammation affecting the valves. The person in whom they were observed died within three hours after his admission to the hospital. He was a stout agricultural labourer, about 47 or 50 years of age. But of his previous state his friends gave no information, except that he had been attacked with difficult breathing and uneasiness in the chest about ten days before he applied for assistance. His pulse was feeble and the surface cold when he was admitted.

5. The surface or margins of the valves may present globular or spheroidal softish dark-red coloured bodies like the granules of cauliflower adhering to them. These are aggregated in masses, so as to form something like fungous or cauliflower growths. They are friable and easily broken off, and most commonly in handling them, many are removed. These bodies seem to be originally masses either of lymph or fibrin, which thus are either effused by, or adhere to the valves in a state of inflammation.

4. *Ossification, Earthy Degeneration of* Scarpa; *Calcareous Deposition.* It has been long known that arteries are liable to deposition of calcareous matter. By De La Sône it was first remarked that this process takes place in the inner membrane only;[*] and Bichat afterwards referred it to the outer or attached surface of the membrane, an opinion in which he is supported by the testimony of Meckel, Scarpa, Hodgson, and others. Scarpa only admits as a possible alternative its deposition in the interval between the inner and proper coat in the delicate tissue termed *second cellular* by Haller.[†] By Jourdan and Breschet, however, the translators of the work of Meckel, who contend that the internal membrane is never ossified, it is positively stated that the calcareous matter is accumulated in the cellular tissue connecting the inner to the proper coat. It is perhaps of no great moment to dispute this point; but I shall mention three facts, which show that the statement of MM. Jourdan and Breschet must be admitted with caution. *1st,* There is no cellular tissue between the two membranes,[‡] and the inner adheres simply to the proper coat. This is established, notwithstanding the authority of Haller, by dissection, and by observing the effects of maceration and boiling. *2dly,* Calcareous deposition is observed to take place at the semilunar

---

[*] Memoires de l'Academie Royale, 1756, p. 199, 12mo.

[†] Sull' Aneurisma, Capitolo v. § 29.

[‡] " La surface externe, foiblement unie à l'autre membrane, comme nous l'avons vu, n'a point un intermediare cellulaire."—Bichat, Tome I. p. 291.

valves, which consist of two folds of inner membrane, when it is found in no other part of the aorta. 3*dly*, Admitting, for the sake of argument, that cellular tissue is placed between the inner coat and the proper arterial tissue, if calcareous matter be deposited in it, it is not analogous to what is observed in this tissue elsewhere. Without relying much, however, on these facts, I shall state the ordinary mode in which the deposition appears, independent of any · opinion as to its precise source.

The calcareous incrustation commences invariably at the outer surface of the inner membrane in the form of minute gritty points, or of small isolated patches. In the former state they appear to be hard and crystalline, and render the inside of the vessel rough; in the latter they are simply firm, and are less earthy or gritty, and without forming asperities in the inside of the vessel, may make it merely firm and unyielding, and deprive it of its elasticity. In either case, these calcareous deposits, confined more or less to one side, may spread along the tube for a considerable extent. They seldom affect the whole circumference of an artery unless in the lower extremities, in which they have been observed to form distinct rings, connected by intermediate portions of sound artery. (Hodgson.)

When the deposition is partial and limited, and of short duration, it is still covered by the inner membrane; and the inside of the vessel, though irregular, is comparatively smooth. When the patches multiply and enlarge so as to coalesce, the inner membrane gives way at one or more points of the margin of the calcareous deposite, which now adheres only to the surface of the proper membrane; and an irregular ragged circumference is exposed. If the artery contains many patches, its entire inner surface presents a series of asperities resulting from the rupture of the thin pellicle of inner membrane with which they were at first covered. Yet these calcareous patches are not known to be detached entirely.

Scarpa represents this morbid change as taking place something differently. But I shall afterwards show that this arises from confounding the calcareous with the steatomatous deposition, a change different in several respects.

In many instances of aged persons, the calcareous deposit appears in the form of rings of bony matter, into which the circular fibres of the middle coat are transformed. It often happens that the arteries of the extremities are thus converted into bony tubes.

This deposition may take place in any part of the arterial system ; and it is said to be equally common in branches as in trunks. It may occur in the radial artery, in the temporal, or in the tibial. By Cowper and Naish it was found in the arteries of the leg in the course of amputation.* I have seen it in the radial and ulnar in tying the vessels of an amputated fore-arm ; and in the femoral and several of the perforating branches of the thigh under the same circumstances. It is, however, most commonly found in the arch of the aorta, or in some of the branches which issue from it. Many cases of its occurrence in the coronary arteries have been recorded. (Crell, Erdmann, Frank, and Parry.) Nor is it confined to the arterial tubes only ; for it is seen in that part of the pellucid arterial membrane which forms the valves, and lines the inside of the left ventricle, and is frequently found to take place in the semilunar and mitral valves.

The nature of this deposition has given rise to various speculations. But this variance has partly arisen from the practice of confounding it with the steatomatous deposition. It is said to differ from osseous matter in two circumstances. *First,* The deposition is earthy from the first, without any previous matrix of animal matter. *Secondly,* It is destitute of the usual fibrous structure, and presents an irregular but homogeneous crust without any obvious arrangement. It consists, however, of the usual combination of animal matter and bone earth. A specimen analyzed by Mr Brande gave 65·5 parts of phosphate of lime, and 34·5 of animal matter in the 100 parts. The latter was chiefly albumen, with traces of gelatine.

Calcareous deposition may take place at any period of life, but is supposed to be most common in advanced age. Portal, Scarpa, and Hodgson, mention instances of its occurrence in young subjects. According to Stevens, it is more common to find the arteries ossified than healthy after the 30th year.† But this statement is probably delivered in too general terms, and from too limited a collection of cases. Baillie restricts its occurrence as a general phenomenon to the period after the 60th year ;‡ and this corresponds with the inference of Bichat, who states, that in ten subjects seven at least present these incrustations after the 60th year.§ Its influence on the circulation varies at different periods of life, and according to its extent and situation. In the aged it is said to

* Philosophical Transactions, No. 285, p. 1391, and No. 369, p. 226.
† Medico-Chirurgical Transactions, Vol. V. p. 433.
‡ Transactions of a Society for the Improvement, &c., Vol. I. p. 133.
§ Anatomie Generale, Vol. II. p. 292.

produce much less inconvenience than in the young and adult. (Bichat.) It is certain that in the latter it almost invariably causes fatal disease of the heart or arteries, or of both.

The most ordinary effect of calcareous incrustation, when extensive, is to induce chronic inflammation and ulceration of the arterial tissue. The earthy matter operates as a foreign body, and by constant irritation destroys the vitality of the inner membrane, which exfoliates, and inflames the proper tissue, which is then eroded. In this state the occasional application of a slight force may be followed by more or less laceration of the proper coat. In arteries covered by a filamentous sheath, the blood thus discharged is injected into the sheath, which is then distended into a spherical sac situate more or less on one side of the vessel. This forms the disease described as true aneurism by Scarpa. In arteries not supplied with filamentous sheath, as in the brain, the blood escapes freely, and may by its quantity induce fatal compression of that organ. (Blane, Hodgson, Bouillaud, and Serres.)

The calcareous deposition renders the arterial tube so brittle, that the application of a ligature invariably cracks it, prevents the usual process of adhesion, and is generally succeeded by ulceration and hemorrhage. In persons advanced in life calcareous deposition in the arteries of the lower extremities is a cause not unfrequent of mortification of the toes, feet, and legs, generally terminating fatally. (Cowper, Naish, and Pott.)

5. *Atheromatous Deposition.* This term has been applied to a semifluid or cheesy opaque substance, which is not unfrequently found between the inner and proper tunics of arteries. Its consistence may vary from that of purulent matter to the tenacity of curd, or the granular firmness of cheese. Observed by the first Monro, by Haller, and others, it appears to be considered by Scarpa as a variety of the same change which I am afterwards to mention as steatomatous deposition. From this certain circumstances show that it ought to be distinguished. 1*st*, Atheromatous deposition appears to arise from a sort of suppuration; for, in general, it is possible to trace the transition from purulent fluid to the concrete matter of atheroma. 2*d*, This account of its origin derives strong confirmation from the fact, that it almost always contains a patch or patches of calcareous matter in its centre. 3*dly*, It is associated much more frequently with the calcareous than with the steatomatous deposite. It is for these reasons not unlikely that the athero-

matous deposition is to be viewed as one of the effects of chronic inflammation, either in the inner or the proper tunic, or in both.

6. *Steatomatous Deposition,* either alone, or with calcareous patches, is often found between the inner surface of the proper membrane, and the outer surface of the internal one. Whether these deposits invariably derive their origin from the former or from the latter of these tissues, is not easy to say. In many instances they appear to be produced rather by the proper arterial tunic. They occur in various forms; but two may be particularly mentioned.

In the first, small irregular patches of yellowish or fawn-coloured matter like wax appear on the inner surface of the proper coat. As the process of deposition advances, these become thicker and broader. They coalesce, and sensibly raise the outer filamentous coat; while, by their prominence interiorly, they diminish the capacity of the arterial tube. At the same time the inner membrane becomes irregular, opaque, and shrivelled; and the connection with the proper tunic being destroyed, it is detached with great facility.*

This deposition constitutes the *steatomatous degeneration* of Professor Scarpa and other authors. The name is not well chosen, for the substance deposited is not adipose, but rather like crude bees-wax. It was applied, however, by Stentzel,† the original writer on this subject, and it is unnecessary to change it, when its exact import is understood. Though it may occur probably in any part of the arterial tubes, it takes place most frequently at the bifurcations of the arteries. It invariably commences in this particular spot of the vessel; and when it occupies any extent of the tube, it will be found to have begun at the bifurcation, and spread thence along the vessel. Thus I have seen this deposition confined to the point common to the common carotid, and its external and internal branches, and this in both sides in the same subject. I have seen it in another person at the same part of the carotids, and at the point common to the internal carotid and the sylvian artery. Lastly, in another instance I have found it affecting at once in the same subject the arch of the aorta, where it gives off the *innominata* and left subclavian artery; the descending aorta, where it gives off the cœliac and superior mesenteric, including the beginning of these vessels; and the cœliac, when it divides into its gastric, hepatic, and splenic branches.

* Morgagni Epist. XXIII. Art. iv. vi.   XLV. Art. xxiii. &c.

† Christiani God. Stentzel de Steatomatibus Aortæ.   Haller Disput. ad Morborum Historiam, &c.   Tomo II. p. 527, Art. lxv.

In describing this morbid state of arteries, Professor Scarpa, I conceive, confounds it with ossification. After noticing the loss of fine polish (*l'intima tonaca dell' arteria perde per certo tratto suo bel liscio,*) which the inner arterial membrane sustains, he represents it as becoming irregular and wrinkled, and successively occupied with yellow spots, which are converted into so many earthy grains or scales, or into steatomatous and caseous concretions. I think they may be justly distinguished, because the calcareous deposite very often exists without the steatomatous; and conversely, the steatomatous may be found without the calcareous deposition. I must not omit to mention, nevertheless, that the circumstance which seems to have led Scarpa to consider these depositions as the same, is, that sometimes in the centre of a steatomatous patch is found a broad scale of hard substance, not so firm as bone, and not so crystalline or gritty as the genuine calcareous deposition. It is generally so soft as to be flexible, and resembles rather a firm piece of cartilage than true bone. It may be designated as the *steatomatous* and *osteo-steatomatous deposition.*

Scarpa represents the steatomatous state as proceeding invariably to ulceration. This, however, is not a uniform result. A large portion of an artery may be affected with it without suffering the smallest breach of continuity or destruction of tissue. It simply distends the vessel mechanically; and if unaccompanied with calcareous deposition, this distension may be considerable without any ulceration or laceration. In this manner probably are produced those simple dilatations of arteries which by many of the French authors are regarded as aneurism. In other instances, more especially when the steatomatous is combined with the calcareous deposition, or when the arterial tunics have been long and much distended, ulceration may take place and terminate in partial or entire destruction and rupture of the arterial tunics. In general, this destruction takes place in the transverse direction, (Hodgson,) and the laceration or fissure is therefore across the tube.

In such circumstances, if the aperture is not large enough to cause fatal hemorrhage, aneurism first by dilatation, and ultimately by rupture, is the consequence.

Of all these changes or deposits, tubercular, atheromatous, steatomatous, or calcareous, the invariable effect is to render the arterial tunics brittle, to impair their elasticity and contractile power, and to render them less pliant and more easily ruptured. Hence in arteries

G

diseased in these modes, as the tunics do not easily become distended, they are liable to give way and burst on any occasion when the blood is either accumulated or delayed within their canals, or when the vessels themselves are exposed to any extraordinary stretching or twisting motion. Sudden or violent motion of any kind, indeed, is liable to produce rupture of arteries diseased and rendered brittle in the manner now specified.

In short, arteries in this state are liable to inflammation, ulceration, and rupture.

7. *Aneurism.* On the nature of the aneurismal tumour some difference of opinion has prevailed. Since it has been the custom to settle points of pathology by reference to dissection, three opinions have been successively entertained. *First,* It was maintained by Elsner, Severinus, Hildanus, Sennert, and others, that aneurism was produced by rupture of the proper coats of the artery. The second opinion, which is that of Fernel, Forestus, Diemerbroek, &c. is, that it consists in uniform dilatation of the arterial tunics. *Thirdly,* From the cases recorded by Lancisi, Friend, Guattani, Morgagni, and especially those described by Donald Monro,* it results that aneurism may arise either from rupture or from dilatation of the arterial tissues, or from both causes jointly.

The first doctrine has been revived and strenuously and ingeniously defended by Scarpa, who infers that aneurism never consists in dilatation, but invariably arises from erosion and laceration of the proper coats, and injection of arterial blood into the filamentous or membranous sheath with which the vessel is invested. By Hodgson, again, this doctrine has been successfully combated, and the third opinion shown to be most consonant with the process of aneurismal disease. The result of his inquiries may be stated in the following manner. 1*st,* In many aneurisms the first step is destruction and partial laceration of the internal and proper coats of the artery ; and when the blood escapes from its cavity it distends the filamentous or membranous sheath into a cyst or sac, between which and the tunics it is found in successive layers. 2*dly,* In several aneurisms the first step of the process is mere dilatation of the arterial tunics, either partial or general. When this has proceeded to a certain extent, varying in different cases, the arterial tissues give way, and the same process of hemorrhage and coagulation in successive layers results.

* Essays and Observations, Phys. and Lit. Vol. III. Art. xii.

It appears, therefore, that in every case of aneurism there is eventually laceration. The only difference is in the mode of origin, which in some is rupture, and in others mere dilatation.* This question M. Breschet investigated anatomico-pathologically in 1832, and drew the following conclusions. 1st, That there exist true aneurisms, that is, aneurisms consisting in dilatation of the arterial walls without any apparent lesion, and without any solution of continuity in the membranes of these vessels. 2d, That arteries of all calibres, from the largest to the most capillary, may undergo this dilatation. 3d, That the arteries of bone are liable to this expansion. 4th, That these true dilatations may be distinguished as to external form, into a. sacciform, b. fusiform, or spindle-shaped, c. cylindroid, and d. cirsoid, or arterial varix ; that there are also mixed aneurisms in which the middle arterial tunic is torn, and in which the inner is protruded through it in the form of a hernial tumour, while the external or cellular coat is dilated and forms the exterior covering of the aneurism ; and that this mixed aneurism depends on lesion of the arterial tunics, and may be multiplied, that is, more than one occurring in the same individual.†

This accords generally with the results obtained by Mr Hodgson. But it must be observed, that, whatever be the amount of experience in France as to the comparative frequency of true aneurism and mixed aneurism, it is certain that the latter is the form of disease most common in England. It may be said that we see fifty cases of mixed aneurism for one of true aneurism. In short, aneurism in England is a disease dependent on previous lesion of the arterial tunics.

In its final result an aneurismal sac bursts in one of two modes. 1st, When it bursts into the cavity of any of the serous membranes, as the pleura, pericardium, or peritonæum, the breach is formed by laceration. 2d, When it bursts through the skin or into cavities lined by a mucous membrane, the breach is the effect of sloughing and ulceration.

Certain divisions of the arterial system are evidently more liable than others to aneurism ; and in general the comparative liability may be traced to the greater or less susceptibility of disease of the tunics, and the situation of the vessel in being exposed to frequent motion. Hence aneurisms are *cæteris paribus* more frequently

---

* Hodgson on the Diseases of Arteries and Veins, p. 74.

† Memoire sur les Aneurismes. Par M. Gilbert Breschet. Memoires de l'Academie Royale de Medecine, Tome troisieme. Paris, 1833. 4to, p. 101.

observed at the flexures of joints than elsewhere. Aneurisms are also more frequent in men than in women. The following table by Mr Hodgson exhibits the comparative frequency of true aneurisms in different arteries, and in the two sexes, in sixty-three cases in which that gentleman either saw the patients during life, or examined the parts after death.

	Males.	Females.	Total.
Of the ascending aorta, the arteria innominata, and the arch of the aorta, · . .	16	5	21
descending aorta, ...	7	1	8
carotid artery	2		2
subclavian and axillary arteries, .	5		5
inguinal artery, ...	12		12
femoral and popliteal artery, . .	14	1	15
	56	7	63

Aneurism in this country is most commonly seen in the arch of the aorta or *innominata*, or both. In the course of eight years I have observed nine cases, and dissected eight of these. Only one was in the abdominal aorta.

8. Cirsoid Aneurism of M. Breschet. *Aneurysma Cirsus. Aneurysma Cirsoideum. Varix Arterialis* of M. Dupuytren. Arterial Varix.

The name Cirsoid Aneurism is applied by Breschet to a tumour of an arterial tube or tubes, called by Dupuytren Arterial Varix, because arteries affected by it may be compared to varicose veins. It consists in dilatation of the vessel in a greater or less extent of its course, often through the whole length of the trunk and its principal branches. The vessel at the same time becomes elongated and tortuous, and describes circuits more or less numerous and considerable. Sometimes, besides these sudden dilatations of the tube, in some parts are seen nodosities or little circumscribed aneurismal tumours, which are true sacciform aneurisms, and occasionally mixed aneurisms.

Most frequently the parietes of the vessel are thin, soft, and flaccid; and when divided, they collapse like those of varicose veins; while in true cylindroid aneurism the parietes are thickened; and if divided perpendicularly to their axis, the diameter (calibre) of the vessel remains open. The artery affected with varix resembles much a varicose vein, and for such it might easily be mistaken if injection or dissection to the principal trunk did not demonstrate the nature of the organ.

. This kind of aneurism has been observed in the arteries of medium calibre, or those of the fourth and fifth orders, as the iliac, the carotids, the brachial, the femoral, the tibial; and in vessels still smaller, or those of the sixth order, as the occipital, auricular, radial, ulnar; in the palmar and plantar arches; and in the ophthalmic **artery.**

Sometimes in arterial varix, amidst a very dilated flexuosity of the artery, we observe a sudden contraction, and for some inches of its length, the vessel preserves its natural volume.

Arterial varix is distinguished from aneurism by anastomosis, by the irregularity of the dilatations which it presents.

It is distinguished from venous varix in the living body by the pulsations of the dilated vessels.

A state quite similar to that of cirsoid aneurism is observed in old varicose aneurism, or aneurism resulting from the simultaneous lesion of an artery and of a vein in the same point by the same instrument, from the interchange of the blood of the two vessels, but especially from the passage of the venous blood into the artery.

Next to the retardation in the artery of the blood below the wound, the dilatation of the whole of that part of the external system, the weakening of the pulsations, the diminution of temperature in the parts below the opening of communication between the two orders of vessels, the violet hue of the same parts; lastly, the less brilliant colour of the blood in the lower end of the artery when it is examined before the application of ligatures, and the entrance of the venous blood into the artery during the diastole of this vessel, are the circumstances which, according to Breschet, leave no doubt on the nature of the disease and its causes, viz. interchange of the two kinds of blood.

This analogical circumstance under the relation of the organic change in the arterial varix and old varicose aneurism, leads naturally to the idea, that in arterial varix there may be a communication between the two orders of vessels and the passage of a certain quantity of the venous blood into the dilated and varicose artery. A case by Pearson would lead to the same inference.

9. *Wounds and their consequences.* An artery may be punctured, perforated, cut longitudinally, divided partially or entirely across, or torn completely asunder.

In the first three cases the blood which escapes is injected into the filamentous sheath, and coagulating, prevents further effusion from the vessel. In a few hours the edges of the wound inflame, and, pouring out lymph, are united by adhesion. In the case of small wounds, especially longitudinal, this union may be effected without obliteration of the canal. ·But when the wound is large or oblique, if the inflammation is sufficient to effect union and prevent further hemorrhage, so much lymph is effused, that in general, with the pressure and rest requisite, the opposite sides of the vessel adhere, and its canal is for some space obliterated. (Jones, Hodgson.)

In most cases, however, of longitudinal or oblique wounds, and in all cases of partial transverse wounds, the process is different. Supposing the external opening to be closed, which it sooner or later is, the blood from the wounded artery is extensively injected into the sheath, where its coagulation prevents as before further effusion. Though inflammation takes place, however, and lymph is effused, it is insufficient to unite permanently the divided edges. Either the wound is never thoroughly united, or at a period after its infliction, varying according to its extent and direction, and according to the size of the artery and its distance from the heart, its edges are rent asunder by the incessant impulse. (Jones, Hodgson, Guthrie.) Blood continues from time to time to escape into the sheath, which it distends into a sac, and in which it is deposited in successive layers. In this manner is formed a pulsating tumour, which has been termed false, spurious, or *bastard aneurism*. (Monro *Primus*.) If the injection is extensive, so as to cause a diffuse swelling, spreading to some distance along the limb, the disease is termed *diffuse aneurism*. If it is more limited, distends the sheath into a globular sac, and assumes the appearance of the usual aneurismal tumour, then it is termed *circumscribed aneurism*. This is the sort of aneurism which takes place when the brachial artery is opened, instead of the vein at the bend of the arm ; (William Cowper, Macgill, Monro *Primus*, &c.) and it is not uncommon in the temporal artery, when that vessel has been opened to discharge blood for affections of the head. It may, however, succeed punctured wounds, especially sword-thrusts in any part of the body. In short, every cause which partially wounds or injures the side of an artery, as a sharp *spicula* of bone, may be followed by false aneurism. At the bend of the arm it is to be distinguished from aneurismal varix and varicose aneurism.

When an artery is entirely divided across, the result varies according to the size of the vessel. The moment the division is completed, a copious gush of blood issues from the vessel, the divided portions mutually recede with more or less force, and the walls of the vessel collapse so as to contract its area uniformly from the circumference to the centre. Of the two latter actions the former is limited by the attachment of the proper arterial tissue to the filamentous sheath. But notwithstanding this limitation, so forcible is the retraction, as it is termed, that the connecting fibres of the filamentous sheath are always rent for some small space from the cut ends of the tube. The annular contraction, or central diminution of the area, is also counteracted by the longitudinal impulse of the blood ; and in large vessels. this resistance to the central contraction is so great, that the latter has little or no sensible influence in suppressing hemorrhage. In such circumstances the chief agents of this process are the pressure of coagulated blood effused into the sheath, (*coagulum externum,*) and a conical or cylindrical plug of the same material (*coagulum internum,*) within the mouth of the divided vessel.* When by the formation of this double clot a temporary check to the transit of blood is given, inflammation and lymphy exudation from the divided edges tend to supply the means of permanent suppression. When this fails false aneurism is the consequence.

In the case of small vessels the annular contraction bears a larger proportion, *cæteris paribus*, to the size of the vessel ; and it exercises a greater influence in arresting the current of blood through the divided orifice. With the pressure of the external and internal clots, and the recession of the divided portions, this annular contraction is in general amply sufficient to stop permanently the effusion of blood from small vessels. Hence in partial wounds of such vessels as the radial, the ulnar, and the temporal arteries, the entire division of the vessel is often the most effectual means of checking the flow of blood from them. In amputation also, in which the arteries are divided transversely, the smaller vessels may be left untied without danger.

The principle now laid down Dr L. Koch of Munich has attempted to carry to a much greater length. Denying that hemorrhage, from arteries entirely divided, is suppressed in the manner now mentioned, denying especially the formation of the double clot

* " The mouth of the artery being no longer pervious, nor a collateral branch very near it, the blood just within it is at rest, coagulates, and forms in general a slender conical coagulum, which neither fills up the canal of the artery, nor adheres to its sides, except by a small portion of the circumference of its base, which lies near the extremity of the vessel."—Jones on Hemorrhage, Chap. I. sect. iii. p. 53.

as a uniform result of transverse division, he has recourse to the supposition of a peculiar force and action to account for the cessation of hemorrhage. · He denies the necessity of ligature in any case, and proposes to leave large as well as small vessels untied. His arguments are manifestly derived from the phenomena of the division of small arteries only, and cannot therefore be justly applied to large ones. I have already shown, that in the case of the former the annular contraction is the main agent of the cessation of hemorrhage; and to this, I conceive, corresponds the peculiar force to which Dr Koch ascribes that process.*

When an artery is lacerated or forcibly rent asunder, the same process of injection, coagulation, retraction, and annular constriction take place, but more powerfully and more speedily than in the case of the same artery divided transversely by a cutting instrument. The external clot especially is formed very rapidly; the internal one is large and extensive; and the annular contraction of the lacerated vessel is much more considerable. (Guthrie and others.) These circumstances afford an explanation of the well-established fact, that any artery, when forcibly rent asunder, bleeds infinitely less than the same vessel completely divided by a transverse incision. So uniform is this fact, that arteries of moderate size have been torn by a transverse laceration without effusing more than a few drops of blood.

10. *Aneurismal·Varix.* It sometimes happens that an artery subjacent to, and in immediate contact with a vein, is punctured by the same instrument with which the vein has been perforated, and the wound thus inflicted establishes between the two vessels a communication, through which the blood passes from the one to the other. Thus, from want of caution on the part of the operator, it may happen that in venesection at the bend of the arm, the lancet may not only transfix the vein, but wound the subjacent artery. The blood flows from the latter into the former with a peculiar hissing noise, and dilates it into a sack which disappears on pressure, but returns when the pressure is removed. The tumour thus formed, which depends on the wound of the arterial and venous tunic remaining open while their sides are in contact, was first distinguished as a peculiar affection by William Hunter,† and is known under the name of *aneurismal varix.* It may occur in any part of

---

* Journal für Chirurgie und Augenheilkunde von Graefe und Walther, p. 9, t. 560.
† Medical Observations and Inquiries, Vol. II. p. 396, 400.

the vascular system in which a vein lies immediately over an arterial trunk. In most of the cases hitherto recorded it has continued for years (five, Hunter, Cleghorn ; fourteen, Hunter, Scarpa, Bell ; twenty-five, thirty-five, Bell, Hunter ;) without serious inconvenience.

· 11. *Varicose aneurism.* In the case of an artery lying beneath, but not in immediate contact with a vein, or in the case of the wound being oblique and the puncture of the vein not corresponding to that of the artery, the same accident is followed with another variety of tumour. The blood from the arterial tube flows partly into the sheath, which is distended into a sac, and partly into the vein, which is morbidly dilated. The tumour thus resulting, the anatomical characters of which are a circumscribed aneurism between the artery and vein, and a varicose state of the latter, has been distinguished as *varicose aneurism.* *

The filamentous sheath, though not proper to the arterial tissue, performs, nevertheless, an important part in the morbid states of arteries, whether spontaneous or resulting from injuries. It has been already shown what is its influence in the production of gennine aneurism, in the suppression of hemorrhage, and in the formation of the several varieties of false or spurious aneurismal tumours. It is liable further to the same forms of inflammatory action as attack this tissue in other parts of the animal frame. But inflammation here is often attended with the bad effect of producing ulceration of the middle coat, and laceration succeeded by hemorrhage more or less violent, according to the size of the vessel. This process, which depends on the destruction of the nutrient vessels (*vasa vasorum*) transmitted in the filamentous coat, may succeed any injury inflicted on the neighbouring parts, as contused wounds, burns, phagedenic sores, especially those in lymphatic glands, the application of improper ligatures, especially broad tapes, and the use of foreign bodies as pads, *presse-arteres* and *serre-arteres* in the neighbourhood of an artery. Removal of the filamentous sheath, partly or entirely, is not unfrequently followed with the same effect. This, however, must be understood to apply chiefly to the human subject. In the lower animals the filamentous sheath may be removed without injuring the proper and inner membrane.

* Park in Medical Facts and Observations, Vol. IV. p. 111. Physick in Medical Museum, Philadelphia, Vol. I. p. 65.

(Hunter and Home.)* This shows that in these circumstances its inflammation is not attended with the bad effects which result in the human subject.

12. Obstruction in the cavity of arteries. *Occlusio arteriarum; oppilatio arteriarum.* The deposits and growths already mentioned, whether tubercular or wart-like, or atheromatous, steatomatous, or calcareous, all tend to diminish more or less the calibre of the artery, and to cause more or less obstruction to the motion of the blood. It is true that soon after deposits of any of these growths have taken place, there appears at their site to be a sort of bulging of the arterial tube, or a dilatation general or partial; and, in point of fact, this often takes place with at the same time a certain degree or dilatation internally. This appears to be the result of the impediment which the blood encounters in passing over diseased portions of an arterial tube; for as the blood meets greater resistance, it is, especially in the aorta, propelled with greater force; and in almost the whole of these cases in which the interior of the aorta is thus diseased, the left ventricle of the heart is more or less hypertrophied.

It also happens, however, that these new growths may by their number and size diminish in a greater or less degree the calibre of the arterial cylinder. Thus in the case recorded by Stentzel, the atheromatous or steatomatous tumour had greatly contracted the dimensions of the canal of the aorta.† In a case given by the elder Meckel, the diameter of the aorta in an aged female was not more than eight lines, from a similar cause.‡ Sandifort mentions the case of a man in whom a similar deposition in the interior of the aorta had contracted much the calibre of the artery. Stoerck states that in inspecting the body of a female, aged 64, who had long laboured under difficult breathing and palpitation of the heart on making any exertion, and who died in syncope, he found the arch of the aorta completely bony, and the tunics thickened, and the canal of the artery so small that it would not admit the little finger. This form of obstruction is generally partial.

In the progress of those changes which take place in aneurism, the calibre of an artery may be so much contracted, and its interior

* Transactions of a Society for improving Medical and Chirurgical Knowledge, Vol. I. p. 144.
† Chris. Gottfr. Stentzel de Steatomatibus Aortæ. Wittembergæ, 1732.
‡ Haller, Dissert. Medico Practicæ, Tom. ii.

3

so much obstructed, as to impede much the motion of the blood through it. The obstruction is caused not only by atheromatous and steatomatous growths adhering to the artery, but by deposits of blood and lymph or fibrin adhering to the internal surface of the vessel previously diseased, most commonly in a state of ulceration.

The obstruction may be partial, and confined to one side of the vessel; or it may be general, extending nearly all round, but not thoroughly closing the canal of the vessel; or it may be complete, closing altogether the tube and preventing the blood from flowing along it.

Partial obstruction is mostly seen in large vessels, as the aorta, the innominata, the thoracic and abdominal aorta, or in the common iliacs, or the common carotid, or the subclavian artery. General obstruction also occurs in these vessels though more rarely; and is usually in vessels belonging to the third class, which are of smaller size. Partial and general obstruction mostly takes place either in consequence of steatomatous deposits in the interior of the artery, or the deposition of blood and lymph in the progressive changes which occur in aneurismal tumours, which pressing more or less completely on the part of the artery on which they take place, retard or interrupt the flow of blood through, cause thus the formation of clots, and thereby tend to diminish much the calibre of the arterial cylinder.

Complete obstruction to the interior of an artery may take place under the same circumstances as partial and general obstruction. That is, the blood and lymph deposited in an aneurismal tumour and within the arterial canal above it, may be so arranged as to compress the vessel and interrupt or obstruct entirely the course of the blood through the artery. Such was the case in the instance recorded by Larcheus, which I have elsewhere described;* in that published by Dr Crampton, and that by Dr Monro. In cases of this nature, one of two effects may ensue. First, the artery distended with blood, which is allowed neither to flow through the trunk nor to escape by collateral branches, may burst, and the accident may prove fatal. This is by far the most common termination when the arterial canal is so much obstructed. Thus I have seen the abdominal aorta burst above an aneurismal tumour, and

* Instance of Obliteration of the Aorta beyond the Arch. Illustrated by similar Cases and Observations. By David Craigie, M. D., &c. Edin. Medical and Surgical Journal, Vol. LVI. p. 427.

the blood escaping tear and dissect away the whole peritoneum from the subjacent muscles. The same appears to have taken place in the case given by Fantoni. Secondly, in consequence of the blood not passing through the arterial tube, the parts to which it is distributed are deprived of their nutrient fluid, and become at first cold, numb, and slightly paralytic; afterwards they become unusually hot; and gangrenous inflammation is rapidly developed and terminates in mortification.

A species of complete obstruction liable to take place in arteries previously diseased, especially in the extremities, is that which takes place in cases of gangrene of the toes in the aged, (*gangræna senilis,*) and which has been described as a form of inflammation of the arteries (*arteritis*) by Dupuytren. The interior of the artery is filled with clots of blood, generally firm and solid, and often extending through the greater part or the whole of the arterial trunk. Thus it may extend through the femoral artery from the ligament of Poupart to the loin, and sometimes the tibial and femoral arteries are filled with solid clots of blood of the same kind. The arterial tube is generally firm, indurated, penetrated or lined by atheromatous or steatomatous specks or osseous matter, indicating that it has been in a state of chronic inflammation. This disease, therefore, is to be considered rather as an effect of chronic inflammation than acute inflammation. In general the first indications of the formation of *coagula*, are pains in the limb, numbness, and then the artery is observed to have ceased to beat. This is followed by the usual symptoms of gangrenous inflammation ;—pain, heat, redness, lividity, *phlyctaenae* or vesications, and death of the limb, followed by general death. In milder cases, one or two toes only, or the foot may be affected, and the limb with life is saved.

A species of obstruction apparently complete, though in several instances temporary in duration, I have seen take place in the arteries of the extremities. A female, between 20 and 25, labouring under rheumatism of the ankles and wrists, with slight indications of affection of the pericardium or endocardium, was suddenly attacked with numbness and loss of power and sensation in the left arm; and when it was examined no pulsation was recognised either in the radial artery or the humeral, to within two inches of the axilla, or in the ulnar artery. These sensations were attended with weight of the arm and occasional pains, pricking and lancinating. Warmth was applied externally. The symptoms, however, continued for about eight days, and after that time gradually subsided. Pulsation returned feebly to the radial artery, but not to the humeral. The patient after some time recovered, and remained well for years, though with some feebleness and numbness in the left arm. Though I have not the evidence of dissection, therefore, yet I infer that this was obstruction in the humeral artery, probably by slight inflammation taking place in its coats and causing effusion of lymph, and the formation of an obstructing clot of blood. A case very similar, illustrated by inspection of the parts, is given by Dr Graves in the Dublin Hospital Reports, Vol. V. p. 1; (case of Patrick Magrath), and one without inspection by Dr Gairdner in the Edinburgh Medico-Chirurgical Transactions, Vol. III.

Obstruction of arteries may also ensue as the effect of external pressure, as the effect of tumours increasing in size and encroaching on the space occupied by the artery. Thus when a small artery, as the temporal, is opened and afterwards subjected to compression, in general its interior is obstructed, sometimes adhering and obliterated. Encephaloid tumours of the chest or abdomen compress and obstruct the abdominal aorta; exostosis of the vertebræ compress the thoracic and abdominal aorta and obstruct the interior; exostoses of the cranium and tumours within the brain have been observed to compress and obstruct the branches of the internal carotid and vertebral arteries; and I have seen in tumours of the uterus and cancerous swellings the posterior iliac artery and its branches closed and its interior obstructed.

13. *Obliteration.* From complete obstruction the transition to obliteration of arteries is easy. The result is the same; but the mode in which it is accomplished is different. In obstruction the closure or impediment is caused by the presence either of new growths or blood and lymph within the artery and the arterial tunics. In obliteration the impediment or arctation of the canal is caused not so much by internal growths as by the approximation of the arterial walls, in consequence of external pressure, or some similar agent. Hence the cases of obstruction which I mentioned at the close of the preceding paragraph may be regarded as examples of obliteration.

Of obliteration of arteries there are several forms and sorts; and the accident may take place in any artery almost, of any class. It is nevertheless more frequent in vessels of the second, third, and fourth class, for very obvious reasons, than in those of the first class. Arteries become obliterated in consequence of pressure of any kind, the presence of coagula in their interior either in consequence of

inflammation or similar causes, and in consequence of the application of ligatures, all arterial canals being obliterated a little above
and a little below, sometimes a good space from the point at which
the ligature has been applied.

14. *Arctation or Obliteration of the Aorta at the definite point.*
The species of obliteration, or sometimes only of ¯obstruction,
which here deserves notice, is one which takes place always at a
definite or fixed point in the aorta. This consists, in a peculiar
arctation or contraction of the aorta, in the arch at its farther end,
or rather at that point of the arch which is beyond the origin of
the left carotid and left subclavian arteries. Of this species of obliteration I met with one case in my own sphere of observation: and
I have collected from various sources other nine cases; and since
that time three or four more cases have been published, so that
thirteen cases altogether have now been recorded and described.
In the whole of these cases the arctation or contraction was observed
at the point specified, viz. where the *ductus arteriosus*, converted
into a ligament, joins the aorta. It appears in the form of a deep
annular indentation surrounding the entire cylinder of the artery,
though sometimes more deep at one side than at another; and in
almost all the cases this indentation is greatest towards the convex.
side of the vessel, and least towards the concave and the attachment
of the *ductus arteriosus*. In general the arch of the aorta becomes
small immediately after giving off the left carotid and left subclavian,
and diminishes greatly, though progressively, to the point of obliteration. In some cases the aorta at the point of obliteration and for
some space around it, is lined or penetrated with osteo-steatomatous matter, and is much indurated. (Otto's Case, Craigie's Case.)

When I published the first edition of this work, and when the
only known. cases were those by M. Paris, Dr Graham, Mr Winstone, M. Otto, and A. Meckel of Bern, though the phenomena
of these cases satisfied me of the peculiar nature of the arctation of
the aorta, yet it would have been premature to have drawn from so
small a number of facts the conclusions which I have since been
enabled to deduce. From comparing the whole ten cases, and
considering what I observed in the case dissected by myself, I infer that the contraction and obliteration when it takes place, depends on the same action which closes the *ductus arteriosus* being
extended into the aorta. It must be remembered that in the fœtus
the pulmonary artery, consists, as it were, of three branches, one
going to the right lung, one to the left, both small, and one to the

aorta, the largest and most capacious of the three. Through the two former little or no blood flows; through the latter a large quantity flows, almost directly from the right ventricle into the abdominal aorta, or that portion of the aorta below the entrance of the *ductus arteriosus.* At birth and after that event, in consequence of the lungs being developed and subjected to the action of respiration, the blood from the right ventricle proceeds along the pulmonary artery and its two divisions, which are now enlarged and daily enlarging, while the third branch, or *ductus arteriosus,* undergoes rapid contraction. The point at which the duct joins the aorta is fixed, and keeps the aorta there as it were immovable. Meanwhile the walls of the duct, in consequence of little or no blood passing through them, mutually approximate, and at length adhere, producing obliteration. The same action may extend into the aorta, the more liable to undergo contraction, that at the very time at which the large current of blood is diverted into the two branches of the pulmonary artery, little passing along the *ductus arteriosus,* little also must flow through this part of the aorta. This action once begun has only to continue. It does not require to be increased. If it continue, while the other parts of the aorta and the arterial system are enlarging, this remains stationary, or in the fœtal condition and dimensions. If this only continue, obliteration at that point is the inevitable result.

Meanwhile the blood is maintaining its old channels which it preserved previous to birth, and rendering them larger and more suited to the exigencies of extra-uterine life. The superior and inferior intercostal arteries, the transverse cervicals, the mammary above; and below, the epigastric and circumflex arteries of the ilium, with the lumbar arteries, are found very much enlarged, and to have constituted the means of conveying blood from the heart to the inferior portion of the trunk and to the lower extremities. These changes are evidently effected in early life, in short, in infancy, and increase with the growth of the individual.

The facts now detailed contain a remarkable example of a defect or impediment in the arterial system, which might be inferred, from our knowledge of that system, to be incompatible with the continuance of life and the enjoyment of good health. They also show the remarkable provision by which the pernicious effects of so great a lesion are very nearly, if not completely, obviated and counteracted. It appears that the lesion has little tendency to abridge the duration of human life; for two persons attained the age of 50 years, one of 57, one that of 60, and one the extraordinary length of 90 years. It appears, nevertheless, that all of the subjects of this lesion had been either exposed to cold, or were labouring under the effects of catarrh, attended with symptoms of dyspnœa, constriction in the chest, sometimes pain and anxiety, with palpitation of unusual violence and severity; and amidst attacks of this nature almost all of them expired. This shows what might *a priori* be expected, that in persons with such a defect or lesion, life is held by a precarious and uncertain tenure. Among the ten cases recorded by me, in four the immediate cause of death was laceration of the heart or aorta; an event attributable to the impediment encountered by the blood in passing out of the left ventricle into the aortic arch.

It is further singular that with so great an impediment to the transit of the circulating fluid, the lower extremities were well nourished: and in several of the cases the persons were strong and robust.

Arteries may be involved in the diseases of muscles, bones, and other parts, and in the progressive invasion of foreign or new productions.

CHAPTER VI.

VEIN, VENOUS TISSUE, Φλεψ.   (*Vena—Tissu veneux.*)

SECTION I.

THE structure of the tubular canals, termed veins, has been much less examined by anatomists than that of the arteries. Some incidental observations in the writings of Willis, Glass, and Clifton Wintringham, comprise all that was published regarding them previons to the short account of Haller. Since that time they have been described with various degrees of minuteness and accuracy by John Hunter, Bichat, Magendie, Gordon, Marx,* and Meckel. In the following account the facts collected by these observers have been compared with the appearance and visible organization presented by veins in different parts of the human body.

· The veins are membranous tubes extending between the right

---

* Diatribe Anatomico-physiologico de structurâ atque vita venarum. Caroliruhæ 1819.

side or pulmonary division of the heart and the different organs in which their minute branches are ramified.

Every venous tube greater than one line in diameter consists of three kinds of distinct substance. The outermost is a modification of the filamentous tissue, (*membrana cellulosa,*) and though less compact, and less thick than the arterial filamentous envelope, is in every other respect quite similar, and is in general intimately connected with it. The innermost (*membrana intima*) is a smooth, very thin membrane. Between these is found a tunic somewhat thicker, which is termed the .*proper venous tissue,* (*tunica propria venæ.*) The structure and aspect of this proper membrane shall be first considered.

1*st,* When the loose filamentous tissue in which the blood-vessels are inclosed, and the more delicate and firm layer immediately contiguous to the veins, are removed, the observer recognises a red or brown-coloured membrane, not thick or strong, but somewhat tough, which is the outer surface of the proper venous tunic. If dissected clean, it is tolerably smooth; but however much so it can be made, a glass of moderate powers, or even a good eye, will perceive numerous filaments adhering to it, which appear to be the residue of the cellular envelope.

According to Bichat parallel longitudinal fibres, forming a very thin layer, may be distinguished in the larger veins; but he admits, although they are quite real, that they are always difficult to be seen at the first glance. In the trunk of the inferior great vein, (*vena cava inferior,*) they are always seen, he observes, more distinctly than in that of the superior; and they are always more obvious in the divisions of the former than in those of the latter vessel, and also in the superficial than in the deep-seated veins. These longitudinal fibres, he asserts, are more distinct in the saphena than in the crural vein, which accompanies the artery. Lastly, he remarks, these fibres are proportionally more conspicuous in branches than in trunks.*

Notwithstanding the apparent correctness of this description, Magendie informs us, he has sought in vain for the fibres of the proper venous membrane; and he remarks, that, though he has observed very numerous filaments interlacing in all directions, yet these assume the longitudinal and parallel appearance only when

* Anatomie Generale, Tom. I. p. 399.

H

the tube is folded longitudinally,—a disposition often seen in the larger veins.

By Meckel, on the contrary, the accuracy of the observation of Bichat is maintained. This anatomist states that he has, by the most minute dissections, assured himself that these fibres are longitudinal ; but he admits that they are not uniformly present in all parts of the venous system, and that in degree and abundance they are liable to great variation. He follows Bichat also in representing these fibres as thicker and more distinct in the system of the inferior than in that of the superior *cava*, and in the superficial than in the deep veins.

In the inferior cava of the human subject, certainly filaments or fibres may be recognised. But, instead of being longitudinal, they may be made to assume any direction, according to the manner in which the filamentous tissue is removed. For this reason probably these fibres are to be viewed as part of the filamentous sheath. In the saphena vein of the leg oblique fibres may be seen decussating each other; but it is doubtful whether these belong to the proper venous tissue, or to the filamentous covering.

I have repeatedly seen and demonstrated the following facts.

If the *vena cava descendens* be cut open by a longitudinal incision and washed in pure water, there is seen first the inner membrane perfectly smooth, very thin, and semitransparent, so much so, that it cannot be detached from the middle coat, without the risk of bringing some of the latter away. Secondly, longitudinal fibres or lines running along the middle coat in its substance parallel to the axis of the vein. Thirdly, when the cellular coat is detached carefully by the forceps, there is seen a moderately thick membranous layer of fawn-colour, presenting longitudinal threads, lines, or fibres.

The same can be seen, though much less distinctly, in several of the large venous trunks, for instance the iliac and common femoral veins.

The nature of this proper membrane or venous fibre, as it is sometimes named, (Bichat,) is not at all known. Its great extensibility, its softness, its want of elasticity in the circular direction, or fragility, its colour and general aspect, distinguish it from the arterial tunic. It possesses some elasticity in the longitudinal direction, and is retracted vigorously when stretched. It possesses considerable resistance, or in common language is tough. The experiments of Clifton Wintringham show that it sustains a considerable weight without breaking, and that this toughness is greater in early life, or in the veins of the young subject, than at a later period.* In short, it may be stated as a general fact, that venous tissue, though thinner, possesses greater elasticity and tenacity than arterial tissue. According to the experiments of the same inquirer this property depends on that of the superior density of the venous tissue, the specific gravity of the matter of the *vena cava* being invariably greater than that of the aorta in the same subject, both in man and in brute animals.

From some experiments Magendie is disposed to consider it of a *fibrinous* character. But it exhibits in the living body no proof of muscular structure or irritable power. When punctured by a sharp instrument, or exposed to the electric or galvanic action, it undergoes no change or sensible motion.

This tunic is wanting in those divisions of the venous system termed *sinuses*, in which its place is supplied by portions of the hard membrane; (*dura meninx.*)

2*d*, The inner surface of any vein which has been laid open and well washed is found to be smooth, highly polished, and of a bluish or blue-white colour. This is the inner or free surface of the inner venous membrane, (*membrana intima.*) It is exceedingly thin, much more so than the corresponding arterial membrane, much more distensible and less fragile. It bears a very tight ligature without giving way as the arterial does; but it also sustains considerable weight, which shows that it is tough and resisting. This is the membrane termed by Bichat *common membrane of dark or modena blood.* According to the views of this anatomist it forms the inner or free surface not only of all the venous twigs, branches, and trunks composing this system of vessels, but it is extended from the superior and inferior great veins over the inner surface of the right auricle and ventricle, and thence over that of the pulmonary artery and its divisions; and through this whole tract it is the same in structure and properties.

This doctrine has not yet been controverted. But perhaps it may be doubted, both with regard to the inner arterial membrane, that the inner tunic of the aorta and of the pulmonary veins is quite the same; and in regard to this inner venous membrane, whether that of the veins in general is quite the same with that of the pul-

* Experimental Inquiry on some parts of the Animal Structure. London, 1740.

monary artery. The subject demands 'further research. Meanwhile strong confirmation is found in the interesting remark of
Bichat, that the osseous or calcareous depositions which are common in various spots of the inner arterial membrane, and especially
at the mitral and aortic valves, are never found in the inner venous
membrane, or at the tricuspid valve, or in the semilunar valves of
the pulmonary artery. Have these depositions been found inside
the pulmonary veins, and not inside the pulmonary artery? This
fact is still wanting to complete even their pathological similarity.

The inner or common venous membrane is, however, the most
extensive and the most uniform of all the venous tissues. It is the
only one which is found in the substance of organs, and is present
where the cellular and proper membrane are wanting. This is the
case not only with venous branches and minute canals as they issue
from the substance of muscles, bones, and such organs as the liver,
kidneys, spleen, &c. but is also very remarkably observed with regard to the venous canals of the brain. I have already noticed
the absence of the cellular and proper tissues in these tubes; and
I have now to remark, that the cerebral veins consist solely of the
inner membrane, while in the brain or membranes, and when in
the sinuses of this inner membrane, placed between folds of the
dura mater. When the jugular vein reaches the temporo-occipital
sinuosity, it loses its proper membrane, while its common or inner
membrane passes into the hollow of the *dura mater*, called *sinus*,
and thus forms the venous canal. This fact is readily demonstrated by slitting open either the lateral or the superior longitudinal
sinus, when a thin delicate membrane, quite distinct from the fibrous appearance of the *dura mater*, will be found to line the interior of these canals.

The inner surface of many veins presents membranous folds projecting obliquely into the cavity of the vessel. These folds, which,
from their mechanical office, have been named *valves*, (*valvulæ*,)
are parabolic in shape, have two margins,—an attached and free,
and two surfaces, a concave turned to the cardiac end of the vein,
and a convex turned in the opposite direction. The attached margin is not straight, as may be imagined, but circular, and adheres
to the inner surface of the vessel. The free margin resembles in
shape an oblong parabola; and the direction of the valve is such,
that a force applied to its convex surface would urge it more closely
to the vein, whereas a force applied to the concave surface would

either obliterate the circular area of the vessel, tear the valve from the vein, or otherwise meet with resistance.

The size of the valves is variable. In some instances they are sufficiently large to fill the canal of the vessel, and in others they are too small to produce this effect. The obliteration of the circular area of the vessel is most perfect when there are two or three at the same point. Bichat ascribed the variable state of this quality to the dilated or contracted condition of the veins at the moment of death. This, however, is denied by Magendie.

In structure these valvular or parabolic folds are said to consist of a doubling, or two-fold layer of the inner membrane; and with this statement no fact of which we are aware is at variance. A hard prominent line, which generally marks their attachment of the fixed margin to the vein, is asserted by Bichat to consist of the proper venous tissue, the fibres of which, he says, alter their direction for this purpose; and when the common or inner membrane reaches this line, it doubles or folds itself (*elle se replie*) to form the valve, which thus consists of two layers of the inner or common membrane. This, however, is denied by Hunter,* who considers them of a tendinous nature, and by Gordon, who made several unsuccessful attempts to split these two layers.†

Valves are not uniformly present in all veins. They are found, 1*st*, In the following branches of the superior great vein;—the internal jugular, the azygos, the facial veins, those of the arms, &c. 2*d*, In the following branches of the inferior great vein; the divisions of the posterior iliac, of the femoral, tibial, internal and external saphena, and in the spermatic veins of the male.

They are wanting in the trunk of the inferior great vein (*cava inferior*,) in the renal, mesenteric, and other abdominal veins, in the portal vein, in the cerebral sinuses, in the veins of the brain and spinal chord, in the veins of the heart, of the womb generally, and of the ovaries, and perhaps in all other veins less than a line in diameter.‡ In the cerebral sinuses the transverse chords are supposed to supply their place.

In situation the valves vary considerably. In general they are found in those parts of venous canals at which a small vein opens into a larger. But even from this arrangement there are deviations. The only valve which is definite and invariable in its situation is

---

* X. Of Veins, p. 182.   † Anatomy, pp. 66, 67.
‡ Haller,'Lib. ii. sect. ii.

the Eustachian, (*valvula Eustachiana, valvula nobilis,*) which is always placed at the cardiac end or beginning of the inferior *cava*, where that vessel is attached to the sinus of the right auricle. Shaped in general like a crescent, the attached margin of which is the arch of a large circle, and the free that of a small one, it proceeds from the left extremity of the sinus downwards, forwards, and towards the left side, where it is insensibly lost on the membrane of the auricular *septum*. At its lower end it generally covers the orifice of the large coronary vein. This membranous production is always larger, more perfect, and more distinct in the fœtus, and in the infant, than in the adult. In the latter it is almost always reticulated; and sometimes the only vestige of its existence is a thin chord or two representing its anterior margin. I have seen it reticulated even at the age of sixteen or seventeen, and almost destroyed beyond thirty. Haller was much perplexed to account for the use of this membranous fold.* The conjecture of Bichat, that it is connected with some purpose in the fœtal circulation, is entitled to regard.

Dr Gordon has mentioned a third partial substance, which is occasionally found in local patches at various parts of veins. This, which I believe to be accidental, or not connected with healthy structure, is, I suppose, the following. Where the veins unite to form a single trunk at the point of union, there is often seen extending from it into the trunk a reddish coloured matter of a triangular shape with the apex turned toward and into the

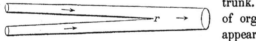

trunk. This seems void of organization, and it appears to me a deposit from the blood exactly at the point where the current is least forcible, upon the same principle as that on which we observe banks of silt, gravel, and sand accumulated under the sterlings of a bridge.

Besides the cellular or filamentous envelope, veins receive capillary arteries, to which there are corresponding veins. The arteries rise from the nearest small ramifying arteries; and the corresponding veins do not terminate in the cavity of the vein to which they belong, but pass off from its body, and join some others from different parts; and at last terminate in the common trunk some way higher.† Nervous branches, or rather filaments, are

---

* Haller de Valvula Eustachii. Extat in Disput. Anatomic. Selec. Vol. II. p. 189.
† Hunter, X. Of Veins, p. 181.

observed in the pulmonary artery and great veins only. Are they derived from the great sympathetic, as is generally said?

In the veins, as in the arteries, the anatomist recognises two extremities, the cardiac or collected, and the organic or the rami-fied. Examined physiologically, however, the terms origin and termination are not of the same import as when applied to the arteries. In reference to the veins, they become convertible terms; and it is the usage even of writers on anatomy to represent the veins as arising where the arteries terminate, and terminating at the organ from which the latter arise. This distinction must be kept in view in the following observations.

The cardiac extremity or termination of the veins is so well known as to render any minute explanation unnecessary.

The organic extremity or origin of the venous system is more obscure and difficult to be understood. It is indeed impossible to trace the origin of the small venous vessels, unless in the manner in which Leuenhoek,* William Cowper,† Henry Baker,‡ Haller and Spallanzani,§ did in their observations on the transparent parts of animals in general cold-blooded. From the experiments of these observers, we know that a very small vessel, evidently tending and conveying blood *towards* a larger, connected with a venous branch, may be seen passing directly from a similar small vessel, as evi-dently conveying blood *from* a larger, which is connected with the arterial system. All that we know from this, however, is, that a vein containing red blood may rise from an artery conveying red blood. This is matter of pure observation, and all beyond is little more than conjectural.

Haller, indeed, admits origins of veins as manifold as the termi-nations of the arterial system, a view in which he has been followed by almost all subsequent authors; and Bichat states it as a leading proposition, that the veins arise from the general capillary system. Neither conclusion is founded on strict observation; and while that of the former physiologist is derived chiefly from uncertain facts

---

* Arcana Naturæ Detect. Opera Omnia, Tom. II. p. 160, 168.

† Philosophical Transactions, No. 280, p. 1179. Cowper saw this communication of arteries and veins not only in cold-blooded animals, as the lizard, tadpole, and fishes, but in the omentum of a young cat and a dog.

‡ On Microscopes, and the discoveries made thereby. Two vols. 8vo. London, 1785.

§ Experiments on the Circulation of the Blood. By Lazaro Spallanzani. Trans-lated by W. Hall. London, 1801.

and loose analogies, the statement of the latter is too hypothetical and general to be either entirely true or wholly false.

Of one fact only are we certain. The blood which is conveyed into the small vessels, and the substance of the tissues and organs, is brought back by the veins. We have seen that the only origin, which is strictly susceptible of demonstration, is that of the red vein from the red artery. The point, then, to be ascertained is, whether colourless veins and absorbent veins arise from the several textures, as colourless and exhalant arteries terminate in them? The proper place for the further examination of this question is the subsequent chapter.

I must not omit to mention, nevertheless, that the veins have been shown to be connected at their ramified extremities with the lymphatics.

When the veins become distinct vessels, branches, and trunks, they become once more objects of sensible examination. In their course or transit from their organic to their cardiac extremities, they present various circumstances which merit attention.

1. In general, every artery is accompanied by a venous tube, which is divided in the same manner, and furnishes or receives an equal number of branches. Thus the descending aorta is accompanied by the *vena cava inferior;* the common iliac arteries by common iliac veins; the anterior iliac, femoral, and popliteal, by anterior iliac, femoral, and popliteal veins. These veins are deep-seated, and are generally named the concomitant veins, (*venæ comites vel venæ satellites.*) In some situations, an artery may be accompanied, either in its trunk or in its branches, by two veins of equal size. Thus, in general, the brachial artery, and its branches the radial and ulnar, are each accompanied by two veins. The only situations in which the number of veins can be said to be exactly equal to that of the arteries, are in the stomach, in the intestinal canal, in the spleen, in the kidneys, in the testicles, and in the ovaries.

2. In the extremities and in the external regions of the trunk we find, in addition to the concomitant veins, an external layer of venous tubes immediately beneath the skin, (*venæ subter cutem dispersæ,* Pliny.) These subcutaneous or superficial veins do not correspond to any artery; but, as they are chiefly destined to convey the blood from the skin and other superficial parts, they open into the deep-seated veins. Thus in the case of the basilic and cepha-

3

lic, two superficial veins of the arm, the former, after passing the bicipital fascia, forms in the sheath the brachial vein, and becoming the axillary in the axilla, receives the latter vessel. In the same manner, the saphena, ($\varphi\lambda\varepsilon\psi$ $\sigma\alpha\varphi\alpha\iota\nu\eta\varsigma$, *vena manifesta*,) the superficial vein of the leg, passes through the falciform process of the *fascia lata* to join the femoral vein. From this it results that the venous canals are on the whole more numerous than the arterial. In a few situations only, a single vein corresponds to two arteries, as in the penis, the clitoris, the gall-bladder, and the umbilical chord. Often also in the renal capsules and the kidneys, two or more arteries have only one corresponding vein. In such circumstances the vein is always large and capacious.

It has been generally stated that the calibre and area of the venous tubes are much larger than those of the corresponding arteries, and, consequently, that the capacity of the venous system is much greater than that of the arterial. I acknowledge that I know not on what exact evidence the former of these propositions, the only one with which the anatomist is concerned, is made to rest. If it be mere inspection in the dead subject, or the effects of injection, little doubt can be entertained that the alleged greater calibre depends chiefly on the laxity and distensible nature of the venous fibre. The arterial tubes appear small in consequence of the tendency which they have to collapse, or annular contraction, when the distending force has ceased to operate. The venous canals appear large by reason of their distension and distensibility during life, from the tendency to accumulation in their branches in most kinds of death, except that by hemorrhage, and from a smaller degree of the physical property of shrinking and annular contraction when empty.

When a vascular sheath is exposed in the human subject, as in the operation for aneurism, or in the lower animals in the way of experiment, the vein, it must be admitted, generally appears larger than the corresponding artery. This, however, is never so considerable as it is represented by most authors, and certainly could by no means afford grounds for the high estimates which Keill, Jurin, and other mathematical physiologists have assigned to the relative capacity of the arteries and veins. It is also to be observed that something of this greater size depends on the increase of dilatation resulting from removing the pressure of superincumbent parts. In young animals, also, the difference between the size of the veins and their corresponding arteries is so trifling as to be scarcely discernible. This would show that something is to be ascribed to the incessant operation of a dilating force increasing uniformly with the duration of life.

Upon the whole, it is chiefly on the ground of their larger numerical arrangement that the veins collectively can be said to be more capacious than the arteries. On this subject some observations of Bichat are entitled to attention.*

3. The veins in general accompany the arteries. The venous trunk placed contiguous to the arterial in the same sheath is divided into branches at the same points, and is distributed into the substance of organs much in the same manner. From this arrangement, however, certain deviations are observed in particular regions. Thus, in the brain, neither the internal carotid, nor the basilar artery, nor their large branches, are accompanied with veins. The small branches only have corresponding veins, which, as they unite to form large ones, pour their blood into the venous canals termed sinuses, the arrangement of which is unlike any other part of the venous system. In the chest also a different disposition of the venous from the arterial tubes is observed. The *venæ cavæ*, though conveying the blood to the pulmonic division of the heart, as the aorta conveys it from it, do not, however, correspond with the latter either in situation or in dependent branches. The *azygos* and the *demiazygos* veins in like manner, which receive the intercostal veins, have no concomitant artery, but open into the *superior cava*, to which it may be viewed as an appendage. *Lastly*, The portal vein, which is formed of the united trunks of the splenic, superior mesenteric and inferior mesenteric veins, corresponds to no individual arterial trunk, and forms of itself a peculiar arrangement in the venous system.

Some anatomists have dwelt much on the more superficial and less sheltered situation of the veins than of the arteries. Upon this point no very positive inferences can be established. In the extremities the former are in general most superficial; but in the interior of the body, especially in the chest, the venous trunks are quite as deep-seated as the arterial.

The course of the venous canals is in general more rectilineal and less tortuous than that of the arteries. In no part of the ve-

* Anatomie Generale, Tome I. p. 378.

nous system is such an inflection presented as that which the internal carotid makes in the carotic canal. The general result of this is, that a set of venous tubes is shorter than a corresponding set of arterial ones. The trunks also are less inflected than the branches.

4. The mutual communications of the venous system, (*anastomoses*, *inosculationes*,) are more numerous and frequent than those of the arterial. 1. The minute veins communicate so freely as to form a perfect net-work. 2. In the twigs, though more rare, these communications are still frequent. 3. In the branches, though less numerous, they are nevertheless observed; and in this respect alone the venous must be greatly more numerous than the arterial inosculations, which are confined chiefly to the smaller and more remote parts of the system. These inosculations, indeed, between the venous branches, constitute one of the most peculiar and important characters of their arrangement, in so far as by their means the communication is maintained between the superficial and deep-seated vessels of the system. Thus the emissary veins are the channel of communication between the cerebral sinuses and the temporal, occipital, and other external veins. The external and internal jugulars communicate by one or two considerable vessels. And the free communication between the basilic and cephalic by the median veins, that between them and the deep brachial vessel, and that between the saphena and its branches and the femoral vein, are sufficiently well known. The application of these anatomical facts to the ready motion of the venous blood is obvious.

But of all the communications between the branches or large vessels of the venous system, the most important, both anatomically and physiologically, is that maintained by means of the *vena azygos* between the superior and inferior *cavæ*. The azygos itself is connected at its upper or bronchial extremity with the superior *cava*, and at its lower extremity it is in some subjects connected directly with the inferior *cava*, in others by means of the right renal vein, and in most by the first lumbar veins. By means of the *demiazygos*, again, it is connected with the left renal vein, or the lumbars of the same side, and in some instances directly with the inferior *cava*. To the azygos and demiazygos, therefore, belong the remarkable property of connecting not only the venous canals of the upper and lower divisions, but those of the right and left halves of the body.

SECTION II.

Venous tissue is liable to inflammation, adhesive or circumscribed, and spreading,—generally suppurative, to *varix*, to osseous deposition, and to the formation of concretions.

1. *Inflammation.* (*Phlebitis.*) Of *circumscribed* or *adhesive inflammation* of veins, a good example is found in the ordinary union
after incised wounds, as in venesection. In this case the lips of the
wound, if accurately applied to each other, adhere sometimes directly by inosculation, in other instances by effusion of lymph,
which becomes organized.

2. *Spreading inflammation* of venous tissue is a much more serious disorder, and appears to belong essentially to the inner venous membrane. Rarely spontaneous, it takes place only after
some violence offered to the vein ; but the degrees of this may be
so various, and even the kinds so different, that it is impossible to
trace much analogy of action between them. Thus it may occur
after a simple clean incision, as in blood-letting ; after the application of a ligature, as occasionally happens in amputation, in the
operation for varix, or in the umbilical chord after birth ; or in
consequence of pressure, as sometimes happens after the use of a
tourniquet. In either case, the inflammatory action originating in
one spot of the inner membrane, spreads along its surface, generally
towards the heart, more or less rapidly, and with much violence.

The pathological effects of this process vary according to its severity and extent. In general the tissue of the affected vein or
veins is swelled, thickened, and indurated to such a degree as make
the vessel resemble an artery. Much pain is felt along the course
of the inflamed vessel. The whole limb is diffusely swelled ; and
the skin is tense, with tenderness of the surface. Upon examination of the parts, it is found that the whole subcutaneous cellular
and adipose tissue are filled with serous fluid. The vein is found
firm and hard, sometimes filled with bloody clots. When laid open,
clots of blood or lymph or both are found adhering to the inner
tunic, which is rough and irregular, and thicker than usual. In
these clots are contained specks of purulent matter. In other instances, the interior is filled with purulent matter, or presents a
series of abscesses along the tract of the canal ; and the inner tunic is generally removed, the middle one not unfrequently injured
by ulceration. This process is always attended with great commo-

tion in the organs of circulation, much general fever, a brownish tint of the complexion, glaring, injected, suffused, or turbid eyes, and more or less affection of the intellectual functions, and if considerable, generally proves fatal.

Inflammation of the inner venous membrane I have represented generally to succeed violence offered to the vessel; but what sort of violence is requisite is not well known. I have in two or three instances thought I could trace it to wound, laceration, or pressure in the site of a valve; but in others this could not be established.

I have seen the disease so often take place after application of the finger to the wound in the vein at the bend of the arm, in the common operation of venesection, that I cannot doubt that it is often produced in this manner. The perspiration on the finger acts like an irritant poison to the cut edges of the vein, and thereby causes inflammation. It was also a very common accident after injecting saline solutions during the epidemic cholera in 1832. In the veins of the womb, after parturition, it may follow the forcible revulsion of the placenta; or the sinuses being left open and patent, air from the atmosphere, or from the decomposition of the blood, or the uterus, may enter these canals and irritate or inflame their coats. In this organ it is most common along the lateral regions of the womb.

The circumstances under which *phlebitis* may take place may be enumerated in the following order.

1*st*, After venesection, especially when the finger is applied to the wound so as to touch the divided edges of the vein; 2*d*, After amputation, especially when there is much fingering, or when a ligature is put on a vein; 3*d*, After laceration of a vein, as in certain lacerated wounds; 4*th*, After any venous tube has been laid open by ulceration or erosion, as in cancer or ulceration of the womb; 5*th*, After laying open the uterine veins, as in child-bearing; 6*th*, After deligation of a vein, as in the operation for varix, the old operation for castration, in which all the vessels were tied in one mass, and after operations on the hemorrhoidal veins.

This process is known to take place spontaneously in the veins of the brain and in those of the womb. The latter Dr Clarke* and Mr Wilson† found filled with purulent matter or lymph in the persons of females cut off by puerperal fever; and in a number of fatal cases of the same disease, I saw these veins containing purulent

---

* Practical Essays on the Management of Pregnancy, p. 63, 72.

† Transactions of a Society, Vol. III. p. 63 and p. 80.

fluid.   Tonellé found among 222 cases suppuration of the uterine veins in 90 cases.   Dr Lee among 45 cases inspected found traces of inflammation of the uterine veins in 24.   Taking both together, we have among 267 cases 114 instances of uterine *phlebitis.*   This is not quite one-half; but it is as near as may be three-sevenths.

The venous tubes of the brain have been found presenting marks of inflammation by Dr Abercromby* and M. Gendrin.†   I have found inflammatory products, as lymph and purulent matter with clots of blood, within the sinuses of the brain, in the following circumstances.

1. In certain cases of inflammation of the internal ear and the petrous portion of the temporal bone, when inflammatory action had spread to the internal jugular vein in the temporal *fossa.*

2. In certain cases of gangrenous inflammation of the lungs, when suppuration takes place in the brain; and when the agents of this process appear to be the venous canals of the lungs opening into the gangrenous or suppurating portion.   Thus, in a child of two years, in whom this affection of the lungs had taken place, I found the convolutions of the brain flattened, the longitudinal sinus filled with lymph and purulent particles and clots of blood, and a similar state of the lateral sinuses, and several of the small sinuses.

3. In cases of hypertrophy of the spleen.   This shall be noticed under its proper head.

It appears, therefore, that inflammation of the inner venous coat rarely terminates in albuminous exudation and adhesion; and it may be stated as a peculiar character of this tissue, as distinct from the inner arterial membrane, that, while the latter is almost sure to assume the adhesive, the former is exceedingly prone to the suppurative form of inflammation.

3. Instances, nevertheless, have occurred in which inflammation of this membrane was followed by deposition of lymph and union of its free surfaces, producing obliteration of the canal of the vessel. Dr Baillie mentions an instance of obliteration of the lower *cava,* from the emulgent veins to the entrance of the *venæ cavæ hepaticæ,* which he ascribes to effusion of lymph and consequent adhesion ;‡ and Mr Wilson records a similar case in which about four ounces of well-formed purulent fluid were found in the *vena cava* imme-

* Medical and Surgical Journal, Vol. XVIII.

† Revue Medicale, Avril 1826.

‡ Transactions of a Society for the Improvement of Medical and Chirurgical Knowledge, Vol. I. Art. viii. p. 133.

diately below the liver, and a considerable quantity of coagulated lymph below the entrance of the three large hepatic veins, (*venæ cavæ hepaticæ*,) which at once united the opposite sides of the vessel, and prevented this fluid from proceeding to the heart.* Similar examples of obliteration are recorded by Haller, Morgagni, and by Hodgson,† and Breschet. In the College Museum collection there is a preparation of a case in which the right *vena innominata* was filled with a solid plug of fibrin or albuminous matter, in consequence of a tyromatous tumour compressing the vessel below, at its junction with the left *vena innominata* and *vena cava*, and in which the left *innominata* was very much contracted at its lower end. The pressure of the tumour in this case had interrupted the current of blood to the heart, and contracted the channel of the vein; and in consequence blood had been coagulated and attached to the walls of the vessel, and so obstructed the interior of the vein.

In 1841, a man under my care in the hospital, with obstinate ascites and indications of liver disease, had undergone the operation of paracentesis twice with relief, when no benefit was produced by internal medicines.

About twelve days after the performance of the second operation, the water was again accumulating, and he died. Upon inspecting the body after death, I found the *vena portæ* in the liver completely obstructed, being contracted and filled with lymph, and the lymph extending into the splenic and mesenteric veins. The lymph was small in quantity, and the trunks of the vessels were evidently diminished in size. The liver was reduced to about one-fourth of its usual size, the whole right lobe almost had become shrunk into a small portion, while the organ was represented by a small left lobe.

A case of obliteration of the *vena cava* is recorded by M. Gely in Gazette Medicale, 7th November 1840.

In other instances, when inflammation in the vein of an extremity takes place, causing permanent obstruction, it produces not only swelling of that extremity, but deposits of lymph in the veins, in the pulmonary artery, and in the vessels of the lungs. Thus I have seen inflammation of the femoral vein with lymphy deposit within the vessel, followed after some time by the deposit of similar lymph and blood in clots in the branches of the pulmonary artery and in various parts of the lungs.

---

* Transactions, &c. Vol. III. Art. vi. p. 63.
† Treatise, p. 10. sect. 3.

All these phenomena, which may be called the secondary effects of *phlebitis,* arise from the inflammatory deposits, viz. lymph and purulent matter, being taken into the veins and circulated along these vessels; and sometimes from purulent matter being carried by the veins directly to the pleura, the veins of the lungs, or the synovial membrane, or the cellular membrane.

4. Purulent matter and lymph may be found within the veins, and prove a cause of death. Thus in a case of hypertrophy of the spleen I found purulent matter and lymph in the sinuses of the brain, and the veins of the chest and abdomen.* In such cases the deposit is not preceded by inflammation.

It is easy to perceive how the pressure of tumours may cause obliteration of these vessels. When any venous tube, under such circumstances, becomes impervious, the collateral communications afford channels for continuing the motion of the blood.

5. Secondary effects of *Phlebitis.* Inflammation of veins, though usually and ordinarily a fatal disease, is neither necessarily so, nor always. But when it has terminated, as it commonly does, in the formation of purulent matter, it occasionally gives rise to a train of very remarkable and dangerous phenomena. This I shall describe in two forms, as it most usually presents itself.

In the ordinary case of inflammation of the vein taking place after venesection, when the patient survives the immediate effects, lymph having been effused, and caused obliteration of part of the vessel, purulent matter is effused at the same time; or rather the effusion is a sort of sero-albuminous matter, the thicker portion of which is the medium of partial and local adhesion, while the more liquid forms purulent fluid. The latter is taken into the circulation; and the original febrile symptoms assume the characters of hectic. Soon after the patient has difficult and laborious breathing, with pain in some part of the chest or side, and purulent matter is formed within the pleura. Or another result may ensue. With the symptoms of great disorder in the organs of respiration, as rapid laborious breathing and cough, without expectoration, the symptoms of hectic fever continue; and after two or three weeks, the patient being much emaciated and feeble, dies. On inspection of the body, the lungs, when divided, present numerous abscesses,

* Case of Disease of the Spleen, in which death took place in consequence of the presence of purulent matter in the blood. By David Craigie, M. D. &c. Edinburgh Medical and Surgical Journal, Vol. LXIV. p. 400.

not larger than peas. When these are examined, they are found to be not abscesses, but the veins of the lungs filled with purulent matter. The veins of the arm are at the same time thickened in their walls, and contain lymph and purulent matter. These appearances I observed in the body of a young man, on whom venesection had been performed three weeks previously for the removal of symptoms of peritonitis. Similar phenomena were seen by Velpeau in a case of amputation.

In other instances the intermuscular cellular tissue, either of an arm or a leg is attacked; and purulent collections more or less extensive are deposited in them. At the same time one or more of the joints, as the shoulder-joint or the knee-joint, may be attacked with acute pain, aggravated by motion and pressure, swelling and heat; and in no long time it is observed that fluid has been formed within the joint. This is most commonly purulent, from inflammation of the synovial membrane. After it has taken place, the synovial membrane is removed by ulceration; the cartilages are partially or entirely destroyed in the same manner; and either the joint becomes ankylosed by the adhesion of the lymphy effusion, or the patient is destroyed by the long-continued severe irritation on the constitution.

When the veins of the womb have been the seat of inflammation, if the morbid action do not terminate fatally, it is occasionally followed by the same train of phenomena as have been now enumerated;—purulent deposits within the pleura, purulent deposits in the intermuscular cellular tissue of the extremities, and purulent deposits within the joints, most usually the knee-joint. The most favourable case is that of purulent deposits among the muscles of the extremities, especially the leg. Yet here, often in the process of healing, adhesions between the muscles take place, and lameness is the result.

6. *Varix.* This consists in permanent dilatation of the venous coats beyond their natural capacity. It is in general, if excessive, confined to one spot; but sometimes a whole vein becomes more or less dilated through its entire course. At the same time it becomes so tortuous, that this may be received as one of the physical characters of varicose veins. We possess no very precise facts on the exact change which takes place in the venous tunics, whether it be mere dilatation or injury of some kind, and rupture of the proper venous coats. By Meckel it is regarded as simple dilatation

I

without injury of texture.   When one part of a vein is dilated into a distinct sac, I believe the inner coat is generally rent.   In some cases of varix one or more valves are lacerated, or detached from the inner membrane.   In others varix has followed a rent or lacerated wound of the outer venous tunic, or a cutaneous ulcer affecting that tunic.

Varix occurs especially in the veins of the lower extremities, for instance in the trunk or branches of the saphena.   It is common in those of the spermatic chord, in which it is distinguished by the name of *varico-cele*, and not unfrequent in the veins of the rectum, where it causes one variety of hemorrhoidal tumours.   In the upper extremities it is rare, one case only by Petit being recorded. I have seen, nevertheless, a varicose tumour of the posterior ulnar vein on the back of the hand, which disappeared under the use of pressure, continued for six or seven months.

Of the internal veins the *vena azygos* and subclavian have been found varicose.   (Morgagni, Portal, Baillie.)   When a cluster of subcutaneous veins becomes varicose, they generally give rise to much pain, swelling and redness of the skin, and if not opposed by suitable treatment, may produce cutaneous inflammation terminating in a bad ulcer.   (*Ulcus varicosum.*)   The same process nearly may result from the inflammation round a single varicose trunk.   Varix sometimes terminates in laceration or rupture; and if the vein be large and not covered by the skin, the hemorrhage may be fatal. (Laurentius, Nebel, Bonet.)   Varix of the *vena azygos* terminating in rupture and fatal hemorrhage was seen by Manfredi.*

Ossification.   Calcareous or osseous matter is very rarely deposited in venous tissue.   Instances of this, however, are recorded. (Morgagni, Baillie, Hodgson.)†

Loose stony concretions have been found in the cavity of veins, which in such circumstances are generally dilated.   These concretions do not appear to be formed and deposited in the venous tissue, but, according to Hodgson, are more likely to have been produced outside by some contiguous tissue, and to have found their way into the venous tube by progressive absorption.   Is it not possible that they are the result of temporary retardation or stagnation of a portion of blood around which, as a nucleus, calcareous matter had been deposited?   They have not been chemically examined; but it is said that they have no appearance of any thing osseous.

* Morgagni, xxvi. 29.   † Treatise, Part iv. sect. 2.

These concretions, which in other respects are very imperfectly known, have been termed *vein-stones.* (Phlebolites.)

CHAPTER VII.

SYSTEM OF CAPILLARY VESSELS,—TERMINATIONS OF ARTERIES,— ORIGINS OF VEINS.

SECTION I.

THOUGH we can scarcely, with propriety, speak of the *capillary tissue*, or the tissue of capillary vessels, we find it requisite to introduce in this place the general facts of the anatomical peculiarities of this important part of the human body.

The term *capillary system*, though much spoken of in physiological and pathological writings, is perhaps not always precisely defined or distinctly understood. According to Bichat it is not only the common intermediate system between the arteries and veins, but the origin of all the exhalant and excreting vessels.[*] If we consider the modes in which arteries have been said to terminate, and veins to take their origin, we shall find, that in this view of the capillary system there are some things which are doubtful, and some which are inconsistent with the rest.

Haller, and most of the physiological authorities since his time, concluded, chiefly from the phenomena of injections, sometimes from microscopical observation, and where these failed, from the obscure and uncertain evidence of analogy, that an artery traced to its last or minute divisions will be found to terminate in one or other of the following modes. 1*st*, Either directly in a red vein or veins; 2*d*, in excreting ducts, as in the lacrymal and salivary glands, the kidney, liver, and pancreas, the female breast, and the testicle of the male; 3*d*, in exhalants, as in the skin, in the membranes of cavities, (serous membranes,) the cavities of the brain, the chambers of the eye, the filamentous tissue, the adipose cells, the pulmonary vesicles, and mucous surfaces and their follicular glands; 4*th*, in smaller vessels, for instance lymphatics; and, 5*th*, in the colourless artery; (*arteria non rubra*.)[†]

---

[*] Anat. Gen. Vol. I. p. 471. *Systeme Capillaire*, Article 1.
[†] Elementa Physiologiæ, Lib. i. sect. 1. p. 22-29.

A similar application of the same facts has assigned to the veins a mode of origin not unlike. If, therefore, we admit the definition given by Bichat, it follows that the capillary system consists, 1*st*, of minute arteries communicating with veins; 2*d*, of excreting ducts; 3*d*, of exhalants; and, 4*th*, of minute arteries or veins containing a colourless portion of the blood. It is obvious, however, that it is absurd to say that the system of capillary vessels at once comprehends and gives origin to the excretories and exhalants. In other respects the whole of this theory, for little of it is matter of strict observation, rests on very hypothetical grounds.

Of the different kinds of terminations assigned to arteries, and of origins assigned to veins, one only admits of sensible and satisfactory demonstration. Arteries, when they have so much diminished as to become *capillary*, are seen by the microscope, in some instances by the naked eye, to pass directly into corresponding capillary veins, or to end abruptly in some organ or membrane unconnected with any other vessel.* It is likewise certain that the microscope shows every capillary vein to arise from a capillary artery; and if there be any other mode of origin, it has not yet been demonstrated or established.† Only one other circumstance requires to be taken into account in this inquiry. This is, that the capillary artery and vein may contain either red or colourless blood; for, according to the size of the vessels, and the nature of the organs or tissues in which they are distributed, the blood which flows through them will be coloured or colourless. This view of the communication of minute arteries and veins, which is perfectly consistent with the known facts, will afford the only explanation which it is possible to give, of the singular division of the capillary system which Bichat has chosen.

This author has considered the capillary system under three general heads. 1*st*, In organs in which it contains blood only; for instance, in the muscles, the spleen, some parts of the mucous membranes. 2*d*, In organs in which it contains blood and other fluids; for example, in bone, cellular tissue, serous membrane, part of the fibrous system, the skin, the vascular *parietes*, glands, &c. And, 3*d*, In organs in which it contains no blood, the instances of which are, tendon, cartilage, ligament, hair, &c.

Now, it is of little consequence to say that the tissues of the two last divisions contain other fluids than blood, when we are also told

* Gordon, p. 56.   † Ib. p. 62.

that the phenomena of injections, which prove that their capillaries communicate directly with arteries conveying red blood, the effect of irritating applications mechanical or chemical, and the phenomena of acute or chronic inflammation, show that they may convey or receive red blood. The conclusion of this in common language is, that the capillary arteries and veins of the second order of tissues do not all contain red blood, but that many of them contain a colourless part of that fluid; and that all the capillary arteries and veins of the third order of tissues convey in the natural state colourless blood only. What, then, is the precise idea which ought to be formed of the intermediate system which Bichat conceived to exist between the minute arteries and veins, or what have been termed the venous *radiculæ?*

It appears that the present state of facts will admit of nothing more to constitute this capillary system than those minute vessels, whether conveying coloured or colourless blood, in which inspection, microscopic observation, and injections show that arterial branches at once terminate, and minute veins (*radiculæ venosæ*) have their origin. It is clear that, physiologically speaking, these vessels can neither be regarded as arteries nor as veins strictly; for the characters on which this distinction is founded are necessarily lost or obliterated in this system of vessels. There is no precise point at which the arterial tissue or structure can be said to terminate, and none at which the venous structure can be said to commence. Microscopic observation shows merely a minute and endless network of interlacing and communicating vessels, in which the blood moves with great velocity. And the vessels are too small to allow their structure to be correctly examined. If, however, we adopt the doctrines of Bichat with regard to the inner arterial and venous tunics forming the ultimate tube of small arteries and small veins, we must conclude that the arterial membrane is lost in the venous, and that the common membrane of red blood is identified with the common membrane of dark or modena blood. In this conclusion there is nothing either absurd or improbable, and, though not founded on actual observation, it is greatly more natural than many similar ideas which have been formed on the nature of this system of vessels. It may be added that it is not at variance with what is observed in these vessels in the living body. It is found that the blood in a minute artery is not of the bright red colour which it possesses in the trunk and large branch from which the minute artery derives its blood, but is gradually acquiring the dark hue which belongs to the blood of the venous branches and trunks.

By some, again, this direct communication of minute arteries and veins is denied. Thus, according to Doellinger, the arteries at their last ramifications are devoid of proper membranous walls; the blood moves in immediate contact with the solid matter of the body, which is in truth the fundamental or penetrating filamentous tissue; and from this it passes into the venous tubes and lymphatics, which also arise from this substance.

According to Wilbrand, again, who equally denies this direct communication of arteries and veins, all the blood is converted into organic fibres and secretions; and these organic fibres becoming gradually fluid are converted into blood and lymph, which continue the circulation.

These notions are too fanciful and too incapable of demonstration to become the object of serious attention to the anatomist. It is of little moment whether the vessels in the ultimate ramifications possess tunics or not. When they cease to possess tunics they cease to be vessels; and to carry observation beyond this point is either impracticable or useless. In other respects the investigation of this point belongs to the subject of the exhalant vessels.

This idea is, however, adopted by Wedemeyer, who founds it chiefly on the fact, that he could not detect by the microscope any membrane interposed between the parenchyma of the tissues and the blood moving in the minuter capillaries, or rather furrows in which it is seen. It must be allowed that this idea receives some confirmation from a fact to be afterwards noticed, that during inflammation, new vessels are observed by the microscope to be formed in inflamed parts.

Bichat has described two great capillary systems in the human body. 1st, The general one, or that which consists of the minute terminations of the aortic divisions, and the origins of the superior and inferior great veins; and, 2d, The pulmonary capillary system, or that which consists of the minute terminations of the pulmonary artery, and the origins of the pulmonary veins. It is evident, that the manner in which the first of these systems is here repre-sented, communicates a very incorrect idea of its true character;

and that there is actually an individual capillary system, not only for every organ, but in some instances for every tissue. The brain possesses an individual capillary system; and that of the membranes is evidently distinct from that belonging to the organ itself. The heart and the kidneys possess each an individual capillary system; and the liver may be said to have two,—one formed by the communication of the hepatic artery and veins, and another consisting of the divisions of the portal vein, with the branches of the hepatic hollow vein. (*Vena cava hepatica.*)

The organic properties of the capillary vessels are as little known as their structure. Many physiological and pathological writers, especially experimentalists, have ascribed to them a power which has at different times been called muscular, tonic, irritable, contractile; and have asserted that, because the larger arteries are provided with a fibrous membrane, which they have called muscular, and to which they have ascribed irritability, or the power of contraction when stimulated, their minute or capillary termina tions must have the same property. This conclusion is completely unfounded for two reasons. 1*st*, I have already shown that the proper arterial tunic is not muscular in structure, and, according to the best experiments, possesses no property of contraction when stimulated. 2*d*, Although it be admitted that the proper arterial tissue is muscular and irritable, it is quite certain that observation has not hitherto shown that this tunic can be recognised in arteries smaller than a line in diameter ; and it is certain that in the capillaries, properly so called, that is, in vessels which partake of the nature of artery and vein, no such structure has yet been observed.

It is not improbable, however, that the capillaries possess certain organic or vital properties; but all that has been taught on this subject is either hypothetical, or derived from an insufficient and imperfect collection of facts. It is certain that the blood which moves through them is beyond the direct influence of the action of the heart, and can be affected by this only so far as it keeps the larger vessels constantly distended with a column of blood which cannot retrograde, and must therefore move forward in the only direction left to it. It has been therefore argued that the capillaries must have an inherent power of contraction by which this motion is favoured. Is it not sufficient to say that they act merely as resisting canals, to prevent their contents from escaping, and to minister to the various tissues and organs those supplies of blood which the several processes of nutrition, secretion, &c. require ?

The experiments of Wedemeyer and Dutrochet show that the capillary vessels are the seat of an action of intro-pulsion and extro-pulsion of fluids, (*endosmosis* and *exosmosis*,) or a force by which fluids may be impelled inwardly into them, or in the opposite direction without them.

The effects which the application of mechanical irritants, or chemical substances, as alcohol, acids, and alkalis, produced in the experiments of Hunter, Wilson Philip, Thomson, and Hastings, have been supposed to demonstrate the irritable nature of the capillary vessels. The conclusion is illegitimate, in so far as the results of these experiments are open to several sources of fallacy. In some instances these effects are to be ascribed to incipient inflammation, in others to shrivelling of the capillary structure, or crispation by chemical action, in others to actual coagulation of the blood of the capillaries; but none of them prove satisfactorily or precisely any peculiar properties in the vessels of which the capillary system is composed.

Section II.

The morbid deviations incident to the system of capillary vessels are of the utmost importance. As they are the main agents of most of the healthy processes of the animal body, so there are few morbid states, in which their operation is not primary, or in which they do not more or less partake. To enumerate these would form a long nosological list, since the diseases of every tissue depend chiefly, if not entirely, on its capillary system. It will be sufficient to consider the influence of the capillary vessels as an individual or *i*solated organic system in the production of morbid action.

1. *Inflammation.* The capillary vessels are believed to be the exclusive seat of the morbid process termed *inflammation*. No tissue, or no substance, rather, destitute of capillaries, is believed susceptible of this process; and its frequency and violence are justly estimated in proportion to the number of capillaries with which the tissue is supplied. Hair, nail, enamel of the tooth, and cuticle, do not undergo inflammation; and their morbid states are to be ascribed to disorder of the textures on which their existence and nutrition depend. Filamentous tissue, on the other hand, mucous and serous membrane, and the substance of such organs as the lung, liver, &c. are very liable to various forms of inflammatory action, which is generally proportional to the predominance of red

4

capillaries in the substance of each. Bichat has justly observed that inflammation is very frequent in the cutaneous, mucous, serous, and filamentous tissues, which injection and microscopic observation show to abound in capillary vessels, but rare in bone, cartilage, and the fibrous tissues in which there are few capillaries, or where the irritable or inflammatory susceptibility, (*la sensibilité organique,*) is more moderate. It is difficult to explain the infrequeney of inflammation in muscular tissue without having recourse to this last property, which this author ascribes to the capillary vessels. Its sensibility to the operation of a stimulus is great. Its susceptibility of inflammatory action is very small.

The change which takes place in the capillary vessels in the state of inflammation has given rise to much speculation, research, and experiment.

But it may be doubted whether the questions which have been agitated on this subject can yet be regarded as decided. On one point only is there any thing like agreement in the various opinions delivered. It appears to be now the general belief, that during the process of inflammation the capillary vessels of the part are dilated, and contain more blood than in the healthy state. (Cullen, Hunter, Vacca, and many other authors.) On the cause of this dilatation, however, the sentiments of pathologists are as much at variance as ever; and not only are the results of experiments made to determine the circumstances on which this distended state of the capillaries depends, variable and sometimes contradictory, but the conclusions to which they have led are very opposite. One opinion is, that the dilatation depends on increased action; according to the other, it is the effect of a weakened state of the capillaries.

The first of these doctrines, which in some form or other has been adopted from Stahl, and De Gorter, by Dr Cullen, appears to have been suggested by the increased number of the arterial pulse in a given space, the hardness and tension of its beat, the throbbing of inflamed parts, and the violent and sometimes rapid changes of structure which attend inflammation. This has led to the conclusion that the blood moves in the capillaries of such parts more rapidly, and with greater force, (*momentum,*) than in the healthy state. (Parry.) With superficial observers this opinion has passed current, as generally consonant with the phenomena and effects of the inflammatory process; and the pathologist has studied to render his notions palpable, by supposing, in the language of the mathematical physicians, an inordinate flow, *morbid afflux*, or *increased determination* of blood to the inflamed parts. Had this opinion ever been subjected to rigid scrutiny, its fallacy must have been manifest.

1*st*, The fact of increased determination is not established. In its present state it is a mere assumption. 2*d*, Increased determination is not necessary to the production of the effect. When the capillaries of any part are unusually loaded, this may take place from the blood not being removed with the same regularity, and in the same proportion in which it is conveyed, with the same facility. as by supposing an increased current. 3*d*, Even admitting the current to be increased through any set of capillaries, it is impossible to discover the agents of such a process. It is clear it cannot be the heart. And to suppose the capillaries capable of this, is to ascribe to them a power which they have not been proved, in ordinary circumstances, to possess.

Against the hypothesis of increased force and increased velocity of circulation, various arguments may be urged ; and several of these depend on the circumstance, that this hypothesis also has been assumed on very insufficient grounds. 1*st*, The increased number of the arterial pulse does not demonstrate that the blood is moving more rapidly than in the ordinary circumstances of health. It merely shows that the heart contracts more frequently in a given time than usual. 2*d*, The increased number, or strength, or tension of the arterial pulse does not indicate that the blood is moving with greater force, or that the arteries through which it is moving are acting with greater power, but rather that the heart is contracting much more frequently in order to overcome some obstacle. 3*d*, It does not appear that the increased number or force of the pulse, as manifested by the contractions of the heart, depends on any other cause, than the vital irritation occasioned by a local stimulus of a morbid nature. 4*th*, The throbbing of inflamed parts proves nothing more, than that the shock communicated from the heart along the arterial tubes is rendered more sensible, first, by their dilated and distended condition ; and, secondly, by the greater quantity of matter deposited in and around these vessels. (Parry.)

On the other hand, it appears to me certain that, from what we see by the microscope in the vessels of cold-blooded animals, as the frog, fish, &c. the blood moves most rapidly in the healthy state; and when it moves slowly, or is retarded, and stops or retrogrades, as is occasionally seen, this is unnatural, and if continued for any time constitutes a morbid state. This is further confirmed by the results of the experiments made by Kaltenbrunner, who ascertained that in inflammation and similar morbid states, the blood not only moved more slowly, but formed what he called *stases*, or points of immobility and stagnation.

The second doctrine, that the distended or dilated state of the capillaries is to be ascribed to weakness or debility in their coats, appears to be more consonant with the usual phenomena of the process, and with the effects which it produces in the different tissues. But although much has been lately done by Wilson Philip, Hastings, and others, to determine this point, it is still beset with some difficulties and objections, and would perhaps require some variation in the experiments, in order to place the subject in the clearest light. This hypothesis first originated with Vacca Berlinghieri, and was supported in this country by Lubbock, Allen, Reeve, Thomson, Wilson Philip, and subsequently by Hastings and Black, and receives some confirmation from the experiments of Kaltenbrunner, who has given the most complete set of observations on this subject. This author regards congestion as a preliminary stage of inflammation, and he therefore considers in connection the phenomena presented by both.

Congestion he considers as a process increasing from an initial point; proceeding to a certain degree of development; and abating and disappearing. In the first stage the following is the state. The congestion accumulated to one point is thence extended to the circumference. Thither the blood flows; its motion is quickened; the walls of the vessels are tense; the globules of arterial blood are no longer changed into venous; they are altered; the parenchyma is swelled.

This state of the vessels takes place at the same time in all points of the organ which is the seat of congestion. Not only is the circulation of the blood altered. The blood itself, the *parenchyma*, and the arterial walls partake in the common affection. The normal functions of the organ are impeded; the formation and absorption of lymph are in general interrupted.

The affection advances to different degrees of intensity according to the nature and severity of the lesion by which it is produced. The afflux of blood is more or less abundant; its motion more or

less accelerated; the vascular walls, especially the arterial, are more
or less tense; the blood is variously altered; the extent of the process varies; in certain cases it is directly proportional to its intensity, and in others it is not.

The extent of congestions is usually limited; and their development is completed within a short time.

When congestion has attained a certain point, it remains stationary. It then attains the second stage.

This is not distinguished by any new phenomenon. The phenomena of congestion are already established; and those that are
essential are, afflux of blood to one point; acceleration in the movement of the blood; extension of the process little beyond its initial
point; the functions of the organ embarrassed; swelling of the
parenchyma; and alteration in the globules.

This condition must not be confounded with certain derangements in the circulation which imitate some of the phenomena of
congestion. These derangements are irregular and proceed from
the local action of any irritant, the effect of which is slight and
temporary. Sometimes, however, these derangements are followed by congestion; and this is when these irritant agents act more
intensely and for a longer time.

The development of true congestion is a successive process, and
takes place only when the immediate action of the irritant cause
has ceased to act on the organ.

When congestion has lasted some time it decreases and terminates in the following manner.

The amount of blood and the velocity of its movement begin to
diminish at the circumference; the blood seeming to flow from this
region towards this centre. The blood during the course furnishes
an exhalation of fluid, which takes place in jets through the capillary vessels, and in general at the surface of the organ. The moment of the exhalation of the liquid is transitory; but it is often
repeated at different points until the congestion disappears. It is
critical, because the congestion subsides in proportion as it is repeated and proceeds. The quality of the secreted matter varies
according to the nature of the affection. It is often bloody, especially in the lower animals. The products of critical exhalation
may always be easily seen. They consist of small red patches dispersed through the parenchyma. In some instances serous fluid is
discharged through the blood-vessels; and in this case the liquid
being transparent is not so easily observed.

It is evident, that, in the phenomena now ascribed to congestion, many would be disposed to see the early stage of inflammation. This, however, Kaltenbrunner distinguishes as a process of greater intensity, with more varied phenomena, and more complex, and presenting greater modifications. The difference, nevertheless, seems more in degree and stage than in any other circumstance, and in the effects which it is liable to produce on the tissues which it affects.

Inflammation like congestion has a period of increase, of establishment, and one of decline, often with destructive effects.

In the period of increase, the phenomena agree in general with those of congestion. The movement of the blood is quickened ; the vessels are distended ; the blood is altered. After this, however, other changes are observed. The blood begins to move less quickly in some capillary vessels, and at length stops completely. Thus are formed in the system of diseased vessels *stases*, statical or stagnating points, which increasing occupy a large space round the part where the cause of inflammation is seated. (An eschar produced by the hot iron.) At the circumference of these statical points the circulation proceeds rapidly. Thus inflammation is established. The same phenomena appear on the application of muriate of soda, alcohol, sal-ammoniac, or corrosive sublimate.

The *stases* are formed in the following manner. At the commencement of inflammation the blood traverses all the vessels with great velocity. Soon, however, its movement becomes slower at first in certain capillaries, situate on the central point of inflammatory action. Then the circulation is disturbed ; its motion becomes unsteady ; the blood seems to oscillate irregularly in the canals ; lastly, its movement is entirely stopped ; and the blood stagnates in different points. These stagnating points progressively increase, and affect even the smaller veins ; but they rarely take place in the arteries.

The blood never stagnates in the canals so as to fill them entirely. It is accumulated in certain points so as to leave void part of the canals. Those in which the blood stagnates are relaxed.

The stagnating points are so much more diffused and dispersed, and occupy a space more extensive, as the inflammation is more severe and has been of longer duration. Their presence is evinced by the redness of the part on which they are situate, which is more intense on the initial point than on the circumference. The inflammatory redness is livid when the inflammation is intense, and the statical points are dispersed and diffused.

The first change which the blood undergoes in an inflamed part is, that it is not converted into venous blood. Next to this the coagulability is increased, so that the globules coalescing form minute clots. Then the globules forming these clots are decomposed; for they are surrounded by serous liquid which exudes from them.

The colour of the blood is in like manner altered. When muriate of soda is used, it gives the blood a purple tint; the use of alcohol imparts a clear colour; that of corrosive sublimate a dull brown colour.

Kaltenbrunner further maintains, that often in the course of the phenomena of inflammation has he observed the formation of new vessels or canals in an inflamed organ. The globules of blood are observed to spring all at once from some capillary canal, to fall into the surrounding parenchyma, pave a path for themselves, and by this reach another canal.* This seems to confirm the idea of Doellinger and Wedemeyer, already mentioned, (P. 134.)

These form the principal phenomena of inflammation in its increasing and to its established periods. After that the phenomena observed relate to an advanced stage, which has been usually considered as that of effects. To these, therefore, I shall revert subsequently.

Upon the whole, two facts may be considered to be established regarding the state of the capillary vessels of an inflamed part. The *first* is, that these vessels are unnaturally and unusually distended, and really contain more blood than in the state of health. This is proved not only by incisions into inflamed parts, but by dissections of every part and organ of the body. The *second* is, that the blood moves more slowly in these vessels than in the healthy state, and even after some time may remain entirely motionless. This is also established by observing the effects of inflammation in the human body, but especially by the phenomena of inflammation excited artificially in the bodies of the lower animals.

It is still a point to be ascertained, whether these two conditions

---

* Experimenta circa statum sanguinis et vasorum in Inflammatione. Auctore Doctore Georgio Kaltenbrunner Monachil, 1826.

Recherches Experimentales sur l'Inflammation, par M. G. Kaltenbrunner, Docteur en Medecine. Breschet Repertoire General d'Anatomie, et de Physiologie Pathologiques, &c. Tome ivtrieme, p. 201. Paris, 1827.

constitute what may be termed the essence of inflammation; and it is still undetermined by what agency these states are induced in the capillary system of any tissue or organ. On this head it may be remarked, that, if by any means the natural velocity with which the blood moves through any set of capillaries be diminished, and continue so, the quantity of blood in these vessels must be gradually and steadily increased, until it becomes very considerable. This appears to be one cause of the accumulation of blood in any part which is in the state of inflammation.

2. *Temporary dilatation of the capillaries not inflammatory.* The capillary vessels undergo a temporary dilatation during the progress of aneurism, whether allowed to go on naturally, or after the application of the ligature to the arterial trunk. When the collateral circulation has been fully established by the enlargement of the anastomosing branches, the capillary system shrinks to its ordinary size.

3. *Extravasation.* When the capillary vessels of any part have been injured, so as to burst or give way, the blood which they contained is effused round them, and into the cellular or other structure of the part, occasioning sometimes considerable swelling, and, if near the surface, a red, blue, or yellowish colour. In such circumstances the blood is said to be *extravasated*, and the change of colour is termed *ecchymosis*.

4. *Mode of repair; union by adhesion and granulation.* When they are divided by simple incision, they pour out first blood, then serous or colourless fluids, lastly, a semifluid, which undergoes coagulation, and which forms the uniting medium of the divided surfaces, (*liquor sanguinis*, or blood-plasma.) This is the *radical moisture* of the older physiologists; (Taliacotius, Ambrose Paré, Phioravant, &c.); *the balsam of Nature,* or *agglutinative balsam* of Wiseman,* the *gluten* of Sauvages, Gaubius, and Cullen, the

---

* " But in regard there is a certain *medium* which answers in proportion to a glue, required in this work, Nature taketh what is next in hand, even the nourishment of the part which is hurt to make it of. *Ubi morbus ibi remedium* is here as an oracle ; where the disease is, there is the remedy. No sooner is the wound made but the balsam is discovered. Blood, at least the serous part of it, is the glue, which she useth both in curing by the first and second intention. The first being performed *per symphysin, i. e.* a reunion of the parts without any medium, by which word I here mean any *callus* or flesh, or other body interposed ; for in another sense the balsam of Nature is the *medium*, the instrument of unity, and puts the parts together ; the second *per cys sarcosin, i. e.* with a medium or interposition of some flesh or callous substance, that

coagulating or *organizable lymph* of Hunter, and the *glutinous or albuminous exudation* of the French pathologists.

According to the observations of Hunter, Baillie, and Home, this lymph is afterwards penetrated with minute arteries and veins, or acquires a capillary system of its own; and in this state it is properly *organized lymph*. This process of formation of new capillaries occurs in every situation in which lymph is deposited; 1*st*, In the exudation of inflamed serous membranes, which afterwards forms the membrane of adhesions; 2*d*, In wounds of skin, cellular membrane, mucous membrane, muscle, &c.; 3*d*, In inflammation of these tissues, whether occurring spontaneously, in consequence of bruise or laceration, or the introduction of foreign bodies. In each of these cases, though suppuration should also take place, still there is lymph effused, and this lymph is penetrated by newly formed capillaries. This formation of new capillaries is termed by the French pathologists, *accidental development of the capillary system*. Is it lymph of a peculiar kind that is effused from the capillaries of fractured bones in the first stage of the process of reunion? The substance named *callus* is not cartilage, as was anciently supposed, and possesses qualities not unlike those of the lymph of soft tissues. Is ʻlymph effused from the fragments of a broken cartilage, or a ruptured tendon? In each of these cases of injury, a soft homogeneous fluid, pale red or bluish, is effused immediately or soon after the injury; and in each it seems to possess the same qualities, and only in the course of the process of reunion to be afterwards penetrated by the peculiar matter of the tissue injured. A preliminary step to this penetration of proper substance is uniformly the formation of new capillary arteries and veins.

In those examples of spontaneous disease or injury in which suppuration takes place, the capillaries in depositing lymph are concerned in another process, the formation of red eminences, hemispherical or hemispheroidal, of various size, and varying in firmness or consistence. This process has been termed *granulation*, a name which has been also improperly given the individual bodies. The simplest, and perhaps the most correct view of this process, shows that it consists of three distinct stages, which it is important for the pathologist to know.

fills up the space between the lips of the wound."—Chirurgical Treatises by Richard Wiseman, Sergeant-Surgeon, Book v. Chap. 1. Of Wounds.

a. The first of these consists in effusion of lymph, or rather sero-albuminous fluid or *liquor sanguinis*, from capillary arteries in the liquid form, and which speedily undergoing coagulation as it exudes, is converted into irregular globules or masses. The extent to which this exudation takes place will depend on the extent of the surface and the degree of inflammation ; and the same principles will regulate the appearance of the globules or masses of lymph in the different points of the granulating surface.

b. After these globules have been effused and coagulated, they are soon penetrated with vessels which, according to Hunter, may be justly esteemed mere prolongations of the capillaries which originally secreted the lymph. This penetration of vessels constitutes what may be considered the second stage of granulation. This process, which must have been observed by many practical surgeons, has been clearly and correctly described by Hunter. " I have often," says he, " been able to trace the growth and vascularity of this new substance. I have seen on a sore a white substance exactly similar to coagulating lymph. I have not attempted to wipe it off, and the next day of dressing I have found this very substance vascular ; for by wiping or touching it with a probe it has bled freely." And, again, " The vessels of granulations pass from the original parts, whatever these are, to the basis of the granulations, from thence toward their external surface, in pretty regular parallel lines, and would almost appear to terminate there."* At the same time the formation or secretion of purulent fluid goes on ; and the surfaces of these bodies themselves acquire the same power of preparing this fluid which the surface from which the granulations were produced, possessed. In this instance we have an example of capillary vessels performing at the same time the effusion of lymph and the secretion of purulent fluid.

In this stage of the process of granulation, Mr Hunter has remarked the disposition to union, ohesion, or adhesion, which granulating eminences possess, and described the mechanism by which this is accomplished. By many it might be deemed a distinct process. But in so far as the capillaries are concerned, the chief object of consideration at present, it is to be viewed as a part of the second stage. The vessels of the granulating eminences continue to secrete lymph, which unites the corresponding surfaces of their new bodies till their capillaries pass into each other, so as to inosculate, and the union is completed.

* II. p. 477.

K

c. The third stage in the process of granulation consists in what he has termed *contraction.* In describing this important part, I fear he has committed two errors—one in looking at the whole granulating surface and contiguous parts, rather than at the individual bodies; the other in ascribing contraction to the elasticity and muscular action of the contiguous parts rather than to a change in the state of the granulations. These circumstances are certainly useful accessory means; but they must not be regarded as the primary and essential cause. Perhaps also some slight differences take place in the time in which contraction occurs, and the extent to which it proceeds, according to the nature of the granulating surface, and the relation which the production of the granulating eminences bears to the part to be restored. The general phenomena of the process appear to be the following.

After the granulating eminence or eminences have been formed, and have united with the contiguous ones, the uninterrupted action of their new capillaries continues to effuse lymph as a basis for fresh granulations, and to give out vascular or capillary prolongations, in order to organize them. Meanwhile the vessels of the granulating eminences near the edges of the surface begin to diminish in size; and as they diminish the eminences themselves become less red and smaller, but more firm. At length, as the eminences become covered with the membrane of cicatrization, they appear to have diminished so much, that little inequality can be recognised, the redness is sensibly diminished, and the whole appears as if it were becoming quite as solid or firm as the contiguous parts. If in this part of the process a granulating surface be injected, the vessels which go to the outer granulating eminences will be found to be, 1*st*, much less numerous; and, 2*d*, to be much diminished in size; and this change will be observed to be most remarkable at the edge, and less at the centre of the sore. It is this diminution in the number and size of the granulating capillaries which is the main agent of the process of contraction. As these vessels become less numerous and smaller, the bodies to which they are distributed diminish and become firmer; and if a wound or part which has been healed by granulation be injected some weeks or months after being healed, the vessels will be actually found less numerous and smaller than in the contiguous parts of the same tissue.

When union by granulation is accompanied with the formation

of a thin membrane, which afterwards assumes the appearance and properties of skin, the last part of the process is called *skinning* or *cicatrization*,—the formation of a scar. The nature and mechanism of this process will be considered in its proper place.

Granulation may be viewed as the means which the several tissues of the human body possess of reproducing themselves, or repairing those losses of substance which result from direct injury, or take place in consequence of disease. Of this process the capillaries of the texture are the agents. But it is uncertain to what extent they possess the power of reproducing the same sort of substance as that of the texture destroyed. The kind of matter which is most generally reproduced is filamentous or cellular tissue. It is certain also that bone is reproduced. But it is uncertain whether skin, that is true skin, muscle, tendon, or ligament, is reproduced, and almost certain that cartilage is not.

5. *Different effects of inflammation.* I have said that granulation is in general accompanied with the formation of more or less purulent matter. This process, which is termed suppuration, generally precedes that of granulation. It has been viewed at one time as a consequence or effect of inflammation, at another as a character of it, and at a third as a cause. The circumstances which justify these distinctions should be understood.

Inflammation is a progressive process, which tends through certain stages to a certain termination. Of the intermediate steps not much is known with certainty; and pathological writers have distinguished chiefly the different modes in which it may terminate. These are resolution, effusion, adhesion, suppuration, granulation, ulceration, cicatrization, induration, and gangrene. This division is more scholastic than natural. The first only can be justly denominated a termination. All the others are to be regarded as effects either immediate or remote of the process.

α. Resolution is that action in which the redness, pain, heat, and swelling of an inflamed part gradually disappear, either spontaneously or under the use of means, with or without sensible evacuation, and in which the part, which had been inflamed, resumes by degrees its natural state, without suffering derangement of structure or properties. This is exceedingly rare. The minute veins are doubtless the great agents of cure in such circumstances.

β. In most cases of inflammation more or less fluid is early effused or extravasated from the capillaries or the exhalants of the part.

No sooner do the vessels become overloaded with blood than part of it either entire, or in the form of serous fluid, is separated from the vessels. Thus in inflammation of filamentous tissue blood or serum may be poured into its interstitial spaces; and the effusion of the latter is one cause of œdematous and anasarcous infiltration. In inflammation of the serous membranes also we shall find that effusion of serous fluid is an early and frequent result.

When this effusion is moderate it may be removed under suitable management by the action of the veins and lymphatics; and in such circumstances this termination would still come under the head of resolution.

γ. In general, however, the fluid effused is of a more complicated nature. The natural tendency of the process of inflammation is to cause the vessels to secrete or exhale, or effuse a fluid which at once contains coagulable lymph and a thinner serum, which, at a later period, at least in the filamentous tissue, corresponds to sero-purulent or purulent fluid. The serum is not converted, as Cullen imagined, into purulent matter. But the same vessels which, at an early stage of the process, secrete serous fluid containing lymph, at a more advanced period secrete purulent matter. This is easily proved by tracing the progressive changes in a large wound; for instance an amputated stump, an incision made into an inflamed swelling, or an incision made on purpose into the soft parts of an animal. The same general conclusion results also from observing the progressive steps in the human body after a seton has been inserted, or an issue established. In the case of part of the surface being destroyed by caustic, actual or potential, the process may be less distinctly observed; but it is still nearly the same.

Upon the whole, the natural course of phenomena in inflammation may be stated in the following order. *First,* vessels dilated and distended with blood, which moves more slowly than natural. *Secondly,* the secretion or effusion from these vessels, or their exhalant terminations, of a fluid consisting of serum and coagulable matter, sometimes with extravasation of blood. *Thirdly,* the secretion of purulent fluid from the same vessels.

The intimate nature of the process by which purulent matter is formed is by no means well known. The notion of Grashuys,* that it arose from a liquefaction or melting of the adipose tissue,

---

* De Suppuratione.

though adopted by Haller,* is too ridiculous to merit the slightest attention. It is sufficient to remark, that purulent matter is prepared by many other tissues which contain no adipose matter; for instance the mucous and serous membranes, and several of the glandular organs, internal and external. The fallacy of the opinion of Cullen, which was derived from the experiments of Pringle and of Gaber, has been already noticed.

The view of Hunter is, on the whole, more correct. In inflammation of the filamentous tissue, where the parts, or more accurately, the vessels lose the power of resolution, they begin to "alter their mode of action, and continue changing till they gradually form themselves to that state which fits them" to prepare purulent matter. This applies, however, only to the case in which lymph is exuded and purulent matter is secreted, simultaneously or successively, or, in other words, to the transition from the adhesive to the suppurative stage. In certain circumstances this transition does not take place, and purulent fluid may be secreted without the previous effusion of coagulable lymph. The first action of the vessels is then to pour forth serous fluid, and the next is the secretion of purulent matter in a more or less perfect form. This is well exemplified in diffuse inflammation of the filamentous tissue.

No doubt can be entertained, from the experiments of Brugmann,† Hunter,‡ and Home,§ and from the daily phenomena of purulent collections, that suppuration is a process analogous to, if not the same as secretion. ‖

This is demonstrated in the case of mucous and serous membranes, in which purulent matter is formed without breach of surface, and in which, therefore, its formation must be ascribed to a new action of the vessels. It does not, however, follow from this that these vessels perform, as Hunter imagined, the office of a gland. This notion appears to be adopted merely to render the conception of suppuration more distinct than-it would be if simply ascribed to the action of vessels.

Suppuration is the direct and exclusive, or the concurrent effect of inflammation. It is generally the direct effect in inflammation of the mucous membranes, often in that of the serous membranes,

* Elementa, Lib. i. sect. 4.   † De Puogenia. 8vo. Groningæ, 1781.
‡ Treatise on the Blood, Inflammation, &c. Chap. v.
§ On the Properties of Pus. 4to. London, 1788.
‖ " This new structure or disposition of vessels I shall call glandular, and the effect or pus a secretion." Chap. v.

and it is so in diffuse inflammation of the filamentous tissue. In circumscribed inflammation in the filamentous tissue, in inflammation of the skin, and occasionally in inflammation of the serous membranes, it is preceded by exudation of coagulable lymph, and is either concurrent or successive to it.

Suppuration is represented by Hunter as always preparatory to granulation. This, however, must be understood to apply to suppuration of cellular tissue, and those textures of which it makes part. In mucous and serous membranes suppuration may, and almost invariably does, take place without granulation. I shall afterwards have occasion to mention another sort of purulent collections, in which granulation never occurs.

Suppuration varies according to the nature of the inflammatory process which it succeeds, and according to the texture in which it takes place.

As inflammation varies according to the nature of the texture in which it takes place, so its effects are different in the different organic textures. The purulent matter formed on the skin differs from that which flows from an abscess of the cellular tissue. That secreted by mucous membranes is different from either ; and even the purulent fluid of serous membranes possesses certain characters by which a careful observer may distinguish it from the same fluid in other situations.

The suppurating process may be varied according to the nature of the inflammation by which it is preceded. A sound principle laid down by John Hunter was to regard every form of suppuration as the result of inflammation. From this, however, he departed in his views of the nature of suppurations of lymphatic glands, of diseased joints, of lumbar abscesses, and of the cold or chronic abscess in general. * It is easy to show, that, with the single ex-

---

* Many indolent tumours, slow swellings in the joints, swellings of the lymphatic glands, tubercles in the lungs, and swellings in many parts of the body, are diseased thickenings, without visible inflammation. And the contents of some kinds of encysted tumour ; the matter of many scrofulous suppurations, as in lymphatic glands ; the suppuration of many joints, viz. those scrofulous suppurations in the joints of the foot and hand, in the knee, called white swellings ; in the joint of the thigh, commonly called hip-cases ; in the loins, called lumbar abscesses ; the discharge of the above-mentioned tubercles in the lungs, as well as in many other parts of the body, are all matter formed without any previous visible inflammation, and are therefore in this one respect all very similar to one another. They come on insensibly, the first symptom being commonly the swellings, in consequence of the thickening, which is not the case with inflammation ; for there the sensation is the first symptom."—Treatise, Chap. iv. IV. p. 391.

ception of pulmonary tubercles, in every one of the instances which he has adduced the formation of fluid matter, is invariably preceded by inflammation, that is, by morbid enlargement of the capillaries of the affected texture.

In the case of lymphatic glands suppurating, these bodies invariably enlarge previously, and are always the seat of dull heavy pain. This enlargement depends either on the vessels undergoing a slow process of dilatation and distension, or on the formation of tubercles in the substance of the gland.

The affections of the knee-joint, hip-joint, and other articulations, have been satisfactorily traced to inflammation either of the synovial apparatus, or of the cartilages, or of both, passing on the one hand to the capsule, and on the other to the bones. During life they are painful, generally swelled or enlarged, and invariably hotter than natural. Dissection shows these parts to be more or less, sometimes highly, vascular.

The collections denominated *lumbar abscess* depend either on disease of the vertebræ, generally of an inflammatory nature, or on slow inflammation of the lumbar cellular tissue and lymphatic glands.

The circumstance in which Mr Hunter trusted, in considering these collections to be independent of inflammation, was the absence of pain as the first symptom. In this, however, I believe that accurate observer was mistaken. In every one of the cases of disease to which he refers as examples, more or less pain is invariably felt in the course, if not from the first date of the complaints. Two circumstances, indeed, distinguish this sort of pain. It is neither severe nor uninterrupted, and may be so moderate as not to attract the attention of the patient, or form a serious subject of complaint. But even admitting the statement of Mr Hunter, that the sensation of pain is not the first, it is doubtless too limited a view of the inflammatory process to imagine, that this can never exist unless when the sensation of pain is the first symptom. In some of the textures, especially mucous membrane, we know that inflammation may be established for some time without much attendant pain. In others, especially the serous membranes, inflammation approaches so slowly and imperceptibly, that both lymph and purulent matter may be effused before the existence of the disease is suspected.

For these and similar reasons it has become requisite to admit the existence of a slow insidious form of inflammation termed *chronic,* corresponding to the inflammation *by congestion* of Paré, Hildanus, Wiseman, and the older surgeons, and causing the *cold abscess* to which I had occasion formerly to allude. But, with the exception of its being attended with little or no pain, and proceeding much more slowly than acute inflammation, little is known regarding the anatomical and pathological characters of this form of the process. From several circumstances it might be inferred that the capillaries begin to assume the suppurative action, at least in filamentous tissue, more readily than in the case of acute inflammation. In other parts chronic inflammation may exist without terminating in the suppurative process.

In cases in which the acute seems to be combined with the chronic, so as to form an intermediate or mixed variety of disease, it has been distinguished by the name of *subacute* inflammation.

Under certain circumstances chronic inflammation may terminate in the acute. Thus an abscess in the cavity of a joint, either by distension or by propagation of action, may induce inflammation in the subcutaneous cellular tissue and in the skin. When a chronic abscess is opened, its whole interior surface is attacked with acute inflammation; and when a lumbar abscess is opened, or is allowed to burst, the same effect results. By carefully excluding the air, indeed, and healing up the wound according to the manner of Mr Abernethy, the severity of this inflammation may be much mitigated; but it always takes place, and sooner or later becomes general and severe. In this sense only can suppuration be said to cause inflammation. But the proper view of the relation of these two processes is, that chronic inflammation may cause the acute form by the capillaries assuming a new mode of action, or by propagating the irritation to those of a new texture. In circumstances of this description, suppuration is in general without granulation or attempt at repair.

δ. Suppuration may be either without attempt at repair, or with absolute destruction of texture; and it is then distinguished as *ulceration*, or the formation of an ulcer. Since the time of Hunter, who gave the first clear idea of this process, ulceration has been generally understood to consist in *absorption with suppuration*. This notion is perhaps more hypothetical than the old one of breach of surface or loss of substance, which simply expressed the fact without reference to its supposed cause. But as loss of substance implies the absorption or resumption of part of the animal texture, and as this must be understood to be effected by the vessels of the part, the chief objection with which this opinion can be charged, is, that not only the lymphatics, but the minute veins must be concerned in the process of resumption.

I do not propose here to consider all the various forms of ulceration, or the circumstances under which it may take place. But I shall mention a few by way of example.

Ulceration occurs in the skin in consequence of inflammation from injury, as wound, tear, burn, &c., death of a part occasioned either by mortification, or by the cautery, actual or potential, or the application of a morbid poison.

Ulceration occurs in the mucous membranes under the same circumstances as in the skin, and also after spontaneous inflammation, that is, inflammation coming on without manifest cause.

Ulceration occurs in the cellular tissue in consequence of the pressure and progressive advancement of a large abscess, in consequence of the presence of foreign bodies, as bullets, sword-points, pins, &c.; or the sharp end of a bone.

Ulceration is not common in serous membranes. In these, however, it takes place in consequence of the continued pressure of large collections of matter. This is seen in empyema and collections of purulent matter in the peritonæum.

Ulceration occurs in bone either spontaneously, or in consequence of the death of part of it. The former is seen in caries, the latter in necrosis and exfoliation.

Ulceration occurs in cartilage in consequence of inflammation. This is seen in diseases of the knee-joint and hip-joint.

In all cases of ulceration, the capillaries of the parts are larger and more numerous than natural, and certainly contain more blood than in the state of health. This is seen very well in the case of ulcers of the cornea, which are invariably surrounded by an annular net-work of small vessels, which in the sound state of that texture are invisible. In the skin it is very well established by incisions made in the treatment of boil and carbuncle. In both cases, if the incision be carried through either tumour, much more blood is discharged from the point where ulceration is established than at any other part. The same fact is demonstrated by the appearance of ulcerated patches of the intestinal mucous membrane.

In the process of ulceration it is generally possible to trace a final intention or definite purpose, after the accomplishment of which it ceases spontaneously. It takes place under circumstances in which it is requisite to remove some part of a texture which is either unsound, or has become foreign to the system, as in the case of dead bones, mortified sloughs, or to procure an outlet for some morbid fluid, as is seen in deep purulent collections, or to expel a foreign body from a situation in which its presence is injurious. Hence it has been justly remarked by Hunter, that every process of ulceration is preceded by adhesive inflammation at one or more points, sometimes round the whole line along which the ulcerating process takes place.   The object of this is to prevent hemorrhage by the closure of vessels, and to prevent the diffusion of purulent fluid in situations where its presence would be injurious.   In several situations, however, it fails to accomplish this purpose.

When the ulcerative process has effected the object for which it was commenced, a new mode of action takes place.   The vessels begin to deposit lymph in rounded masses, which become vascular, and all the phenomena of granulation succeed.   In such circumstances, are we to suppose that the absorbing process has given way to that of deposition,—the action of veins and lymphatics to that of minute arteries?

In certain situations, this process of deposition may be observed going on in one part of a sore, while that of removal, destruction, or absorption is proceeding in another.   Thus in an eschar occasioned by a burn, or by cautery, actual or potential, while the process of ulceration is detaching the margin of the slough, a crop of granulations may be observed rising with equal rapidity and steadiness, and pushing off, as it were, the dead substance.   The phenomena of these and similar processes present objections to the theory of Hunter.

ε. Softening (*Malacismus ; Enallaxis ; Sphacelismus ;*) or preternatural diminution of consistence, is an effect of inflammation, which in different tissues is liable to ensue.   The tissues in which it is most frequent are the brain, spinal chord or nerves, the lungs, the uterus, and the bones.   It consists in the more or less complete separation of the component atoms of these tissues, whether fibrous, globular, or amorphous, by the destruction or dissolution of their filamentous tissue, and occasionally, if not constantly, with the substitution of serous, sero-albuminous, sero-sanguine, or sero-purulent fluid.   The characteristic organization of the tissue is, indeed, more or less completely destroyed.   Its elasticity and tenacity are destroyed; and it is rendered lacerable. In certain tissues, especially that of the lungs, and perhaps that of the brain occasionally, softening is analogous to mortification of other tissues. In the brain, however, it is most usually analogous to suppuration.

One variety of softening is often observed in parts or new structures, originally hard, and consists not so much in the process now mentioned, as in the slow solution or liquefaction of the tissue or substance, partly by disruption of its particles, partly by death of their individual atoms, with the admixture of blood, serous or seropurulent fluid. This softening, which takes place in encysted tumours, tyromatous or scirrhous tubercles, and in most of the adventitious tissues, is a spurious variety of suppuration.

ζ. Induration (*Scleroma*, V erhartung), or preternatural firmness, is a usual concomitant and effect of the process of inflammation. The process rarely, indeed, exists for a few hours or days in any tissue without rendering it considerably harder and more resisting than natural. In the external parts of the body this is seen in inflammation of the skin and filamentous tissue, in which the inflamed parts are much harder and firmer than natural; and every inflammation of the filamentous tissue is accompanied with hardness more or less extensive. This hardness, which is also accompanied with swelling and enlargement, depends partly on the excessive distension of vessels by blood, and partly on the effusion of sero-albuminous fluid.

The latter circumstance explains the presence of induration as a consequence of the inflammatory process. The sero-albuminous fluid, though first,, when effused, liquid, and homogeneous, is speedily separated by virtue of its property of spontaneous coagulation into two parts,—the serous, liquid, or non-coagulable, and the albuminous, consistent, or coagulable. The former is the cause of the œdematous swelling already mentioned as often accompanying inflammation, and, after remaining for some time in the interstices of the filamentous tissue of the part, may be removed by the absorbent property of the capillaries and minute veins. The latter, in the form of minute amorphous masses, disposed between the filamentous fibres, or the component atoms of the tissue, augments its volume, and the space which it occupies, agglutinates contiguous parts, and, eventually contracting and becoming consolidated, increases much the natural consistence and density of the tissue in which it has been deposited. In this manner induration takes place in the subcutaneous and intermuscular cellular tissue after an abscess, in the female breast or male *testis,* and the liver of both sexes, after inflammation, and in the pulmonic tissue after an attack of peripneumony. In the glands now mentioned, and even in the prostate gland, inflammatory induration has been repeatedly mistaken for scirrhous induration. This error the accurate pathologist will avoid. Inflammatory induration occasionally disappears, and is never attended with acute pain. Scirrhous induration never disappears, but proceeds to disorganizing softening, and atomical mortification, and is always attended with stinging darting pain, and flushes of burning heat.

Along with the state of induration, the textures are often rendered brittle and lacerable. This is seen in the arteries, the tendons, and the bones.

η. *Gangrene or Mortification.* This is much less frequent than has been supposed. It may occur in the skin, in mucous membranes, in fibrous structures, especially tendons, in bone, in cartilage, and in the substance of the lungs. In dry gangrene, (*necrosis, ustilago, mal des ardens,*) which is the most perfect specimen of the death of parts. It affects skin, cellular membrane, muscle, tendon, ligament, artery, vein, periosteum, bone, and cartilage indiscriminately and generally. Its anatomical character consists in coagulation of the blood in the vessels, always the capillary, sometimes the larger branches. But whether this be the cause or the effect of the death of the parts is uncertain. A fact formerly mentioned regarding the influence of ossification of the arteries in producing gangrene of the toes, feet, and legs in old persons would seem to show that it is the cause. The phenomena of the dry gangrene, or that produced by spurred rye and bad food, on the other hand, might favour the notion, that coagulation of blood is the effect. The gangrene produced by tight ligature, and in the case of tumours, may be referred to either head.

6. *Fever.* In this disease, whatever be its form, intermittent, remittent, or continued, the capillary vessels are the principal seat of disorder. Nor is the affection confined to the capillaries of one region, of one organ, or of one tissue. The seat of fever is to be sought neither in the capillaries of the brain and spinal chord, nor in those of the lungs, nor in those of the alimentary canal, but it is diffused over the minute ramifying communications of the aortic

and venous branches in whatever part of the body these communications are found.   To establish the truth of this statement, it is requisite merely to consider the phenomena of fever in the living body, and its traces and effects in the dead.

a. I presume that the affection of the capillary system of the brain, both cranial and vertebral, is too generally admitted to require being formally demonstrated.   In point of fact, the pain of the head in the beginning of all fevers, the derangement of thought during their progress, and the tendency to stupor, and absolute coma towards the conclusion, are sufficient alone to prove disorder of the cerebral capillaries.   But when blood or serous fluid is found effused into the ventricles, when the vessels of the brain are found turgid, distended with blood, and more numerous than natural, it is impossible to resist the inference as to the overloaded state of the cerebral capillaries during life.   I am aware that cases of fever are sometimes adduced, in which neither pain of the head nor deranged thought are observed.   I can only say, that, among a very great number of cases which I have observed, though in a few the patient did not complain of headach, it was always possible to recognize more or less derangement of thought.

In all cases, pain is felt when the patient coughs or stoops, or when the head is slightly shaken, and when no pain is said to be felt, it indicates that the stage of natural sensation is passed, and that he complains not, because he does not feel.

In ague, the oppression of the cerebral capillaries may be so great as to constitute inflammation (*Siriasis Ægyptiaca,*) or phrenitic ague, or in various degrees the sleepy quotidian, the sleepy, lethargic, hemiplegic, carotic, and apoplectic tertian, and the comatose quartan of practical authors, (Werlhof, Torti, Lautter, Morton, Sydenham, &c. ;) the same disease which has been named by Lancisi, Baglivi, and Morgagni, epidemic apoplexy. (*Apoplexia febricosa, Carus febricosus.*)

The disorder of the capillaries of the spinal chord is indicated by pain and weight in various parts of the column, by the derangement in the muscular motions, especially local palsy, *e. g.* of the arms, legs, &c. by the tetanic spasms and convulsions taking place in many fevers.   After death, much serous fluid flows from the *theca ;* the vessels of the chord are distended and numerous ; in all instances, serous fluid is effused, and sometimes pure blood issues from its capillaries.

β. That the capillary system of the lungs is overloaded and oppressed in all fevers, is one of the most certain points in pathology. During the ague fit, the respiration is invariably quicker than natural, sometimes to the amount of thirty or thirty-six in the minute; the patient complains of a sense of weight in the breast, cannot breathe fully, pants, and has frequent cough. In continued fever, the respiration is invariably quicker and more laborious than natural, a deep breath cannot be drawn easily, and more or less sense of oppression and weight is felt. I have found the respiration in continued fever so quick as thirty-six in the minute, while, in ordinary cases, the application of the stethoscope indicates an embarrassed state of the circulation in the pulmonary capillaries. In persons predisposed, expectoration streaked with blood, (*hæmoptoe,*) is not unfrequent during continued fever.

The same conclusion is clearly established by examination of the lungs of persons cut off either by intermittent or by continued fever. In many instances of the former it induces bronchial inflammation, or proceeds to actual peripneumony or pleurisy, constituting the catarrhal, pneumonic, or pleuritic tertian respectively. (Werlhof, Torti, Lancisi, &c.) In the latter, the bronchial mucous membrane is always more or less red, sometimes crimson or purple, or of a deep brown colour, rough, and much thickened; the submucous tissue is brown and loaded with serous fluid; and the minute vessels are much distended with dark-coloured blood. The bronchial tubes are very commonly, in fatal cases, perfectly filled with thick viscid mucus, which adheres to the inner surface of the bronchial membrane. The serous surface of the organ is generally livid or marbled from this cause; but the pleura itself is not much changed, save from bloody serum discharged into its cavity. The lungs in totality are generally dense, and firmer than in the natural state.

These changes arise from the minute ramifying vessels at the termination of the pulmonary artery, and the origins of the pulmonary veins being unusually loaded with blood. As they are more so than can be readily affected by the ordinary quantity of air admissible in such a state, imperfect respiration and undue change of venous blood contributes powerfully to the bad symptoms and the unfavourable termination of the disease. In such a state of the organs of respiration the bronchial arteries are less able to counteract the bad effects of imperfectly respired blood, in so far as they

3

receive from the aorta, blood which has not been sufficiently arterialized.

γ. In the capillary system of the chylopoietic and assistant chylopoietic viscera traces of the same condition may be recognized, both from the symptoms during life and the appearances after death. In these organs two capillary systems may be distinguished, a primary and a secondary one. The primary is that which consists of the ultimate divisions of the splenic, gastric, and duodenal arteries, and of the superior and inferior mesenteric arteries, and their corresponding veins, which afterwards terminate in the splenic and superior and inferior mesenteric veins. The secondary capillary system is that which results from the union of the minute extremities of the portal vein, and of the hepatic artery with those of the *venæ cavæ hepaticæ.*

It is unnecessary to dwell on the proofs of the loaded state of the capillary system of the alimentary canal. It is sufficient to remind the student that the furred or brown tongue, the thirst, the sense of internal heat, the loathing, squeamishness, and sometimes sickness, with weight, oppression, and tenderness of the epigastric region, sufficiently demonstrate the morbid state of the capillaries of the œsophagus, stomach, and duodenum ; while the constipation of the bowels at the commencement, insensibility to cathartic medicine throughout, and occasional looseness at the conclusion, indicate the deranged condition of those of the intestines. After death the minute vessels of the whole of these parts are found much distended with blood, generally dark-coloured. (Hamilton, Mills, Bateman, Percival, &c.)

In one form of fever, the abdominal or intestinal typhus, the ileum and its mucous follicles, are very much affected. The follicles become enlarged, elevated, and prominent, and swelled in consequence of their proper tissue being attacked, and perhaps their secreting pores being obstructed. The apices become dead, and are thrown off in the form of sloughs ; and in their place are left small ulcers, which in no long time enlarge, spread, and increase in depth. These changes may take place either in the isolated follicles or in the aggregated patches, or in both orders of glands. They shall be considered more fully under the proper head.

In certain forms of fever there are pain, distension, and uneasy sensations in the right iliac region ; and when percussion is employed, the sound emitted is dull, while a peculiar croaking noise is heard, and a gurgling movement is felt beneath the fingers, as if produced by air and liquid moving within the intestine. These symptoms continue the greater part of the duration of the fever; and though they are abated by local depletion, by means of leeches and the use of laxative medicines, they do not disappear until the fever itself either abates or altogether retires.

The portal vein constitutes, among the vessels of the digestive organs, a secondary capillary system, in which the blood is not less accumulated than in the primary one. It may be thought, that, as the blood is accumulated in the first, it ought not so readily to find its way into the trunk, branches, and ramifications of the second. But this objection will vanish, when it is remembered that at the same time both the primary and the secondary system of capillaries become overloaded. This state of the capillaries of the portal and hepatic system is established by the appearance of the liver in persons cut off by fever.

The spleen may suffer so much from this capillary distension as to resemble a mass of clotted blood without trace of organization.

This morbid and extraordinary distension of the primary and secondary capillary systems of the chylopoietic organs, though distinct enough in the fevers of temperate countries, is most conspicuously demonstrated in the agues and remittents of warm climates, and especially in the severe and exquisite form termed *yellow fever*. In the former great sickness and epigastric tenderness, with more or less vomiting, are frequent, and in the latter constant symptoms. The vomiting, nevertheless, is not bilious, as has been too generally imagined. It is at the commencement always a watery fluid, evidently derived from the capillaries of the gastric, and perhaps the duodenal mucous membrane. (Dr John Hunter, Jackson, &c.) After some time it begins to be mixed with bile, expressed in all probability from the gall-bladder by the pressure of the stomach in the act of vomiting. A much more uniform occurrence, however, if the disease does not subside spontaneously, or is checked by art, is the gradual admixture of blood somewhat darkened with the watery fluid. This blood issues from the capillaries of the gastric and intestinal tissues by a process analogous to exhalation in the sound state, but differing in so far as in the capillaries, from which it proceeds, a degree of disorganization has taken place. As the blood escapes into the cavity of the canal originally not highly scarlet, it is rapidly blackened by the action of the carbonic acid and sulphuretted hydrogen gases, at all times present in greater or less quantity. This bloody exudation is at first scanty, but gradually increases as the disease goes on, until it constitutes the greater part of what is discharged both by vomiting and by stool. In the former case it forms the black vomit, (*vomito prieto*,) or coffee-ground matter, so frequent in fatal cases of remittent or yellow fever. In the latter it forms the dark, tarry, or treacle-like stools mentioned by practical authors in the same disease. (Jackson, Hunter, Physic, Cathrall, Bancroft, &c.)

The description now given is general, and applies to this capillary disorganization, as it takes place both in bad agues and remittents, and in yellow fever. In the former it is less frequent, but nevertheless takes place sufficiently often. In the latter it is seen in its most exquisite form, and is almost invariable in fatal cases. Its origin and formation have been traced in the most satisfactory manner by repeated dissections.

The idea of black vomit being morbid or vitiated bile deserves no attention. In some instances of severe yellow fever a dark-coloured fluid of the same physical characters as those found in the intestinal tube, may be traced coming down the biliary and hepatic duct from the *pori biliarii*. This, however, instead of being bile, is blood which has oozed from the hepatic capillaries in the same manner as that from the intestinal ones.

δ. The capillaries of the urinary system are much affected during fever. Both in intermittents and in continued fevers bloody urine has been discharged.

ε. In the same manner the capillaries of the muscles, of the filamentous tissue, and of the skin are morbidly distended. One of the most common symptoms of fever is pain, soreness, and a sense of bruising in the muscular parts and limbs in general. In fatal cases, when these parts are examined by incision, unusual vascular distension and extravasation of blood are frequently seen. The livid spots and patches, (*molopes ; vibices ; ecchymomata*) are proofs of the same state of the capillaries of the filamentous tissue, as petechial eruptions denote this in the skin.

In short, there is scarcely a texture or organ of the animal body, the capillaries of which are not disordered in the different forms of fever; and this disorder, instead of being confined to the capillaries of a single organ, is extended throughout the capillary system at large.

It is doubtless true that in individual cases this disorder may be greater and more distinct in one set of capillaries than in another. In one set of patients the capillaries of the brain may appear to be most disordered; in another those of the lungs; in a third those of the intestinal canal; and in a fourth those of the urinary organs. It is always found, however, in such cases, that the affection of one organ does not entirely exclude that of another; and while the capillaries of the one are very much affected, though those of the others are less so, they are by no means in the healthy state. In all cases of severe and exquisite fever, whether intermittent, remittent, or continued, the capillaries of the brain, of the lungs and heart, of the chylopoietic organs, of the urinary organs, of the muscles, of the cellular tissue, and of the skin, are affected nearly in the same degree. (Macartney, Cooke, &c.)

ζ. An important question is to ascertain the precise nature of this affection. The dissections of Pringle, Home, Ploucquet, Mills, &c. as to the brain, those of Schenck, Morgagni, Lieutaud, Sarconi, and others, as to the thoracic organs, and those of Lieutaud, Petit and Serres, Broussais, Lerminier and Andral, Louis, Chomel, and Bright, as to the intestinal canal, might favour the supposition that the morbid process of fever consists in inflammation. Against this conclusion, however, various facts and arguments may be adduced. 1st, In fatal cases of fever unequivocal traces of inflammation are not uniformly or invariably found. The proportion in which these marks, as albuminous effusion, suppuration, ulceration, &c. are observed, is small compared with the number in which accumulation of blood in the capillaries, and more or less disorganization of these vessels are observed. 2d, In cases of pure, genuine, and unmixed inflammation of the internal organs, whether spontaneous or from injury, the concomitant symptoms, though febrile, are totally different from those which distinguish either intermittent or continued fever. 3d, The marks or effects of inflammation which are found in the bodies of persons cut off by fever are accidental complications, and may almost invariably be traced to inflammatory reaction supervening on the febrile process, in consequence either of the physical peculiarities of the individual, the local weakness of the parts, or the influence of external morbific causes. 4th, Inflammation is a local action confined to the capillaries of one tissue, or at most of one organ and contiguous tissues; and while the structure and functions of the

3

organ may be completely impaired, those of others remain un-
altered. In fever, on the contrary, the capillaries of all the tissues
and of every organ are affected ; and while no individual organ is
much affected at the commencement, every organ suffers a little in
the general disorder of the capillary system. *5th*, Inflammation
gives rise to albuminous exudation, suppuration, ulceration, and in
certain parts to serous or sero-purulent effusion. In fever the
morbid state of the capillaries terminates in complete destruction
or disorganization of their organic extremities, and the consequent
oozing of blood from the surface of the several membranes and organs.

In conclusion, though it may be regarded as established, that
during the morbid process of fever the whole capillary system is
unduly distended and loaded with an inordinate quantity of blood,
which really moves more slowly and imperfectly than during health,
we have no facts which enable us to determine what induces this
peculiar and excessive accumulation. Much has been lately said
of congestion, and especially venous congestion. The state of the
capillary system which I have attempted to describe is that of congestion or accumulation ; and so far the hypothesis of congestion
is intelligible. Of the existence of venous congestion, however,
unless as an effect of that in the capillary vessels, there is neither
proof nor probability. It is not a primary but a secondary, or
rather remote consequence. (Marsh.)

η. Changes in the blood in Fever. (Hæmatopathia.) Another question belonging to a different head, nevertheless, in this
place may deserve some consideration in explaining this universal affection of the vascular system. This is the state of the
blood itself, and to what extent and in what manner it influences
the formation of these phenomena of deranged action in the vascular system. Though this has been already in part noticed under
the head of the blood, yet it may render the pathological views
on fever more complete and more intelligible to advert shortly to
certain facts on the subject in this place, and the necessary inferences from these facts.

All observers agree in representing the blood to be more or less
changed in its properties and constitution in the different varieties of
fever, whether intermittent, remittent, or continued. To the principal views of the old pathologists it is unnecessary to advert. But by
all observers during the 18th century, when it was supposed import-

ant to attend much to the state of the blood and its appearances, it is commonly described as dissolved, and deficient in *crasis*.

What this dissolved state consists in we are not informed; neither do we at present possess means of knowing. In many of the continental schools, however, the term *dyscrasia* of the blood has been and is now employed to express a morbid state of that fluid.

The following facts, which I have repeatedly observed in continued fever, appear to me deserving attention.

If a person attacked with fever (*synochus* or *typhus*,) be blooded at the commencement of the attack or within three or four days therefrom, the blood coagulates very much in the usual time, and, with a moderately firm coagulum, shows an average proportion of serum. If in a person labouring under fever blood be drawn about six or seven days after the commencement of the symptoms, it coagulates more slowly, and less perfectly. The coagulum is loose and soft, and the quantity of serum small. If blood be drawn at a period still later in the disease, the coagulum is yet more loose and soft, and the serum still smaller in quantity. In the majority of cases of fever at this stage, the serum sometimes does not exceed one drachm, or at most two, and in some cases no serum at all is separated. At the same time, the coagulum is soft, flaccid, tremulous, and when divided, evidently consists of the coagulum, properly so called, and the serum involved and retained within the clot: This I have seen so often, and after trials made with attentive observation of the fact, that I cannot doubt its accuracy as a general fact.

The conclusion which I conceive naturally flows from the facts now stated, is, that in fever the coagulating power of the blood is progressively impaired in the course of the disease, and it may in extreme cases be altogether gone. The quantity of serum produced is in general in the direct ratio of the coagulating power. If the blood coagulates vigorously and energetically, the serum is expressed from it in large quantity. If the serum is separated in small quantity, it shows not that little serum is in the blood, but that the coagulating power being impaired and weakened, it does not force the serum out of the fibrin in due quantity. When no serum appears at all, it shows that the coagulating power is so far destroyed, that it is unable to separate the blood into clot and serum.

That this loss of coagulating power in the blood takes place in fever, and increases gradually as the disease advances, is rendered certain, not only by the facts now stated, but by the condition of the blood found in the vessels after death. That fluid is then found filling the arteries, as well as the veins, not scarlet, but of a dark-brown colour, and viscid, grumous, and very imperfectly coagulated.

There appear, therefore, here, two remarkable circumstances; one, the diminution or loss of coagulating power; the other the diminution or loss of arterialization.

What is the cause of these changes? It is reasonable to think that for this cause we ought to look chiefly in the lungs. The lungs, I have already observed, are in all cases of fever more or less disordered, their vessels are congested and oppressed; their action is impaired; and there is proof of great derangement in the action of the bronchial membrane, imperfect admission of air to the bronchial tubes and their membrane, and, accordingly, inadequate arterialization, or it may be the lowest possible degree of that function. These may be regarded as matters of fact, capable of demonstration. Does this morbid state of the blood, then, begin in the lungs, or in some other part, or set of vessels? When we consider the large extent of the bronchial membrane, the fact that upon it are ramified the capillary divisions of the pulmonary artery and veins; the fact that through these vessels passes the whole blood of the body, and the further fact of the manifest disorder of the whole blood of the system in fever, it is impossible to resist the conclusion, that it must be chiefly, perhaps solely, on the blood of the lungs, that the cause of fever begins to display its primary and initial operation.

On the nature of this cause it is not possible to speak with confidence or certainty. But if the general opinion, that it is a poison diffused through the air, be well founded, it is not difficult to perceive at least some traces of its mode of operation. Whether that poison be extricated in the form of a vapour or exhalation from the surface of the earth, and is telluric in origin; or is eliminated from vegetable matters in certain circumstances of decay or change; or from vegetable and animal matters conjoined; or is given off as a subtile effluvium from the bodies of living human beings, in circumstances unfavourable to ventilation and the healthy performance of the functions; or is the result of some unknown and unappreciable state of the atmosphere;—it must equally be inhaled with the air in inspiration, and thus thoroughly mixed with the blood of the lungs in successive acts of the function of respiration. If it be so mixed, it must be circulated with the circulating blood, and in this manner distributed through the whole vascular system to every organ of the body. In doing so, however, this poisonous material must have so altered the blood in the lungs, as to produce in that blood and in these organs a more decided effect than elsewhere. The shock first inflicted on the blood in these organs appears, it is natural to think, the great cause of the loss of coagulating power and the impaired arterialization. We know that one of the great uses of the lung next to, or along with the arterialization of the blood, is to maintain the coagulating power, and to restore it when impaired. It is, therefore, natural to infer, that when the coagulating power is diminished, it depends on some impediment to the function of respiration, and that when the function of respiration is imperfectly performed, that should evince its effects in a diminished proportion of coagulating power.

If these views be well founded, it follows, that, when the blood thus altered is circulated, however imperfectly, it must operate hurtfully on the organs to which it is transmitted. It must act, in truth, as a poison; and many of the phenomena of fever are similar, certainly, to the effects of poison, especially a poison at first irritant, and then sedative and narcotic. This appears to be the mode in which, towards the latter stage of fever, its cause acts on the brain and spinal marrow.

7. *Hemorrhage.* In all cases of Hemorrhage, whether by rupture or by exhalation, the capillaries are unusually loaded with blood. This is established by the appearance of the brain in apoplexy, of the lung in *hemoptysis*, (pulmonary apoplexy of Laennec,) *pneumonorrhagia* of Frank and Latour, of the prostate gland in chronic enlargement, (Home,) and the state of the mucous surfaces in general. In the two first cases, especially in that of the lungs, the pulmonic capillaries are large, numerous, and distended with blood, the pulmonic tissue more or less injected and firm, and blood is found oozing from the surface of the bronchial membrane. (Stark and Laennec.) With this, however, is conjoined a friable or lacerable and imbrowned state of the bronchial membrane and pulmonic tissue.

8. *Excess of Nutrition.* (*Hypertrophia.*) Hypertrophic augmentation. That every unusual increase in the size of parts is to be ascribed to the agency of the capillaries is well established by

the phenomena of morbid enlargements and preternatural growths. Every instance of unusual or anormal size is of three kinds.

α. A texture or organ becomes enlarged in consequence of a uniform increase of its proper organic substance. Thus the heart becomes thicker, firmer, and larger in all its dimensions. Its muscular substance, and perhaps the intermuscular filamentous tissue, are actually augmented. They are redder, firmer, and contain more blood than natural; and their blood-vessels are increased in size and number. The bladder in like manner undergoes the same change; and in its thickened and indurated tissue also dissection shows a more copious supply of blood, and a more abundant distribution of vessels than in the natural state.

Of this preternatural increase of bulk and density the capillaries of the organs are the sole agents. In some instances this hypertrophy appears to be of the nature of a chronic process of inflammation. This is exemplified in the case of the liver, the testicle, the prostate gland, the female breast, and even the heart.

β. Any individual texture may undergo a preternatural or anormal enlargement by local deposition of matter similar to itself. Thus a bone may become enlarged, as in *exostosis*; a gland may become enlarged, as in various instances the testicle and the female breast do. That the skin is liable to a particular species of hypertrophic augmentation is well ascertained from cases given by many authors, but especially from one recorded by Mr John Bell.* In mucous membrane, lymphatic gland, and secreting glands, similar local augmentations take place.

γ. In any tissue or organ a deposition of new matter altogether foreign to that tissue may take place. This new matter may be either similar to that of some natural tissue of the animal body; for example, it may be serous membrane, or bone, or cartilage; or of a nature entirely dissimilar, and never seen unless in the morbid state; for instance, the several varieties of tubercular deposition of scirrhous deposition, of fungoid deposition, and several of the forms of *sarcoma* enumerated by Mr Abernethy.

In whatever mode these new productions vary in intimate structure, all agree in being connected with more or less augmented development of the capillary system. In many the growth, if not the origin, can be traced to the increased number, or at least enlarged size, of the capillary arteries. In most of these tumours

* Principles of Surgery, Vol. III. Discourse ii. Case of Eleanor Fitzgerald.

the vessels are large, numerous, and well filled with blood; and if divided in the living body they are the source of abundant hemorrhage. In some instances these vessels penetrate from the adjoining tissue all round the tumour in the form of numerous minute arteries, which afterwards are ramified in the tumour. In others, which are perhaps more numerous, they enter at one point in the shape of three or four large trunks, which are afterwards divided in the substance of the growth.

As these new or foreign growths, therefore, are known to abound in capillaries, it is inferred, that, if this abundance of vessels be not the direct cause, they furnish the materials of growth. The difficulty in the theory of their formation is to ascertain the circumstances which first determine this local development of the capillary system. In some instances it can be distinctly traced to mechanical injury, (John Bell and Abernethy.) After a bruise, for example, blood and lymph being poured forth, instead of being absorbed, become penetrated with vessels, which conversely are stimulated by the presence of this substance to convey more blood, and thus enlarge in size. In others this local capillary development commences without obvious cause. Upon the whole, the growth of tumours is to be viewed as the result of an aberration or anormal action of the usual nutritive process to which the capillary vessels are subservient.*

The theory of tumours or morbid growths depending on inordinate local development of the capillary system was understood by Valsalva, Morgagni, Pohl, and others, but was first fully illustrated by John Bell and Mr Abernethy,† and afterwards by Sir Everard Home and Mr Macilwain.

---

* " As wounded parts are healed by adhesion, so are dilated or strained parts by increased nutrition."—" Tumour and various modifications of disease follow from the same law of vascular action and nutrition which maintained health. If each individual vessel, whether artery or vein, have its coats thickened by dilatation or partial laceration, the same must be presumed of each minuter vessel in the distended womb, of each lesser vein and petty artery in a piece of distended skin, or in a diseased gland. The enlargement, then, of each blood-vessel by deposition of nutritious matter along its sides makes not a mere distension of vessels, but a solid and permanent bulk. The more vessels are enlarged consistently with their healthy action, the more particles are they able to secrete ; whence the increment of tumours is perpetually accelerating unless when opposed by peculiar causes."—The Principles of Surgery, by John Bell, Surgeon. Vol. III. Discourse ii.

† An Attempt to form a Classification of Tumours according to their Anatomical Structure, by John Abernethy. London, 1811.

ERECTILE TISSUE,—(*Vasa Erigentia,—Vascula Erectilia,—*
Tissu Erectile.

Section I.

The peculiar arrangement of vessels constituting the erectile tissue was very early anticipated by our countryman William Cowper, who states, that he demonstrated the direct communication of arterial and venous canals, not only in the lungs, but in the spleen and penis, " in which," says he, " I have found these communications more open than in other parts."*

The system of capillary arteries and veins does not present the same arrangement in all situations or in all the tissues of the human body. Among the terminations of arteries enumerated by Haller, one which he referred to the head of exhalants was that of a red artery or arteries pouring their blood into the spongy or cellular structure of the cavernous bodies of the nipple, the clitoris, and the penis, that of the wattles of the turkey, and the comb of the cock.† His detailed examination of these parts shows, that, with a correct knowledge of their anatomical structure, he had not a very distinct conception of the manner in which their vesels are disposed.

Bichat remarked that the spleen and the cavernous body of the penis, instead of presenting, as the serous surfaces, a vascular or capillary net-work, (*reseau vasculaire,*) in which the blood oscillates in different directions according to the impulse which it receives, exhibit only spongy or lamellar tissues, still little known in their structure, in which the blood appears often to stagnate instead of moving. As this peculiar structure was known in the cavernous body to be the seat of a motion long known by the name of *erection*, MM. Dupuytren and Richerand distinguished this arrangement of arteries and veins as a peculiar tissue, under the name of *erectile,*—a distinction which, though partly understood before, nas only now been admitted as well-founded in the writings of anatomical authors. According to the arrangements of M. Beclard, this tissue comprehends not only the structure of the ca-

* Philosophical Transactions, Vol. XXIII. No. 285, p. 1386. 1703.
† Elementa, Lib. ii. sect. 1. sect. 24. III. p. 102.

vernous body, but that of the spongy substance, (*corpus spongio-sum*,) which encloses the urethra, and forms its two extremities, the bulb and gland, the *clitoris*, the *nymphæ*, and the nipple of the female, the structure of the spleen in both sexes, and even that of the lips.* Some are disposed to add the structure of the *iris*, and the peculiar plexiform network of vessels in the vagina of the female.

It is somewhat unfortunate that the researches of anatomists on this erectile tissue have been restricted chiefly to the spongy body of the urethra and the cavernous body of the penis; and it is rather by analogy than very direct proof, that similarity of structure between them and the other parts referred to the same head is maintained. I shall state here what is most satisfactorily known on the subject.

The cavernous body of the urethra, or what is now termed its *spongy body*,† is represented by Haller to consist of fibres and plates issuing from the inner surface of the containing membrane, and mutually interlacing, so as to form a series of communicating cells,‡ into which the proper urethral arteries pour their blood directly during the state of erection.§

The cavernous body of the penis is in like manner represented to be a part of a spongy nature, or to consist of innumerable sacs or cells separated by plates and fibres, which, at the moment of erection, are distended with blood poured from the arteries, and which was afterwards removed by some absorbing power of the veins.

This opinion, which was that of many subsequent anatomists, even Bichat himself,‖ was derived apparently from the facility with which the blood so deposited escapes, not, as it was believed, from divided vessels, but from *areolæ*, or interlaminar spaces. It appears, however, to have been at variance with what had been anciently taught by Vesalius, Ingrassias, and Malpighi, and more positively stated regarding these vessels by Hunter; and modern

---

* Additions à l'Anatomie Generale de Xav. Bichat, par P. A. Beclard, p. 118.

† Haller applies the name of *cavernous body* not only to the structure of the penis, but to that of the urethra.—Elem. Lib. xxvii. Sect. 1.

‡ Elementa Physiologiæ, Lib. xxvii. sect. 1, § 33.

§ " Sed et in pene, et in clitoride, et in papilla mammæ, et in collo galli indici, nimis manifestum est, verum sanguinem effundi, neque unquam ejus color totus de iis partibus evanescit, quæ ab effuso sanguine turgere solent."—Elementa, Lib. xxvii. sect: 3, § 10.

‖ Systême Absorbant, § 3, p. 598.

researches have shown it to be completely erroneous. Cuvier and Ribes in France, Mascagni, Paul Farnese, Moreschi in Italy, and Tiedemann in Germany, have shown that there are no cells or spongiform structure in the erectile tissue of the cavernous body. The first correct view of the structure of parts of this description in the human subject was given by Mascagni in his account of the arterial and venous communications in the Spongy Body of the Urethra. In 1787 he announced in his work on the Lymphatics, that the parts called cavernous bodies, both in the *penis* and in the *clitoris*, were simply fasciculi, or accumulations of arterial and venous vessels without interruption of canal; but that between the arteries and veins of the spongy bodies a dilated cavity or minute cell was interposed. In 1795 repeated minute injections led him to doubt the existence of this sort of cell; and about the close of 1805 he publicly demonstrated the fact, that many veins of considerable calibre collected in the manner of a plexus, with corresponding arteries, but small and less numerous, really form the outer and inner membranes of the urethra, the whole of the *glans penis*, and the whole substance of the spongy body. In each of these parts, and also in the spongy structure inclosing the orifice of the vagina, he ascertained by repeated injections that there are no cells, as was imagined, and that the arteries, reflected, as it were, give origin to numerous veins,[*] which, forming an intimate plexiform net-work, constitute the whole glans, and the entire vascular body which surrounds the urethra and the entrance of the vagina.

In the cavernous bodies of the penis and clitoris he had not sufficient facts to ascertain the existence of the same structure, as he had never succeeded in injecting these parts so completely as the *glans* and the spongy part of the urethra. Eventually, however, he succeeded, especially in children, in injecting fully these cavernous bodies of the penis and clitoris. He found in their interior nothing but *fasciculi* of veins, with corresponding arteries, though rather smaller. He inferred, therefore, that these vessels, collected and ramified in various directions, constitute a vascular texture capable of expanding and shrinking, according to the quantity of blood conveyed to it.[†]

---

[*] " Le arterie vi si ritorcono, et danno origine alle vene, e queste formano in seguito alcuni plessi, i quali accumulati in varia maniera, instituiscono tutto il glande, e tutta quella massa vascolare, che trovasi intorno al' canale dell' uretra, e all' ingresso della vagina." Prodromo della Grande Anotomia di Paolo Mascagni. Folio, Firenze, 1819. Capitolo, II. p. 61.

[†] Prodromo del Paolo Mascagni, *loco citato*, p. 61.

The general accuracy of this description has been since confirmed by the researches of Paul Farnese and Moreschi. The latter especially has shown, 1*st*, That the glans consists of arteries and a very great number of minute veins, which pour their blood into the cutaneous dorsal vein ; 2*d*, That the urethra, and especially its posterior part, may in like manner be shown to consist of numerous minute veins, which terminate in a posterior branch of the dorsal vein, and communicate with the veins of the bulbous portion of the urethra; and 3*d*, That in the cavernous bodies, though also receiving blood-vessels, these are much less numerous, and are chiefly derived from the urethral vessels.*

The same arrangement was recognized by Cuvier in the penis of the elephant, and by Tiedemann in that of the horse.

Upon the whole, the facts collected by different anatomists on this subject furnish the following results.

If the arteries, on the one hand, be injected, they are found to terminate in very fine ramifications, the disposition of which is exactly the same as in other parts. If, on the other, the veins be injected, it is easy to perceive the two following circumstances. 1*st*, That they are much dilated at their origin, that is, that the venous *radiculæ* are really more dilated than might be anticipated from the other characters of these vessels. 2*d*, That the tubular dilatations to which they are accessory, form very numerous inosculations or anastomoses, precisely as the capillary system of which they constitute a part. The effect of this arrangement is to give these vessels the appearance of being penetrated with sieve-like openings, which makes them resemble *areolæ*, or interlaminar spaces mutually communicating. As the whole difference, therefore, between the capillary vessels of this and other parts of the human frame, consists in the minute veins (*radiculæ venosæ*) being dilated or distended in a peculiar manner, M. Beclard concludes, that the erectile tissue of the cavernous body consists simply of minute arteries and dilatable veins interwoven in the manner of capillary nets. These distended venous cavities are indeed so remote from being cells, that they are truly continuous with veins, the inner membrane of which may be easily recognised among them.†

* Commentarium de Urethræ Corporis Glandisque Structura 6to Idus Decembris 1810 detectâ Alexandri Moreschi, Eq. Coron. Ferreæ in Ticinensi primum, tum Bononiensi Archigymnasio, Anatomes Professoris. Mediolani, 1817.

† Additions, p. 119.

During erection the blood accumulates in this tissue; but the cause and mechanism of this accumulation are completely unknown. Since these observations were made, M. Müller of Berlin has, by injecting the arteries of the penis, been enabled to give a more detailed and satisfactory account still of the peculiar arrangement of the erectile vessels.

By injecting the principal artery of the penis before its subdivision, and dividing longitudinally one of the *corpora cavernosa*, the ramifications of the nutrient arteries are then seen upon the inner side of the venous spaces, the arteries becoming smaller and smaller, until they pass into the capillary network, where their divisions cannot be seen by the naked eye. Besides these nutrient ramified arteries, there is seen on careful inspection another set of arterial branches of different size, form, and disposition, which are given off nearly at right angles from both the larger and smaller trunks. These arterial processes are about one-hundreth of an inch in diameter, and one-twelfth long, and are easily seen by the naked eye. They project into the cavities of the spongy substance, and terminate either bluntly or by dilated extremities, without undergoing any ramification. These short arterial processes are turned round at their extremities into a semicircle or more, and present a spiral appearance like the extremity of a screw. This disposition suggested to M. Müller the name of Helicine, or spiral or screw-like arteries; (*Arteriæ Helicinæ.*)*

The helicine arteries of the penis are more easily seen in man than in any other animal which Professor Müller has examined. He has found them in all the animals in which he has sought for them; they are to be seen at the posterior part only of the penis in the stallion, but in the dog exist throughout the whole organ.

In man, the helicine twigs of the penal arteries sometimes come off singly, and at other times they form tufts or bunches, consisting of from three to ten branches, and having in general a very short common stem. The swelling at the extremity, when it occurs, is gradual, and is greatest a little way from the end. The helicine branches given off from large arteries are not of a greater size than those coming from smaller ones, and even the smallest capillary arteries of the *profunda penis*, which can be seen with the help of a glass only, give off helicine twigs of a much greater size than themselves.

* Ueber die Arteriæ Helicinæ. Von Johann Dr Müller. Archive fur Anatomie und Physiologie, Heft II. 1835.

Each helicine branch projecting into a venous cavity is covered by a thin membrane, which Professor Müller regards as the inner coat of the dilated vein, and when there is a tuft of helicine twigs, the whole tuft is covered with one envelope of a gauze-like membrane. This covering is considerably thicker on the helicine arteries in the posterior part of the *corpus spongiosum urethræ* than in the *corpus cavernosum;* but it is probable that this is in some measure connected with the state of repletion of the arteries; for when the injection has run well, it becomes difficult to distinguish the external covering.

Professor Müller could not discover any apertures either in the sides or in the ends of the helicine arteries; but he seems to regard it as probable that there are minute apertures, which may be of a nature to allow the passage of blood in some states and not in others.

The helicine arteries are not, as some may suppose, loops of vessels which have been incompletely filled, and which, after making a coil, pass into venous spaces, as E. H. Weber discovered to be the case with the arteries of the maternal portion of the placenta. They are merely branches projecting from the arterial trunks containing blood.

The helicine arteries are more numerous towards the root than near the point of the penis. They are observed in the *corpus spongiosum urethræ*, especially towards its bulb, but they are not so easily seen there as in the *corpora cavernosa.* They have not yet been observed in the glans. Their structure is nearly the same in all the animals in which they have been observed; those of the ape bear the nearest resemblance to those of man, and in most animals they are less obvious than in the human subject. In the horse and dog they give off small nutrient twigs from their sides, which render them more difficult to be seen in these animals than in man.

It seems not doubtful that the accumulation of blood in these helicine arteries is the physiological cause of the phenomena of erection.

The spleen, M. Beclard thinks, may be said to resemble the cavernous body both in structure and phenomena; and he considers it as at once consisting of erectile tissue, and to be the seat of a species of erection more or less similar to that of the cavernous body. This organ, he argues, becomes the occasional seat of a motion of expansion and contraction; and he adduces the three following conditions in which it takes place. 1*st*, In experiments; when in a living animal the course of the blood in the splenic veins is arrested, the spleen swells, but returns to its former dimensions as soon as the circulation is restored. *2d,* In diseases; the paroxysms of intermittent fever are accompanied with obvious enlargement of this organ, which subsides at the conclusion of the paroxysm. *3d,* It appears that the same phenomenon takes place during digestion.

Sir Everard Home, with the assistance of the microscopic inspection of M. Bauer, has made many observations on the structure of this organ. But his purpose appears to have been more particularly directed to ascertain the phenomena of its function and uses; and I cannot discover that his ideas on its intimate structure, and the arrangement of its capillary system, are very precise or distinct.

The most distinct examples, in short, of erectile tissue are to be found, according to Beclard, in the spongy texture which surrounds the *urethra,* in the cavernous body of the *clitoris,* the vascular structure of the *nymphæ,* and in the nipple of the female. The structure of the lips in both sexes is not unlike. The veins of these parts may be shown to be well-marked and largely dilated at their origin, so as to give the appearance of cellular net-work. The same disposition is observed in the pulp of the fingers. It has been attempted to explain the motions of the iris by supposing it to be formed of this erectile tissue; but the justice of this conjecture seems doubtful.

In the tissue now described it is manifest that the physiologist ought to place the phenomena of the process distinguished by the name of vital turgescence (*turgor vitalis*) by Hebenstreit,[*] Reil,[†] Ackermann,[‡] and Schlosser.[§] Though these authors suppose vital turgescence in different degrees in almost all the textures of the animal body, their most distinct examples are taken from those parts which consist of erectile vessels. After the explanation of the anatomical structure above given, it is superfluous to seek for any other cause except the arrangement of the minute vessels, their helicine termination, and the disposition of the veins.

[*] Brevis Expositio Doctrinæ Physiologicæ de Turgore Vitali. 1795. Ab Ernesto Benjamino Gottlieb Hebenstreit, M. D., &c., extat in Brera Sylloge Opusculorum Select. Vol. II. Opusc. vi.

[†] Archiv. für die Physiologie, I. Band, 2. Heft, S. 172.

[‡] Ackermann Physische Darstellung der Lebenscraft, 1797. 1. Band, S. 11.

[§] Georgii Eduardi Schlosser Dissertatio de Turgore Vitali ext. in Brera Sylloge, Vol. VII. Opusc. ii.

SECTION II.

Little is known regarding the peculiar pathological states of this tissue.

1. *Rupture* of its vessels occasionally occurs, but is not attended with peculiar phenomena, unless there is an external communication, when hemorrhage takes place.

2. It is liable to a peculiar species of enlargement or swelling, in which the parts are very tense, and resemble a swollen bladder. They have an œdematous appearance, yet it is not œdema. This is often seen in *phimosis* and *paraphimosis,* in enlargement of the *nymphæ* and *labia* in females, and in a swelling incident to the eyelids after the application of leeches in both sexes.

This swelling, I think, is most usually connected with some morbid state of the surface of the parts; either inflammation, as in gonorrhœa and leucorrhœa, or an abrasion, an ulcer, or laceration, or some similar lesion.

3. *Priapism* is a morbid state of the erectile tissue of the cavernous body. The painful and anomalous mode of erection termed *chordee* appears to depend on the erectile tissue of the *corpus spongiosum* being unduly irritated by the presence of the inflammatory stimulus in the urethral membrane and its submucous tissue. There is at the same time, however, a spasm of the erector muscle, (*ischio-cavernosus,*) which, Haller justly remarks, instead of erecting the penis, ought to depress it.

4. Is the erectile tissue more prone to hemorrhage than others? Is this hemorrhage more frequently venous than arterial? These are points on which we have almost no certain information. Urethral hemorrhage, when violent and copious, may depend on rupture of the erectile tissue of the spongy body, or those vessels of the urethra which have been well delineated by Mr Shaw.* When it is so copious as to be restrained with difficulty, there is reason to believe that a communication is opened between the urethra and the communicating veins of the spongy body.

It may here be mentioned that hemorrhage from the vagina, whether intentionally or accidentally inflicted, is always most profuse and copious, and difficult to be restrained. From this cause various females in this country have died, before adequate means

---

* Medico-Chirurgical Transactions, Vol. X. p. 342 and 357.

to suppress the hemorrhage could be adopted. This is manifestly dependent on the plexiform arrangement of the multiplied venous vessels by which the vaginal mucous membrane is surrounded.

5. The disease described by John Bell and Mr Freer* under the name of *aneurism by anastomosis*† (*aneurysma per anastomosin*), termed by Meckel *angiectasia*, (Αγγειον εκτασις, *vasorum dilatatio*,) and by some of the German pathologists, *telangiectasis*, (*vasorum ultimorum distensio*,) appears to be an accessory or morbid form of erectile tissue occurring in parts naturally provided with simple capillary tissue. In some circumstances it is a congenital disease, and appears at birth like a *nævus maternus*. In its early stage the tumour is a mere pimple, and appears to consist of a congeries of arteries and veins.‡ In this state it is firm, and the throbbing is indistinct; but as the cellular net-work, which ultimately forms the bulk of the swelling, is developed, it becomes more compressible, and the pulsation becomes more evident. At last it appears to consist of a cluster of sacs of a purple or livid colour, which burst from time to time, and bleed profusely. Anastomotic aneurism may occur in any part of the body in which the capillary vessels are numerous. Mr Bell saw it in the face, near the angle of the eye. Mr Freer saw it within the mouth, between the gums and the cheek. I have seen it on the skin of the nose and on the gum.

In two instances in which I saw it on the skin of the nose, the body resembled a small reddish mark on the skin, about the size

---

* Observations on Aneurism and some Diseases of the Arterial System. By George Freer, Fellow of the Royal College of Surgeons, London, &c. Birmingham, 1807, p. 34.

† The Principles of Surgery, in Two Volumes, &c. by John Bell, Surgeon, Discourse XI. p. 456, Vol. I. 4to Edition. 1801.

‡ "The tumour is a congeries of active vessels; and the cellular substance through which these vessels are expanded resembles the cellular part of the penis, the gills of a turkey cock, or the substances of the placenta, spleen, or womb. It is apparently a very simple structure that enables those parts, (the womb, the penis, the spleen,) to perform their functions; and it is a very slight change of organization that forms this disease. The tumour is a congeries of small and active arteries, absorbing veins, and intermediate cells. The irritated and incessant action of the arteries fills the cells with blood; from these cells it is reabsorbed by the veins; the extremities of the veins themselves perhaps dilate into this cellular form. There seems to be a perpetual circulation of blood; for there is incessant pulsation. The tumour is permanent, but its occasional variation of bulk is singular. It swells like the penis in erection, or the gills of a turkey-cock in a passion. It is puffed up by exercise, drinking, or emotions of the mind. It is filled and distended with blood upon any occasion which quickens the circulation, as by venery, menstruation, the pleasures of the table, heated rooms, or the warmth of the bed."—Principles of Surgery, p. 457.

M

of a split pea, without elevation, but presenting, when closely examined, a cluster of minute vessels proceeding from a circumference to a point, in the asteroid form. In both cases they were
liable to become red and uneasy on exposure to external heat,
during blushing, and on any excited state of the circulation. When
pressed, the vessels seemed to be for one moment emptied and then
to be immediately filled, giving the part a deeper red colour than
before. In the instance, in which I saw the tumour on the gum,
(*parulis aneurysmatica*,) the form of the disease was greatly more
distinct. It appeared in the form of a tumour of the size of a
large pea, situated in the gum of the upper jaw. It pulsated
strongly and distinctly, and was the seat of a disagreeable sensation of heat and throbbing. When situate on the mucous surfaces,
these tumours are liable to attacks of hemorrhage; and occasionally this accident takes place in those of the skin.

When it occurs on the surface of the body, its covering is so
thin as to appear destitute of the usual corion. The pulsation in
the tumour is increased by all those causes which accelerate the
action of the heart.[*]

The arterial disease found often affecting the branches of the
temporal, posterior aural, and occipital arteries, as described by
Mr Maclure, Mr Maclachlan, Mr Syme, and M. Lallemand, is
manifestly the same affection as that already noticed under the
head of arterial varix and cirsoid aneurism. The arteries are
dilated, tortuous, and serpentine; the tunics of the vessels are thin,
flaccid and feeble, and pulsate strongly; while occasionally after
death these vessels are observed, like veins, to have undergone the
suppurative inflammation.[†]

6. *Osteo-aneurism.* Not dissimilar to the anastomotic aneurism
is a species of throbbing tumour observed by Pearson,[‡] and fully
described by Scarpa.[§] In the latter instance a pulsating tumour,
which had gradually attained the size of the fist, was formed in the
substance of the anterior part of the tibia, beneath the periosteum,
which had become thick and fleshy, and formed a sort of containing membrane. Its inner surface was villous and irregularly

[*] For further details on this subject the reader may consult Warren on Tumours,
section viii. Boston, 1837.

[†] Breschet, Memoires de l'Academie, Tome III. p. 161.

[‡] Medical Communications, Vol. II. p. 95 and 100.

[§] A Treatise on the Anatomy, Pathology, and Surgical Treatment of Aneurism.
By Antonio Scarpa. Edinburgh, 1808, Case x. p. 439.

spongy, like the uterine surface of the placenta; and wax injected into the popliteal artery escaped from it, and was deposited between layers of coagulated blood, which must have proceeded from vessels opening on this surface. The substance of the tibia at the bottom of the cavity was rough, corroded, and partly destroyed.

After the limb was removed the patient remained well for five years, when the stump, and eventually the whole thigh, was attacked with painful pulsation. At death, which soon took place, the substance of the thigh-bone was found to be removed by absorption from the cut end to near the neck; and the periosteum, which was much thickened, was interspersed with largely dilated vessels, and formed a sort of capsule or inclosing membrane to the diseased parts.

This disease differs from anastomotic aneurism in its pulsation and distension being at all times the same, and in not presenting the phenomena of erection. Though it is mentioned in this place from its general resemblance to that disease, it may be more justly regarded as genuine aneurism of the capillaries, or rather aneurism of the arteries of bone.

Morbid States of the Spleen as an erectile organ.

1. *Softening.* The most common morbid state of the splenic tissue is that of softening. This may be various in degree. In the least severe the texture of the spleen is lacerable; and when torn, the surfaces present a good deal of the natural structure of the organ in the form of fibres and vessels, and filaments of some firmness. In the next stage, the softening is more complete and the organ may be crushed between the fingers. When a stream of water is directed on the surface, it washes away much wine-red-coloured fluid, leaving shreds and filaments. In the third and most complete degree of this lesion, the spleen is converted into a soft semi-fluid pulpy mass, of a dark-red or deep pink colour, like thick wine-lees, with nothing but a few shreds and filaments left.

This change of consistence takes place in ague, remittent fever, yellow fever, typhus, occasionally in puerperal fever, and sometimes in diseases of the stomach and alimentary canal.

The nature and origin of softening of the spleen is not perfectly known. If not an effect of inflammation, it must be regarded as one of excessive vascular distension. It is associated with that state in which the internal vascular system in general, and that of the abdomen in particular, is for a long time inordinately distended. Inflammation, it must be remembered, has the effect of destroying the cohesion of tissues, and thereby causing softening. It seems to be in fever a mortal lesion.

2. *Splenia; Splenitis; Lienia.* The spleen appears to be liable to four forms of inflammatory action; 1*st*, proper inflammation, terminating in resolution or suppuration; 2*d*, suppurative inflammation; 3*d*, simple enlargement from vascular distension; and, 4*th*, enlargement, with induration of its tissue.

Simple inflammation, though not common, does take place. In two cases of inflamed spleen examined by Dr William Hunter, where the inflammation had advanced to suppuration, the patients could not define accurately the seat of the pain, which seemed to travel over the general cavity of the abdomen. In another case, in which Anthony de Haen found the spleen distended with a large quantity of thick white purulent matter, the symptoms had, during the inflammatory stage, been ascribed to pleurisy.

Both Schmidt, Heusinger, and Grottanelli record, in like manner, instances in which suppuration had taken place in the spleen without the production of any manifest symptom or local uneasiness, sufficient to lead the circumstance to be suspected, except general bad health and wasting. A remarkable case of this kind is recorded by Dr Abercrombie, in which the patient, after slight catarrhal symptoms, pined away without distinct local uneasiness for six months, and died wasted and weakened, latterly with diarrhœa of two days' standing; and upon inspection the spleen contained several ounces of purulent matter. Similar instances of purulent collections in the spleen, where no indication of previous disorder was afforded, have come under my notice in the course of inspecting bodies at the Royal Infirmary.

These facts show clearly that suppuration of the spleen may take place without being attended with evident or urgent external symptoms. In this case it may become a question whether the suppuration is the effect of acute inflammation, or rather of a peculiar chronic suppurative action,—connected probably with that convenient and ill-defined abstraction, the strumous diathesis. It must not be imagined, nevertheless, that no symptoms are produced by this disorder. There are always wasting or pining, considerable weakness, sometimes a thin unhealthy look, sometimes slight dyspeptic symptoms, and sometimes, though more rarely, a sense of uneasy fulness deep in the left hypochondriac region. The most perplexing part of the semiography and symptomatology is this, that these purulent collections cause almost no uneasy feelings, till by their size they induce distension or painful stretching of the organ, or pressure or tension of some of the surrounding parts.

In such circumstances, it is chiefly by negative signs that the practitioner can infer the existence of disease, in the shape of inflammation or abscess of the spleen; and, if he meets with a case in which the patient pines away, without cough, expectoration, cavernous respiration in the chest, or the signs of empyema in the side, or indications of enlarged liver, or ulceration of the intestinal mucous membrane, he may then infer the probable existence of suppurative or other disorder of the spleen.

This disease is rare, and therefore not well known; but the practitioner must not expect, like Pemberton, never to meet with it. Abscess of the spleen is sometimes found to be the only morbid appearance in sundry cases of long ill health, with wasting and hectic fever.

3. It is not perfectly ascertained whether the form of simple enlargement of the spleen, or the enlargement with induration ever proceeds to suppuration, or whether suppuration and abscess of the spleen is in certain circumstances the result of one peculiar form of inflammation. From the testimony of Grottanelli suppuration of the spleen seems a lesion not unfrequent in Tuscany and other aguish districts in Italy. * M. Raikem of Volterra records in a young book-keeper of 21, a case of *splenitis* ending in an extensive collection of fetid purulent matter, in which, from the progress of the symptoms, there is reason to believe that the organ had been affected at first with simple enlargement from vascular distension. The whole duration of the disease appears to have been rather more than three months; the acute symptoms for which the patient was under the care of M. Raikem, two months; and the tumour of the left hypochondre, which was at first hard and resisting, and extended to the *linea alba* and navel, became about the sixth week soft, increasing in size, and afterwards diminishing remarkably.

Inspection of the body disclosed the following facts. The left pleura contained more than two pounds of citron-yellow serous fluid, with albuminous flakes floating in it. The pleura of that side was covered by a thin coating of concrete puriform matter, and was

* Ad Acutæ et Chronicæ Splenitidis in humilibus præsertim Italiæ locis consideratæ eidemque succedentium Morborum Historias Animadversiones. Auctore Stanislao Grottanelli, Philosoph. Med. et Chir. Doctore. Florentiæ, 1821. 8vo.

reddish, and had the appearance of being slightly thickened. The corresponding lung was crepitant and void of tubercles. Its pleura adhered to the costal pleura by means of soft recent albuminous bridles; and the lobes were connected in the same manner.

The upper portion of the descending colon and the large end of the stomach adhered closely to the spleen. This organ was twice its ordinary size, and was of a crimson red colour at the margins. The portion of the abdominal peritoneum, corresponding to the posterior splenic surface, was raised by a white, thick, purulent, very fetid liquid, proceeding from the interior substance of the spleen, which was hollowed into a large abscess with purulent-lined walls. The contents had been effused between this serous membrane and the adjoining muscular layer, the vertebral column, and left kidney, and had extended to the crural arch. *

It seems probable that this is an example of suppurative inflammation from the commencement.

In some instances of suppuration or abscess of the spleen, instead of one large abscess, several small ones are observed. These are probably of a more chronic character, and perhaps are indications of the strumous diathesis. A case, in which, in a young woman of 20, the spleen contained two circumscribed abscesses, is given by Dr Tweedie in his Illustrations of Fever. In this case there were ulcers in the intestinal mucous membrane.

Do these collections ever find their way to the surface by means of progressive absorption? Fantoni gives an instance of one which had opened at the navel in a female, and who recovered her health and afterwards bore a child. Five years afterwards she died, and upon inspecting the body after death no trace of spleen was found.

The following case is given by Grottanelli. A Franciscan monk, aged sixty-seven, a sufferer from ague, was attacked, in the autumn of 1812, with pain in the region of the spleen, where was a hard painful swelling. At the end of eighteen days the pain was abated; but there appeared in the abdomen, near the *linea alba*, a considerable convex swelling with fluctuation. Three days after, under the use of anodyne plasters, an opening spontaneously took place; and there was discharged a fluid partaking of the character of steatomatous and albuminous matter. Of this forty-eight ounces were discharged the first day, and as much on each of the three following days. At the end of thirty days the patient was well; the spleen was a little larger than natural, but without pain and un-

---

* Breschèt, Repertoire General d'Anatomie et de Physiologie, Tome vii. p. 115.

easiness. This person lived about two years afterwards. He was again attacked with ague, *œdema* of the feet, and died. *

The external opening is doubtless the most favourable. That into the stomach or colon, when it is followed by purulent vomiting or diarrhœa, is next favourable. That through the diaphragm into the pleura or lungs is much less favourable, and must be considered as peculiarly dangerous. And when the outlet is made within the peritoneum, or without that membrane, it is necessarily and very speedily fatal.

It is necessary to mention, nevertheless, that Grottanelli gives two cases, (IX. § 53, § 56,) in which he states that, notwithstanding this kind of outlet within the peritoneum, recovery took place. In the first, in consequence of a kick on the abdomen, an abscess of the spleen had burst into its cavity ; and though the immediate effects bore all the characters of speedily approaching death, yet, after twenty hours, the patient began to rally, and after voiding a large quantity of urine-like fæces for the space of three weeks, finally recovered, and was seen perfectly well seven years after. In the second, the person received a kick from a horse in the region of the organ ; yet, after diarrhœa and bloody hypostatic urine lasting for many days, he eventually recovered.

4. *Simple or indolent enlargement from vascular distension.* — Almost all authors have noticed enlargement of the spleen, supervening either spontaneously or after ague and other bad fevers. Morgagni relates an instance in which the spleen of a slender woman of twenty-eight, who had undergone chronic fever, occupied the whole of the left side of the belly, and weighed eight pounds and a-half, without change of its interior structure, but apparent dilatation of the vessels and development of its lymphatics ; and Pemberton mentions one weighing three pounds two ounces, yet with perfectly natural structure. Mr Elliot describes one weighing eleven pounds thirteen ounces, with natural structure,† and Bree states it to vary from one to twenty or thirty pounds after ague and chronic diseases of the viscera. The natural weight of the spleen is from nine to fourteen ounces. Baillie remarks, that this simple enlargement with structure perfectly healthy, happens to the spleen more commonly than to any other organ, and regards it rather as a monstrous growth than as actual disease. It appears to me that this is correct only to a certain extent ; and that simple

---

* Ad Acutæ et Chronicæ Splenitidis, &c. Art. V. Hist. XI., quoted by Raikem, but carelessly.

† Med. Com. Vol. XVII. p. 497. Stoll, Ratio Med. i. 163, 251.

enlargement is an incipient morbid state, which will progressively terminate in another morbid state, which is distinguished by less equivocal organic characters. Pemberton formed a just notion of this enlargement or swelling of the splenic substance, when he said it might perhaps arise from a larger quantity of blood being conveyed to it by the arteries, without, however, these arteries taking on that action, which is the essence of inflammation. In short, whatever be the remote cause or the material agent, the disease consists in unusual accumulation of blood in the organ, whether conveyed by arteries or not removed by veins; and if this accumulation continues long, it will, under certain circumstances, render the organ unusually soft. When the capsule, which in such circumstances is very tender, is broken, the substance of the spleen seems to consist of little else than a very soft brownish red mucus, intermixed with a spongy fibrous texture. This softening, as it may be named, appears to be caused by the immense quantity of blood in the vessels, producing a slow but severe disorganization or breaking down of the proper splenic tissue. (See Dr Bree's paper.) Baillie thinks it is hardly to be considered as a disease; but this opinion, I fear, rests on no good foundation. In some circumstances, to be afterwards specified, the structure of the spleen not enlarged is unusually soft, apparently from some cadaverous change; but the true softening of the enlarged organ is effected in the manner represented. *

The symptoms of simply enlarged spleen are not well known. The patient usually complains of a sense of fulness rather than pain in the left side; in some instances pain is felt when the left side is examined or pressed; in others the pain is not perceived in the seat of the spleen, but at the lower part of the left side, inclining towards the back;† and in others, the swelling may proceed to a very large size without causing any uneasiness whatever. In most cases the left hypochondriac region bulges out, and in some the enlargement may be distinctly felt by the hand. The patient can only lie on the left side; the countenance is sallow, but not jaundiced; hemorrhages from the nose take place; and if it continues long, it may cause watery effusion within the peritoneum; (ascites.)

Indolent enlargement of the spleen may terminate in resolution, by subsiding spontaneously or under medical treatment, in softening with emaciation or death, or in induration and incurable dropsy of the belly.

* See note on Cooke's Morgagni, Vol. II. p. 176.   The spleen, a mass of gore.
† Morgagni, lxv. 10.

The causes of indolent enlargement are little known. A long residence in districts infested by intermittent fevers, especially quartans, and repeated attacks, or the prolonged continuance of these disorders, give the spleen a tendency to swell; and the disease is common in fenny and aguish districts, both in this island and on the continent. Thus in Lincolnshire, Essex, Kent, Cambridgeshire, &c. it is not uncommon ; it assumes its most formidable appearance in the department of the lower maritime Alps in France ; in Hungary it is endemial ; and in the Carolinas and other southern states of the American Union, it is rare to find persons who have attained thirty or five and thirty years, without more or less enlargement of the spleen. In some instances the disease succeeds a blow on the hypochondre.

5. *Indurated enlargement of the Spleen.* This is perhaps more common than enlargement with softening ; for every enlarged spleen may in process of time become hardened. In this state the organ may be five or six times its natural size, yet, when divided, presenting its natural structure, only much more dense and compact than natural. This is sometimes considered as scirrhus, but it is unlike to this in other parts of the body, and its real nature is not well understood. It is not improbable that it is the effect of chronic inflammation. It is generally attended with dropsical effusion within the peritoneum. It can seldom be recognised till the disease has made such progress that the enlarged organ is felt externally, when it protrudes the false ribs, and the anterior edge or top of the organ can be felt by the hand applied to the belly under the margin of the ribs. It is sometimes notched. Even in this state the only symptoms are an unhealthy sallow look, wasting of the fleshy parts, and swelling of the belly, dry skin, and at length the usual signs of dropsy of the belly.

The disease is a common effect of residence in aguish districts. According to Grottanelli it is endemial in the territory of Pitigliano and other low districts in Italy.

The size and weight of the spleen, when affected with hypertrophy and induration, are seldom so considerable as when the disease is simple induration. The spleen weighs, then, in this country, from three to seven pounds. In one remarkable case which I have published for other reasons, the indurated spleen weighed seven pounds three ounces and a-half; and in another case which had also been under my care, and in which death took place in the same manner, the spleen weighed seven pounds twelve ounces.

Hypertrophy of the spleen with induration presents occasionally a singular mode of termination.   When the swelling has attained a great size, the patient is attacked rather suddenly with symptoms of inflammatory fever of considerable intensity, accompanied with marked disorder in the circulation of the brain. The skin is hot, the pulse quick, from 100 to 110 ; the face is of a deep-red or brown colour ; the eyes are suffused and injected ; and the patient complains of thirst and pain in some part of the head. The breathing is also a little hurried and oppressed. The symptoms, in short, are very similar to those of *phlebitis*. After this has proceeded for one or two days, delirium comes on, the breathing is more oppressed, and the patient expires.

Upon inspection all the large veins of the chest and abdomen, and the sinuses and veins of the brain are found filled with masses of clotted blood mixed with lymph and purulent matter.   The tunics of the veins, however, are not thickened, nor are the lining membranes roughened.

This result I have seen take place in two cases, both of which were so carefully observed, that no error appears to me to have been committed: The occurrence it is not easy to explain.   All that we can do is to note the fact, that in such cases of splenic disease, a severe lesion is liable to take place with lymphy and purulent deposits in the venous blood of the chest, abdomen, and brain.*

6. *Tubercles* of the spleen or tyromatous bodies are occasionally met with.   The organ is generally enlarged ; and its interior presents disseminated through it a number of whitish-gray or cream-coloured bodies, globular or spheroidal, varying from the size of small peas to that of moderate sized beans.   Their substance is very much like that of tyromatous matter in other parts of the body, that is, a sort of albuminous or caseous matter without organization.   The splenic tissue is at the same time in general a little more consistent than usual.

An important circumstance to be observed is the early period at which tubercles of the spleen may be generated. I have seen them in infancy before the termination of the first year of life. This I observed in the body of an infant in 1832, who had been cut off by intestinal disorder. Tubercular deposits were found also in the lungs.

* Case of Disease of the Spleen, in which death took place in consequence of the presence of purulent matter in the blood.   By David Craigie, M. D., &c., Edin. Med. and Surgical Journal, Vol. LXIV. p. 400.

CHAPTER IX.

SYSTEM OF EXHALANTS, (*Vasa exhalantia.*)—EXHALANT SYSTEM,—
(*Systeme exhalant.*)

SECTION I.

ARE there such vessels as the exhalants described by physiological authors? Is their existence proved by observation or inspection? If not, what are the proofs from which their existence has been inferred?

The existence of minute arteries, the open extremities of which are believed to pour out various fluids in different tissues of the human body, has long been a favourite speculation with physiological anatomists. The decreasing vessels, (*vasculorum continuo decrescentium multi sibique succedentes ordines,*)* and exhalant orifices of Boerhaave, are, or should be known to almost all. Haller ascribes to the skin, membranes of cavities, (*serous membranes,*) ventricles of the brain, the chambers of the eye, the cells of the adipose membrane, the vesicles of the lung, the cavity of the stomach and intestines, an abundant supply of these exhalant arteries or canals, which, according to him, pour out a thin, aqueous, jelly-like fluid, which, in disease, or after death, is converted into a watery fluid susceptible of coagulation. The existence of these vessels, he conceives, is established by the watery exudation which appears in these several parts after a good injection of the arteries.†

As these minute canals, however, through which this injected fluid is believed to percolate, have never been seen, or rendered capable of actual inspection, their existence was denied by Mascagni, who ascribed the phenomena of exhalation to the presence of inorganic porosities in the arterial parietes, through which he imagined the fluids transuded to the membranes or organs, in which

---

* Haller, Elementa, Lib. ii. sect. i. and his Notes on Boerhaave, Prælectiones, Tome II. p. 245.

† " Aqueum humorem de arteriis perinde exhalare, olei terebinthinæ, aliorumve pigmentorum et vivi argenti iter persuadet, quod anatomica manu impulsum, aut omnino vivo in homine a consuetis naturæ viribus eo deductum, in ejus humoris, quam vocant cameram, depluit."—Elementa, Lib. vii. sectio 2, § 1.

they were found. This mechanism, which was equally invisible with the Hallerian, was, for obvious reasons, denied by Bichat, who resolved to reject every opinion not founded on anatomical observation, and to determine the existence of the exhalants by this evidence alone. Obliged, however, to avow the difficulty of forming a distinct idea of a system of vessels, the extreme tenuity of which prevented them from being seen, he undertook to attain his object by what he terms a rigorous train of reasoning.

This consists in nothing more than the effects observed to result from fine and successful injections of watery fluids, or of spirit of turpentine containing some finely levigated colouring matter, from the phenomena of active hemorrhage, which Bichat considers merely as exhalation of blood instead of serous fluid, and from a multitude of considerations which are to be unfolded in the course of further examination of the subject. In this manner he believes himself warranted to conclude, that the only things rigorously ascertained are, 1st, The existence of exhalants; 2d, Their origin in the capillary system of the part in which they are distributed; and, 3d, Their termination on the surfaces of serous and mucous membranes, and the outer surface of the corion or true skin.

The exhalant vessels, the existence, origin, and termination of which he thus proved, he distinguished into three classes. The first contains those exhalants which are concerned in the production of the fluids, which are immediately removed from the body,—the cutaneous and the mucous exhalants. The second contain those exhalants which are employed in the formation of fluids, which, continuing a given time on various membranous surfaces, are believed to be finally taken again into the circulation by means of absorption. And the third class consists of the exhalants concerned in the process of depositing nutritious matter in the different tissues and organs of the human frame. This arrangement is more distinctly seen in the following table.

Exhalants may be
1. Exterior, opening on natural surfaces or canals.   { Cutaneous.
                                                        { Mucous.

2. Interior, opening on membranes, or within cellular   { Serous.
   textures.   { Synovial.
                                                        { Cellular.
                                                        { Medullary.

3. Nutritious.

Each organic tissue is in this system supposed to have its appropriate exhalant arteries, from which it derives the material requisite for its nutrition.

It is undeniable that this arrangement is at once clear, and possesses a sort of interesting regularity, which would prompt the wish, that the existence of these vessels was actually demonstrated with certainty. It is evident, however, that the regularity of arrangement is the only advantage which it possesses over the views of those authors, whose method and opinions Bichat professed not to follow. The existence of exhalants is as little proved in the rigorous reasoning of Bichat, as in the fanciful theories of Boerhaave, the generalizing conclusions of Haller, or the bold supposition of lateral porosities by Mascagni. This defect in his system has therefore been recognised by Magendie and Beclard, the first of whom, though he admits the existence of exhalation as a process of the living body, allows that no explanation of its mechanism or material cause has been given, and asserts that Bichat has created the system of vessels termed exhalants;—while the second thinks that anatomical observation furnishes no evidence of their existence.

The colourless capillaries, he observes, which are admitted by all, and the existence of which is satisfactorily established by the well-known experiment of Bleuland, proves nothing whatever concerning the existence of exhalant vessels; for these colourless arteries are observed to terminate in colourless veins, and there is no proof hitherto adduced of their proceeding further, or terminating by open mouths. He admits that the fact of exhalation in the living body, of nutrition, of transudation by arterial extremities, shows that these extremities possess openings through which the fluids of exhalation, the materials of nutrition, and the matter of injection escape. But whether these openings are found at the point, at which the capillary arteries are continuous with veins, or belong to a distinct order of vessels continued beyond these arteries, is a question which observation has not yet determined, and which it perhaps is unable to determine. Meanwhile, that the existence of a process such as exhalation is believed to be, is carried on in the animal body, appears to be proved by the phenomena of *endosmosis* and *exosmosis*. Such is the present state of knowledge in relation to the existence of exhalant arteries. While the process of exhalation is admitted and believed, we must avow, as Cruikshank did long ago, that we are unable to prove satisfactorily the existence of any set of vessels, or any mechanism by which it might be accomplished.

This difficulty, however, need not prevent us from observing, that this is the proper place for noticing those morbid changes, which are referred to the process of exhalation.

SECTION II.

The exhalations, properly so called, may be morbidly augmented or diminished, or quite changed. ·

1. The best examples of morbid increase of exhalation is conceived to be found in those of the serous membranes, giving rise to the disease termed *dropsy*, (*Hydrops.*) It is most frequent in the peritoneum and in the general cellular membrane ; less so in the pleura and pericardium, and in the arachnoid membrane or its divisions.   In a local form it is very frequent in the vaginal coat of the testicle.   Recent observations on this morbid change, and on the state of the system when under its influence, lead to the conelusion, that it is rarely a primary process, but is generally to be considered as the effect of another,—as the symptom of a peculiar condition of the system of capillary arteries going to the tissue which is the immediate seat of exhalation.

The conditions of the capillary system in which exhalation is preternaturally augmented are referable to two general heads. The first of these is the state of distension which takes place during inflammation, fever, &c.· The second is the distension which results from any mechanical impediment to the free motion of the blood in a venous trunk or trunks, or in the arteries.

α. That the distended or overloaded state of the capillaries which occurs during inflammation may cause a great and disproportionate increase in the fluid exhaled, is established by the phenomena of inflammation of the filamentous tissue, and especially of the serous membranes.   In the former, œdema and anasarca are results by no means unfrequent.   In the latter, one of the first effects of inflammation, under certain circumstances, is effusion of fluid more or less copious, and containing various proportions of coagulable matter.   If the proportion of the latter be great, its coagulation forms organizable lymph, which is the medium of adhesion, while the serous part disappears, apparently by absorption.   If it be small, its coagulation gives rise to mere loose flakes, which, with the constant increase of the quantity of fluid effused, are unable to maintain their attachment to any part of the membrane; while the thin serous part is so copious, that as it is not removed by the veins and lymphatics, it remains in the form of a serous, a sero-sanguine, or a sero-purulent fluid, constituting genuine dropsy. The detailed examination of this morbid accumulation belongs to the chapter on the serous membranes.

That the capillary distension which takes place in fever is a frequent cause of anormal exhalation, is shown by the collections of limpid serum often found in the brain and spinal chord, by that sometimes seen in the pericardium, and by the brownish watery fluid often found in the pleura in the bodies of persons cut off by any of the varieties of that disease.

β. The influence of impediment to the return of the venous blood in the production of extraordinary effusion has been known from the earliest periods of medicine. In proof of this I shall not adduce the experiment of Lower, who by tying the *vena cava* in a dog, produced dropsy in a few hours; for the injury in such a case may produce inflammation of the peritoneum, and consequent effusion; and Hewson has justly objected to its competency, that the ligature might have included lymphatics along with the venous trunk.* Nor is it requisite to notice the experiments of Peyer, Bontekoe, and others. It is sufficient to say, that the fact is established by the effects of deranged circulation, as they take place, *first*, in veins; *secondly*, in arteries; and, *thirdly*, in both sets of vessels jointly, or in the capillary system.

To the first head are to be referred tumours in the vicinity, or affecting the substance of veins; various diseases of the right auriele and right ventricle of the heart; hard disorganization or tubercles of the liver; *cirrhosis* of the liver; hepatization or tubercular disorganization of the lungs; hard disorganization or scirrhus of the pancreas; induration and hypertrophy or tubercles of the spleen; and compression of the ascending *cava* by the gravid womb during the latter stage of pregnancy. Of a more local character are the œdematous swellings which appear in the neighbourhood of tumours and abscesses. Thus in abscess, aneurism, or tumour of the arm-pit, and in scirrhus or cancer of the female breast, the whole arm becomes œdematous from the top of the shoulder to the tip of the fingers. One of the earliest symptoms of lumbar abscess is in some instances an œdematous enlargement of the leg of the side on which the abscess takes place; and almost all deep-

---

* Experimental Inquiries, Part ii. by William Hewson, F.R.S. London, 1774. p. 142.

seated collections of matter give rise to considerable œdema of the superior cellular membrane and skin.

The operation of the several circumstances now mentioned, though well understood by many pathologists, has been happily illustrated by M. Bouillaud, who has shown that in many instances tumours in the neighbourhood of venous trunks compress them so much, as to produce obliteration of their canal. The interior of the vessel is then occupied with a clot of blood, solid, fibrinous, and more or less friable, manifestly produced by the blood being stopped in its course along the vein.* To obstruction of this description M. Bouillaud traced several instances of partial dropsy.

Of the influence of the second cause in producing dropsical effusion, we have examples in that which results from enlargement of the right side of the heart, ossification and contraction of the mitral or semilunar valves, ossification of the coronary arteries, aneurism of the aorta or innominata, or even of the cœliac artery, all of which give rise to more or less serous effusion in the pleura, or a symptomatic dropsy of the chest.

The third condition is perhaps the most common origin of the symptomatic or secondary dropsies. Whatever retards the free circulation of blood through the minute arteries and veins of any organ or texture will produce one or other of the following effects ; viz. inflammation, injection with effusion of red blood, or effusion of serous fluid from the exhalants, according to circumstances. In subjects where the structure of the parts is somewhat lax and yielding, the last will be the most likely result ; and it may be regarded as the mere consequence of the mechanical obstruction which the blood encounters in its transit from the capillary vessels to the larger trunks. " The compression of a vein," it is judiciously remarked by Hewson, " may, by stopping the return of the blood, not only distend the small veins, but the small arteries ; and the exhalants may be so dilated, or so stimulated as to secrete more fluid than they did naturally."† It is in general, however, a remote consequence, and is observed to take place only after the cause of deranged circulation has subsisted for some time. Thus tumours, tubercles, and other foreign growths of the brain give rise to watery effusion within its ventricles. Hepatization and tu-

---

* De l'obliteration des veines et de son influence sur la formation des hydropisies partielles, &c. Par M. Bouillaud. Interne des hopitaux civils de Paris.—Archives Generales de Medecine, Tome II. p. 188.

† Experimental Inquiries, Part ii. &c. p. 142.

bercles of the lungs, chronic inflammation of the bronchial membrane, ossification, cancer, tubercles, and other morbid changes in the pleura, produce a symptomatic water within the chest. And in dysentery, tubercular disease of the peritoneum, and enlargement of the mesenteric glands, (*tabes mesenterica*), symptomatic ascites is a very frequent occurrence.

2. Unusual increase of exhalation may take place in the synovial membranes, either articular or tendinous. In the former case it constitutes one form of disease of the joints, to which perhaps the name of *hydrarthrus* ought to be restricted. To this head also belongs the effusion which takes place in articular rheumatism and in synovial rheumatism. In the latter, inordinate exhalation producing effusion forms the elastic hemispheroidal tumour known under the denomination of *ganglion.*

3. Diminution of exhalation is rare, unless in consequence of an unnatural augmentation of it elsewhere.

4. *Hemorrhage.* The only example of complete change of exhalation is that termed by Bichat *preternatural exhalations,* and the most common of these is when the matter exhaled consists not of the usual watery fluid, but of pure blood, constituting several forms of the disease termed hemorrhage. This bloody exhalation may take place either in the exhalations termed excrementitial, or in those termed recrementitial.

a. To the first head are to be referred those hemorrhages from the skin which are sometimes observed, and those from mucous membranes, which are very frequent, during congestion of their capillary system. In the lungs for example, nothing is more common than exudation of blood from the bronchial membrane during catarrh or bronchial inflammation. In such circumstances it is generally small in quantity, (*hæmoptoe,*) and unlike the copious and irresistible discharge of pulmonary apoplexy.

It is still more distinct in *hæmoptysis,* in which considerable quantities of blood issue from the surface of the bronchial membrane without breach or laceration, and consequently from the orifices of vessels by a process analogous to exhalation. (Bichat.) Is it also by exhalation that the copious discharge of pulmonary apoplexy takes place? On this point facts are wanting.

In hemorrhage from any point of the gastro-intestinal membrane the blood is exhaled in the same manner. The researches of Portal,* and Abernethy† especially, as well as those of Bichat, establish the point as to the stomach and small intestines in *hæmatemesis* and *melæna*. In dysentery the blood, however copious it may appear, oozes from a large extent of the surface of the lower end of the ileum, and from that of the colon, without ulceration or gangrene, and evidently from the vessels of the villous membrane, which during health secrete mucous and intestinal fluid. The same is to be understood of hemorrhages from the rectum, indiscriminately known under the name of *hæmorrhois* and hemorrhoidal discharges, and erroneously supposed to proceed, in all cases, from the hemorrhoidal veins. The true source of many of those bloody discharges is the vessels of the villous membrane of the bowel, which is usually observed to be reddened or embrowned, thickened, softened, and covered with blood-coloured mucus.

In the exhalants of the genito-urinary mucous system the same condition takes place. Hemorrhage from the kidney, unless caused by *calculus*, is the result of exhalation. Menstruation, both in the sound state and when excessive, is equally so. (William Hunter apud Cruikshank,‡ Bichat.)

In all these cases of hemorrhage two conditions of the capillary and exhalant system may be remarked. *First*, In the capillaries an unusual proportion of blood is accumulated, so that the small ones conveying red blood become large and distended, and those conveying the colourless part are injected with red blood. *Secondly*, After this state has continued for some time, red blood is observed to ooze in minute drops from the surface of the membrane, and progressively to increase in quantity and superficial extent.

---

* Mémoires sur la Nature et la Traitement de plusieurs Maladies. Par M. Antoine Portal. Tome II. Paris, 1800, p. 108.

† On the Constitutional Origin and Treatment of Local Diseases. By John Abernethy. London, 1811.

‡ " It happened that a woman died when her menses were flowing. Dr Hunter examined the internal surface of the uterus, found it exceedingly red and loaded with blood ; that the principal redness was from the distended and convoluting arteries. He pressed forward the blood, which was fluid, and which, he asserted, never coagulated, and saw it appear on the surface near the extremities of these arteries. As this discharge happened instantly, and from the gentlest pressure of the finger, it could not be transudation, which always requires time ; it could not be rupture of vessel. I have had several opportunities of repeating this experiment, which always succeeded in the same manner."—The Anatomy of the Absorbing Vessels of the Human Body, by William Cruikshank. London, 1786 and 1790, Chapter xi. p. 55: The same fact has been satisfactorily established by observation in cases of prolapsed or retroverted uterus, when the blood is seen oozing from the villous surface of the organ.

3

The cause of this accumulation and consequent exudation is not known. To assert, as Bichat has done, that a change in the organic sensibility of the exhalants opens a passge through them to are unchanged blood, is to describe the fact in a different mode without explaining its reason. The hemorrhagic effort of Stahl, and the *error loci* of Boerhaave, are equally true and not less intelligible.

β. In the recrementitial exhalants, and first in those of transparent or serous membranes, though less frequently, the same anormal condition may be often recognised. In the pleura or the pericardium, and in the peritoneum, it is not unusual to find bloody fluids of various tints, evidently the result of exhalation. The fluid effused may be simply bloody serum if little blood is exhaled, very red if more is poured forth, or even, as I shall show afterwards, it may be pure blood. In several of the cases in which blood is found in the ventricles of the brain, it cannot be traced to any other source save the exhalants of the choroid plexus; and blood may be shown to be effused occasionally from the outer division of the arachnoid membrane, and also from that which covers the spinal chord.

In each of these cases, whether the fluid is merely sanguinolent or is pure blood, it issues from the same vessels which, in the healthy state of the membrane, prepare its proper secretions. No rupture or breach can be recognised by the most accurate scrutiny. Bichat is disposed to view the sanguinolent effusions as the effect of inflammation, acute or chronic, or like dropsy, as the consequence of organic disease. The few cases hitherto accurately recorded show, that, whatever be the remote cause, the state of the capillaries of the serous membranes is much the same as those of mucous surfaces under similar circumstances.

I formerly spoke of hemorrhage occurring in cellular membrane. The blood is in this case derived from the exhalants of that tissue exactly as it issues from those of the serous membranes. As an active hemorrhage, it is not unfrequent in severe *phlegmon*, and in the bloody abscess, as it is named, with which the practical surgeon is familiar. As a passive hemorrhage, it occurs in land-scurvy and in sea-scurvy.

In some instances the synovial membranes, both in joints and in the tendinous sheaths, are found to contain blood or bloody fluid, which must have issued from their exhalant arteries.

5. *Elephantia.* Another example still of disease to be referred to the head of anormal exhalation, is presented in the unshapely

enlargement of a member, which has been termed elephant-leg, (*Elephantiasts,*) the glandular disease of Barbadoes by Hendy, and which is known in the East under the name of the Cochin-leg. Though most frequently seen in the lower extremity, it is not peculiar to this part ; and authentic instances of its occurrence in the upper extremity are not wanting. Thus, Fabricius Hildanus relates a case of enlargement of the arm, (*brachium monstrosum,*) in a poor woman of Champs d'Or.* Henseler records and delineates an example of the same in the arm of a woman at Ulm ;† and mentions an instance in the arm and leg at once in a woman at Dresden. And an instance not dissimilar in the person of a Hindoo was given not long ago by Mr Kennedy of Madras.‡ According to Dr Graves, it is most frequent in the upper extremity in Ireland.§ Cases of the same kind from Caithness, Ross-shire, and, if I remember right, from the Shetland Islands, are occasionally seen here. The instances in the lower extremity are doubtless most common in tropical countries.

Though it has been the general practice since the time of Hendy to regard this disease as resulting from obstruction of the lymphatic vessels and glands, the phenomena of its formation and progress, with those of its morbid anatomy, show clearly, I think, that the inordinate enlargement arises from a quantity of albuminous or sero-albuminous fluid, being effused from the exhalants into the cellular tissue of the limb, and which is not removed by adequate absorption. That the enlargement is effected in this manner, and that the effusion is the result of some form of the process of inflammation recurring periodically, may be inferred from the following considerations :—

1*st*, In all the cases of the disease which have been accurately observed, the first attack of enlargement is preceded by general inflammatory action affecting the whole limb, described as similar to rose (*erysipelas,*) and distinguished by heat, pain, general swelling, and more or less redness. Of these symptoms the effusion and enlargement are a sort of natural crisis.

2*d*, In most, if not all the cases, this inflammatory attack recurs

---

* Joannis Henseler, Historia Brachii Prætumidi. Extat in Haller Disputat. Chirurgicis, Vol. V. p. 445.

† Centuria IV. Observ. 69, with a good wooden cut.

‡ Case of diseased arm, by Alexander Kennedy, Esq. Edinburgh Medical and Surgical Journal, Vol. XIII. p. 54.

§ Dublin Hospital Reports, Vol. IV. Clinical Observations, by Robert Graves, M. D.

after certain intervals, which are progressively shorter, and always with the effect of increasing the enlargement.

3d, In all the cases in which the enlarged limb has been examined by dissection, the subcutaneous and intermuscular filamentous tissue is hardened, thickened, and condensed, and contains a quantity of granular matter, viscid and gelatinous in consistence, but like fat in appearance. This has not been analyzed ; but little doubt can be entertained that it contains a good proportion of albuminous matter. That this is the essential change, is established by the testimony of many observers. (Jaegerschmidt, Henseler, Kennedy, Graves, Hull.) The distension of the skin, the enlargement of its papillæ, the slender blanched appearance of the muscles, and the enlargement of the inguinal glands, are effects only of the state of the subcutaneous and intermuscular cellular tissue. In short, until new facts be adduced, the description given by Dr Graves, and the case of Mr Hull, establish the inference, that the elephantine enlargement of the extremities is the result of gelatinous or albuminous exudation from the arteries of the subcutaneous filamentous tissue. Dr Musgrave considers it as migratory inflammation.

6. *Accidental Development or Morbid Formation of the Exhalant System.* In several instances a process of exhalation takes place in certain textures in which it did not originally exist, at least under the same form; or a process of exhalation may go on without a corresponding one of removal by absorption. Of this abnormal development of the exhalant system, which constitutes the tumours called encysted, (*tumores cystici, tunicati,* Salzmann, Heister,) several varieties have been noticed by practical authors, as Ingrassias, Severinus, Tagault, Paré, Schelhammer, Astruc, Meek'ren, Heister, &c. ; and the division of Celsus into *meliceris, atheroma,* and *steatoma,* has been repeated by the generality of writers, from Hildanus to Monteggia, Abernethy, and Boyer. This division, to which I have already adverted in speaking of encysted tumours in the cellular tissue, is nevertheless imperfect; and indeed no distinct and connected arrangement of all the varieties of encysted tumour has yet been given, unless the seventh genus of the system of Plenck be entitled to this character.[*] Without attempting to specify the individual defects of the classification of

_____

[*] Josephi Jac. Plenck, Novum Systema Tumorum, quo hi morbi in sua genera et species rediguntur. Viennæ, 1767.

this surgeon, I conceive I am justified in asserting, that one more
strictly pathological may be given.

Considered as examples of inordinate exhalation without corresponding absorption, the species of encysted tumour may be enumerated in the following order.

α. *Acephalo-cysts* or *Hydatids* are cysts secreting limpid watery
fluid. They have been commonly believed to be living animals. And
since the full account of their origin and nature by Laennec, this
opinion has been almost universally received. They therefore do not
properly belong to the present head, and should be arranged with
that of parasitical productions. By Plenck the hydatid is regarded
as a variety of the next species—the *hygroma*. Combined with
atheromatous or steatomatous matter, hydatid-cysts are occasionally
found in the subcutaneous cellular tissue. (Heunden *apud* Tyson,
sixty hydatids in a cyst in the neck.)

β. *Hygroma.* The serous cyst. Cysts secreting sero-purulent,
or even a sero-sanguine fluid. This epithet Plenck applies to a
spherical tumour containing coagulable lymph, evidently meaning
fluid; and regards it as differing from the hydatid in size only,
and from lymphatic (serous) tumours, by the possession of a membranous covering, or proper cyst. It is more expedient to apply
it to all encysted tumours not manifestly hydatoid, which contain
serous, sero-purulent, or viscid glairy fluid, or even reddish serum,
in whatever situation they are found. The best example of this
tumour is the cyst or cysts often found in the female ovary, in
which they vary in size, and in the colour and consistence of their
contents, from mere serum, with more or less albumen, to reddish,
bloody, or even tar-like fluid. They occur in the brain, *e. g.* its hemisphere,[*] and in the pineal gland. The cases delineated by Hooper
as vesicles and encysted tumour, are evidently of this description.
Plenck admits the serous hygroma in the cellular membrane.

γ. *Hæmatoma.* A cyst secreting, or containing a bloody fluid.
Severinus, Ingrassias, and more recently Monteggia, John Peter
Frank, Scarpa, and Montini, mention examples of globular or
spheroidal tumours containing blood more or less fluid within a
membranous sac or covering. Under the name of *bloody abscess*,
indeed, Severinus[†] assembles aneurisms, as well as the blood-cyst.

[*] The Morbid Anatomy of the Human Brain. By Robert Hooper, M.D. Plate
XIII. XII. Fig. 8. and XIV.

[†] Matei Aurelii Severini apud Neapolitanos Medici ac Philosophii Regii, de Abscessuum Recondita Natura, Libri viii. Lugduni Batavorum, 1724. Lib. iv. cap. vii.

Frank, I believe, first (1786) distinguished one of these tumours on the chin of a girl of nine, of the size and shape of a goose-egg, as of the encysted kind, and first applied to it the denomination of *hæmatoma*.* About the same time (1789) Monteggia described the bloody tumour similar to that of Severinus, as occurring in the arm-pit, and attaining a great size, and, when opened, speedily proving fatal.† An example of the disease was afterwards seen by Scarpa in the same situation in the person of a priest about fifty, in the thyroid gland and neck of other subjects, and in the breast of a lady ;‡ and Montini saw it in the thigh of a woman in childbed at Lodi.§

An example of this species of tumour was in 1843 given by the late Dr Hannay of Glasgow. It occurred in the lateral and posterior region of the neck of a child of fourteen months, in other respects healthy. It appeared first on the left side of the neck, half-way between the jaw and collar-bone, in the form of a small hard body about the size of a gooseberry. It remained stationary for months. When seen by Dr Hannay, it had attained the size of a goose's egg, consisted of two or more lobules, was smooth, something glistening, and of a very indistinct shade of blue or venous blood colour. The long diameter was horizontal. It was elastic, and gave a sense of fluctuation ; and touching or handling seemed to cause pain. It was punctured by the lancet, and three ounces of grumous but fluid blood were discharged. After this the cyst seems to have contracted.

Dr Hannay adds, that previous to this he had seen four cases. Of these, one was presented by Mr Brookes to his pupils as a case of abscess ; and some alarm was caused, when the puncture by the lancet was followed by blood apparently pure. Against mistakes of this kind, if not to be obviated, surgeons would be prepared, by informing themselves of the nature of the *hæmatoma* or blood-cyst. Of the other three cases, Dr Hannay had seen two within six months ; one in an infant, the other in a woman between forty and fifty years of age.‖

* Joannis Petri Frank, Med. Clinic. in Ticinensi Academia, Prof. Discursus Academic. mense Junii 1786, habitus, Observationem de Hæmatomate, &c. exhibens-Delectus, Vol. III. Ticini, 1787.

† Monteggia, Fasciculi Pathol. p. 88. Mediolani, 1789.

‡ Treatise on the Anatomy, &c. Appendix, p. 456. See also Richter *de raro tumore mammæ*. Works of Else, and J. E. Pohl de Varice, § XI.

§ Montini, Saggio di Osservazioni et Riflessioni Chirurgico-pratiche. Lodi, 1808.

‖ Pathological Gleanings ; or Cases in Dispensary Practice. By A. J. Hannay, M. D. &c. Edinburgh Medical and Surgical Journal, Vol. LX. p. 319, October 1843.

From the united testimony of these observers, it appears that the blood-cyst (*hæmatoma,*) is a tumour consisting of a membranous sac, the inner surface of which is liberally supplied with blood-vessels, from which blood, or a bloody fluid, is incessantly oozing or distilling by exhalation. In some instances this fluid contains a proportion of fibrin sufficient to effect coagulation ; and the interior of the cyst then resembles the spleen or a mass of clotted blood. From aneurism it may be distinguished by the following marks ; that it does not throb ; that it contains a fluid ; that it is surrounded by bluish tortuous veins ; and that it is dark or purple-coloured, while the investing skin is transparent. When seated in the neck, however, near the carotid artery, it may derive from it, or from the subclavian, a pulsating motion, which may give it the appearance of aneurism.

There is no reason to believe that these tumours are in any way malignant, or •of the character of heterologous growths. They seem to be cysts, the inner surface of which secretes either blood or a bloody liquid for some time, until by their size and position they cause inconvenience. When the fluid has been evacuated, the cyst contracts, its opposite walls adhere, and the action ceases.

The ordinary locality of *hæmatoma* is easily understood from what has been already said. It occurs most usually in the filamentous tissue of the arm-pit and neck, in the substance of the thyroid gland, and at the knee. (Monteggia.) Zeller describes it as it appears in the brain of infants, under the name of *cephalæmatoma.* Dr Hooper has represented an example of what he refers to this head in his tenth engraving. But from the description, the justice of this appears questionable.[*] It is also mentioned by Dr Monro.[†]

δ. *Meliceris.* An indolent tumour, generally small, with smooth uniform surface, communicating a sense of fluctuation, and containing viscid matter of the aspect and consistence of honey. Seated always in the skin or its attached surface, meliceris consists in the enlargement of one of the subcutaneous glands or follicles, arising from obstruction of its excretory duct. The mechanism of its formation from this source was understood by Plenck[‡] and Monteggia,[§] and was, in 1819, brought under notice by Sir Astley

[*] Morbid Anatomy of the Human Brain, p. 27.
[†] Morbid Anatomy of the Brain, p. 56.
[‡] Josephi Jacobi Plenck, Novum Systema, Classis vii.
[§] " Alcuni cisti si formano per la chiusura del orificio escretore dèi follicoli sebacei e mucosi." Instituzioni Chirurgiche di G. B. Monteggia, edizione seconda. Milano, 1813. Vol. II. capo xiii.

Cooper.* It must not be forgotten, however, that it is to this variety only of encysted tumour, that this mode of explanation is applicable. Meliceris is in short the only example of the *folliculated* tumour.

Meliceris may occur in any part of the person where sebaceous follicles exist. When on the scalp, they are distinguished among the older surgeons by peculiar epithets (*talpa et testudo ;*) and *natta* when on the face. In such situations they often contain hair. Those which Severinus mentions at the wrist appear to have been *ganglia;* a mistake which enables us to understand why he doubted whether the meliceris was an encysted tumour.

ε. *Atheroma.* A wen or cyst, indolent, uniform on the surface, firmer than the *meliceris*, of the same colour with the skin, and containing granular semifluid matter like boiled meat or saw-dust. It is always confined to the cellular tissue. The mechanism of its formation is unknown, unless that proposed by Monteggia be admitted. According to this pathologist, the tumour may originate in slight adhesive inflammation of any definite portion of cellular tissue, in consequence of which one cell, being obstructed and prevented from communicating with others, is progressively distended by deposition of matter, which, pressing on the surrounding tissue, gradually condenses it into a membrane as it extends. To this idea objections have been already stated from Bichat; and it must be admitted that facts are still wanting to explain this otherwise than by saying, that the cyst is formed, and secretes its proper contents.

ζ. *Steatoma.* A wen or cyst, containing adipose matter like lard, or fat void of its natural yellow colour, and become white, firm, and granular like suet, (Boyer,) with more or less albumen, approaching to the nature of adipocire. In the first case it is soft, compressible, and generally small, and is not unfrequent in the eyelids and on the scalp. In the second case it is more common on other parts of the body; and the size which it then attains is enormous. In all surgical works almost instances are given of the extraordinary size of steatomatous tumours.† In some instances

* Surgical Essays, by Astley Cooper, F. R. S., and Benjamin Travers, F. R. S. Part II. London, 1819. Essay iii. On Encysted Tumours, p. 220.

† *Vide* Joannes Philip. Ingrassias de Tumoribus. Severini, de Abscessum Natura Recondita, Lib. iii. Cap. xxii. Gulielmi Fabricii Hildani, Opera omnia. Francof. 1646. Gabrielis Fallopii. Op. Lib. de Tumoribus, p. n. c. 24. Fabricii ab Aquapendente, Lib. i. Ambrose Paré, Book vi. c. xix. one of twenty-six pounds. J. Langius ;

osséous matter is deposited either in the cyst, or with the sebaceous matter; a circumstance which has procured it from Plenck a separate place with the title of *osteo-steatoma*.* (Scheuzer, ·Hundtermarc, and Haller.) It is merely a variety of the steatom. The appearance of steatomatous cysts in bones and bony tumours, as seen by Kulm and Weidmann,† belongs to another place.

η. Lipoma. This name was first applied by Littre to a wen or cyst filled with soft matter possessing the usual properties of animal fat.§ The matter of steatom, according to this surgeon, is either not, or imperfectly inflammable, by reason of its degeneration or commixture with some other animal secretion. The propriety of this distinction has been denied by Louis and others, who maintain that these tumours differ in nothing, unless perhaps in degree. It has been favoured, nevertheless, by Morgagni, and adopted by Plenck, Desault, Bichat, and various foreign surgeons, and is defended by Boyer, who represents the steatom as differing from *lipoma*, in the matter being white, firm, and changed from its original character, and in possessing the tendency to degenerate into cancer.‡ Plenck had previously distinguished the lipoma, by being destitute of cyst, a circumstance not required by Littre.

Though thus admitted to differ, the anatomical character, as given by Morgagni,‖ and confirmed by Boyer, is in both nearly the same. A cyst containing unchanged fat, or granular adipose matter, ín cells formed by the original fibres of the adipose membrane, according to Morgagni, or those of the filamentous tissue, according to Boyer. At the base or stalk in the case of pendulous steatoms, the cells are compressed, but loose in the body of the tumour.

—one said to weigh sixty pounds. Papers in Haller's Disputationes Chirurgicæ, Vol. V. by Elsholz, Kell, and Friesse. Fred. Ruysch, Epist. ad Boerhaave. J. Palfyn. Anatomie du Corps Humain, B. ii. chap. ii. Two of great weight, one by Schroeck, from Morgagni in the Ephem. Nat. Curios. Cent. 5. Ob. 27, and others in the same work. In the Phil. Transactions, Mémoires de l'Academie Royale de Chirurgie, &c. Edinburgh Medical Essays, Vol. III. Medical Com. I. 190. Ed. Med. and Surg. Journal, Vol. IX. J. P. Weidmann de Steatomatibus, 4to, Moguntiæ, 1817.

* Breslau Sammlungen, 1722, p. 319. Tittmani Dissert. Osteo-steatomatis, cas. rar. Halleri Opuscula Pathologica, Obs. 6.

† Joan. Adami Kulm, Disputatio Medico-Chirurgica de Exostosi Steatomatode, &c. Haller, Vol. V. p. 653. Weidmann, p. 6, and Fig. 5.

‡ Histoire de l'Academie Royale des Sciences, Anno 1709. Observat. Anatom. 3.

§ Traité des Maladies Chirurgicales, Tome II. Chap. i. Art. 12.

‖ De Sedibus et Causis Morborum, Lib. ix. Epist. I. Art. 24 and 25, and Lib. v. Epist. lxviii. Art. 6 and 8.

This description, with the alleged cancerous tendency, accords more with the characters of the adipose *sarcoma* than those of the genuine wen. Personal examination enables me to say, that, in the case of small steatoms of the scalp, eyelids, face, &c. no fibres of this kind are recognised; and to such if any distinction be adopted, the name of *lipoma* should be confined. In the case of such large steatoms as I have seen in other regions of the body, though the contents are firmly connected together, and some filamentons threads may be seen here and there, or the tumour may be even separable into masses, I have not been able to trace the distinct arrangement of cells mentioned by Morgagni and Boyer. Wiedmann mentions, that in one case the matter of steatom was a sort of liquefied fat, and in another firm and dense, and not divided into lobes or cells.

The chemical history of steatomatous and lipomatous tumours is imperfectly known. Many years ago Dr Bostock analysed a stearoid tumour without obtaining any precise result. The effects of the agents employed indicated the presence of neither fat, jelly, nor adipocire; nor was any change accomplished by potass. From its general intractability, however, and the effects produced by sulphuric acid, he infers that it is composed chiefly of carbonaceous matter.*

I attempted some years ago to examine the chemical nature of the matter contained in a steatomatous cyst removed from the eyelids. This matter was of a lemon yellow colour, not absolutely opaque, yet not translucent, and like a mixture of fat and wax. It communicated a stain to paper, and liquefied on exposure to heat. Though it was perfectly soluble in oil of turpentine, I found that no method which I could devise could make it unite with *potassa*. It was also soluble in ether. From the experiments of Chevreul, it is not improbable that they contain stearine, cetine, or adipocire. But it must be admitted, that precise information is still wanting.

θ. *Lupia.* This term, which has been often applied generally to wens, (*loupes,*) is used in a more limited sense by Plenck, to designate a cyst containing a spongy substance in the cellular tissue, of which it is conceived to be a degenerate form. It is convenient as a head to which certain rare and anomalous cystic tumours may be referred.

* Edin. Med. Journal, Vol. II. p. 14 and 17.

ι. Melanoma. In many instances the melanotic matter, already mentioned, is deposited in a cyst. In such circumstances, therefore, it is referable to this head.

CHAPTER X.

LYMPHATIC SYSTEM, *Vasa Lymphatica,—Vasa Lymphifera,— Lymphæ-Ductus* of GLISSON and JOLYFFE.—SYSTEME ABSORBANT. Die Saugadern.

SECTION I.

IN most situations of the human body, and especially in the vicinity of arterial and venous trunks, there are found long, slender, hollow tubes, pellucid or reddish, which present numerous knots, joints, or swellings in their course, and to which the name of lymphatics or absorbents has been given. It is most expedient to employ the former appellation only, as the latter implies the performance of a function, the reality of which has been much questioned of late years.

Though Eustachius had seen the thoracic duct in the horse, and some slight traces of a knowledge of vascular tubes, different either from arteries or veins, are found in the writings of Nicolaus Massa, Falloppius, and Veslingius, the merit of establishing their existence is generally ascribed to Caspar Asellius, a physician of Pavia. This anatomist, who had, in 1622, seen the white-coloured tubes, then first named *lacteals,* issuing from the intestines of the dog, observed also a cluster of vessels less opaque near the portal eminences of the liver,—an observation which he afterwards repeated in the horse and other quadrupeds. The same vessels were also described and delineated by Highmore.

Passing over the uncertain and obscure hints given by Walaeus and Van Horne, the first exact information after Asellius is that which relates to Olaus Rudbeck, who, in 1650, is said to have seen them in a calf, and to have demonstrated the thoracic duct, and the dilated sac, afterwards termed *receptaculum chyli.*

Glisson informs us that Jolyffe had, in 1652, imparted to him the knowledge of a set of vessels different from arteries and veins; and it appears from the testimony of Wharton, that Jolyffe had demonstrated these vessels in 1650.* In short, the discovery of lymphatics, and the correction of some errors of Asellius, is ascribed to the English anatomist, not only by Wharton and Glisson, but by Charleton, Plott, Wotton, and Boyle.

The existence of these vessels, thus partially demonstrated, was afterwards more fully established by the researches of Bartholin, Pecquet, Bilsius, Nuck, the second Monro and Haller. It is chiefly to the exertions of William Hunter and his pupils, Hewson,† Sheldon,‡ and Cruikshank§ in this country, and to those of Mascagni‖ in Italy, that the anatomical world are indebted for the complete examination and history of this system of vessels.

The lymphatic vessels consist, in the members, of two layers, a superficial and a deep-seated one. The first is situate in the subcutaneous cellular tissue, between the skin and the aponeurotic sheaths, and accompanies the subcutaneous veins, or creeps in the intervals between them. A successful injection of these superficial lymphatics will show an extensive network of mercurial tubes surrounding the whole limb.

The deep-seated layer of lymphatics is found chiefly in the interspaces between the muscles, and along the course of the arterial and venous trunks. In tracing both layers of lymphatics to the upper, fixed, or attached end of the members, we find they increase in volume, and diminish in number. At the connection of the members with the trunk, they are observed to pass through certain spheroidal or spherical bodies, termed lymphatic glands or ganglions. The lymphatics of the upper extremity, after passing through the glands of the arm-pit, terminate in trunks, which open into the subclavio-jugular veins, one on each side of the neck. Those of

* Francisci Glissonii Anatomia Hepatis, Cap. xxxi. Thomæ Wharton, Adenographia, Cap. ii. p. 98.

† Experimental Inquiries, Part the Second. By William Hewson, F. R. S. London, 1774, 8vo. Also the Works of William Hewson, F. R. S. Edited by George Gulliver, F. R. S. By Sydenham Society. London, 1846.

‡ The History of the Absorbent System, &c. by John Sheldon, Surgeon, F.R.S., &c. London, 1784. Folio.

§ The Anatomy of the Absorbing Vessels of the Human Body. By William Cruikshank, London, 1786, 4to. The Second Edition, London, 1790.

‖ Pauli Mascagni Vasorum Lymphaticorum Corporis Humani Historia et Ichnographia, folio, Paris, 1787. See also Prodromo, &c. Capitolo, i.

the lower extremity, after passing through the glands of the groin, proceed with the common iliac vein into the abdomen, where they unite with other lymphatics.

The lymphatics of the trunk consist in like manner of two layers, a subcutaneous and deeper seated one, distributed in the chest between the muscles and pleura, and in the abdomen between the muscles and peritoneum. In the chest and belly, each organ possesses a superficial layer of lymphatics distributed over its surface, and pertaining to its membranous envelope ; the other ramifying through its substance, and pertaining to the peculiar tissue of the organ. This twofold arrangement is most easily seen in the lungs, the heart, the liver, spleen, and kidneys.

In a similar manner are arranged the lymphatics in the external parts of the scull, on the face, where they are very numerous, in the spaces between the muscles, and on the neck, in which they pass through numerous glands. No lymphatics, however, have been found in the brain, the spinal chord, their membranous envelopes, the eye, or the ear.

All the lymphatics hitherto known terminate in two principal trunks. One of these, termed from its site *thoracic duct*, (*Ductus thoracicus* ; die Milch-bruströhre ; *le canal thoracique*) is situate on the left side of the dorsal vertebræ. It receives the lymphatics of the lower extremities, of the belly, and the parts contained in it ; those of great part of the chest, and those of the left side of the head, neck, and trunk, and left upper extremity. The other lymphatic trunk, which is situate on the right side of the upper dorsal vertebræ, is formed by the union of the lymphatics of the right side of the head, neck, right upper extremity, and some of those of the chest. Both of these trunks, it is well known, open into the subclavio-jugular vein of each side.

That lymphatics terminate in branches of the venous system has been asserted on the authority of various observers. Steno, for instance, states that he traced the lymphatics from the right side of the head, the chest, and pectoral extremity in animals into the right axillary vein ; and he gives delineations of anastomotic connections of several lymphatics with the axillary and jugular veins. Similar facts have been reported by Nuck, Richard Hale, Bartholin, and Hartmann. Ruysch traced the lymphatics of the lung into the subclavian and axillary veins ; Drelincourt those of the thymus gland in animals into the subclavians ; and Hebenstreit saw those of the loins pass into the *vena azygos*.

Haller, though unwilling to deny the testimony of these observers, regards it liable to various sources of fallacy, and doubts the direct communication of the lymphatic and venous systems. John F. Meckel, the grandfather, maintained in 1771 the communication, from the circumstance, that he injected the lymphatics from the veins.* Hewson, though not doubting the fact, regards it as an exception to the general rule. Cruikshank, again, states that he never saw a lymphatic vessel inserted into any other red veins than the subclavians and jugulars. The termination remarked by Steno and his successors constitutes in truth the common trunk or lymphatic vein admitted by Cruikshank,—a *thoracic duct* of the right side.

This mode of termination was afterwards in 1821 revived by Tiedemann and Fohman,† who, in the seal, state that the lactiferous vessels communicate with veins arising from the mesenteric glands, and pass thence into the venous trunks without proceeding through the thoracic duct. This, however, was shown by Dr Knox to be a mistake, resulting from the decomposed state of the animals examined by the German anatomists.‡ M. Lauth Junior of Strasbourg, again, conceives that he has demonstrated, that lymphatics communicate with veins within the substance of organs, and in the interior of the lymphatic glands;§ an inference which at present requires further verification. The statements of Lippi of Florence, that every lymphatic almost communicates freely with venous tubes, is still more improbable, and has been rendered exceedingly doubtful by the researches of Rossi;‖ and Panizza shows that there is no communication between the minute arteries and the lymphatics.

The connections of the ends of lymphatics with the organs and tissues from which they arise, termed their *origins*, are completely unknown. In some favourable instances the lymphatics of the intestinal canal are so filled with a reddish or whitish fluid after the process of digestion has continued for some time, that not only are their larger branches easily seen, but by the aid of the miscroscope

---

* Jo. Fr. Meckel, Nova Experimenta et Observationes de finibus Venarum ac Vasorum lymphaticorum, &c. § I. p. 4.   Lugduni Bat. 1772.   8vo.

† Anatomische Untersuchungen uber die Verbindung der Saugadern mit den Venen. Heidelberg, 1821.

‡ On the Anatomy of the Lacteal System in the Seal. Edin. Med. and Surgical Journal, Vol. XXII. p. 25, &c.

§ Essai sur les Vaisseaux Lymphatiques. Strasbourg, 1824.

‖ Cenni sulla comunicazione dei vasi linfatici colle vene ; di Giovanni Rossi Doctore, &c.   Annali Universali di Medecina, Anno 1826. Vol. XXXVII. p. 52.

some of the smaller may be traced to their commencement. This, which was ascertained by Cruikshank, (p. 55 and 58,) and confirmed by Hewson, Bleuland, and Hedwig, has been contradicted by the observations of Rudolphi and Albert Meckel. In all other parts, however, though a successful injection may show the course and distribution of many of the smallest lymphatics, yet no orifices are perceptible at the point at which they seem to stop, and we are uncertain whether these points are their origins. (Cruikshank.) Mere observation is here as unavailing as in regard to the termination of exhalants. The continuation of lymphatics with arteries, unless in the case of those which arise from the interior of arterial tubes, (Lauth,) is not satisfactorily established. It has been conjectured, however, that their ends or imperceptible origins are connected to the tissues to which they are traced, and that the lymphatics arise in this manner from these tissues.

The lymphatics are distinguished by being in general cylindrical in figure, and by varying in calibre at short spaces. In this respect they differ from the arteries and veins. It has been further justly remarked by Gordon, that the middle-sized lymphatics are remarkably distinguished from the corresponding parts of the arterial and venous system by three peculiarities. 1st, When two lymphatics unite to form a third, the trunk thus formed is seldom or never larger than either of them separately; 2d, their anastomoses with each other are continual; and, 3d, they seldom go a great space without first dividing into branches, and then reuniting into trunks.*

The outer surface of a lymphatic is filamentous and rough, the inner smooth and polished, like that of small veins. It is impossible to observe the structure of these tubes in the middle-sized, or even in the large lymphatics; and anatomists have generally been satisfied with supposing that the structure of all of them is similar to that of the thoracic duct, or some other large vessels equally susceptible of examination. According to the observations of Cruikshank, (Chap. xii.) which have been verified by Bichat, the thoracic duct presents, 1st, a layer of dense firm filamentous or cellular tissue, exactly similar to that found inclosing arterial and venous tubes, which the latter regards as foreign to the vessel, but giving it a great degree of support and protection; 2d, a proper membrane, delicate, transparent, and moistened inside by an unctu-

---

* System. p. 71.

ous fluid, which he seems inclined to ascribe to transudation. Muscular fibres, of which Sheldon speaks positively, Cruikshank represents, though seen in some instances, (Chap. xii.) yet to be more generally not demonstrable. Their existence, though admitted by Schreger and Soemmering, is denied by Mascagni, Rudolphi, and J. F. Meckel, and I, may add, by Bichat and Beclard. This account differs not much from that of Dr Gordon, who could not recognize distinctly more than one coat, similar to the inner coat of veins. The filamentous layer noticed by Bichat, and considered by Mascagni as an external coat, is of course excluded.

The knotted or jointed appearance of lymphatics is occasioned chiefly by short membranous folds in their cavity called *valves*. These folds are thinner than the venous valves; but they are equally strong, and have the same shape and mode of attachment to the inside of the vessel. They are generally found in pairs, but never three at the same point. A single valve is sometimes found at the junction of a large branch with a trunk, or of a trunk with a vein. According to Cruikshank there is considerable variety in the distribution of valves; but in general a pair of valves will be found at every one-twentieth of an inch in lymphatics of middling size. In the larger lymphatics they are less numerous than in the small. The structure of these valvular folds is as little known as that of the inner membrane, of which they appear to be prolongations. According to Mascagni they sometimes contain a small portion of fine adipose substance.

The tissue which forms the lymphatic tubes is strong, dense, and resisting ; and, from the weight of mercury which they bear without rupture, it has been generally concluded, that they are stronger in proportion to their size than veins. This tissue also possesses considerable elasticity.

The opposite states of lymphatics during digestion and after long fasting, and the phenomena of mercurial injections, prove that the tissue of which they consist is distensible and contractile. Though it does not exhibit appearances of muscular structure, it has been long supposed to be endowed with a property analogous to irritability. Such is the inference which Hunter, Hewson, Crnikshank, and others have derived from various phenomena in the living and recently dead tissue.

Though Bichat doubted what he termed organic sensible contractility, yet he admitted the insensible contractility as necessary to the functions ascribed to lymphatics. Previous to his time

o

Schreger, in different experiments, observed the first of these qualities in consequence of the application not only of acids, butter of
antimony, and alcohol, but even of hot water and cold air.   Similar contractions and relaxations have been induced by mechanical
irritation.* Such phenomena are observed not only during life,
but even after death ; and if we add to this, that the thoracic duct
is often after death large and flaccid, though empty, but in the living body is almost always contracted and scarcely visible, and that
a portion of it included between two ligatures and punctured,
quickly expels its contents, it may be inferred, according to Tiedemann and Beclard, that the lymphatic tissue possesses a considerable
degree of this vital or organic property.

SECTION II.

The lymphatic vessels have been supposed to perform an important part in the formation of the diseases incident to the animal
body.   In addition to the ordinary causes of disease which affect
all organic substances, the several derangements of property or
function to which they are liable have been supposed to exert a
powerful influence on other tissues and organs, and on their functions.   On this principle Hewson, Cruikshank, Thomas White,
Nudow, Isenflamm, Johnstone, and Maanen, have ascribed to different forms and degrees of disorder of the lymphatic system a very
large proportion of the diseases incident to the human body.   All
of these authors, nevertheless, have been exceeded by Soemmering,
and more recently by Alard, both of whom represent the lymphatics as mainly concerned in every morbid state of the human
body.   The former has delineated an extensive picture of diseases,
in the production of which the lymphatics are believed to be more
or less concerned.   Besides immediate morbid states of the lymphatics themselves, he enumerates upwards of sixty diseases and
morbid states of the human body, in which, according to one or
another pathologist, the lymphatics have an influence, direct or
indirect, immediate or remote.† The latter reasons most strenuously for the universal influence of the lymphatic system in every
disease almost of the animal frame.

* Schreger de Irritabilitate Vas. Lymph. Lips. 1789.
† S. Thomæ Soemmering de Morbis Vasorum Absorbentium Corporis Humani sive
Dissertationis quæ prœmium retulit Societatis Rheno-Trajectinæ, anno 1794, Pars
Pathologica. Trajecti ad Mœnum, 1795. 8vo.

Little doubt can be entertained, that by these authors the influence of the lymphatic vessels has been very much overrated. Notwithstanding the authority of their names, it is certain that neither anatomical inspection, nor the observation of the phenomena and effects ·of disease, justify the views advanced by these authors. It further requires little argument to show, that this mode of explaining the formation and nature of diseases does not tend to the advancement of accurate pathological knowledge.

All the diseases to be referred to this head come naturally under two divisions. The first consists of disordered states occurring in the lymphatic vessels themselves. In the second are included morbid states of other textures or systems, arising immediately from disease of the lymphatics.

1. *Inflammation,* — (*Angioleucitis.*) The first morbid state to be mentioned as incident to the lymphatics is inflammation. As a spontaneous occurrence it is little known, and perhaps is exceedingly rare. Hendy, indeed, undertook to show, that inflammation of the lymphatics was the pathological cause of Barbadoes leg;* and this view, which has been almost implicitly adopted by every subsequent observer, has been strenuously maintained and illustrated by M. Alard.† I have already adduced such facts and arguments as I conceive are sufficient to show that this disease depends on a peculiar inflammation of the filamentous tissue of the limb, recurring periodically, and terminating in albuminous exudation; and that the affection of the lymphatic glands, vessels, &c. on which the hypothesis of Dr Hendy is founded, is an effect of this diseased state. It is unnecessary, therefore, to give the subject more consideration.

Not less objectionable is the notion advanced by Charles White,‡ that inflammation or obstruction of the lymphatics is the cause of the swelled leg, (*phlegmasia dolens,*) of puerperal women. Observation and dissection concur in showing that this malady arises from inflammation of the uterine and pelvic veins terminating in albuminous or sero-albuminous exudation, and causing obstruction to the venous circulation.

Angioleucitis Uterina puerperarum. Inflammation has been

* Treatise on the Glandular Disease of Barbadoes, proving it to be seated in the Lymphatic System. By John Hendy. London, 1784.

† Histoire d'une Maladie particulière au Systeme Lymphatique, &c. 1806 ; et Nouvelles Observations sur l'Elephantiasis des Arabes. Par M. Alard, 1811.

‡ Inquiry into the Nature and Cause of that Swelling in one or both of the Lower Extremities in Lying-in-Women. By Charles White, Surgeon. Warrington, 1784.

observed to attack the lymphatic vessels of the womb in puerperal fever, and then it too often proceeds to suppuration. The uterine lymphatics are then seen extending over the surface of the organ jointed and knotted, and distinctly presenting purulent matter in their interior, and sometimes along their exterior. Tonellé found among 222 fatal cases of puerperal fever, that in 32 purulent matter was contained in the lymphatics.* This shows that in about one-seventh of the cases of puerperal fever, inflammation and suppuration of the lymphatics may take place. This doctrine has been forcibly illustrated by Cruveilhier.†

Inflammation of lymphatic vessels may almost invariably be traced to irritation, or an irritating cause at their organic extremities. Thus a sore in the finger or hand, whitloe, or other inflamed states of the fingers, are often attended with painful red streaks or lines, extending up the arm to the arm-pit. These red streaks indicate inflammation of the subcutaneous lymphatics. In like manner I have seen a blister applied to the surface of the belly cause inflammation of the lymphatics leading to the inguinal glands.

The inflammation when not violent terminates in resolution. In more severe cases it may cause effusion of lymph into the cavity of the vessel, so as to effect adhesion and obliterate its canal. This was probably the cause of the obstruction which Mascagni states he found in the lymphatics of several subjects after the use of blisters. Suppuration, as a consequence of inflammation of lymphatics, is little known.

2. *Wounds* of lymphatics must occur frequently. In truth, scarcely an incision dividing the skin and cellular membrane can fail to involve several lymphatics, and every deep incision divides many of them.‡ They appear to unite easily. Is the cavity obliterated? The frequent anastomoses render this event of no consequence. Hewson observed that in several instances lymphy coagulable fluid continued to ooze from the wounded vessel for days.

3. *Cirsus* (Κιϱσος) *or Varicose Dilatation.* This name is applied by Meckel to denote a dilated state of lymphatics similar to varix in veins. Schreger and Tilesius delineate what they conceive to be varix in the lymphatics of the conjunctiva ; Mascagni repre-

---

* Des Fievres Puerperales observées a la Maternite de Paris pendant l'année 1829. Par M. Tonellé, Archives Generales, XXII. p. 345.

† Anatomie Pathologique.

‡ Monro in Edin. Medical Essays, Vol. V. Art. xxvii.

sents the same condition in those of the lungs; and Soemmering describes those of the intestines as varicose in hernia. The same condition was observed by Bichat in the lymphatics of serous membranes. In dropsical subjects they are always much distended with fluid; and hence the anatomist finds their demonstration much more easy in such circumstances.

4. *Rupture* of the lymphatics has been assumed as a probable **cause** of consumption by Morton, of scrofula in general by Ackerman, of Barbadoes leg by Hendy, of puerperal swelled leg by White, of dropsy by Van Swieten, Haase,[*] Assalini,[†] Metzler,[‡] and Soemmering,[§] and of white swelling of the joints by Brambilla.[||] Yet in neither of these diseases has the existence of rupture of the lymphatics been demonstrated; nor has the accident been shown to be one of ordinary frequency. Baillie admits that the thoracic duct may have been ruptured. But Guiffart is the only person who is said to have seen this accident in the person of a boy of fourteen.[¶]

5. *Dilatation with Obstruction.* Soemmering repeatedly found the lacteals of the small intestines near the duodenum filled and distended with a thick curdy matter like soft cheese. Of the same deposition in the lacteals of the jejunum with much induration, Walter delineates an example in a man of about thirty. Edward Sandifort represents the lacteals in an infant of a few weeks much thickened, approaching to varicose, with swelled mesenteric glands.[**] And Ludwig saw them in a similar state in a girl of seven, with induration of these glands.

6. *Osseous Deposition.* Callous hardness, with osseous matter, was seen in the coats of the lymphatics in the pelvis by Mascagni, Cruikshank, and Walter found them ossified, and of stony hardness. The thoracic duct was found filled with caseous or tyromatous matter by Poncy, all the neighbouring glands, both thoracic and mesenteric, being enlarged and tyromatous;[††] and with earthy

[*] J. Gottl. Haasius de Vasis Cutis, &c. Absorbentibus. Leip. 1786.

[†] Essai Medical sur les Vaisseaux Lymphatiques, &c. p. 56.

[‡] Dissertatio de Hydrope, &c. p. 23.

[§] De Morbis Vasorum Absorbentium, p. 132.

[||] Acta Acad. Medico-Chirurg. Militaris Viennensis, Tome I. p. 16.

[¶] Apud Bartholini Opuscula nova de vasis Lymphaticis, &c. Hafniæ, 1670.

[**] Observation. Anatom. Pathologic. Lib. ii. cap. 8.

[††] Nouveau Recueil D'Observations Chirurgicales Faites par M. Saviard. A. Maitre-Chirurgien de l'Hotel Dieu et Jeuré à Paris. Paris, 1702. Obs. CXI. p. 500.

or osseous matter by Assalini.* Cheston found it obstructed with a solid substance resembling calcareous matter ;† Bayford found it much obstructed by the pressure of an aneurismal tumour ;‡ and Scherb is said to have met with an actual concretion.§ All these phenomena, excepting that of the aneurismal tumour, are the effects of strumous disorder.

The lymphatics have been long supposed to be the agents concerned in the formation of king's evil, (*struma, scrofula*,) and in the development of the disease when latent. What are the proofs of this opinion? Have the lymphatics been actually found disorganized in cases of strumous disease, and does scrofula never take place without traces of this disorganization? Do they act as the cause, or do they partake in the effects of another morbific agent more general in operation? In answering these questions much will depend upon the meaning attached to the term scrofula. If this be a disease appearing in the lymphatic glands only, there may be some ground for the opinion. But to assemble the numerous disorders termed *strumous*, under the head of the lymphatics, implies conclusions which are not supported by anatomical facts.

It seems more natural and more consistent with the known phenomena of diseased action, to place the *genesis* of *struma*, whatever that may be, in the process of digestion, in the lacteal vessels that arise from the *jejunum*, and in the blood of the small capillary vessels generally. From what is most generally observed, the process of arterialization in the lungs appears to be defective.

Since the arguments which have been adduced against the absorbent power of the lymphatic vessels by Mayer, Magendie, and others, their influence either in the production of dropsy, or in removing it, seems to be very doubtful.

How far can they be admitted to explain the process of ulcerative absorption so ingeniously contrived and ably maintained by John Hunter? and what share can they be supposed to possess in the removal of other matters, either proper or foreign to the system, as that pathologist believed? Upon these questions accurate facts are still wanting.

* Essai Medical sur les Vaisseaux Lymphatiques, &c. Par Paolo Assalini. Turin, 1787-8.

† Philosophical Transactions, Vol. LXX. 1780. And Pathological Inquiries ; and Observations on Surgery, from the Dissections of Morbid Bodies ; with an Appendix containing three Cases on different subjects. By Richard Browne Cheston, Surgeon to the Gloucester Infirmary. 4to. Gloucester, 1766.

‡ Medical Observations and Inquiries, Vol. III. p. 18.

§ Apud Haller, Dissertation. Patholog.

CHAPTER XI.

LYMPHATIC GLAND OR GANGLION, KERNEL.—(*Glandulæ Lym
phaticæ,—Glandulæ Conglobatæ.*—Die Saugader-Dreusen.)

·SECTION I.

THIS is the proper place to consider the structure of those bodies
which are in common language termed *kernels*, to which anatomists
have applied the name of *lymphatic glands*, and the French anatomists have more recently given that of lymphatic ganglions. The
general appearance, figure, and usual situation of these bodies, are
well known and described in the common treatises on anatomy. In
general they are spheroidal, seldom quite globular, and most commonly their shape is that of a flattened spheroid. In different subjects, and in subjects at different ages, they vary from two or three
lines to an inch in diameter. The medium rate is about half an
inch. Their surface is smooth; their colour grayish-pink, sometimes pale red, bluish, or of a peach-blossom tinge,—varieties which
seem to depend on degrees of bloody transudation; for when washed and slightly macerated, they assume the gray or whitish-blue
colour. In a few instances they are jet black,—a peculiarity
which seems to depend on a degree of black infiltration, or on the
incipient stage of that change which has been termed *melanosis*, or
melanotic deposition. The idea that it may be derived from the
carbonaceous matter suspended in the atmosphere of great cities,
has been shown by Cruikshank to be absurd. Its anatomical possibility may be justly questioned.

They are always situate in the celluloso-adipose tissue found in
the flexures of the joints. They are found in small number at the
bend of the ham, and that of the elbow; they are more numerous
in the arm-pit and groin; in considerable number in the cellular
tissue of the lumbar region, before the *psoas* and *iliacus* muscles;
and they are most abundant round the neck. The posterior mediastinum, and the cellular tissue between the mesentery and vertebral column, abounds with lymphatic glands mutually connected
in clusters.

Each gland may be said to consist of a peculiar substance, in closed in a thin membrane like a capsule. The capsule is a thin pellucid colourless substance, which is resolved by maceration into fine whitish fibres. It is very vascular; and Mascagni appears to have detected absorbents in it. It is connected to the proper sub-stance by fine filamentous or cellular tissue. The capsule is con-sidered by Beclard as a fibro-cellular membrane. The proper sub-stance of lymphatic glands consists of a homogeneous pulp, in which injections have shown numerous ramifications of minute ves-sels. As these vessels are injected from the lymphatics which are seen to enter the body of the gland, they are believed to be conti-nuous with them, and to be lymphatics arranged in a peculiar man-ner. These vessels are of two kinds, one entering the gland called *vasa afferentia or inferentia*, entrant lymphatics; the other quitting is called *vasa efferentia*, egredient lymphatics. This distinction is founded on the direction of the valves. In the *vasa inferentia* the free margins of the valves are turned toward the gland; in the *vasa efferentia* they are turned from it.

The number of entrant lymphatics varies from one to thirty, and, what is more remarkable, almost never corresponds with that of the egredient lymphatics, which are in general much fewer. Cruik-shank says he has injected fourteen entrant lymphatics to one gland, to which only one egredient vessel corresponded. When the en-trant lymphatic reaches the gland it splits into many radiated branches, which immediately sink into its substance. The egredi-ent lymphatics are generally larger than the entrants.

The arrangement of these vessels in the interior of the glands is best described by Mascagni, whose observations are confirmed by Gordon. To see this well, it is requisite to inject the entrant lym-phatics of two glands in two different modes; one with mercury, the other with wax, glue, or gypsum. After a successful mercu-rial injection, the entrants are seen, before sinking in the gland, to divide into two orders of branches. One of them, which belongs chiefly to the surface or circumference of the gland, consists of large vessels, bent, convoluted, and interwoven in every direction, communicating with each other, and swelling out into dilated cells at certain parts, and of smaller vessels, which form a minute net-work on the surface, and which seem to terminate in the cells or distended parts of the larger vessels.

From these distended parts or cells, again, arise many minute vessels, which, after winding about on the surface of the gland, unite gradually, and form the egredient vessels of the gland.

The wax, glue, or gypsum injection is employed to show the deep-seated or central vessels of the gland. The distribution of these is found to be quite the same as that of the superficial vessels. The cells delineated by Cruikshank, I am disposed to regard as mere dilated parts of the lymphatic vessels which constitute the intimate structure of the gland.

These minute tubes are connected by delicate filamentous tissue, which is more abundant in early life than afterwards.

Injections show the existence of blood-vessels, which accompany the convolutions of the lymphatics in the glands. But no nerves have been found either in the glands or their capsules.

The white matter described by Haller and Bichat is not contained in the cellular substance, but in the cells of the lymphatic vessels themselves.

SECTION II.

1. α. The lymphatic glands as organized bodies, may be supposed to be liable to ordinary inflammation. Yet on this subject no very precise facts are given. The swelling called *bubo*, (βουβων, Hippocrates) appears to be in most cases inflammation of the capsule and surrounding cellular substance.

β. *Adenosis.* ¯ *Strumous Inflammation.* The glands, however, appear to be liable to a slow chronic inflammation, which does not readily suppurate, and which, when it does suppurate, always forms a bad and tedious disease. They are believed to be often affected in scrofulous subjects; and the definition of the *evil* (*struma, scrofula, les ecrouelles,*) has been directly taken from this pnenomenon. In such affections these bodies undoubtedly become the seat of a slow inflammatory action, which is attended with gradual enlargement, without much pain or change of colour in the integuments. At length, the gland is found to become softer than it had been, and an opening takes place in the skin, through which a fluid is discharged, not homogeneous, but in general consisting of a thin serous water, in which thicker pieces like curd are mixed. This fluid, which is generally most completely formed in suppuration of the lymphatic glands, is what has been termed scrofulous, or strumous matter. Simple strumous enlargement in these glands may proceed to such an extent as to interfere with, and even impede the functions of important organs. In those of the neck they have, by compressing the windpipe, caused fatal suffocation. (Soemmering and others.) Bleuland saw them in an infant impede deglutition by pressing the œsophagus, *

γ. *Adenitis. Irritative Enlargement.* The lymphatic glands are liable to become painful and enlarged, in consequence of causes not originally resident in themselves. A sore or wound, especially if punctured or lacerated, on the hand or foot, may be succeeded in a few days by an enlarged painful swelling of one or more glands in the arm-pit or groin. A wound of the scalp may be followed by a glandular swelling of the neck; and a spoilt tooth, or a sore of the mouth, will often give rise to a painful enlargement of the glands under the jaw. I have repeatedly seen a whole chain of them enlarge, and continue so for months, in consequence of the use of mercury carried to salivation, and especially after enlargement and ulceration of the muciparous follicles of the ileum, whether isolated or aggregated. It is particularly to be observed, that when these follicles of the aggregated glands become prominent and swelled, or affected by ulceration, which usually takes place towards the lower end of the ileum, then the mesenteric glands opposite and corresponding to these intestinal follicles become enlarged and swelled often to a great degree. The enlargement and swelling seem at first to be simple enlargement of the glandular parenchyma; but after some time this appears to contain a new deposit, which appears to be what I have called tyromatous matter. The tracheo-bronchial glands become enlarged in inflammation of the bronchial membrane of the pulmonic tissue, and other diseases of the lungs; and those of the mesentery increase in consequence of disease of the intestinal canal. In such instances it is obvious that irritation at the organic end of the lymphatics is the cause of morbid action in the glands, at the glandular end of these vessels.

In other instances, for example, when a sore on the penis is followed by enlargement of the inguinal glands, or a cancerous breast is attended with swelling and pain of the axillary glands, it has been concluded, that, as the primary diseases depend on a peculiar or *specific action,* as it was termed, peculiar matter is absorbed, and conveyed to the gland, in which it gives rise to the morbid changes. We now know that it is unnecessary, in the majority of cases, to suppose absorption, which indeed is rendered very doubtful; and

---

* Observationes de sano et morbosa Œsophagi Structura. Lugdun. Bat. 1785.

it is sufficient to ascribe the glandular enlargement in such instances to mere irritation at the organic ends of the lymphatics.

2. *Enlargement from the Operation of Poisonous Matter. Pestilential Bubo.* In plague the glands of the arm-pit and of the groin generally become enlarged as the disease advances. The period at which this takes place is uncertain, but seems to vary from the first twenty-four hours to the seventh or eighth day. (Russel, de Mertens, Orraeus, &c.) This enlargement, which soon proceeds to a bad open sore, accompanied with sloughing and the discharge of foul, dirty-coloured fluid, has been generally ascribed to the absorption of the pestilential poison, and its direct operation on the glandular system. This is probably in general the true account of the pestilential bubo. As, however, they are almost invariably accompanied with carbuncles, it is not unlikely that in some instances the bubo may be the result of irritation from the presence of a carbuncle.

3. *Enlargement with Death of the Glandular Tissue. a. Strumous Mortified Bubo.* Of strumous bubo there are many varieties well known to the practical surgeon. To this head, however, I refer a peculiar disease which I have seen in the glands at the bend of the arm. The glands become enlarged, painful, and hard; and, notwithstanding all efforts to procure resolution, the skin first gives way, chiefly by sloughing, and matter with some membranous shreds is discharged. A sore of a peculiar character is formed. Its edges consist of skin cut very sharp, and notched or serrated, as it were, into angular slips. From these margins the sore descends deep and rather foul to an ash-coloured, solid, convexly-rounded body, which is evidently a diseased gland. Round this the process of suppuration and ulceration proceeds, with the occasional discharge of sloughs, till the gland is expelled either in fragments or in a mass. After which the hollow is filled with granulations, and cicatrization is easily effected.

This process is attended with pain at first in the skin chiefly, but afterwards it seems to cause no more uneasiness than an ordinary abscess. Its duration varies according to the size and number of the glands to be ejected. In the most distinct cases which I have seen, it occupied between three and four months. This disorder I regard as arising from a gland being suddenly smitten, as it were, with death in its intimate structure, from previous disease of its membranous capsule and proper vessels. I have seen it only in those at the bend of the arm; and to Cruikshank it appears to have occurred in the same situation.* It may occur, however, and probably has been seen by others elsewhere.

β. *Phagedenic Bubo.* Seen principally in the inguinal glands in persons labouring under the operation of the syphilitic poison, or who have been subjected to repeated courses of mercurial medicines. The skin first becomes hard, painful, hot, and dull red, with circumscribed edge, but diffusely swelled. The transition to a dirty grayish-brown indicates that the skin has become dead; and the process of ulceration, alternating with sloughing, is established. As the skin, and successively the cellular tissue, are thrown off in this manner, one, two, or more glands come into view, somewhat swelled, and of a brownish-red colour, but equally distinct as if they had been carefully dissected. The surface of the sore is generally a deep-red brown, covered with a foul blood-coloured serous fluid, without appearance of granulations, and with the sensation of burning or searing pain. The process of sloughing proceeds in the cellular tissue, while the gland or glands remain as so many brownish masses, with small marks of vitality, until they are detached entirely from the cellular substance, in which they are imbedded, and are thrown off dead. In effecting this object, the process of sloughing may proceed to such extremity as to affect first the superincumbent cellular coat, and next the sheath of the femoral artery, which, in such circumstances, inevitably gives way; and the patient is suddenly destroyed by hemorrhage. An instance of this accident in a soldier of the guards used to be mentioned by Dr Hunter.† In a case which occurred some years ago in the military hospital of the Castle, it was deemed requisite to avert the impending danger by tying the femoral artery. Subsequent gangrene of the foot and leg, however, rendered amputation indispensable; and recovery at length took place.

In more favourable circumstances, after great destruction of parts, and the expulsion of one, two, or more mortified glands, the phagedenic action stops spontaneously, granulation takes place, and the sore is gradually healed.

I have described the progress and phenomena of this disease, as I have witnessed them in several instances which have fallen under

* " I have known the last mentioned glands (the brachial) die, and slough out in scrofula without any great inconvenience."—The Anatomy of the Absorbing Vessels, p. 132.

† The Anatomy of the Absorbing Vessels, p. 122, p. 134, second edition.

my observation. It appears that the active symptoms manifest themselves first in the skin and cellular membrane; and it may therefore be thought that the disease belongs properly to these tissues. Their affection, nevertheless, is so far as can be determined, the result of the previous state of the glands, which appear to be directly killed either by the syphilitic poison, or the mercurial action, and thus to give rise to the violent process of disorganization, which then takes place in the skin and cellular membrane.

Enlargement of the mesenteric glands has been supposed by most authors to be the anatomical characters of the disease termed mesenteric wasting—(*Tabes mesenterica. Tabes glandularis.* Wharton, Baglivi, Richard Russell.) Without absolutely denying this, I shall afterwards show, that, in most instances of that disease, the enlargement of the glands is secondary to some morbid state either of the intestinal villous membrane, the muciparous follicles, or of some of the intestinal tissues.

4. *Enlargement and Induration.* (*Vascular Sarcoma.*) Either after repeated attacks of inflammation, alternating with resolution, or with a slow and indistinct form of the disease, a gland, or a cluster of glands gradually enlarges, and, resisting all means of resolution, becomes unusually hard. This continues, or is liable to slight occasional aggravations, with dull pain in the substance, or in the neighbourhood of the gland. Though such enlargement may be termed *strumous*, and may have originated in what is termed strumous action, the structure of the gland or glands is so much changed as not to be distinguished from *vascular sarcoma.* A tumour of this kind, when divided, presents a firm homogeneous substance of a bluish-gray colour, somewhat elastic and compressible, traversed with more or fewer vessels which may be injected from the neighbouring arteries, and consisting in its intimate structure of amorphous granular masses united by dense filamentous tissue. The great hardness, and the malignant tendency of this growth, have procured for it from most authors the ominous names of *scirrhus* and *cancer.* Though correct enough for all practical purposes, these epithets are not justified by the anatomical characters.

Sarcomatous enlargement may occur in any of the lymphatic glands. It is frequent in those of the neck, and may often be traced to strumous inflammation, or to the irritation of spoiled teeth. Cruikshank mentions an instance in which the tracheo-bronchial lymphatic glands were affected with this morbid change to such extent as to cause fatal suffocation.* In the internal iliac glands it is not uncommon, so as to form large indurated masses; and in the female may operate as a cause of difficult parturitipn equally fatal to the mother and the infant. (Hunter *apud* Cruikshank.)† The same disease occurs in the mesentery either primarily, or in consequence of ulceration of the intestines.

5. *Tyroma glandularum. Tyromatous deposition. Tubercular deposition.* The lymphatic glands are liable to become the seat of a deposit of matter different in all appearances from their own tissue. The gland or glands so affected may either be enlarged or not; but in almost all cases they are eventually enlarged, sometimes to three, four, or even six times their natural size. Their shape they sometimes retain, sometimes not, becoming irregular on the surface, lobulated, and generally projecting considerably in the free or unattached direction. When divided by incision, the section presents not the usual bluish or pale-red tint of the healthy lymphatic gland; but a colour cream-yellow, gray, or whitish gray. Nor is this colour always uniform; for in one lymphatic gland in a cluster it is cream-yellow, or grayish, and in another it is of white colour, and sometimes this difference is seen in different parts of the same gland. In this material few or no vessels are recognised. The whole is more or less a homogeneous matter of gray or cream-yellow colour, like soft cheese, pretty firm and resisting; and it presents to the glass no arrangement of cells or vessels, but a confused mass of substance with no trace or mark of organization. This has been called cheesy or caseous substance; and in those cases in which it is deposited in the form of small spherical or spheroidal globules, it has been named tubercle, and tubercular. I think that the term *Tyroma* (Τυρος, caseus,) is most suited to express its nature and most obvious characters.

This tyromatous substance is effused in the fluid or semifluid form, and then gradually acquires the consistent character. It appears in several instances to be effused at different points of the gland; and hence the consistence and colour is different at different points. In the most fluid form it is like thickish cream, or a mixture of chalk and water. In others more consistent the matter contained is like soft putty, or consists of consistent granules diffused in a whey like or milk like fluid. This is what is often called

---

* Anatomy of the Absorbing Vessels, p. 129.   † Ibid. p. 123.

pultaceous matter and atheromatous matter. In some of these ty-romatous deposits are observed portions much firmer, sometimes as hard as cartilage, and in some as solid as earthy or stony matter.

This deposit of earthy or bony matter also takes place in the liquid or semifluid form, and gradually becomes thick and consistent by the absorption of the serous or most fluid part; and the earthy or gypseous portion shows its true nature by becoming solid and its particles coalescing.

This deposit is liable to take place in any of the glands. It is, however, most common in the bronchial lymphatic glands and in the mesenteric lymphatic glands, and in the lymphatic glands of the neck. In the bronchial lymphatic glands it is mostly a disease of infancy, certainly of early life. I have not seen it much in adults; but I have repeatedly met with it in dissecting the bodies of infants and children; and many of the thoracic and tracheal affections to which children are liable may either be traced to or are associated with the presence of enlarged and tyromatous bronchial glands. This may be caused by the fact, that most children, in whom the bronchial glands are tyromatous, die in childhood.

Enlargement of the bronchial and tracheal glands gives rise to great dyspnœa, and sometimes to symptoms of crowing inspiration.

In the glands of the neck it is less hurtful, not being a cause of disease in the lungs or trachea; and hence it continues longer without influencing much the duration of life.

In the abdomen, on the other hand, it is different. For there it evidently compresses the lacteals proceeding from the intestinal tube. At the same time it is there seldom alone, but is preceded by more or less disease, often enlargement and ulceration of the intestinal follicles, as was mentioned when speaking of common glandular enlargement.

This species of deposit takes place chiefly in those in whom the habit called strumous predominates. It is supposed, indeed, to be the effect and an indication of the strumous disposition; and such probably it generally is. Though not a heterologous deposit, and consisting entirely of crude albumen insusceptible of organization, yet it is in its consequences sufficiently hurtful. When large tyromatous glands compress the bronchial tubes and lungs, and cause cough and difficult and laborious breathing, they may also by their size and position compress important blood-vessels and seriously derange the circulation.

Tyromatous glands, after becoming consistent, are liable to undergo an ulterior stage of softening, and apparently almost ulcerative sloughing. Thus we find them soften and suppurate in the neck and groin; and after a tedious process of suppuration subside and disappear, leaving bad and indelible scars with much irregular contraction of the skin. In the bronchial glands, when tyromatous, I have seen them in like manner softened and converted into a sort of cream-like sero-purulent matter; and others presenting deep ragged ulcerated cavities. Lastly, in the mesentery, where they are often allowed to pass through all their stages before the death of the patient, it is not uncommon to find the glands in different stages of softening. One or two are firm and consistent; others present softening, taking place at different points; others present portions of cream-like or soft caseous purulent matter; and others are represented by bags of puriform atheromatous semifluid substance, which is the tyromatous matter dissolved or liquefied, contained within the capsule or tunic of the gland, the only persistent portion of the whole structure.

The tubercular disorganization is represented by Laennec, Dupuy, and others, as exceedingly frequent in lymphatic glands. By some authors these bodies are regarded as constituting the anatomical character of the strumous or scrofulous gland. In many instances of scrofulous enlargement and induration, the glands are indeed found to be occupied with minute bodies, somewhat firm, which undergo a slow liquefaction or mollescence. But it is perhaps too limited a view to restrict to this only the characters of scrofula. In some instances these tubercles appear to consist of the original cells of the gland, filled with albuminous or albuminocalcareous matter.

6. *Ossification, Calcareous Deposition.* The lymphatic glands are liable to become ossified, or to be penetrated with deposition of calcareous matter. The diseased action commences at one or more points, and is progressively extended, till the gland is converted into a bony mass.* This change was observed by Cruikshank in the tracheo-bronchial glands, which he represents as in that state producing ulceration through the trachea, and being coughed up as osseous concretions.† Baillie, adopting the same view, regards the calcareous deposition as more common in these bodies than in any other of the same texture.‡ Lastly, Rayer has observed this

---

* A Practical Essay on the Diseases of the Vessels and Glands of the Absorbent System, &c. By William Goodlad, Surgeon, &c. p. 74. London. 1814.

† Anatomy, &c. p. 129.   ‡ Morbid Anatomy.

change not only in the tracheo-bronchial glands in subjects which he terms phthisical, but in the cervical glands in laryngeal consumption, and occasionally in persons cut off by mesenteric scrofula, (*carreau*,) and in the inguinal glands in persons who have had buboes. This change he considers the effect of inflammation.*
To the same head are to be referred the earthy or calcareous depositions (*matiere platreuse, gypseuse*) observed by Dupuy in these glands.

7. *Melanotic deposition* is common in the tracheo-bronchial lymphatic glands, and in those of the groin. Of the former, an example is at the present moment before me in the lungs of a woman much occupied by tubercular masses.

CHAPTER XII.

THE three orders of tubes or canals, the anatomical characters, and pathological relations of which have now been completed, constitute what has been termed the VASCULAR SYSTEM, (*Vasa ; Systema Vasorum*. Das Gefass System. *Le Systeme Vasculaire.*) The great extent of its distribution, and the part which it performs in all the processes of the living body, both in health, and during disease, must be easily understood. In every texture and organ arteries and veins are found; and in all, except a few, the art of the anatomist has demonstrated those colourless valvular tubes denominated lymphatics. The arrangement of the former, especially in the substance of the several textures, essentially constitutes what is termed the *organization* of these textures. Many anatomists have imagined that each texture has a proper matter, or *parenchyma*, by which it was supposed to be particularly distinguished, and which was conceived to consist of minute inorganic solid atoms. Whether this opinion be well founded or not, it is perhaps of little moment to inquire. At present it is certain that it is not susceptible of demonstration.

The phenomena of injections, in which he was eminently successful, led Ruysch to entertain the opinion, that every substance

---

* Memoire sur l'ossification morbide, considerée comme une terminaison des phlegmasies. Par P. Rayer. Archives Generales, Tome I. p. 439.

of the animal frame consisted of nothing but vessels. This idea,' though opposed by Albinus,* on the same grounds on which it was advanced, was nevertheless revived by William Hunter, who believed that the inorganic parts of animal bodies are too minute for sensible, or even microscopical examination. In every part, however minute, always excepting nails, hair, tooth enamel, &c., vessels could be traced; and even a cicatrix he demonstrated is vascular to its centre.†

By the aid of the microscope the researches of Lieberkuhn tended still more powerfully to favour this opinion.‡ But repeated observation of the effects of injection in every part and texture almost of the body by Barth and Prochaska has led the latter to conclude, that this opinion, understood in the ordinary mode, is not tenable. Prochaska, who has investigated this subject with much attention, thinks he is justified in dividing all the substances of the animal frame into two,—those which may be injected and those which cannot. In this manner he regards skin, especially its outer surface, muscle, various parts of the mucous membranes, the *pia mater*, the lungs, the muscular part of the heart, the spleen, the liver, kidneys, and other glands as very injectible; but tendon, ligament, cartilage, &c. as not injectible.§ Without entering minutely into the merits of this distinction, or the inferences which Prochaska makes to flow from it, it is sufficient, so far as all useful knowledge is concerned, to infer, that blood-vessels are an essential constituent of every organic texture, however different; and, if there be any other matter inherent in such textures, it must be derived from these as a secretion. Muscle, brain, nerve, osseous matter, and cartilage are depositions or the product of nutritious secretion from the respective arteries of these organized substances.

To apply these distinctions to pathological anatomy, therefore, two leading facts are presented as principles. The first of these is the arrangement of the vessels in the substance of the organic textures ;—their organization. The second is the great result of organization, the principal duty performed by the vessels in each tissue;—the formation of each organic substance, or the process of

* Annotationum Academicarum, Lib. iii.
† Medical Observations and Inquiries, Vol. II.
‡ De Villis Intestinorum.
§ Georgii Prochaska Disquisitio Anatomica-Physiologica Organismi Corporis Humani ejusque Processus Vitalis, 4to. Vienna, 1812.

nutrition. To changes in one or other of these two circumstances almost all morbid actions which become the subject of pathological anatomy may be referred; under the two general divisions, 1*st*, of *changes in organization;* and, 2*d, changes in nutritious deposition, or intimate structure.*

It is unnecessary to render this division more complex, by admitting, as has been done by several pathological writers, a third head in the changes which take place in the process of secretion. That process is to be viewed in general, nay, in almost all circumstances, as a complementary effect of nutrition; and the morbid changes which it occasionally undergoes may, without violence, be referred to one or other of the two foregoing heads.

It is different, however, with a third form or source of disease. I allude to those errors in the formation and relative situation of parts, especially the integrant parts of organs, which have been termed malformations, (Missbildungen.) These have been shown by Oken, Meckel, and others, to depend on the accidental interruption of the process of development, and misapplication of the component parts of organs during the early stage of that process.

In the subsequent chapters of this work, though it is unnecessary to abandon the simple arrangement hitherto observed, the morbid changes incident to the several textures shall be enumerated in reference to the two first distinctions,—those in minute organization and its products, and those in nutrition and intimate structure. The various forms of malformation constitute a distinct family by themselves.

BOOK II.

THE NERVOUS SYSTEM.

THE nervous system of the animal body includes, according to the most rational views, two general divisions. The first of these is collected in a single and indivisible mass, and contained in a peculiar cavity, formed by part of the osseous system of the animal. In the less perfect tribes this is limited to the vertebral column, or something analogous to it; but in man, and the more perfect animals, we find a large cavity at the superior extremity of this column superadded. The second division of the nervous system is found in the form of long chords or threads mutually connected, and running in various directions through the body in the mode of ramification. To these the name of nervous trunks or chords, or simply nerves, has been long applied.

CHAPTER I.

A. THE CENTRAL PART OF THE NERVOUS SYSTEM.

SECTION I.

BRAIN, CEREBRAL SUBSTANCE, *Cerebrum,*—BRAIN, CRANIAL AND SPINAL. Μυελον εγκεφαλον και μυελον νωτιαιον;—*Marrow of the Head and Marrow of the Back,* GALEN.

Of all the works which have been composed on the anatomy of the brain, the subjects may be referred to two general heads;—those which treat of the configuration of the organ, and those which undertake to investigate its minute structure. The authors themselves, however, do not always distinguish accurately between these two departments of anatomical science. As it is chiefly the latter which is to occupy attention at present, I may mention, that after the epistle of Varoli on the base of the brain and the origin of the optic nerves, the writings of Willis, Malpighi, and Vieussens, are the first which claim much notice. The works of Ridley,[*] and of Glaserus,[†] contain some good observations; and that of Santorini[‡] deserves to be mentioned for the first good description of the optic *thalami* and the *corpora geniculata.* Father Della Torre,[§] Prochaska,[‖] and Monro, are the first after Lewenhoeck who treat of the structure of the brain after microscopical observation. The essay of Vicq-D'Azyr, and his elaborate engravings are sufficiently well known.[¶] About the same time, 1780, Vincenzo Malacarne described the component parts of the organ with more accuracy than had hitherto been attempted.[**] Reil followed, and communicated much new information on the minute structure of several parts of the organ.[††] The work of Rolando, which appeared in 1809,[‡‡] has been little known till of late. Better fortune awaited the elaborate treatise of John and Charles Wenzel,[§§] which is highly appreciated by every anatomical inquirer in Europe. Lastly, the description of Gordon,[‖‖] the microscopical observations of Sir Everard Home,[¶¶] who has confirmed many of the facts observed by Della Torre, and the microscopical observations of Ehrenberg, who has examined every part of the brain with much care, and those of Treviranus, Valentin, and Weber, are entitled to attention.

The brain may be considered as a continuous organ consisting of three divisions;—the convoluted, the laminated, and the smooth or uniform portions. Of these divisions, which are framed according to the peculiar external configuration of each, the first part

---

[*] Anatomy of the Brain. By Henry Ridley. Lond. 1695.

[†] J. H. Glaserus de Cerebro. Basil, 1680.

[‡] Jo. Dom. Santorini Observationes Anatomicæ. Lugdun. Bat. 1739.

[§] D. Giovanni Maria Della Torre, Nuove Osservazione Microscopiche. Napoli, 1776.

[‖] Georgii Prochaska, De Structura Nervorum Tractatus Anatom. Viennæ, 1779, et apud Op. Min. 1800.

[¶] Recherches sur la Structure du Cerveau. Mémoires de l'Academie des Sciences. Paris, 1781-83.

[**] Encefalotomia Nuova Universale di Vincenzo Malacarne Saluzzese. Torino, 1780.

[††] Fragmente Ueber die Bildung des Gehirns im Menschen. Vom Professor Reil. Archiv. fur die Physiogie. 8ter Band, &c. et various papers in 9ter Band.

[‡‡] Saggio sulla vera Structura del cervello dell' uomo. Sassari, 1809.

[§§] J. et C. Wenzel, De Penitiore Structura Cerebri Hominis et Brutorum. Tubingæ, 1812.

[‖‖] Observations, &c. and Outlines of Human Anatomy. By John Gordon, M. D. &c. Edinburgh.

[¶¶] Phil. Trans. 1821, p. 25, 1824, p. 1, and 1825, p. 436.

corresponds to what is called the brain proper, (*cerebrum ;*) the sècond to the small brain, (*cerebellum ;*) and the third to the oblong cylindrical body contained within the vertebral column, and known under the name of *spinal churd.*

The convoluted portion presents two surfaces, an outer or convoluted, and an inner or figurate.   The laminated portion in like manner presents two surfaces, an outer or laminated, and an inner or central.   The third has only one exterior surface.

The exterior surface of the convoluted division of the organ is formed into eminences longitudinal and rounded, but directed in various ways, and separated from each other by deep hollows. These eminences have been named convolutions or circumvolutions, (*gyri,* Soemmering, Wenzel,) and the depressions *sulci* or furrows. This surface of the organ is most properly termed the. *convoluted surface.*   To see it distinctly, the vascular membrane termed *pia mater,* (*meninx* tenuis,) (Das Gefasshaut,) must be cautiously removed by dissection.

The convoluted surface communicates with another interior surface at two parts; 1*st*, on the middle plane, under the posterior end of the middle band or meso-lobe, (*corpus callosum ;*) 2*d*, on each side of the middle plane, at the outer margin of the fluted masses termed *limbs* of the brain, (*crura cerebri*); (Diè Hirnschenkel); between these limbs and the posterior end of the optic chamber or couch, (*thalamus opticus*); (Der Sehhugel.)   This surface of the organ may be termed the central or figurate.

The exterior surface of the cerebellum is differently disposed. Instead of presenting convoluted eminences, it consists of thin portions of cerebral substance, placed contiguously, and either parallel or concentric.   These portions, which have been named plates (*laminæ,*) or leaves (*folia,*) are separated from each other by furrows of various depth.   This surface, which may be named the *laminar* or *foliated* surface of the small brain, communicates also with the figurate surface; 1*st*, at its superior part on the middle plane, between the semilunar notch (Der halbmondformige Ausschnitt; Reil); behind, and the white cerebral plate termed Vieussenian valve, before.   2*d*, At its inferior surface between the parts termed almonds by Malacarne, or spinal lobules by Gordon above; and the upper end (*medulla oblongata*) of the spinal chord, below.

The. convoluted surface of each hemisphere may be conveniently divided into the following five regions; 1. The commutual or dichotomous; 2. The lateral-superior, or convex; 3. The antero-inferior, or frontal; 4. The medio-inferior, or spheno-temporal; 5. The posterior or cerebellic region of the convoluted surface. The first of these regions of the convoluted surface is easily understood. Plane in its surface, of a shape nearly semicircular, it forms the central boundary of each hemisphere, corresponds to the falciform or dichotomous portion of the hard membrane, (μη·ιγξ σκληρη, *meninx dura*,) by which it is separated from the similar surface of the opposite hemisphere. Before and behind it extends from the superior to the inferior surface of the brain; but a considerable portion of its middle is terminated by the upper surface of the object named middle band, (*mesolobe, corpus callosum*,) which lies between the two hemispheres. It is contained between the semicircular and the rectilineal margins.

The second region of the convoluted surface is extensive, and occupies the whole of the anterior, upper, lateral, and posterior parts of the hemisphere, from their anterior to their posterior extremity, and from the semicircular margin to a line which extends between these extremities along the lateral borders of the organ.

The antero-inferior, or frontal, is that region of the convoluted surface which rests on the horizontal part of the frontal and ethmoid bones, and commencing before with a curved outline,—the anterior end of the hemisphere is bounded behind by the curvilinear hollow, which has been named the pit or fissure of Sylvius. It is slightly uneven, and is bounded at its inner or mesial margin by the great fissure which separates the hemispheres. This inner margin always presents one convolution, which is quite uniform in direction, extent, and configuration. It consists of a longitudinal eminence, which extends in the adult brain about 1½ inch from the beginning or posterior end of the notch, towards its anterior extremity. The inner margin of the eminence, which is about four lines broad, forms the side of the fissure; and its outer margin or border is separated from the contiguous part of the convoluted surface, by a furrow or hollow equally uniform in direction and figure with the eminence,—about the same average length (1 inch 5 lines.) This furrow contains the cerebral portion of the first pair or olfacient nerves.

The medio-inferior, or spheno-temporal, is situate immediately behind this region, from which it is separated by the curvilinear hollow. (*Fossa Sylvii.*) In the ordinary descriptions, this forms what has been named the *middle lobe* of the brain; while the posterior part of the convoluted surface, or that which corresponds to the cerebellum, though distinguished by no evident mark or limit, has been with equal impropriety named the *posterior lobe.* If the whole region be examined from the curvilinear hollow to the posterior tip of the hemisphere, it affords no mark, line, or boundary on which to establish this popular and much used division; and the whole presents one uniform region of convolutions, which resemble in every respect those found on other parts of this surface. The whole region, therefore, ought to be viewed as a single division of the convoluted surface; but as its posterior part rests not on the cranium, but on the horizontal portion of the hard membrane which covers the small brain, while the division of lobes must be discarded as artificial, it may be expedient to subdivide the surface into two, the medio-inferior and postero-inferior regions of the convoluted surface, according as they correspond to different containing parts.

The first, which near the curvilinear hollow, is slightly convex or rounded, is lodged in a considerable cavity of the cranium, formed by the sphenoid and temporal bones, bounded before by the spheno-frontal arch, and behind by the pyramid or petrous portion of the temporal bone. This part of the convoluted surface, which may be named the *spheno-temporal,* is one of considerable importance, and should be accurately known by the anatomical student.

The posterior division of this region, which is plane, corresponds to the horizontal or cerebellic part of the hard membrane, and, though not to be distinguished by any innate or organic limit, may, however, for the sake of more precision, be marked by this adventitious character.* It may be named the *cerebellic region* of the convoluted surface.

The ordinary appearance of the convoluted surface is well known. It is formed of cerebral matter, of a gray or dirty wax colour, the surface of which is smooth and polished, where it has not been rent by the removal of the membranes and their attachments. The convolutions consist of longitudinal eminences, rounded transversely, running in various directions, and separated from each other by deep furrows. If these be examined when the membranous cover-

---

* Lest the use of these terms be objectionable by their obscurity, I may observe that, in describing parts of the human body, it is not unfrequently requisite to have recourse not only to marks on the organ described, but also to certain characters belonging to the contiguous parts. The first of these may be named the *organic or innate,* as they belong to the organ; the second, which do not belong to it, should be named *adventitious or esoteric.* This is indispensable in relative anatomy.

ings are removed, they are observed to present many minute orifices, into which the soft membrane (λεπτη μηνιγξ, *meninx tenuis*, *pia mater*,) transmits filamentous bodies, most of them minute bloodvessels. They are neither arteries nor veins exclusively, but seem to consist of both.

Neither the eminences, nor the hollows or depressions, are uniform in number or distribution; and in no two brains is it possible to trace any similarity in the figure, presence, or direction of these objects. This must be understood of the whole upper, lateral, and posterior part of the convoluted surface, and, in short, all its divisions, unless where it approaches the central or figurate surface. In the latter situation, this want of uniformity disappears; and a number of important objects are presented to the attention of the observer. The points at which this approach of the two surfaces takes place, are, 1*st*, Along the rectilinear margin of the commutual region, where it is contiguous with the upper surface and the posterior end of the middle or central band; 2*d*, From the last of these situations, on each side over the protuberance and cerebral limbs; 3*d*, From this again by the outer margin of the cerebral limbs, to the curvilinear hollow and along its course. In the last of these situations chiefly the convoluted surface becomes important, and exhibits objects which distinguish these regions from the others.

The outer surface of the cerebellum, or small brain, differs from that of the brain proper. It cannot be said to be convoluted; for it does not present the tortuous eminences and furrows which constitute the convolutions of this part of the organ. But the cerebral matter of which it consists, is disposed in the manner of plates (*laminæ*) or leaves (*folia*), parallel to each other, or at least concentric, and separated by parallel or concentric furrows. It is scarcely requisite to say, that this definition is not meant to imply, that the direction of all these objects is the same throughout the whole organ,—but merely that the cerebellic plates, of which certain groups consist, observe the same direction;—and that any one or two plates or leaves have several of the contiguous ones parallel or concentric with them, while those of the next group, though disposed differently, observe the same direction in relation to each other. By this peculiarity the various regions of the laminated or foliated surface of the small brain may be distinguished. The plates of the hemispheres are curvilinear and concentric, and pursue in various regions of the organ certain definite directions;

those in the middle between the hemispheres are straight, transverse, and parallel; and at one spot they are oblique and parallel. By means of these invariable characters of the cerebellic plates, the surface of the organ may be conveniently distributed into several divisions.

To the cerebellic plates or their peculiarities, little attention was given before the time of Vincenzio Malacarne, professor of surgery in the city of Acqui, in the duchy of Montferrat. This learned person, the most diligent descriptive anatomist of his time, published in the year 1780 three treatises on the Anatomy of the Brain;* in the third of which he describes with much precision and minuteness, the anatomical characters of the outer or laminated surface of the cerebellum. Some knowledge of his distinctions, which were adopted by Reil, is requisite to comprehend distinctly the configuration and structure of this part of the organ.

Commencing with the well-known division of the whole organ into two hemispheres, Malacarne remarks, that, if the whole upper surface of the organ be presented to the eye, the outline of each hemispherical surface is found to describe three-fourths of a circle; and as these circular segments mutually meet towards the mesial plane, where they are respectively adapted to different parts, the mode of union varies according to the figure of these adjoining objects. 1st, As the hemispherical border approaches the anterior part of the organ, it is found to be suddenly interrupted, where the cerebellic branches or peduncles (crura cerebelli) are connected with the protuberance, and, pursuing a retrograde direction on each side towards the mesial plane, forms a species of re-entrant curvature. The hollow thus formed, which corresponds to the lower of the four eminences on the upper surface of the protuberance (corpora quadrigemina, Die Vierhugel,) is named by Malacarne the semilunar curvature,—(der halbmondförmide Ausschnitt; Reil.) 2d, Again, as the hemispherical borders approach the posterior part of the small brain, advancing nearer to the mesial plane, they proceed, by an acute circular turn, almost straight backwards, so as to form, at the posterior edge of the organ, a deep rectangular notch,) (not unlike the figure of the ancient lyre. This posterior hollow, in which is lodged the cerebellic vertical portion of the hard membrane (falx cerebelli,) is named by Malcarne the common perpendi-

* Encefalotomia Nuova Universale di Vincenzo Malacarne, Saluzzese. Torino, 1780.

cular fissure (incurvatura,) and by Reil, to whose fancy this epithet seems to have been deficient in expression, *the purse-like fissure* (Der beutelförmige Ausschnitt.) Between these two well-marked boundaries the cerebellic plates, of which the hemispheres consist, are united in the middle by a confused interlacing junction, (*un intreccio confuso ed irregolare di sostanza,*) to which the Italian anatomist gives the name of suture (*raffe,* raphe) of the cerebellum. I find that the careful removal of the soft membrane, (*pia mater,*) renders this more distinct, and shows the mesial termination of the hemispherical plates. On the surface, a large hollow between the hemispheres, and extending backwards from the semilunar to the purse-like fissure, previously called by Haller (*vallecula,*) the little valley, received from Malacarne the corresponding term (*valletta*) in his own language.

The divisions of the cerebellic surface made by Malacarne, and adopted by Reil, are founded entirely on the groups of plates, and the comparative depth of the furrows by which these groups are separated. Groups of plates, separated by the deepest furrows, are named lobes, (*lobi,* M. Lappen, R.); and those separated by furrows of less depth are named lobules, (*lobetti,* M. Läppchen, R.) In some situations the lobules present divisions formed by furrows of less depth, between which the groups of plates are of greater or less size. To such clusters Malacarne gives the name of laminar leaflets, (*foglietti laminosi.*)[*]

Each hemispherical surface consists of five lobes. 1. The anterior-upper. 2. The posterior-upper. 3. The posterior-lower. 4. The slender, rarely exceeding three lines in breadth. 5. The two-bellied or biventral. The two first belong to the upper or flat hemispherical surface; the three latter to the lower or convex hemispherical surface. Besides these, a sixth lobe may be mentioned as common to the two hemispheres. It is situate on the mesial plane of the upper surface, between the anterior end of the middle line (*raffe,*) and the middle or apex of the semilunar fissure. This situation is not an improper reason for the name by which Malacarne has distinguished it,—the central lobe.

In the bottom of the purse-like notch are many bundles or clusters of plates, which unite the posterior lobes of the upper and lower surfaces to those of the opposite hemispheres. These Malacarne names *transverse laminar chords (cordoni laminosi traversali,)* or commissures of the cerebellum.

---

[*] Encefalotomia, nuova, &c. Parte iii. Articolo i. No. 13.

The anterior-upper lobe, with four sides and four angles, named therefore by Malacarne the *quadrilateral* or *four-sided* lobe, (*vier-seitige*, Reil,) approaches somewhat to the figure of the trapezoid. It is bounded by three curved margins and one straight one. Of the former, the most anterior forms one-half of the semilunar fissure; while the posterior, which is also the longest, and parallel to this, is a curvilinear or circular tract (the great furrow,) extending from the bottom of the purse-like fissure behind to the anterior outline of the hemisphere before, where it terminates about one inch from the end of the semilunar fissure. This last space between the anterior end of the great furrow forms the third curved margin of the four-sided lobe; while its straight margin is made by the middle line, which here is common to the two lobes. Malacarne further divides this lobe into five lobules, and describes the limits of each with minuteness and accuracy. For the details of these distinctions I refer to the original.

The posterior-upper lobe—the second division of the upper hemispherical surface—may be defined in the following manner. The circular tract or great furrow, which I have already said forms the posterior margin of the four-sided lobe, is its anterior boundary. The hemispherical outline of the upper surface, if traced from before backwards, will be found to coincide about $1\frac{1}{2}$ inch, sometimes more, from the purse-like notch, with a considerable furrow (the horizontal,) which turns round at the purse-like notch to meet the great furrow already mentioned. The curved outline thus continued is the outer boundary of the posterior lobe; and it is easy to perceive, that, in consequence of the direction which this line observes, and its meeting with the great furrow, the lobe is contained between the horizontal and great furrow, or between two curved lines. This lobe is subdivided by Malacarne more minutely than the former. It is found, however, that the number of lobules is not the same in both,—those of the left being most uniformly about eight, while those of the right are more numerous, but in general less distinctly marked.

These with the central lobe, the general situation of which has been already noticed, form the several divisions of the upper region of the cerebellic laminated surface. The inferior region presents divisions more numerous, more complicated, and more interesting.

The first of these, the posterior-lower, is contiguous, at its outer or greater boundary, with the posterior-upper lobe, where a small segment of it is seen, when the cerebellum is examined from above. Its anterior or inner boundary is marked by a curvilinear furrow of moderate depth, by which it is separated from the slender lobe, and the posterior end of which terminates, not in the purse-shaped notch, but, after a sigmoid turn towards the laminar pyramid,* is insensibly lost among a cluster of transverse plates, which shall be afterwards noticed.

Immediately anterior to this is found the slender lobe, (*il lobo sottile*, Malacarne; Der zarté Lappen, Reil;) which is not above three lines broad, and being contained between two concentric furrows, is not unlike the segment intercepted by the truncated arcs of two small circles of a sphere.

The space of the hemispheric surface within the slender lobe, or between this and the peduncle or arm, is inclosed by three circular lines, two of which, the exterior and interior, correspond to so many furrows; while the third, which is anterior, is formed by the horizontal or marginal furrow. The space thus inclosed is similar to a spherical triangle, and is occupied by a group of plates which Malacarne denominates the *biventral lobe*, (der Zwey-bauchige Lappen, Reil.) Its contiguity with the cerebral end of the pneumogastric nerve led Vicq-D'Azyr to give it the name of *the lobule of the eighth pair*, (*lobule du nerf vague;*) and its situation at the posterior corner of the peduncle, and under that body, is the reason why it was called *sub-peduncular lobule* by Dr Gordon. Of these plates the arrangement is peculiar, since they are neither so exactly concentric as in the other lobes; nor yet is their direction different from each other. The plates at its outer margin are the largest, as they extend the whole length from the marginal furrow to the end of the slender lobe, at which, however, they are contracted to a narrow point. The next set are shorter, and are more contracted or acuminated at their posterior end, where they are contiguous to the almonds or tonsils. The third and last set are the shortest, and are more twisted down, as it were, next the almonds. These contracted or acuminated ends of the cerebellic plates are named (*code*,) tails by Malacarne.

The disposition now described renders the posterior corner of the biventral lobe very pointed, and its margin very concave; and between this margin and the parts which occupy the valley is placed a group of plates somewhat convex, rounded, and disposed also in

* Encefalotomia, &c., Articolo i. No. 20, ed Articolo ix. No. 77. See p. 318.

a peculiar manner. This group Malacarne names the tonsil, or tonsils, (*tonsille*,)* a term which Reil, regarding it synonymous with *amygdalæ*, renders literally almonds, (Die Mandeln); *the spinal lobule* of Dr Gordon. If the cerebellum be examined before the head of the spinal chord is cut from the protuberance, the inner margin of the almond will be found contiguous to the oval eminence (*corpus olivare*,) and even pressed by it. It is best, however, to examine the almonds after the chord (*medulla oblongata*) has been removed. It will then be perceived that each almond is bounded on the outside by a well-marked circular furrow, which separates it from the biventral lobe on the inside by a free surface directed to the corresponding surface of the opposite almond; and before, by a continuation of this directed outwards toward the biventral lobe. I have already said that the direction of the constituent plates of this body is peculiar. In general they observe a direction opposite to that of the biventral plates; so that, if produced, they would cross. Its apex or most pointed corner is contiguous to that of the biventral lobe; and altogether, each almond presents the appearance, on a cursory glance, of two similar bodies directed inversely to each other.

The last body which I shall notice here is the Flock or Flocks. The description of its situation, as given by Malacarne, is by no means clear; but perusal of the context, with examination of the parts described, can leave no doubt on the certainty of the object which he has in view. The flock (*il fioccho, il fiocchi*, Die Flocken,) is a minute body, of a shape not easily defined, situate in the angular hollow between the biventral lobe and the branch or peduncle (*crus; gamba; braccia*; Die Arme) of the small brain. The lower or free surface of the latter object (the branch) possesses an anterior and posterior margin or corner. The latter is contiguous to the biventral lobe, from which it is separated by a small furrow, out of which the flock seems to issue. Each flock consists of six or seven plates (*laminæ*) starting directly, as it were, from the beginning of the peduncle, and with the concave margins directed towards the protuberance.

Ruysch has represented in their site objects to which he applies the name of vermiform prominences; a circumstance which is in some measure to be ascribed to the vague manner in which this term has been used.

* Encefalotomia, Articolo ix.

The valley, (*vallecula*, valletta, das Thal) or hollow between the two hemispheres, is occupied by a numerous series of plates, which lie transversely, are parallel to each other, and which form a sort of uniting medium of the cerebellic plates of each side. The appearance of this region in the brain of the dog and monkey, the animals which the ancient anatomists chiefly dissected, might furnish them with some reason for applying to it the name of worm, or worm-shaped body ; (σκωληξ, επιφυσις σκωληκοειδης.) But the modern anatomists are not bound to apply it to the corresponding part of the human cerebellum, which certainly by no means justifies the appellation. The confusion which has arisen from this practice of imitating the ancients is a sufficient reason to abandon the term for ever; since scarcely two anatomists agree in giving the name of vermiform process to the same part of the organ.

With a view to obviate all misconception on this point, Malacarne has recourse to distinctions completely new. Beginning with the back end of the valley at the purse-shaped notch, where are seen the plates afterwards named by Reil the *short exposed crossbands*, (Die kurzen und sichtbaren-Querbänder;) and the long *covered cross-bands*, (Die langen verdeckten Querbänder;) and proceeding forward, he distinguishes a group of parallel plates, or laminated leaves, to which he applies the name of *pyramid*. This body, which is bounded behind by the purse-shaped notch, and before by another cluster of plates called by Malacarne the *uvula*, consists of twenty parallel plates, of which six, he observes, are very short; and a triangular termination in the longer, forms the summit of the body. The *uvula* (*ugola*) (Der Zapfen,* Reil,) which is anterior, he found to consist of twelve laminated leaves, to have six lines of longitudinal extent, and four of breadth. It is smaller than the pyramid, and conical, with its base turned to that body, (Reil). Lastly, anterior to the uvula, and separated from it by a furrow, is the laminar tubercle,† (*tuberculo laminoso*,) consisting of about ten thin leaves or transverse plates. This body, which is the smallest in the row, is the *nodule* or knot, (Das Knotchen) of Reil.

The second surface of the brain is very different from the first. In situation it is interior or central; and its configuration is such,

---

* Mr Mayo, by translating this term *spigot*, makes it appear to be a different part from that meant by Malacarne, and understood by Reil. Though the word der Zapfen signifies *spigot*, it is also used to denote the uvula, and in this sense it is employed by Reil.

† Encefalotomia Nuova, &c. Parte iii. Articolo x. p. 61.

that it may be named the *figurate or symmetrical surface* of the
brain.   Instead of presenting the uniform eminences and hollows
which distinguish the convoluted surface, it is disposed or moulded
into definite shapes, which correspond with each other, as they are
situate on opposite sides of the middle plane,—or the parts of which,
when situate on this plane, are exactly symmetrical.   The surface
formed by these variously figured objects, bounds what are termed
in the common descriptions the *ventricles* or *cavities* of the brain.
They cannot justly be termed cavities any more than the hollows
between the convolutions, but ought to be viewed as continuations
of the exterior or convoluted surface.   As the several objects of
the figurate surface are well known, I shall at present, avoiding
minute description, notice those circumstances only which have not
been sufficiently studied, or correctly represented, or which are
necessary to establish the general principle,—that the convoluted
surface of the brain and the laminated surface of the cerebellum
communicate directly with the inner, central, or figurate surface of
these organs.

The commutual or dichotomous region of the convoluted surface
is terminated below by a sinuosity, which is formed chiefly by a
part of the brain, remarkable in appearance and organization.   This,
which was named by the ancient anatomists the smooth or polished
body (σωμα τιλλοειδες, *corpus læve*),* to distinguish it from those surfaces which were formed by a cutting instrument, appears in the
form of white fibrous matter, passing transversely between the hemispheres; but is also marked by certain longitudinal lines, first
correctly represented by Vicq-DAzyr.   The most conspicuous of
these is that which lies exactly in the middle plane, and which is
formed by the meeting of the transverse fibres, of which this body,
termed *middle or central band*, (*mesolobe* of Chaussier, the beam
(der Balken) of Reil,)† consists.   These fibres, which issue like

* This is the literal translation and the true meaning of the term used by the Alex-
andrian school.   The name *corpus callosum*, which is adopted by modern anatomists,
is a bad translation made at the revival of literature.   In defence of the error, Vicq-
D'Azyr contradicts nature by the assertion, that this is somewhat harder or firmer than
the other parts of the brain.   " Cette production a *plus de consistence* que le reste du
cerveau.—Ce corps un peu plus dur que le reste de la substance blanche du cerveau."
Of many brains examined, with a different object, certainly, from that of proving the
learning or ignorance of the translators of the Greek physicians, I never could perceive
any difference in the consistence of this and other parts of the brain.

† Archiv. für die Physiologie.   Neunter Band.   Erstes Heft. 3. b. p. 172.

white parallel lines, exceedingly minute, from the substance of the hemispheres, either stop suddenly, or change their direction at this point. Their sudden termination gives rise to an appearance, to which the expressive but erring epithet of suture (*raphe*) has been given. On each side of this other lines are remarked following the same direction. In general, they are situate about three or four lines from the median plane; but are in a few instances observed to be very regular in their disposition at the anterior end of the middle band. About its middle, however, a very distinct appearance of lines collected into a considerable bundle, may be observed proceeding backwards to its posterior end. As they advance they become more distinct, are about $1\frac{1}{2}$ line broad, and of a grayish colour; at the posterior end of the middle band, they diverge somewhat, and, passing over this, proceed in a lateral direction downwards, till they are lost about the spot where the limbs of the brain (*crura cerebri*, Die Hirnschenkel) issue from the optic eminences. This forms the inner, central, or gray portion of the cylindroid eminence.

The posterior extremity of this body is rounded; and when the membranes have been removed, the surface which forms this rounded end is found to communicate directly with the chamber named third or middle ventricle. This surface is in truth continued forward, and forms the vault or ceiling, (*fornix*, Die Zwillingsbinde, *the twain band*, Reil,) a point which, though sufficiently obvious, is never noticed in description, or perspicuously demonstrated. The names of *callous body* and *vault* are applied in the ordinary works, as if they were denominations of different objects, or rather of different bodies. If they are still to be retained, it ought to be stated that they are names applied to opposite surfaces only of the same object.

The relations of the round or posterior end of the middle band are worthy of examination. The handle of a scalpel inserted beneath it will be found to be in the middle ventricle, with the vault above, the *conarium* or pineal body, and four eminences of the upper surface of the protuberance (*corpora quadrigemina*) below, and a part of each optic chamber on each side. I find it convenient to remove the posterior part of the hemispheres by a transverse section following the plane or level of the hinder end of the central band. A distinct view is thus given of this communication of the convoluted with the figurate surface; and it may be observed, not only in the middle, but on each side. The middle one is bounded above by the posterior end of the middle band and the back part of the vault; below, by the pineal body and the four eminences; before, it is continuous with the middle ventricle; behind, it looks to that space between the convoluted surface of the brain and the laminated surface of the cerebellum, which is occupied by the horizontal part, (*tentorium cerebelli*), of the hard membrane.

On the sides,—that is beyond the margin of the body with the four eminences, a different arrangement is observed. The posterior end of the middle band penetrates into the substance of the hemispheres; but the gray chords which have been already noticed, in pursuing their lateral course, are immediately enveloped in white plates, derived, as we shall see, from the sides of the vault, assuming thus a cylindrical appearance. Thus is formed exactly opposite to the cerebral limbs, a body with a free rounded surface, which bends in a curvilinear direction laterally and downwards, and is found to be the great *hippocampus* or cylindroid process. (Chaussier.) In observing this curvilinear course, it rests on and corresponds to, the upper margin of the cerebral limb, as it issues from the optic chamber. It must not, however, be imagined that it adheres to this body. The surfaces both of the beginning or upper end of hippocampus, and of the cerebral limb, are free and unconnected. They are indeed covered with vascular membrane, (*pia mater*,) which keeps them in apposition; but if this be removed, as it ought always to be, the two surfaces will be found quite distinct, and in no manner connected, unless in corresponding with each other. The whole of this communication may be seen, and is best examined by keeping the organ in its natural position, and viewing it from behind, after the posterior parts of the cerebral hemispheres have been removed. It forms what was described by Bichat under the name of *the great cerebral fissure*.* This denomination does not accurately express the idea intended; nor does the idea itself, it may be remarked, present a correct view of the natural arrangement. The conformation which I have attempted to describe does not form a fissure, but a regular symmetrical opening, by which the convoluted surface communicates distinctly and directly with that which is figurate.

. The next step of the process in the further exposition of this opening or communication, requires the inversion of the brain, and

_____

* Anat. Descriptive, Tom. III.

the exposition of the inferior regions of the convoluted surface,—the base of the brain. We have seen the manner in which the convoluted passes into the figurate surface, above and behind the middle band. At the inferior regions this transition is effected in a mode somewhat different;—and the channel or means by which it is made, is the curvilinear hollow. To understand clearly the relations by which this is established, the demonstrator should remove in small portions the membrane which covers the optic commissure and tracts, the pituitary peduncle, the pisiform eminences, and which binds together the adjoining convolutions, and especially those which are connected by it to the limbs of the brain.* When the convolutions are thus exposed, the furrows on each side of the hollow will be found to be very deep, and the eminences proportionally high from the more solid part of the encephalic organ; and the hollow itself will appear almost like the furrow of a convolution on a large scale. Its peculiarity indeed is, that the bottom of the hollow is not convoluted, but presents an extensive uniform space of grayish cerebral matter, on each side of which, but especially behind, the convolutions are very large and distinct. This convoluted part begins insensibly at the outer or lateral edge of the hemisphere, where it is narrow; becomes broader as it advances forwards and inwards; and about one inch from the mesial plane, is particularly distinct, broader, and more spacious than at any other part of its course.

It here presents an infinity of holes or orifices of various size in the cerebral substance, not arranged in any regular order, but uniformly found in this situation. Some of these orifices are sufficiently large to admit the point of a small silver probe; but the greater number are more minute, and do not exceed the calibre of a common-sized bristle. The space over which they extend is various, and its figure cannot be accurately defined; it is generally equivalent to the half of a square inch. In numerous dissections, I have found it uniformly at this part, and of this size, as nearly as it is possible to estimate, in measurement of objects so variable as those of the organs of the animal body. I have not been able to recognize any difference in the colour of this and other parts of the convoluted surface. I suspect, therefore, that Vicq-D'Azyr,

---

* This process is best performed by the scissors and forceps, with the occasional use only of the scalpel, and with the aid of an assistant with delicate fingers and forceps.

who in noticing this part has called it the *white perforated substance,* (*substance blanche perforée*), applied the term of colour without examining the contiguous parts, when denuded of their membranous investments. The same name nearly, (*lamina perforata*), has been given it by Reil. The orifices which characterize this part of the brain admit, from the Sylvian or middle artery, an infinity of blood-vessels, which here penetrate the part denominated the *hook-shaped cerebral band* (Der Haaken-förmige Mark-bündel) delineated by Reil. This circumstance renders the adjoining part the most vascular of the whole organ,—a fact which will be shown to be important in the pathology of the brain.

Anterior to the perforated spot at the extreme verge of the unconvoluted substance, is situate a small pointed eminence, of gray colour, shaped like a triangular pyramid, most conspicuous when cleared of the membrane which covers it. Proceeding backward from this, we remark two slender white lines of different lengths, and following different directions. The inner of these is short; and after a course seldom exceeding four or five lines in the adult brain suddenly ceases to be visible. The outer one is much longer, follows a curved direction, with the concave part of its course directed anteriorly, and is of a more vivid white colour. These two lines are the generating or initial filaments of the first pair of nerves.

Within the perforated spot the curvilinear hollow is generally conceived to be terminated. The unconvoluted space, however, in which it consists, is here directly continuous with the figurate surface of the brain. This space indeed makes here a sharp turn backwards; and having on the inside the long cerebral band termed the *optic tract,* may be conceived to be bounded by the limb of the brain. This body, with that of the opposite side, will be imperfectly seen at first; and though the end which unites each with the bridge or protuberance is sufficiently conspicuous, the opposite extremity cannot be distinctly perceived. It is indeed covered by a portion of the convoluted surface, the inner and prominent surface of the medio-inferior or spheno-temporal region. This must therefore be gently moved outwards or laterally, and also raised; and with the aid of the handle of a scalpel and the fingers of a dexterous assistant, the cerebral limb may be shown to be here crossed or surrounded by the optic tract of the side. The purpose of this part of the exposition is to show the *geniculate bodies,* or posterior eminences of the optic chambers.

But the attention of the demonstrator is to be directed to that part of the convoluted surface which covers the anterior end and outer margin of the cerebral limb, and which has been raised on the scalpel-handle. When gently everted, it is found to present the thin white body named the *tape or fringe* (*tænia*) of the hippocampus; and if the portion of convoluted brain most anterior or next to the curvilinear hollow be raised and everted in the same manner, the anterior end of this object termed the *foot* (*pes hippocampi*) will come into view. If this operation be properly performed, no part will be torn, broken, or displaced; the objects exhibited are free surfaces, not adhering to each other but only in apposition. The white plate or tape of the hippocampus forms, in the natural position of the organ, the outer and lower border of the opening, while the limb of the brain, and after that the outer and lower surface of the optic chamber, forms its inner border.

To obtain an idea yet more clear and distinct of this communication between the convoluted and figurate surfaces of the brain, it is convenient to follow the direction of the opening with the scalpel handle backwards and upwards, until it reach the upper margin of the brain-limb, where it is shown to be merely a continuation of the lateral part of the posterior opening. This step of the exposition requires cautious and gentle management; and the peculiar curvature which the parts forming the outer border of the communication follow, renders it difficult to avoid laceration or displacement. In general, it is best accomplished on a single hemisphere, from which the cerebellum has been previously removed; but it is desirable to preserve also the whole of the central band, which shows not only the relative connection of the several parts, but serves also to demonstrate a curious fact in the configuration of the parts forming the outer border of the communication. This is the hippocampus through its entire course, or the body which its figure has led Professor Chaussier to name the *cylindroid process*.

This body consists essentially of two parts. The first is an inner or central portion, gray in colour, notched or indented in appearance, and though free at the indented edge, adhering to the cerebral substance by its opposite margin. This is *the gray indented band;* (Gordon;)—*le corps godronnée,* Vicq-D'Azyr.) It is as thick as a large crow-quill. This is covered by the outer or second part, which is a broad thin plate of white cerebral matter rolled or folded over the gray indented band, precisely as a map is rolled

rover a cylinder of wood, and covering it unless removed by art.
This last part of the cylindroid process is what is well known, and
always described under the name of the *tape or fillet* of the hippocampus. Its arrangement with regard to the gray indented band
is less generally understood, and is indeed never noticed in the ordinary descriptions. A correct idea of it may be formed in the
following manner.

Divide, by successive transverse sections, the hippocampus from
the part named the foot upwards, as far as it can be traced. It will
be found that each section presents a central portion of gray matter,
enveloped in a thin curled plate of white matter, which is free at
one edge,—the concave one,—and hangs over the gray band like
a veil, but adheres, by its opposite, to the cerebral substance. It
will be perceived, also, that the white plate does not adhere to the
gray band, unless at its fixed margin, and that a probe or scalpel
handle may be introduced into the angular furrow between them.*
As the sections approach the upper end of the cylindroid process a
new arrangement is observed. The white plate becomes unusually
broad, and is less bent or rolled over the gray band; while the
latter, thus less completely covered, instead of following the same
direction with the white plate which it does below, is much separated from it, and leaves a considerable angle between the plate and
itself. This arrangement is most conspicuous where the process
corresponds to the upper part of the optic chamber and the cerebral limb. The white plate of the hippocampus traced further is
found to coalesce with the margins of the vault, and tapering as it
approaches the anterior end of that body, is finally identified with
its substance. The upper termination or connection of the gray
band is different. When it begins to recede from the white plate,
which it does nearly opposite to the optic eminence, it proceeds directly to the rounded posterior end of the central band, (*corpus
callosum,*) over which, and along the upper surface about one inch,
it may be traced; and beyond this it is seldom capable of being
distinguished from the white matter of which the central band consists.† The *gray indented band*, therefore, which forms the inner

* This last fact may also be demonstrated without transverse sections, by simple
elevation of the white plate by the handle of the instrument.

† The importance of this object in forming the outer border of the great communication, will render it not improper to glance at the history of its discovery. Vicq-
D'Azyr is supposed to have been the first anatomist who observed and described its
site and appearance with accuracy ; and we find him, in a Memoir of the Royal Aca-

3

or central part of the cylindroid process, is continuous, or connected with the upper surface of the central band of the organ ; and
if the terms of origin or derivation be admitted, may be said to be
derived from it; while the thin white plate which is rolled over the
gray band, and gives the hippocampus its cylindrical figure, is connected with the under surface of the same central band, or that
part which the usual nomenclature styles the vault (*fornix*) of the
brain.

Such, as nearly as language can represent, is the configuration
of the cylindroid process,—an object which it is impossible to know
too accurately, if we reflect, that it forms the entire outer border
of the great communication between the convoluted and figurate
surfaces of the brain. If, by the method now described, a clear
idea of this disposition is not communicated; it is expedient to use
another contrivance, which I have rarely found to fail in demonstrating the facts which I wish to impress. Let a brain, divested
of its membranes, be inverted ; and when the opening behind the
outer margin of the cerebral limbs has been exposed, let a deep
transverse incision between the feet of the hippocampus of each side
be made. This incision must not touch the cylindroid process, but
going deep into the substance of the organ, will detach the whole
of that part which contains the several objects of the figurate surface from the anterior part of the hemispheres. The portion thus
separated will, however, still adhere by the sides to the substance
of the hemispheres; and other incisions must be made, following
the direction of the outer or lateral margin of the striated bodies

demy of Sciences in 1787, detailing its peculiarities with some minuteness, under the
name of " Bord externe et dentelé de la Corne d'Ammon." He subsequently represented it in his great work in the year 1786, under the name of gray, cortical, external
notched portion of the Horn of Ammon, and speaks of it familiarly enough by the
term of *corps godronnée.* Bichat, however, whose descriptive anatomy was published
in 1802, though his accurate manner prevented him from overlooking it, and
led him to give a sufficiently minute account of it, boldly asserted, that it had
been entirely neglected by authors. Dr Gordon of this place, who was quite aware of
this oversight in Bichat, took special care, in demonstrating it, to notice the merit of
Vicq-D'Azyr ; and this fact he mentions shortly in a note, in his description of
the gray band. None of these eminent anatomists have been altogether right in this
matter ; and the truth is, that Vicq-D'Azyr is not the first who delineated this body.
The gray indented band is distinctly represented by Pierre Tarin, in the second engraving of his Adversaria ; and although this had been published in 1750, thirty years
before the engravings of Vicq-D'Azyr, yet it was requisite for the latter writer to make
it the subject of a particular memoir, and Bichat to write a description of it, before it
seems to have been known as part of the organ.

(*corpora striata*) and the optic chambers (*thalami optici,*) until the whole be completely insulated.   If these incisions be properly managed, the whole of the middle band, the vault, the cylindroid process, and the white tape, will be left uninjured, and will present a large hollow surrounded by an extensive border, the posterior part of which is made by the posterior end of the central band, while lateral divisions are formed by the cylindroid process of either side. The observer will likewise form a very just idea of the situation and connections of the middle band, and will perceive that its inferior surface is the same as that named *vault* or *ceiling*.   He will further remark, that the thin white plates (*tæniæ*) which are attached to the margins of this object, and between which is the space improperly named the *lyre*, extend in a circular and revolute direction outwards and downwards, so as to cover, in the mode described, the gray band of the cylinder, and give this object its cylindrical aspect.

The correct understanding of the outer border of this communication should be followed by an equally just idea of those parts which form what we must name its inner border.   These are more numerous and rather more complicated ; but frequent examination, with a little attention, will enable the student to overcome all the difficulties with which they may be attended.   The parts contained in the mass of brain removed, as we described in the last section, will contribute also very much to render the knowledge of this border easy and intelligible.   I have already said, that at the posterior end of the middle band the inner or lower border is formed by the four eminences (*c. quadrigemina*) situate on the upper surface of the thick mass named *protuberance*.   On each side of these the inner border is formed by successive portions of the optic chamber, until it has reached the inferior region of this body, where the outer and lower margin of the limb of the brain becomes the border of the opening.   To render this arrangement more intelligible, I shall here state some circumstances of the figurate surface, which are either omitted or indistinctly mentioned in the ordinary descriptions.

Its principal objects are familiarly known ; and none can be ignorant of the situation of the striated bodies, the optic chamber, the semicircular chord between them, and other similar objects.

The posterior eminences, or the optic chambers, hold the most important place; and their connection and relative situation render them much more interesting, than they are usually made in works of descriptive anatomy. Connected before and on the outside to the striated body by means of the double semicircular chord (*centrum semicirculare geminum*, Vieussens,) each optic eminence presents four free surfaces,—the upper, the inner, the posterior, and the lower. The upper, the first, is gently rounded and of white colour. Its figure and limits are not easily defined. The outer margin is bounded by the circular band, which even passes on anterior to it, so as to form its boundary in that direction also. Behind, it is less distinctly limited, unless by the appearance of a considerable prominence, which has been generally named the posterior tubercle of the optic couch. The inner margin of the upper surface is most distinctly marked by a small sharp gray line, which, beginning insensibly at the anterior part of the body, becomes more distinct as it extends backwards, and is ultimately found to bend gently toward the median plane. There it unites with a similar elevated line of the opposite optic eminence; and to the point of union is attached a small conical body with a minute point, of a gray colour, and of a shape like that of the pine-apple. This is the object improperly termed pineal gland; (*glandula pinealis, conarium*; Die Zirbel-drüse; Reil); and the minute linear eminences or tracts, which form the inner edge of the upper optic surface, have been named *peduncles* of the pineal gland. The inner surface of the optic couch or chamber presents nothing important, save the small portion of soft cerebral matter, which unites it to the similar surface of the opposite body. Its posterior edge, however, is terminated by the cerebral limb of that side; and the lower edge meets that of the opposite one, and is connected to it by a portion of brain, which, examined in this manner, has received no name, but forms the lower part of the middle ventricle. The portion of brain which corresponds to it on the outside (base of the brain) has been named the *bridge of Tarin.* (*Pons Tarini.*) This is the triangular space between the limbs of the brain which has been called by Vicq-D'Azyr *the pit of the oculo-muscular nerves.* It may be named the *triangular intercrural hollow.*

The posterior surface of the optic eminence is the most important, but the least understood. It is so intimately connected with the inferior, that in description they cannot be easily distinguished. Santorini, I believe, was the first who observed that the posterior

part of the optic couch was terminated by a projection or process,
which he named the *jointed or geniculate body*, and which, he had
likewise the merit of observing, gives rise to the optic nerve.*
More recently Malacarne remarked that this region is rendered
unequal by a tubercle, from which the nerves seem partly to rise.†
About the same time it was noticed by Vicq-D'Azyr, that on the
side, a little behind and below, there are three superficial tubercles of a rounded figure, and disposed in a triangle ; and that one
of them must have been the body mentioned by Gunz and Bon-
homme, and of which Haller avowed his ignorance.‡ He afterwards mentions a slight prominence near the upper of the four
eminences, of a white colour, but gray exteriorly, communicating
with the optic tract ;§ while the external-lateral region of the optic
couch presents several similar eminences, but less considerable.
The notice given by Bichat is still more brief and less satisfactory
" Tout a fait en arriere cette parti inferieure offre une ou deux
saillies, et se continue avec les tubercules quadrijumeaux."
    The inaccurate manner in which these authors seem to have exa-
mined this part of the organ, the vague and unprecise terms in
which they speak of it, as if its existence were apocryphal,—show
the necessity of more correct researches. Soemmering and Gordon describe in this situation two eminences, termed the outer and
inner geniculate bodies. The description of the former author is
brief and precise, but not quite so satisfactory as could be wished.
That of the latter is more minute ; but in some respects it is either
not clear, or it does not apply generally.

* " Quod tamen per repetitas diligenterque institutas disquisitiones ab eadem potius
membrana eos non proficisci, sæpius vidisse vissus sum ; verum tum ab eorum Thala-
morum interiori parte, tum a *quodam velut geniculato corpore circa eorundem Thala-
morum posteriora locato adjunctoque*, cujus corticalis seu cinerea interior substantia
est, medullaris et candida exterior facies luculentius prodire, sum assecutus : Ad ho-
rum tamen exortus locum a latere prominentiarum quod natiformes nuncupantur,
conspicuus medullaris tractus transversim sic Thalamis conjungitur, ut vel in eorum
substantia disjiciatur, vel inflexus cæterisque fibrillis involutus ad Nervorum opticorum
exortum accedat, conjicere quidem, decernere autem minime vaiui." Observat. Anatomic. Joan. Dom. Santorini, cap. iii. § 14.   See also a more minute description in his
posthumous *Tabulæ Anatomicæ*, Tabula iii. fig. 1. p. 32. Parmæ, 1775.
    † " La stessa faccia superiore—è coperta d'una lamina midollare tenuissima ed ha
disuguale la posteriore estremità per un *bernacolo irregolare*, da cui sembra che in
parte usscono i nervi ottici." Articolo, vii. 68.
    ‡ Elementa Physiologiæ, Tom. IV. lib. x. sect. 1. § 24.
    § Recherches sur la Structure du Cerveau, &c. ix. Mémoires de l'Academie
Royale des Sciences, Année 1781.

The confusion and uncertainty which prevails on this part of cerebral anatomy, induced me to adopt a method which I find to be more certain in unfolding the objects in question, and which may be safely recommended to the practical anatomist. Let the brain be examined from below, and let the examination commence with the optic tracts. That the acceptation of this term may be definite, I observe that the optic nerves should be in accuracy counted from the commissure only. The cerebral extremity or origin, as it is named, of a nerve, should ·be reckoned from that point only at which it.is quite free in its whole circumference from the organ. This happens to the optic nerves at the anterior part of the commissure only; for behind this body the longitudinal bands called *tracts* adhere by one side (the outer) to the cerebral substance. A narrow angular sinuosity, admitting the point of a small probe, is found at the inner or mesial edge of the tracts; but beyond this they adhere indissolubly. As they pursue their course backward and outward, they reach the limbs of the brain, the inferior surface of which they cross, still adhering by their outer edge, but more extensively. Here likewise they are sensibly broader than at their anterior end.

When they have passed completely the limbs of the brain, at which they are about the breadth of three lines, they begin to present a linear furrow or depression, which extends in their long direction about one-half or three-fourths of an inch, and thus divides the tract into an *outer* and an *inner* limb. This depression, however, does not divide the tract equally, but leaves the outer broader than the inner limb. It is insensibly terminated at the upper surface of the optic eminence or chamber; and its last part, (about three or four lines,) contemplated with care, will be found to separate two spheroidal eminences which are respective terminations of the outer and inner limbs of the tract. The outer of these eminences is the largest and most prominent, and is the body mentioned by authors as the posterior tubercle of the optic chamber. It is the body which Santorini named the geniculate, (*corpus quiddam geniculatum ;*)—an epithet for which it is not easy to account, unless we suppose that his fancy had likened it to the appearance of a bent joint, especially that of the knee, to which, if viewed laterally in connection with the tract, it bears some remote resemblance. It is broader, larger, and more convex than the inner eminence, and is evidently the chief origin of the optic tract. The eminence on the inside of the linear furrow is much smaller, and often less distinctly marked than the outer. In ordinary circumstances it may be described as an eminence of cerebral matter contained between two circular segments, in such manner that its longitudinal extent, which is nearly vertical, is greater than its transverse. It is obviously connected with the smaller limb of the optic tract. Whether this body actually takes its origin from the four eminences (*corpora quadrigemina,*) depends on evidence of a different description.

The inner or mesial side of the geniculate bodies is contiguous to the four eminences, and is separated from them by a linear furrow. These eminences occupy the upper surface of the protuberance, and partly that of the limbs of the brain, and the linear furrow marks the point at which the limbs issue from the substance of the optic couches. The lower surface, indeed, of these bodies presents the long thick cylinder of the limbs; and while they occupy this conspicuous situation, and a considerable proportion of the ‧ lower surface, it is impossible to assign them more cerebral space above, than that occupied by the upper two of the four eminences (*nates,*) and the adjoining part of the optic couch.

This view of the objects occurring in this region of the figurate surface, will show the formation and arrangement of the inner border of the communication. It will be seen that it consists of successive portions of that figurate surface, proceeding from the mesial line, on each side to the lower and outer margin of the cerebral limbs. It will be seen, that, if we begin at the longitudinal furrow of the four eminences, we find first the upper eminence of one side; then the contiguous part of the optic couch; then the greater geniculate eminence; after this, as the cylindroid process pursues its winding and revolute course, the outer part of the cerebral limb; and, lastly, the outer and lower angle of that limb.

Not only, however, does the convoluted surface of the brain communicate with the figurate one, but the laminated surface of the cerebellum communicates with the analogous surface of that organ, and thus with the great figurate surface. This communication takes place on the middle plane, below the transverse or middle plates which form the pyramid, uvula, and nodule, and between these bodies and the restiform processes. This is the fourth ventricle of anatomical writers; and as it has never been denied that it communicates with the outer surface of the cerebellum, it is noticed here merely as an integrant part of those views which I apply to the organ at large. The central or figurate surface exposed in the manner now explained is smooth, polished, and possesses a degree of firmness and closeness of texture which prevents it from being readily broken or abraded. These qualities are ascribed by Reil to a thin membranous pellicle, which he terms *Epithelion*, and with which he conceives the proper matter of the brain is covered.* Trusting to ordinary inspection, aided by a good glass, I do not think there is any sensible proof of the existence of this covering. It is more natural to regard it as cerebral matter modified for its situation. In point of fact, the deep cerebral matter may be rendered equally firm with this by immersion in alcohol or dilute acids. But nothing can give the smooth, polished, close-grained surface which belongs to every spot of this part of the brain. After this explanation, I shall not scruple to use the term *Epithelion*, not in the sense given by Reil, but merely as a name to the firm smooth substance which forms the figurate surface of the brain.

In certain situations this surface is unusually firm, for instance in the narrow winding hollow between the striated bodies and the optic eminences. (*Centrum semicirculare geminum*, Vieussens; *tænia semicircularis*, Haller.) Of the central surface, not only does every division mutually communicate, but the whole central surface of the convoluted brain communicates with the central surface of the laminated part of the organ. Thus the lateral divisions, called *ventricles*, communicate freely and directly with each other below the vault or twain-band; (*fornix*, Die Zwillingsbinde;) the surface of which lies free over the top of the *thalami*. These again communicate with the intermediate space called the third ventricle, from which it is well known there is a passage to the space between the *medulla oblongata* and the cerebellum. The communication with the posterior and inferior divisions, (*cornua*), is well known.

The whole of this surface is covered by a vascular membrane, which is a continuation of that (*pia mater*) of the convoluted surface. One part of this which lies over the objects in the lateral ventricles has been long known under the name of *choroid plexus;* and an intermediate portion by which those of the two sides are united, has been distinguished by the term *velum interpositum*. Not only are each of these parts of the same membrane, and con-

* Archiv. für die Physiologie, 9ter Band, 3. Untersuchungen, &c. p. 143.

nected with the *pia mater ;* but individual portions of vascular membrane or choroid plexus, all continuous, are found in every division of the figurate surface of the brain.   This membrane sustains the vessels going to and issuing from the cerebral substance. Between the two surfaces now described is placed the proper matter of the brain, which in different regions of the organ is arranged differently.   The intimate arrangement peculiar to individual parts, and the manner in which the arrangement of each is mutually connected, are now to become the object of examination. The convoluted surface first claims attention.   The colour of this is well known to be of an ash-gray, passing in certain parts to pale brown.   In whatever part the substance of the convolutions be examined, they never present any appearance of linear or fibrous arrangement.   I have often examined the convoluted substance of the human brain after induration in alcohol and dilute nitric acid ; and I never could recognize the distinct fibrous disposition observed in other parts of the organ.   A portion of brain, hardened in the manner now mentioned, breaks with a small conchoidal fracture, and an uneven granular subordinate surface.   The surface thus exposed presents, however, a very determinate aspect, which it is easy to recognize after repeated trials.   It is ash-gray and without lustre.   It is rough, and consists, when minutely examined, of roundish grains aggregated together.   The direction of the fracture is more at right angles to the convoluted surface than obliquely or parallel to it.   In some instances even it is possible to recognize depressed marks perpendicular to the surface, sending off angularly like branches smaller depressed marks, meeting similar ramifications from other perpendicular depressions.

I have often attempted to determine, by breaking portions of brain in every direction, whether this appearance is uniform ; but I cannot say that I have obtained satisfactory proof of the point. I am not unaware that Reil represents the intimate structure of the convolutions to be distinctly fibrous.   So far as I understand his description, I admit the fact of the conchoidal fracture which I have often verified ; but I am not prepared to allow that this arises, as he imagines, from the fibrous matter being arranged in plates or leaves, which are folded and rolled together.*   Upon the whole, the convoluted substance I regard as chiefly granular, but so arranged as to be more frangible in the direction perpendicular to

* Archiv. für die Physiologie neunter Band, p. 145.

its surface than otherwise. It is said to be more abundantly supplied with vessels than the white matter; (Ruysch, Albinus, Prochaska, Soemmering, and Ehrenberg;) and indeed a great number of large vessels enters it all over, and especially at certain parts, *e. g.* the perforated space of the Sylvian fissure. It is not, however, absolutely and at all points more vascular than the white matter. The transition from the gray convoluted matter to the white inclosed, is in all parts of the hemispheres sudden and distinct. It is more distinct, however, after induration by immersion in alcohol or dilute acid than in the recent brain.

The only part of the convoluted surface which presents a distinct fibrous arrangement is that part of the Sylvian fissure which has been named by Reil the unciform bundle; (der haakenförmige Markbündel). This, however, can scarcely be said to belong to the convoluted surface. It is situate on the outside of the perforated spot, and corresponds with a short smooth convolution, which passes between the middle and the anterior lobes. The unciform bundle, in short, unites these lobes, and is intimately connected* with the internal arrangement of the *nucleus* and its capsule, parts immediately to be noticed.

The white cerebral matter is arranged in various parts of the organ, in the form of inconceivably minute parallel lines, lying in juxtaposition. It is unnecessary to enumerate all the parts in which this arrangement may be observed; and greater advantage will result from a short view of the mutual relation and connection of the fibrous parts of the organ, so far as they are well ascertained.

In tracing this part of the intimate structure of the brain, several anatomists have imbibed the notion that one part of the brain gives rise to or generates another. From this assumption even Reil is not wholly exempt. Without entering on the subject of organogenesy, or the question of, which part of the brain in the fœtal existence is first, and which subsequently formed,—which will be considered in its own place—I begin with stating, that in the adult every part of the organ is supposed to be coeval; that the idea of one part generating or reinforcing another is an effort of fancy which must not be admitted in strict science; that when a bundle of fibres, or a fibrous arrangement, is seen proceeding *from* one part *to* another, it is imagination only which suggests that the former produces the latter, or conversely; and that from this nothing

Archiv. für die Physiologie, 9ter Band, pp. 184, 197, and 201.

more can be inferred than that the parts so arranged are mutually and generally connected.

The inner fibrous part of the brain proper is divided by Reil into the system of the brain-limbs (*crura* ;—Das Hirnschenkel-system ;) the system of the beam or mesolobe, (Das Balken system ;) and the striated ganglion (das gestreifte Hirnganglion ;), and to one or other of these he refers the arrangement of all the other parts of which the organ is composed. I do not adopt all his views, nor is it requisite to follow his distinctions minutely. But I shall attempt to trace briefly what I conceive admits of demonstrable proof.

The beam or mesolobe, (*corpus callosum*, Der Balken) consists of white cerebral matter disposed in transverse fibres, which meet on the mesial plane, and thus give rise to the longitudinal lines seen on its upper surface (*Raphe externa et interna*, Reil). They appear to change direction, and bend down at right angles, parallel with those of the opposite half. At the distance of from four to five lines on each side, these transverse fibres undergo a similar interruption or change of direction, so as to form the *covered bands* (die bedeckten Bänder), which appear also in the form of long, firm, fibrous lines, extending longitudinally along the upper surface of the beam. Between these bands and the inner margin of the olfacient groove a connection may be traced over the *knee* (das Knie), or anterior end of the beam.

Beyond the covered bands the transverse fibres pass directly into the white matter of the hemispheres, where they are connected in different modes with different parts. The general direction is that of expansion, like the rods of a fan, or radiation, like the rays of a luminous body. The fibres which compose the knee or anterior end, sinking into the hemisphere near the anterior *cornu*, meet those forming the first and anterior staff of the brain-limb, which lie in the anterior knotty end of the striated body, and wind round the adjoining edge of the staff-wreath ; (der Stabkranz). In the intermediate substance, which is knotty before, and spreads into a brush-shaped expansion behind, the middle rods of the staff-wreath unite with their anterior extremities, and with the fibres of the beam. This forms the *first* or *anterior* junction of the beam with the limbs.

The middle fibres, passing immediately into the hemisphere, meet more abruptly with those of the limbs Suddenly contracting, as it were, they coalesce with those of the *tœnia*, and are covered by the gray matter of the brush-like termination above-mentioned, and epithelion, which is here very thick. The radiating fibres of both systems are here shortest. The deep layers form in some parts immediate mutual communications, especially in the posterior *cornu;* and at this point alone the inner layer of the beam descends directly on the fibres of the limb. In expansion, these radiating fibres receive between them white matter from the hemispherical circumference; and in this manner form connections, as remarked by Reil, with the peripheral or convoluted part of the hemispheres, and especially with those which form the Sylvian fissure.* This may be considered the *second* connection of the beam with the brain limbs.

The hinder part of the beam is something firmer than the fore part reckoned towards the centre ; a circumstance which depends on the closeness with which its fibres are here compacted in mass. After forming the elevated ridge which constitutes the hinder crossbar of the vault, they plunge into the hemispheres in the form of thick bundles, which, running horizontally backwards over the posterior *cornu,* are expanded in the posterior parts of the hemispheres. The inner layer of these fibres, which falling on the outer wall of the *cornu* over the radiation of the limbs, covers it and part of the outer wall, is named by Reil the *tapestry*, or *hanging*. (Die Tapete.) This may be viewed as a *third* point of junction between the beam and the brain limbs.

I am now to trace the direction of the component fibres of the latter parts. These are connected below, above, and behind, with so many important parts, that it is requisite to comprehend several parts under the general denomination of *System of the limbs.* After the example of Reil, we begin from the head of the spinal chord ; (*medulla oblongata.*)

This part consists in the human adult of six eminences, three on each side of the mesial plane ; the *pyramidal* or *pyriform* eminences before and below, the *restiform* bodies behind and above, and the *olivary* eminences on each side. Of these the olivary eminences are to be viewed as the most important, since by each containing a ciliary or moriform nucleus, (*corpus ciliare, c. dentatum, c. moriforme, c. rhomboideum,*) they make an approach in structure to the character of the cerebellum.

The pyriform or pyramidal bodies are important in another light.

* Archiv. für die Physiologie, Neunter Band, p. 179.

R

Varoli, who has the merit of first examining with attention what is termed the *base* of the brain, traced in these bodies longitudinal fibres passing upwards through the body, named after him *Pons Varolii*, the *annular protuberance*, (*protuberantia annularis ;* Willis; *nodus cerebri;* Rau ;) towards the limbs and substance of the brain. By Vieussens and Morgagni the fact of this arrangement was afterwards verified; and it has been confirmed by the observations of Reil on the adult brain, and by those of Tiedemann in the fœtal organ.

The pyramidal bodies, situate on the anterior part of the *medulla oblongata*, and mutually separated by the median furrow, consist entirely of bands or rods of whitish fibres, (Die Mark Stabchen,) extending longitudinally through them. Becoming thicker, but not less compact at the upper end, where they are connected with the part named bridge, (*pons Varolii;* die Brucke;) or annular protuberance; (*nodus cerebri ;*) these longitudinal fibres undergo a new arrangement. *First,* They are covered with a firm layer of transverse fibres, which proceed, as it were, from the middle line on each side circularly round. These fibres are white, firm transversely, and abundantly distinct. When peeled off to the depth of about 1½ line or two, the longitudinal fibres of the pyramids begin to appear ; but no longer collected in mass as below. Numerous transverse or circular-transverse fibres are interposed between them, so as to separate them into layers. Hence results the complex structure of the bridge, which externally appears to consist of circular-transverse matter, but internally presents many longitudinal bands. It is worthy of notice, that in transverse and longitudinal sections the part which appears gray on the transverse section, is white on the longitudinal, and conversely. The closeness with which the circular fibres are compacted render the bridge decidedly the firmest part of the whole brain.

Proceeding from the lower to the upper surface of the bridge, this combination of long and cross bands is less distinct. Part, if not the whole of the transverse fibres, sink into the peduncles or *crura* of the cerebellum ; and they evidently predominate here over the longitudinal.

The posterior-upper part of the *medulla oblongata* consists of two longitudinal bodies separated on the median line by a deep furrow. These, which are the *restiform* or rope-like processes, *chordal-processes* of Ridley, (*corpora restiformia*) (*processus restiformes,* Mor-

3

gagni,) are described in most works as the pyramidal eminences. (Haller, Malacarne, Reil.) As there is no doubt that this part of the spinal chord presents six eminences, three on each side, as above stated, with the view of avoiding the confusion with which anatomists speak on these bodies, I adhere to the plan originally adopted by Willis, Ridley, Ruysch, and Morgagni, of distinguishing the anterior eminences as *pyramidal*, and the posterior as the *restiform processes.**

Stretching in the form of thick strong bands between the peduncles of the cerebellum above, and the spinal chord below, the restiform processes are mutually parted by a deep furrow, (*calamus scriptorius*,) in the bottom of which, when slightly separated, white chords proceeding from the process of one side are observed to be plaited or crossed with those of the other. This arrangement was first observed by Dominico Mistichelli,† a physician at Rome, in 1709, and shortly after by Pourfour de Petit‡ at Namur. Though subsequently verified by the observation of Santorini,§ Win-

---

* " The third descends from this part (the cerebellum) backwards upon the upper side of the *medulla oblongata*, like two longish thick chords on each side, making the *medulla* look somewhat thicker and broader in that place, and not unfitly styled the *chordal process.*" The Anatomy of the Brain, &c. By H. Ridley, Coll. Med. Lond. Soc. London, 1695, chap. xiv. p. 136. Of this the term *processus restiformis* is a literal translation, given by his Latin translator, and in the collection of Mangetus. It is remarkable, that, though thus early noticed by Ridley, and afterwards distinguished as posterior pyramidal eminences by Ruysch, the restiform processes have been completely neglected, and are scarcely known even by name. It is not uncommon both in books and in demonstration to see them pointed out as the *corpora pyramidalia*. By those who wish to avoid the confusion resulting from this oversight, they are termed *posterior pyramidal bodies ;* and in support of this, the authority of Ruysch, Prochaska, and Soemmering* may be adduced.

† Trattato dell' Apoplessia. Roma, 1709. Lib. i. Cap. vi. ix.
‡ Lettre d'un Medecin des Hospices du Roi. Namur, 1710.
§ " Nos autem sic eam luculenter conspeximus, sic evidenter, ubi apta incidere cadavera demonstravimus, ut nulla amplius nobis de hac re supersit dubitandi ratio. Id autem triplici potissimum in loco animadvertere potuimus ; in utraque scilicet priore posterioreque annularis protuberantiæ crepidine, atque maxime in imo medullaris caudicis, qua in spinalem abit. In priore itaque annularis protuberantiæ parte, qua superius reflexa pro comprehendendis oblongatæ medullæ cruribus in anguli formam interius producta tenuatur, sic ex concurrentibus fibris, strictiorique agmine coeuntibus, altera alteram scandit, ut præter mirum implexum, decussatio luculentissime appareat. Id ipsum ferme in postica ipsius crepidine occurrit. Eo iterum in loco, qui quarto ventriculo subjicitur, (the space between the restiform processes,) præter varios fibrarum

---

* Frederici Ruyschii Responsio ad M. E. Ettmuller de Corticali Cerebri Substantia, &c. p. 25. Amstel. 1721. Georgii Prochaska De Structura Nervorum Tractatus, &c. Sectio 3. tabula i fig 1. S. T. Soemmering De Basi Encephali, &c. Tab. II. sect. 3. § 18. Apud Ludwig, Tom. II.

slow,* Lieutaud, and Soemmering,† it had escaped the notice of Haller, Vicq-D'Azyr, Monro, and others, and was, therefore, doubted till revived by M. Gall. Independent of the testimony of the above authors, it is easy to demonstrate by slight separation of the restiform bodies the fact, that whitish chords are seen lying obliquely across the linear depression, and that those connected with the right process cross to the left, while conversely those of the left cross to the right. It is to the inner or mesial fibres of the restiform processes only that this cross plaiting is confined. Neither the pyramidal, nor the olivary, nor even the whole of the restiform bodies partake of it. It is sufficient, however, to establish a communication between the right and left halves of this part of the spinal chord. It was seen by Tiedemann in the fourth and fifth weeks of uterine life.

The interior fibres of these bodies are longitudinal, and proceed partly to the cerebellum, partly to the protuberance. The deep-seated layer is partly interwoven with the transverse circular fibres of this body, in the same manner in which those of the pyramidal eminences are, partly bends up to the peduncles of the cerebellum, with the bands of which they are then combined. The superficial layer is connected chiefly with the substance of the *corpora quadrigemina*, (Die Vierhugel,) which constitute the upper surface of the protuberance.

The structure of the olivary body is more complex. Though its surface consists of longitudinal fibres, which, like those of the other eminences, are lost in the protuberance, these form a sort of superficial covering to a capsule of gray matter arranged in a serrated form, inclosing a nucleus of white. This arrangement constitutes a ciliary or moriform body, (*corpus ciliare, c. dentatum, c. rhomboideum*,) precisely similar to that in the white trunks of the cere-

ordines et colores, in adversum latus productas, et decussatas fibras commodé spectavimus. Si ea tamen evidenter uspiam conspicitur, profecto quam evidentissime duas vix lineas infra pyramidalia, atque adeo olivaria corpora conspici potest. Qua enim in longitudinem producta linea, seu rimula pyramidalia corpora (the restiform processes) discernuntur, si leniter diducantur, probe prius eo potissimum loco artissime hærente tenui meninge nudata, non tenues decussari fibrillas sed *validos earundem fasciculos in adversa contendere*, quam apertissime demonstravimus." Observ. Anatom. J. D. Santorini. Lug. Bat. 1739. Cap. 3, § 12. p. 61. Also Tab. II. apud Girardi, p. 28, 29.

* Exposition Anatomique, &c. Par J. B. Winslow. Paris, 1732. Traité de la Teste, 110, p. 626.

† S. T. Soemmering de Basi Encephali, lib. ii. sect. 3. § 18.

bellum, to which, therefore, the olivary eminence approaches in organization.

All these parts may be viewed as external markings on the bulb of the spinal marrow, (*medulla oblongata.*) It is to be observed, that in the foetus, the infant, and in young subjects in general, they are more distinct, than in the brains of adults and especially of the aged. In the brains of infants and the young, all the markings both separating furrows and elevations are most distinct; and the restiform bodies or posterior pyramidal bodies present each a longitudinal furrow, parting them in two portions, one lying close on the median line and furrow, the other lying between their median and most posterior portions and the olivary bodies. To these sometimes the name of posterior pyramidal bodies is applied, and the name appears sometimes to be applied to the restiform bodies, while that of restiform bodies is given to these anterior portions of the posterior masses, still regarded as posterior pyramids.

As life advances this longitudinal furrow becomes less distinct, and at length is so small as to be imperceptible in many adult and aged persons. This is the reason of the discordance in the statements of different anatomists.

In the infant brain, therefore, and in that of the young, the *medulla oblongata* is marked or distinguished externally into eight bodies, or four on each side of the mesial plane. At this period of life also, each of the four lateral bodies is more strongly figured, and appears in more distinct relief than in the brain examined at a subsequent period.

In the brain of the young, also, the internal structure is if possible more strongly marked than in that of the aged. It is then seen, that the longitudinal fibres of the bulb are interlaced or interwoven with numerous transverse fibres; that the *corpora restiforma* are closely connected with the peduncles of the cerebellum; that the anterior pyramids are connected or continuous with the *crura* of the brain; and that the olivary bodies, by presenting a *corpus dentatum*, form a repetition of the *cerebellum* in the spinal marrow.

The longitudinal fibres of these several parts passing through the protuberance are observed beyond this body to be in direct continuation with those of the cerebral limbs. (*Crura*, Die Hirnschenkel.) These are cylindrical masses, stretching obliquely between the protuberance behind and the optic chambers or eminences before. The longitudinal bands of which they consist give their lower surface a fluted appearance, at least to the inner margin of the optic tracts, by which they are obliquely crossed. Connected before with the posterior-inferior region of the *thalami*, they may be traced into the substance of these parts, where they undergo an arrangement new and peculiar.

Though the name couch or *thalamus* be still applied to these bodies, it conveys an erroneous idea of their anatomical relations. With the striated bodies, they form the central portion and most perfectly organized nucleus of the organ.

Each optic thalamus may be said to be united behind with its fellow by means of the quadrigeminous eminences. These consist superficially of epithelion or capsular cerebral matter, below of a semilunar stratum of fibres derived from the cerebral limbs, while a similar production forms the deep layer of the *corpus geniculatum internum*.

In each optic thalamus may be distinguished, according to Reil, four layers, each consisting of gray and white matter. The uppermost is merely the epithelion or condensed matter which forms the covering. The second is connected with the inner *corpus geniculatum*, from which fibres appear to spread or expand in the manner of rays, over the outer edge of the limb, and embracing the part to be mentioned as the nucleus of the brain. The third layer consists of a set of fibres which, issuing from the upper layer of the brain-limb at their entrance into the thalamus, are firmly tied as it were into a loop or knot, (die Schleife,) and are then expanded like a brush into the substance of the thalamus. The lower is formed chiefly by the cerebral limb. It is partly in the former, partly in the latter, that the dark-coloured matter constituting the *locus niger* is placed.

The *thalamus* is so intimately connected with the limbs, that they must be viewed as essential parts of the same organized whole. The component rods or fibrous bands (seine Markstabchen) of the latter, partly combining with the former, but chiefly receiving them, spread out near the outer edge of the thalamus circularly, and constitute the radiated expansion called by Reil the Staffwreath. (Der Stab-Kranz.) These rods, at first obliquely horizontal, gradually, as they expand, assume a more vertical direction. Inwards, or towards the mesial plane from the first band or rod ascends the anterior pillar of the Twainband (*fornix*) to the knobs of the beam.

Then follow the first band or spoke of the wreath, and the rest in succession. The anterior rods are long, slender, numerous, and thickly crowded on each other. The middle or lateral are short, thick, roll-like, and form a sort of crest or comb. The posterior are long and of fibrous structure. As they expand they form nearly a complete circle, which radiates through all the lobes. The *radii* of this circle are connected in the anterior lobes with the knee of the beam, cross the *fossa Sylvii* near the anterior and posterior *cornua* to the outer edge of the thalamus, and terminate in the lateral *cornu* in the apex of the middle lobe, at the beginning of the Sylvian furrow. In this course the anterior rays of the Staffwreath are longer than the middle and lateral rays, the interruption of which forms the *comb* or crest. (Der Kamm.) The posterior, which go to the border of the outer wall of the capsule, are the longest; and shorter ones are again seen below in the region of the lateral cornu.

The last part, the organization of which can be here made the subject of short consideration, is the striated body. When observed, this part presents a singular arrangement of white and gray matter in the form of alternate streaks. This arrangement, though constant, it is unnecessary to describe minutely, unless so far as it is connected with the appearances already mentioned. The parts which chiefly claim attention on this head are the *cerebral nucleus*, its *capsule*, and the *walls of the capsule*.

The striated part of the brain may be regarded as a· nucleus, (Der Kern) or organized central mass,* which is contained within a capsule consisting of three walls or enclosing plates of white matter; a *lower*, an *outer*, and an *inner wall*.

The lower wall of the capsule, which is accidental, consists chiefly of the *tractus innominatus*, (Die ungenannte Marksubstanz,) the perforated spot, and that part of the convoluted space from which the olfacient nerve issues.

The outer wall is the most remarkable. It rests on the unciform band (Der haakenförmige Markbündel) at the entrance of the Sylvian fossa, which connects the convolutions of the anterior lobes by the perforated spot with the middle lobe. From this unciform band as a centre, the fibres of the whole outer wall radiate; and as the

---

* Reil considers it a ganglion, (Das Gestreifte grosse Hirnganglium.) But this idea is hypothetical; and while I use the term *nucleus*, I wish to convey no idea but that of one part contained within another.

deep ones are beneath the level of the cerebral limb, Reil regards them as connected neither with this nor with the beam or mesolobe. He represents, nevertheless, the radiation of the outer wall as too much detached from the unciform band. Frequent examination of this part leads me to represent the outer wall and the unciform band as parts of the same system of fibres. The unciform band is situate not on the same vertical plane with the rest of the outer wall, which not only radiates in every direction forward, upward, and backward, but swells out laterally, or towards the convoluted region of the hemispheres. The result of this arrangement is, that the section which shows the unciform band most distinctly shows only the peripheral or marginal fibres of the outer wall. A section more external or lateral, however, shows the radiating fibres of the part between the centre, (the unciform process,) and the circumference; and in order to see them distinctly all at once, and to have a correct conception of their assembled disposition, it is requisite to pare off from its outer surface the exterior white matter, or to excavate externally, so as to form a spherical segment.

The outer wall of the capsule is, in short, a spherical shell, consisting of fibres radiating from a point above the *fossa Sylvii.* So far as I have been able to observe, it has no connection with the limbs of the brain.

The inner wall of the capsule is composed, on the contrary, of the stem of the limb, and the fore-part of the staffwreath, which sends fibres under the round part of the inner portion of the nucleus. Joining the outer wall above by means of an arched margin, and at acute angles, it gives the capsule the shape of an inverted boat.

In this capsule is lodged the outer part of the large striated nucleus of the brain; the inner, usually named *corpus striatum,* being covered only by epithelion within the ventricle. Both are parts of one organ which should not be separated.

Of the cerebellum, the internal arrangement is nearly the following.

The restiform processes I have already mentioned as connected partly with the protuberance, partly with the four eminences, (*corpora quadrigemina*), situate on its upper surface. The circular transverse fibres of the protuberance, which enclose the longitudinal ones produced in a lateral-posterior direction, plunge into the cerebellic hemispheres in the form of thick, strong, white chords, named *stalks* or *peduncles* of the cerebellum. At the point at which they take this direction, they further receive a considerable accession from the restiform processes, the fibres of which are here seen to make a slight bend upwards, in order to follow the direction of the peduncles. Thus is composed a thick strong trunk of white matter, which on each side forms a sort of central pillar, (Die Marksäule, Der Pfeiler,) to each cerebellic hemisphere. The interior arrangement of this pillar or trunk is distinctly fibrous longitudinally, at its origin, or parting from the protuberance, and for a considerable distance from this point through the hemisphere. Unless I am misled by optical deception, the part derived from the restiform processes is also fibrous, and changes direction, to accord with that of the peduncular bands.

In the centre of the white fibrous pillar thus formed is contained a body consisting of a capsule of fibrous matter enclosing a nucleus of white. The serrated or indented form in which both the nucleus and its capsule are arranged gives it the name of ciliary or moriform body; (*corpus ciliare* v. *dentatum, c. moriforme* or *rhomboideum.*) The capsule is incomplete at one end, that turned towards the base or root of the trunk. Each trunk or stem (Stämm) divides into a certain number of branches, (Aestc); each branch into a number of twigs (Zweige ;) and to each twig is attached a number of leaves. (*Folia ;* Blättchen.)

Of these plates or leaves the structure is uniformly the same,— white matter internally, covered with a thicker layer of gray. Whether the white is really fibrous or not, as Reil describes, is not easy to say, in consequence of its extreme tenuity and small quantity. It is certainly fibrous in the stems and branches, in which the linear appearance can be seen almost by the eye, and always by a glass. I cannot say that it is so evident in the twigs, in which it is in very small quantity; and in the leaves the intimate disposition is still more difficult to recognize. In the gray matter it is impossible to trace any thing like fibrous structure.

The ramification (die verzweigung, die zerastelung,) in the cerebellic hemispheres is connected with the circular-transverse fibres of the protuberance and the restiform processes exclusively. Some would say that from this, this ramification is derived,—the precise meaning of which I have already endeavoured to determine. In the middle of this organ, however, or on its mesial plane, is found a ramification which appears to be connected with a different source.

This is the structure of the upper and lower worm. Between the lower of the quadrigeminous eminences and the cerebellum is a thick semicylindrical band on each side, known under the name of *pillars of the valve*, and *processus a cerebello ad testes*. These a little below the lower margin of the valve seem to sink directly into the cerebellic substance, mutually join, and form a whitish stem, which is ramified in the middle of the cerebellum. About four lines or half an inch from their first entrance into the organ, a branch set off almost straight upwards is the vertical branch, (Der Stehende Ast,) which, after giving off its first twig (der erste zweig) to the central lobe, divides into other seven, which are distributed to the anterior or mesial lobules of the quadrilateral lobes, as they meet on the mesial plane. The white stem of this vertical branch is thick and large.

A more slender stem, the continuation of the original white band, proceeding horizontally backwards towards the purse-shaped notch, is the horizontal stem (Der Liegende Ast,) which constitutes by ramification a number of important parts on the mesial plane of the cerebellum. After giving three or four twigs generally small, and also vertical, to the last leaves of the quadrilateral lobes, the branches are parted in the following order :—1*st*, A twig under the cross commissures of the posterior-upper lobes, forming the *short exposed cross-bands* (die Kurzen und sichtbaren Querbander,) and the *long covered cross-bands ;* (die verdeckten und langen Querbander ;)—2*d*, A branch dividing into three strong twigs, forming the leaves of the *pyramid ;*—3*d*, A long branch dividing into three twigs, forming the leaves of the *uvula* (der Zapfen ;)— 4*th*, The last generally a single twig, constituting the *laminar tubercle* or *nodule* (das Knötchen.)

The spinal chord is the last part of the central class of organs coming under the head of brain. It may be viewed as two longitudinal bands united by the middle. Both are fibrous internally throughout their entire length ; and in the lumbar region of the canal these fibres are separated and expanded into a true brush-like arrangement, named *cauda equina*. Some anatomists have imagined they could recognize cross fibres in the chord ; but, with the exception of what has been stated regarding the connection of the restiform processes, nothing of this nature can be regarded as established.

Some anatomists have also thought it possible to demonstrate the existence of a longitudinal cavity or canal in the spinal chord. In the adult this never exists in the normal state. The canal of the chord is part of the fœtal structure only; and in this respect it is to be viewed as one of many peculiarities of formation belonging to the lower animals, through which the human fœtus passes in the early stage of development. A longitudinal canal is found in the spinal chord, during the whole course of existence, in reptiles, fishes, and birds. In mammiferous animals in general it is always found in the fœtus, and continues in several for some time after birth. (Sewel, F. Meckel, and Tiedemann.) As the animal grows, however, it ceases to be found; and the only trace of its previous existence is a longitudinal depression on the anterior part of the chord. In the young of the human subject it has been found after birth by Charles Stephen, by Columbo, Piccolhomini, Bauhin, Malphighi, Lyser, Golles, Morgagni, Haller, and Portal. No doubt can be entertained, however, that in such cases it was part of the fœtal structure continued to an unusual period by the slow progress of growth, or in consequence of some interruption to the usual process of development. The chord, in short, is formed in two portions; and when these are incomplete, the longitudinal cavity exists between them. As by progressive enlargement they mutually approximate on the mesial plane, this canal necessarily diminishes until it entirely disappears.

I am now to consider shortly the minute anatomical structure of cerebral matter in the several parts of the organ. The three divisions of brain, small brain, and vertebral prolongation, and their constituent parts, do not present every where the same aspect or obvious qualities, but appear to consist of substances which are distinguished chiefly by their colour.

The outer convoluted part of the first division (*cerebrum*) consists of peculiar substance of a gray or ashen colour. Its convoluted surface, which is covered by the adherent surface of the soft or vascular membrane, (*meninx tenuis, pia mater*), is smooth and uniformly gray, without spots or streaks. At various situations it presents minute holes or orifices, which correspond to arterial or venous branches. It is not easy to apply accurate terms to denote the kind of colour; but, according to Gordon, this surface is of the wood-brown or lead-gray tinge;[*] and the substance so coloured

* Syme's Nomenclature of Colours.

extends only one-eighth or one-tenth of one inch in depth, and is then succeeded by a tinge of orange-white substance. Of the correctness of this observation, I am not assured. If sections of the convoluted part be made, no difference can be observed in the recent brain; and the cut surface appears to consist of homogeneous and uniform gray matter, from the outer or free margin to that which adheres distinctly to the white substance. The consistence of the convoluted cerebral substance is considerable; but it is less than that of the white matter.

If we trust to the observations of Father Della Torre, the gray and the white substance of the brain, *cerebellum* and spinal chord, consist of an accumulation of transparent globules, floating in a transparent *crystalline*, but somewhat viscid fluid.* These globules, he imagined, are largest in the brain, smaller in the cerebellum, and still smaller in the spinal chord.

According to the observations of Prochaska, however different in colour the gray cerebral substance be from the white, no difference in minute structure can be recognized by the most powerful lens. Each appears to consist of an infinite multitude of globules, connected by a peculiar, elastic band; and he observes that this cerebral globule does not float in a fluid, as Della Torre imagined, but is connected to the contiguous ones by a thin and transparent cellular web, (*tela cellulosa subtilissima et pellucidissima,*) which is a series of membranous partitions derived from the soft membrane and minute vessels. This last conclusion is not quite certain, and would require to be made the subject of further researches.†

On the structure of these globules nothing is known with certainty. They are not exactly spherical, but are said to be irregularly round. The observation of Della Torre, that they are largest in the convoluted brain, (*cerebrum*,) smaller in the laminated, (*cerebellum*,) and most minute in the vertebral portion, is fanciful, and perhaps unfounded. Prochaska, however, admits that the globules are not all of the same size, but that it is impossible to ascribe their variable magnitude to a regular principle, unless the proximity or remoteness of the lens.‡

The accuracy of these observations is confirmed in general by

* Nuove Observazione Microscopiche. Napoli, 1776. Osserv. 16, 17, 18, 19, &c.

† Georgii Prochaska De Structura Nervorum, &c. Viennæ, 1779. Sectio 2, caput iv.

‡ Ibid.

the testimony of Soemmering, whose inferences, derived from the observations of Lewenhoek, Della Torre, Malacarne, Metzger, and Prochaska himself, are found in the conclusion of his description of this organ.*

From thirty-one experimental observations on the cerebral matter of the human subject, in various mammiferous animals, fowls, and fishes, Joseph and Charles Wenzel of Tubingen have drawn the conclusion;—that the gray and white (cortical and medullary) matter of the human brain, the substance of the *colliculi*, (optic chambers and striated bodies,) that of the conarium, spinal chord, and nerves; in short, the mass of brain in mammiferous animals, birds, and fishes, consists of the same small roundish bodies, mutually cohering, of which the substance of muscle, liver, spleen, and kidney is composed; that as these minute bodies derive their shape from the cells of the cellular tissue, the substance of brain, spinal chord, and nervous matter, appears to consist of the same roundish minute bodies; but that the relative size of these cells cannot be determined.

These conclusions throw little light on the point at issue,—the minute structure of the cerebral matter in general; and it must be said that the microscopical observations and chemical experiments of these anatomists do not communicate information proportioned either to their number, or to the elaborate assiduity with which they appear to have been conducted. Subsequently the atomic constitution of different parts of the brain and cerebellum was investigated by Sir Everard Home, aided by the powerful microscopes of M. Bauer.

According to this observer, white cerebral matter consists of innumerable globules, aggregated or connected in rows, so as to constitute fibres, by means of a transparent, colourless, jelly-like matter, somewhat viscid, elastic, and readily soluble in water. The globules are whitish, semitransparent, and vary from $\frac{1}{2400}$ to $\frac{1}{4000}$ of an inch in diameter, the average being $\frac{1}{3200}$.

Upon different proportions of these two constituent elements, and partly upon differences in size of the component globules, the chief peculiarities of structure in the several sorts of cerebral substance depend. Thus the gray matter of the convoluted surface of the brain, and the laminated surface of the cerebellum, consists chiefly of globules from $\frac{1}{3200}$ to $\frac{1}{4000}$ of an inch in diameter, the smaller

* Samuelis Thomæ Soemmering De Corporis Humani Fabrica, Tom. III. Trajecti ad Moenum, 1800.

globules being most numerous, of a large proportion of the gelatinous, elastic, viscid substance, and a yellowish fluid resembling the serum of the blood, probably albuminous. In the white matter, on the contrary, the large globules ($\frac{1}{4000}$ of an inch) predominate; the connecting jelly is more tenacious, but less abundant in proportion to the globules; and the latter are more distinctly arranged in rows, so as to constitute fibres.

The mesolobe contains the greatest quantity of the small globules ($\frac{1}{3400}$ of an inch;) and the viscid jelly is said to be at least equal to the globules in quantity. In the limbs of the brain and peduncles of the cerebellum, the jelly is said to be in greater proportion than the globules. The annular protuberance is chiefly composed of globules of the average size ($\frac{1}{3200}$,) with abundant viscid matter. In the restiform processes, the pyramidal bodies, and the olivary eminences, the fibrous structure consists chiefly of the large globules, with abundant viscid jelly, which is rapidly soluble in water.*

When the brain by immersion in alcohol is hardened, the elastic jelly is coagulated and rendered opaque, and the appearance of globules is lost.†

These observations partly verify those of Della Torre, partly explain those of Prochaska. They show, that, so far as the microscope can be trusted, the globules of which cerebral matter consists vary in size and proportion in different parts; and that the white cerebral matter generally consists of larger globules, or at least contains a larger proportion of these globules than the gray.

The observations by Ehrenberg in 1833‡ on this subject next deserve attention.

This observer, by using the compound microscope, found the following forms of organic structure in the brain and nerves:—

1. A substance consisting partly of very minute fine grains, with some coarser grained matter, disseminated, as is said in the language of mineralogy, through the fine-grained matter. The latter is entirely confined to the gray matter of the convoluted surface of the brain, and the laminated surface of the cerebellum.

* The Croonian Lecture. Microscopical Observations on the Brain, &c. By Sir Everard Home, Bart. V. P. R. S. Philosophical Transactions, 1821, Part i. v. p. 25.

† The Croonian Lecture. On the Internal Structure of the Human Brain, &c. By Sir Everard Home, Bart., V. P. Philosophical Transactions, 1824, p. 3.

‡ Ehrenberg employed a microscope manufactured by Chevalier of Paris, and augmented in Power by Pistor and Schick of Berlin ; and the powers varied from 260 to 360 diameters.

2. A set of tubes presenting at definite intervals globular or spheroidal expansions, so as to resemble a string of beads, which do not touch each other, but have a short communicating space interposed between each bead. To these tubes he gives the name of *varicose*, from their resemblance to the *varices* of a vein, and *jointed* or *articulated* tubes, because of the slight resemblance to a set of joints. These tubes, which present to the microscope the appearance of parallel fibres, he shows by various proofs to have an internal cavity or canal, and to contain a peculiar matter, to which he assigns the name and qualities of nervous fluid. These are confined chiefly to the white matter of the brain. They may be termed *moniliform* tubes.

3. A set of tubes straight and uniform, without the alternate spheroidal enlargements, also hollow, and to which he applies the name of *simple cylindrical tubes*. These are found chiefly in the nervous chords and trunks. They are generally larger and coarser than the articulated tubes. But at certain points the latter pass into the former by gradually losing their bead-like enlargements. These tubes Ehrenberg represents to be distinguished from the cerebral jointed tubes, by containing in their interior a viscid, white, but less transparent matter, to which he applies the name of *medullary*.

The substance of the circumference or the convoluted part of the brain consists of a thick, very delicate, vascular network, conveying often numerous blood-globules, and traversed by serpentine tendinous fibres. Besides the thick delicate vascular net of the first substance, Ehrenberg saw in the same, near its utmost edge and its remotest circumference, a very fine-grained soft substance, in which here and there are imbedded larger grains or *nuclei*. These large grains are free, and consist of granules or *nucleoli* which are connected in rows by means of slender threads to the fine small grains of the substance singly. In the neighbourhood of the medullary substance, the fibrous character of the cortical matter always appears more distinctly ; and in the same substance the blood-vessels are larger and less numerous.

The white or medullary matter of the brain shows more distinctly the arrangement of fibres, which proceed in the form of direct and enlarging continuations of the delicate cortical fibres, from certain eminences, that is, the linear or band-like origins of the convoluted surface, in a radiated manner, towards the brain. These are not simple cylindrical fibres; but resemble hollow strings `of pearls, the component parts of which are not in contact, but are connected by a canal for a small space; or they resemble tubes or cylindrical canals dilated at intervals into minute bladders. These bladders or *ampullulæ* of the tubes were known to Leeuwenhoek, who regarded them as globules of fat, which constituted the greatest part of the brain. The connecting canals also he has obscurely indicated. These tubes, uniformly straight, are generally parallel in direction, sometimes, however, crossing each other. Four times Ehrenberg recognised ramification in such individual canals; but anastomoses he never observed. These tubes vary in diameter from $\frac{1}{90}$ to $\frac{1}{3000}$th part of one line.

In the neighbourhood of the base of the brain and in the matter surrounding the ventricles, there are always seen between these bundles of nodulated or jointed tubes, individual tubes much thicker than the rest. In these thick tubes it is often possible to recognise in their walls an external and internal boundary; or they present, besides their two external boundary lines, other two inner lines, which enable the observer to distinguish the width of the area of the internal cavity of the tubes. These nodulated linear parts of the brain are VARICOSE ARTICULATED TUBES OR CANALS.

The large cerebral tubules of the cerebral matter converge towards and pass into those parts of the base of the brain, where the peripheral nerves arise. Some of the large jointed-tube-matter appears to terminate in or be connected with the cerebral cavities, in the walls of which it is well developed. Many jointed or varicose tubes pass into the spinal marrow, and thence immediately proceed to the spinal nerves.

In the spinal marrow the arrangement now described is in some respects reversed. In the brain the most vascular and delicate structure is placed at the exterior; while the least vascular, but perhaps more organised, viz. the varicose tubular structure, is placed at the interior. In the spinal chord the most vascular and delicate part lies in the centre; while it is covered externally by the coarse medullary matter.

Both substances are quite like those in the brain. From the external medullary matter, consisting of large varicose or moniliform tubes, the spinal nerves immediately proceed; and these varicose or jointed tubes, as they emerge from the investing *dura mater*, assume suddenly the form of nerve-tubes, becoming thicker and passing into the pure cylindrical form. These transitions are easily recognised in the posterior part of the spinal marrow.

The optic, the auditory, and the olfactory nerves are immediate continuations of, or productions from, the varicose medullary tubes of the brain. All the other nerves, excepting the sympathetic in the middle of its course, differ from the cerebral matter.

All these other nerves also consist only of cylindrical parallel-lying tubes, about $\frac{1}{120}$th part of a line in diameter, normally never anastomosing. These are the elementary nerve-tubes, which, united in *fasciculi* or bundles, again form larger bundles, which constitute the nerve-chords.

These are the chief facts ascertained by Ehrenberg regarding the minute structure of the brain and spinal chord. These have been mostly confirmed by Berres and Müller. By others again the accuracy of these results has been called in question. Thus the observations of Treviranus, Valentin, and Weber tend to show that all the primitive cerebral fibres or tubes are cylindrical, and that the varicose or moniliform appearance is an effect of compression; or the violence employed in subjecting them to microscopic observation. Müller, nevertheless, admits that the primitive cerebral tubes have great proneness to become varicose or beaded.

The only points which, amidst the discordance of the results of different microscopical observers, from Leewenhoek and Fontana to Ehrenberg, Berres, Treviranus, and Müller, can be regarded as established, are the following; that the convoluted portion of the brain consists of very minute granules or *nucleoli* arranged in rows so as to form fibres, which radiate from the periphery to the inner boundary of the convoluted portion; that near the inner boundary, and as they approach the white cerebral matter, this fibrous arrangement becomes more distinct; and that the white cerebral matter forming the walls of the ventricles and the base of the brain is composed of tubular cylinders, mostly of large size, and having a cylindrical cavity; but whether these are varicose or not seems undetermined.*

* C. G. Ehrenberg in Poggendorff's Annalen der Physik und Chemie, Jahrg. 1833. Band XXVIII. § 449–65, und 1834. Band XXXIV. § 76, 80. Also Beobachtung einer bisher unbekannten auffallenden structur des Seelenorgan bei Menschen und Thieren. Von C. G. Ehrenberg. Gelesen in der Akademie der Wissenschaften am 24 October 1833. Gedruckt im, Feb. 1836. Abhandlungen ; seite 665. Translated, with Additions and Notes. By David Craigie, M. D. Edinburgh Medical and Surgical Journal, Vol. XLVIII. p. 257. October 1837.

G. Valentin uber die Dicke der varicosen Faden in dem Gehirn und dem Ruckenmark des Menschen. In Müller's Archiv. 1834. § 401–410.

The sources from which the brain derives its blood are well known. It is highly vascular throughout. These vessels, first divided in the productions of the *pia mater*, are afterwards subdivided to an incredible degree of minuteness, in the substance of the organ. They never anastomose. (Home.) They are accompanied with very minute veins, provided, it is said, with valves. Of these the most delicate branches are found, according to Sir Everard Home, in the gray convoluted matter, contrary to the statements of Ruysch, Albinus, and others ; and conversely in the white matter they are much larger.*

The substance of brain has been examined by several chemists ; but the analysis most to be trusted, is perhaps that of Vauquelin, who found that 100 parts of cerebral substance consist of 80 of water, 7 of albumen, 4.43 of a white adipose matter, 0.70 of a red adipose matter, 1.12 of osmazome, 1.5 of phosphorus, and 5.15 of acids, salts, and sulphur. Upon the presence of the albuminous matter depends the solidification which the brain undergoes when immersed in alcohol, acids, or solutions of the metallic salts, which coagulate that substance. Upon the presence of the white adipose matter depends the formation of those brilliant white crystalline plates, resembling cholesterine, observed by M. Gmelin in the brains preserved in the anatomical cabinet of Heidelberg.† The opinion of this physician, that it pre-exists in the brain, in the form of the adipocerous or cholesterine matter (waxy brain-fat,) is improbable, and requires more decisive experiments than those on which he has founded it.

The development and growth of this organ was, in 1816, investigated with much care by Tiedemann, who has ascertained the following points. In the embryo of six weeks, the spinal chord is represented by a flat long substance, the upper end of which is slightly enlarged. In the second month, when the brain is little developed compared with the spinal chord, it may be said to consist, 1*st*, of a cerebellum, with considerable transverse extent ; 2*d*, of brain proper, exceedingly small ; 3*d*, of a third portion placed

G. R. Treviranus Beitrage zur Aufklarung der Erscheinungen und Gesetze der Organischen Lebens Band I. Heft. II.   1836–8, § 24.   H. und Heft. IV.   1836'

E. H. Weber in Schmidt's Jahrbuchern der in-und-auslandischen Medicin. Bd. X X. § 5. und Henle ebendaselbst.   § 339.

* Philosophical Transactions, Lond. 1821, pp. 29 and 30.

† Zeitscrift für Physiologie, Von Tiedemann, Treviranus, und L. C. Treviranus, Band I. 1 Heft, 1824.

between these two, and the size of which exceeds that of the brain. This third portion corresponds to the protuberance, or rather to that part of the organ, the upper surface of which is formed by the four eminences, (*corpora quadrigemina*,) and the lower surface by the annular protuberance.* According to M. Serres, it is formed in man and animals before the brain and cerebellum, and immediately after the spinal chord. In the fifth month the brain covers a part of the protuberance; it advances to the cerebellum, and in the seventh exceeds it. At the same time, the other parts, and especially that, which we have mentioned, as the third or central portion, do not grow at the same rate.

At the beginning, that is about the seventh week, the brain is found to be divided in two portions by a longitudinal fissure. Each half mutually approaches as growth continues, and are at length united, so that at the third month the only parts found separate are the middle ventricle, the aqueduct or canal, which is at this time a large cavity continuous with it, and the fourth ventricle. The development of the cavities called lateral ventricles is closely connected with that of the contiguous parts of the organ. These appear nearly in the following order.

The lateral lobes appear first about three months after conception; and about the same time the mesolobe, (*corpus callosum*,) is formed by union of the hemispheres; and the cylindroid processes, (*cornua ammonis*,) vault, (*fornix*,) mammillary eminences, posterior commissure, and cerebral limbs or peduncles, may be recognized. Shortly after may be seen the *ergot*, or small hippocampus, and the anfractuosity from which it issues, and the *conarium* and its peduncles; then the anterior commissure, the thin partition (*septum lucidum*) and its cavity, which at this time communicates with the middle ventricle; lastly, the semicircular fillet, (*tænia semicircularis*,) and the infundibulum, which correspond to the seventh month; and about the same time the outer surface of the brain begins to present the eminences denominated convolutions, and the cerebellum its laminated or foliated appearance.

In the early weeks of existence the brain is fluid, soft, and homogeneous. The white matter and its fibrous structure is first seen; and the cross structure of the fibres of the pyramids are observable about the eighth week, according to M. Serres. About the sixth month the cerebral substance appears, when microscopically exa-

* Anatomie und Bildungs-Geschichte des Gehirns im Fœtus des Menschen u. s. f. Von Dr Fredrich Tiedemann, Professor der Anatomie, u. s. f. Nurnberg, 1816, 4to.

mined, to consist of globules immediately beneath the *pia mater,* and of fibres at a greater depth. In the seventh month a section of the ventricles shows very distinct layers of radiating fibres. After these are seen new ones, which form convolutions, and which are termed converging fibres. At the ninth month the organization is complete.

The gray substance appears a long time after the white. At the end of the sixth or seventh month this substance is formed in the olivary eminences, which then assume their proper appearance; about the end of gestation the spinal chord is also filled with gray matter, and about the ninth month this substance is distinctly seen in the convolutions, the plates of the cerebellum, &c. These results are much like those of Serres, unless as to what regards the brain proper, in which, according to this anatomist, the optic chambers and striated bodies consist originally of gray substance entirely, to which white cerebral matter is afterwards added.

Of the process of growth, the principal, indeed the sole agent is the vascular membrane; (*meninx tenuis, pia mater et plexus choroides:* das Geffasshaut.) The two divisions of this, viz. the external, or that belonging to the convoluted surface, and the internal, or that pertaining to the figurate, may be distinguished previous to the formation of any part of the brain, and when the two portions, which are afterwards destined to be separate, are the same, and indistinguishable from each other. The formation of the organ appears to commence at once upon two orders of vessels mutually looking towards each other; that which is to be the central (*plexus choroides*) being merely a mesh of vessels looking to that which is to be peripheral, (*pia mater.*) The first portions of newly deposited cerebral matter form the barrier between these extremities, which continue to be more widely parted, as the process of development advances. This membrane is then more vascular than at any subsequent period. The cerebral matter is first deposited soft, and firmly adherent to these vessels, which are ramified in every direction through its substance. It becomes firmer afterwards and less vascular the longer the period from deposition. Hence the two surfaces, the outer and inner, are much softer and more pulpy, and more firmly attached to the vessels, than the intermediate deep matter. Tiedemann appears to regard the process of development as proceeding from the centre to the circumference. This is correct, but not in the exact sense in which he understands it. The centre is not in this case the figurate surface of the brain, but the centre of the optic and striated bodies which is first deposited, and from which the process of deposition advances to both surfaces at the same time, and nearly at equal rates. These inferences are established by the phenomena observed in the development of the organ in the young of mammiferous animals in general.

Section II.

Cerebral substance is liable to inflammation, acute and chronic, to hemorrhage, to effusions of serous fluid, to alterations in its natural consistence, and to tumours.

1. *Encephalia Acuta; Encephalitis.* (Frank, Costantin.) Acute inflammation of the brain is a rare disease, and, perhaps, if always carefully investigated, would be found never to take place spontaneously or primarily. As the effect of accidental violence, and the result of morbid poisons, it is much more frequent; and it is chiefly under such circumstances that its phenomena and effects are known. (Pott, Dease, Hill, Malacarne, Desault, J. Bell, M. A. Petit, O'Halloran, Abernethy.) As the effect of mechanical injury, the disease is found to be generally circumscribed. Part of the brain becomes very vascular, acquires a red colour of various shades of intensity, and eventually becomes brownish or green, and much softer than natural. The formation of matter in a distinct cavity appears not so common in this form of the disease as in another, which I am soon to mention. An abscess is not very frequently remarked under such circumstances, unless when a foreign body, as a bullet, a stone, or a piece of bone has been driven into the brain. This process gives rise to intense headach, delirium, and intolerance of light, quickly succeeded by convulsions, coma, and death.

Of the effect of morbid poisons in inducing cerebral inflammation more or less acute, an example is found in the severe form of fever prevalent in jails and camps. In several examples of this disease abscesses of the brain have been found, (Pringle); and it is often possible to trace the process from the first marks of injection to the complete formation of purulent matter.

2. *Encephalia Subacuta.* (Pulpy destruction; *ramollissement,* Rostan, Lallemand, &c.) Subacute or chronic inflammation of the brain is greatly more common. Its anatomical characters are much the same as those of the acute form; but the longer duration of the process gives rise to modifications which the pathologist should dis-

tinguish. At first a part of the brain becomes more, or less red and vascular. As this goes on, it passes successively into crimson, violet or purple, brown, or claret colour, while the consistence of the part is much diminished. A shade of green announces the formation of purulent fluid; and in proportion as this process continues before life is extinct, the part becomes yellow, or gray, or grayish brown, (*subfusca*) very soft and pulpy, or even semifluid. It is perhaps equally rare in this as in the former case, to find perfeet purulent matter in a distinct cavity. This change, which is often mentioned by Morgagni,* is one form of the disease described by Rostan † and Lallemand,‡ under the name of *softening* (ramollissement) *of the brain*, and since that time by Bouillaud, Bright, Durand-Fardel, and other authors. The softening is a mere effect of the process of inflammation, subacute or chronic. In some instances the softening is attended with effusion of serous fluid, without much discoloration of the part.

˙. Subacute or chronic inflammation, terminating in softening of the brain, may take place either on the convoluted surface of the organ, when it generally occupies an extent of two or three square inches; or at the figurate surface, when it is most common on the middle portion, (*septum lucidum*,) and extending along the twainband; or in the substance of the organ, when it affects most frequently the striated bodies, the optic *thalami*, the central part of the hemispheres, the cerebellum, and the cerebral prolongations, (*crura cerebri*,) in the order now enumerated. Its occurrence in the spinal chord, in which the same series of changes takes place, has been described by M. Pinel the younger,§ M. Olivier,‖ and M. Velpeau.¶

What is the intimate nature of this disease, and wherein does it

* Epistola, V. 6, 7. IX. 16, 18, 19. In the brain of Marchetti, the anatomist, who, after two epileptic attacks, died apoplectic, the gray matter was so tender, that on the slightest touch it was converted into a fluid substance, as if it never had co. hered.—L. vii. 14, 15.

† Recherches sur une maladie encore peu connue, qui a reçu le nom de ramollissement du Cerveau. Par L. N. Rostan, Medecin de la Salpetriere, &c. A. Paris, 1820.

‡ Recherches Anatomico-Pathologiques sur l'Encephale, et ses dependances. Par F. Lallemand, Prof. de Clinique, &c. Paris, 1820–1821.

§ Sur l'Inflammation de la Moelle Epiniere. By M. Pinel, Fils. Journal de Physiologie Experimentale, Vol. 1i. p. 54.

‖ De la Moelle Epiniere et de ses Maladies. Par C. P. Ollivier. Paris, 1824.

¶ Memoire sur une Alteration de la Moelle Allongée, &c. Par M. A. Velpeau. Archives Générales, Tome VII. p. 52 and 329. Paris, 1825.

differ from suppuration of the organ ? This question must be determined by considering the anatomical characters of the lesion, and the circumstances under which it takes place. In the part affected, the portion of brain is never entirely removed. The cerebral substance is separated, broken down, and mixed either with serous, with bloody, or with purulent fluid.

It may succeed at least four morbid states of the organ. 1. It may be the consequence of the blood-stroke, (*coup de sang,*) or injection of the vessels of a given region of the organ. The softened part is then reddish, rose-coloured, amaranth, crimson, or brown. 2. It may follow the effusion of red blood, which nearly in the same manner separates and breaks down the delicate substance of the organ in which it is effused. The softened portion is then generally brown, or a wine-lee colour ; but if a considerable time has elapsed after effusion, it may be of a dirty or ashy colour, tending to green, and not unlike softened bread. 3. It may either accompany or follow the process which terminates in hydrocephalic effusion. It is then of a milk-white colour. (Rostan, Lallemand.) 4. It may take place in the cerebral substance surrounding tumours, (Meckel, Blane, Powell, &c.) when its colour varies from pale-red to green, yellow, and brown.

From these facts it may be inferred, that *softening*, or *pulpy disorganization* of the brain is not so much a proper disease as the effect of a morbid process, which takes place in different conditions of the brain.

When it occurs in the first manner, it is the result of a species of diffuse inflammation, in which there is no tendency to limit the action of the disease by the effusion of lymph, or the formation of a vascular cyst. This is well illustrated in those cases recorded by Morgagni, in which parts of the brain had become yellowish or greenish, with much diminution of consistence, (Epist. iii. 2. ix. 20. xxv. 10. lii. 23); and in the eighth delineation of Dr Hooper, (p. 23.) In cases of this description, a sero-albuminous or semi-purulent fluid is infiltrated into the cerebral substance, portions of which are thus separated and detached from each other. The process is allied to inflammation ; but it is an abortive form, in so far as it fails to concentrate the action to a definite spot.

That it takes place in the inflammatory or disorganizing process which succeeds mechanical injury is established by the necrological appearances found in the brain in such circumstances. (Fantoni,

Morgagni, Louis, Le Dran, Schmucker, O'Halloran, Dease, Abernethy, Thomson, Hennen, &c.)

When softening takes place in connection with serous effusion, .
it is partly the concurrent effect of inflammation, partly of the effused fluid. This is well illustrated in those cases in which the
septum lucidum is attenuated, reticular, and perforated, or at length
ruptured. This form of destruction, accompanied with more or less
softening of the twain-band, *(fornix)*, is repeatedly mentioned by
Morgagni, and has been noticed by most authors who have described
cases of watery effusion within the cerebral cavities. I have seen it
in three sorts of cases; first, in the true hydrocephalic effusion;
secondly, in that which takes place in continued fever; and, thirdly,
in the course of chronic meningeal inflammation, with thickening
of the *dura mater*, after injury.

Not only does pulpy disorganization occur in this part of the
organ in continued fever, but it takes place in the substance of the
hemispheres. Of this pathological fact good instances are given by
Jemina, as they occurred in an epidemic at Montreal, in the territory of Turin, in 1783-84. In one the white matter of the hemisphere (*centrum ovale*) was soft, pulpy, *(fracidum,)* of an ash-colour,
passing into yellow, and pasty; in another it was soft and tawny-
coloured, like spoilt fruit; and in a third the cerebellum was simi-
larly changed.* The same change was observed by Dr Black of
Newry in the cerebral hemisphere. (Transactions, Vol. II.)

When pulpy disorganization is connected with effusion of blood,
it has been supposed by M. Rostan to be the cause of that effusion.
That this supposition is inadmissible, I infer from the following
facts, which I have witnessed more than once. 1*st*, That the portion of brain inclosing the clot is soft and pulpy all round, but
sound in proportion to the distance from the clot. 2*d*, That in
some instances in which partial recovery takes place, part of the
red clot has disappeared, and its place is supplied by serous fluid.
3*d*, That in cases in which death takes place early, the pulpy disorganization is less complete than those in which it takes place at
a later period. In short, the extent of the disorganization is proportionate to the interval which elapses between the effusion of the
blood and the period of death.

When pulpy disorganization accompanies tumours of the brain,

* De Febre, Anno 1783-84, Monteregali Epidemica, auctore Marco Antonio Jemina,
M. D. &c.   Extat in Brera Sylloge, Vol. X. p. 218, 247.

that it is the effect of the presence of these tumours, and the chronic congestion which they cause, is sufficiently obvious to render super-fluons any minute induction. It is enough to say, that, though not constant, it is a very general effect. (Morgagni, Meckel, Sandi-fort, Powell, Yellowly, Blane, &c.) The morbid change now described was supposed by Morgagni and Lieutaud, to the former of whom it was well known, to be of the nature of gangrene in other parts. This idea, which is also that of Jemina* and of Baillie, has been revived by Dr Abercrom-bie.† Though unwilling to dissent from the opinion of a pathologist distinguished for accurate induction, it appears to me exceedingly doubtful, for the reasons above stated, how far this analogy can be demonstrated.

A part of the brain changed as above described is indeed disor-ganized, may be said to be dead, and in this sense the change may be termed *gangrene of the brain.* But when it is found in different degrees, and in so many different morbid states of the brain, some of them of long continuance, it is difficult to be satisfied that every one of them must be viewed equally as gangrene. In the present work I avoid as much as possible whatever is hypothetical or doubt-ful. Upon this principle I conceive it improper to offer, on the nature of this .change, any further opinion than can be collected from the circumstances above stated of its history and connections.

One form of softening, nevertheless, there is, which is more justly entitled to the character of gangrene than the others. In a certain proportion of cases the arteries of the brain become steatomatous and opaque and inelastic, or osteo-steatomatous and more or less rigid. Thus the Sylvian artery or its branches, the basilar artery or its branches, the posterior and middle cerebral, and the cerebellic, may all be affected with this transformation. In such circumstances, it is observed that softening comes on very suddenly, and, apparently without any preliminary inflammatory or hemorrhagic stage, pro-ceeds instantly or speedily to complete brown or green-coloured disorganization of a portion of the brain. The entire duration of this form of softening seldom exceeds three or four days. It is

---

* "Aliud etiam ex hoc morbo defuncti caput aperui ; et memini inter cætera ob-servata substantiæ cerebri pulposæ portionem magnitudine nucis avellanæ, colore, et consistentia vitiatam, ita ut esset coloris *tane* et mollior, non secus ac poma vel pyra cum intus marcescere incipiunt. Annon gangræna hujus visceris? De Febre, annis 1783–84. Monteregali Epidemica, auctore Marco Antonio Jemina, M. D. &c. Apud Brera Syllogen, Tom. X. p. 247.

† Pathological and Practical Researches, p. 25.

most common in the *corpus striatum*, or that and the optic *thalamus*, and in the *crura* of the brain.

This affection resembles in some respects gangrene of a member from disease and obstruction of its arteries.

Pulpy softening presents different characters in different regions of the brain. On the convoluted surface in many brains there are seen depressed orange-coloured spots about the size of a split pea, and sometimes larger. These spots, which are slightly depressed or hollow, are the remains of previous attacks of softening affecting the convoluted surface. In some instances, especially where they have succeeded injury or violence inflicted on the skull, they are more extensive and deeper; and, while the depressed surface is of the orange-colour, it is also softened, pulpy, not presenting the usual structure; and there has been a manifest loss of substance.

Persons, in whose brains these appearances are observed, are unsteady or tottering in gait, paralytic, and speak inarticulately and thick. Their memory is feeble, sometimes greatly impaired; their intellect is sometimes disordered; and in certain cases they are fatuous.

When softening affects the central portions of the brain, it converts them into a soft, white, cream-like substance. The fornix is either much softened or destroyed; its posterior and lateral limbs are softened; the *septum lucidum* is perforated by many holes, or completely broken down, and converted into one large aperture.

When softening affects either of the *corpora striata* or *optic thalami*, it usually assumes the reddish-brown colour, showing that there had been effusion of blood; and sometimes the reddish-brown is mixed with yellow, or greenish-yellow softening, or the wine-lee softening passes into the greenish-coloured softening, showing that blood had been effused, and that suppuration was proceeding.

Lastly, in either of the *crura*, softening is commonly what is called hortensia-red, that is, of the deep crimson imitating the colour of the flower of the *hortensia*; in short, it is blood recently effused, breaking down and mixed with the cerebral matter. The reason of this is, that hemorrhagic softening in the *crura* is in general speedily fatal, that is, it is followed by death within three or four days, and the life of the individual is rarely prolonged to the sixth day.

Hemorrhage within the substance of the protuberance is still more rapidly fatal; and in that body accordingly softening, properly so called, is almost never seen.

Lastly, it is proper to observe, that, in a large proportion of cases, softening of the brain is preceded by the steatomatous or osteo-steatomatous degeneration of the cerebral arteries, which are either specked, or opaque, or rigid and brittle, and by an unsound and irregular state of the circulation within these vessels. The effects of this disease on the system are not very well distinguished. They may be divided into common and proper. The common effects are dull pain, or sense of weight in the head, dullness, impaired memory, frequent drowsiness, and occasional peevishness at trifles, and paralytic affections of the face, head, and members. The proper effects are sense of formication, numbness, and rigidity, or occasional involuntary contractions of the muscles of the upper extremities, followed by delirium or fatuity, and a peculiar odour about the head, not dissimilar to that of the mouse. In the spinal chord it gives rise to numbness and rigid contraction of the muscles of the lower extremities, and eventually palsy more or less complete.

These symptoms, which are chiefly those given by the French authors already mentioned, apply to the acute form of the disease. In more chronic states it seems not to affect the muscular motions considerably, but rather to induce fatuity and other forms of impaired intellect. This inference at least results from some of the observations of Morgagni,* and those of Dr John Hunter.† This is the state of brain which takes place in cases of fatuity succeeding coup-de-soleil.

3. *Suppurative Inflammation, Apostema Cerebri.* Collections of purulent-matter have been often found in the substance of the brain. That these collections may take place spontaneously, as a consequence of previous inflammation, is established by the testimony of Morgagni,‡ Lieutaud,§ Baader,|| Baillie,¶ Powell,** Brodie,†† Hooper,‡‡ and Abercrombie.§§ Of the observations of these authors the result is, that, though a collection of purulent fluid to a greater

---

* Epist. viii.   † Apud Baillie, Morbid Anatomy.

‡ Epistola v.   § Historia Anatomico-Medica.

|| Josephi Baader, Observat. Med. Obs. 22. Extat apud Sandifort Thesaurum, Vol. III. p. 28.

¶ Engravings to illustrate the Morbid Anatomy, &c. X. Fasciculus, Plate vi. p. 221.

** Some Cases illustrative of the Pathology of the Brain. By Richard Powell, M. D. Transactions of the College of Physicians, Vol. V. p. 198, Case 6 and 8.

†† Case of Abscess in the Brain. By B. C. Brodie, Esq., F. R. S., &c. Transactions of a Society, Vol. III. p. 106.

‡‡ The Morbid Anatomy of the Human Brain. By Robert Hooper, M. D. London, 1826. Plate ix. p. 25.

§§ Abercrombie, Cases 31, 32, 33, and 34.

or less extent may take place in either of the hemispheres, and in almost any part of these hemispheres, its situation is influenced much by the kind of abscess. The ordinary abscess, consisting of an irregular cavity containing purulent matter, sometimes mixed with flakes of lymph, and rendering it curdly, may take place either in the anterior lobe (J. Earle,* Hooper,) or in the centre of the hemisphere (Chizeau,† Baillie). An abscess, consisting of several small communicating cavities, takes place in the anterior lobe, and occasionally in the substance or in the vicinity of the striated nucleus of Reil. The abscess consisting of a firm cyst, containing purulent matter, is generally found in the centre of the hemispheres. (Powell, case 8 ; Hooper, Pl. 9, Fig. 3 ; Abercrombie, cases 16, 17.)

Collections of purulent matter have been found in the lobes of the cerebellum by Bianchi,‡ (often Latinized Janus Plancns,) Stoll,§ Weikard,‖ and Abercrombie.¶ In general they are contained in a cyst more or less distinct, the walls of which are membranous and vascular. In the case of Weikard he represents the whole white matter almost of the left lobe to be converted into a millet-like, something foul, purulent matter, by which I understand it to have been flocculent and lymphy. Suppuration, less distinctly defined, and deposited generally in small irregular cavities, takes place in the *medulla oblongata*, especially in that part of the olivary body which contains the *corpus dentatum*. Abercrombie mentions a case at the junction of the protuberance (39.) In the chord itself, though more rare, and generally confined to the surface, yet it has been seen in the form of infiltration by Brera ;** and in a distinct cavity in the cervical portion by Velpeau.††

The origin of these collections is not well known. That they are the result of a form of inflammation cannot be denied ; but that it is not ordinary inflammation, is to be inferred from the slow progress which they generally observe, and from the vari-

---

* Med. and Phys. Journal, Vol. XXIII. p. 89.

† Recueil Periodique, No. xxxiv.

‡ Giovan. Bianchi Storia d'un Apostema nel lobo destro del Cerebello. Rimini, 1751. And Jani Planci Storia, d'un Apostema nel Cerebello. Rimini, 1752.

§ Maximil. Stoll Rationis Medendi, Pars i. 178, et iii. 159.

‖ Vermischte Schriften von M. A. Weikard fürstl. Fuldisch Leibartz. Frankfort am Main, 1782. Viertes St. p. 74.

¶ Pathological and Practical Researches, case iii. and xl.

** Cenni sulla Rachitide.

†† Revue Medical, 1826.

able effects to which they give rise. They are said in general to be connected with the strumous diathesis; and they are most commonly found in subjects who present the usual marks of this diathesis. This, however, is only expressing, in different terms, an obscure fact, the real cause of which is quite unknown. The encysted abscess, especially that such as is delineated by Dr Hooper, is of the kind called by old pathologists *abscess* by *congestion*, or *cold abscess.*

One form of suppuration of the brain I think there is strong reason to believe depends on the presence of previous disease, inflammatory, suppurative, or gangrenous, in the lungs, and probably in other organs. This is when suppuration takes place in the brain, either in one abscess, or diffusely, or in the sinuses of the brain after suppuration or gangrene of the lungs. This connection was observed in the two following cases.

In the summer of 1836, I was requested to see a child of about two years, labouring under apparent affection of the brain. Symptoms of this I indeed observed in the heat of the head, the restlessness, the spasmodic movements of the eyes, a little enlargement of the head, constant tossing backwards and to each side, the uneasiness of the stomach, and the insensible state of the intestinal tube. But besides these symptoms, the child was greatly emaciated, coughed much, and occasionally expectorated. There was much general feverishness. On examining the chest, I found considerable cavernous destruction of the upper lobe of the right lung, with some flattening and depression of the ribs. Two days afterwards, death took place. I found the upper lobe and part of the middle lobe of the right lung hollowed into a rugged cavernous abscess, with irregular cavities, and walls covered with a little purulent matter, emitting an offensive odour. In the brain the convolutions were much flattened, indeed their eminences were almost effaced; a little turbid sero-purulent fluid was contained within the ventricles; the longitudinal sinus, the *torcular*, the lateral sinuses, and the small sinuses at the base were filled with blood half-coagulated, and containing lymph and purulent matter; and even the large veins of the *pia mater* opening into these sinuses contained half-clotted blood and purulent matter.

It appears to me nearly certain, that the lymph and purulent matter were conveyed by the veins of the lungs into the circulation, and thence into the venous canals of the brain.

I have elsewhere published in detail the circumstances of a case
of abscess in the right hemisphere of the brain, immediately on the
outside of the ventricles, in which this lesion accompanied or followed an attack of gangrene of the right lung. The matter was
here contained within a distinct cavity ; was opaque, consistent,
greenish-yellow, like well-formed purulent matter ; and the progress
of the symptoms had been carefully watched. The abscess was
about two inches and a-half long antero-posteriorly, and one inch
broad transversely,* and about one inch at its greatest vertical depth.

I am aware that in both cases it may be argued there was merely
coincidence in the two circumstances. And by some it may be even
said, that the evidence is as strong for the affection of the lungs
having followed that of the brain, as the affection of the brain following that of the lungs. All this may be correct. The main
point is to remark the fact of coincidence or simultaneous existence,
and the anatomico-pathological fact, that in other instances the
veins appear to act as the channels for conveying, through various
parts of the human body, lymph, purulent matter, and other substances presented to their orifices.

One variety of cerebral abscess, that connected with discharge
from the ear, originates in a more obvious manner. Purulent discharge from the ear-hole is indeed generally connected with inflammation, subacute or chronic, of the *dura mater,* or vascular
membrane, or both ; and in some instances the disease takes an
unfavourable turn in this manner, and speedily proceeds to a fatal
termination. (Morgagni, Powell, case 5 ; Itard, Duncan Junior,
Abercrombie.) In other circumstances, however, either with or
without this meningeal inflammation, a similar affection strikes suddenly a part of the cerebral substance, and, proceeding rapidly to
the suppurative stage, forms a distinct cerebral abscess. Cases of
this description were early noticed by Ballonius, Gontard, and
more recently by an anonymous writer,† Mr Brodie,‡ Dr O'Brien,§
Mr Parkinson,‖ and Dr Duncan Junior:¶

---

* Cases and Observations illustrative of the Nature of Gangrene of the Lungs. By
David Craigie, M.D., F.R. S. E., &c.   Edin. Med. and Surgical Journal, Vol. LVI.
p. 1, case 1.

† Medical Commentaries, II. 180. The History of a Suppuration of the Brain, &c.
‡ Transactions of a Society, &c. Vol. III. p. 106.
§ Trans. of King and Queen's Coll. Dublin, Vol. II. p. 309.
‖ Medical Repository. London, 1817.
¶ Edinburgh Medical and Surgical Journal. Contributions to Morbid Anatomy,
No. ii. Vol. XVII. p. 331. By A. Duncan, Jun. M. D., &c. Cases 4th, 5th, and 6th.

By Bonetus this affection of the cerebral substance was believed to precede and to cause the discharge from the ear. Although this idea was refuted by Morgagni, who regards the cerebral abscess as consecutive to the ear-discharge, especially its suppression, it has been revived by Mr Brodie, who seems to think the affection of the brain coeval with that of the ear. I shall afterwards show that the internal affection, to which Bonetus and Mr Brodie ascribe this character, and which they think causes the ear-discharge, is disease either of the tympanal cavity, or of the *dura mater* investing the temporal bone. The inflammation which terminates in abscess of the cerebral substance is the effect of inflammation of the membranes, and in some instances of the discharge being suddenly checked, and the chronic external inflammation being suddenly converted into an acute internal disease. 1*st*, It is generally remarked to succeed quickly the suppression or the disappearance of the external discharge. This, which was the opinion of Morgagni, is proved by the cases of Mr Brodie, Mr Parkinson, Dr O'Brien, and Dr Duncan. 2*d*, That it does not exist from the origin of the discharge may be inferred when the patient is suddenly attacked with acute deep pain in the head, intolerance of sound, and delirium, quickly followed by insensibility and coma. 3*d*, It is improbable that a disease, commencing with the acute symptoms to which the formation of this abscess can generally be traced, should be going on for years without deranging more considerably the faculties of sensation, thought, and motion.

This disease is generally observed in young subjects of the habit named *strumous*. So far as I have observed or read, though it takes place in one of two modes, either as an extension of the original disease of the ear and cerebral membranes, or an alternating and vicarious result, the latter is most frequently its genuine character. The abscess is contained in an irregular cavity, surrounded by lymph and cerebral matter, which is very vascular. It is in all cases attended with inflammation, thickening, and suppuration of the membranes. The *pia mater* is highly vascular, and more or less covered with lymph. The *dura mater* is thick, opaque, dark-coloured, and detached from the bone.

The variety of abscess now mentioned is understood to depend upon the operation of internal causes only. At least no external cause can be recognized; and if it were, it would be such as in other subjects would perhaps be inadequate to the effect. There

is, however, a class of purulent collections in the brain which in
general it is possible to trace to mechanical violence inflicted on
the head; and it is remarkable how long a period may elapse between the date of the injury, and that destruction of the organ
which renders the continuance of life impossible.

Pigray gives a case in which an abscess, the size of a nut, proved
fatal at the end of six months;* and Morand mentions one in which
a soldier, who had received a shot in Italy, after slight treatment
of the wound, proceeded thence to Paris; and nine months elapsed
before suppuration and total destruction of the right lobe terminated life.†

In a case mentioned by Prochàska, the first foundation of the
disease appears to have been frequent beating on the head for years,
finally carried to intensity by a blow on the forehead, five months
after which death took place.‡   In a case by Sir E. Home, nearly
nineteen months elapsed between the receipt of the injury and the
fatal termination.§   In one by Dr Denmark, the interval between
the supposed injury and the period of death was twelve months.||
Many similar cases are found in the writings of surgeons.¶   The
result is, that a portion of brain more or less extensive is converted into purulent matter, contained in general in a membranous
cyst, more or less thick and vascular, according to the interval between the infliction of the injury and the time of examination.

Between suppuration of the brain, from internal and external
causes, a distinction has been drawn by Baillie, in the circumstance, that in the former it is generally in the substance, and in
the latter on the surface of the organ.   This distinction does not
hold good in several respects, and requires modification.   1st,
Where a long interval elapses after the infliction of the injury, the
collection of purulent matter is almost invariably deep seated.   2d,
In like manner, when the injury operates in the manner of counter-
stroke, the collection is also often within the substance of the or-

* Libre IV. chap. ix.
† Opuscules de Chirurgie, l. c. p. 159.
‡ Obs. Patholog. Section iv. apud Opera Minora, p. 304.
§ Transactions of a Society, Vol. III. p. 94.
|| Medico-Chirurgical Transactions, Vol. V. p. 24.
¶ See especially several cases of this kind in the writings of Louis, Le Dran, Rava-
ton ; and by Volaire, Journal de Med. Vol. XX. p. 503.   Thilenius, Med. und Chir.
Bemerkungen.   Walther, Obs. 33.   Thulstrup Physicalks Bibliothek. für Danmark 1
Band. April.   Bailey in Med. and Phys. Journal, Vol. XXIII. p. 376.

gan. (Pigray, Quesnay, Petit, Chopart.* For example, several weeks or months after a blow on the upper or fore part of the head, from which the patient never perfectly recovers, but is more or less paralytic, perhaps occasionally lethargic, deaf, blind, or fatuous, death takes place, and an abscess is found in the substance of the hemispheres, in the *corpus striatum*, or even in one of the lobes of the cerebellum. 3*d*, In some instances of suppuration after injury, the collection does not take place at the part at which the blow struck the skull, but either in the line of the force passing through the brain, or in some of the lines into which this force may be resolved. 4*th*, It is chiefly when the force has been directly expended on the part, *i. e.* when the bone has been immediately broken, and its membranes injured, that suppuration takes place on the surface of the brain. This suppuration is then the result rather of the affection of the membranes, especially of the *pia mater*, than of the cerebral substance itself.†

Suppuration may take place in any part of the brain; but it is most frequent in the hemispheres. The effects which it produces vary according to the situation and the extent of the purulent collection. They are much the same as from the presence of blood, tumours, or other unusual substances.

In the circumstances now mentioned, purulent collections are the result of primary inflammation, spontaneous or traumatic. I must further repeat explicitly what has been already said, that they take place in a secondary manner in fever. Collections of purulent matter within the brain after fever were first distinctly found by Pringle, afterwards by Borsieri and Eisfeld,‡ and more recently by Jackson and Mills. These are doubtless the effects of inflammation, which, however, is, in this case, a secondary and adventitious circumstance in the progress of the disease.

These, nevertheless, and similar phenomena, have been conceived to afford evidence that fever consists in inflammation of the brain. It is unnecessary to examine the origin of this theory; the first traces of which may be found in the writings of Willis, Werlhof,

* Mémoire sur les contre coups dans les lesions de la tete. Par M. Chopart. Mémoires pour le Prix. de la Academie Royale de Chirurgie, Tom. XI. 12mo.

† Traité des Plaies de Tete, et de l'Encephalite, principalement de celle qui leur est consecutive, &c. Par J. P. Gama, Officier de la Legion d'Honneur, Chirurgien en Chef, &c. Paris. 1830. 8vo.

‡ J. F. A. Eisfeld Meletemata, Quædam ad Historiam Naturalem Typhi Acuti Lipsiæ æstivo tempore, anni 1799, grassantes pertinentia. § xviii. p. 72, &c. apud Brera, Vol. VI. p. 1.

Torti, Donald Monro, and a paper of M. Marteau de Grandvilliers.* Riel appears to have entertained the idea, that cerebral inflammation, though not the cause of the symptoms, takes place in fever. The first attempt, however, to connect the phenomena of fever with those of inflammation, was made by Ploucquet of Tubingen in 1800,† and this was more expressly undertaken by Costantin of Leipzic in the same year, in consequence of an epidemic typhus which had prevailed at Leipzic in 1799. According to the latter author, *Encephalitis,* by which he understands that form of fever which happens to the cerebral and cerebellic vessels and membranes, comprehends three *genera, Synocha, Typhus,* and *Paralysis ;*—the first distinguished by increased irritability, with normal or increased reaction ; the second by increased irritability, but impaired reaction ; and the third by irritability and reaction being equally impaired, inert, and more or less abolished.‡

These ideas, though carried to an extreme, derive some support from the phenomena of fever, and the morbid changes left in the brain. They were afterwards more fully developed by Clutterbuck § and Mills‖ in this country, and by Marcus¶ and others in Germany. The merits of this theory I have already attempted partially to appreciate. Though autoptic examinations prove that the capillaries of the brain, in common with those of other organs, are much overloaded with slowly moving blood, this state differs from inflammation in several respects. Suppuration, especially, is not a constant, or is rather an exceedingly rare occurrence, and is to be regarded as adventitious, or depending upon accidental peculiarities and idiosyncrasies, and not essential. The overloaded state of the capillaries, though taking place in those of the organ itself, is nevertheless more remarkable, according to my observation, in those of the proper cerebral membrane. The principal character of that blood is, as I have above shown, that it is non-arterialized, and consequently poisonous.

* Description des Fievres Malignes avec une Inflammation sourde du Cerveau, &c. &c. Par M. Marteau de Grandvilliers, Medecin de l'Hopital à Aumale, Journal de Medecine, Tome VIII. 1758. p. 275.

† G. F. Ploucquet Expositio Nosologica Typhi. Tubingen, 1800. Tubing. Anz. 1800.

‡ Caroli Fred. Costantin, M. D. Dissertatio de Encephalitide. Lips. 1800. Ext. in Brera Sylloge, Vol. VI. p. 72.

§ An Inquiry into the Seat and Nature of Fever, &c. By Henry Clutterbuck, M.D. &c. Lond. 1807, and second edition, London, 1825.

‖ On the Utility of Blood-letting in Fever. By Thomas Mills. Dublin, 1819.

¶ Ephemeriden der Heilkunde. Band I. Heft. 1.

5. Ulceration; Erosion. From the various forms of pulpy destruction and abscess, the transition to ulceration is easy. By this is understood destruction of part of either of the surfaces of the brain, so as to present a hollow or depressed surface, rough, irregular, and covered partially either with bloody or albuminous exudation. In the former case its claim to the character of a genuine ulcer may be doubtful, since it may be viewed as the residue of a partial effusion of blood. It is possible that this may have been the origin of the case of erosion of the *corpus striatum* described by Morgagni, in which that body is said to have been entirely detached from the brain;* and I think it is next to certain this was the cause of the *ulcerous cavity,*† which he shortly after states was found in the base of the left ventricle of another case. This is almost admitted by Morgagni himself, who regards these ulcers as ruptured cavities or cells, originally formed by effused serum. (Ibid. art. 8.)

So far as accurate observation hitherto goes, the genuine ulcer is found chiefly at the convoluted surface of the brain; (Ridley, p. 212; Powell, case 6;) or the foliated surface of the cerebellum (Haller, Vol. iv. p. 351,) and is always connected with an unsound state of the proper or vascular membrane. Of this sort of ulcer, Stoll found an instance on the cerebellum of a young man of twenty-six, accompanied with redness, thickening, and erosion of the *pia mater.* ‡ Two cases of the same nature are recorded by Scoutetten. In one, the lower part of the right anterior lobe presented a hard, dry, irregular surface, thirteen lines long and seven broad, with irregular indented edges, with the contiguous cerebral substance sound. In the other, the extremity of the posterior lobe presented two small ulcerated patches, one oval, six lines long, and covered with deep gray pulpy matter; the other a linear depression,—both with wine-lee colour of the adjacent brain. In both cases, the investing proper membrane was red, injected, and somewhat eroded. § From these facts, it results that ulceration of the brain is an effect of circumscribed inflammation of the *pia mater.*

The instances of erosion, or ulceration from the penetration of foreign bodies, mentioned by Morgagni and various surgical authors, are rather examples of suppurative destruction.

6. Encephalæmia. Hemorrhagia Cerebri, Hoffmann. *Hemorrhage. Apoplexia Sanguinea,* Sauvages, Cullen, &c. *Apoplexie Ce-*

---

* Epist. xi. 2. † Ibid. 4.

‡ Ratio Medendi, pars tertia, p. 122.

§ Memoire sur quelques cas rares d'Anatomie Pathologique du Cerveau, &c. Par Scoutetten, D. M. P. &c. Archives Generales, Tome VII. 31.

rebrale of Serres. One of the great uses of the proper or vascular
membrane (*pia mater*) is to sustain and convey, as it were, the minute
arteries into the substance of the brain. No artery, however minute, enters this organ without previously passing through the *pia
mater* ; and if the carotid and vertebral arteries be injected, the cerebral matter may be washed away entirely ; while all the vessels,
by which it was traversed, are seen issuing from the attached surface
and numerous processes of this membrane. The vessels thus demonstrated consist of minute arteries and veins, through which, in
the sound or normal state, the blood moves uniformly and easily
without undergoing any permanent retardation. Dissection, however, shows, that from various causes, either the whole of these vessels, or a certain cluster or set of them, may become inordinately
distended with blood ; while others, which, in consequence of conveying colourless fluid previously, eluded observation, now becoming injected with red blood, are rendered visible. The existence
of this state is proved by cutting into thin slices the brains of persons cut off in this condition, when numerous blood-drops follow
each incision, and each part is penetrated by a much greater number
of vessels than natural.* The exquisite or most perfect degree of
this state is when the blood-drops enlarge immediately after incision,—a circumstance from which a very inordinate quantity of fluid
blood in the cerebral vessels is indicated. †

This state of the cerebral vessels is similar to that of inflammation. The patient is highly sensible to transitions of heat and cold ;
the skin is hot and dry ; the tongue foul ; the stomach disordered,
and the urine high-coloured and sedimentous. The pulse is full
and strong, sometimes hard, but not frequent. The local complaints
are dull pain and weight of the head, occasional giddiness, indistinctness of vision, or dazzling of the eyes, and more or less abolition of memory. When blood is drawn, I have found it present a
thick, tough, buffy coat ; an observation in which I find I am anticipated by Stoll ‡ and Sir Gilbert Blane.

When the above phenomena have continued for a few hours,
sometimes a day or two, according to circumstances, the individual
falls down destitute of sense and motion, and continues so for a
short time. After a little, recollection gradually returns, and with
it sensation and the power of moving the limbs, though not with
such freedom as before. A sense of tingling and numbness may

* Morgagni passim, especially iii. and iv.
† Morgagni epist. x. 17 and 18.
‡ Ratio Med. Pars v. p. 31. Viennæ, 1789.

remain in an arm or leg for some time. This is the simplest and mildest form of the apoplectic seizure. (*Cataphora*.) It has been thought that this could not happen unless blood is effused ; but various instances have occurred to competent observers in which the cerebral vessels are loaded only, and in which effusion had not yet taken place. It may further be inferred, that the instances in which persons recover from complete apoplectic seizure without suffering palsy depend upon vascular injection only. That fatal cases even may result from mere accumulation, is admitted by Morgagni,* afterwards by Baillie,† without being aware that the observation had been made, and by Rochoux, who thinks, however, that it is not uniform.‡ I observe, nevertheless, that M. Rochoux forgets that the cases in which it occurs being less frequently fatal, are more rarely the subject of inspection.

According to M. Serres, indeed, cases of apoplectic seizure without palsy depend on injection of the membranes exclusively.§ This point shall be afterwards considered when speaking of the cerebral membranes. In other respects, however, the researches of this physician tend to establish the general inference, that extravasation is not necessary to apoplexy. 1*st*, From experiments made on living animals,‖ from the phenomena of effusions of blood either spontaneously, or from wounds and injuries of the head, it appears that a considerable quantity of blood or other fluid may be effused in various parts of the brain without causing apoplectic symptoms. (Wepfer, Valsalva, and Serres). 2*d*, From various cases it appears that the apoplectic symptoms connected with extravasation disappear, while the extravasated blood remains. (Serres's cases, 7, 8, 7, 10, 11, 12, and others.) 3*d*, It results from cases recorded not only by Morgagni, Baillie, and Rochoux, as above mentioned, but by the physicians of Breslau,¶ by Quarin, by Stark,** and

* Epist. iii. 25 and 26.

† "The milder forms of apoplexy depend upon a distension of some of the vessels of the brain from undue accumulation of blood in them. I have known, however, one instance of fatal apoplexy, where many of the blood-vessels were found, upon examination after death, to be much distended with blood ; but no blood had been extrava-sated in any part of the brain."—Lectures and Observations on Medicine. London, 1825, p. 167.

‡ Recherches sur l'Apoplexie. Par J. A. Rochoux. Paris, 1814.

§ Nouvelle Division des Apoplexies ; par M. Serres ; Chevalier, &c. Annuaire Medico-Chirurgicale des Hopitaux et Hospices Civiles de Paris. A Paris, 1817. 4to, p. 246, 277.

‖ Annuaire Medico-Chirurgicale, 260, 261.

¶ Historia Morborum Vratislaviensium.

** Clinical and Anatomical Observations, Part iv. § 4, p. 73. This appears, howmore recently, I may add, by Dr Abercrombie, that complete symptoms of apoplexy may result from mere general injection of the cerebral vessels. The same phenomenon appears to have been witnessed by Cheselden. (Book iii. chap. 14, p. 224.) If, on this point, my own observation be entitled to any weight, I may add, that in 1817 I had occasion to examine the body of a young woman who died with all the symptoms of well-marked apoplexy; and though every part of the brain was cut into minute portions with the utmost care, no effusion of red blood could be recognized. The only abnormal appearance was some injection of the vessels going to the annular protuberance and *medulla oblongata.** 4th, Though in several cases of persons cut off with well-marked apoplectic symptoms, I have found extravasated blood, it bore no proportion to the severity of the disease. Instead of being in the shape of clots in distinct cavities, it consisted simply of long linear streaks of blood stretching through parts of the brain, sometimes in the neighbourhood of blood-vessels. In such cases, however, the blood-vessels were much injected, especially in the vicinity of the membranes. In other instances capillary injection is observed in the *corpora striata* or substance of the hemispheres. This is the capillary apoplexy of M. Cruveilhier.

Upon the whole, I conceive it legitimate to infer, that the essential anatomical character of apoplexy is injection of the vessels of the brain more or less general. This may terminate in one of two modes, both of which are accidental and accessory. The first is effusion of serous fluid; the second is effusion of red blood.

Serous fluid exhaled from the capillaries has been supposed to constitute a peculiar form of apoplexy entirely distinct from that termed sanguine, and depending on extravasation of blood. In the writings of morgagni and others are cases in which the effusion of serous fluid was associated with distinct and general vascular injection. Cases of this description are referred by Stoll to the head of *sanguine* apoplexy, in which the pathological character is injection or *accumulation*, which is at once the cause of the serous effusion and of the apoplectic symptoms.† It was afterwards demonstrated

---

ever, to have been a case depending on vascular injection of the *medulla oblongata* and spinal chord.

* Case of Ann Dinwiddie. Clinical Ward.

† *h* In apoplecticorum secto cerebro frequenter leguntur *vasa cerebri sanguine turgida, et serum multum effusum.* Hujus generis apoplexiæ plerumque *serosæ* audiunt. Verius *sanguineæ* appellarentur; accumulatus enim intra caput sanguis, et seri effusi, et apoplexiæ causa est; serum ipsum effusum *ad concausas pertinet serius accedentes,*

4

by Portal, that serous infiltration and effusion invariably arise from the same state of the vessels as hemorrhage;[*] and this inference has since been confirmed by the observations of Dr Cheyne, Dr Abercrombie, of M. Serres, and others. In short, if from any cause the circulation within the head becomes unusually slow, and the vessels of the brain become inordinately distended, either red blood or serous fluid is poured out from the extremities of the arteries. The latter process, if we admit the testimony of Cheselden,[†] Morgagni,[‡] and Willan,[§] takes place in the slow and gradual drowsiness and stupefaction which distinguish the form of the disease termed lethargy ; (*veternus.*)[||] The cause of the symptoms, however, is not the effusion, as Willan imagined, but the general vascular distension and injection from which the effusion arises.

Hemorrhage, nevertheless, takes place in a considerable proportion of cases. Howship says in nine of ten ; but this is evidently a general assertion founded on no accurate elements. From the distended vessels blood escapes, though whether by exhalation or by actual rupture is not agreed; and, forcing its way through the cerebral substance, breaks it down, and forms a sort of hollow or cavern, in which it coagulates. If the quantity be considerable ; if it be effused suddenly, and in certain parts of the brain ; (optic thalamus, annular protuberance, brain-limbs, and *medulla oblongata ;*) if the cerebral injection continues, notwithstanding the discharge and the use of remedies, complete coma very soon terminates in death ; and on dissection more or less blood is found in some part of the substance of the brain, and the vessels are much, sometimes exceedingly injected with fluid blood.

When the effusion is not copious, or dependent upon very general injection of the cerebral vessels, nor take place suddenly, or in a vital part of the brain ; or if the injection is thereby, or by other means moderated ; then further changes take place, and continue until the natural structure of the organ is so much altered that life can no longer be continued. The effused blood, both

quæve morbum ipsum non produxere, attamen productum augent." Rationis Medendi, Pars i. p. 138. . Lugduni Bat. 1780.

[*] Sur la Nature et le Traitement de Plusieurs Maladies, &c. Tome I. p. 280 ; et Sur l'Apoplexie, et Sur les Moyens de la prevenir. Paris, 1811. Tome II. p. 216.

[†] The Anatomy of the Human Body. Book iii. chap. 14.

[‡] Epist. vi.

[§] Reports on the Diseases in London. By Robert Willan, M. D. &c. 1799, p. 338, 8vo edit. 1821.

[||] Thomæ Willis, De Anima Brutorum, Pars Pathol. Cap. 14.

when fluid, and especially after coagulation, acts as a foreign body, —breaks down, softens, and disorganizes the part with which it is in contact. After some time the clot begins to change, assumes a brown or brownish-black colour, and is separated into fragments floating in a wine-lee fluid. The further dissolution of these forms a homogeneous chocolate-coloured matter, which is eventually removed more or less perfectly ;* while the part, which the extravasation converted into a hollow, is filled with serous fluid, and softened or pulpy cerebral matter. In some cases of complete recovery this is gradually converted, by a slow process of adhesive inflammation, into a membranous substance, harder than the surrounding brain, which, however, is generally softer than sound cerebral matter. (Lerminier, cases 1, 2.) In this manner are formed the cavernous sacs described by Wepfer and Morgagni, (Epist. iii. 7, 8, 9, lx. 2, 6,) and the cavities described by Baillie, (450, 455,) Wilson, Abernethy,† and others.

The contiguous enclosing cerebral matter also undergoes peculiar changes, which vary with the interval between extravasation and death. The portion in immediate contact with the clot is generally dark red, wine-lee colour, or, at later periods, of a chocolate brown, and rather pulpy. The portion exterior to this is paler, and of an orange colour, but generally much penetrated by distended vessels. Exterior to this again may be in general distinguished a layer of bluish-white or bluish-yellow matter, gradually terminating in sound brain, but all more or less traversed by blood-vessels. In other cases, in which a longer period elapses between extravasation and death, the portion of brain enclosing the clot is pulpy, of a dun-red or orange-colour, passing to yellow, and terminating gradually in brain of natural colour and consistence. In both cases minute shreds of cerebral matter and filamentous threads may be traced in the pulpy matter and in the bloody clot, either recent or dissolved into the chocolate-coloured fluid. By some these filamentous threads are supposed to be the fine cellular tissue of the brain; but I think it impossible to doubt that they are

* " The appearance of the effused blood differs according to the duration of its effusion. When death ensues quickly, at the end of three or four days, for example, it is in the form of soft blackish clots. After a month or six weeks it becomes firmer, assumes a deep brown colour, and resembles the blood of aneurismal tumours. At a more remote period it becomes still more compact and of a pale red colour, bordering on ochreous yellow. Lastly, it is entirely absorbed."—Rochoux, p. 86.

† Surgical Works, Vol. II. On Injuries of the Head, pp. 18, 19, and 20. London, 1811.

minute capillary vessels. This general description I have derived partly from the description of Rochoux,* but especially from those of Lerminier and Serres,† and partly from personal observation. The change in the structure and consistence of the brain surrounding the clot forms one variety of softening (*ramollissement,*) or pulpy disorganization; and notwithstanding the opinion expressed by Pariset, Recamier, Rochoux,‡ and others, that it is the cause of the effusion, it is invariably the effect either of this or of the preliminary injection. This is established not only by the facts already mentioned, but by the cases of Morgagni, of M. Dan de la Vauterie,§ and especially by those of Lerminier and Serres.∥

Vascular injection, with or without bloody effusion, may take place in any part of the brain; but certain parts are much more commonly the seat of this discharge than others. Thus Morgagni, treading in the steps of Bonetus, justly remarked, that either bloody effusion, or the caverns formed by it, are found almost always in the striated bodies, or in the optic *thalami,* or in both, while the anterior part of the hemisphere was very rarely, and the posterior part almost never affected.¶ The general accuracy of this conclusion is in some degree confirmed by modern observation, which, in a majority of cases, has found the striated and optic bodies diseased. Rochoux particularly shows, that of forty-one cases of bloody effusion terminating fatally, twenty-four were found in the *corpus striatum,* two in the optic thalamus, one in the *corpus striatum* and optic thalamus, and one beneath the *corpus striatum;* while only thirteen, not more than one-half, were found in other parts of the brain. The reason of this is to be found in the anatomical relations of this part of the brain. Near the beginning of the fissure of Sylvius is situate the *white perforated spot* of Vicq-d'Azyr ("substance blanche que j'appelle *perforée.*") Through these orifices the Sylvian or middle artery of the brain, which lies in the fissure, transmits a great number of arteries of various sizes into the substance of the brain, and through the cerebral nucleus (*corpus striatum,*) which lies immediately over this perforated spot. This arrangement renders the striated body, or rather the striated nucleus, the most vascular part of the whole organ, and the most liable, when the cerebral vascular system is overloaded, to effusion of blood.

* Recherches. Cases, passim. Article vi. pp. 87, 88. Section ii. art. 2.
† Annuaire Medico-Chirurgicale. Lerminier, Cases 4, 5, 7, 8. Serres, various cases in § 12. *Apoplexie Cerebrale.*
‡ Recherches, &c. pp. 88 and 89.   § These soutenue, &c.
∥ Annuaire, loco citato.   ¶ Epistola iii. 18.

This doctrine is not, however, altogether free from objection. By M. Serres especially it has been said that hemorrhagic cavities are formed in the fore part, the middle, or the posterior part, of the hemispheres, without affecting the *thalami* or striated bodies, much more frequently than is represented by Bonetus, Morgagni, and Rochoux. I find from examining the cases of Howship, Lerminier, Serres, Tacheron, and others, that this is not entirely without foundation. Of 6 cases of cerebral hemorrhage given by Lerminier, 3 are in the hemispheres, 1 in the right optic *thalamus,* one in the left optic thalamus, and 1 in the left *corpus striatum.** Of 7 cases of cerebral hemorrhage given by Serres, two are in the centre or posterior part of the left hemisphere, 1 in both hemispheres, 1 in the left hemisphere and in the mesolobe, and 3 in the annular protuberance.† Among 19 cases of cerebral hemorrhage or its effects, recorded by Tacheron, 5 were in the right hemisphere, and 4 in the left, 2 were in the posterior part of the right hemisphere, 2 in the substance of the optic eminences, 2 in that of the striated bodies, 1 in the mesolobe and adjoining part of the left ventricle, 1 in the annular protuberance, 1 in the optic eminence and striated body at once; and in one, in which the last extravasation took place in the right optic thalamus, one cyst was found in the neighbourhood of the cylindroid eminence, another in the centre of the left optic thalamus, and a third in the annular protuberance.‡

Upon the whole, we are in possession of few very accurate elements to determine this question. From the authentic cases, however, which I have perused, for it is in vain to draw conclusions from individual observation only, I think there are grounds to infer, that, next to the striated nucleus, the hemispheres are the most frequent seat of cerebral injection and hemorrhage. It is worthy of remark, that the extravasation, when it takes place, does so chiefly on the outer side of the lateral ventricle, generally towards its posterior end, and in that portion of brain which forms the external-lateral boundary of the optic *thalamus,* separated from the ventricle by a thin plate. Into the ventricle it rarely takes place primarily; and when blood is found there, it is the result either of bloody extravasation in the hemisphere breaking down the floor,§

---

* Annuaire Medico-Chirurgicale, p. 213, et ensuite.

† Ibid. p. 324, §. xi. et ensuite.

‡ Recherches Anatomico-Pathologiques, &c. par C. F. Tacheron, Doct. à Medecine, &c. Tome IIIme.   Paris, 1823.   Ordre 4trieme, 2ieme genre.   Case 31st.

§ Howship, Case 15, 19.

the wall, or the ceiling of the ventricle, or, as shall be afterwards shown, it issues from the choroid *plexus.* The same remark applies to blood on the surface of the brain.

In this process the hemorrhage produces extensive laceration of the substance of the hemisphere attacked ; and if the blood effused be copious, and the laceration of the hemisphere great, the lesion proves speedily fatal. This fact I have verified by several cases carefully observed and examined after death ; and, in order to illustrate more clearly the nature of the lesion and its attendant effects, I shall mention shortly the condition of the brain in one extreme case. A quantity of dark-coloured blood, spread over the surface of the brain, was found on the anterior, superior, and lateral regions of the right hemisphere. This was thin at the posterior and superior part of the hemisphere, that is, about the thickness of a half-crown piece, diminishing to that of a shilling. At the anterior lobes it became much thicker, and at their lower surface and the anterior end of the mesolobe (*corpus callosum*), it was at least one-fourth of an inch thick. It was spread, much to the same extent and of the same dimensions, over the olfactory nerves and inferior surface of the anterior lobes, over the optic *chiasma,* pisiform eminences, and most of the whole lower surface of the middle lobe. A lacerated opening had taken place at the inner margin of the right hemisphere where it is joined to the mesolobe, and by this, which had forcibly torn up the mesolobe from its connections with the hemisphere, the blood had escaped, and gradually spread itself over the lower, anterior, and superior surfaces of the hemisphere.

It was then found that a large lacerated cavity had been formed in the substance of the right hemisphere, about three inches long, tapering at each end, but about two inches or one inch and a half in diameter at middle ; that from this the blood had escaped by one lacerated opening anteriorly to the surface of the brain ; and by a lateral one into the ventricle, which was also filled with blood.

Cases of the kind now specified are of extreme violence, and not only fatal, but very speedily fatal. It has been said that apoplexy, that is, cerebral hemorrhage, is not a speedily fatal disease ; and, under certain restrictions, this is correct. It is indeed not instantaneously fatal, like the bursting of an aortic aneurism, or the sudden death following on disease of the valves of the aorta or the heart. According to Rochoux, the shortest time that, in the most rapid cases, elapses between the first appearance of the symptoms and the occurrence of the fatal termination, is sixteen hours. I am satisfied, nevertheless, from several facts, as well authenticated as these can, under the circumstances, be, that, in the cases now adverted to, the interval between the first attack and the cessation of life is much shorter. In one case, in which my attention was particularly directed to this point, the interval between the first symptoms and the extinction of life might be six hours, but did not exceed eight hours. In other cases there is good reason to believe that the interval was not more than five hours.

The cause of this speedy extinction of life, compared with other cases, is to be found in two circumstances; 1st, the large quantity of blood effused, and consequently compressing a large extent of the brain and suspending its functions; and, 2d, the great injury inflicted on the brain by laceration of its substance, disorganization of its structure, and consequent disorder and suspension of its functions. The amount of effused blood, in short, and the great extent of brain injured, place this lesion as to fatality and speedy influence on the same footing with effusion of blood into the substance of the annular protuberance.

Next to the hemispheres in hemorrhagic tendency may be placed the protuberance, the limbs of the brain, the *medulla oblongata*, and the *cerebellum*, in the order now enumerated.

When hemorrhage takes place into the annular protuberance, the blood is generally deposited in layers in the interstices between the transverse fibres. In one fatal case I observed this so distinctly, that the blood and cerebral matter formed alternating layers. When it is very abundant, however, the transverse fibres are broken through, and the effused blood is contained in irregular cavities. (Cheyne, case 9, Serres, Tacheron.) The proximity of the protuberance to the large transverse branches of the basilar artery affords some reason for the readiness with which it may be affected with vascular injection and hemorrhage.

Of effusion into the cerebellum little is accurately known. Morgagni records two cases, one in both hemispheres, most in the left; and it is interesting to remark, that he lays particular stress on the pulpy state of the surrounding substance of the cerebellic hemisphere.* In the other, it appears to have been more recent. In a case by Dr Abercrombie a clot was found in the right hemisphere.

* " Ea autem portio cerebelli quæ corpus ejusmodi circumstabat, *fracida* erat." Epistola ii. 22. Epist. lx. 6.

Howship furnishes a curious case of extravasation into the *medulla oblongata*, in which parallel layers of blood were deposited transversely in the substance of the part.* (Case 20.)

· Genuine hemorrhage of the brain, as now described, though issuing from the capillaries, is thought not to take place by exhalation.† It is never possible to trace it to a single vessel; and hemorrhage from rupture of an arterial trunk, though producing the same symptoms, belongs anatomically to a different head. Cheyne,‡ and more recently Lerminier and Serres, appear to have found always many minute capillaries opening into the hemorrhagic cavity.

On the greater frequency of affection of the right side of the brain nothing very satisfactory has been ascertained. Morgagni believing it, ascribes it to the greater frequency with which the muscles of the right side are used than those of the left. In 41 cases, however, given by Rochoux, the number in the left was 18, that in the right 17, and that in both sides 6, which proves that this cannot be established with any precision.

It is important to ascertain the influence which bloody effusion in different parts of the brain, exerts on the functions of sensation, voluntary motion, and the muscles of respiration. For there is reason to believe, that, according as congestion or hemorrhage takes place in the hemispheres, in the striated bodies, in the annular protuberance, in the cerebellum, or in the *medulla oblongata*, the effects produced will be palsy, or apoplexy more or less violent, and with different degrees of lethargic or comatose affection. The inquiry is beset by this difficulty, that not the extravasation, but the injection, is the essential cause of death. Scarcely a part of the brain has been found unaffected in fatal cases. It is certain that effusion into the white matter of the hemispheres, and into the striated nucleus, is not essentially and invariably fatal, unless from the size of the rent in the brain and the amount of blood effused. For from cases of this kind temporary recovery has taken place. Neither is the inference of Bichat, that effusion into the protuberance is invariably fatal, well-founded. Tacheron records a case in which temporary recovery was effected. It must be admitted, nevertheless, that effusion into this part is more likely to be fatal than into any other. The cases of Serres afford the explanation of this fact, by showing, that injury done to the protuberance causes a severe and permanent

* Practical Observations on Surgery and Morbid Anatomy, &c. By John Howship. London, 1816.
+ Bichat, Anatomie Generale, Tome II. article iii. p. 279.
‡ Cases of Apoplexy and Lethargy. 8vo, London, 1812.

lesion of the function of the lungs, the vessels of which become distended with unrespired blood, while the air-vesicles are ruptured, and death is effected by asphyxia. The state of the cerebral vessels which terminates in hemorrhage may occur, perhaps, at any period of adult life. But these blood-vessels are liable to a peculiar state which predisposes to impeded motion, accumulation, and extravasation. This consists in deposition of earthy matter between the coats of the internal carotid arteries, and of the basilar artery and their branches. In consequence of this deposition, they lose much of their contractile and distensile powers, and some of their tenacity; become rigid, brittle, and less able to perform their functions as transmissile tubes; and whenever blood is accumulated in unusual quantity, as they do not so readily admit of distension, rupture is the consequence. (Baillie, 454.) Hodgson also shows how generally this morbid state of the cerebral arteries is connected with extravasation.*

This cause, however, is predisponent only. A fit of apoplexy may occur and prove fatal in persons in whom neither ossification of the arteries of the brain, nor any other state, except mere vascular injection, is found. And, on the other hand, the cerebral arteries may be ossified or steatomatous, in many persons who have never had a single fit of apoplexy. The general result of the cases observed by Vater, Morgagni, Cheyne, Howship, Rochoux, Serres, and Tacheron, is, that disease of the arterial coats is connected with vascular injection, which may terminate, according to circumstances, in serous effusion, pulpy destruction, or bloody extravasation. It is a well established fact, however, that the extravasation does not take place from the diseased arterial trunks, but from the minute capillaries in which these arteries terminate.

Old age has generally been regarded as a predisponent cause of apoplexy; and it is attended with two circumstances, which are perhaps not altogether without reason regarded as of some moment. The first of these is the venous plethora, so ingeniously maintained by Cullen. The second is the tendency which the arterial system more especially betrays to become diseased after the meridian of life. The proofs of the existence of venous plethora, and the theory of its operation, may be found in Cullen, who, perhaps, overrated its influence. There is little doubt that the circulation in the veins, either in consequence of diminished pressure and tension of the skin and other coverings, does not go on with the same perfection and

---

* A Treatise on the Diseases of Arteries and Veins, pp. 25 and 26.

facility with which it does in early life. But whether there is a greater venous plethora in the head at that period than before or not seems doubtful. There is reason to believe, that the fulness resides as much in the arteries as in the veins. It is manifest also that the main cause of this venous plethora in advanced life, viz. the frequency of disease of the heart, especially its mitral valve, and of the aortic valves, Cullen altogether overlooked. Of the effect and reality of arterial disease I have already spoken.

In point of fact, cases of apoplexy occur at all ages, but are most frequent between the 50th and the 65th, or 70th year. Willan informs us he has seen young persons from 12 to 18 years of age affected with apoplexy and hemiplegia. In Bonetus and Morgagni, instances of apoplexy are found occurring in persons below the age of 30 ; but in general they were induced by external violence or organic diseases. I have seen an instance of cerebral hemorrhage terminating in hemiplegy in a young man of 19, labouring under disease of the left auriculo-ventricular orifice. The young woman to whose case I have already alluded, was, I think, about 22 ; and in general when the disease takes place between 18 and 30, it is in consequence of disease of the heart or its valves, or of the aorta. Of eighteen cases described by Bonetus, five occurred in persons above 60, and six in persons below 40. Morgagni relates the cases of thirty apoplectic persons, seventeen of whom were above the age of 60, and five below that of 40. Of thirty-one cases of bloody extravasation in the ventricles or the substance of the brain, recorded by Lieutaud, one was at the age of 25, eight between the ages of 30 and 41, eleven between 41 and 51, six between 51 and 61, two between 61 and 71, two between 71 and 81, and one only above 100. Of twenty-nine cases seen or dissected by Portal, two were between 19 and 23, four between 30 and 41, seven between 41 and 51, eight between 51 and 61, four between 61 and 71, and the same number between 71 and 81. Of 6 cases of cerebral hemor. rhage given by Cheyne, three were between 30 and 35, two at 50, and one at 63. Rochoux, however, has given the fullest and most accurate results on this point. Among sixty-three cases of apo_ plexy, two occurred between the age of 20 and 30, eight between that of 30 and 60, seven between that of 40 and 50, ten between that of 50 and 50, twenty-three between that of 60 and 70, twelve between that of 70 and 80, and only one between that of 80 and 90. According to this view apoplexy is extremely rare before the 30th year ; from that period to the 50th it is not common but may occur; after 50 it becomes more common; between 60 and 70 is more frequent; becomes of the same rate of frequency after 70 as before 60, and is very rare after the 80th year. Of the cases given by Lerminier and Serres, though two are between 30 and 35, the great part are between 60 and 75.

The state of the cerebral circulation now described is understood to depend exclusively on the vessels of that organ, and to constitute, therefore, primary apoplexy. The same state, or a near approach to it, may take place secondarily in at least two different states of the system; first, as a consequence of injuries of the head; and, secondly, in the course of fever intermittent, remittent, or continuous. The first shall be considered afterwards. The second, or the febrile apoplexy, belongs to this place.

α. *Apoplexia Febricosa.* The best example of this occurs in certain forms of ague, accompanied with marks of great accumulation in the head. It takes place chiefly at the termination of the cold stage, and the commencement, or in the course of the hot. In a slight degree the paroxysm is attended with drowsiness or lethargy, from which the patient may still be roused. When this recurs once or twice, the insensibility is more complete, till the phenomena of perfect apoplexy are induced. In other instances after dull heavy pain of the head, dizziness, impaired vision, and some affection of the urinary secretion, the individual falls down suddenly with the mouth open, the eyelids fluttering, and other marks of relaxed muscles; and continues during the rest of the paroxysm in a stertorous sleep. This may cease spontaneously, or terminate in death, unless the paroxysm, which is generally protracted to twenty-four hours, and follows the tertian type, is finished. Though this is most frequent in the tertian, it is not uncommon in the quartan and quotidian.

The cases examined necroscopically show the cerebral vessels to be much distended with blood, sometimes bloody extravasation. In other instances which belong to a different head, the distended vessels are accompanied with serous effusion between the membranes, or within the cavities. The anatomical character of soporose ague is therefore inordinate injection of the cerebral and cerebro-meningeal capillaries.

This constitutes in various degrees the *sleepy quotidian* (C. Piso, Obs.*178,) the *sleepy, lethargic, hemiplegic, carotic, and apoplectic tertian,* (Werlhof, Torti, Lautter, Morton,) and the *comatose quartan* (Piso, Werlhof;) and is the disease which has been named by

3

Baglivi* and Lancisi† epidemic apoplexy (*apoplexia febricosa, carus febricosus*), and which Morgagni‡ and Casimir Medicus§ represent as periodical and intermitting. When it is known that the apoplectic symptoms are regulated by the motions of the ague, which alone is epidemic, or rather endemial, the nature of the periodical and epidemic apoplexy is easily understood.

These soporose agues may be sporadic or general; prevail mostly in the summer or autumnal months in warm countries; and after a few paroxysms, sometimes the second or third, are generally fatal. Their mortality is so uniform that they have been named *death-fevers* (Todten-fieber) in Germany and Hungary, where they used to be very common. They were observed at Rhodes by Praxagoras, the master of Herophilus; afterwards at London in 1678 by Sydenham; at Rome and in various parts of Italy by Baglivi in 1694 and 1695, and by Lancisi the same year, and at Bagnarea in 1707; at Hanover by Werlhof; and by Cleghorn in Minorca.

The extravasations into the cavities of the brain, observed by Jackson in yellow fever, belong to the head of meningeal hemorrhage.

In continued fevers of this and other countries, apoplectic death is so common, that I need only refer to the works of Stoll, Mills, Bateman, Cheyne, Barker, and Harty. It appears to be at once cerebral and meningeal.

In purpura and sea-scurvy death not unfrequently takes place from hemorrhage within the brain, or on its surfaces. The latter is most common, and as such belongs to the head of meningeal hemorrhage.

β. *Apoplexia Traumatica. Traumatic Apoplexy. Apoplexy from violence. Hemorrhage from the Cerebral Membranes. Traumatic Apoplexy. Meningeal apoplexy of Serres.* The effects of injury on the skull, especially in the form of repeated blows, are very peculiar. One blow, of course, or a fall, in which the skull lights on a stone or other hard body, may, as it often does, fracture the skull, and prove fatal either by the concussion, or by blood effused afterwards. But there is another class of cases in which a series of blows has been inflicted on the head, proving fatal, yet without fracturing the skull. In the class of cases, also, to which I now refer, the patient falls into a

---

* G. Baglivi Dissertatio, 8vo. De Observationibus, &c. Appendix de Apoplexiis fere epidemicis proximo elapso biennio in Urbe et per Italiam Observatis. Op. Om. Antwerpiæ, 1715, p. 683.

† De Noxiis Paludum Effluviis.　　　　　‡ Epist. iii. iv. and v.

§ Geschichte Periode-haltender Krankheiten. Erstes Buch; Erstes Capitel, § ii. Peode-haltender Schlagfluss, p. 5. Frankfurt und Leipzig, 1794.

U

state of insensibility from which he never recovers; and this, after lasting from 40 or 50 minutes to two, three, or more hours, terminates in death.

The state of the brain is in such cases the following.

The whole surface of the brain under the site of the blows, and not unfrequently all over, is covered with a layer of what appears to be blood of considerable thickness. At first sight this appears to be outside the membranes. But on examination it is found that the blood is effused or infiltrated into the subarachnoid or inter-membranous tissue, and that it has escaped from the lacerated vessels of the *pia mater*. The thickness of this layer varies. Sometimes it is pretty uniformly spread as thick as a crown piece all over the upper and lateral parts of the hemispheres. It generally increases in amount and thickness at the lateral and inferior regions of the brain. •The whole posterior lobes and the cerebellum may be covered by it. Most usually, however, it is thickest over the *crura*, the intercrural *fossa*, the annular protuberance and the *medulla oblongata*. Over these parts, in two fatal cases in which death followed almost immediately repeated blows on the head, I found the blood effused into the intermembranous tissue over the base of the brain, to the thickness of half an inch.

This, therefore, is a meningeal hemorrhage.

In the same class of cases blood is effused within the ventricles often to a great amount. It is coagulated, and the clot is surrounded by bloody coloured serum. This escapes in like manner from the vessels of the choroid plexus and the internal *pia mater*. These appearances are so uniformly the result of violence, that the circumstance of their situation and appearance may, along with other circumstances, be justly inferred, in doubtful cases, to prove that death is the result of violence. The fact, therefore, forms a valuable piece of evidence in medico-legal inquiries, to prove that such hemorrhage and such death could not have taken place from internal causes. Attempts are often made either by ignorant or designing persons, or by counsel, to prove that this intermembranous or meningeal hemorrhage is sanguineous apoplexy. The answer is very simple but decisive. In sanguineous apoplexy the hemorrhage always takes place in the substance of the brain and lacerates the brain. In traumatic apoplexy, or that from violence, it takes place on the surface from the vessels of the membranes, and compresses the organ.

By M. Serres, indeed, a species of meningeal apoplexy has been recognised as taking place spontaneously. It is a very rare occurrence, and the hemorrhage is in general on the free surface of the arachnoid membrane; in other words, within the arachnoid membrane. Collateral circumstances will here be available. •

γ. *Apoplexia Neonatorum.* Among the cases of infants expelled from the womb lifeless, or in such a state that they soon cease to live, in a considerable number the appearances are the following. A layer of blood, mostly coagulated, but with some bloody serum oozing from it, is spread uniformly over the whole of the superior, anterior, posterior, and lateral surfaces of the hemispheres. A similar layer of blood is found extending over the laminated surface of the *cerebellum,* and less frequently, perhaps, over the base of the brain. Within each lateral ventricle, and sometimes within the third and fourth, are found clots of blood with bloody serum. At first sight, it might be thought that these infants had been born alive, and had died in consequence of violence inflicted on the head. This inference is not quite correct. Violence has been in some degree inflicted; but it is the violence resulting from the efforts of the uterus in forcing a large head, or a wrong presentation through the pelvic outlet; and the infants were either not born alive, or vital action speedily ceased. Life was extinct before the head was expelled, in consequence of blood effused from the meningeal vessels into the subarachnoid tissue, all over the brain, and from the choroid plexus within the ventricles. The cause is most commonly protracted and tedious labour, during which the head is forcibly compressed against the pelvic bones; and the hemorrhage from the membranes takes place.

This is the *apoplexia neonatorum,* or apoplexy of new-born infants, a lesion almost necessarily and invariably mortal. To me it appears to be the most frequent cause of still-births, as they are termed; for at least 17 instances in 20 that I have inspected, in the course of a long series of years, presented the appearances now specified. To understand the true nature of this lesion is important in a medico-legal point of view; for rash and ignorant persons have often inferred, that it was the effect of violence intentionally inflicted on the head of an infant born alive. Cruveilhier gives good illustrations of the lesion, and the history of several cases in proof of its true nature and origin.* He shows that all infants with this lesion are not still-born, but may die soon after birth; that it is impossible, in all cases, to determine the cause of death; that is, the cause of the hemorrhage; but that cases take place after presentation of the vertex, of the hips, of the chord; and after long

* Anatomie Pathologique, Livraison **xv.**

and repeated attempts at turning. In general the head has been too slowly born, or the presentation has been unfavourable.

δ. On a form of apoplexy termed *nervous* much has been said by Zuliani of Brescia,* Kortum of Dortmund in Westphalia,† and Kirkland of Ashby de la Zouche ;‡ and the subject. has been re-vived by Mr Abernethy,§ and Dr W. Philip. In this, apoplectic symptoms are said to take place without any abnormal state of the brain or its vessels, and from some disorder in the chylopoietic organs, which is supposed to induce a torpid condition of the brain, or suspension of its proper energy. It may be doubted whether satisfactory proof of such a state has yet been adduced. 1*st*, A fallacy results from the doctrine that hemorrhage is in all instances requisite to give rise to apoplectic symptoms. I have shown that congestion, injection, or distension of the cerebral vessels is adequate to produce this effect ; and whether this state is to disappear, remain unchanged, or produce serous effusion, or bloody extravasation, so as to remain after death, will depend much on the constitution of the individual and the treatment employed. No satisfactory conclusion can be drawn from the absence of hemorrhage or serous fluid. 2*d*, Disorder of the chylopoietic organs is an accessory remote cause, which may operate on the meningeal and cerebral circulation. 3*d*, The instances adduced as examples of this disease are at least ambiguous. The fourth case of Kirkland cannot be admitted. The case of Stark (§ iv. p. 73,) I have already mentioned as one of injection either of the spinal chord or its membranes. The first case of Dr Powell might have been similar, for the spinal chord was not examined.‖ In other instances, as in that recorded by Morgagni, (Epist v. 17 and 19,) one in the meningeal vessels, and in the vascular system in general, might have been the cause of death. 4*th*, It has been shown by M. Serres, that many of the cases of supposed nervous apoplexy must have been examples of what he terms meningeal apoplexy, *i. e*, injection of the meningeal vessels with or without effusion or extravasation. 5*th*, In other instances a very slight and incipient degree of the state which is

---

* F. Zuliani De Apoplexia presertim Nervea. Lipsiæ, 1780.

† C. G. Theod. Kortum Tremoniæ Westphali dissertatio de Apoplexia Nervosa. Gœttingæ, 1785. Ext. in Frank. Dilectu, Vol. IV. p. 1 ; et Ludwig Scrip.-Neur, Tom. IV. p. 379.

‡ A.Commentary on Apoplectic and Paralytic Affections, &c. By Thomas Kirkland, M. D. 1792.

§ On the Constitutional Origin of Local Diseases.

‖ Medico-Chirurgical Transactions, Vol. III. By Thomas Chevalier.

to proceed to pulpy destruction may cause death. When it affects a whole hemisphere, which it may sometimes do, (Morgagni, Epist. v. 15, 16; li. 7, 11,) it may alter the appearance so little as readily to escape observation. 6*th*, The first and fourth cases of Dr Abercrombie I am unable to explain; but I think they may have taken place in persons with granular disease of the kidney, which not unfrequently causes apoplectic death, yet without leaving any traces of vascular injection or hemorrhage.

For the reasons now assigned, it may be justly questioned whether there is ground for admitting such a state of the brain as the *nervous apoplexy* of Zuliani, Kortum, Kirkland, and Abernethy. According to the present state of evidence, it is wisest to adopt the side which does not recognize this form of apoplectic disease.

7. In the foregoing account of the state of the brain giving rise to apoplectic symptoms, I have said nothing of that loss of voluntary muscular power known under the name of palsy, (*paralysis; paresis; resolutio nervorum;*) because I suppose it to depend on the same state of the cerebral capillaries which causes the general apoplectic affection, which it either precedes, accompanies, or follows; or on that state of the brain or spinal chord which I have already described as terminating in pulpy destruction. In attempting to establish clearly the anatomical characters of palsy, two circumstances merit particular attention.

First, several cases of apoplectic death are preceded by paralytic affection of one side, more or less extensive, in the successive forms of distortion of one side of the face, loss of speech, loss of power in an arm, a leg, or the entire side. When these phenomena are followed by coma and death, necroscopic inspection shows, as in apoplexy, capillary injection with or without extravasation, and generally more or less destruction of brain. The commencement of the morbid process in this instance is doubtless the same capillary injection of part of the organ, which in a more exquisite degree produces the comatose state. *Secondly*, Though there are not a few instances in which an attack of loss of consciousness, sensation, and motion, is not followed by loss of voluntary motion, these, I have already attempted to show, depend on that capillary injection which is removable by the use of remedies. When the capillary injection proceeds to destruction either by hemorrhage, by soften-ing, or by ulceration, *i. e.* by superficial pulpy destruction of cerebral substance, consequent on hemorrhage, it almost invariably leaves after it more or less loss of voluntary motion, generally on the side of the body opposite to that of the brain which has sustained the lesion.   One of the most frequent effects of cerebral hemorrhage and its consequences, indeed, is palsy of the hemiplegic form ; and in the brains of such persons as have laboured under this disease, either a broken down and softened spot, or one or more hemorrhagic cavities or cysts are found after death, (Wepfer, Willis, Morgagni, John Hunter, Baillie, Wilson, Abernethy, Rochoux, Serres, Lerminier, Tacheron, Abercrombie.)   The general accuracy of these conclusions is confirmed not only by the necroscopic appearances of the brains of those who die of coma succeeding to palsy, but of those who die of the effects of injuries of the head, of abscess of the brain and cerebellum, and of tumours and other organic changes taking place either in the brain or in its membranes.

I have said that palsy occurs generally in the side opposite to that in which the lesion of the brain is found, because in some cases it has been observed in the same side.

Though this singular phenomenon early attracted the attention of pathologists, it cannot be said that the circumstances, under which it takes place or does not take place, are determined.   The fact was early demonstrated by Molinelli ; and, in order to obtain a satisfactory explanation of it, much inquiry and experiment was undertaken by Pourfour de Petit, Saucerotte, and others, members of the Academy of Surgery ; and the phenomenon has since been the subject of occasional inquiry to several from Morgagni, Haller, and Prochaska, to Dr Anderson and Dr Yellowly.   The mutual interlacement of the cerebral chords between the restiform bodies has been supposed at various times, from Mistichelli and Pourfour de Petit, adequate to explain it.   To this the principal objection is the fact, that palsy of the opposite side, though frequent, is not an invariable result of injury of the brain.

The situation of these destroyed spots and hemorrhagic cavities, when inducing palsy, corresponds much with that of the cerebral injection or hemorrhage from which they arise.   The region most generally affected is that already described as the striated *nucleus* of Reil. Willis, for example, states, that in several dissections of persons dead after long-continued and obstinate palsy, he invariably found the *corpora striata* unusually soft, discoloured like wine-lees, and with the usual alternation of white and gray streaks much obliterated.[*]   The accuracy of this inference regarding the part of the

* Thomæ Willis, Cerebri Anatome, cap. xiii. p. 43, et De Anima Brutorum, cap. ix. p. 144 et 145.

organ most frequently affected is confirmed by cases given by
Petit; by several of those given in the Essay of M. de la Peyro.
nie* by Antonio Caldani; by Morgagni in repeated observations
both of paralytic cases terminating in coma, and of those originally
apoplectic, accompanied with distinct palsy ; (Epist. xl. 2, 4, 6,
11 ; li. 12 ; lxii. 7, 9;) by three cases given by Prochaska ;† by
Cheyne, by Rochoux, by Lallemand, by Tacheron, (26, 27, 28, 29,
30,) and by Abercrombie, (p. 252, cases 112, 113, 114, 115.)
On this point, however, the remarks already made on the seat
of cerebral hemorrhage are applicable. Though the striated nucleus and the contiguous part of the hemisphere forming the outer
and upper walls of the capsule, are the most frequent seat of hemorrhagic cavities and pulpy destruction, other parts of the brain
are not exempt. In the work of Dr Abercrombie are given cases
in which the diseased spot was nearer the surface of the organ.
(111, 116, 117, 118.) I met with one instance in which hemiplegia was connected with pulpy disorganization of the posterior part
of the hemisphere, so near the convoluted surface, that the lesion
could be immediately recognized after removing the *dura mater,*
by the unusual change of colour and consistence. Dr Duncan
Junior records two excellent examples in which pulpy destruction
of the anterior and middle lobes of the brain caused hemiplegy,
and that of the *cerebellum* gave rise to palsy of the paraplegic form,
without disorder of intellect.‡ It appears also from the testimony
of Dr Cheyne, that the form of disease which he terms *creeping*
palsy depends on the progressive softening of the substance of the
hemispheres. In the only example of this lesion recorded by the
author, the morbid change was vascular injection, and pulpy destruction of the white matter of both cerebral hemispheres, which
was of the consistence of thick cream.§

The circumstances of cases, in which this change takes place,
show that it is not so much the destruction of the cerebral substance as the capillary injection or inflammation, with which it is
attended, that produces the loss of power in the muscles of volun-

* Observations par lesquelles on tache de decouvrir la partie du Cerveau où l'ame
exerce ses Fonctions. Chez Memoires de l'Academie Royale des Sciences, 1741.
† Georgii Prochaska Op. Minorum, partem ii. Viennæ, 1800. Observat. Patholog.
sect. iv. *Casus tres complectens, &c.*
‡ Contributions to Morbid Anatomy, No. II. By A. Duncan Jun. M. D., &c.
Ed. Med. and Surgical Journal, Vol. XVII. 328, 329.
§ Dublin Hospital Reports, Vol. IV. p. 270.

tary motion. In some instances of paralytic disorder lasting for a considerable time, instead of finding hemorrhagic cavities or destroyed spots in the brain, it is impossible to recognize any thing but some vascular injection and effusion of serous fluid, which doubtless proceeded from the overloaded vessels. This injection is not confined to one spot, but is diffused in different degrees through the brain, and is in some instances strongly marked in the cerebellum, annular protuberance, and the meningeal vessels towards the base of the organ. The effects which this state of the brain produces vary somewhat from genuine apoplectic palsy. They constitute a double but unequal hemiplegy approaching very gradually, and very often simulating paraplegia. From this, however, they differ, in the lower extremities being seldom affected in the same degree and at an equal rate. It is often attended with some loss of memory, or sensation, and some slight degree of mental imbecility. The anatomical character of the disease may be represented as a chronic congested state of the cerebral capillaries. It may terminate either in serous effusion from the meningeal vessels, in softening of the cerebral substance, or in induration. In the first instance, it belongs to the head of meningeal injection, to be afterwards noticed. In the second case, it will often correspond with the *creeping palsy* of Dr Cheyne ; or it may give rise to epileptic attacks. (Morgagni, ix. 16, 18, 20, 23 ; Greding, No. 49, p. 494 ; No. 42, p. 524 ; Wenzel, Portal.) In the third, it is one of the morbid states of the brain causing insanity.

8. The spinal chord is liable to the same species of vascular injection and hemorrhage which takes place in the brain. The capillaries, which, in the sound or normal state, are small, and convey almost colourless fluid, become enlarged and penetrated with red blood. In a stage of the process, which is to be regarded as further advanced, drops of blood, and occasionally clots of some magnitude, are found deposited in the substance of the chord. These undergo and give rise to the same changes which have been already described as taking place in the brain, and are a cause by no means unfrequent of pulpy disorganization of the chord. In the case given by Gaultier de Claubry, which is the most distinct on record, the chord opposite the seventh cervical vertebra was of a deep red colour from vascular injection, but still unbroken in structure ; from the seventh cervical vertebra to the third dorsal it was not only deep red on the surface, but on the substance, and

so soft as to sink under the knife or finger ; and from the third dorsal vertebra to the lower part of the sacrum, it was a red blood-coloured pulp destitute of organization.* The cases of Chevalier, which belong rather to the head of meningeal hemorrhage, shall be noticed afterwards.

Pulpy softening of the spinal chord may arise either spontaneously or as a consequence of injury, more especially if that injury causes fracture or even concussion of the vertebræ. When it takes place spontaneously, often the arteries of the chord are previously diseased. Most commonly the appearance of the chord is that of a pulpy softened mass, falling entirely down on the membranes being divided. In extreme cases, the chord is converted into a soft semifluid diffluent mass, not unlike cream. Sometimes in recent cases, considerable vascularity and injection are observed. But in chronic cases, the vessels are in general scanty. When the disease arises spontaneously, it may affect a large portion of the chord.

When softening is the result of injury, as contusion, concussion, or fracture of the vertebræ, it is in general limited to the spot where the injured bones are situate. The anatomical and physical characters are the same.

The effects produced by capillary injection and hemorrhage in the spinal chord vary according to the stage of the process and the region of the chord in which it occurs. In the stage of injection it produces irregular involuntary twitches of the muscles of the trunk and extremities, numbness and coldness of the skin about the back, and occasionally of the limbs, and more or less of muscular power. In the advanced stage, whether that of hemorrhage or of pulpy destruction, numbness and palsy of the paraplegic form are complete.

In some instances the state of capillary injection appears to give rise to tetanic symptoms. This fact, which was observed by Dr Robert Reid in Ireland,† Duchatelet,‡ Martinet, and Ollivier,§

* Journal General de Medecine de Chirurgie et de Pharmacie, &c. 12ieme année, Tome XXXII. A Paris, 1808. P. 129.

† On the Nature and Treatment of Tetanus and Hydrophobia. By Robert Reid, M. D. Dublin, 1817.

‡ Recherches sur l'Inflammation de l'Arachnoide cerebrale et Spinale, &c. Par M.M. Parent-Duchatelet et L. Martinet. Paris, 1821.

§ De la Moelle Epiniere et de ces Maladies, &c. Par C. P. Ollivier d'Angers. A Paris, 1824. Pp. 307, 308, 317, 349.

in France, and by Dr Duncan Junior, in the stage of suppuration,* has led to the recent revival of an opinion originally proposed by Galen, and reproduced in modern times by Fernel, Willis, and Hoffmann,—that tetanus depends on a morbid state of the spinal chord or its membranous coverings. This inference, nevertheless, is not in its present state susceptible of that degree of accuracy which entitles it to a place among the established principles of pathology. Though in some instances capillary injection of the chord, and the origins of the spinal nerves is attended with tonic spasms of the muscular system, in a great number, perhaps a larger proportion, no contractions of this kind take place, notwithstanding every morbid change from vascular injection to pulpy destruction or suppuration. Tetanic spasms, Ollivier infers, are connected with the advanced and intense forms of the disease; but the cases collected, not only by this author himself, but by Pinel, Velpeau, and Abercrombie, show, that in some of the most aggravated forms of the disease no spasms had taken place till the last few hours of existence. In short, the circumstances under which tonic spasms occur in connection with vascular injection and inflammation of the chord, have not yet been distinctly indicated. From the cases observed by Reid, Duchatelet, and Martinet, Jones, Ollivier, and Duncan Junior, tetanic spasms appear to be more frequently connected with injection of the membranes than of the substance of the chord.

The variation of effects according to the region of the chord affected may be distinguished into three heads;—as the morbid process affects the longitudinal extent, the transverse breadth, or the antero-posterior thickness of the chord.

α. When it is seated in the upper or cranial portion of the chord, (*medulla oblongata*,) the effects are more or less disorder of the senses, locked-jaw, gnashing of the teeth, impaired articulation and deglutition, respiration oppressed, disordered, and panting, palsy, and death by asphyxia.

When it is seated in the cervical portion it gives rise to tetanic rigidity, convulsion, or palsy of the muscles of the neck, more or less palsy of the intercostals, and muscles of the trunk and extremities in general, paralytic weakness of the diaphragm, and eventually, as this advances, death by suspension of the mechanical agents of respiration.

* Contributions to Morbid Anatomy, Case 5th.   Medical and Surgical Journal, Vol. XVII. p. 332.

In the dorsal region it induces convulsive throes of the trunk, palsy of the intercostal muscles, with short, languid, diaphragmatic respiration, palpitation, and irregular throbbing of the heart, hiccup, squeamishness, vomiting, and eventually death, partly by impaired respiration, partly by failure of the action of the heart.

In the lumbar region, palsy of the lower extremities is always a prominent symptom; but to this are added paralytic retention of urine at first, afterwards incontinence and involuntary voiding of the contents of the rectum.

β. The transverse diameter of the chord is so small, that in general the capillary injection and its consequences are not confined to one side only. When this happens, however, which is rare, it produces hemiparaplegia, or palsy of the lower extremity of one side. Though this has been so frequently observed to occur on the same side with the lesion of the chord, that it may be stated as a general result, it is nevertheless requisite to mention, that to Portal we are indebted for a singular case, in which capillary injection and pulpy destruction of the right side of the lumbar division of the chord, gave rise to palsy of the left inferior extremity.*

γ. To the antero-posterior diameter of the chord the same observations nearly apply; and it is rare to find the anterior part diseased without affection of the posterior, and conversely. Instances of this, nevertheless, have been observed; and it is interesting to remark, that the effects which respectively result from lesion of either singly, tended to confirm those inferences which Charles Bell and Magendie have drawn regarding the anterior and posterior roots of the spinal nerves. Thus when the anterior part of the chord is affected without the posterior, the effect is loss of muscular power more or less complete, while sensation remains. Conversely, when the posterior part of the chord is injured without the anterior, sensation is more or less obliterated, while voluntary motion is little affected. Thus in a case recorded by Dr Jones, vascular injection of the posterior surface of the chord impaired sensation remarkably, but left motion little affected.† In like manner, in a case communicated by Royer-Collard to Ollivier, (Obs. 47, p. 334,) pulpy destruction of the anterior part of the chord, from the restiform and olivary eminences, down to the lum_

---

* Anatomie Medical, Tome IV. p. 116.
† Medical and Surgical Journal, Vol. XXI. p. 81, 83.

bar portion without affection of the posterior, caused palsy of the trunk and lower extremities without impairing sensation.

9. *State of the Brain in Fever.* A singular state of the brain is observed in fever, whether *typhus* or ordinary *synochus*, which usually ends in *typhus*. The whole of the convoluted portion of the brain, and the laminated portion of the *cerebellum*, indeed the whole gray matter of the organ acquires a peculiar deep colour, as if the gray matter had been tinged of a reddish-brown, or slight pink-colour. The white matter is also redder than usual, and presents when divided numerous dark-red points effusing semifluid dark-coloured blood. The white matter of the *crura* of the brain, of the protuberance, and the bulb of the spinal marrow (*medulla oblongata*), acquires a peculiar pink-colour, totally different from that observed in death by other diseases, and similar only to the state of the brain, in persons destroyed by acute or chronic asphyxia. The membranes are generally loaded with serous fluid, which is also found in the cerebral substance and within the ventricle. Brains in this state are not easily preserved. They are soft, and lacerable, and generally undergo decomposition early and speedily.

This state is manifestly the result of the brain being supplied only with dark-coloured or non-oxygenated blood. With this its arteries are filled during life and after death. The organ is indeed poisoned with unrespired blood, much as if the individual had breathed carbonic oxide gas. These appearances, which depend on the quality, not the amount of blood, in the cerebral vessels, have been ascribed to turgescence, to inflammation, to venous congestion, and everything but the true cause, which is the state of the lungs and blood, already noticed in Chapter VII. Section II. p. 164. Unarterialized blood is sent to the brain, and by poisoning suspends and annihilates its functions. Death is in such cases preceded by stupor and coma, more or less deep, and on some occasions by fits of convulsions.

10. *Malakencephalon.* Diminished consistence of the brain. The change above described in the consistence of the brain is always accompanied with more or less destruction of its texture. Under certain circumstances, nevertheless, its consistence may be diminished without change of texture.

The natural consistence of the recent adult brain, though well known, it is difficult to describe in exact terms. In general it possesses a degree of toughness which prevents it from being easily

4

divided, unless by a very keen instrument; and after incision minute fragments are left on the sides or edge of the knife. A very thin slice of white cerebral matter is sufficiently tenacious and consistent to sustain its own weight, and to admit of considerable stretching without being broken or lacerated. If put into pure water it continues unchanged for at least eight, ten, or sometimes twelve hours, and without any portion of it being either dissolved, or rendering the water in any degree turbid. A newly cut surface of brain communicates to the finger a peculiar clammy or viscid sensation, in consequence of which it moves with less facility over the skin of any opposite surface.

These qualities, the existence of which may be easily demonstrated, pertain especially to the white substance of the adult brain, when death takes place either accidentally or by an acute disease, without direct lesion of the organ. The consistence of the gray matter of the convoluted surface is inferior to that of the white. The white matter of the twain-band (*corpus callosum*) is firm and tough in the direction of its cross fibres, and may be pulled to a considerable degree without giving way. The cylindrical fluted masses forming the *limbs* of the brain, (*crura*,) which consist chiefly of white matter, are much firmer than the substance of the striated nucleus, which is mostly gray; and the annular protuberance, which is chiefly white matter, is the firmest and most tenacious part of the organ. The cerebellum, which consists chiefly of gray matter, is invariably less firm than the brain; and the firmest part of the former is the substance of the peduncles and the white matter of the cerebellic hemispheres. Of the spinal chord, the cranial part, especially the olivary eminences, are the firmest; and the consistence, though less than that of the brain, is tolerably uniform to the lumbar region, in which it undergoes a distinct diminution, and finally becomes very loose in the caudiform expansion.

The degree of consistence now attempted to be defined, varies at different periods of life, and under different circumstances of health and disease.

In early life the substance of the brain is very different in consistence and tenacity. In the fœtus and at birth its softness approaches to semifluidity. Some weeks after it passes from a soft pulpy substance to a state of greater firmness and tenacity; but at the distance even of many months after birth, it is still much inferior in these qualities to the brain of an individual, who has attained the fourteenth or fifteenth year. In three cases of infants cut off by different acute diseases, between the ages of 20 months and 2½ years, I found the brain soft, compressible, elastic, but not tough; of the consistence of custard-pudding; but not quite so firm as to bear much handling or stretching without being broken or torn. In several cases of children dead between the 7th and the 11th year of scarlet-fever or measles, the brain was firmer, and had acquired greater tenacity, but was still considerably softer and less tough than the brains of adults who had attained the 18th, 20th, or 22d year. Between 12 and 15 the brain in general acquires a decided degree of firmness and tenacity ; for, though still highly elastic, it is much less compressible, and much more distensible without laceration than before. This increase of firmness and tenacity is particularly conspicuous in the twainband and mesolobe, in the limbs, in•the optic *thalamus*, in the annular protuberance, and in the olivary eminences. It is impossible to say when the organ may be said to attain its maximum of firmness. But after the 22d year I have not been able, in a very considerable number of human brains, to recognize much variation of .consistence not connected with some morbid state, either of the system at large, or of the or_gan itself.

In extreme old age, it has been said the brain generally becomes firmer, harder, and drier than in the meridian of life. This, I believe, is not altogether without foundation ; though it is doubtful how far this is to be regarded as a uniform change, independent of disease or morbid effects. It is further exceedingly difficult to define the time at which this change in the consistence of the brain commences or is accomplished. In persons between 50 and 60, I have seen the brain as firm as in others between 70 and 80, or above that age. Conversely, the brain is found sometimes soft, even in persons much advanced in life.

The brain of the adult is liable to lose its normal consistence, and become preternaturally soft in chronic diseases of emaciation, as dropsy, pulmonary consumption, and other pulmonary disorders, mesenteric wasting, marasmus, diabetes, and organic diseases in general. The diminished consistence now remarked is most frequently observed in dropsy, diabetes, and pulmonary disorders.

In the first the brain is almost invariably soft and flaccid throughout.• It cannot sustain itself, but falls down much more quickly than in the ·natural state. It is not easily.cut, but rather gives way before the knife; and a portion of such a brain is easily lacerated, and falls down quickly in water. This diminished consistence, which, though greatest at the centre, extends through the whole organ, depends partly on the deposition of the proper cerebral matter being interrupted, and partly on the admixture of serous fluid with its minute atoms. The texture or atomic constitution of the organ is not altered.

In diabetes a similar change takes place, chiefly from the former cause.

In pulmonary consumption, whether depending on chronic bronchial inflammation, chronic pleurisy, or on tubercular disorganization, the brain is invariably found softer than natural. When the disease which induces death has continued long, this softness is very considerable, and amounts almost to semifluidity. It may then constitute a true cause of adventitious disease. This state of the brain, combined with a languid and retarded motion of the blood through the cerebral capillaries, may be the pathological cause of the delirium, which, either alone or alternating with coma, not unfrequently precedes the death of phthisical patients. The cerebral capillaries in such subjects I have found large and numerous. Is the density of the brain diminished? Meckel states that he found a cube of six lines of the brain of a man of 24, cut off by phthisis, to be $1\frac{1}{4}$ grain lighter than the same bulk of sound brain.

Confinement, with inactivity and low diet, tend to impair the firmness of the brain. Thus in condemned felons and others, who have been imprisoned for some time previous to death, either violent or natural, the brain is found unusually soft. Dr Monro, *tertius*, formerly Professor of Anatomy in the University of Edinburgh, who has had numerous opportunities of examining the brains of persons cut off under these circumstances, states that in criminals in general he found the brain unusually soft; and in a young man otherwise healthy, who was put to death for piracy, the brain was so soft that it gave way at the *corpus callosum*. The softness appears, from the account of Dr Monro, to be greater internally than externally, so that it was impossible to demonstrate the deep-seated parts of the organ.* In opposition to this, however, I must not omit to mention that Littre found the substance of the brain, cerebellum, and *medulla oblongata*, unusually compact

* The Morbid Anatomy of the Brain. By Alexander Monro, M.D., &c. &c. Vol. I. Edinburgh, 1827, p. 35 and 160.

and dense in a felon, who, to avoid public punishment, killed himself by dashing his head against the wall of his cell. *

To the same head probably is to be referred a form of diminished consistence, without change of texture, which is occasionally observed in the brains of persons in whom chronic encephalo-meningeal congestion caused mental derangement. The brain in fatuous persons appears to have been early observed by Tulpius, Kerkringius, King, and Scheide, to be soft and flaccid. This fact, which was repeated by Morgagni, was afterwards verified by John Ernest Greding of Waldheim, who, in 1771, in an elaborate description of the abnormal changes found in the brains of epileptic maniacs, states, that in more than one-half (fifty-one cases) the brain was either universally or very generally, especially in its central parts, unusually soft and flaccid ; and that though this may not be a uniform cause of deranged intellect, it is a frequent accompaniment of the state of the brain on which this depends.† In twelve cases the vault and *septum* were so soft, that spontaneously or by a slight touch they were reduced to thin pulp.

Among thirty-seven cases of this form of cerebral disorder inspected by Haslam, in seven the substance of the brain was soft, very soft, or doughy with abundance of red points, the usual indications of capillary injection, and effusion of serous fluid, the effect of meningeal injection.‡ Among the dissections of Dr Marshall, not more than one belongs to this head,§ (case, 6th p. 202.) This change depends on chronic injection of those capillaries of the vascular membrane (*pia meninx*) which are distributed through the brain.

11. *Sclerenkephalia.* Induration of the brain.—That the brain may acquire an unnatural degree of firmness, and perhaps of density, is well established from the observations of Morgagni, Meckel, Greding, Haslam, Marshall, Serres, Lallemand, Lerminier, Pinel Jun., Bouillaud and Gaudet. Instead of 'the usual compressible elastic character which it presents in the sound state, it may be-

---

* Histoire de l'Acad. Royale des Sciences, An. 1705.

† Melancholico-Maniacorum et Epilepticorum in Ptochotropheo Waldheimensi demortuorum sectiones tradit Joannes Ernestus Greding. Cent. 2*da*, Apud Ludwig Adversaria, &c. Vol. ii. partem 3tiam, p. 533.

‡ Observations on Madness and Melancholy, &c. By John Haslam, 2d edition, London, 1809. Cases 4, 10, 18, 25, 28, 30, 37.

§ The Morbid Anatomy of the Brain, &c. London, 1815.

come like coagulated or boiled albumen, or may approach in consistence to that of the brain which has been immersed in strong alcohol or dilute acid. From the facts hitherto collected, this in-duration appèars to be of two kinds, according as it takes place in a shorter or longer period.

α. According to the facts collected by Bouillaud, a general in-duration of the brain may take place within ten or fifteen days be-fore death, with more or less redness and injection of the cerebral substance. By M. Gaudet this change is conceived to be one of the material causes of ataxic, (typhoid) fever.* This is not very widely different from the view of Bouillaud, who, like M. Brons-sais, regards it as the result of meningo-encephalic inflammation.†

Notwithstanding the authority of these observers, I think it doubtful whether this change can be supposed to take place in the short period assigned for it. Is it not more reasonable to think that this change had pre-existed for some time, and that it ter-minated in a more acute disorder of the organ or its membranes, which proved fatal?

β. The chronic induration of the brain has been long known. Originally observed by Littre, Geoffroy, Boerhaave, Lancisi, and Santorini, it was recognized by Morgagni as a morbid change which occasionally caused more or less mental derangement.‡ J. F. Meckel afterwards undertook to establish this doctrine more fully, and to show that the organ is harder and more elastic than natural. With this change, however, he rather paradoxically con-nects another, diminution of specific gravity, and finds that a cube of six lines of. indurated brain is from $1\frac{1}{2}$ to 2 grains lighter than a cube of the same size of sound brain. In six among fifteen cases given by this author, the brain was much firmer than natural; in some as hard as indurated white of egg, and always elastic.§

This result, though not entirely, is partly verified by the re-

---

* Recherches sur l'endurcissement general de l'encephale, considerée comme une des causes materielles des fievres dites ataxiques, par M. Le Docteur Gaudet. Paris, 1825.

† Observations et Reflexions sur l'induration generale de la substance du Cerveau, considerée comme un effet de l'encephalite generale aigue, par M. Bouillaud. Ar-chives Generales, Tome viii. p. 477.

‡ Epistola Anatomico-Med. viii. 4—18.

§ Recherches Anatomico-Physiologiques sur les causes de la Folie qui viennent du vice des parties internes du corps humain, par M. Meckel. Mem. de l'Academie Royale de Berlin, Tome vii. p. 306, art. 92. Avignon, 1768.

searches of subsequent inquirers. Greding, whom I have already mentioned as having found the brain in a large proportion of cases softer than natural, found it in thirty-nine cases natural in consistence, firm, or even exceeding the natural firmness.* He thinks, however, that this difference is more in word than reality. Of the thirty-seven cases inspected by Haslam, in nine the brain was unusually firm, in one (24) remarkably so, and in one (29) elastic.† In all the cases given by Dr Marshall, except two, again, amounting to fifteen, the brain was unusually firm and generally elastic.‡

The cause of this change, and the means by which it is effected are entirely unknown. It is conjectured that it is a result of inflammation; and it may be admitted as a proof of this, that the brain is almost invariably penetrated with numerous loaded capillaries, and that more or less effusion of serous fluid is found beneath the arachnoid membrane and in the cavities. These, however, might be effects of the induration, or at least of the concomitant capillary injection. M. Serres has seen cases of cerebral injection and hemorrhage causing apoplectic symptoms terminate in induration;§ and Lallemand,‖ Bouillaud,¶ and Pinel,** have found portions of the brain indurated in connection with chronic inflammation. But whether this is to be viewed as the result of capillary injection or of some derangement in the process of nutrition, it is at present impossible to determine. It would be desirable to ascertain chemically the exact nature of the change which takes place, and in what respect the indurated cerebral matter differs from that of the normal state. It is possible that the albuminous substance may be either changed, or in greater proportion; but on this point no accurate observations have hitherto been made.

Whatever be the agent or means of this change, nevertheless, enough is known to show that when it exists, it is in general accompanied with an injected state of the cerebral capillaries, and

---

* Adversaria Medico-Practica. Ludwig, Tom. ii. p. 3tiæ, p. 533.
† Observations on Madness and Melancholy, &c. Lond. 1809.
‡ The Morbid Anatomy of the Brain, &c. Lond. 1815.
§ Annuaire Medico-Chirurgicale.
‖ Recherches Anatomico-Pathologiques, &c. Lettre 2xieme, cases 30, 31, p. 305 and 313.
¶ Traité Clinique et Physiologique de l'Encephalite, Obs. 40, p. 198.
** Recherches d'Anatomie et de Physiologie Pathologiques sur les Alterations de l'Encephale. Bulletins, &c. chez Revue Medicale, Tome vi. Paris, 1821, p. 298 and 315.

that it gives rise to loss of memory, confusion of thought, and derangement of the mental faculties. It appears, indeed, to be a frequent cause of insanity, especially when permanent, without lucid
interval; and if long continued, it may cause that complete obliteration of the intellect which constitutes fatuity ; (*dementia.*) The
cerebral arteries are generally found opaque, and affected with
steatomatous deposition. (Marshall.)

From slight induration of a great part or the whole of the cerebral mass, to considerable induration of particular regions, the
transition is easy. According to the researches of M. Pinel the
younger, who has examined the subject with particular attention,
in the change from sound brain of natural consistence to that of
final, compact, and apparently inorganic induration, two distinct
stages may be recognized.

a. From the observations of MM. Foville and Pinel-Grand-
Champ, it results that in certain persons the exterior or peripheral
part of the brain is liable to a state of capillary injection or chronic
inflammation; in other words, that the meningeal and encephalo-
meningeal capillaries may become the seat of a process of injection
partly chronic, partly intermittent, or variable, according to the
state of the vascular system in general, and the operation of various exciting causes. One of the effects of this encephalo-meningeal injection is to tinge of a red colour more or less deep, the gray
colour of the convoluted surface ; and while the injection produces
more or less mental derangement, this red tint is connected almost
invariably with furious and maniacal paroxysms. When it proceeds to fatuity, albuminous deposits take place on the surface, or
on the membranes of the brain ; and the gray substance becomes
very pale, and softer or firmer than natural.*

I have above said that the subacute or chronic cerebral inflammation which terminates in pulpy destruction is a frequent pathological cause of mental derangement.. In general the disease is
then of shorter duration, and terminates sooner either in convales-
cence or in death. A more chronic form, however, is connected
with this encephalo-meningeal congestion, the duration of which
may vary from twelve or fifteen months to as many years. At the
termination of these periods the cerebral substance is compact, remarkably white, appears void of blood-vessels and capillaries, is

* Recherches sur les Causes Physiques de l'Alienation mentale. Par M. Pinel
Fils, D. M. P. Journal de Physiologie, Tom. vi. p. 44. A Paris, 1826.

diminished in volume, no longer falls under the fingers, but is torn with difficulty, and recoils with elasticity when stretched. It assumes a horny hardness under the action of fire or nitrous acid. These circumstances show that it contains altered albuminous matter. The gray matter also is thinner and paler than natural, and seems to be confounded with the white.

The effects observed to accompany this change are defect and progressive loss of memory, inattention to momentary impressions, apathetic indifference to the present and the future, and slight difficulty of articulation, followed by abolition of appetites, desires, and ideas, increased loss of speech, palsy, or at least want of command over the muscles, fatuity, wasting, and death.

That this change in the consistence of the brain is the result of a slow organic process succeeding to inflammation, M. Pinel infers from the symptoms during life, from the collateral effects after death, and from the state of the meningeal and cerebral vessels which is known to precede the change. That this is not remote from the truth many circumstances tend to show. I have above mentioned the relation between hemorrhagic injection of the brain and induration as noticed by M. Serres and Bouillaud. A proof still more unequivocal is found in the fact, that inflammation, both in the membranes and in the cerebral substances, is known to be followed by induration of the latter. Thus Abraham Kaawe Boerhaave mentions the case of a soldier cut off by an epileptic attack, in the head of whom, besides firm adhesion of the *dura mater* to the inner table and the *pia mater*, with tubercular deposition, the subjacent convoluted gray substance was *hard* and *scirrhous* in various places.* The cheese-like induration recorded by Lallemand in the thirtieth case of his second letter is adduced elsewhere. Here, however, I may mention, that in a man of 55, in whom fixed pain of the forehead, slight palsy of the face, and confusion of memory were soon followed by death, he found the membranes firmly matted together for the extent of a thirty sous piece at the outer† end of the left hemisphere, and the subjacent cerebral matter, also adhering to the membranes, hardened to scirrhous or cartilaginous firmness.

Lastly, M. Bouillaud records a case, in which a man of 68, who,

* Commentarii de Rebus in Scientia Naturali, Vol. i. Pars i. p. 234.

† Recherches Anatomico-Pathologiques sur l'Encephale et ces dependances, par F. Lallemand. Paris, 1820, p. 313.

after cerebral disease, regarded as chronic softening, laboured under impaired memory, headach, and difficulty of expressing ideas, terminating in muscular weakness, and fatal convulsions. In this, with injection of the cerebral substance, was induration passing from the striated body of the left hemisphere through the nucleus, at the upper region of which it formed a cavity with hard yellow walls, and a similar hardened portion in the posterior lobe.*

The disease is not very frequent in this country. One very well marked case, however, came within the sphere of my observation, and was inspected by me after death. The following was the state of the brain. A considerable portion of the outer part of the left hemisphere was unusually firm and hard, not dissimilar to cheese. The space so changed was a sort of crescentic segment of the hemisphere, being about three-fourths of an inch, or one inch broad in its middle, which corresponded with the middle of the hemisphere, and tapering away to a narrow line or point before and behind. The induration ascended to the upper part of the hemisphere to within one inch of the mesial plane and mesial fissure, and below it approached close on the *hippocampus major*, part of which was involved in the induration. The indurated segment thus formed, was bounded, as it were, between the segments of two spheres of unequal diameter, the external one being the smallest or of greatest curvature. The portion when divided cut firm, and did not fall down or dissolve on exposure to air. The *pia mater* adhered to it most firmly, and seemed to be thickened over the indurated portion. The convolutions were flattened and depressed, and presented in this respect an obvious difference from those of the opposite hemisphere. At the internal margin of the indurated portion was a band or zone of cerebral substance distinctly softened, while within that again the rest of the brain presented its natural consistence. The indurated portion, both gray and white, presented, I thought, very few small vessels, but a few large ones dispersed through the mass.

Serous fluid, to a small extent, was effused into the subarachnoid tissue, mostly at the apex and base of the organ, and also within the ventricles.

To the best of my remembrance, this is the only case of induration of the brain, in which that lesion was associated with softening

* Traité Clinique et Physiologique de l'Encephalite, Observ. xl. p. 200.

inside. The latter I ascribe to a secondary orgasm or vascular action caused by the presence of the indurated portion, nearly as the presence of tumours is occasionally observed to induce softening.

In this case the individual, a young man about 30, had long laboured under bad health, latterly with epileptic fits of frequent recurrence. The last time I saw him alive, he was dragging his legs in a semiparalytic manner, had an expression approaching to fatuons, did not readily comprehend what was said to him, and looked thin, pale, and haggard and stupid. He had consulted or been under the care of different physicians, all of whom differed more or less in opinion as to the exact cause of his symptoms. Between three or four weeks after I saw him, he fell into a stupid and comatose state and died.

From these and similar facts, no doubt can be entertained of the tendency of the process of inflammation to indurate the brain under certain circumstances. The difficulty consists in ascertaining what are the conditions under which a process usually terminating in softening should give rise to an opposite change. It is probably premature to attempt any explanation of a process so contradictory in appearance. I shall merely say, that induration seems in general to be occasioned by the encephalic capillaries having their nutritive action so much injured by the inflammatory process, that they cease to deposit healthy cerebral substance.

The induration now described commences generally in the base of the brain by the *hippocampus major*, (*cornu ammonis*,) and these extends to the neighbouring parts. If confined to the brain only, it causes, according to M. Pinel, mere fatuity, (*dementia*,) with more or less palsy. But if it affect the annular protuberance, the limbs, or the olivary bodies, or the chord itself, epilepsy, general palsy, and death by marasmus, are the usual consequences.

b. The change which produces fatuity is the early stage of a more serious lesion of the cerebral substance, atrophic hardening, (*sclerenkenphalia*,) an extreme state of induration found in the brains of idiots. From that already described, it differs chiefly in degree. A portion of brain so changed becomes a compact inorganie looking mass, resembling in colour, consistence, and density, indurated egg or even cheese. The cerebral substance is depressed, shrunk, and condensed, and seems utterly void of vessels or capillaries. When exposed to the action of fire, instead of swelling up without odour, and leaving a brownish light residue, it assumes a horny hardness, emits a strong heavy smell, and leaves a compact shining blackish residue. This hardening affects the white matter more than the gray, in which M. Pinel has not yet recognized it.*

This change is connected with idiocy either congenital or observed soon after birth, in some instances with fatuous stupidity and palsy. In one of the cases, however, the individual appears to have possessed faculties of the ordinary degree of intelligence, till the age of 49, after which repeated attacks of palsy terminated in calm but complete fatuity, (*dementia.*)

That the spinal chord·is liable to the same change in consistence is proved by the case of Count de Lordat, (Med. Obs. and Inq. Vol. III. p. 270,) and that of M. de Causan, recorded by Portal, ·in which the cervical portion was so hard as to resemble cartilage, and the membranes were red and injected. This change gave rise to palsy, proceeding from the fingers up the arms of the right side, and from the feet, till the legs lost power, and the whole side became atrophied, and eventually the same phenomena in the left side. Similar examples are given by Bergamaschi.†

12. *Hypertrophy of the Brain.* (*Hypertrophia.*) Though among the writings of authors on morbid anatomy slight notices are found of the lesion characterized as hypertrophy of the brain, and it was mentioned by Bouillaud, as a peculiar lesion, it was not made the subject of special observation, until M. Dance‡ and M. M. Laennec,§ cousin of M. R. T. Laennec, and M. Scoutteten in 1828,‖ all within a short period, gave examples of it. And in 1835, Dr Sims communicated to the Medico-Chirurgical Society of London a memoir, containing much information on the characters and nature of hypertrophy and atrophy of the brain. From the facts given by these authors, it results, that the brain is liable to undergo a morbid

---

* Recherches de l'Anatomie Pathol. sur l'Endurcissement, &c. par M. Pinel Fils. Journ. de Physiol. Tome ii. p. 191.

† Sulla Mielitide Stenica, &c. Pavia, 1820. 2d, 4th, 8th.

‡ Observations pour servir à l'Histoire de l'Hypertrophie du Cerveau. Par M. Dance. Breschet, Repertoire Général d'Anatomie et de Physiologie Pathologique, Tome V. p. 197. Paris, 1828. (Four cases in adults of 26, 24, and 30 years of age.)

§ Observations sur l'Hypertrophie du Cerveau. Par Meriadee Laennec, M. D Revue Médicale, Decembre 1828. (Five cases, a woman of 32, a woman of 22, a girl of 13 ; and two men of 43 and 44, both white-lead manufacturers.)

‖ Observation sur une Hypertrophie du Cerveau. Par M. Scoutteten, M. D. Archives Générales de Médecine, Tome VIII. p. 31. (Case of a boy aged 5½ years.)

increase in nutrition, distinguished by flattening and approximation of the convolutions, narrowing and diminution of the dimensions of the ventricles, universal firmness and whiteness of its gray and white substance, remarkable dryness of its parenchymatous matter, and of the cavity of the arachnoid membrane; while the texture of the organ appears not to be sensibly changed; 2d, that this hypertrophy is constantly observed over the whole encephalic mass, excluding the *cerebellum;* and, 3d, that, instead of increasing the energy of the cerebral action, it tends, on the contrary, to diminish, pervert, and suspend that action, by reason of the compression which it necessarily establishes within the cranium.

The leading anatomical and physical characters of hypertrophy, therefore, are the following. Increase in the volume of the brain, such that its internal substance presses forcibly the convolutions against the inner surface of the skull and against each other, and thereby flattens and depresses these bodies, and causes them to approximate; while the same internal substance, by pressing the ventricles, diminishes their cavity. Increase in weight and density, which is said to have been ascertained in all the cases, the specific gravity being increased. The substance of the brain is also firm, as much as boiled white of egg, pale, and void of blood-vessels, while it is unusually dry. From all these circumstances, it results that this lesion consists in the deposition or addition of new matter in the interstitial tissue of the brain; in short, a great increase in nutrition.

The effects and symptoms of this lesion, though always present, are not uniform. It is usually preceded or attended by intense headachs, subject to aggravation; an obtuse or weakened state of the intellectual faculties, perversion of these faculties, and fits of giddiness accompanied with stupor. Afterwards accessions of convulsion repeatedly take place, or all at once the patient suffers a general loss of sensation and motion. The pulse is slow; the temperature of the skin natural. Lastly, the patient is unexpectedly cut off in the course of an epileptiform accession.

The circumstances, under which this disease is developed, are not well ascertained. According to M. Dance, it appears to take place very slowly under the influence of very obscure causes. M. M. Laennec, again, thinks that it is developed much more rapidly than any other hypertrophy; and in this respect he allows that it resembles the lesions of inflammatory character. All the cases given by M. Dance took place in adults. One case given by Laennec was in a young girl of thirteen. The case given by Scoutteten took place in a child of five and a-half, with a head so large and heavy, that whenever the child attempted to run, he fell forward from the great weight of the head. Three of the cases given by Laennec took place in persons employed in white-lead manufactories, and liable to lead colic; and of the four cases given by M. Dance, two occurred in house-painters. The disease had not then been observed in persons above 50. In most of the cases, the patients were between 20 and 30; in two cases among fourteen, the individuals were 37 and 39 years of age; and in two men 43 and 44 years of age.

Andral thinks that the lesion takes place, as it were, in two stages or periods; that in the first the disease appears like a chronic affection, with headach, hebetude of the intellectual faculties, and similar phenomena; and that in the second, which is attended with epileptiform convulsions, it presents all the characters of an acute and speedily fatal lesion.*

Dr Sims gives the details of fifteen cases, which tend partly to confirm, partly to modify the results now stated. Among these fifteen cases, in the first place, the ages of the subjects were as follow. One at 11 months; one at 3 years; two at 10 years; one at 16; one at 22; one at 24; two at 29; two at 40; one at 48; two at 60; and one at 70. Of none of the cases is the occupation stated, all having been occupants of the St Mary-le-bonne Charity Workhouse. Eleven were females and four males. Though in most of the cases portions of the brain were unusually firm and consistent, Dr Sims extends the term hypertrophy to cases also, in which the brain is unusually large, without increased consistence. Dr Sims further recognizes two forms of hypertrophy; one a state of mere enlargement or addition of particles, without appreciable difference. from the ordinary state of the organ, congenital or connected with rickets, and early evincing its presence; the other connected with increased weight of the brain, the flattening of the convolutions, the white and albuminous appearance, and the bloodless state of the organ. It is chiefly the latter form of the disease which corresponds with that described by Dance, Laennec, and Andral. He confirms the con-

---

* Clinique Medicale. Par G. Andral, M. D., ou Choix d'Observations, &c. Livre premier; 4trieme ordre; 3ieme edit. 1834. Paris. (Three cases; a female of 27, a man of 29, and a man of 39.)

Case of Hypertrophy of the Brain, with Spontaneous Obstruction of the Humeral Artery, &c. By Dr Christison: Edin. Med. and Surgical Journal, Vol. XLII. p. 257. (A female aged 37, Edin. 1831,) published 1834.

elusion of these authors that the change affects, so far as is hitherto known, the brain alone, and not the cerebellum ; but he modifies their inference, that it affects the whole organ. Though this does take place, yet hypertrophy may be partial, affecting only one hemisphere, one lobe, one *corpus striatum*, or one optic thalamus. He finds, lastly, that the brain may be, in certain circumstances, unusually large, yet not amounting to hypertrophy, in persons dying of various diseases ; for instance, extensive pneumonia and other diseases of the lungs and heart ; and then the brain is generally very much loaded with blood.[*]

From this account it appears that cerebral hypertrophy differs little, if at all, from what is above described as induration of the brain.

13. *Atrophy of the Brain.* (*Cerebrum Ebriosorum; Cerebrum Bibacium.*) *The Spirit-drinker's Brain.* The term atrophy is employed in two senses, something different. In one sense, it is employed to indicate diminution in the size of the brain, and especially of its convoluted surface. The convolutions are shrunk, small, narrow, and occasionally soft; the *sulci* are large and open; and the brain recedes from the interior of the skull; while the subarachnoid tissue is very much loaded with serous fluid, which has the appearance of a jelly investing the whole brain. This is observed, not only along the superior and lateral regions of the hemispheres, but all over and at the base of the brain. This shrinking of the brain and the supplying of the place by fluid, may amount to the thickness of about one crownpiece, or even two crown-pieces, all over ; and in some extreme cases the shrinking and the filling with serous fluid in the subarachnoid tissue amounts to the extent of half an inch in thickness.

The brain is, at the same time, very soft and watery ; large quantities of fluid escaping both from the convolutions, when the membranes are cut, and from the white substance of the hemispheres. The ventricles also are enlarged and capacious, and almost constantly contain serous fluid in considerable quantity. Much also is found in the lower part of the brain, and escapes from the cavity of the spinal chord.

This is general atrophy of the brain, or atrophy of the convolutions; and it is supposed to depend on wasting and actual loss of the cerebral substance, both white and gray, while the place of the lost matter is supplied by serous fluid.

* On Hypertrophy and Atrophy of the Brain. By John Sims, M. D. Medico-Chirurgical Transactions, XIX. 315. London, 1835.

This is one mode of accounting for this sort of atrophy; and it is probable that to many examples of the disease it correctly applies. It may be quite true, for instance, of the atrophy taking place in old age and in various enfeebling diseases, in which all the organs suffer more or less waste and loss of substance from imperfect nutrition; and in general steatomatous and osteosteatomatous disease of the arteries of the brain. This form of atrophy is nevertheless so frequent in persons who are much addicted to the use of spirituous liquors, to whisky-drinkers, gin-drinkers, and brandy-drinkers, and is so common in those who have either had *delirium tremens*, or who, after a long course of moderate but steady drinking, have died either of that or some similar affection, that the shrunk convolutions and watery state may be regarded as characteristic of the drunkard's brain. I do not say that atrophy of the brain does not take place in the temperate. But it is so constantly observed in connection with the habit of incessant drinking, that it may, in a large proportion of cases, be considered as the effect of that habit.

Local forms of atrophy are also observed. Thus portions of the convoluted surface may be depressed, and yellowish and covered with fluid within the membranes. These are the remains of some former congestion of the part. The surface or substance of one *corpus striatum* may be depressed and, as it were, abraded; or the surface of one optic thalamus may be less developed than that of the opposite side. These are mostly the effects of some previous attack of capillary congestion, sometimes with effusion of a little blood, or an attack of softening which had stopped spontaneously.

This local form of atrophy has been examined by Dr Sims; and it seems quite certain, that these local losses of substance were the effects of previous attacks of disease. Among four cases fully detailed, and eleven cases noticed by this author, nine took place in persons above 70 years of age, and in whom they were associated with, or preceded by, attacks of cerebral disease of different kinds; and two were observed in persons above 60, both with marks of diseased brain. In the other four also, though young persons, very considerable morbid changes of different kinds had taken place in the brain and its membranes.*

Lastly, the term atrophy has been employed by Cruveilhier to designate that extensive deficiency of portions of the brain which

---

* On Hypertrophy and Atrophy of the Brain. By John Sims. Medico-Chirurgical Transactions, London, Vol. XIX. p. 364. London, 1835.

takes place in the fœtus, in consequence of diseased action during intra-uterine life. This is altogether different from the sense in which the term, as above explained, has been employed; for the atrophy in the cases here considered is not congenital, but acquired in the progress of life. The atrophy of Cruveilhier, on the other hand, is congenital, and is the most common cause of idiocy. As such it is considered under the head of Anencephalous Malformation or Deficient Brain, (*Enkephalelleipsis.*)

14. *Organic changes, morbid growths, or tumours.*—Of these various forms have been observed by different authors. But they have not in all instances distinguished accurately between tumours originating in the cerebral substance, and those which, originating in the membranes, affect the substance of the organ secondarily. As this distinction must be observed, at least in pathological anatomy, I shall not be liable to the charge of futile innovation, if I attempt to trace the distinction in the following sketch.

The different forms of tumour occurring in the brain may be referred to the following heads: α, the simple cerebral tumour; β, the adenoid or fleshy tumour; γ, strumous tumours, comprehending tubercles and tubercular deposits; δ, the gelatiniform tumour, (*colloma ;*) ε, the adipose, lardaceous, or wax-like degeneration, (*ceroma ;*) ζ, the cholesterine tumour, (*margaroides ;*) η, the cartilaginous tumour, (*chondroma ;*) θ, calcareous or bony deposits; ι, encysted tumours, including a, the hydatid-cyst or vesicular tumour, b, the blood cyst, (*hæmatoma,*) c, the fungoid tumour, and d, the melanotic cyst.

α. Simple cerebral tumour. (*Scleroma.*) Of considerable induration of particular regions of the brain, I have already spoken. When the indurated portion is definite in limits, and the rest of the organ preserves its usual characters, these indurated portions have been vaguely described under the general name of *tumours.* It is more correct, however, to regard them as portions of brain indurated to an unusual degree, and perhaps changed in intimate structure. As the simplest form of tumour incident to the brain, this claims the first place.

Of this change the most authentic examples have been recorded by Platerus, Meckel, Roederer, Perotti, and Greding. From the descriptions given by these authors, part of the cerebral substance appears to acquire unusual firmness, and to become somewhat like coagulated albumen. It is not much changed in colour, unless in losing some of its whiteness, and assuming a pale yellow or orange-gray tint. The surrounding cerebral substance is almost invariably softened. Water is effused into the ventricles; and if the indurated mass is seated near the convoluted surface, the membranes become opaque and thick, and morbidly adherent. The following references to the cases will communicate some idea of the nature of this change.

Felix Platerus, lib. i. p. 108.—In the fore part of the left hemisphere of a man of 24, who had headach, amaurosis, and mental imbecility, a globular tumour like a gland, as large as a hen's egg, but irregular, and like a pine cone ; its interior substance white, firm, and uniform, like boiled egg, but harder, inclosed in a firm vascular membrane. Weight 14 oz.

Buonaventura Perotti in Raccolta d'Opuscoli Scientifici e Fisiologici in Venezia, Tom. xlvii. p. 339. 1751.—A woman of 25, who had headach for several years, died lethargic. The convoluted gray matter of the left hemisphere was destroyed. In the right hemisphere, though externally sound, a hard body as large as a nut penetrated from the gray to the white interior substance.—Commentar. de Rebus in Scientia Naturali et Medicina observatis, Vol. iii.

Meckel, Mémoires de l'Academie Royale de Berlin, 1761. Tom. vii.—In a man of 50, right hemisphere externally harder, more resisting and more elastic than natural. Left hemisphere before the same ; posterior lobe soft ; upper posterior part of left hemisphere firm ; pia mater opaque and thickened; arachnoid adhering to dura mater ; substance of the hemisphere posterior to corpus striatum soft, diffluent, and moist with fetid serum. In the posterior part of the left hemisphere, behind the ergot, a hard body, the size of three nuts, consisting of three spherical protuberances, aggregated together, weighing 2 oz. and 2 drs.; surrounding substance soft and pulpy.

In a child of 4, the white matter of the posterior lobe of the left hemisphere a scirrhus (hardened mass) the size of a nut ; surrounding part vascular and injected.

Roederer, J. G. Programma de Cerebri Scirrho, Goettingæ, 1762. This after some search I have not been able to see.

Vincenzio Galli negli atti dell' Academia della Scienzi di Siena detta Fisico-critici, Tom. ii.—A man of 40, who had laboured under severe cephalalgia, which was relieved by venesection, but afterwards recurred with giddiness and delirium, terminating in death. Inflammation of the membranes ; effused serum in the cavities ; in the right ventricle, stretching from the optic thalamus to the corpus striatum, a tumour as large as a hen's egg, with irregular surface, and external substance dense, firm, and ash-coloured.

M. Marcot, chez Mémoires de la Société de Montpellier, Tom. i. p. 334. Lyon, 1766.—A man of 47, attacked with giddiness, headach, impaired vision, palsy of right side, followed by paraplegia, convulsions, lethargy, and apoplectic death. The posterior part of the brain corresponding to the tentorium, to the branches and limbs of the vault (fornix), was scirrhous and almost cartilaginous, requiring to be divided by good scissors, and grating against the cutting instrument.

F. Lallemand, Recherches Anatomico-Pathologiques. Paris, 1820. Lettre 2xieme, No. 30. 1820.—A girl of 14, with right hemiplegy, followed after four months by paraplegy, insensibility of the skin, palsy of the sphincters, and paralytic dyspnœa advancing progressively to fatal asphyxia. The white matter of the left hemisphere, immediately above the lateral ventricle, for the space of 1½ inch long, 1 inch broad, and 2 or 3 lines thick, converted into a hard substance like Gruyere cheese, and resisting the knife.

Dr Abercrombie, Researches, &c. p. 431. Notes.—In a child of 4, unable to walk, with imperfect articulation, deficient intelligence, difficult deglutition and respiration, and frequent convulsions, terminating at the end of eighteen months in death, the olivary bodies, peduncle of the cerebellum, and mammillary eminence, were in a state of cartilaginous hardness.

M. Andral Fils, Journal de Physiologie, Tome ii. p. 111.   1822.—In a girl of about 20 months, with alternate motion of the head to the right and left, terminating in fatal coma, without convulsion or palsy, several of the convolutions of both hemispheres had become extremely hard, and assumed the colour of ivory: When pressed between the fingers they resisted like fibro-cartilage ; when drawn, they recoiled.   Similar indurations were found in the substance of the hemispheres to their base.   The right hemisphere of the cerebellum contained a round cyst with smooth walls, of the capacity of a nut, containing minute, hard, irregular shaped concretions, of strong consistence, and similar to the spiculæ of a fractured bone.

M. J. Bouillaud, Traité de l'Encephalite.   Paris, 1825.   P. 161, Obs. 33.—A man of 57, with impaired speech, after a cerebral disorder ; in the anterior lobe of the left hemisphere an albuminous mass, the size of an egg, sprinkled with drops of blood, and drops of purulent fluid.

Ibid. Observat. 36, p. 183.—A man of 57, with right hemiplegy, intellectual imbecility, and involuntary repetition of the last words spoken to him, after an apoplectic attack, terminating in complete fatuity and death, with injection of the membranes and cerebral substance, in the anterior third of the left hemisphere was found an indurated nut, the size of an egg, surrounded by bloody clots and distinct injection.   A longitudinal section presented yellowish colouring and red-brown points, depending on the presence of blood coloured with the substance in which it was effused.   The substance of the indurated mass resembled concrete pus mixed with blood, grating under the knife, and containing minute bloody effusions with filamentous substance, and, though much firmer than the rest of the brain, falling easily under the finger.   It was separated from the surrounding brain by a circle of well injected capillaries.   In the middle lobe of the same hemisphere was a similar mass, less extensive, and rather softened than indurated.

This appears to be an albuminous tumour in its early stage.

In the following cases the diseased change was found in the cerebellum.

Joannis Harderi, Apiarum Basileæ, 1687.   4to.   Observat. 58, p. 238.—A girl of 17, of scrofulous habit, who suffered severe lancinating pains of the head, followed by fatal convulsions.   The membranes containing much yellow serum ; vessels minutely injected ; in the cerebellum, near its termination, three hard globular bodies, (scirrhi,) one as large as a nutmeg in the beginning of the spinal chord.   They contained yellowish matter of considerable consistence.

Ephemerides Naturæ Curiosæ.   Decade iii.   Ann. iv. p. 148.—In a hydrocephalic subject, the cerebellum indurated, adhering to the dura mater and skull without intermediate cavity.

J. Mar. Lancisi, De Noxiis Paludum Effluviis, Lib. ii.   Epid. iii. c. vi. 218.—In the cerebellum of a man subject to convulsions, cut off by intermittent fever, was a hard white body, two inches broad and three long, composed of several globular masses aggregated, invested with membranes.

Mémoires de l'Academie Royale des Sciences, 1705, No. 13.—In a boy of $4\frac{1}{2}$, who was stupid for two years before death, the cerebellum, with the posterior half of the medulla oblongata, (the restiform bodies?) was changed into a hard white homogeneous mass.

Morgagni, Epist. lxii. 15.—A man aged 48, pursuing the occupation of a cook, and exposed to charcoal fumes, laboured, for a year before death, under a$_c$ute pains of the head, and weakness of the lower extremities, which terminated in paraplegy, without affection of the arms, finally became soporose during the day, with slight raving at night, and with lucid intervals, and died. The cerebellum was hard to the knife. Instead of the usual appearance of ramified arrangement, which had disappeared, was one of parallel white streaks, firm, (*scirrhosa*,) of a uniform colour, approaching to pale carnation ; and when minutely examined appearing to consist of roundish atoms, mutually aggregated, without membrane or blood-vessel. This change, which affected the whole left hemisphere, encroached a little only on the right.

La Peyronie, Memoires de l'Academie Royale des Sciences, 1741. P. 208, 4to, 283, 12mo.—A man of 30, who for ten years passed for a melancholy hypochondriac, complained during the three last months of life of weight and pains of the head, towards the occipital region and neck ; had convulsions about half an hour in all the members ; and two days after perished in a fresh attack, lasting only a quarter of an hour. Attached to the fourth ventricle was a hard tumour as large as a hen's egg, occupying the place of the cerebellum, which was reduced to a glairy membrane as thin as a line, investing the tumour. This tumour, which compressed the *tubercula quadrigemina*, appears to have been attached to the choroid plexus of the fourth ventricle, and probably grew from it originally.

Brisseau mentions a hard tumour, as large as a pigeon's egg, in the middle of the cerebellum, producing palsy.—Obs. iii. p. 27.

From this list, which contains, if not the whole, at least the most authentic cases of this form of cerebral tumour, it may be inferred, that it consists in a portion of brain becoming unusually hard, assuming a white or yellow white tint, and in losing much of its appearance of organization, especially fibrous structure and vascular ramification. The hardness of these tumours varies from that of granular cheesy matter to firm indurated albumen. Of some the structure is said to be fibrous; but in such cases the fibrosity of sound cerebral substance is not meant. In the presence of a capsule or a vascular spherical shell there is some variation, which seems to depend on the stage of growth which the tumour has attained. If recent, it is generally surrounded by such a vascular cyst. If of long standing, it is generally surrounded with a layer of softened brain, the result of the vascular irritation established in the confines of of the tumour.

β. *Adenoid or flesh-like tumour.* (*Adenoidea.*) To the second head may be referred a sort of tumour which has been described sometimes under the vague name of scirrhus ; sometimes under that of scrofulous tumour ; but which cannot be admitted to possess unequivocal characters of either. It is generally described as similar to a mass of flesh, or an enlarged absorbent gland. Its colour is light pink or pale flesh-colour; its firmness is considerable; and in some instances it is compared to the kidney. To this head belong the following cases :—

Felix Platerus Observation. Lib. i. p. 13.—A military man of equestrian rank, who had for two years laboured under mental derangement, with much loss of memory and natural appetites, and with frequent somnolence at table, at length expired. Upon the mesolobe, upon separating the hemispheres, was found a remarkable globular tumour, fleshy like a gland, hard, but spongy *(fungosus)*, of the bulk of a moderate pippin, enclosed in a proper tunic, vascular, and free from all connection with the brain.

Did this originate in the *pia mater*, in which it appears to have been enclosed?

Joannes Rhodius, Centuria i. Observat. 55.—In the ventricle of the brain of a noble Bolognian a fleshy tumour gave rise to epileptic fits.

Miscellanea Curiosa.—In the substance of the brain a tumour like a strumous gland.

Johan. Jac. Wagner, Miscellan. Curios. Dec. ii. Ann. 10.—A boy of 14, suffering pain in the forehead and occipital region near the junction with the vertebræ, coming on in paroxysms, relieved by vomiting ; epileptic symptoms and death. In the white matter of the posterior part of the brain (occipital,) a preternatural hard sebaceous gland, friable ; in the convolutions of the anterior lobe two glands ; in the end of the cerebellum, near the *calamus scriptorius*, one as large as a walnut.

Mémoires de l'Academie Royale.—In the right *corpus striatum* a glandular substance the size of a bean.

Joh. Gottfr. Zinn. apud Comment. Soc. Reg. Scientiarum Gottingensis, Tom. ii. 1752.
—In an infant affected with enlarged lymphatic glands a hard substance as large as a walnut. Of this, however, he neglected to preserve an accurate account.

In another infant, part of the left hemisphere of the cerebellum, to the extent at least of two inches, was converted into five hardish bodies of different sizes, yellow, like hardened lymphatic glands, mutually adhering. In some parts the traces of the circular leaflets of the cerebellic plates was left ; in others they had disappeared, and left a uniform inorganic mass. The *pia mater* was readily detached, except at the middle of the hard mass, where it adhered so firmly that it could not be removed without laceration. The contiguous vessels were injected.

In an adult female, he observed beneath the parietal bone in the convoluted part of the brain three similar hard bodies, each as large as a nutmeg. They adhered to the *dura mater* ; and, in all probability, they originated in that membrane.

Haller, Opusc. Pathol. Obs. 1.—In a beggar girl of six years, with enlarged mesenteric, inguinal, and bronchial glands, the left hemisphere of the cerebellum was found adhering to the occipital *dura mater* ; the whole substance, white and gray, changed into a hard mass two inches in diameter on both sides, uniformly thick, fibrous like the kidney, fissile, destitute of vessels, and without remaining trace either of gray matter or of white ramification.

John Jac. Huber, Nova Acta Physico-Medico Academ. Cæsareæ Leopoldino-Carolinæ, Tom. iii. p. 533 ; also Comment. de rebus in Scientia Naturali, Vol. xviii. p. 335.
—In the brain of a boy of 3, cut off by decay *(tabes)*, a hard glandular tumour of the size of a filbert, in colour, hardness, and other qualities like a lymphatic gland. When divided it was found to consist of a thin coat enclosing a hard nucleus, which, though compared to purulent matter, was firm and coloured.

Jo. Ernest. Greding, apud Ludwig Adversaria Medico-Practica, Vol. ii. p. ii. p. 492. 1771.—A woman of 30, of delicate constitution, unmarried, labouring under mania, with paroxysms of great violence ; apoplectic attack followed by palsy of left side ; death in about twenty days after. In the right hemisphere, about one inch below the convoluted surface, an ovoid mass, five inches long, three broad, convex-shaped like a lens, one-fifth of an inch thick at middle, resting on the *centrum ovale* and mesolobe, consisting internally of dark-red (*atro-rubens*) hard granular substance, like half-rotten sandy pear, enclosed all round in gray, soft, inodorous puriform matter, (*ramollisse-ment.*)

Mr Henry Earle, in Medico-Chirurgical Transactions, Vol. iii. p. 59. 1812.—A boy, 2 years and 9 months old. Dilated pupil ; palsy of lower extremities and sphincters, followed by convulsions of the face, and palsy of the upper extremities and trunk ; death by paralytic asphyxia. In the anterior lobe of the right hemisphere a large dusky red tumour, rather tough. In the posterior lobe of the same hemisphere, and in that of the left, a tumour each. In the cerebral substance, on a level with the mesolobe, four more tumours ; the largest the size of an orange, the smallest not less than a chestnut. They were very firm, of a dusky red colour, and with streaks of white interposed.

Dr Powell, in Medical Transactions, Vol. v. Case xi. p. 241.—A man of 30, with excruciating pain of the head more or less constant, followed by impaired vision, dilated pupil, and at length an apoplectic attack, which in two days terminated life. From the inferior part of the anterior lobe of the left hemisphere projected a firm mass, of the size of a large walnut, and when cut into resembling a large absorbent gland. It was surrounded by softened cerebral substance, which was of a light brown colour, and so pulpy as to give the sensation of a semifluid.

γ. *Tubercular Deposition.* (*Tyroma.*)—Under the head of tubercles and scrofulous growths of the brain, various changes, some not very similar, have been described. Though the terms tubercle and scrofula have been perhaps applied too vaguely, these differences, however, if well examined, will be found to consist more in the external form in which the tubercular matter is deposited, than in any essential change in its intimate characters. The term *tubercular deposition,* therefore, I adopt for the purpose of designating matter of a white or pale-yellow colour, firm, like soft cheese, but less tough, sometimes granular and friable, and consisting chiefly of a large proportion of albuminous matter. The substance thus defined may be deposited in various forms. In the brain these seem referable chiefly to two ;—1. one, two, or more homogeneous individual masses of considerable size ; and 2. several, sometimes many, minute spherical or spheroidal bodies separate from each other.

a. One or two homogeneous masses of considerable size. Mangetus is among the first who notices near the *corpora quadrigemina* a body like a sebaceous gland, hard and friable, which there is reason to believe was one solitary tubercular mass. The two similar which he found in the same brain between the convolutions, if not belonging to the membranes, were examples of the same growth in the convoluted substance.

I have already mentioned under another head the case of Huber, which is probably an example of the same nature. The second one of Merat, if really tubercular, is also an instance of this form

Y

of the tubercular deposit. Many others are recorded by different authors. Thus Rochoux gives an instance of a tubercular tumour in the cerebellum, in all respects similar to those of the lungs.* Dr Powell's seventh case is an instance of large tubercular masses in the white matter of the right hemisphere.† To the same head also belong the cheese-like tumour described by Sir Gilbert Blane;‡ the white tubercle represented by Baillie, (Plate VII. Fascic. 10;) and the instance given by Coindet in the annular protuberance;§ the instance of an albuminous mass as large as an egg in the anterior lobe of the left hemisphere by Bouillaud;‖ that recorded by the same author as a steatomatous tumour in the left hemisphere, containing an opaque homogeneous substance like white paste or thick starch, (*l'empois blanc*, p. 195;) the 76th, 77th, and 78th cases of Dr Abercrombie; perhaps that of Dr Chambers;¶ a very good instance recorded by M. Piedagnel;** another by M. Berard in the anterior lobes,†† and perhaps those given by Dr Hooper (Plate XI. Fig. 1.)

The physical characters of this form of tubercular deposit are tolerably uniform. Varying in number from one or two to four, five, or six, and in size from that of a pea to a walnut, they consist of opaque white matter, with a tint of pale-yellow, of the consistence of soft, cheese, sometimes granular, but always without vessel or trace of organic structure. It is chiefly albuminous and friable. In general they are surrounded by a vascular cyst of variable thickness. Of the manner of their formation little is known. Several of the cases of Dr Abercrombie would lead to the idea, that the white albuminous matter of the tubercle is deposited in a fluid or semifluid shape, which afterwards undergoes slow coagulation.‡‡ M. Bouillaud adduces various facts and arguments to show that they are the result or product of an inflammatory process; and, if the idea attached to this term be sufficiently comprehensive, the opinion may not be remote from the truth. The tendency of this process is to produce albuminous secretions or depositions in va-

* Recherches sur l'Apoplexie, Obs. xxxix. p. 151.
† Transactions of the College of Physicians, Vol. v. p. 222.
‡ Transactions of a Society, Vol. ii.
§ Mémoire sur l'Hydrencephale, p. 106 and 107.
‖ Traité Clinique et Pathologique, p. 161.
¶ Medical and Physical Journal, Vol. lvi. New Series, Vol. i. 1826, p. 5.
** Journal de Physiologie, Tome iii. p. 247.
†† Ib. Tome v. p. 17.
‡‡ Pathological and Practical Researches, &c. Cases 83, 84, and 85, in which the cysts contained soft or semifluid albuminous matter, coagulable by heat. Pp. 176-181.

3

rions forms; and it is not improbable, that, under certain circumstances, it may be so modified as to cause the deposition of this substance in an indivisible mass, in a limited situation, and from a proper cyst.* Often, however, the formation of these bodies is the result of derangement in the process of nutrition.

Whatever be the origin of these bodies, it is understood, that, sooner or later, they undergo a change in their interior, which sometimes at the centre, sometimes in several points, simultaneously begins to soften and become fluid. It is at least known, that such bodies are found to have fluid or semifluid contents, consisting chiefly of serous liquor with albuminous flakes or curd-like masses in it. Of this description are the tumour of the protuberance represented by Dr Yelloly as in a state of imperfect suppuration;† the cerebral *vomicæ* described by Coindet as similar to tumours of meliceris; the seventy-fifth case of Dr Abercrombie; that in the protuberance given by Dr Kellie, (Monro, p. 178,) and by Dr Moncrieff in the same work, (pp. 50—53.) When the softening or liquefying process is complete, the tubercular mass assumes the form of an encysted abscess. Of such abscesses, it may indeed become a question whether the fluid or the solid state is the incipient one. The principal facts in favour of the latter idea are, the circumstances of the fluid being found in the centre while the circumference is solid, and the larger bodies being found soft while the small are firm. According to this, which is the general opinion at present, in the incipient stage the tubercle is said to be *crude*, in the more advanced to be softened or dissolved.

b. The second form in which tubercular deposition takes place is when it is found in numerous minute spherical or spheroidal bodies, disseminated through the substance of the brain. Of this the best examples with which I am acquainted are recorded by Reil and M. Chomel. In the case given by Professor Reil more than 200 oblong spherical bodies were found in the gray matter of the brain and cerebellum. They were a little firmer than the brain itself; mostly of a pale yellow; some few of a very pale blue colour; of the size of a lentile or a pea; and when divided, showed internally an adipose-like substance, resembling in colour and consistence boiled or beaten potatoes. From some, which were marked in the centre with a dark point, and seemed to be covered by a thin cyst, the slightest incision discharged a matter like vermicelli. These

* Traité Clinique et Pathologique, p. 181.
† Medico-Chirurgical Transactions, Vol. i. p. 182.

bodies were confined to the gray or external matter, none being found in the white cerebral substance.* Not dissimilar were the bodies found by M. Chomel in the brain of a woman of 30, who, with obstinate vomiting and epigastric pain, had headach at first slight and confined to the hind head, latterly extending to the frontal region, when it was constant and severe. Though the intellectual powers are stated to have been unimpaired to the last, death was preceded by sudden aggravation of her sufferings and loss of consciousness. In the brain were found about thirty or forty small round bodies, resembling the human crystalline lens in colour, size, and consistence. In the cerebellum were two similar, and in the spinal chord, opposite the last dorsal vertebra, one. In several parts of the organ also were minute abscesses, supposed to be produced by the softening of similar tubercles.†

The two cases now noticed are considered as of a strumous nature by the authors under whose observation they fell. It is unfortunate that they have given almost no information on the physical and chemical qualities of the matter thus deposited in the substance of the brain. Though its nature is thus left undetermined, I have ventured to refer them to the present head, because they seem to be deposits of albuminous matter slightly modified, and because they doubtless present some alliance with certain of the forms of tubercular deposition in other textures.

From the researches of Dr H. Green, it results that *Tyroma* of the brain is a disease principally of early life. Among 30 cases inspected, all were between the ages of 19 months and 12 years; and 13 cases occurred between the ages of two and four years inclusive. As to sex, 14 cases took place in boys and 16 in girls. It is a chronic disease, and causes few symptoms until it has encroached much on the cerebral substance.‡

δ. *The Gelatiniform tumour.* (*Colloides.*) To this head I refer a peculiar sort of new growth which I have seen extending over the base of the brain from the optic chiasma backwards to part of the protuberance, and on each side over the hemispheres. The body was soft and jelly-like, not dissimilar to white currant jelly or thin glue, tremulous, and easily lacerable. It varied in thickness, being in some

* J. C. Reil, Memorabilia Clin. Vol. ii. Fasc. i. No. 2. 1792.

† Nouveau Journal de Med. Mars 1818, p. 191-196. A similar is given in the supplement to Dr Abercrombie's work, from Prof. Nasse, p. 431. The case of Dr Hawkins, (Med. and Phys. Journal, Vol. lvi. p. 8,) may probably be of the same description.

‡ Observations on Tubercle of the Brain in Children. By P. H. Green, M. D., Medico-Chirurgical Transactions, Vol. XXV. p. 192. London, 1842.

parts as thick as half an inch, in others not more than the thickness of two crown pieces or even one. Its outline was irregular. It had produced softening of the brain on the part where it pressed, and the base of the cranium on which it rested was absorbed, rough, and carious. The *dura mater* corresponding was thin, and detached from the inner table. I do not think that this substance, which was void of organization, resembled any other sort of tumour which I have seen either in the brain or elsewhere. It was too soft and too lacerable to be compared to the colloid tumour. It was contained within a thin arachnoid membrane, different, as it appeared to me, from the arachnoid membrane of the brain.

The individual in whose brain this production took place had been long in state of infirm health; two years at least. The first symptoms were epileptic seizures; then loss of memory of that kind, that with every wish and effort to recall either a name or objcet, or an event, he was quite unable to do so. Latterly the fits became more frequent; the memory more thoroughly impaired; and for some time before death he became blind and paralytic. Death was preceded by great debility and slight stupor. But the epileptic attacks had ceased to recur. This person's intellect was originally good; his memory was powerful; and his disposition was mild, gentle, and amiable. On these mental qualities, excepting the memory, his disease seemed to make no impression. I was assured, that a day or two before his death his intellect was clear; and it was merely the remembrance of past transactions in which he was confused. He could by no means be said to be insane or even fatuous.

ɩ. *Adipose tumour, lardaceous degeneration.* (*Keroma.*) Peter Borelli is the first who notices the existence of much fat-like matter in the brain of an epileptic subject. The adipose tumour described by the Wenzels seems to be the same with that which was previously mentioned by Merat, and which has since been noticed under the name of *lardaceous degeneration* by M. Hebreart formerly of the Bicetre. The first author describes, under the name of tuberele behind the upper part of the *medulla oblongata,* a fatty, reddish, or rose-coloured body, the size of a nut, consisting internally of homogeneous substance traversed by minute red lines, probably blood-vessels. It was contained in a fine thin envelope. A similar one, though somewhat less, was found in the middle of the left cerebellic hemisphere. By the Austrian anatomists it is represented as externally smooth, and of a yellow colour, and internally, when divided, as consisting of adipose ash-coloured solid substance, tending in some parts to bony.* Among the many brains which these anatomists examined two only presented this change of structure. Though found near the exterior or convoluted surface, they penetrated pretty deep into the substance of the organ.

According to the cases given by M. Hebreart this change may occur either under the shape of a conversion or degeneration of the cerebral substance into matter of a yellowish colour and lardaceous consistence, or in the formation of a distinct tumour in the substance of the organ. Though from his account it appears to be by no means so rare as might be expected from the observations of the Austrian anatomists; he gives only two cases of its occurrence in the brain, and two in the cerebellum. In the first of the former, a distinct tumour, consisting of matter of a yellow-colour and lard-like consistence, the size of a nut, in the anterior part of the anterior lobe of the right hemisphere, gave rise to idiocy. In the second, a square inch of the posterior lobe of the left hemisphere was converted into a yellowish pulpy substance, which was separated from the contiguous sound brain by hardened cerebral matter. This in a man of 40 caused epileptic paroxysms once or twice a month, terminating in asphyxia, which at length proved fatal. In the first of the cerebellic cases, in a young man, who had been idiotic for six years, the cerebral substance forming the walls of 'the fourth ventricle had, for the depth of more than one line, been converted into yellowish lardaceous matter. In the second, that of an incurable maniac, a space six lines in diameter of the lower part of the right hemisphere of the cerebellum had become hard, lardaceous, and of a yellowish colour, not only in the gray lamellated matter, but penetrating for some lines into the white substance. In this change the membranes also participated.† A similar case is related in the Bulletins de la Faculté de Medecine, May 1816.

I know not whether to these cases should be added the third,

---

* " Tumor exterius lævis erat, *colore luteo*, (couleur jaunatre, of M. Hebreart,)" &c. " Persecantes tumorem, intrinsecus inveniebamus quandam adiposam, (" une degenerescence de consistence lardacée" of M. Hebreart,) subcineream, admodum solidam, (" substance devenue dure, lardacée, de couleur jaunatre") substantiam quæ parvo quodam loco tactu velut ossea erat." Josephus et Carolus Wenzel de Penitiori Structura Cerebri Hominis et Brutorum. Tubingæ apud Cottam, 1812. Fol. p. 104 et 105.

† Observations sur quelques maladies du cervelet, du cerveau, et de leurs membranes, recueillies à l'hospice de Bicètre ; par M. Hebreart, Medecin ordinaire des Alienés, &c. Annuaire Medico-Chirurgical, &c. Paris, 1819, p. 579.

given by the same author. In this a man of 50, who became maniacal, with lucid intervals, however, lost judgment, speech, memory, and finally became paralytic and idiotical. These symptoms were found to depend on the conversion of the lower surface of the left cerebellic hemisphere into a jelly-like matter, separated from the sound part of the organ by walls of hard polished cerebellic substance. It is possible that this jelly-like matter may have been either the result of the process of softening in a part previously hard, or the incipient stage of what was afterwards to acquire the lardaceous consistence.

ζ. *Margaroid and Cholesterine tumour.* (*Margaroides.*) Cruveilhier describes and illustrates with figures a tumour consisting of white glistening globular masses, like pearls; and indeed the tumour appears to consist of minute or middle-sized pearls aggregated together. These bodies vary in magnitude, from the size of vetches to that of peas. The colour was that of dead silver, pearl, or whitish-gray wax. The tumours thus formed varied in size, from that of a nut to a walnut, or a small pippin. In general the tumours had greater latitudinal extent than thickness. They were irregularly round; but seemed in some instances to consist of two or more tumours aggregated together.

These bodies were situate mostly on the base of the brain, over the protuberance, or that and the limbs of the brain, or the lower surface of the cerebellum.

This sort of tumour is formed in the subarachnoid cellular tissue, that is between the arachnoid membrane and the *pia mater.* As it increases in size, however, it encroaches on the base of the brain, and it may, as in one case given by Cruveilhier, destroy the floor of the third ventricle and the contiguous parts, and present itself immediately beneath the *fornix.*

This tumour presents no trace of organic structure. It is a secreted product or deposit formed within the cells of the cellular tissue; a sort of adipose matter having the consistence of marrow or suet, covered by a layer of more coherent matter imitating the brilliancy of silver or pearl.

When this substance was examined chemically, it was found to consist almost solely of cholesterine.

Of the cases given by Cruveilhier, one occurred in a young woman of 18 years; another took place in an old soldier of 40 years.[*]

The effects produced by tumours of this kind are very similar to

[*] Anatomie Pathologique. Deuxieme Livraison. Pl. VI.

those resulting from other tumours developed in the substance or on the surface of the brain. Hebetude of the intellectual faculties, loss of memory, epileptic seizures frequently recurring, a fatuous and vacant expression of countenance, sometimes blindness or squinting, then stupor and palsy, and finally death, are the ordinary consequences of the presence of this deposit.

The same cholesterine deposit in scales is occasionally found on the spinal chord.

η. *Cartilaginous induration ; Scirrhus ; (Chondroma.*) This is probably to be regarded either as a variety of the first kind, or as intimately connected with it. Unhappily the term *scirrhus* has been so vaguely applied to every kind of tumour, if a little hard, that no precise idea is communicated by it. In the brain especially all authors have comprehended, under this general appellation, every change of texture which was harder than that of the surrounding organ, without much regard to the anatomical characters of the new substance. Hence we find all the instances already adduced recorded as examples of scirrhus, though in many of them no proof of this structure is given, and in none is there any other proof than the greater consistence of the part.

Without attempting to define the character of scirrhus when occurring in the brain, I refer to the present head those instances of morbid structure in which, with hardness approaching to that of cartilage, there is a fibrous arrangement, and more or less tendency to cancerous ulceration. Even with this limitation it may be doubted whether this disease occurs primarily in the cerebral substance. Meanwhile, however, for want of more satisfactory elements in the arrangement of the organic changes incident to the brain, to this head may be referred the following examples :—

M. Jean Cruveilhier, Essai sur l'Anatomie Pathologique, Tome ii. p. 80. Paris, 1816.—A woman of 40 was brought to the Hotel-Dieu in a state of idiocy, in which she was stated to have been for six months after severe mental distress. She lived a month without much sign of intellect, became comatose and died. In the right hemisphere, beneath the mesolobe, corresponding to the striated body on the outside, and projecting into both ventricles, was found a hard tumour of a triangular shape, the posterior angle elongated, the right anterior angle advancing to the anterior extremity of the right lobe. It consisted of two sorts of structure;—one in the centre, as large as a pigeon's egg, had the consistence of fibro-cartilage, and resembled fibrous substances proceeding to the cartilaginous state; the other exterior, grayish, was confounded with the cerebral substance from which it appeared to be formed.

L. N. Rostan, Recherches sur une Maladie encore peu connue. Paris, 1820. P. 84. Observ. 20ieme. 1820 —A woman of 62 had during the course of life been deranged several times, during which she committed extravagant acts, though rare and of short duration. She had now constant headach, with occasional raving, giddiness, and vemiting, followed by palsy of the right side, and complete derangement. In a few days more she became comatose, and, with complete right hemiplegia and stertorous respiration, she expired. In the upper middle of the left hemisphere, which was softened all round, a little beneath the convoluted substance, was a small yellowish granular nut. Anteriorly in the striated body was a cancerous tumour as large as a nut, compressing the ventricle. In the right hemisphere, which was sound and consistent in its anterior three-fourths, but injected towards the posterior-inferior region, was a cancerous tumour as large as a small nut, with pulpy destruction of the surrounding substance.

This account is deficient in failing to state the physical characters of the several tumours. A record more instructive is found in the following :—

M. Andral Fils, Cancer du Cerveau, from La Charité, in the wards of M. Lerminier, Journal de Physiologie, Tome ii. p. 105, 1822.—A man of 58 felt fifteen years before acute pain of the right temple, radiating in the right side of the head and face, and lasting for six weeks. During subsequent years it returned at irregular intervals, and continued for periods of various duration till two months previous to admission, when it became so intense, as to oblige the patient to give up his usual employments. Without affection of sensation, intellect, or motion, he suffered severe tearing pain in the whole right side of the head, and slight convulsive motions of the face, followed after eight days by palsy of the lower limbs, and soon after by coma, which continued in a greater or less degree for a few days, when he died. In the centre of the right hemisphere, outside of the optic *thalamus* and *corpus striatum*, the space of four finger-breadths long, and two or three wide, was a reddish-gray, knotty, rough, unequal surface, which when cut resisted like the scirrhous masses of the stomach or liver. In the resisting points was a substance of areolar texture, bluish-white colour, semitransparent, very hard, presenting here and there minute cavities containing a fluid like apple-jelly ; (scirrhus proceeding from the crude to the softening stage). In other points was a firm texture of dirty white colour, traversed by reddish lines crossing in various directions (supposed to be encephaloid texture in the crude stage.) In other points was seen a reddish-purple, which appears to have been simply softened brain.

Bouillaud, Traité Clinique et Physiologique de l'Encephalite. 1825.—A lady of 77, with convulsive motions of the left arm, followed by palsy of that and of the left leg, impaired speech, complete hemiplegia, and death by exhaustion, without loss of consciousness, a firm, yellowish, lardaceous, bulky, many-lobed mass, occupying the greater part of the posterior lobe, almost the whole of the middle lobe, and part of the anterior lobe of the right hemisphere. Contiguous to the optic thalamus, which was entirely softened, a lobule penetrated below the striated body, and reached the exterior of the middle lobe, where it was connected with the membranes and the bone. Softening all round.*

Ibid.—A man of 66. Right hemiplegy twice, followed by raving, unintelligible speech, insensibility, coma, and death. In the central and posterior part of the left hemisphere a hard irregular mass, internally of a saffron-yellow colour in some parts, of a rust-yellow in others, jaspered, marked by numerous small white bodies varying from the size of a lentile and a pea to that of a filbert, furrowed in various directions by minute filaments. The hardest of these bodies M. Bouillaud regards as scirrhous matter in the crude stage. Others resembling a white concentrated glue, he thinks, might

---

* This case is stated to be already published in the work of M. Rostan. This, however, appears to be a mistake. The only example of cancer in the brain recorded in that work is the case above mentioned of *Marie Gerard*. With this it evidently does not correspond, either in age or in other circumstances. A case of tumour called cancerous is also given in the " Observations" of M. Lermi. nier.—Annuaire Medico-Chirurg. p. 225.

be the *colloid* or glue-like cancer of M. Laennec. While the greater part of this body
was hard, its centre was reduced to a yellow diffluent pulp.

    Mr R. Wade, Medical and Physical Journal.—In the upper part of the left lobe
(hemisphere) of the brain, a hard body of the size of a small hen's egg, like medullary
sarcoma, but as firm as scirrhus of the female breast. The greatest part consisted of
yellow-white striæ, as hard as cartilage, the remainder dark-gray and less firm, not very
distinguishable after maceration. Pulpy destruction around.

    Under his fifth head, Dr Monro has shortly noticed seven speci-
mens of this change of structure preserved in the University
Museum. Its hardness, irregular surface, and cartilaginous structure, with a resemblance to a section of the kidney, are the circumstances principally remarked.

    From the above accounts, which I consider to be the most au-
thentic on record, a general idea of the anatomical characters of
what is meant by scirrhus of the brain (*chomdroma*) may be obtained. A mass generally of irregular shape, distinguished from
the surrounding cerebral substance by its firmness, sometimes a
lobulated structure, by its interior substance consisting of a proportion more or less considerable of yellowish matter as hard as
cartilage, arranged sometimes in streaks or bands, in other cases
in round nodules, constitutes the principal characters of this morbid growth in its crude or early stage. At a more advanced period cavities begin to be formed, in which is contained a fluid or
semifluid matter sometimes jelly-like, at other times thinner, and
occasionally tinged with blood. Before this process of softening
has advanced far death takes place in general by suspension of the
functions of the organ.

    The cartilaginous tumour may be deposited in a tubercular form,
and perhaps consisting partly of tubercular or albuminous matter.
Of this a good instance is given by Bayle in his Treatise on Pulmonary Consumption. A printer of 58, with complete paraplegy,
and obliteration of the intellect almost to idiocy, followed by weakness of the arms and sudden loss of speech, died with lethargy and
paralytic dyspnœa. In the anterior part of the right hemisphere
was a tubercular and cancerous mass the size of a turkey's egg,
nearly spherical, and of considerable consistence and specific gravity. With a reddish-gray surface irregularly knobbed, traversed
by blood-vessels, it consisted internally of a canary-yellow, thick,
granular, pasty matter, void of vessel or trace of organization, resembling scrofulous tubercles beginning to soften, with this difference, that in some points it was humid and infiltered with serous

fluid. This was the case in the walls of an anfractuous irregular cavity without membrane, and containing two spoonfuls of clear yellowish fluid. The tubercular matter formed the centre and the three upper fourths of the tumour. The rest was what is described as cancerous,—a firm grayish-white shining tissue, traversed in all directions by blood-vessels, and presenting even a minute bloody effusion. Though the tumour was without cyst, its surface was covered by a celluloso-vascular tissue, which sent numerous irregular productions into the substance. It was surrounded by a layer of cerebral matter, reduced as usual to the consistence of thick cream.*

θ. Calcareous or Bony deposits, and Concretions.—This morbid deposition is by no means so common in the brain as in its membranes; and a large proportion of the cases termed ossification or petrification of the brain are doubtless examples of ossific tumours originating in the membranes. It appears, nevertheless, that some instances have occurred to different observers. Kerkringius mentions as a cause of fatuity, a concretion weighing thirteen grains in the right ventricle.† Kentmann notices an ash-coloured one, the size and shape of a mulberry ;‡ Deidier found the left *corpus striatum* osseous;§ and Tyson mentions the case of a man who died of the effects of a blow on the head, in whom one of the inferior *corpora quadrigemina* was as large as a nutmeg, and contained a chalk mass like a cherry-stone, with pulpy destruction of the organ.‖ Blegny saw a stone as large as a bean at the union of the optic nerves in the brain of a lady, who, after violent pains of the head with fever, became blind, and died.¶ In the brain of a man who had suffered long from acute pain of the hind head, notwithstanding the use of blisters, setons, &c. M. Boyer found a hard plaster-like concretion as large as a filbert.** In the brain of a boy of 16, an idiot from birth, Sir E. Home found the protuberance, cerebellic peduncles, and part of the cerebellum, containing so much earthy matter as to be with difficulty cut by the knife.†† Professor Nasse found in the left

---

* Recherches sur la Phthisie Pulmonaire, &c. Par G. G. Bayle. A Paris, 1810. P. 305.

† Observat. Anatom. 35.

‡ De Calculis Libellus.

§ Des Tumeurs, p. 351.

‖ Philosophical Transactions, No. 228.

¶ Zodiacus Gallicus, Obs. xiv. p. 81.

** Cruveilhier, Essai sur l'Anatomie Pathologique, T. ii. p. 84.

†† Phil. Trans. 1814.

lobe of the cerebellum a body one inch long and ten lines broad, composed of alternate layers of chalky matter, fluid albumen and solid albumen.* Lastly, Andral in a phthisical subject found, in the substance of the left hemisphere, near its upper anterior extremity, a granulation the size of a large pea, with the consistence of the calcareous concretions of the lung.†

In such cases a minute portion of brain appears not to be converted into bone, but to be infiltrated with chalky matter, void of animal substance so far as can be discovered. Of these earthy deposits no analysis has yet been made. It is, however, not improbable that they consist chiefly of lime, united either with carbonic or phosphoric acid, or both. Dr Hooper has delineated in his twelfth engraving a bony tumour, or what he names a tubercle, which is said to consist of the same materials as healthy bone, with a little more animal matter. It is not stated whether this was found in the cerebral substance or connected with the membranes. From its appearance, however, and the fact now stated of its chemical character, I think it next to certain that it was of the latter description. Upon the whole, it may be inferred that the substances denominated *concretions of the brain* consist of infiltrations or depositions of calcareous matter in the substance of the organ.

To this head may be referred the concretions found in the *conarium* or pineal gland. In this body small sabulous or calcareous particles have been very often found; and it was long supposed, partly in consequence of the hypothetical opinions of Descartes, that this change could not fail to affect materially the functions of the entire organ. For correct information on this point, we are indebted to Soemmering, who showed by the collation of numerous cases, that scarcely any person arrived at the age of puberty, though in the best health and the most perfect enjoyment of his faculties, could assure himself that his conarium did not contain calcareous matter. He regards it as part of the natural structure.

Though Soemmering states that sabulous deposition is found in the conarium of infants as well as adults, he nowhere specifies the exact authority for this fact; and the youngest subjects on which he records its occurrence were 14 and 16.‡ The Wenzels assert

---

* Abercrombie, Pathological and Pract. Researches, p. 426.
† Journal de Physiologie, Tome ii. p. 110.
‡ S. T. Soemmering de Acervulo Cerebri Dissert. Apud Ludwig, Scriptorum Neurolog. nunc Delect. p 322, 329.

that they have seen stony particles so early as the 7th year, and a substance very similar a few months after birth.* I am satisfied that I have seen in the pineal glands of young children, whose ages I could not ascertain, but who certainly did not exceed 9 or 10, small sabulous particles; but my personal observation does not enable me to say how far the statement of the Austrian anatomists as to earlier periods is correct.

The conarium itself consists chiefly of firm reddish gray cerebral matter, at the basis or posterior end of which are two whitish threads, which proceed on each side to the optic thalamus, and form what are termed the *peduncles* of the gland, from which they are separated by a small linear depression. Behind the union of these peduncles, covered here by part of the choroid web, is placed invariably an irregular-shaped mass, varying in size from that of a small pin-head to a grain of hemp-seed. When seized by the forceps this is found to grate like sand or grains of stone; and when examined it actually consists of minute granules aggregated together by membranous filaments of animal matter. This irregular-shaped sandy mass is what is termed by Soemmering *acervulus conarii*. The granules in the centre are generally larger than those at the surface; and its irregular shape depends on the number and size of the small superficial granules. They are generally yellow or citron-coloured, hard, rough, semitransparent, and distinctly grating on a steel instrument.

Besides the situation now mentioned,—the union of the peduncles,—sandy particles are occasionally found anterior to the peduncles close on the basis of the gland, or disseminated in its substance. In infants before the 7th year, it is never found in the substance of the conarium, but generally in the plate which connects it to the *thalami*. The most ordinary place for it in adults is the pit between the conarium and its peduncles; and in aged subjects it may be found in all the three situations. It has been found in natives of every European nation almost, and in Africans.

According to the analysis of Muller these stones contain calcareous earth; and from some experiments of Müneb it appears that the lime is united with oxalic acid.

Whatever be the quantity of this deposition, it is well ascertained that it exercises no influence on the cerebral functions. It is nevertheless difficult to imagine it to be a natural or healthy product.

* De Penitiori Structura Cerebri, pp. 155—157.

From its situation I have often been inclined to think that it is a secretion from the vessels of the choroid web.

Petrifaction, or osseous induration of the whole brain, has not been seen in the human subject. Instances, however, of this in the lower animals have been recorded by Duverney, Simson, Pitchell, and Renauld.

ι. Encysted Tumours.—Of these any of the forms may probably be found in the brain. Hitherto, however, those actually said to occur may be referred to one or other of the following heads.

a. Hydatoid or vesicular tumours. It may be justly doubted whether the genuine animal hydatid, (*Cysticercus cellulosus,* Rudolphi,) has ever been found in the brain. Though stated generally by Bremser, he mentions no authority ;* it is never noticed by Rudolphi ;† and seems to be denied entirely by Blainville. None of the social hydatids (*Coenuri* and *Echinococci*) were found in that situation, till M. C. Rendtorff discovered, in 1811, a cluster of the latter sort in the right ventricle of a girl of 8, who, after remaining hemiplegic for some months, died lethargic.‡

Notwithstanding this, instances of bodies described as *hydatids* occurring in the brain have been mentioned by Scultetus, Panaroli, Paw, Borelli, Lancisi, Wepfer, Home, Rostan, Headington, and Morrah. In the case of Scultetus, a cyst as large as a hen's egg, not unlike a hydatid, was found in the left hemisphere.§ In that of Panaroli, several whitish round bladders, containing pituitous fluid (*hygroma?*) were found in the mesolobe.‖ In that of Paw, a bladder containing half a pound of limpid fluid was seated over the commissure of the optic nerves.¶ The case of P. Borelli was a cyst containing watery fluid, attached to the nates and infundibulum.** That of Lancisi is styled a hydatid as large as a pigeon's egg, thin, yellowish, jelly-like lymph, in the posterior part of the right hemisphere.†† The case of Wepfer, which was a cyst as large as a hen's egg, containing a turbid brownish liquor, appears to belong rather to the head of *hygroma.*‡‡ Those of Home,§§ Ros-

---

* Traité Zoologique, &c. Paris, 1824, P. 141, chap. ii.
† Entozoorum Synopsis. Mantissa, Gen. 28, p. 546.
‡ De Hydatidibus præsertim in cerebro repertis.
§ Armamentarium, Obs. 10 and 11.
‖ Pentecoste I: Obs. 17.   ¶ Petri Pawii, Observat. 2.
** P. Borelli, Obs. Medico-Physicæ.
†† De Mortibus Subetaneis, Lib. i. cap. xi. 13.
‡‡ Historiæ Apoplecticorum.
§§ Phil. Trans. 1814, p, 483.

tan,* Headington,† and Morrah,‡ though more recent, are not more unequivocal, since their authors give no description of the physical characters by which their claim to the title of hydatids might be determined.

Upon the whole, though the occurrence of the genuine solitary animal hydatid in the brain may not be impossible, it is not clear that any of the cases hitherto recorded belong to this head. They are to be regarded rather as serous or vesicular cysts, (Portal, Anat. Med. Tome IV. p. 72,) or examples of the tumour called (*hygroma*). Of this kind also are the case described by Forlani of Sienna, containing glutinous matter like white of egg,§ and the globular cysts so beautifully represented by Dr Hooper in his fourteenth engraving. The cases mentioned by Fischer, Zeder, and others, belong to the membranes.

b. Steatoms are mentioned by Drelincurtius, Thomann, Home, and Bouillaud.

c. The blood-cyst, (*hæmatoma*). The occurrence of this in the brain, though not common, has been observed. Like hæmatoma in other regions, it consists of a membranous cyst, sometimes containing small cysts, the inner surface of which is composed of a vascular tissue, from which blood or bloody fluid exudes by exhalation, forming a mass resembling layers of coagulated blood. Of this disease the most distinct example is given by Rochoux. A man of 65, about twenty months after a violent blow on the head which stunned him, began to feel pain and weight of the head, with occasional moments of forgetfulness. These symptoms became more severe and more frequent, were followed by embarrassed speech, palsy of the left side of the face, great general weakness, coma, and death. In the anterior and external part of the left hemisphere was found a firm red-brown tumour, the size of an egg, round, flattened, filled with blood, which in certain places appeared to be contained as in the spleen, in others in small clots of a line diameter of an areolar-cellular tissue, grayish, dense, and analogous in appearance to the matter of tubercles. Adhering without to the dura mater of the arachnoid, which was red and much thick-

---

* Recherches, &c. Chap. x. Acephalocystes, p. 166.
† Medical and Surgical Journal, Vol. XV. 504.
‡ Medico-Chirurgical Transactions, Vol. II. p. 262.
§ Caspar M. Forlani, Obs. Med. Pract. Anat. Senis, 1769.

ened, it was lodged in a depression of the hemisphere. The contiguous cerebral matter was in the state of yellow ramollissement.*
In his tenth engraving Dr Hooper gives a good delineation of
an example of this disease. In this case the tumour, which was of
an irregular oblong spheroidal shape, about 3½ inches long and 2½
broad, arose by a broad base from the white cerebral substance of
the left hemisphere near the ventricle, but not communicating with
that cavity. Externally it was of a pink-red, or pale carmine colour, and of an irregularly lobulated arrangement. Though soft
to the touch, it was elastic and cut firm, exposing a vascular mottled surface of a reddish-yellow colour, with portions of blood-like
structure here and there. Besides the *pia mater,* which it raised,
it was covered by a delicate and very vascular membrane, laminated and shaggy.

A tumour of similar characters is described under his sixth head
by Dr Monro *Tertius,*† formerly Professor of Anatomy. In a
young man who had suffered from headach, impaired vision, and
nausea, followed by epilepsy terminating fatally in a few hours, in
the middle lobe of the right hemisphere was a body the size of an
orange, somewhat soft, but elastic, and of the colour and consistence of clotted blood. The surrounding brain was in a state of
pulpy destruction.

These two last cases are regarded as similar to the tumour named
hæmatoid fungus. I am not prepared to prove that they do not
belong to this head; but their general resemblance in anatomical
characters to that described by Rochoux, induces me to refer them
to the head of *Hæmatoma.*

To the same head may be referred that described by Dr George
Gregory,‡ who, in a man labouring under headach, irritable stomach, and epileptic fits, and finally destroyed by epilepsy, found
within a cyst in the anterior *cornu* of the left ventricle, before the
striated nucleus, a body as large as a nutmeg, hard and fleshy, laminated interiorly an inch thick like coagulated blood, with a cavity
in the centre.

d. Fungus Hæmatodes. Encephaloid or Cerebriform tumour.—
This morbid growth has been often found in the brain either exclusively or in common with other textures. Enclosed almost in-

* J. A. Rochoux, Recherches sur l'Apoplexie. A Paris, 1814. Obs. 38, p. 149.
† The Morbid Anatomy of the Brain. By Alex. Monro, M. D. &c. p. 56. chap. i.
‡ Medical and Physical Journal, Vol. LIV. p. 462.

variably in a cyst, it consists of soft, compressible, spongy matter, of the consistence of fœtal brain, and not dissimilar in colour to gray cerebral matter, with a tinge of red, a shining aspect, divided in lobulated masses, which move on each other when slightly touched. Though found chiefly in young subjects, it may occur in the brains of adults; but is rarely seen in the aged.[*]

e. *Melanosis*. The melanotic deposit has not been very often found in the brain. Streaks of dark matter along the blood-vessels were seen by Dr Alison and Mr Fawdington;[†] and Dr Hooper delineates melanotic masses of small size in the substance of the organ.[‡]

Of these several changes now enumerated, the effects, in general uniform, may be said to vary only according, 1*st*, to the morbid changes induced in the contiguous cerebral substance; 2*d*, according to the extent which the organic change occupies; and 3*dly*, according to its relative situation in the organ.

1. All the tumours above enumerated, independent of the changes proper to their own structure, agree in producing certain common changes in the contiguous cerebral substance. All of them tend to derange the capillary circulation of the brain and its membranes. In the former they induce not only a general injection of the cerebral capillaries, but a local action in the immediate confines of the tumour, and pulpy destruction of the cerebral substance. It often happens also that the whole organ is, in consequence of the capillary injection, infiltrated by pale or bloody serous fluid. In the membranes these tumours also induce injection, terminating in infiltration of the subarachnoid tissue, and effusion from the choroid web into the ventricles. The effects on the cerebral functions are then precisely similar to those which result from derangement of the capillary circulation taking place primarily. If local and intermittent, that is, recurring on the operation of certain causes, the irritation from the tumour and its disturbance on the capillary circulation induces chronic headach, with epileptic attacks. When the vascular orgasm becomes more general and constant, loss of memory, and sometimes of judgment, irregular contractions of the members, and more or less palsy, are the consequences. As it advances to pulpy destruction, the involuntary contractions of the muscles are followed by palsy; the abolition of sensation, recollection and in-

---

[*] Observations on Fungus Hematodes, by James Wardrop. Edinburgh, 1809. To this belongs the case of Dr Latham, in Medical and Physical Journal, Vol. lvi. p. 1.

[†] A Case of Melanosis, &c. by Thomas Fawdington.

[‡] The Morbid Anatomy, Plate XII.

tellect, give rise to fatuity; and life may be terminated either by coma, with or without convulsion, or by a sudden apoplectic attack.

2. Most of these organic changes, if small or limited in extent, exercise little influence on the functions ascribed to the brain. Even when large, their influence seems to be referable chiefly to the morbid changes in the capillary circulation now mentioned. In many instances no change in sensation, intellect, or locomotion is induced till within a few days before death, when the convulsions, palsy, and coma, which preceded this event, must be ascribed chiefly to vascular injection taking place a little before these external effects become manifest.

3. The situation of the morbid substance and of the disordered action is certainly of some moment in modifying the effects produced. To determine the influence of local situation in this respect attempts, direct and indirect, have been made by La Peyronie, Zinn, Lorry, Haller, and Saucerotte, and more recently by Rolando, Flourens, Serres, Bouillaud, and others. Without attempting to inquire into the merit of the experimental and argumentative investigations of these authors, I shall merely state some of the most important conclusions, which they have thought their researches justified.

1. Injury done to the anterior lobes of the brain causes, according to M. Bouillaud, more or less loss of speech, depending either on disorder or abolition of memory, or on that of the muscular motions of the organs of speech.[*]

2. According to the observations of M. Serres[†] and MM. Foville and Pinel Grandchamp, when the *corpus striatum*, that is, the anterior part of the striated nucleus, is injured, the motions of the legs are disordered and impaired; and when the optic *thalamus*, or the posterior region of the striated nucleus, is injured, the motions of the arms are impaired.

3. Though M. Serres has endeavoured to demonstrate the position of M. Gall, that lesions of the middle lobe of the cerebellum have a particular influence on the generative organs, this is rendered very doubtful by the researches of Rolando, Flourens, and especially Bouillaud. M. Flourens endeavours to show that the cerebellum regulates, influences, or co-ordinates the voluntary motions.

---

[*] Recherches Cliniques, &c. Par M. J. Bouillaud, D. M.   Archives Générales, Tome viii. p. 25.   Traité Clinique et Physiologique, p. 157-161.   Paris, 1825 ; and Note sur une article de M. Pinel Fils, &c. Journal de Physiol. Tome vi. p. 19.

[†] Annuaire Medico-Chirurgical et Journal de Physiologie, Tome III. p. 123-128, et ensuite.

Bouillaud shows that, though it cannot be said to regulate the whole of these motions, it co-ordinates those concerned in equilibrium, the state of rest, and the different forms of locomotion. It seems further to be the seat of a modification of memory, that of voluntary motion. When disordered, the memory is obliterated, the motions are impaired or disordered, and the patient exhibits all the phenomena of imbecility, in willing any regular or steady motion, or in preserving any sensible attitude of rest.*

15. *Anencephalous Malformation. Deficiency of the whole Brain or of its parts.* (*Enkephalelleipsis.*)—This should be noticed elsewhere, under the head of affections dependent on the membranes and blood-vessels. But it may render the history of the abnormal states of the brain more complete, to introduce here a short account of a species of malformation arising from interruption of the process of development.

Instances of acephalous fœtuses, as they have been named, are numerous from the first records of anatomy to the present time. They vary in degree from deficiency of the whole brain to that of more or fewer of its parts. All of them depend, so far as is hitherto ascertained, on the same general cause, a sudden check given to the process of growth in this organ or some of its parts, while the others continue to increase. The general accuracy of this conclusion is established by the researches of Meckel,† of Duncan, Junior,‡ of Breschet,§ and of Serres.‖ In 1835 I collected from different sources several cases, in order to illustrate the nature of the malformation, and the mode in which it is effected;¶ and subsequently the subject has been elucidated by Cruveilhier.**

The mode in which the growth of the brain is arrested may be understood from the history of the progressive development of the organ, which I have above stated is formed by deposition from the vascular membrane, commencing near the centre of the

* Recherches Experimentales, &c. Par J. Bouillaud, Membre-Adjoint, &c. Archives Générales, Tome xv. p. 64.

† Handbuch der Pathologischen Anatomie. Von J. F. Meckel. Leipzig, 1812.

‡ Case of Hydrocephalus with Bifid Brain, in Medico-Chirurgical Trans. Edin. Vol. i. p. 205.

§ Note sur deux enfans nouveaux-nés hydrocephales et manquant de cerveau Par J. Breschet, Journal de Physiologie, Tome ii. p. 269. IIde Note sur des enfants Nouveaux-nés, &c. Par G. Breschet, Jour. de Phys. Tome iii. 232.

‖ Essai sur une Theorie Anatomique des Monstrosités Animales. Revue Medicale, Tome vi. p. 180. Paris, 1821.

¶ Edinburgh Medical and Surgical Journal, Vol. XLIV. p. 527, Oct. 1835.

** Cinquieme Livraison et Huitieme Livraison. Paris, 1833.

hemispheres, and proceeding in both directions towards the convoluted and the central surfaces. When the process of nutritious deposition is arrested at an early period, the brain is entirely wanting, and one or two imperfectly shaped tubercles only denote the site of the *corpora quadrigemina*, the *thalami*, or the protuberance. If at a later period, the cerebellum and the lower part of the brain, with several of its objects, may be completed. But separating the two hemispheres above, there is found a large chasm, filled by water, and in which neither mesolobe, vault, septum, nor thalami can be recognized. This interruption M. Serres ascribes to imperfect development of the arterial system going to the brain. But this is only a collateral effect.

In some instances a hemisphere is wanting; in others the anterior lobe is deficient; in others both anterior lobes are wanting; and in others there is a general diminution in the size of one whole hemisphere, and the magnitude of its component convolutions, while the other presents its normal dimensions and proportions.

All these phenomena are produced in the same way and proceed from the same cause. An attack of meningeal inflammation or hydrocephalus in the womb, before birth, or immediately after that event,—not sufficient to extinguish life,—arrests the nutritive action of a certain order of the cerebral capillaries. The nutritive action is employed in secreting serous fluid. The growth of part of the brain affected is suddenly stopped; and while the growth of the rest advances, that remains stationary.

This interruption of normal action of vessels depends on a sudden change somehow effected in them, in consequence of which they no longer continue the nutritious process. The proof that the imperfect development of the arterial system is only a collateral effect, is found in the fact, that the development of these vessels is always equal and sometimes superior to the progress of the abnormal action and its effects.

It is manifest that, in cases of this nature, the atrophy of the brain is not a primary or idiopathic lesion, but is indeed the effect partly of the excessive distension of the walls of the brain by an extraordinary quantity of fluid, and partly of mechanical compression by the fluid inducing sometimes condensation of the parts, sometimes softening, but always more or less destruction of the proper structure. Atrophy, indeed, is one of the effects of great effusions of fluid. It cannot be denied that in cases of this class the brain is not nourished, or is even deprived of nourishment. But it must be borne in mind that the suspension or interruption of nutrition is the effect of a preceding morbid state, in which the blood-vessels, the natural nutrients of the organ, are made to assume a new and perverted action.

From the cases now recorded it further appears that the atrophied parts of the brain are diminished in size or shrunk, and that they also cease to possess their characteristic physical and physiological properties, and to perform their functions duly. Thus in all the cases with the diminution in size of the parts, there is more or less loss of motion and sensation in some of the voluntary organs. Loss of memory appears occasionally to take place; but loss of intellect is not invariable. This, however, may depend on the part of the brain atrophied, and on the extent of the atrophy. The mental energy is generally enfeebled; but the most characteristic feature is that one faculty may retain considerable force, while others are disproportionately weak. The intensity of the intellect is unequal.

This is a frequent cause of congenital idiocy, surd-muteness, palsy of one side or various parts of the body; and unequal development of several organs.

Often one or more members may be shrunk, withered, and paralytic; and occasionally one side is hemiplegic.

As to the intimate nature of the change induced in the parts so shrunk and diminished we have as yet no precise information. It may arise either from arrest of the growth of the parts, or from the removal of parts by absorption, or rather by disruption and breaking down. The pressure increased by the presence of a new fluid may be adequate to prevent growth of the parts compressed, and even to break down and disorganize.

Atrophy of the brain, therefore, may differ according as it takes place during the process of development or after that process is completed. If it take place during the process of formation, then that process is suddenly interrupted, and the brain presents more or fewer of its parts in an incomplete or rudimentary state. Thus in cases in which the process is interrupted previous to the formation of the convolutions, and in which serous fluid more or less copious is effused from the nutrient vessels, the brain resembles a shapeless uniform bladder of membranous and cerebral matter enclosing serous fluid. This is perhaps the most complete example of the atrophy of the brain, and corresponds with the *agenesia* of M. Cazauvieilh (Archives de Med. xiv.)

The parts which next to these are most generally wanting are the meso-lobe, *fornix* and *septum lucidum*.   Reil observed the want of this part in an idiotic female who had attained the age of thirty years.

Independently or along with the meso-lobe and fornix, the upper region of the hemispheres may be wanting as far as the ceiling of the ventricles.   But it is difficult to distinguish the atrophy of this part from atrophy of the convoluted surface of the brain.

Atrophy may next affect the *corpora striata* or optic *thalami*, in the form of diminished bulk and general dimensions, proceeding to such extent that these bodies may be altogether wanting.

The same lesion may occur in the cerebellum, the annular protuberance, or in the peduncles and the spinal bulb.

The spinal chord or vertebral portion of the brain is in like manner liable to atrophy, both during the process of development and after its completion.

In the first case the chord is entirely or partially wanting, and its place is supplied by serous fluid, more or less copious, contained within the membranes.   Thus in many cases of *spina bifida*, as it is denominated, that disease is the effect of some interruption given to the process of growth in the spinal marrow, by reason of which the arterial action is expended in the effusion of fluid, which fills and distends the -membranes, prevents the further deposition of cerebral matter, and preventing also the union of the spinal plates on the mesial plane, gives rise to a soft elastic tumour at the most yielding and dependent part of the spinal column.   In general the spinal marrow is either partially or entirely wanting in some part of its course in cases of this kind.   Its continuity is interrupted either without a single trace, or with a few streaks of cerebral matter on the one side, or at the anterior part of the column, while the vacancy is supplied by serous fluid or shreds of cerebral matter.

In other instances of this species of atrophy, each lateral half of the chord is in a very slender and imperfect form of development, and is separated from that of the opposite side by the interposition of serous fluid.   In cases of this kind, it is not uncommon to find the median canal persistent long after birth, imitating in this respect the structure observed in the spinal chord of the lower animals.

It may be doubted whether it be quite correct to apply the term atrophy to those lesions of the spinal chord, in which the breaking down, the softening or shrinking of the parts, is evidently due to inflammatory action excited in them from disease of the membranous investments or the bones.   Thus, in cases of disease of the *vertebræ*,

3

inflammation of a chronic character is very soon propagated to the membranes and the chord, and part of it is softened and disorganized. The injury may not be sufficient to extinguish life; and after some time, when the active part of the inflammatory process has subsided, part of the spinal marrow is contracted in size, and compressed by the new products; and this constitutes, according to the strict understanding of the term, the anatomical characters of atrophy. In admitting this application of the term, therefore, it ought to be distinctly understood, that the term atrophy designates, not a primary lesion, but a lesion which is the effect of another previous action. Several cases of the kind are recorded by Ollivier and others.

CHAPTER II.

B. The Distributed Part of the Nervous System.

Section I.

NERVE, NERVOUS TISSUE.—(Νευρον,—*Nervus,*—*Tissu Nerveux,*— *Systeme Nerveux.*)

The structure of the nerves has been examined with different degrees of accuracy and minuteness by a great number of anatomists. The more ancient authors, who wrote at a period when observation was much corrupted by fancy, and most of those who give descriptions in general systems, may be without much injustice passed over in silence. It is sufficient to say, that some good facts are given in the works of Willis,[*] Vieussens,[†] Morgagni,[‡] and Mayer;[§] that Prochaska,[||] Pfeffinger,[¶] and the second Monro,[**] are the first who professedly wrote on the structure of the nerves; that the

[*] Thomas Willis, Cerebri Anatome Nervorumque Descriptio et Usus. Amsterdam, 1682.

[†] Raymundi Vieussens Neurographia Universalis. Lyon, 1684.

[‡] Adversaria Anatomica, 4to. Lugduni Bat. 1723.

[§] J. C. Mayer Abhandlung vom Gehirn, Ruckenmark, und dem Ursprunge der Nerven. Berlin, 1779.

[||] Georgii Prochaska de Structura Nervorum Tractatus Anatomicus. Viennæ, 1779 and 1800, *apud* Op. Minora.

[¶] Jo. Pfeffinger, de Structura Nervorum. In Ludwig, Scriptorum Neurolog. Select. Tom. I.

[**] Monro on the Structure and the Functions of the Nervous System. Edinburgh, 1783. Folio.

works of Reil,* Bichat, and Gordon, contain the most accurate information on the nervous chords in general ; and that the treatises of Scarpa† and Wutzer‡ contain the most satisfactory information on the arrangement of those parts named ganglions and plexus. Lastly, by the microscopic researches of Ehrenberg, Treviranus, Müller, Valentin, Weber, and Remak, some facts, though rather discordant, have been communicated on the minute structure of the nervous filaments.

Each nerve forms connections in three different ways ; 1*st*, A nerve must be connected to some part of the central mass by one of its extremities,—the cerebral or spinal end ; 2*d*, It must be connected to some texture or organ, or part of an organ by the other extremity,—the organic end ; and, 3*d*, It may be connected to other nerves by a species of junction called anastomosis, (*ansa*)— anastomosing or uniting point. By means of the two first connections, it is supposed to maintain a communication between the central mass and the several organs ; and by the latter it is understood to be subservient to a more general and extensive intercourse, which is believed to be necessary in various functions and actions of the animal system.

Every nerve consists essentially of two parts ; one exterior, protecting and containing ; the other interior, contained, and functional, forming the indispensable part of the nervous structure.

The first of these, which has been known since the time at least of Reil by the name *neurilema*, (νευρον, ειλεω, ειλημα, *nervi involucrum*,) or nerve-coat, (Nervenhaut, Reil ; Nervenhülle, Meckel ;) has the form and nature of a dense membrane, not quite transparent, which is found on the outside of the nervous chord or filament, and invests the proper nervous substance. It must not, however, be imagined that the *neurilema* forms a cylindrical tube, in the interior of which the nervous matter is contained. This latter disposition, if it actually exists, applies to the smaller nerves only, and to some of those which go to the organs of sensation,—a peculiarity which we shall notice subsequently.

Any large nervous trunk, for example, the spiral or median of the arm, or the sciatic nerve of the thigh, is found to be composed

---

* J. C. Reil, Exercitationes Anatomicæ de Structura Nervorum.   Haller, 1797

† Anatomicarum Annotationum, Lib. Prim. de Nervorum Gangliis et Plexibus. Auctore Antonio Scarpa.

‡ De Corporis Humani Gangliorum Fabrica atque Usu, Monographia.   Auctore Carolo Gulielmo Wutzer, Med. Chirurg. Doct. &c.   Berolini, 1817.

of several small nervous chords placed in juxtaposition, and each of which, consisting of appropriate *neurilema* and nervous substance, is connected to the other by delicate filamentous tissue. These, however, do not, through their entire course, maintain the parallel disposition in respect to each other, but are observed to cross and penetrate each other, so as to form an intimate interlacement of nervous chords and filaments, each of which, however minute, is accompanied with its investing neurilema. The neurilema, in short, may be represented as a cylindrical membranous tube, giving from its inner surface many productions forming smaller tubes; (*Canaliculi,* Die Nervenröhre; primitive cylinders of Fontana ;*) in which the proper nervous matter is contained.

Of this arrangement the consequence is, that each nerve or nervous trunk, enveloped in its general neurilema, is composed, nevertheless, of a number more or less considerable of smaller chordlike nervous threads (*funiculi nervei,* Prochaska; *chordæ, funes,* Nervenstraenge, Reil,) into which the nerve, by maceration and suitable preparation, may be resolved. Each chord, again, or *nerve-string,* as Reil terms it, though invested with a proper nurilem, may be further resolved into an infinite number of minute filiform or capillary filaments, (*Fila, fibrillæ,* Nervenfasern, Reil,) which, invested in a delicate covering, are understood to constitute the ultimate texture of the nerve.

This threefold division may be easily observed in the brachial and spiral nerves of the arm, and still more distinctly in the sciatic in the thigh. The utility of understanding the internal arrangement from which it results will appear forthwith, when the structure of those parts termed ganglions and plexuses comes under examination.

Of this arrangement in different nerves, and in different regions, this membrane undergoes great modification; and all opinions on its nature derived from thickness or transparency are liable to considerable fallacy. Scarpa seems to view it as connected, in anatomical origin and character, with the hard membrane, (*meninx dura, dura mater.*) Reil, who devoted more care and time to the examination of its nature and structure than any other inquirer, represents it as consisting of cellular substance, many blood-vessels, and some lymphatics.† Bichat thought it resembled the soft mem-

---

* Observations sur la structure des Nerfs, &c. apud Traité sur le Venin, &c. par M. Felix Fontana.

† De Structura Nervorum, cap. i. p. 3.

brane of the brain, ((*pia meninx, pia mater,*) and was derived from it.* Gordon considers the neurilema of the cerebral nerves as consisting of soft membrane, (*pia mater*) at their origin, but in all other situations as a species of cellular membrane.

By Mayer the neurilema is accounted a fibrous tissue, for the following reasons. 1*st*, It consists almost entirely of tendinous fibres, and is cellular only where it is very thin. 2*d*, The transverse folds presented by most of the nerves, and which give them a dentilated form, are derived from the neurilema, are of fibrous character, and are similar to those observed in tendinous sheaths. 3*d*, Several nervous productions are actually converted into tendinous or fibrous filaments; for example, the brain of the snail tribe, (*limaçons,*) and the spinal chord both in these and other animals at the *cauda equina*. 4*th*, The neurilema is either a continuation of the proper cerebral membrane, (*pia mater,*) or very similar to it ; and this membrane is fibrous and aponeurotic at the spinal chord, and even at its upper end, and, according to Mayer, forms the denticulated ligament, which is a fibrous tissue.†

These views, which are the result, not of observation, but of hypothesis, it is impossible to adopt. Its connection with the *pia mater* was disproved by Reil ; and though its analogy with the denticulated ligament were established, it would prove nothing regarding the neurilema. Upon the whole, the idea communicated by Reil is the most probable. According to the observations of this anatomist, who examined the neurilema after fine and successful injection, it is liberally supplied with blood-vessels. These derived from the neighbouring arteries penetrate the filamentous sheath of the nerve ; and, immediately on reaching the neurilema, divaricating at right angles, generally run along the nervous threads, (*funes,*) parallel to them, forming numerous anastomotic communications, and divide into innumerable minute vessels, which penetrate between them into the minute neurilematic canals. So manifold is the ramification, and so perfect the distribution, that in these canals not a particle of nervous substance is found which is not supplied with a vessel.‡ The arrangement of the veins is analogous.

It appears, therefore, that the neurilema is a tissue of membra-

* Anatomie Generale, p. 137, &c.

† Discours sur l'Histologie, par le Docteur Mayer. Bonn, 1819, Journal de Medecine, Vol. XIII. p. 99. 1822.

‡ Joannis Christiani Reil, Exercitationum Anatom. de Structura Nervorum, cap. 5, p. 19.

nous form, with a multiplied mechanical surface, liberally supplied with blood-vessels, from which the nervous matter is secreted and nourished. It is impossible, indeed, to doubt, that of the two parts which compose the nervous chord, it is the most perfectly organized; and that, though it may not be similar in structure to the *pia mater*, it is quite analogous in the use to which it is subservient. Like that membrane, it sustains the vessels of the nerve; it presents a multiplied surface, over which the vessels are distributed; and by penetrating deep into the body of the nerve, it conveys the nutritious vessels in the most capillary form to the inmost recesses of the nervous substance.*

The arrangement which has been above described is the only one which can be regarded as general. It varies in particular regions; and these varieties in the neurilematic disposition occur principally in the nerves which are distributed to the proper organs of sensation.† 1*st*, The olfactory nerve is soft, pulpy, and destitute of neurilema, from its origin in the sylvian fissure, to the gray bulbous enlargement which terminates its passage in the cranium; but as soon as it reaches the *canaliculi* or grooves of the ethmoid bone, and begins to be distributed through the nasal anfractuosities, it is distinctly neurilematic. 2*d*, The optic nerve is still more peculiar in this respect. The instant it quits the optic commissure, (*commissura tractuum*,) it begins to be invested by a firm general neurilema, which sends into the interior substance of the nerve various membranous *septa* or partitions, forming separate canals, in which the nervous matter is contained. These partitions, however, are so thin, that at first sight the optic nerve seems to consist merely of one exterior membranous cylinder inclosing the proper membranous substance. 3*d*, *Lastly*, we remark, that the auditory nerve, or the soft portion of the seventh pair of most anatomical writers, the eighth pair of Soemmering, is the only nerve in which this covering cannot be traced.

The neurilema is much thinner and more delicate in the nerves which are distributed to the internal organs, as the lungs, heart, stomach, &c. (nerves of the organic life, great sympathetic and pneumogastric nerves, *par vagum*), than in those belonging to the muscular system.

The second component part of the nervous chord or filament is

---

* Reil, ibid. chap. i.

† By the term " proper organs of sensation" is understood those of sight, hearing, smell and taste, which are confined to a fixed spot in the system.

the proper nervous matter which occupies the cavity of the neurilematic canals. Little is known concerning the nature or organization of this substance. It is whitish, somewhat soft, and pulpy; but whether it consists of aggregated globules, as was attempted to be established by Della Torre and Sir Everard Home, or of linear tracts disposed in a situation parallel to each other, as appears to be the result of the inquiries of Monro, Reil, and others, or of capillary cylinders containing a transparent gelatinous fluid, as Fontana represents, seems quite uncertain. It has been presumed, rather than demonstrated, that it resembles cerebral substance. But this analogy, though admitted, would throw little light on the subject; for at present it is almost impossible to find two anatomical observers who have the same views of the intimate nature of cerebral substance itself. Whatever be its intimate arrangement, it appears to be a secretion from the neurilematic vessels. (Reil.)

The structure of the nervous chord may be demonstrated in the following manner. When a portion of nerve is placed in an alkaline solution, the whole, or nearly the whole, of the nervous matter is softened and dissolved, or may be washed out of the neurilematic canals, which are not affected by this agent, and the disposition of which may be then examined and demonstrated.* Aqueous maceration may likewise be advantageously employed to unfold this structure; for it separates and decomposes the cellular tissue by which the neurilematic canals are united, and subsequently occasions decomposition of the nervous substance, while it leaves, at least for some time, the neurilema not much affected. When, however, the maceration is too long continued, it is separated and detached like other macerated textures.

Lastly, If a large nerve be placed in diluted acid for the space of one or two weeks, the neurilema is gradually dissolved, and the nervous matter becomes so much indurated and consolidated that it may be separated from the contiguous chords in filaments with great facility.* In undergoing this change the portion of nerve becomes much shorter and considerably contracted,—is subjected, in short, to the process of crispation; so that unless a large nerve like the sciatic be employed for the experiment, it may be impossible

---

* J. C. Reil de Structura Nervorum, cap. i. p. 3 and 5.

† According to the experiments of Reil, nitrous acid diluted with water answers best. Muriatic acid, though equal or even superior in effecting solution of the neurilema, softens the nervous matter too much, and separates the component filaments too completely.—De Structura, cap. iii. p. 16.

to obtain the result in the most satisfactory form. These experiments, with many others of the same nature, were first performed
by Professor Reil, and afterwards repeated and varied by Bichat
and by Dr Gordon. Personal repetition of them enables me to
assert, that, when correctly conducted, they never failed to give the
results as described by these authors.

Nervous tissue, like all others, receives a proportion of what may be
denominated the systems of distribution,—cellular tissue and blood-
vessels. In the substance of the former, the disposition of which
we have already remarked, we find the more conspicuous branches
of the latter distributed. In a more minute and divided form they
penetrate the neurilema and nervous substance. Reil, who derived
his conclusions from the result of delicate and successful injections,
perhaps overrated the quantity of blood which in the sound state
they convey; for it is quite certain, that, in the healthy state, hardly
any red blood enters the nervous tissue, as may be easily shown by
exposing the sciatic nerve of a dog or rabbit.

No good chemical analysis of nervous matter has yet been published. Every chemical examination of it has been conducted on
the assumption that it is analogous to cerebral matter. Of this, however, there is no direct proof. In the analysis by Vauquelin the
neurilematic covering appears not to have been detached,—a proceeding always necessary to obtain correct results in this inquiry.
The effects of acids and alcohol show that it contains albuminous
matter; but beyond this it is impossible at present to make any precise statements.

This description may communicate an idea of the structure of the
nervous chord in general. In particular situations this structure is
considerably modified. The modifications to which we allude occur
under two forms—ganglions (Die knoten;) and plexuses (Die Ner-
vengeflechte.)

Every ganglion consists essentially of three parts; 1st, an exterior covering; 2d, a collection of minute nervous filaments; and,
3d, a quantity of peculiar cellular or filamentous texture, by which
these filaments are connected, and which constitutes the great mass
of the ganglion.

The ganglions are of two kinds, the spinal or simple, and the
non-spinal or compound. These two kinds of bodies differ from
each other, 1st, in the situation which they respectively occupy; 2d,
in the kind of envelope with which they are invested; 3d, in the
mode in which the nervous filaments pass through them and from

them.   By Wutzer, who considers the ganglion of Gasserius, the
ciliary and the maxillary of Meckel, as cerebral ganglions, they are
divided into three sets, those of the *cerebral* system, the *spinal* system, and the *vegetative*, or those connected with the organs of involuntary motion.*

Void of the dense strong coat with which the others are invested,
the cerebral ganglions consist of soft secondary matter, connected
to the filaments of one, or at most two branches, and are arranged
with less complexity.   (Wutzer.)

The spinal ganglions are said to possess two coverings, one
of which resembles the hard cerebral membrane, (*meninx dura,*)
the other the soft cerebral membrane, (*meninx tenuis, pia mater.*)
The non-spinal, or compound ganglions, have also two coverings,
which are merely different modifications of filamentous tissue less
dense and compact than in the former.   Both these sets of ganglions
being by maceration stripped of their tunics, and deprived of the
soft pulpy cellular matter, are resolved into an innumerable series
of nervous threads, most of which are minute and scarcely perceptible; all are continuous with the nerve or nerves above and below
the ganglion.   It appears that the nervous chord, when it enters
the one apex of the ganglion, begins to be separated into its component threads, which diverge and form intervals, between which
the delicate cellular tissue is interposed; and that these filaments
are subsequently collected at the opposite extremity of the ganglion,
where they are connected with the other nerve or nerves.   Scarpa,
to whom we are indebted for the most of the knowledge we possess
on this subject,† compares the arrangement to a rope, the component cords of which are untwisted and teased out at a certain part.

Lastly, In the simple ganglions, the filaments of which they consist, invariably follow the axis of the ganglion; but in the compound
ones they are found to rise towards the sides and emerge from them;
and upon this variety in the direction and course of these filaments
depends the variety of figure, for which these two orders of ganglions are remarkable.   These nervous threads (*stamina s. fila nervea*) described by Scarpa, correspond to the medullary filaments
(*fila medullaria*) of Wutzer.   According to this anatomist these
filaments, when about to enter the ganglion, lay aside their neurilem;
yet they are sufficiently tough to resist a certain degree of tension.

* De Corporis Humani Gangliorum Fabrica, &c. cap. i. ii. § 41, p. 52.
† Anatomicarum Annotationum Liber Primus de Nervorum Gangliis et Plexubus.
Auct. Ant. Scarpa.

Wutzer mentions a cluster of vesicles or cells (*cancelli*) in the filamentous tissue of the ganglion. But he was not enabled by any means, mechanical or chemical, to ascertain their exact nature. The ganglions are well supplied with blood-vessels, derived in general from the neighbouring arteries. The intimate distribution is represented by Wutzer to be the following. The artery proceeding to a ganglion gives vessels to the filamentous tissue; and, perforating the proper coat, is immediately ramified into innumerable minute canals, the first order of which forms vascular nets on the inner surface of the tunic; while the residual twigs penetrate the flocculent texture, and the individual vesicles of the secondary or filamentous matter of the ganglion.*

This short exposition of the structure of the ganglions shows the mistaken notions of Johnstone, Unzer, Bichat, and others, on the structure and uses of these bodies. 1*st*, The idea first advanced by Johnstone,† and Unzer,‡ adopted by Metzger,§ Hufeland,‖ Prochaska,¶ Sue, and Harless,** and afterwards applied with much ingenuity by Bichat, that the ganglions are so many nervous centres or minute brains, is disproved by strict anatomical observation. 2*d*, That they are connected with the order of involuntary actions, and influence these actions, appears to be the only inference that can at present be admitted regarding them. Ganglions are not observed on any of the nerves proceeding to organs of voluntary motion. Sensation, circulation, nutrition, and secretion are the functions, over which they preside. 3*d*, Lastly, we remark, as a circumstance of some importance, that the only difference between a ganglion, and any other part of a nervous chord, is, that in the former the minute nervous filaments appear to be uncovered with neurilema, and lodged in a mass of cellular tissue, which is then inclosed in the neurilematic capsule; while in the latter each nervous filament has its appropriate neurilema, and the cellular tissue, instead of being within, is on its exterior, and connects it to the contiguous filaments.

---

* De Corporis Humani Gangliorum Fabrica, &c. cap. ii. § 41.

† Philosophical Transactions, Vol. LIV. LVII. and LX. and Essay, &c.

‡ J. A. Unzer, Physiologie thierischer Körper. Leipzig, 1771, p. 66.

§ I. D. Metzger Opuscula Anatomica et Physiolog. Gothæ, &c. 1790.

‖ C. W. Hufeland Ideen über Pathogenie, &c. Jena, 1795.

¶ G. Prochaska Lehrsatze der Physiologie, &c. I. ter Band. Wien, 1797.

** J. J. Sue, Recherches Physiologiques, &c. Paris, an. vi. German Translation by I. C. F. Harless, 1797, p. 2. Nurnberg, 1799, p. 3.

In various situations two, three, or more nervous trunks or chords mutually unite by means of some of their component threads, and after proceeding in this manner for a short space, again separate, but not in the same number of original trunks, or preserving the same appearance. In general, the number of chords into which they finally separate is greater than that of which they consisted before union. Three or four nervous trunks, for example, after uniting in this manner, will form on their final separation five or six nerves or nervous chords; and it is quite impossible to determine which of the latter order was derived from any one or two of the former, or what number of individual chords it has received from each. Between the two points also, the first point of union, and the last of separation, many of the more minute component threads are detached from two or more of their trunks, and after first uniting with each other in an indistinct network, are again united to two or more of the nervous chords near the point at which they finally separate from the further end of union. This arrangement has been termed a *plexus, plait,* or *weaving,* in consequence of the manner in which the nervous chords are interlaced or plaited together. The arrangement which we have noticed as consisting of the more minute nervous threads has been called a *smaller plexus; (plexus minor.)* It is a subordinate plexus within a larger one.

The best and most distinct example of a plexus is that commonly named the brachial or axillary.* This, as is well known, is situate in the space contained between the broad dorsal muscle (*latissimus dorsi*) behind, and the great pectoral muscle before, and is formed in the following manner. The fifth, sixth, seventh, and eighth cervical nerves, and the first dorsal, after forming the usual connections, (*ansae,*) pass downwards from the vicinity of the vertebræ between the middle and anterior *scaleni* muscles, and nearly opposite

---

* Imo nullibi fortasse clarior atque evidentior est hæc multarum conjugationum nervearum consociatio atque commixtio, quam in hac nervorum spinalium implicatione *plexum brachialem* appellata. Ibi enim quinque memorati nervi spinales cervicales una convenientes, qua primum cohaerent, aut tribuunt aut mutuo dant et accipiunt a sociis stamina, quæ demum in plures ramos consociata de plexu exeuntes brachiorum nervos faciunt ex omnibus illis quinque conjugationibus spinalibus, aut ex earum plerisque, compositos. Atque exinde sequitur, ut nervi brachiales dicti, qui a plexu ad brachium, manum digitosque ejus omnes derivant, minime ad unam, sed ad plures spinalium conjugationes, nempe ad quatuor cervicales inferiores et dorsalium primum pertineant.—Anatom. Annotation. cap. iii. § 9. pp. 4.

the lower margin of the seventh cervical *vertebra,* or about the level of the first rib, begin to be united by the component threads of each nerve. Threads of the fifth and sixth cervical unite,—sometimes to form a single chord; in other instances to be connected a short space onward with threads of the seventh cervical in a similar manner. The seventh and eighth form two kinds of union. When the seventh is large, it divides almost equally into two chords or branches, one of which is connected first with the fifth and sixth, afterwards with the eighth, and with the first dorsal by interlacement of minute nervous threads. The other either passes downward to form one of the separate brachial nerves, or is also connected with the eighth cervical and first dorsal in a plexiform manner.

From this arrangement immediately arise the individual nervous branches which form the nerves of the arm, and which are named brachial nerves. The interlacement of minute nervous threads between the seventh and eighth cervical, and the first dorsal, is what Scarpa has termed the *plexus minor.* He says it is peculiar, in being quite uniform, and in connecting those nervous branches which, from their subsequent destination, are called Median and Ulnar.

This description, though not generally applicable, will communicate some faint idea of the nervous unions and interlacements termed *plexus* or weavings. For more minute information on the distribution, arrangement, and configuration of this part of the nervous system, I refer to the work of Scarpa already quoted.*

Plexiform arrangements are not confined to the exterior regions of the body. They are more numerous internally; and almost all the organs of the chest and belly have each a plexus, sometimes two, from which they derive their nervous chords.

Plexiform arrangements are generally situate in the neighbourhood of blood-vessels, and in some instances inclosing considerable arterial trunks more or less accurately. Thus the axillary plexus surrounds the axillary artery. The cœliac artery is surrounded with the solar plexus; and the coronary, hepatic, splenic, superior mesenteric, and renal, are also surrounded with plexiform nervous filaments. In some instances these nervous filaments are so intimately connected with the arterial tubes as to lead some

---

* Annotation. Anatom. § 9. cap. iii. pp. 94, 95.

A a

anatomists to consider them as forming a peculiar net-work surrounding the vessel, and to exercise great influence on the circulation. (Wrisberg, Ludwig, and Haase.)

It is remarkable that the structure of the nervous chords which form a plexus, has either appeared so simple as not to demand particular attention, or is so obscure as to be never noticed. Have the nervous chords and threads in such situations their usual envelope? Is the nervous matter in the chords quite the same as in other situations? Is there any other means of union, save the nervous substance itself? We believe there is no doubt that every chord in a plexus is provided with its neurilema as in other places ; but this neurilema is generally thinner and more delicate ; and the general neurilema seems to be wanting. Its mechanical properties of cohesion and resistance have not been examined.

The view which has been given of the structure or arrangement of the nervous plexus has led Scarpa to consider them as nearly allied to ganglions. The same separation of the component threads or filaments of the nerve or nerves, the same interlacement, and the same or similar formation of new chords, appear to take place in both orders of structure. A ganglion, indeed, he conceives, is a condensed or contracted plexus; and a plexus is an expanded or unfolded ganglion. The great anatomical purpose of both appears to be simply a new arrangement or disposition of nervous branches, previous to their ultimate distribution in the tissues or organs to which they are destined. This is nothing but the expression of a fact,—the interpretation in intelligible terms of an arrangement of organized parts without reference to any supposed uses.

The minute structure of the nerves has been examined by Fontana, Prochaska, Bauer, Ehrenberg, Valentin, Muller, Wagner, and Remak.

M. Bauer found the optic nerve to consist of many bundles of very delicate fibres, connected together by means of a jelly-like, transparent, semifluid, viscid substance, easily soluble in water. These fibres consisted of globules, which are from $\frac{1}{3800}$th to $\frac{1}{2000}$th part of an inch in diameter, with a few at $\frac{1}{2000}$th part of an inch in diameter, the latter being the size of the red globules of the blood deprived of colouring matter. The retina appeared like a continuation of the bundles composing the optic nerve, consisting of the same sized globules connected into fibrous lines, and forming bundles radiating from the end of the nerve to the circumference of the retina, where they disappear, terminating in smooth membrane.*

The olfactory, optic, and auditory nerves, Ehrenberg found to consist of varicose or moniliform medullary tubules, directly continued from the moniliform tubes of the white cerebral matter. The moniliform tubules of the olfactory nerves are the thickest known, and vary from $\frac{1}{160}$th to $\frac{1}{300}$th part of a line in diameter. Those of the optic nerve are smaller, being from $\frac{1}{300}$th to $\frac{1}{500}$th part of a line in diameter; and tubules of the same dimensions are observed in the *chiasma* or decussation, in which the tubes are represented crossing each other; while the retina consists of articulated tubules $\frac{1}{2000}$th part of a line in diameter, traversing medullary grains about $\frac{1}{300}$th part of one line in diameter. It contains also mace-like or club-shaped bodies.

The structure of the auditory nerve is also peculiar. The simple tubules of this nerve Ehrenberg found considerably thicker than those of the others, and the spheroidal enlargements or *ampullulæ* flatter and less prominent, yet everywhere distinctly seen. In other respects it was similar to the olfactory and optic nerves.

The great sympathetic nerve, in like manner, consists of articulated cerebral tubules; but there is a mixture of simple cylindrical tubes at each extremity.

The nerves now specified, the olfactory, optic, auditory, and great sympathetic, are *articulated or moniliform nerves.*

All the other nerves consist, not of articulated or moniliform tubes, but of simple cylindrical tubules, somewhat larger, being from $\frac{1}{120}$th to $\frac{1}{110}$th part of one line in diameter. These tubules are surrounded and inclosed by vascular networks, and contained within ligamentous or neurilematic partitions; and they contain a medullary substance, semifluid, but capable of expression from them, and coagulation within their interior. These are *tubulated nerves.*†

The ganglia vary in structure. All consist of articulated or bead-like cerebral tubules, which, either alone, as in the *chiasma*, form the knot, or, as in all the ganglia of the sympathetic examined, are mingled with large cylindrical nervous tubules, inclosed within a close slender vascular network, between the meshes of which are deposited granules similar to those observed in the retina.

* Philosophical Transactions, 1821 and 1824.

† Beobachtung einer auffallenden bisher unbekannte structur des Seelenorgan im Menschen und Thieren ; and Edin. Med. and Surg. Journal, Vol. XLVIII. p. 282.

The tubules and cylinders now specified, which correspond with the primitive cylinders of Fontana, are merely in juxtaposition, and do not intermingle in substance with each other. The general accuracy of the facts now stated has been confirmed by Müller, Krause, Wagner, and Remak. Neither Ehrenberg nor Müller have been able to recognize in the roots of the sensiferous and motiferous nerves any essential difference in microscopical structure.

In the hypoglossal and glossopharyngeal nerves are seen only cylindrical tubes.

I have already shown what is meant by the organic end or termination of a nerve. Although the nervous trunks are distributed in every direction through the animal body, they do not terminate in all the tissues or organs indiscriminately; and have been observed to be lost in the following only. 1st, the proper organs of sensation, the eye, ear, nose, palate, and tongue; 2d, the muscles, whether subservient to voluntary or to involuntary motion, as the heart, stomach, intestines, &c.; 3d, the mucous surfaces; 4th, the skin; 5th, glands, salivary, liver, kidneys, &c.; 6th, bones.

Nerves, therefore, are not, strictly speaking, organs of general distribution. According to Bichat, they have never been traced to the following tissues:—the cartilages; both articular and of the cavities; fibrous textures, viz. periosteum, dura meninx, capsular ligaments, aponeurotic sheaths, aponeurosis in general, tendon and ligament; fibro-cartilaginous textures; those of the external ear, nose, trachea, and eyelids, (cartilages of other authors); the semilunar cartilages of the knee-joint; those of the temporo-maxillary articulation; those of the intervertebral spaces; marrow; the lymphatic glands.

To this we may add the testimony of a professed anatomist of the nervous system, whose reputation for patient and industrious research cannot fail to sanction every thing which he has advanced. " In every subject," says Walter of Berlin, " in which I was desirous to trace the nerves, I injected the arteries with red-coloured wax, the veins with green, and even the lymphatics with quicksilver, so that I was able to distinguish the nervous filaments from each of these orders of vessels. By this contrivance, though it occupied much time and labour, yet I was satisfactorily convinced that the pleura, the pericardium, the thoracic duct, and the peritoneum, receive no nerves. Nay, that, contrary to the opinions of the most eminent recent anatomists, no nerves terminate in the lymphatic or conglobate glands. Sometimes, indeed, these organs are perforated by one or two twigs, as I have often had occasion to observe; but they instantly proceed to the next place assigned to them, and in which they are finally lost."* If after this conclusion of Walter personal testimony can be of any use, I may add, that I have examined the *dura mater*, the periosteum, and most of the synovial membranes repeatedly, to discover nervous filaments in them, and always without success; and I may say the same regarding the absence or non-appearance of nerves in the peritoneum and pleura.

The nerves have different uses in the different organs and tissues to which they are distributed. 1. In the organs of sensation they receive the mechanical impressions made on the mechanical part of the organ. In the eye, the retina receives the last image formed by the transmitting powers of the transparent parts. In the ear, the terminations of the auditory nerve are affected by the oscillations or minute changes in the fluid of the labyrinth, occasioned by the motions of the tympanal bones. In the mucous membrane of the nasal passages, the filaments of the olfactory nerve are affected by aromatic particles, dissolved or suspended in the air. In the palate, tongue, and throat, the gustatory nerves are affected by sapid bodies dissolved in the mouth, or applied in a fluid state to the mucous membrane of that cavity. 2. In the system of voluntary muscles the nerves retain the action of the muscular fibres in a state of uniformity and equality, and keep them obedient to the will. In the involuntary muscles they appear merely to keep their action equable, regular, and uniform; and in both they maintain a communication, or consent or harmony of action between different parts of the same system of organs, or even between different organs concurring to the same function. 3. In the glandular organs the nerves certainly exercise some influence over the process of secretion; but what is the exact nature of this influence, or in what degree it takes place, is quite uncertain.

When we observe the nerves distributed to organs of sensation and organs of motion, it is a natural thought to inquire whether the nerves minister to both functions, and whether different nerves or different sorts of nerves minister to each function. It seems to have been an idea of considerable antiquity, that one set of nerves are sensiferous, and another set motiferous. Erasistratus derives the

* Praefat. Tab. Nerv. Thoracis et Abdominis, J. G. Walter.

nerves of motion from the brain and cerebellum, and those of sensation from the membranes; and Galen distinguishes the nerves into Νευρα Αισθετικα and Νευρα Κινητικα, the former, soft, from the brain, the latter, hard, from the spinal marrow. This distinction was not altogether lost sight of among the anatomists and physiogists of the eighteenth century; but it was rather maintained as a probable speculation, than elucidated and enforced as an established doctrine, pregnant with important results. It was recognized by Glisson, and taught by Boerhaave,* and received and promulgated by his pupils, Tissot and Van Eems;† but opposed by Haller‡ and Cullen. The distinction was, nevertheless, maintained by Lecat, Morin, and Pouteau, the last of whom was led from various examples of persons, who, after injuries, had lost sensation, but retained the power of movement, to espouse it with considerable energy.§

In 1784 George Prochaska, Professor of Anatomy at Vienna, published on the functions of the nerves a commentary, in which he gave, after Haller, Caldani, Whytt and Unzer, a more precise and correct view of the uses, properties, and powers of these organs, than had hitherto been formed. In this commentary he fully recognizes the distinction between sensorial nerves or those devoted to sensation, and motific nerves or those ministering to motion; he shows that sensorial impressions or impressions made on the sensitive nerves, are reflected or transmitted in a reflex direction to the motific nerves; that the latter nerves are thereby excited to action ; that the purpose of this reflex operation is the preservation of the individual; and that the whole are under the influence of the *Sensorium Commune.* He distinctly states, that this reflected action is

* Prælectiones Academicæ in proprias Institutiones Rei Medicæ, Editæ et Notis Auctæ, ab Alb. Haller. VII. Tomi. 12mo. Goettingae, 1745

† Hermanni Boerhaave, Phil. et Med. Doct., &c. Prælectiones Academicæ de Morbis Nervorum, Quas ex Manuscriptis collectas edi curavit Jacobus Van Eems, Medicus Leydensis. Tome I. and II. Lugduni Batavor. 1761. " Omnes (nervi) inserviunt motui vel famulantur sensui ; sed in illis qui cordi, pulmoni, hepati, aliisque partibus vitalibus destinati sunt, sensus non deprehenditur. Qui motui inserviunt, abeunt ad musculos, et in iis ita mollescunt, ut in verum quasi cerebrum degenerent. Ramuli, qui sensibus famulantur, in ipsis organis mollitie fere diffluunt, uti patet in expansione nervi optici, olfactorii, ubi se applicat ad os ethmoides, et acoustici in labyrintho," p. 261.

‡ Elementa Physiologiæ, Liber X. Sect. VIII. § xxii., Tomus Quartus, p. 389.

§ Memoire et Recherches sur la difference a etablir entre les nerfs du sentiment et les nerfs du mouvement, a l'occasion de quelques observations sur cette espece rare de paralysie, qui prive un membre de tout sentiment, sans lui oter l'usage du mouvement   Oeuvres Postumes de M. Pouteau, Docteur en Medecine et Chirurgien en Chef de l'Hotel-dieu de Lyon. Tome II. p. 480. Paris, 1789.

not regulated by physical laws, where the angle of reflection is equal to the angle of incidence, but obeys peculiar laws impressed by nature, as it were, on the sensorium, and which laws we can understand from their effects alone. This reflex action further takes place either without or with the consciousness of the soul. The motion of the heart, stomach, and intestines, is independent of the cognizance of the soul; and in many other instances of sensorial impressions being transmitted to motific nerves, though the soul is conscious, it can neither prevent them nor promote them.[*]

The commentary of Prochaska is the first precise view of the functions of the nervous system in modern times; and the first in which the automatic and instinctive phenomena enumerated by Whytt are referred to a reflex operation.

In 1811, Sir Charles Bell, in a tract containing *the Idea of a New Anatomy of the Brain*, stated that he had proved experimentally that " the posterior *fasciculus* of spinal nerves, which are gangliophorous, might be detached from its origin without convulsing the muscles of the back ; whereas, on touching the anterior *fasciculus* with the point of the knife, these muscles were immediately convulsed." From this it seemed a probable inference that gangliophorous nerves had no concern in motion, and that nerves void of ganglion ministered in some way to that function.

In 1818, Charles Francis Bellingeri published at Turin,[†] a Dissertation treating, among other subjects, of the anatomy and physiology of the fifth and seventh pairs of nerves. In this he showed that the great portion of the fifth pair or trifacial nerve, which forms the large semilunar plexus called Gasserian ganglion, is a nerve, not of motion but of sensation; that its three branches are distributed to certain parts of the eye, the nasal cavities, the palate and tongue ; ministering in these parts not to motion, but to sensation, and probably to circulation, nutrition, and secretion ; and that the small branch of that nerve (*nervus masticatorius*), is distributed to muscles, (*temporalis, masseter, pterygoideus, buccinatorius,*) and is a

---

[*] Georgii Prochaska, M. D., Professoris Anatomiæ, Physiologiæ et Morborum Oculorum in Universitate Vindobonensi, Operum Minorum. Pars II. Viennæ, 1800. 8vo. Commentatio de Functionibus Systematis Nervosi.

[†] Caroli Francisci Bellingeri E. S. Agatha Derthonensi. Phil. et Med. Doct. Amplessim Med. Collegii Candidati Dissertatio Inauguralis quam publicæ defendebat. In Athenaeo Regio Anno MDCCCXVIII. Die IX. Maii ; hora IX.na. matutina. Augustæ Turinorum. 8vo. 1818. Ex Anatome ; De Nervis Faciei ; Ex Physiologia ; Quinti et Septimi Paris Functiones, &c.

nerve of motion. He also showed that the seventh pair, or lateral facial, presides over sensation and motion in the functions of the head, face, and neck, but mostly over motion.

In 1821, Sir Charles Bell undertook to establish the principle, that of the two nervous trunks distributed to the face, viz. the *trigeminus*, or fifth cerebral nerve, and the *portio dura*, or seventh cerebral nerve, the lateral facial, the former presides over the sensations or common sensibility of the head and face; that it also possesses branches going to the muscles of mastication; whereas the latter nerve regulates the muscular motions of the lips, nostrils, and *velum palati*, and especially in associated action with the motions of respiration.

About the same time Magendie claimed the merit of showing experimentally the fact of the distinction between nerves ministering to sensation and nerves ministering to motion, and of proving that, of the double row of nervous roots issuing in parallel lines from the lateral regions of the spinal chord, the anterior are destined for motion, and the posterior for sensation.

Lastly, Mr Mayo, partly by dissection, partly by experimental inquiry and reasoning, arrived at the conclusion that almost all the branches of the large or gangliophorous portion of the trifacial nerves are nerves of sensation, while those of the small fasciculus, which is void of ganglion, are nerves of motion.

In this manner, by successive steps, has been established one of the most important doctrines on the functions of the nervous chords in modern physiology; and its justice has been confirmed by the labours of many observers. The distinction is most clearly proved by the original experiment of Sir Charles Bell. If the spine be laid open, especially in a cold-blooded animal, as a frog, and the posterior or gangliophorous roots alone be irritated, no movement is produced; but the moment the anterior roots are touched, the extremities are agitated by active convulsive motions.

Of the cerebral nerves, the first or olfactory, the second or optic, and the eighth or auditory, are pure nerves of proper sensation, and are distributed to the sensitive parts of the eye, the nasal cavities, and the cochlea and labyrinth respectively. The third, fourth, and part of the sixth, or abducent, are motific nerves connected with the movements of the eye. The fifth or trifacial is a very peculiar nerve. The gangliophorous, or rather plexiform part of it, communicates with all the organs of proper sensation,—the eye, the ear in a small degree, the nasal cavities largely, and the palate, mouth, and tongue largely ; and it is distributed extensively along with the minute arteries of the face. Of this arrangement the result is, that it is a nerve neither of vision, nor of hearing, of smell nor of taste, or deglutition nor of touch, or physiognomical expression, exclusively, but over the whole of these faculties and their proper organs exercises a general modulating power. It maintains between them a mutual consent or harmony of action, absolutely necessary to the due separate exercise of each and the conjoined exercise of all. Lastly, by accompanying the arteries of the face, it regulates the circulation of that region, and may be the means of maintaining between the brain and the facial circulation those conditions and expressions which arise from various mental emotions ; as paleness, blushing, indignation, the sense of joy, triumph, the sublime, and similar emotions.

Not less peculiar is the seventh, the small sympathetic of Winslow. Though mostly a motiferous nerve, yet it ministers to mo tions of a particular order. It is, however, as a nerve distributed to the skin of the face, a nerve contributing to, if not regulating animal sensation and involuntary motion. It is, in fact, as shown by Wrisberg, a double nerve, the large portion of which is devoted to the purposes of animal life, and the small one to those of organic life. It is a musculo-cutaneous nerve of the head and face.

In proceeding further in explaining the respective functions of the nerves, it is requisite to keep in view not only their gangliophorous character and the reverse, but their position as anterior and as posterior nerves, and nerves consisting of anterior and posterior roots.

The ninth pair, (*nervus glosso-pharyngæus*,) consists of two parts, one large, completing sensation to the root of the tongue and pharynx, the other smaller, moving the pharynx, and connected, notwithstanding, with the tenth pair, pneumogastric, and the great sympathetic.

The tenth pair, (*nervus vagus*,) or pneumogastric nerve, is chiefly a sensiferous nerve, regulating the sensations of the larynx, the œsophagus and stomach, and the lungs, and placing these organs in harmony as to function. One particularly, the recurrent branches, appear to be motiferous. All the other branches appear to regulate circulation and secretion.

To the accessory nerve, or eleventh pair, seems to belong the function of placing the pulmonary and laryngeal divisions of the pneumogastric in harmony and relation with the external muscles of the back and lateral regions of the neck.

Lastly, the hypoglossal, or twelfth pair, having mostly an anterior origin, are motiferous. They form the motiferous nerves of the muscles of the tongue.

It is to be observed, nevertheless, that though this distinction in functions belongs to particular nerves, yet nerves ministering to sensation, and regulating organic or involuntary functions, and nerves ministering to motion, and regulating either voluntary motions, instinctive motions, or involuntary, but associated and necessary motions, are often closely connected, and proceed together in the same sheath, or in close apposition to the same organ. This, which is observed in the fifth, the seventh, the ninth, tenth, and eleventh, is rendered necessary by the offices which the organs have to perform. The impulse or impression is communicated to the organ, and received by its sensiferous nerves. By these the proper sensation is transmitted, and the motiferous nerves are excited to action. This appears to be the mode in which such actions as sneezing, coughing, yawning, deglutition, and numerous other instinctive and associated actions are called into operation.

Of the spinal nerves it is almost superfluous to speak after the explanations now given. The splanchnic or great sympathetic appears to be a nerve of organic sensibility and impression, and as such regulates the circulation of the abdominal organs, and transmits their impressions to the central connections. The further continuance of these by its spinal connections establishes a harmonic action with the spinal marrow, always for good purposes, but often under disease producing painful and destructive effects.*

This may be said to comprehend all that is accurately known regarding the uses of the nerves. Every other doctrine relating to sensibility, sympathy, irritability, &c. is either unfounded, not proved, or altogether imaginary and hypothetical.

In the fœtus the nerves are developed with remarkable perfection. I cannot speak from personal observation much earlier than the sixth month, when I have found the nerves of the extremities

---

* For further information and illustrations of the principles now stated, I refer the reader to Arnold's Illustrations of the Nerves of the Head and Face,* and an account of the same work in the forty-third volume of the Edinburgh Medical and Surgical Journal, January 1835, p. 225.

---

* Frederici Arnoldi Icones Nervorum Capitis. Heidelbergæ, 1834. Folio.

and voluntary muscles large and distinct. At the eighth month they are still more conspicuous. The anterior crural nerves are in the form of flat white cords one and a-half line broad, and their branches like good sized threads. The sciatic is still more distinct. In the form of a thick cylindrical cord, fully a line in diameter, and not unlike a piece of whip-cord, it is tough, stringy, and resists tension, and its constituent threads are well marked. I immersed a portion of this nerve three and a-half inches long in *aqua potassæ*, when it first became much firmer and denser than before, assumed in two days the satin fibrous appearance first described by Fontana, and at length by solution of the nervous matter was separated into chords and neurilematic canals. In this state, preserved in spirit of turpentine, it conveys a tolerably correct idea of the arrangement of the neurilematic canals.

The nerves of the involuntary muscles are equally distinct in proportion. Those of the lung, heart, and splanchnic system are distinct and manifest at the eighth month.

The neurilem is much more vascular in the fœtus than in the adult. In the same fœtus of about eight months I found the neurilem of the sciatic nerve, from the ischiatic notch to its divarication in the ham, covered with a thick net-work of minute vessels, all injected with dark blood.

Section II.

1. *Inflammation, spontaneous and from injury,—Nerve-ach, Neuritis. Neuralgia. (Neurilemmia.)* Various observers, as Boerhaave, have doubted the spontaneous occurrence of inflammation of a nerve (*neuritis;*) and certainly the disease is not very common. Others, on the contrary, have gone to the opposite extreme, and thought that it was a frequent affection. Peter Frank, for instance, and Joseph Frank, maintain that there is no doubt that *neuritis* arises spontaneously, and that it is a lesion not uncommon ; and in this they are supported by the testimony of Nasse, Nicod, and other authorities. It is nevertheless as a primary affection, and not induced by injury, or previous disease of the bones, or of the soft textures, not very frequent.

When it takes place, the morbid action may affect either the nerve-coat or the nervous matter, or both. In the first case the neurilema is thickened, hardened, and rendered rigid. The ner-

vous matter is also enlarged ; and often a perceptible enlargement
is formed at the point at which this morbid orgasm is established.
Lymph and blood are also effused; and to this, indeed, the enlargement is owing. Inflammation of the neurilema is certainly a common accompaniment, if not a cause of neuralgic pain.

When inflammation affects the nervous matter, it may produce
softening from slight effusion of serum or suppuration, or induration from the effusion of lymph. Our knowledge of these effects
is obtained mostly either from injuries of nerves, as when they are
torn, bruised, or divided, or from observing the results of experiments on the lower animals. In this point of view, I shall have
occasion to recur to the subject afterwards.

Nervous tissue, therefore, is liable to inflammation. This may
arise spontaneously, or in consequence of injury, as contusion, wound,
laceration, ligature, &c. It is accompanied first with gnawing pain,
which is oftener periodical than constant, spreading along the course
of the nerve, sometimes its branches, with a sense of heat often very
disagreeable, and a peculiar tenderness of the surface. After some
time the pain is less violent, but more constant; and more or less
derangement in the functions of the parts to which the nerve goes
takes place. The skin becomes numb, cold, and insensible. Of
muscular parts the motions are variously disordered, becoming irregular, spasmodic, and little under the influence of the will, so as
to constitute convulsions, and finally being lost in different degrees,
so as to cause palsy more or less complete. This constitutes one
form of *neuralgia* or nerve-ach. It is most frequent in the sciatic,
partly in consequence of its exposed situation, and sometimes in
consequence of actual violence locally inflicted, as in falling. (*Is-
chias nervosa* of Cotunnius.) I have, however, seen this affection
arising in other nerves; for example, the median or spiral, in the
arm, and sometimes the posterior tibial, in the leg, in consequence
of similar causes. In one instance it was confined with accuracy
to the anterior branch of the radial nerve, which goes to the thumb
and index finger. In such cases the inflammatory action is confined pretty accurately to a part of the neurilematic coat, which becomes firm, vascular, and more or less tender.

In neuralgia of the face (*tic douloureux*, Fothergill,) (*prosopalgia*,
Frank, Weisse,) it is not easy to say what is the pathological cause.
It is undoubted that it is seated in the nerve ; and though some
forms of this malady evidently depend on inflammation of the neu-

rilema, yet others of them, which are of long continuance, and are attended by other peculiarities, are not perhaps to be ascribed to this cause. It is not requisite to suppose that the long continuance of this action, without producing suppuration or other changes, is an argument against its inflammatory character. The inflammation may be, like those in fibrous tissue, of long continuance, without inducing any other effect save that of thickening and stiffening by effusion of lymph.

One of the most painful and least managable forms of nerve-ach is that which is produced by previous disease either of a bone or its periosteal covering. Chronic periosteal inflammation, for instance, attacks the bones of the face, and affects some one of the *foramina*, through which a nervous chord emerges. The periosteum becomes thickened as the periosteal disease proceeds; the bone itself is affected, and *exostosis* is formed. This tumour compresses the nerve and its covering, which are also perhaps inflamed; and if the newly formed bone is sharp, rough, or spicular, by lacerating and stretching the nerve, it causes to the patient acute pain and much suffering.

Neuritis should be distinguished from *Neurilemmia*, though often they are associated and consequently cannot be distinguished. Joseph Frank, nevertheless, thinks that the constancy of the pain in the former, and its occasional remission and periodical recurrence in the latter, may serve to distinguish the two affections.

An idea has been advanced by Reil, that general inflammation of the neurilema takes place in typhus fever, and is the pathological cause of that disease.* That the vessels of this tissue may be gorged, and their blood poisoned and rendered hurtful, in common with those of every other, is exceedingly probable, and may be often the case. But it is manifest that this is one only of many simultaneous effects; and it is further evident, that neither observation nor anatomical inspection can justify the conclusion, that inflammation of the neurilema is the pathological cause of fever.

2. *Neurilemmia Chronica.* Inflammation of nervous tissue may terminate, 1*st*, in resolution; 2*d*, in effusion of lymph; 3*d*, in ulceration; or, 4*th*, it may induce a low chronic action, accompanied with enlargement of the nerve, or morbid growth by deposition of new matter. These phenomena are most distinctly seen in the changes which follow wounds of nerves. In this case effusion of lymph is common, and is not unfrequently succeeded either by lo-

* Fieberlehre, Band. IV. p. 56.

cal palsy, or by a train of symptoms similar to nerve-ache. (*Neuralgia.*)

Dr Denmark saw a contused wound of the radial nerve produce neuralgic symptoms requiring amputation.* Charles Bell saw the same result succeed contusion without wound in the popliteal nerve, and the inflammation occasioned by the application of quicksilver to the same nerve.† Mr Wardrope saw neuralgic symptoms succeed a puncture of the finger, in which he thinks a nerve was injured;‡ and in another instance similar effects from wound of the thumb, in which a branch of the radial nerve close to the digital artery was punctured.§ In venesection it sometimes happens when the cutaneour nerves are pierced, that numbness and tetanic stiffness, with spasmodic twitches, are felt in the arm or fore-arm for some time after. These symptoms it is justifiable to ascribe to chronic inflammation, with thickening and induration of the nerve.‖ (Denmark.) This thickening depends partly on extreme and undue distension of the neurilematic vessels, partly on exudation of lymph, which proceeds from the same source.

In the remarkable case described by Mr Pearson, in which he ascribes severe and complicated neuralgic and paralytic symptoms to "a morbid condition of the nerves distributed to the extremity of the thumb,"¶ this morbid condition was probably chronic inflammation of some part of their neurilematic covering.

Patients who have undergone amputation sometimes complain of acute pain in a single point of the stump, liable to aggravation when touched, and spreading up the limb in the course of the nerves. It is usual to ascribe such complaints to implication of the nerve in the cicatrix; but it is more likely that a minute branch has been included in the ligature of some of the vessels. In such circumstances it is manifest that a cause is given for the most severe and obstinate form of neurilematic inflammation. *Lastly,* I may notice, that to the same head is to be referred a painful gnawing sensation of contraction ascending up the arm from the finger, which I have

---

* Medico-Chirurgical Transactions, Vol. IV. p. 48. London, 1813.

† Surgical Observations, &c. By Charles Bell. London, 1816, p. 440. Case of Baron Driesen.

‡ Medico-Chirurgical Transactions. Lond. Vol. VIII. p. 246.

§ Medico-Chirurgical Transactions, Vol. XII. p. 205.

‖ "The nerve was found thickened to twice its natural diameter, and contracted."— Transact. Vol. IV. p. 51.

¶ Account of Remarkable Symptoms, &c. By John Pearson, Esq. &c. Medico-Chirurg. Trans. Vol. VIII. p. 252.

seen follow the cõmmunication of the inflammation of whitloe to one
of the small branches of the radial nerve.

3. *Ulceration* of nervous tissue, though rare, may occur either
after wound, laceration, or contusion of a nerve, as in the case of
ligature, or in consequence of an ulcer of the contiguous parts
spreading to the nerve. It does not appear to occur spontaneously
after inflammation.

4. *Division and Re-union; Excision or Removal, and Reproduction.* When a nerve is cut across, no doubt can be entertained
that it is again reunited. But it is questionable whether it is reunited by simple adhesion, by the growth of new nerve, or by the
growth of new matter entirely different. The latter point has been
a particular subject of inquiry to many anatomists and physiologists
in the case of excision, or removal of portions of a nervous trunk.
Though the nerves have been divided by many, the first accurate
experiments made with a view to ascertain their reproductive power
were performed by Cruikshank. This anatomist found, that, when
a portion of nerve is removed by incision, its place is supplied by
blood and lymph, which first becomes vascular and organized, and
is afterwards converted into a substance of the same colour as
nerve; and which, though not fibrous, he regarded as nervous.*
These experiments were repeated by Fontana, who, after much
hesitation, came to the conclusion that nervous matter is reproduced;† by Arnemann, who denied that the new-formed matter is
nerve;‡ by Haighton, who inferred that this substance is really and
truly nerve;§ by Baronio,‖ Michaelis,¶ and Meyer,** who have
arrived nearly at the same general result, and assert that nervous
filaments may be traced through the new matter of the cicatrix.

According to Arnemann, who describes the process of reunion
particularly, shortly after section, the end of the upper portion of
cut nerve inflames and swells, forming a grayish, long, and hard

---

* Experiments on the Nerves, particularly on their Reproduction. By William
Cruikshank, F. R. S. &c.   Phil. Transactions, 1795.   Part I. p. 177.

† Experiences sur la Reproductions des Nerfs, apud Traité sur la Venin de la Vi-
pere, &c. Par Felix Fontana. Tom. II.   Florence, 1781, p. 177.

‡ Ueber die Reproduction der Nerven.   Goettingen, 1786.   Versuche Ueber die
Regeneration der Nerven.   Ibid. 1787.

§ An Experimental Inquiry on the Reproduction of Nerves.   By John Haighton,
M. D.   Philosophical Transact.   Lond. 1795.   Part I. p. 190.

‖ Memorie de Matematica e Fisica, Vol. IV.

¶ Fr. Michaelis Ueber die Regeneration der Nerven.   Cassel, 1785

** Meyer apud Reil Archiv. für die Physiologie, II. Band. p. 449.

knot; the end of the lower portion undergoes the same change, but in less degree; the knotty parts unite; and the substance which thus connects the cut portions of nerve, though it continues hard and large, is considered as either nervous matter, or as containing a considerable portion of that substance, for the sensations and motions of the parts are in most cases restored shortly after union.

This process, according to Bichat, therefore, consists of four stages. 1st, After incision the cut ends inflame, and the capillaries of the divided portions effuse coagulating or organizable lymph, which is penetrated with blood-vessels. 2d, This effusion, which takes place chiefly from the neurilema, forms a sort of cellular tissue, in which nervous matter is afterwards deposited. This cellular tissue, and the new matter in general, is in quantity according to the spaces to be filled up. If it be large, the new matter is augmented by successive effusion and granulation; and when small, the connection by deposition appears to be very speedily effected. 3d, The adhesion of the individual granulating bodies and consolidation of the part. 4th, The deposition or exhalation of nervous substance in the new matter.* Is this, which is said to be the last stage of the process, not co-existent and simultaneous with the effusion of new matter in general? What are the proofs which show that the proper nervous matter is last deposited?

When a nerve has been divided under circumstances which prevent it from uniting in any manner with its detached segment, as in amputation, the extremity enlarges and becomes vascular, from the neurilematic vessels assuming the inflammatory action; blood and lymph are effused both from the cut extremity and into the interstices of the neurilematic canals; more or less adhesion is contracted with the contiguous textures; and when the active state of this process has subsided, a hard knotty tubercle is left in the site of the cut extremity. This tubercle is at first rendered vascular, afterwards grayish, solid, and so firm that the knife may be blunted in dividing it. (Arnemann.) The changes now mentioned I have often traced in the surface of stumps during healing. The size and shape of the tubercle vary according to circumstances not well ascertained. When situate not exactly at the extremity, as observed by Van Horne,† it merely shows that the inflammatory process had spread farther up the nerve than usual.

* Anat. Gen. Tom. I. Art. iii. sect. 3, p. 176.

† De iis quæ in partibus membri amputatione vulneratis notanda sunt. Lugduni Batav. 1803.

It was at one time supposed that the morbid growth called *blood-like fungus (fungus hæmatodes)* was peculiar to the nervous tissue. This idea is now known to be incorrect; and it appears that there is no process of disorganization peculiar to nerve, and not occurring in other textures.

Nervous texture is sometimes unnaturally soft; as in dropsy, fatal hemorrhages, and diseases of long wasting. (Autenrieth.) Is it ever unusually soft primarily, and without being the result of another disease? It undergoes mollescence (*ramollissement*) in consequence of mechanical injury; but it is exceedingly doubtful if this takes place spontaneously.

4. Local forms of palsy, that is, loss of mobility in an order of muscles, or in a limb, is a common result of injury done to a nerve or nerves. The effect of such injury is in general to produce inflammation or extravasation, and subsequent destruction of the proper nervous matter. It becomes soft, pulpy, and disorganized. In this state the nerve is no longer fit to perform its usual functions, and it loses the influence which it possessed over the muscles to which it is distributed. In the course of this process irregular motions, or what are termed spasms, not unfrequently occur.

5. *Tetanus.*—Punctured or lacerated wounds of nervous tissue may be followed by tonic spasms, (*tetanus,*) or by convulsive motions in general. It is uncertain in this case whether the irregular motions depend on injury of the nerve, or its neurilematic sheath.

The following facts I have ascertained in several cases in which tetanus followed fracture of the fingers with contused wounds of the soft parts.

In two cases I may mention, in which the injuries were very similar, viz. fracture of the middle phalanges of the finger, the symptoms of tetanus came on about three weeks after the infliction of the injury, and proceeded in the course of a few days to the fatal termination. In the first case, the body of a cart, which had been emptied, and for this purpose had been raised, fell on the hand of the person, and caused fracture of the bones of the finger with contusion. In the second case, the mast of a boat which had been raised, and was standing not securely, fell on the hand of the person, and in like manner produced fracture of the phalanges of the thumb.

In both cases the nerve-coat connected with the injured part was reddened, vascular, and injected, and manifestly thickened, while the nervous matter of the nerve was reddened, swelled, and softened.

In the first of these cases, which took place in the person of a young man, who had been brought from Musselburgh to the Edinburgh Royal Infirmary, I examined the whole spinal chord with care. I found it quite sound, except in the cervical portion, where the envelopes were reddened, and had evidently been the seat of inflammatory injection. Beneath these envelopes, the spinal chord in the cervical portion was reddened and softened for the space of between one inch and a-half and two inches. So far as I could determine, this was the point which gives origin to, or is connected with those branches of the cervical nerves which proceed to and chiefly form the brachial plexus.

In this case, therefore, I inferred, that the injury done the finger, and the subsequent inflammation, especially of the digital nerve and its nerve-coat, had been reflected, as it were, to the spinal origins of these nerves, and thus induced inflammation and irritation of the spinal marrow, then softening; and that these were the efficient causes of the tetanic symptoms and their fatal termination.

In the second case, in which the patient died under the care of my friend, Dr Paterson of Leith, and by whose attention I was present at the inspection, we found the contused ends of the nerve red and softened, and its tunic in like manner red, injected, and thickened; and in the same manner, on inspecting the spinal marrow, a portion of that organ in the cervical region not less than two inches in length, very distinctly reddened and softened, indeed, quite creamy, while the rest of the chord was firm and of normal consistence.

The spot thus affected with softening corresponded very accurately with the origins or spinal connections of the cervical nerves which contribute to form the brachial plexus.

It is proper to say, that I had mentioned to Dr Paterson what I expected to find in the spinal marrow, and my reasons for this expectation as founded on the facts of the previous case. The discovery of the connection between the inflamed nerve and the reflected irritation and inflammatory softening of the spinal chord was not the effect of accident.

I have repeatedly seen the nerve or nerves of parts injured and contused in tetanic cases, presenting redness, vascularity, thickening of the neurilemma, and softening of the nerve. But I have not had opportunities of examining the spinal chord in any other case.

I think, nevertheless, that it is reasonable to infer, that the irritation is propagated from the injured parts in the reflex direction to the

3

spinal connections of the nerves; that there it is followed by another irritation and by inflammation of the spinal marrow; and that the last is the cause of the tetanic symptoms. This further seems most probable when we consider that some time always elapses between the date of the infliction of the injury, and that of the development of the tetanic symptoms; that is to say, the establishment of the inflammatory irritation of the spinal marrow.

At the same time, to render this theory of the cause of tetanus complete, it would be requisite to inspect in the same manner cases in which fractures or other injuries of the lower extremities had been followed by tetanus. This I have not had opportunities of doing.

Traumatic tetanus is almost invariably a fatal disease; and the reason of this is, that it follows or is caused by a severe lesion of the spinal chord at parts essential to the continuance of life.

6. *Tumours.* A. (*Neuroma* of Odier.) Tumours of various size and structure have been found in nervous trunks. These may be either common to nerve with other tissues, or proper.* Of the former an example is given in the encysted tumour (*hygroma*) which Cheselden† found in the centre of the cubital (*ulnar*) nerve. Of that met with by Gooch in the axillary nerve, the account is not so distinct.‡ Sir Everard Home mentions a tumour removed from the middle of the right arm by John Hunter, and in which the musculo-cutaneous nerve was found imbedded, divided into two portions, each much flattened.§ This tumour appears to have originated in the neurilem. In another instance Sir E. Home removed a tumour, in which one of the large nerves of the axillary plexus was encased.

Lastly, Odier describes, under the name of *neuroma*, in the person of a member of his own family, an instance of tumour in the radial nerve, in which its component threads were separated from each other in the manner of a fan, or like the ribs of a melon,

---

* It is singular to remark with how little precision pathological writers speak of these tumours. Odier compares the one mentioned by Cheselden to a firm one noticed by Gooch, and to the yellow-whitish tumour which he met in the radial nerve of a relative. Meckel also refers to Cheselden's case in speaking of tumours, considerably hard, roundish, yellow-whitish, of fibrous structure, and approaching to fibro-cartilage. The case of Cheselden should have been carefully distinguished from the tumours intended to exemplify this description. For that surgeon states specifically, that " it was of the cystic kind, but contained a transparent jelly." It was in truth an instance of *hygroma*, and, as I have stated in the text, it was common to the nervous and other tissues.

† The Anatomy of the Human Body, p. 256. London, 1778 and 1784. 12th Edit.
‡ Cases and Practical Remarks in Surgery, Vol. II.
§ Trans. of a Society, &c. Vol. II. p. 152. An Account, &c.

while the centre was filled with white and yellow matter, effused in the intervals of an infinite number of transparent vessels, mutually interlacing.* Examples of similar tumours are mentioned by Marandel,† Neumann,‡ Von Siebold,§ Spangenberg,‖ Alexander,¶ Mojon, and Covercelli.**

Of the cases recorded by Von Siebold, one occurred in the person of an aged female with varicose veins of both legs and feet. Two small nervous tumours were situate near each other at the instep, between the ankles. They caused severe pains, which were alleviated neither by narcotics nor stimulants. His father applied caustic, and the disease disappeared, but soon returned. Von Siebold himself again employed caustic more efficaciously, and extirpated the disease.

The case recorded by Neumann took place in an old man of 70, on the middle and lower part of whose fore-arm a tumour as large as a pea, very painful on being touched or sustaining the slightest pressure, had continued for thirty years. It was ascribed to a violent blow received on the arm. The skin covering it was healthy and movable, though the tumour itself was immovable, in consequence of attachments to muscles. Neumann recommended excision. But the surgeon was afraid, lest, in dividing the nerve he should injure the artery, and he attempted to remove it by exciting suppuration produced by the application of caustic. Meanwhile the patient was destroyed by apoplexy.

Of the cases described by Spangenberg and Alexander, two occurred to Dubois. One as large as a walnut, was situate on the patella. Another, as large as a middle-sized melon, was connected with the median nerve of the right arm. It was slightly movable without discoloration of the skin. Both were extirpated.

The great evil of these tumours is, that from their relations they cause much pain. Thus Nicod states, that in 1816 he removed from the chest of a female aged 40, a lenticular tumour from six to seven lines in diameter, movable in the subcutaneous cellular tissue, apparently covered by the skin, which was attenuated so

---

* Manuel de Medecine Pratique, &c. Par Louis Odier, Doct. et Prof. a Paris et Geneve, 1811. Cl. IV. Ord. v. 17, p. 362.

† Bulletin apud Journal de Medecine continue, Vol. XI.

‡ In Von Siebold Sammlung Chirurg. Beobachtungen.

§ Von Siebold I. Band. p. 80, 82.

‖ In Horn Archiv. V. Band, 2 Heft, St. 2. 306.

¶ F. S. Alexander, Dissertatio de Tumoribus Nervorum. Lugd. B. 1810.

** Chiron, Band 1. St. 3; and Memorie della Societate di Genova.

much as to present a faint brownish tint. This colour, with the severe pains which totally prevented sleep for months, made it be taken by several medical men for cancerous. It was encysted, and its removal was followed by sound sleep, which lasted that day and the ensuing night and day.*

Some years ago I saw, in the arm of a woman about thirty, an oblong pyriform hard body, extending along the inner margin of the *biceps flexor*, in the site of the brachial vessels and nerves, to the anterior tuberosity of the *humerus*. It was attended with prickling pain, and alternating with numbness of the arm, fore-arm, and fingers. From these symptoms (Home,) the absence of pulsation and its situation, no doubt could be entertained that it implicated the brachial nerve. The woman refused, however, to submit to have it removed; and I have not since heard of her. The evidence of dissection as to its precise nature is therefore still wanting.

It is not easy to determine which of these tumours are to be regarded as common, or proper to the nervous chord or the neurilematic tissue. It is manifest that the case of Cheselden, and perhaps that of Gooch, and the second one of Home, were common. That of Odier, and the first of Home, appear to have been seated either in the neurilema, or its cellular tissue, and probably consisted in deposition of new matter in the interstices of the neurilematic canals. In the former case the filaments of the nerve are more or less expanded and separated. In the latter they pass through the body of the tumour in a mass.

The anatomical structure of these tumours is probably most fully illustrated by a case recorded by Alexander, in which a tumour as large as a hen's egg was removed from the left arm of a soldier of 19 years of age, and in whom it was believed to be seated in the ulnar nerve. In this case the neurilema formed an external capsule. The ulnar nerve divided longitudinally for nearly half an inch above the tumour was found sound, to the point where it was dilated; as it was also sound below the tumour, where in like manner about half an inch of the nerve was removed by the incisions, which embraced the longitudinal extent of four inches.

The colour of the tumour was the same as that of the nerve, though more brilliant. The naked eye distinguished longitudinal fibres, invested by some transverse fibres. It was hard to the touch, elastic, and it was then observed to enclose a liquid.

When divided longitudinally, the external wall was more resist-

* Nouveau Journal de Medecine, Nov. 1818.

ing than that of the nerve, and of a consistence about tendinous, but not cartilaginous. By a small opening there escaped a limpid fluid similar to serum, and coagulating; and when this was forced out by the elasticity of the external tunic, the volume of the tumour diminished one-third.

The external wall or neurilematic tunic of the tumour was hard and thicker than in the sound state of the nerve. At the middle of the tumour this capsule was expanded into a thin though consistent membrane. The inner surface of the capsule, when examined by a lens, presented fine parallel fibres.

The cavity formed within the neurilema was lined all over by a dense pulpy plate; leaving in the centre of the tumour an oblong cavity like that of an egg, in which was contained the sero-albuminous fluid.

In the interior of the tumour, the pulp, differing from that in the sound state, presented a morbid aspect, well marked, was half an inch thick, presented no straight parallel fibres, but a mass of numerous small round bodies, firm and covered by an envelope, similar to fibres twisted in the spiral direction, aggregated, resembling those which Fontana recognized, by the aid of the microscope, in the medullary matter of the nerves, and in the cortical matter of the brain.

In another case recorded by Alexander, in which a very painful neuromatic tumour was extirpated by Reich from the right elbow of a gentleman of 44, in whom it had been growing since the eleventh year of his age; though it was not so easy to ascertain the anatomical characters, it was observed, that the nervous fibrils were enlarged, and filled with serous fluid at the place of the tumour; that their neurilema was indurated and contained a fluid; and that in this investment were seen firm tendinous fibres.[*]

Cruveilhier represents a spheroidal tumour the size of a small nut, which was formed in the substance of the radial nerve, where it passes between the *supinator longus* and the *brachiaeus anticus*. The long supinator was thinned, and thrown outward by the tumour on which it was moulded. The substance of the nerve seemed interrupted at the site of the tumour; yet most of its filaments were continuous though separated, and could be traced, some before and others behind the tumour. Several were lost in the fibrous covering; none traversed the tumour. Cruveilhier considers this a carcinomatous tumour, and the effect of secondary cancerous infection.[†] If that view be correct, it should not be regarded as *neuroma*.

---

[*] Observatio secunda.   [†] Livraison xxxv.

' The gangliophorous or organic nerves, as well as those of animal life, are liable to the formation of tumours. Cruveilhier represents in the cervical ganglions of the great sympathetic oblong spheroidal tumours of fibrous character, which had been formed in these ganglions. These tumours he considers as instances of the fibrous development with hypertrophy; a statement from which little is to be learned.* It is certain that the ganglions are much enlarged, and that their substance is indurated; that these swellings are contained within a tumour or capsule of some thickness and firmness; and that the substance enclosed presents a fibrous arrangement, yet with some remains of the original matter of the ganglion. They seem, indeed, to be examples of *neuroma.*

' On the whole, it seems probable that the neuromatic tumour is not in all cases the same; that sometimes it is the result of sero-albuminous fluid effused interstitially in the texture of the nerve at one point in consequence of chronic inflammation, and afterwards coagulating; that sometimes, from the operation of the same cause, a cavity or cavities are formed, containing sero-albuminous fluid uncoagulated; that the nervous fibrils are seldom destroyed, but are often separated and stretched, irritated, and compressed; and that never in the proper neuroma is new or heterologous matter deposited.

B. *Neuromation,* (Νευρομάτιον.) (Subcutaneous tubercle of Mr Wood.) By this name may be distinguished those pisiform tumours or hard tubercles which form beneath the skin, and of which I had already occasion to speak when enumerating the morbid states of the filamentous tissue. I then had occasion to remark, that there is strong reason for thinking that this painful disease consists in the hard body being seated in some of the nervous twigs beneath the skin. I am now to advance such evidence as may show, that little doubt can be entertained that this is the true pathology of the subcutaneous tubercle.

Valsalva had early observed an instance of a small hard tumour at the ankle of a lady, in whom it continued from the 16th year, and gave rise to pain so intense, that she would herself have attempted extirpation, had she not been prevented by her domestics. It was removed and the pain returned no more.

Hard, painful, pisiform tumours beneath the skin are next mentioned by Cheselden, who met with three cases in which he employed excision, without being aware that they might be seated in the nerves or their coverings.† The next recorded case is that given by

* Livraison I. Planche iiiieme.
† Anatomy of the Human Body. By William Cheselden, p. 136.

Dr Short, who in 1720 found in the leg one causing epilepsy, and which he removed by excision.* Camper is, so far as I am aware, the first anatomist, who remarks the occasional occurrence of minute hard tubercles, not larger than a pea, in the cutaneous nerves; where he represents them as giving rise to excruciating darting pains night and day, admitting of no alleviation from external remedies. Of this kind he met with one in the musculo-cutaneous nerve of a woman at Franequer, and another in the knee of a woman at Amsterdam. Both he removed by excision, and found them white internally, of gristly hardness, elastic, and seated within the neurilema.†

The next notice of this disease is by Dr Bisset, who observed it in the form of an irregularly-oval tumour, the size of a filbert, on the outside of the left leg, six inches above the outer ancle, also in a woman of twenty-nine years.‡ Soon after it was observed by Mr Pearson in the subcutaneous nerve which accompanies the saphæna vein, in the leg of a woman of fifty-one; in the back of the leg, near the *tendo Achillis ;* and at the bend of the arm, near the median vein,§ in a young married woman. Since this time the disease was fully and accurately described by Mr William Wood of this city ;‖ and occasional cases have been published by other authors.¶

Mr Wood questions the justice of the opinion of Camper, that the tubercle is seated in the nerve-coat, or is a nervous tumour; and thinks that it is a distinct or peculiar species of tumour, situate in the subcutaneous cellular membrane. It may not perhaps be possible to prove that every little subcutaneous tubercle is of this description. But the observations of the authors above mentioned, and those of A. Petit,** Tissot, Lassus, Jacopi,†† Monteggia,‡‡ and Alexander,

* An Epilepsy from an Uncommon Cause. By Dr Thomas Short, Physician at Sheffield. Medical Essays and Observations, Vol. IV. art. xxvii. p. 416. Edinburgh, 1738. A tumour the size of a pea in the posterior tibial nerve, near the lower end of *gastrôcnemii.*

† Petri Camper Demonstrationum Anatomico-Pathologicarum, Lib. i. Caput 2. § 5. p. 11. Lugduni Bat. Folio Imp.

‡ Memoirs of the Medical Society of London, Vol. III. p. 58. Case of Irritable Tumour. By C. Bisset, M. D. &c. London, 1792.

§ Medical Facts and Observations, Vol. VI. p. 96. Account, &c.

‖ Medical and Surgical Journal, Vol. VIII. p. 283, 429. Edinburgh Medico-Chirurgical Transactions, Vol. III. Edinburgh, 1829.

¶ Ibid. Vol. XI. XVII. XVIII.

** Essai sur la Medecine, &c. A Lyon, 1806.

†† Prospetto della Scuola di Chirurgia Pratica, &c. Vol. I. cap. 9. Milano, 1813.

‡‡ Istituz. Chirur. Vol. II. Capo xiv. p. 197. Milano, 1813.

show manifestly that the nerves are liable to tubercles of this kind. The proofs, in short, which may be adduced in favour of this idea, are the following. 1. In many instances of subcutaneous tubercle the lenticular body has been formed in the substance or coat of a nerve. (Short, Camper, Bisset, A. Petit, Tissot, Lassus, Jacopi, &c.) 2. In the majority of cases the tubercle can be traced distinctly to the branch, twig, or filament of a subcutaneous nerve. 3. The painful sensation of which it is the seat, though severe and constant, is always aggravated by handling or pressing the tumour, and may be always traced along nervous branches.

In the cases in which the neuromatic tubercle has been dissected, it has been found hard, cartilaginous, and slightly vascular. It seems in general to consist in morbid change of the neurilema, by deposition of albuminous matter in the neurilematic interstices. (Jacopi.) It is much more frequent in women than in men, in the proportion nearly of from seven to one, and from ten to one. Monteggia states that he found the entire nervous system occupied with numerous (*centinaia*,) neuromatic tubercles, which would indicate, as he observes, in some instances a neuromatic diathesis.* The cause of their formation is not known; but from the effects of ligature, division, and other injury, it may be in some manner conceived.

It is important to observe, that in both classes of cases, the presence of these tumours gives rise to various remarkable effects. Thus they may, by the irritation which they cause in the nerve, induce not only intense pain, but give rise to epileptic motions. This is shown by the remarkable case given by Dr Short so far back as in 1720,† by the cases recorded by Mojon and Covercelli,‡ and by one mentioned by Portal.§ Is it not probable that, of the cases described as preceded by *aura epileptica* several belong to this head, and are cases in which there is in a nerve either a tubercle or some similar source of irritation?

In other instances, these tumours are attended with anomalous and sometimes severe nervous symptoms. Pain and prickling or the feeling of the electric shock from the tumour along the limb.

* Istituzione Chirurgiche, Vol. II. p. 197.

† An Epilepsy, &c. Med. Essays and Observ. Vol. IV. p. 416.

‡ Memorie della Societate di Genova. Und Von Siebold, Chiron, Band I. St. 3, where the Memoires of Mojon and Covercelli are translated.

§ Anatomie Medicale. Par A. Portal, Tome IV. p. 246. A body like a hard corn near the articulation of the first with the second phalanx on the palmar surface of the thumb.

Occasionally spasmodic motions take place; and in certain cases the functions of the part are destroyed. Thus a man of 36 years of age lost his sight in consequence of the formation of a neuromatic tumour in the optic nerve, (Sedillot,) a little larger than a hempseed.* In a man of 60, who suffered from symptoms of asthma, a tubercle the size of a pea was found in the right diaphragmatic nerve.†

The causes of *neuroma* and *neuromation* are little known. In several of the cases, the formation of the tumour was preceded by violence or injury. In others it arose spontaneously. The circumstances of the following case show the effect of chronic inflammation arising from causes operating on the system at large, and probably on the digestive functions.

A student in medicine, an internal pupil at the Hotel Dieu of Angers, occupying an apartment situate several feet below the level of the court, and sleeping in a recess formed in the substance of the wall of the hospital, suffered, at the end of some months' abode in this unhealthy place, an attack of *arthritis* in the great toe; and, shortly after, there was formed, beneath the skin covering the internal saphena vein and nerve in the leg, a hard tumour, of the size of a grain of wheat, and, whenever it was touched by the patient, either in dressing or undressing, or under any other circumstances, caused pain, shooting like an electric shock upon the foot, in the direction of the ramifications of the nerve.

Having obtained from the administrators of the hospital another apartment, he was at the end of some months cured of the neuralgia and the neuromatic tubercle. The same individual, when some years afterwards at Paris, had under the chin a little boil, the cicatrix of which continued for several months the seat of acute pain, caused by the friction of the razor, and which spread in a radiating direction over the neck and chest. The subject of this case was the late M. Beclard.‡

7. Considerable wasting and shrinking were seen in the optic nerves by Spigelius, Riolan, Rolfinck, Morgagni, Santorini, and Benninger; and complete destruction in the olfacient nerves by Falkenburg. These changes, which take place generally at the cerebral end of the nerve, are accompanied with diminution or loss of function.

* Journal de Medecine, Tome L.

† Dissertation sur les Affections Locales des Nerfs. Par Pierre Jules Descot, D. M. Paris, 1825. P. 257.

‡ Ibid. p. 212.

BOOK III.

STEREOMORPHIC TEXTURES. KINETIC TEXTURES.

THE textures which next come under observation are those which give solidity and figure to the body, or the STEREOMORPHIC TEXTURES; and as in general they are the agents of movement, they may be called KINETIC TEXTURES. These are muscle, sinew, or tendon, white fibrous system, yellow fibrous system, bone, cartilage, and fibro-cartilage.

CHAPTER I.

SECTION I.

FLESH, THEW, MUSCLE. Μῦς,—Μυες.—*Musculus,—Lacertus,— Tori.*—MUSCULAR TISSUE.—*Tissu Musculaire.*

THE ordinary appearance of the substance named flesh or muscle must be familiar to all; and it is unnecessary to enumerate those obvious characters which are easily recognized by the most careless observer. A portion of muscle, when carefully examined, is found to consist of several animal substances. It is traversed by arteries and veins of various size; nervous twigs are observed to pass into it; it is often covered by dense whitish membranous folds, (*fasciæ,*) or by serous or mucous membranes, all which will be examined afterwards; and it is found to contain a large proportion of filamentous tissue. But it is distinguished by consisting of numerous fibres disposed parallel to each other, and which may be separated in the same manner by proper means. The appearance, arrange- ment, and characters of these fibres demand particular notice.

According to Prochaska, muscle in all parts of the body may be resolved, by careful dissection, into fibres of great delicacy, as mi- nute as silk-filaments, but pretty uniform in shape, general appear- ance, and dimensions. Their diameter appears not to exceed $\frac{1}{40000}$

part of an inch, whatever be their length. They seem all more or less flattened or angular, and appear to be solid diaphanous filaments. Prochaska appears not to doubt that these muscular threads, (*fila carnea*) are incapable of further division; and he therefore terms them *primary muscular fibres.*

The microscopical examination of the atomic constitution of the muscular filament, which was first attempted by Lewenhoeck, and afterwards prosecuted by Della Torre, Fontana, Monro, and Prochaska, was in 1818 and 1826 revived by M. Bauer, the indefatigable assistant of Sir E. Home. From the observations of this accurate inquirer, each muscular filament appears to consist of a series of globular or oblong spheroidal atoms, disposed in a linear direction, and connected by a transparent elastic jelly-like matter. *

The primary muscular fibres are placed close and parallel to each other, and are united in every species of muscle into bundles ; (*fasciculi; lacerti;*) of different, but determinate size ; and, according as these bundles are large or small, the appearance of the muscle is coarse or delicate.   In the deltoid the bundles are the largest. In the *vasti, glutæi,* and large pectoral muscles the bundles are greatly larger than in the *psoæ.* In the muscles of the face, of the ball of the eye, of the hyoid bone, and especially in those of the perinæum, these bundles are very minute, and almost incapable of being distinguished. The number of ultimate filaments which compose a bundle varies in different muscles, and probably in different animals. In a muscular fibre of moderate size in the human subject, Prochaska estimates them to vary from 100 to 200; and in animals with larger fibres, at double, triple, or even four times that number. † There is reason to conclude, from correct microscopic observation, that the largest do not exceed the $\frac{1}{8}$th of an inch, and that the smallest are not less than $\frac{1}{16}$th.

By cutting a muscle across, these bundles are observed to differ not only in size but in shape. Some are oblong and rhomboidal ; others present a triangular or quadrangular section; and in some even the irregular pentagon or polygon may be recognized.

These bundles are united by filamentous tissue of various degrees of delicacy, as may be shown by the effects of boiling; and the

---

* The Croonian Lecture. On the changes the blood undergoes in the act of coagulation. By Sir Everard Home, Bart. V. P. R. S. Phil. Trans. 1818, p. 175.—The Croonian Lecture. On the structure of a muscular fibre, from which is derived its elongation and contraction. By Sir E. Home, Bart., &c. &c. Phil. Trans. 1826, Part 2d, p. 64.

† De Carne Musculari, Sect. i. Chap. iii.

muscle thus formed is penetrated by arteries, veins, and nervous twigs, and is enclosed by filamentous tissue, which often contains fat.

This fascicular arrangement appears to be confined to the muscles of voluntary motion. It is not very distinct in the heart or diaphragm; and in the urinary bladder and intestinal canal I have not recognized it. Nor is the parallel arrangement of the ultimate filaments always strictly observed in the involuntary muscles. The component fibres of this order of muscles are often observed to change direction, and unite at angles with each other. This fact, which was observed by Lewenhoeck, has been verified by Prochaska.

Among microscopical observers it has been recently the practice to distinguish muscular fibres into three sorts. 1st, Muscular fibres with cross striæ, or articulated, moniliform fibres, containing the voluntary muscles; 2d, Muscular fibres with the characters of the fibres of the middle arterial coat, the examples of which are found in the fibres of the stomach and intestinal tube, and the muscular coat of excretory ducts, for instance, the vas deferens; and, 3d, Muscular fibres with the character of ligamentous tissue, of which the iris and the tunic of the lymphatic vessels are understood to be good examples.

The fibres of the voluntary muscles, as seen in the flesh of animals and the human body, are separated by maceration or boiling into smaller or more slender fibres, which are the primitive fibres. The course of these is either straight or curled, rarely spiral. The individual inflections of the curled fibres, (fibræ cirrosæ,) are mostly in sharp angles opposite each other, in a zig-zag direction; and the angles of the zig-zag inflections are more or less acute.

The diameter of the primary fibres in man and the mammalia varies. The most are from $\frac{5}{10000}$ to $\frac{6}{10000}$ of a Paris line, though some attain not the size of $\frac{1\,75}{10000}$ of a Paris line, and others again are so thick that they are from $\frac{2}{10000}$ to $\frac{3}{10000}$ in breadth. Only the smallest approach the cylindrical shape. The largest are flat, but they are never so flat as inarticulated muscular fibres. The large primary fasciculi are by dark, frequent but interrupted longitudinal striæ again divided into smaller fasciculi.

Many, and especially the fine primary fibres, have a feebly granulated membranous covering, void of structure, and distinguishing them from the fibrous content.

The surface of a primary fasciculus is often covered with more or less numerous nucleated cells, which become distinct by immersion in vinegar.

These are either broad, oblong oval, with nucleated cells, or collected in long or short, small *striæ*, acuminated at both ends, which are incurvated in the semilunar or serpentine form, like the corpuscles in the roots of the hair; or they may be in rows of three, four, or six small dark *nuclei*. The nuclei lie sometimes detached; sometimes alternating, or placed with their edges opposite each other; sometimes on the surface of the fasciculi in great quantity. Most of them are straight, with their long axes parallel; but sometimes they are oblique or transverse.

The circumstance that principally distinguishes the animal muscles from the other two sorts of muscular fibres, and from all other tissues, is the striated arrangement of the *fasciculi*, which run both transversely on the fasciculi, and in the longitudinal direction, and preferably sometimes in one, sometimes in the other direction. Only in the heart, especially in the neighbourhood of the external and the internal covering, are seen *fasciculi*, which are sometimes small-grained, like the smooth muscular fibres, but are also undulating and curled, like ligamentous tissue, and even intermediate between the two. Others are observed in the heart, and sometimes also in the muscles of the trunk, which appear to have a fine-grained content; but the granules or *punctula* of which are not arranged in determinate lines.

It would exceed the limits within which these notices must be confined, were I to describe the whole as represented by the microscope. It is enough to say that the fibres of the voluntary muscles are distinguished by this character of being varicose, like a string of very minute beads, or moniliform, that is, consisting of granules or nuclei arranged in rows, so as to form a beaded filament; that in some of these longitudinal striæ predominate, in others transverse striæ; and in others, the appearance of the longitudinal striæ is such that they seem to be cirrose or curled; and in others, again, the transverse beading is so strongly marked, that it seems to obscure and disguise the longitudinal arrangement.

2. The second order of muscular fibres is that of the muscles formed after the type of the middle arterial coat. If the muscular layer of the stomach or bowels, or that of an excretory duct is separated into fibres, there are similar, often long flat *lamellæ*, as in the annular tissue of arteries, or the longitudinal fibrous coat of

veins, with the same *nuclei*, and the same transformation of nuclei to dark *striæ*. Over the middle of the *lamellæ*, in their long direction, passes sometimes a longer or shorter and proportionally broader granular patch, sometimes a long slender fine dark streak, sometimes an interrupted row of fine dark *punctula*.

Besides these lamellæ, which are most abundant in the neighbourhood of the serous coat, are individual fragments of broad, very flat, stiff fibres. These lie in the muscular coat, in general parallel to each other, united in greater or smaller numbers in bundles. They seldom pass by oblique anastomoses into each other. Between and over them run the nucleated fibres, which often form a similar net-work, as the nucleated fibres of the middle arterial coat. They are more translucent, more slender, and less numerous than in the middle arterial coat. The breadth of the granulated muscular fibres is from $\frac{24}{10000}$ to $\frac{56}{10000}$ of one line; the breadth of the fibrils about $\frac{8}{10000}$ of one line.

This species of muscular fibres, which are known as flat, inarticulated organic or involuntary fibres, belong chiefly to the viscera, or organic and internal muscles.

Of the third species, embracing the iris and lymphatic vessels, it is unnecessary to speak here.

The colour of muscle varies. In man and the mammiferous animals, at least adult, it is more or less red; in many birds and fishes it is known to be whitish; in young animals it is grayish or cream-coloured; and the slender fibres which form the middle coat of the intestines in all animals are almost colourless. The colour of the muscles of voluntary motion in man is red or fawn; but repeated washing or maceration in alcohol or alkaline fluids renders them much paler.

The examination of the physical properties of muscle has occupied the industry of Muschenbroek, Croone, Browne Langrish, Wintringham, and others of the iatro-mathematical school. I cannot perceive that minute knowledge of these properties is of much moment to the elucidation either of its sound or its morbid states. Amidst the variable results necessarily obtained in such an inquiry, the only point which is certain is, that muscular fibre has much less tenacity and mutual aggregation than most other tissues. It sustains much less weight and force of tension without giving way.

Chemical analysis has not yet furnished any satisfactory results on the nature of muscular tissue; but the general conclusion of the numerous experiments already instituted show that muscle contains fibrin, albumen, gelatine, extractive matter (osmazome,) and saline substances. It is difficult to say how far the gelatine is to be regarded as proper to muscle, or derived from the filamentous tissue, in which it certainly exists. The saline matters are common to muscle with most other organic substances. There is reason to believe that fibrin in considerable quantity, and albumen and osmazome in smaller proportion, are the proper proximate principles of muscle. Though the various proportions of these principles have been stated in numbers by chemists, there can be no doubt that in the present condition of animal chemistry it is impossible to place on them any reliance. It is also to be remembered, that the relative proportion of the proximate principles varies at different periods of life. In early life the muscular fibre contains a large proportion of gelatine, and very little albumen, fibrin, or osmazome. In adult age, however, the gelatine is very scanty, and the fibrin is abundant. The albumen and gelatine found in muscle seem to be derived chiefly from the filamentous tissue, and the aponeurotic intersections.

During life the muscular fibre possesses the property of shortening itself or contracting under certain conditions. These may be referred to the following heads. 1*st*, The will in the voluntary muscles. 2*d*, Proper fluids in the involuntary muscles, as the blood to the heart, articles of food or drink in the stomach, chyme in the small intestines, excrement in the large intestines, urine in the bladder, &c. 3*d*, Mechanical irritants in all muscles. 4*th*, Chemical irritants; and, 5*th*, Morbid products generated in the course of disease.

This property of contracting has received various names; contractility (*vis contractilis* of L. Bellini), irritability (Glisson), (*vis vitalis* of De Gorter and Gaubius), excitability, mobility, *vis insita*, *vis propria* of Haller, and the organic contractility of Bichat.

It is peculiar to muscular fibre, and is found in no other living tissue.

The influence of the brain and nerves over muscular contraction, and the inquiry of the properties peculiar to muscles, form an interesting subject of investigation, on which many facts have been communicated since the time of Haller and Whytt, and especially by Nysten, Le Gallois, Wilson Philip, Brodie, Bell, Magendie, Mayo, Flourens, Fodera, Rolando, and Marshall Hall. But it is too extensive to be considered in this place; and, for information on the subject, I refer to the ordinary physiological works, and to those journals in which these researches are detailed.*

The muscles have been divided according to the manner in which the phenomena of contraction take place,—into, 1*st*, muscles obedient to the will, or voluntary; 2*d*, muscles not under the influence of the will, or involuntary; and, 3*d*, muscles of a mixed character, the motions of which are neither entirely dependent or independent of the will.

The first order comprehends all the muscles of the skeleton; the second comprehends the hollow muscles, as the heart, stomach, and intestinal canal; and the third comprehends such muscular organs as the diaphragm, intercostal muscles, bladder, rectum, &c.

Section II.

1. *Myositis.*—Muscle is liable to inflammation, which may be acute or chronic in duration, and may differ according to its kind. One form of muscular inflammation seems to constitute a species of rheumatism (Carmichael Smyth),† and when this continues long, it terminates in loss of power, constituting a local palsy.

α. Myositis Purulenta.—Another form, equally serious and more certainly injurious, is the suppurative form of muscular inflammation. In this the muscular structure suppurates and sometimes sloughs extensively; and, whether acute or chronic, is generally a fatal disease. The most familiar instance of the chronic form of suppurative inflammation in muscle is that which constitutes lumbar abscess,—inflammation of the great psoas muscle.‡ Of this Schoenmezel records a good example in the person of a muscular young man of 28, in whom the whole of the *psoas magnus* and *iliacus* of

---

* Elementa Physiologiæ, Tome iv. Lib. xi. Sect. ii.

Physiologie de l'Homme, par N. P. Adelon, 4 tomes, 8vo. Paris, 1823–1824.

Outlines of Human Physiology. By Herbert Mayo, F. R. S. &c. 3d Edition. London, 1833. 4th Edition. London, 1836, 8vo.

Handbuch der Physiologie des Menschen für Vorlesungen. Von Johannes Müller, Ordentlich Offentl, Prof. der Anatomie und Physiologie U. S. W. in Berlin. Zwey Band. Coblenz, 1835 und 1840, 8vo.

Journal de Physiologie, Tome i. ii. &c. &c. Archives Generales, *passim*.

† Medical Communications. Vol. II. p. 217, 218.

‡ "The most remarkable and complete destruction of muscle which occurs from suppuration is that which is seen in the disease called psoas abscess, where the whole or the greater part of the muscle often disappears, and its capsule is filled with the matter of suppuration."—Thomson on Inflam., p. 152.—Lectures, p. 159.

the right side was destroyed and converted into purulent matter, forming a sac extending from the last lumbar vertebra along the surface of the *ilium* to the small trochanter.* Three similar cases described by Mr Howship form the clearest account of the anatomical characters of this disease.† In such instances, since there is either no affection, or at least no primary affection, of the bones of the spine, it must be inferred that the disease consists in suppurative inflammation either of the muscular tissue, or at least of the filamentous tissue of the muscles. The structure of these muscles, especially that of the psoas, is greatly more delicate than that of any other large muscle, and may have some influence in the destructive sero-purulent secretion which follows. Is the muscular texture destroyed or merely separated? I have seen discharged along with the fluid of lumbar abscess capillary filaments, brownish, firm, and evidently the remains of the muscular fibres. At the same time, in the dissections above quoted, no fibres are mentioned in the purulent cyst. In a case by Mr Milroy fibres are stated to have been discharged.

The acute form of muscular inflammation is more rare, but sometimes occurs in the muscles of the abdomen, of the chest, of the thigh or leg, in persons of broken constitution and diseased habits. By some authors, however, the muscular fibre is believed to be incapable of inflammation; and the instances ascribed to it are by them said to be inflammation of the intermuscular cellular tissue. On this head, I refer to the section on Diffuse Inflammation of the Cellular Membrane.

β. *Carditis.*—Another example of inflammation of muscular tissue is presented in that of the heart. The testimony of Dr Baillie shows that this is a rare disease, and is almost never primary, but the result of inflammation of the pericardium, from which it spreads to the filamentous tissue, and partly to the muscular fibres of the organ. The general accuracy of this statement is confirmed by Laennec, who contends, that though partial inflammation in minute spots is not uncommon, yet general inflammation of the cardiac substance, either acute or chronic, is a thing almost unknown in the records of medicine. The cases adduced by Corvisart he regards as examples of pericarditis; and the same may be said of those of

* Francisci Schoenmezel, Med. Prof. Heidelbergensis Observatio de Musculis Psoa et Iliaco suppuratis. Heidelbergæ, 1776. Frank Delectus, Vol. V. p. 169.

† Practical Observations on Surgery and Morbid Anatomy.

Dr Davis.* The possibility of the fact, nevertheless, he admits on the evidence of the case of Meckel.† Stronger proof he might have found in a case by Mr Stanley, in which the cut substance of the heart was exceedingly dark-coloured from injection of the capillaries; the fibres were soft, loose, easily separable, and compressible between the fingers; while sections of each ventricle exhibited numerous small distinct collections of dark-coloured purulent matter among the muscular fasciculi,—some deep, approaching the cavity of the ventricle, others superficial, raising the pericardium. The muscular substance of the auricles was softened and loaded with blood; but without purulent deposits.‡

In this case, which took place in a boy of 14, the chief symptoms were those of intense inflammatory fever, with great heat, delirium, and feverishness, and some frontal headach. On one day the patient complained of pain in the thigh and knee; but at no time in the whole course of the symptoms, which lasted only four days, did he give any indications of pain within the chest. Death was preceded by difficult breathing. The case, indeed, was one of great acuteness and rapidity in progress.

It cannot be denied that in this case the muscular tissue of the organ exhibited marks of inflammation; but the purulent deposits might be seated in the intermuscular filamentous tissue, which, though delicate, is abundant.

In 1828, Dr P. M. Latham, after remarking the rarity of finding purulent matter as a proof or effect of inflammation of the substance of the heart, added that, nevertheless, he had met with two examples of this lesion. In one instance the whole heart was deeply tinged with dark-coloured blood, and its substance was softened; and upon section of both ventricles, innumerable small drops of purulent matter oozed from various parts among the muscular fibres. This was the result of a most rapid and acute inflammation, which terminated in death, after an illness of only two days' duration.

In another instance, after death, which terminated an illness of long duration, and characterized by symptoms referable to the heart, a distinct abscess was found in the substance of the left ventricle, closed externally by a portion of adherent pericardium, and con-

* Inquiry into the Symptoms, &c. of Carditis. By J. Ford Davis, M. D. Bath 1808.

† Mémoires de l'Academie de Berlin.

‡ Medico-Chirurgical Transactions, Vol. VII. p. 323.

nected internally with an ossified portion of the lining membrane.*

In the descriptive catalogue of Mr Langstaff's museum, are several preparations in which the muscular substance of the heart is said to have been inflamed. No. 298, a female of 46, 303, a boy of 8. (The muscular structure showed all the signs of *carditis.*) 303, a man of 47. No specific details, however, are furnished.†
In the Morbid Anatomy Collection of the University of Edinburgh is a preparation of a heart, (P. 12,) in which a large abscess with an irregular inner surface, which contained lymph and purulent matter, occupies the whole extent of the *septum cordis,* and communicates, by a small orifice the size of a quill with the left ventricle. In this case inflammation must have affected the *septum,* perhaps the neighbouring parts of the left ventricle, and may have eventually been concentrated on the *septum,* in which it induced suppuration, confined within the walls of a distinct cavity. Twelve months previous to death the patient laboured under symptoms of pneumonia, and at last died suddenly.

An instance not less decisive is recorded by Mr Salter of Poole, in the person of a man of 50 years. The disease appears in this case, however, to have been at first slow in progress, and chronic in duration, as the symptoms continued for about six weeks. These were dull, heavy, but not lancinating pain, in the lower part of the chest, rather inclining to the left side; much distressing oppression in breathing, aggravated at intervals, and never quitting the patient; frequent small pulse; considerable uneasiness in the left arm frequently recurring, and a feeling as if he could not live. No cough nor any sign of pulmonary affection was observed. All the symptoms assumed an aggravated form with great orthopnœa, anxiety, and restlessness, for sixty-five hours only before death.

In this case the heart was rather larger than natural and of moderate firmness. Large white and yellow clots were contained within the chambers of the organ, and marks of incipient ossification were observed in the ascending aorta, but no disease in the *endocardium* or in the valves. The muscular substance of the heart

---

* Pathological Essays on some Diseases of the Heart ; being the substance of Lectures delivered before the College of Physicians. By P. Mere Latham, M.D., Physician to St Bartholomew's Hospital. London Medical Gazette, Vol. III., p. 119. London, 1829. Essay III.

† Catalogue of the preparations illustrative of Normal, Abnormal, and Morbid Structure, constituting the Anatomical Museum of George Langstaff, F. R. C. S., &c. London, 1842. 8vo.

was of a light yellow colour, yet preserving the fibrous texture of muscle; and it presented purulent matter at the surface of the various sections made in it. In some parts were observed small cavities filled with purulent matter, varying from the size of a pin-head to that of a small pea.

The pericardium was unusually vascular; a state ascribed by the author to inflammation, but its surface presented no lymph.* It is probable that the inflammatory state of the cardiac muscular fibres had spread to the investing membrane.

All these cases, it must be admitted, afford examples of inflammation either of the muscular substance of the heart, or of the connecting filamentous tissue, or of both. Indeed, it is not easy to conceive the one tissue to be inflamed without the other; and whether we say that the inflammatory process begins in the filamentous tissue, and thence spreads to the muscular, which is probable, or begins in the muscular tissue and spreads to the filamentous, the result is the same.

It is impossible therefore to doubt, that the muscular substance of the heart is liable to be affected by inflammation, and its most common product suppuration; and from the cases now recorded it seems to result, that the inflammation is often very acute and rapid in progress, and in other instances is slow and more chronic. The process also appears sometimes to attack the whole organ; in other instances only one part of it, or after attacking the whole, to become concentrated on one point.

Lastly, Bouillaud gives various examples of what he denominates Inflammation of the substance of the heart. His views, however, on this subject are so peculiar, that I think they may be more properly introduced under a different head. Aneurism of the heart he considers as the effect of inflammation.

Abscess and ulceration of muscular tissue are the result of local or punctuate inflammation. In the former case, a cavity, with smooth walls, containing purulent matter, is formed in one region of the muscular substance. In the latter a rugged irregular surface, produced by ulcerative absorption or erosion, takes place near the surface of the muscle. The examples of both forms, as they take place in the heart, are the most interesting to the pathologist. Of abscess in this organ, instances are given by Poterius, Benivenius, Cornax, Nicolaus Massa, Fantoni, and Laennec. Of ulcers

---

* Case of Carditis by Thomas Salter, Esq. Surgeon, Medico-Chirurgical Transactions, Vol. XXII. p. 72. London, 1839.

on the outer surface, instances were seen by Olaus Borrichius,[*] Riverius,[†] Job à Meekren,[‡] Peter de Marchettis,[§] Malpighi,[||] Peyer,[¶] Graetz, and Morgagni.[**]   The ulcer occurring in the inner surface of the heart was seen by Morgagni, (Epist. xxiv. 17,) and by Laennec, who found one an inch long, half an inch broad, and more than four lines deep in the centre, in the inner surface of the left ventricle, which was hypertrophied, and at length rupured.

γ. *Myositis emolliens.*—To this head may be referred the softened or pulpy state occasionally observed in the substance of the heart in weak extenuated subjects liable to fainting-fits, and also in those cut off by fever.   The muscular fibres then assume a light fawn colour or pale yellow, like the dead leaf, become flabby and friable, and so easily lacerable as scarcely to sustain handling.   By Laennec this is regarded as the result of error of assimilation or defective nutrition ; while Bouillaud ascribes it to inflammation.   One variety of softening appears to be the consequence of inflammation, and may be considered as gangrene of the heart.   Most usually, however, it is the result of imperfect nutrition of the organ during disease, either chronic or subacute.

2. *Hypertrophy.*—There is reason to believe that the condition described as hypertrophy of muscles is mere enlargement with thickening and induration of the constituent fibres, depending on chronic inflammation.   It is certainly quite different from the enlargement occasioned by exercise, to which it has been erroneously compared.   In the heart and bladder, in which it has been most frequently found, not only is the muscular substance thickened and enlarged, but it is rendered hard, firm, and in some parts almost cartilaginous.   In the early stage the colour is simply brown; subsequently it acquires in certain parts a leaden-gray tint, which seems to depend on parts of the muscle assuming the cartilaginous induration.   The substance of the organ then cuts firm, and resists the knife.   The change seems either to depend on, or to be connected with, a process of chronic injection ; for the vessels are large, distended, and abundant.   In the deltoid and biceps of the fencer, and the *glutaei* and *gastrocnemii* of the dancer, though large and

---

[*] Bartholini, Acta Med. Haf. Vol. I. Obs. 69.
[†] Cent. i. Ob. 87.   [‡] Obs. Chirurg. 35.
[§] Observ. Med.-Chir. 46.   [||] Morgagni, Ep. xxv. 17.
[¶] Method. Hist. Anat. c. vi. in Schol.
[**] Epist. xvi. 17.

well developed, no change of this description can be recognized. They are indeed firm and tough, like the muscle of entire male animals, but present nothing of the morbid enlargement, congestion, and induration found in the hypertrophied heart and bladder. In proof of the justice of these views it may be added, that the instances in which the muscular coat of the stomach is admitted to be hypertrophied, are those in which scirrhus, or some similar chronic inflammatory state, affects the collateral tissues. (Louis.)

Hypertrophy of muscular organs takes place most commonly in connection with some permanent resistance opposed to their action. Thus hypertrophy of the heart is connected with permanent contraction of the aortic orifice and disease of the valves, or with an unnaturally irritant state of the blood, as in rheumatism and disease of the kidney. Hypertrophy of the bladder, in like manner, usually takes place as an effect of stricture of the urethra, and sometimes of chronic inflammation or other disease of the mucous coat, or enlargement of the prostate gland.

3. *Atrophy* of muscles, or diminution of size, is more frequent, and may arise either from general disease, as in consumption, dropsy, &c. or from local debility, as in rheumatism, palsy, &c. ; or, in short, from defective local nutrition, or, as after unreduced luxations, from want of exercise of particular muscles. The best example of complete atrophy is that which takes place in muscles poisoned by lead, which become small, shrunk, pale, and void of irritability.

4. *Steatosis ; Adipification.*—I cannot understand upon what grounds the fatty degeneration of muscle is denied by Beclard ; for there is no doubt that authentic instances are recorded of this change occurring in the muscles both of man and of the lower animals, under certain diseases. Independent of its being seen in the muscles of the sheep by Vaughan,* it has been observed in those of the human subject by Haller, Louis, Maugre, Vicq-D'Azyr, Dumas, Emmanuel, Laennec, and Adams. Louis, so early as 1739, in amputating the right leg, found the *gemelli, plantaris, poplitaeus, solaeus,* the long common flexor of the toes, the proper flexor of the great toe, and the *tibialis posticus* converted into fat.†

---

* Some Account of an Uncommon Appearance, &c. By W. Vaughan, M. D. London, 1813.

† Rapport sur une Observation, &c. Journal General de Medecine, Tome XXIV. p. 5.

Maugre found the muscles of the same region, excepting the *gemelli*, which were greatly diminished in size, converted into an adipose mass easily divisible by the knife.* Vicq-D'Azyr, in an old subject, saw the *psoas* and *iliacus*, the *glutæus medius* and *minimus*, the adductors, the deep posterior muscles of the leg, and the plantar muscles, completely changed into fibro-cellular fat, without traces of remaining fibre. In the sciatic portion of the *semitendinosus* and biceps, the *gemelli*, the extensors of the toes, that of the great toe, and the *tibialis anticus* only, was it possible to recognize fibres with distinct direction. The *sartorius* presented the gradual transition from muscle to fat, being muscular above and adipose below. The fat into which these muscles were changed is described as white, firm, contained in numerous minute cells; the uniting cellular tissue whitish, looser, and more separable than usual; and the fat is not deposited between its filaments, but forms part of their substance. Examined by a good glass, it presents a mass of soft transparent fibres of various diameters, in different parts of their length.† Dumas saw the muscles of the fore part of the chest, and those of the posterior region of the shoulder and arm, reduced to an adipose mass, contained in condensed cellular membrane; those of the abdomen and the *triceps adductor* much changed; and the *glutaeus maximus* and first adductor half changed into fatty matter.‡ Emmanuel, in the person of a woman of 38, dead of childbed fever, found the abdominal muscles entirely changed into fat.§

Lastly, this transformation was seen by Laennec and Adams in the human heart. The changed portions assumed a pale-yellow colour, which is most distinct externally, and approaches to the natural tint as it proceeds inwards, at which the muscular fibres are less changed. According to an analysis by Cruveilhier, it consists of solid adipocerous fat, oily fluid, (*elaine*), and a little gelatine.

5. Elongation and shortening of muscular fibres are mentioned among morbid changes.

6. *Rupture or laceration.*—Of this occurrence in muscular organs, the most important example is that of rupture of the muscular substance of the heart. Instances of this have been collected by

* Rapport sur une Observation, &c. Journal General de Medecine, Tome XXIV. p. 6.
† Journal General de Medecine, Tome XXVI. p. 11.
‡ Ibid. Tome XXIII. p. 61.
§ Ibid. Vol. XXIV. p. 4.

Morand,[*] Morgagni,[†] Haller,[‡] Portal,[§] Brera,[||] Baillie, Rostan,[¶] Bland,[**] Rochoux,[††] and Adams.[‡‡] According to the results obtained by these observers, rupture of the heart is most frequent in the left ventricle, which gives way by a longitudinal fissure near the base and middle of the ventricle. In most of the cases, this rupture may be traced to previous ulceration, (Morgagni, Haller, Portal, Brera, &c.) and appears to be the result of the ulcerative process advancing from one surface of the ventricle to the other. Of rupture of the right ventricle too little is known to determine whether it be also the result of ulceration or not. So far, therefore, as is hitherto known, laceration of the muscular substance of the heart is not so much the consequence of being violently or forcibly torn, as of its being previously wasted, extenuated, and weakened.

Transverse laceration of muscular fibres, or forcible detachment from the tendons, may happen in consequence of external violence. This was seen by Wolfius,[§§] Wynandts,[||||] Cheselden,[¶¶] Portal,[***] Deramé,[†††] Bichat,[‡‡‡] and Wardrop.[§§§]

Rupture of the muscular coat of the stomach, which is not unfrequent, is in like manner the consequence of ulceration or erosion of its villous membrane, and shall be noticed under that head.

7. *Bony induration or deposition.*—This, though not very frequent, is not unknown. Morgagni mentions in his first case of ulcerative rupture a bony mass an inch thick, shaped like a half ring, being found in the muscular substance of the left ventricle, adhering, however, to the mitral valves, also ossified. A similar case is recorded by Haller; and to such instances it may be justly objected, that they are not so much examples of conversion of muscular fibre into bone as deposition of bony matter in collateral tissues progressively encroaching on the muscular layer. One of the most distinct examples of seeming conversion of muscular fibre into

* Mem. de l'Acad. Roy. des Sci. 1732.
† Epist. xxvii. 2, 5, 8 ; lxiv. 15. ‡ Elem. Physiolog.
§ Mem. de l'Acad. Roy. des Sci. 1784.
|| Sylloge Vol. X. Opusc. vi. p. 202.
¶ Nouv. Journ. de Med. Avril, 1820. Tome VII. p. 280.
** Bibliotheque Med. Aout, 1820.
†† Sur les Ruptures des Cœur.
‡‡ Dublin Hospital Reports, Vol. IV.
§§ Haller Bibl. Chir. I. p. 223. |||| Verhand. von Haarlem
¶¶ Anatomy, p. 207. *** Anat. Med. II. p. 412.
††† Mem. de la Soc. Med. I. p. 159. ‡‡‡ Anat. Gen. Tome III. p. 234.
§§§ Medico-Chirurgical Transact. Vol. VII. p. 278.

calcareous matter is given by Renaudin in the person of a man of 33, subject to violent palpitation. The substance of the left ventricle was infiltrated with sabulous and crystalline grains. This calcareous deposition must not be confounded with ossified pericardium,—the usual example of ossified heart.

8. *Accidental productions and tumours.*—Muscular structure is liable to tubercular deposition, to scirrho-carcinoma, to lardaceous degeneration, (*keroma*), to encephaloid tumours, and to the melanotic deposit, (Cullen.) Serous cysts (*hygroma*) are said to be rare; but they have occasionally been observéd.

9. Parasitical animals have been observed in the muscles of the human subject. The solitary hydatid (*cysticercus cellulosæ*) is not uncommon.* The latter especially has been seen in the *trapezius, serratus posticus, psoas, iliacus, glutaeus,* and other large muscles, (Werner, Rudolphi,) and in the heart by Morgagni, (xxi. 4.) Portal, Mr Price, and Mr Evans.

Mr D. Price found in the muscular substance of the heart of a boy of ten years, who expired suddenly, a large hydatid, of the character of which no details are given. There is good reason, nevertheless, for believing that it was an acephalocyst.† More satisfactory information is given in the history of another case recorded by Mr Herbert R. Evans. In this case, which took place in a female aged 40, of slender frame and weakly appearance, the individual became languid and feeble, and unable to ascend an acclivity or a staircase without breathlessness. Occasionally she felt a sort of sharp pain darting, as it were, through the heart. These feelings lasted for five or six months; when, in consequence of attempting, on the 20th April, to run up stairs quickly, she was attacked with a paroxysm of great dyspnœa, accompanied with throbbing and pain in the region of the heart. These symptoms continued with little intermission for six weeks; and death took place on the 1st of June. The cavity of the pericardium contained about one ounce of fluid. The membrane was covered by lymph over part of the anterior surface. The apex of the heart was lost or rendered round and obtuse in a considerable tumour, which communicated to the touch a sense of fluctuation. This tumour, which formed a consi-

---

* Bremser, Traité Zoologique, xi. p. 280.

† Case of Sudden Death, in which a. large Hydatid was found in the Substance of the Heart. By David Price, Esq. Medico-Chirurgical Transactions, Vol. XI. p. 274. London, 1821.

derable projection encroaching on the cavity of the right ventricle was globular and about three inches in diameter; and when laid open it was found to be a cyst containing a number of small cysts or hydatids, varying in size from that of a pea to the bulk of a pigeon's egg, the interstitial spaces between them being filled by a soft curd-like substance of a yellow colour. These hydatids were of the irregular spheroidal shape, and resembled in all respects the acephalocyst.* The muscular substance of the heart was attenuated.

Trichina Spiralis.—There is also found in certain circumstances in the muscles of the human subject, a small capillary or hair-like worm coiled up in the spiral form. It has from these circumstances received the name of *trichina spiralis.* At the same time it must be observed, that all cylindrical worms are in general coiled up in the spiral or spherical form, so as to constitute little balls contained within membranes. This is probably the fœtal or oviform stage of these animals. In the case of the *trichina,* its presence is indicated at first sight by the appearance of little vesicles or bags ; and when these are brought under the field of the microscope, it is found that they contain hair-like worms of extreme minuteness and delicacy, coiled up in the spiral shape.

It is not well known under what peculiar circumstances these parasitical animals are found in the animal body. In one body in which I saw them, the person had died of pulmonary consumption, that is, tuberculation and *vomicæ* in the lungs. In others it appears in the bodies of persons in a bad state of general health, emaciated and enfeebled with disease of the liver, or the intestinal tube.

The zoological and physical characters of the animal have been very accurately described by Mr Owen, to whose work I refer for more ample details.

* Case in which a Cyst containing Hydatids was found in the Substance of the Heart. By Herbert R. Evans, Esq. Surgeon. Medico-Chirurgical Transactions, Vol. XVII. p. 507. London, 1832.

CHAPTER II.

SECTION I.

SINEW, TENDON, *Tendo.*

SINEW or tendon was united by Bichat with ligament, fascia, aponeurosis, and periosteum, under the general name of *fibrous system;* and the substance of this arrangement has been adopted by Gordon, Meckel, and Beclard. I am inclined, however, from personal observation, to regard tendon as essentially distinct, at least in the present state of knowledge, from these substances. Examined anatomically, it does not bear a very close resemblance to any of them, and in its known chemical properties, it is considerably different.

The appearance of this substance must be familiar to all. Almost cylindrical in shape, but flattened at the muscular end, and tapering where inserted, a tendon consists of numerous white lines as minute as hairs, of satin-like glistening appearance, placed parallel and close to each other. A tendon is easily divided, and torn into longitudinal or parallel portions, and by the forceps very minute fibres may be detached and removed with ease, its whole length. These facts show the great tenacity of this tissue, and the regular parallelism with which the component fibres are united. The last circumstance distinguishes them completely from ligaments and periosteum, in which the fibres cross in all directions, and in consequence of which these tissues cannot be so easily split or separated. These fibres are united by filamentous tissue.

Tendon is softened and more easily separable by maceration in water or alkaline fluids; it is crisped by acid fluids, and rendered translucent by immersion in oil of turpentine. It has not been injected, but it is presumed to have blood-vessels and absorbents. No nerves have been traced into it.

Tendon when boiled becomes soft and large, assumes the appearance of a transparent gelatinous substance; and finally, if the boiling be continued, is dissolved and converted into gelatine. This fact, which is well known to cooks, who prepare jellies from tendinous parts of young animals, shows that tendon consists principally of gelatine, disposed in an organized form.

A species of flattened tendons, to which the name of *aponeurosis* has been given, may justly be united with this tissue. The best examples are in the aponeurotic or tendinous expansion of the external oblique muscle of the abdomen, the aponeurotic part of the occipito-frontal muscle of the head, and the upper or broad end of the *tendo-Achillis*. The anatomical structure and the chemical properties of each of these varieties of animal substance are quite similar, and somewhat different from that which has been termed *fascia*.

Section II.

In tendon inflammation is rarely spontaneous, and is generally the result of wound, tear, bruise, twist, wrench, or burn, when the effects vary according to the nature of the injury. Simple division of tendon may unite without much difficulty, though the medium of union appears to be filamentous tissue with some gelatino-albuminous matter. In laceration complete reunion will depend upon the extent of the injury. That of the *tendo-Achillis* is the most frequent. I have seen complete rupture of the extensor tendon of the middle finger unite in the course of four months without perceptible trace of the accident, and with complete restoration of the functions of the finger in about four or five months more. Twists or wrenches of the joints often injure not only tendons, but ligaments, fasciæ, and even cartilage, and occasion inflammation of all these textures at once. Of this the injury termed sprain is an example. Tendinous texture readily sloughs under inflammation, either spontaneous or from injury. In whitloe the tendons of the flexor muscles of the fingers are often killed and thrown off by ulceration; and when tendons are injured by burns or gunshot wounds death of their texture is almost invariable. In this state tendon loses its silvery white appearance and lustre, assumes a dull leaden gray aspect, and becomes thick and doughy.

The process of inflammation is most distinctly seen in wounds of the extremities, and in lacerations or ruptures of the tendons. They become enlarged, sometimes expanded in various affections of the joints. Punctured or lacerated wounds of tendinous structure are sometimes succeeded by tetanic motions, which terminate fatally. Ossification, so common in the tendons of birds, is almost unknown in the human subject; unless the sesamoid bones be admitted as examples of this transformation.

CHAPTER III.

Section I.

WHITE FIBROUS SYSTEM. *Ligament,*—Δεσμος, οι δεσμοι; *Periosteum;*
Dura Mater; Fascia.

AGAINST the formation of this order of tissues fewer objections
can be urged, though ligament and periosteum undoubtedly furnish
its most perfect examples; and it may be doubted whether *fascia*
ought to be referred to it, or arranged with tendon and aponeurosis. The *dura mater,* the *tunica albuginea,* and the fibro-synovial
sheaths, are to be regarded as compound membranes.

Ligament and periosteum are easily shown to consist of strong
whitish or gray fibres, as minute as threads or hairs, interwoven together in various directions, and thus forming an animal substance
which is not to be split or torn asunder as tendon; but when ruptured by extreme force presents an irregular ragged surface or
margin. Maceration in water or alkaline fluids separates the component fibres, and shows their irregular disposition more distinctly.
They are crisped by affusion of boiling water, or immersion in
acids; and they become translucent by immersion in oil of turpentine.

The properties of this tissue are chiefly physical. Those which
are vital are referable to its organization and nutrition. It is
powerfully resisting, and is one of the toughest and strongest tissues in the animal body, as is shown by the numerous experiments
recorded in the writings of the iatro-mathematical physiologists.
It is supposed to possess the exhaling ends of arteries and colourless veins. No nerves have been recognized; and Bichat expresses
his ignorance of absorbents being traced into it.

Ligament when boiled yields a small portion of gelatine, but
obstinately resists the action of boiling water, and retains both its
shape and tenacity or cohesion. The crispation which it undergoes
in boiling water, alcohol, and diluted acids, seems to indicate that
albuminous matter forms its chief chemical principle.

As to their mechanical shape, the ligaments are divided by Bichat into two sorts; those in regular and those in irregular bundles.

The former comprehends all the distinct clusters of ligamentous structure, which sometimes in a cylindrical, sometimes in a flattened shape, connect the articulating ends of bones, and form the lateral ligaments of the various articulations. The latter consists of those loose parcels of ligamentous fibres which are found in various regions of the skeleton, not in regular cylindrical or longitudinal bands, but irregularly connecting bones not admitting of articular motion; for instance at the *symphysis pubis* and the sacro-iliac junction. The division of Beclard into articular, non-articular and mixed, is more comprehensive and more natural. The first are those which connect the articular extremities of different bones. The second are those which, attached to different parts of the same bone, convert notches into foramina, as in the orbitar arch and the supra-scapular hollow, or close openings, and give attachment to muscles, as the obturator ligament. The last are those which, like the sacro-ischiatic or the interosseous ligaments of the fore-arm and leg, connect bones susceptible of little or no motion, and especially give attachment to muscles. The two latter species of ligaments approach closely in their characters, physical and anatomical, to periosteum, and are probably to be regarded as modifications of this membrane.

The articular or perfect ligaments are naturally divisible into two subgenera,—the capsular and the funicular.

The capsular ligaments or the fibrous capsules, (Bichat), consist of cylindrical ligamentous sheaths attached all round to the ends of the articulating bones, and intimately interwoven with the periosteal tissue. Consisting essentially of fibro-albuminous matter strongly compacted, they are surrounded by cellular tissue, or rather celluloso-adipose tissue, and are lined internally by synovial membrane. Though the most perfect examples of the capsular form of ligament are presented in the scapulo-humeral and coxo-femoral articulations, less complete ones, nevertheless, are seen in the other joints. In those of the knee and elbow, an arrangement of this kind may be demonstrated; and minute capsules may be shown to connect the oblique articular surfaces of the vertebræ with each other.

The funicular ligaments, which consist of round chords or flat bands, are employed in connecting the articular ends of bones either without or within the cavity of the joint. Of those of the former description, the best examples are seen in the elbow and knee-joints, and in the wrist and ankle, where they are termed *lateral* ligaments, (*l. lateralia, accessoria.*) Of the latter instances, are the round ligaments, (*ligamenta teretia,*) of the shoulder and hip-joints, and the crucial ligaments of the knee-joint. These receive an investment of synovial membrane.

Of the white fibrous tissues one of the most important is that denominated *fascia.* Consisting in intimate structure of long fibrous threads placed in parallel juxtaposition, sometimes obliquely interwoven, and closely connected by filamentous tissue, it forms a whitish membranous web, variable in breadth, of some thickness and great strength. Fascia is perhaps, not excepting the skin, the most extensively distributed texture of membranous form in the animal body. It not only covers, if not the whole, at least by far the greatest part of the muscles of the trunk and each limb, but it sends round each muscle productions by which it is invested and supported, and even penetrates by minute slips into the substance of individual muscles. Of several of the large muscles it connects the component parts, as is seen in the *recti abdominis ;* to many it affords points of origin or insertion ; and to all it furnishes more or less investment and support. Most of the tendons, especially the flexor and extensor tendons, are enclosed by it ; and their synovial sheaths derive from it their exterior covering. At the extremities of the bones it is connected with the ligaments and periosteum, with which it is closely interwoven ; and it forms a general investment to the articular apparatus.

Though fascia may thus be viewed as one membranous web consisting of many parts all directly connected with each other, it is the practice of anatomists to distinguish its divisions, according to the region which they occupy. Thus in the fore part of the neck and chest is found a fascia, the relations and uses of which have been well described by Mr Allan Burns.* In the cervical region we find a firm fascia descending from the occipital bone along the vertebræ, covering and connecting the muscles of each side till it reaches the loins, where, in the form of a thick strong membrane, it forms the *lumbar fascia, (fascia lumborum.)* It may further be traced over and between the *glutaei* muscles ; connected afterwards with the broad femoral fascia, (*fascia lata ;*) and thence over the knee and leg to the foot. Much in the same manner a membranous web, thinner and more delicate, but of the same structure, may be

* Surgical Anatomy, pp. 33, 36.

traced from the chest along the upper extremity, till at the wrist it is identified with the annular ligament, and in the hand with the palmar fascia. In all these situations the general fascial envelope sends slips or productions (*fasciæ intermusculares*) between the muscles, and into their substance.*

SECTION II.

The morbid relations of this system are important. But in consequence of their being often combined with other tissues, it is difficult to distinguish them properly.

1. Inflammation in various forms is not uncommon, and may take place either spontaneously, or as the effect of accident.

α. *Desmodia.*—Inflammation of ligament may be spontaneous or the result of injury. In the former case it is generally chronic, and is attended with much thickening of the desmoid tissue. The morbid action spreads to the synovial membrane on the one side, causing it to thicken and effuse morbid fluid, and on the other, to the peridesmoid cellular tissue, which is then infiltrated with jelly-like fluid, and becomes separated and somewhat indurated and granular. These changes take place in those forms of articular disease commonly known under the vague name of *white swelling ;* (*tumor albus ; fungus articuli ;* der Gliedschwamm.) After some time this morbid state of the extra-articular cellular tissue may proceed to suppuration, but without necessarily opening the cavity of the articulation. The capsular ligament, however, and even the funicular ones, may be so much changed in structure as to become unfit for their functions.

Though the process now described is that which takes place in inflammation of ligament when primary, it is necessary to mention, nevertheless, that inflammation in these tissues is much more frequently the consequence of previous disease in the synovial membrane or the articular cartilages. This is particularly the case in the knee-joint and elbow.

β. *Ulceration* of ligament is the result either of traumatic inflammation proceeding to suppuration, or of suppuration within the articular cavity. Even in the latter case the desmoid tissue itself is rarely destroyed; and the opening takes place between its fibres,

---

* Surgical Anatomy, by Abraham Colles. Dublin, 1811.

which are loosened and separated. The most frequent instances of ulcerated destruction of this tissue are seen in destruction of the round
ligament and part of the capsule in the coxo-femoral articulation,
and in that of the crucial ligaments in the femoro-tibial articulation.

γ. *Periostitis.* Periosteum is liable to inflammation either from
injury, spontaneously, or from the operation of the syphilitic or the
mercurial poison. In fractures of the extremities the periosteum
may be seen reddened, thickened, and depositing semifluid substance, which appears to coagulate and unite the broken or wounded portions. When it takes place spontaneously, it is said to depend on the strumous diathesis, of which it is believed to be an indication. The membrane becomes thick, painful, unusually vascular, and, unless the action subsides, or is controlled by art, semifluid lymph is effused beneath it, and even bloody, sanious, purulent matter may be formed. If the inflammation be confined to
one spot, the thickened membrane, with the lymphy induration beneath it, gives rise to the swelling termed node; (*nodus*). When
suppuration takes place, it is too often followed by caries of the
subjacent bone if of soft spongy texture, as in the sternum; or
death (*necrosis*) if in one of more compact structure, as in the
skull. The distinction, however, is not invariably observed; for
caries of the *tibia* or *ulna* is seen to follow periosteal inflammation
in these bones.* The appearances produced in the bones by this
process belong to another head. Though any part of the periosteum may be attacked by inflammation, certain regions seem more
liable to it than others. Node, whether from strumous, syphilitic,
or mercurial origin, generally takes place in parts of the periosteum
where that membrane approaches the surface. Thus the anterior
surface of the tibia, the posterior internal surface of the ulna, the
outer surface of the radius, and the anterior surface of the clavicle
and sternum, are usual situations for periosteal inflammation.
Strumous periosteal inflammation in the phalanges of the fingers I
have seen only in young children. The phalanges are then rough
and denuded; and the discharge of fetid sanious matter gives rise
to sinuous ulcers not easily healed. These effects are to be attributed to the suspension of the nutritious powers of the periosteal
vessels.

In some instances inflammation of the periosteum terminates in

* Practical Observations in Surgery and Morbid Anatomy, &c. By John Howship,
London, 1816, p. 176.

a bony swelling, or a deposition of hard osseous matter on the surface of the bone. (*Exostosis.*) The exact nature of the process is not well understood. But there is reason to believe, that what is originally a deposit of lymph as in node, becomes eventually penetrated by calcareous matter.*

The perichondrium is not very dissimilar in morbid relations to the periosteum. Its inflammation may cause in like manner thickening, morbid deposits, and ulceration, or even death of the subjacent cartilage. Such is the course of phenomena occasionally observed in the cartilages of the larynx and those of the ribs.

δ. *Sparganosis. Rheumatismus.* Rheumatism. Fascial inflammation. Though I have above admitted, on the authority of Carmichael Smyth, inflammation of muscular tissue as a cause of rheumatism, I doubt whether it is entitled to the character of a genuine or uniform pathological cause of that disease. Independent of the fact, that the rheumatic pains occur often round joints, in which there are no muscles, the theory is at best only an ingenious assumption, and is not supported by any strong facts or arguments.

Though rheumatic pain is often referred to muscular parts, it is less frequently so than to joints and parts covered by aponeurotic sheaths and *fasciæ.* Of 520 cases, Haygarth observed in 388 the rheumatic action to be seated in joints, in 118 in muscular parts, and in 14 wandering, general, or migrating through the limbs. Of 170 cases, in 154 one or more joints were inflamed; in 33 cases, both joints and muscles were simultaneously affected; and in some cases only were the muscles affected without the joints.

Though from these facts Dr Haygarth infers that acute rheumatism is seated chiefly in the joints, he does not attempt to ascertain the particular texture, in the affection of which the disease consists. It is further manifest, that while it is impossible to exclude affection of the muscles entirely, it results that this affection is only secondary. The proof adduced by Dr Scudamore from pressure of the whole course of a muscle, and grasping its substance during severe rheumatism, to show that the fleshy part is not the seat of complaint, is entitled to attention. Combined with those already mentioned, and with other considerations to be adduced immediately, it results that the rheumatic action is seated in a texture, which, confined neither to the site of the joints, nor to that of the muscles exclusively, is common to both, and which, from its extensive distribution and complicated arrangement, accords best with the phenomena,

* Medico-Chirurgical Transactions, Vol. VIII. p. 90.

progress, and effects of the disease. It is unnecessary to repeat
the considerations above adduced from the anatomical relations and
characters of fascia and its various divisions. That they are the
chief seat of acute rheumatism may be inferred from the following
circumstances.

· 1. When the rheumatic action is seated in muscular parts, instead of· being confined to the muscular fibres, it may always be
referred to the aponeurotic membrane which covers or penetrates
them.. 2. The peculiar pains of rheumatism are always most dis-
•tinct in those situations in which several folds of aponeurotic membrane meet; and their migrations may be traced from one extremity to another of an aponeurotic membrane, and along the course
of its principal divisions. 3. The kind of pain which attends rheumatism resembles that of the fibrous tissues in general when inflamed
in undergoing aggravation under the influence of external heat and
during the night. 4. This view of the seat of rheumatic disorder
affords the most probable explanation of the effusion which takes
place in the tendinous sheaths (*bursæ mucosæ ;*) and even occasionally within the joints; for since each sheath is partly enveloped in
aponeurotic membrane, and every articulation is covered by fasciæ inserted into the capsules or periosteum, the inflammatory process which takes place in the *fasciæ* soon gives rise, as in analogous
cases, to effusion, critical or non-critical, from the contiguous synovial membrane. 5. This view also affords the most rational explanation of·the fact remarked by all authors, that rheumatism almost
never terminates in suppuration.   To suppose that muscle does not
suppurate, is perhaps erroneous from what has been above adduced.
That fascia and fibrous tissue in general is little disposed to suppurate, unless when mechanically injured, is manifest from a number
of circumstances; and this may perhaps be regarded as the true
explanation of the fact now noticed. 6. It must further be remarked,
that inflammation in this tissue renders it thick, hard, and rigid,
and occasionally causes between its fibres effusion of lymph, which
increases this thickening, induration, and rigidity. On these changes
depend the immobility of rheumatic parts, and the loss of power
which follows long and obstinate, or neglected and repeated, attacks
of the disease.

The question, whether there be any thing peculiar in the nature
of rheumatic inflammation is not undeserving attention. This, however, is not the place for discussing it; and if the views now advanced

be well-founded, it may be inferred that its peculiarities consist in the anatomical and physical qualities of the texture in which I have attempted to show it is seated.

Though in acute rheumatism the inflammation affects a large proportion, if not the whole of the fascial system, local forms of the disease may occur, in which it is confined with more or less accuracy to one or two fasciæ. Thus inflammation of the fascia of the temporal and masseter muscles produces rheumatism of the temple and rheumatic locked jaw; that of the occipito-frontal fascia rheumatism of the head; that of the cervical fascia crick in the neck; that of the pectoral fascia and the intersections of the intercostal muscles spurious pleurisy (*pleurodyne ;*) that of the abdominal fasciæ a rheumatic belly-ach; that of the lumbar fasciæ *lumbago ;* and that of the aponeurotic parts of the glutael muscles genuine *sciatica* or hip-gout.

2. *Fascia* is liable to undergo, in consequence of the operation of certain agents, a peculiar degree of thickening and rigidity of its tissue, with contraction, which has the effect of impeding much or abolishing entirely the motions of the parts with which it is connected. Thus the fascia covering the joints is liable, in consequence of articular rheumatism, or that affecting the capsule and synovial membrane, to be affected by more or less thickening, rigidity, and contraction. The most usual situation, however, in which this change is seen is the palmar aponeurosis, which becomes thickened, crispated, and shortened, and the effect of which is to inflect forcibly the ring-finger into the palm of the hand, preventing it from being extended, then the little finger, and afterwards the index and middle fingers.

This change is most usually observed in those who have to make efforts with the palm of the hand in handling and compressing hard bodies; for instance, the hammer, the oar, or the whip. Hence wine-dealers, who have to pierce wine-casks, and coach-drivers, who have to handle the whip, masons and similar workmen, are liable to suffer from this disorder.

Patients feel the approach of this malady by a sense of stiffness in the palm, and difficulty in extending the finger. Soon the fingers remain incurvated one-fourth, one-third, or one-half; in some instances the tips of the fingers are forcibly incurvated into the palm. At first is felt on the palmar surface of the fingers and hand the sensation of a cord, which is more tense when any effort to stretch the fingers is made, and which almost entirely disappears when the fingers are completely bent. This cord is rounded in form; and its most prominent point is at the top of the articulation of the finger with the metacarpal bone supporting it. There this cord forms a sort of bridge.

Little pain is felt in the course of this disease, which is confined entirely to the fascia, and in which the prominent feature is stiffness and inextensible incurvation of the fingers.*

3. *Tyroma.*—The tyromatous deposition in the tubercular form may take place in the periosteum. The tubercles, which in colour and physical qualities resemble tyromatous matter in other situations, are minute, irregularly spheroidal, and occupy the substance of the membrane. Their presence gives rise to chronic inflammation of the membrane, which becomes thick, spongy, and vascular, and is at length detached from the bone by effusion of purulent fluid; and their liquefaction eventually forms a bad suppuration. This is one of the forms of what is usually termed strumous disease of the bones.

4. *Chondroma.*—Cartilaginous induration of the white fibrous tissue is so common that it scarcely requires separate notice. The ligaments are often affected with this, especially in stiff and ankylosed joints, and appear then to acquire the properties of genuine cartilage. This, which may be regarded as one of the effects of chronic inflammation, with long disease of the articular tissues, I conceive, is what is meant by inordinate *rigidity* of the ligaments, much dwelt on by practical authors. It never occurs, I am satisfied, unless under the circumstances now mentioned. In the periosteum I have seen the same change resulting from the same causes. It takes place after compound fractures, occasionally after amputation, and, in short, in all circumstances in which the membrane is inflamed.

5. *Ossification.*—Partial or general conversion into bone, though not uncommon in the white fibrous system, is nevertheless restricted in a peculiar manner. It is, for instance, much less frequent in ligament than in periosteum; and in fascia it is scarcely known. Ossification in ligament commences at the point connected with the periosteum; and it is uncommon to observe it extend over the

* Leçons Orales de Clinique Chirurgicale Faites à l'Hotel Dieu de Paris. Par M. le Baron Dupuytren, Chirurgien en Chef. Recueillies et Publiées par MM. le Docteurs Brierre de Boismont et Marx, 2xieme edit. Tome IV. Paris, 1839. Article xi. p. 473.

whole ligament, unless in cases of anchylosis and stiff joint, in which it is rather a sort of cartilaginous rigidity and induration than actual conversion into bone. The former appears to be the origin of the bony nodules or sesamoid bones occasionally found in the substance of the funicular ligaments. In the irregular filaments, especially the sacro-ischiatic, it is not unusual to find ossification in aged subjects.

That the periosteum may be converted into bone is a point which has been alternately admitted and denied during a whole century. While the numerous experiments of Du Hamel * and Troja† tend to establish it in the affirmative, it is rendered very doubtful by the facts and arguments of Leveillé and Richerand. From the experiments of the former authors it results that the periosteum becomes thick, highly vascular, very firm, and eventually acquires a bony hardness in its inner layer under either of the following circumstances ;—1st, when it is detached from the bone ; 2d, after fractures during the process of reunion ; and 3dly, when the marrow or its membrane is destroyed. That in the two former instances the inner layers of the periosteum truly undergo conversion into bone, may be regarded as established, not only by the experiments of Du Hamel and Troja, but by those of Dupuytren,‡ Cruveilhier,§ Breschet,‖ and Villermé,¶ and especially by the phenomena of reunion after fractures by gunshot wounds. The third case, that of injury of the marrow and its vessels, is perhaps more ambiguous. It appears, nevertheless, from the experiments of M. Cruveilhier, that only when the medullary membrane is destroyed, with the permanent continuance of a foreign body in the canal, ossification at the surface of the bone takes place at the expense not only of the periosteum, but even of the muscles. The condition necessary for the ossification of the periosteum after injury appears to be, that the concomitant inflammation produces albuminous effusion only ; for when the membrane is in contact with purulent matter, effusion of albuminous or coagulable fluid is precluded ; and in this sense only, perhaps, are the inferences of Leveillé to be admitted.

* Mem. de l'Acad. des Sciences, 1741, &c.
† Mem. de la Societe Roy. de Med. 1776.
‡ Journal Univers. des Sci. Med. T. xx. p. 131.
§ Essai sur l'Anatomie Pathologique, Tome ii. p. 25, &c. Paris, 1816.
‖ Quelques Recherch. Hist. et Exper. sur le Cal. Paris, 1819.
¶ Quart. Journ of Foreign Medicine, No. ii. London, 1819.

On this subject, however, I shall have occasion to make some observations in the fourth chapter, when treating of Nekrosis.

In fascia, I have said, and I may add tendinous aponeurosis, ossification is almost unknown. To this head, however, may perhaps be referred the instance recorded by Hoernigk of alleged ossification of the tendinous centre of the diaphragm and part of the intercostal muscles;* that of chondro-osteoid induration of the right half of the diaphragm by Lieutaud from the Petersburgh Transactions;† a similar case seen by Leveillé in 1793; and that of ossification of the tendinous centre of the same muscle mentioned in the body of Collalto by Cruveilhier. The instance of cartilaginous induration of the deep-seated muscles of the leg, found by Dupuytren in the body of a man affected with Arabian elephantiasis, though considered by Cruveilhier as ossification of the muscles, is probably with greater justice to be viewed as of the same description.‡

A singular instance of ossification of the fibrous *septum* of the *corpus cavernosum,* so complete as to requre excision, occurred to Dr M'Lellan of Baltimore in the United States.§

6. Some of the forms of *osteo-steatoma* and *osteo-sarcoma* appear to originate in the periosteum. The former is generally an encysted tumour, and, according to the observation of Meckel, may primarily affect this membrane. The latter, from its anatomical characters, bears a greater affinity with this source; and I think, in several cases, I have been able to trace osteo-sarcomatous tumours to the periosteum.‖ Of neither, however, are the local relations, when examined, so simple or distinct as to enable the pathologist to determine the question positively. Does true cancer (*scirrho-carcinoma*) ever originate in the periosteum? The tumours to which this name has been applied are rather examples of *osteo-sarcoma* than of genuine scirrhus. Such at least is the character of most of the tumours of the maxillary sinus.

7. When the encephaloid degeneration (*fungus hæmatodes*) appears in the periosteum, it may often be traced to the contiguous muscles, or to some of the adjoining articular tissues, or to the bone itself. In the latter case, however, it is almost impossible to de-

* Haller, Disputationes Medico-Pract. Tom. VI. p. 344.
† Historia Anatomico-Med. Tome II. p. 99.
‡ Essai sur l'Anatomie Pathologique, Tome II. p. 73.
§ Philadelphia Monthly Journal, Nov. 1827. Vol. I. No. 6, p. 256.
‖ Mr Howship in Medico-Chir. Trans. Vol. VIII. p. 95 and 99 ; where the same conclusion is formed.

termine whether the bone or periosteum were the original seat of the disease.

8. Punctured and contused wounds of the white fibrous system, especially of the ligaments and periosteum, are liable to be succeeded by tetanic motions, more or less general; and wounds with much laceration in subjects of all ages are too often followed by gangrenous inflammation terminating fatally. This I have seen several times, not only in compound dislocations of the larger joints, but in contused wounds of the feet, in which the white fibrous system is much injured. Partial laceration of the capsular ligaments occasionally takes place in dislocation. (A. Bonn, Desault, Howship, Sir A. Cooper.)

9. *Desmectasis.* *Excessive relaxation* is mentioned as an abnormal state occurring in ligaments. It is the result of repeated overdistension, as in luxation or subluxation, or in consequence of the weakness sometimes left after local inflammation, or long-continued disease. Though this may happen to the ligaments of any joint, it is most frequently seen in those of temporo-maxillary and scapulo-humeral articulations. Distortions of the spine are ascribed by Dr Harrison to relaxation of the vertebral ligaments. But if this be the cause, it is merely as the effect of previous disease; and it is quite inadequate to produce the extreme deformity so frequently observed in the vertebral column of young persons.

On the new or accidental production of the fibrous system in other tissues, much has of late years been written by Bichat, Bayle, Laennec, and other foreign authors. Without positively denying the principle, that the fibrous system may be accidentally developed, I think with Meckel, that in general these products partake of the cartilaginous character. The notice of them, therefore, will more conveniently be introduced under that head.

CHAPTER III.

YELLOW FIBROUS SYSTEM.   *Ligamenta Flava ; Ligamentum Nuchæ.*
Tissu Fibreux jaune, Beclard.

THE yellow ligaments (*ligamenta flava*) which connect the spinous
processes of the vertebræ to each other differ considerably from the
articular ligaments and the periosteum, and suggested to Beclard
the necessity of establishing a particular order of fibrous tissues, to
which he applied the denomination of *yellow or tawny fibrous system.*   Under this he includes also the proper membrane of the arteries ; that of the veins and of the lymphatic vessels ; the membranes
which form excretory ducts ; that of the air-passages ; the fibrous
covering of the cavernous body of the urethra, and perhaps that
of the spleen.   The actions and occasional distensions of which
these parts are the seat require, it is said, a tissue, the resistance
and elasticity of which may at once counteract any extraordinary
effort, and cause them to resume their original state, when the distending cause ceases to operate.   In the lower animals this purpose is more conspicuous than in the human subject.   The posterior
cervical ligament (*ligamentum nuchæ,* Arab. ; *cervicis,* Lat.) coun-
teracts the tendency to inclination of the head ; and a similar membrane strengthens the abdominal parietes, and resists the weight
and distending power of the *viscera.*   In the feline tribe, an elastic
ligament inserted into the unguinal phalanges retains them extended so long as the muscles do not alter their direction.   The
shells of the bivalve molluscous animals, as oysters, mussels, &c.
are opened by a similar fibrous tissue as soon as the muscles which
close them are relaxed.

The disposition of the component fibres is the same in the elastic
as in the common white fibrous system.   Their colour, which is
yellow or tawny, is generally more distinct in the dead subject.
They are said to be less tenacious, but more elastic than those of
any other tissue.   In respect to chemical composition, they appear
to contain a considerable quantity of fibrine in a peculiar condition,
combined with some albumen and a little gelatine.   Their other
properties are not very conspicuous.

The morbid changes incident to them are quite unknown.

CHAPTER IV.

Section I.

Bone, οϛεον.   *Os,—Ossa,—Tissu Osseux*, die knochen.

No animal substance has been more frequently or thoroughly examined than bone ; and the greatest difficulty in describing its general anatomy consists in selecting and concentrating information.*

Several attempts have at different times been made to ascertain the atomic constitution of bone, but without much success. Malpighi, though he corrected the extravagant fiction of Gagliardi regarding the osseous plates and nails, fancied bones to be composed of filaments, which Lewenhoeck represented as minute hollow tubes; (*tubuli.*) By Clopton Havers, again, the ultimate particles of bone were imagined to be fibres aggregated into plates (*laminæ*) placed on each other, and traversed by longitudinal and transverse hollows or pores, (*pori.*)† This view was adopted by Courtial,‡ Winslow,§ Palfyn,‖ Monró,¶ and Reichel,** the last of whom was at some pains to demonstrate this arrangement of plates and minute tubes by microscopical observation.

The justice of these notions was first questioned by Scarpa, who, in 1799, undertook to show, by examinations of bone deprived of

---

* The principal authors on the structure of bone are Dominici Gagliardi, *Anatome Ossium, novis inventis illustrata.* Romæ, 1689.

Malpighi, *De Ossium structura ex Op. Post.* who corrected the fictitious views of the former. Marcelli Malpighii Opera Omnia Tomis Duobus Comprehensa. Londini, 1686. Folio. Opera Posthuma. Londini, 1697.

Clopton Havers, *Osteologia Nova*, or Some New Observations of the Bones and the Parts belonging to them. London, 1691.

De La Sone, *Memoire sur l'organisation des os*, Mem. de l'Academie, 1754.

G. C. Reichel, de *Ossium ortu atque structura.* Lips. 1760.

Ext. in Sandifort Thesaur. Vol. ii. p. 171.

Antonii Scarpa, *de Penitiori Ossium Structurâ Comment.* Lips. 1799. Republished in *De Anatome et Pathologia Ossium, Commentarii*, Auctore A. Scarpa. Ticini, 1827.

Papers by Mr Howship in the sixth and seventh volumes of the Medico-Chirurgical Transactions.

† Osteologia Nova. London, 1691, p. 34, 37, 41, 46.

‡ Nouvelles Observations sur les Os. A. Leide, 1709.

§ Exposition Anatomique.   ‖ Anatomie Chirurgicale.

¶ Anatomy of the Bones.   ** De Ossium Ortu, &c. § v.

its earth by acid, and long macerated in pure water, that it consists, both externally and internally, of reticular or cellular structure.* So far as I understand what idea this eminent anatomist attaches to the terms *reticular* and *cellular*, I doubt whether this opinion is better founded than any of the previous ones. After repeating his experiment of immersing in oil of turpentine, bone macerated in acid, I cannot perceive the reticular or cellular arrangement which Scarpa describes as demonstrable in bone. It must, I conceive, be the result of the mode of preparation. Recently bone has been submitted to microscopic examination by Mr Howship, who has been led to revive the opinion of the existence of minute longitudinal canals, as maintained by Lewenhoeck, Havers, and Reichel, but with Scarpa maintains the ultimate texture not to be laminated but reticulated.† *Lastly,* the existence of fibres and plates, which is admitted by Blumenbach, Soemmering, Bichat, and Meckel, apparently on insufficient grounds, is to be viewed as an appearance produced by the physical, and perhaps the chemical qualities of the proper animal organic matter of which bone consists. Though it does not demonstrate, it depends on, the intimate structure of this body.

The minute structure or atomic constitution of bone is probably the same in all the pieces of the skeleton, and is varied only in mechanical arrangement. When a cylindrical bone is broken, and its surfaces are examined with a good magnifying glass; or when minute splinters are inspected in a powerful microscope, it appears to be a uniform substance without fibres, plates, or cells, penetrated everywhere by minute blood-vessels. Its fracture is uneven, passing to splintery. In the recent state its colour is bluish-white; but in advanced age the blue tinge disappears. Delicate injection, or feeding an animal with madder, shows the vascularity of this substance.

To have a clearer and more accurate idea of the minute structure of bone, it is requisite to break transversely a long bone, and examine its fractured surface by a good glass, or to examine in the same manner the transverse fracture of a long bone which has been burnt white in a charcoal fire. The broken surface presents a multitude of minute holes, generally round or oval, which are larger towards the medullary cavity, but become exceedingly minute towards the outer surface of the bone. Of these minute holes

---

* De Penitiori Ossium Structura, 4to. Lips. 1799.

† Experiments and Observations, &c. Medico-Chir. Trans. Vol. vi. p. 287, and Microscopic Observations, &c. Vol. vii. p. 392, &c.

no part of the bone, however compact in appearance, is destitute; and the only difference is, that they are more minute, and more regularly circular towards the outer than towards the medullary surface. These circular holes are transverse sections of the *tubuli* of Lewenhoeck, the longitudinal pores of Havers, (*Osteologia,* p. 43 and 46,) the pores and *tubuli* of Reichel, and the longitudinal canals of Howship. They communicate with each other by means of their great multiplicity and slight obliquity and tortuosity. They contain not blood-vessels exclusively, but divisions of the vascular filamentous tissue, which secretes the marrow. They are seen very distinctly in bones which have been burnt. After many careful examinations, I have never been able to observe holes in longitudinal fractures of bones; and I therefore infer that there are no transverse pores.

These capillary pores are seen in the flat bones of the skull. I find them in the compact matter of the outer and inner tables of the occipital bone when well burnt, in which they seem to pass gradually from the lattice-work of the *diploe* to the distinct pores of the tables. I doubt, however, whether these pores can be said, as in the long bones, to indicate canals. They seem rather to belong to a very delicate cancellated structure.

These pores are most numerous and distinct in the bones of young subjects. In the humerus of a child burnt to whiteness, I find them to be large, numerous, and distinct, even at the periosteal surface of the bone. In that of a young man of 28, they are larger, more numerous, and more distinct than in bones of older subjects. In a very dense ulna before me, though distinct through a good glass, they are exceedingly minute, and quite imperceptible to the naked eye.

Though these circular pores are most distinct in calcined bones, and might therefore be thought to be the result of the burning, yet that they are not, I infer from the circumstance that they are seen by a good glass in the transverse fracture of splinters of the femur and other large bones.

If a portion of bone be immersed in sulphuric, nitric, muriatic, or acetic acid properly diluted, it becomes soft and pliable, and when dried, is found to be lighter than before; yet it is impossible to discover that any particle of its substance has been mechanically removed, or that its shape and appearance are changed.

If a portion of bone be placed in a charcoal fire, and the heat be gradually raised to whiteness, it burns first with flame, and at length becomes quite red. If then it be removed carefully and slowly cooled, it appears as white as chalk, is found to be very brittle, and to have lost something of its weight. Yet neither in this case does any part of its substance appear to be removed, nor is its mechanical figure or appearance altered.

Chemical examination, however, informs us that in the first case a portion of earthy matter (phosphate of lime) is removed by the agency of the acid, and held suspended in the fluid, while the pliant, but otherwise identical piece of bone consists chiefly, if not entirely, of animal matter ; and that, in the second case, this animal matter is removed by destructive decomposition, while the earthy matter is left little changed by the action of fire. It is therefore to be concluded, that every particle of bone, however minute, consists of animal or organic, and earthy or inorganic matter intimately united; and that it is impossible to touch with the point of the smallest needle any part of bone which is not thus constituted. A piece of bone consists not of cartilaginous fibres varnished over, as Herissant imagined, with earthy matter, but of a substance in which every constituent atom consists essentially of animal and earthy matter intimately combined.

There is therefore no rational ground for dividing osseous tissue into compact and spongy, as the older anatomists did ; for though the middle or solid parts of long bones are denser and heavier than the ends of these bones, or the bodies of the vertebræ, the difference consists not in chemical composition, but in mechanical arrangement and structure. On dividing the head of a long bone, the lattice-work or *cancelli*, as they are named, are formed by many minute threads of bone, crossing and interlacing with each other. But each thread is quite as dense, and consists of the same quantity of animal and earthy matter as the most solid part of the centre of the same bone. These threads, however, instead of being disposed closely and compactly with each other, so as to take a small space, are so arranged that they occupy a large one, and present a considerable bulk.

The minute anatomical structure of bone was again investigated by Deutsch in 1834, and by Müller and Miescher in 1836.

The former observed the pores or tubules of Havers, (*canaliculi Haversiani*) to be surrounded with concentric *lamellæ*, and the medullary canal in the cylindrical bones to be inclosed by another order of *lamellæ*, and the same canals in the flat bones proceeding from the parallel of the surface. These tubules he describes as crowded and passing across from one lamella to the next. He also mentions the oblong corpuscula, which have been discovered by Purkinje to be everywhere dispersed through their texture.

In many circumstances, the observations of Müller and Miescher agree. Both admit the existence of *lamellæ*, of *corpuscula*, and of *canaliculi* or tubular canals, the pores of Havers.

The *lamellæ*, says Müller, are so translucent, that, when laid on written paper, the characters may be easily read through them. When these lamellæ are examined under the lens on a dark ground, it is seen that the whiteness of bones depends on the *corpuscula*, and that their intermediate substance is entirely transparent.

Laminæ or *lamellæ* are not observed in the bones of infants. But they are distinctly seen in the compact tissue of the cylindrical bones of adults, in which they form the external surface or compact tissue. Near the medullary canal, where the number of intersecting *canaliculi* increases, they gradually, and at length completely vanish.

The thickness of these *laminæ* is estimated by Deutsch at $\frac{1}{480}$th part of an inch. This Miescher thinks the result of typographical error, and he makes them $\frac{1}{4440}$th part of an English inch, or ·0027 of one line. In the thigh-bone of the ox, in which the *laminæ* may be separated into *lamellæ* much more easily and more distinctly than in human bones, the component *lamellæ* appeared as it were to be separated or united by fibres interposed; and in parts where the *lamellæ* were most closely united, Miescher observed slender, tapering *fibrillæ* following the longitudinal direction, of a brown colour, and firm, which, throughout, penetrated the *laminæ*, and which he regards as certainly the same with the nails or *claviculi* of Gagliardi, and the fibres described, in 1818, by Medici. The lamellæ may be divided by needles into several very slender *foliola* or leaflets.

The *canaliculi* are found in all the compact osseous tissue, and, in general, their direction follows that of the process of ossification in the fœtus. Thus, in the cylindrical bones, they proceed from the middle of the shaft to the articular extremities; and in the frontal and parietal bones, from the centre to the circumference.

The interior of these canals is cylindrical, and it is smallest in those near the surface; conversely, near the medullary canal, they become larger, so that they may be three or four times more ample than those at the compact surface of the bone. The intersection of these canals, also near the medullary cavity with their enlarged size, produces the formation of cells, which communicate with several of the *canaliculi.*

The wall of the canaliculi is composed of from 10 to 15 concentric lamellæ, and is from $\frac{1}{300}$th to $\frac{1}{400}$th part of an English inch broad. These canals contain marrow or a substance like it.

The *corpuscula,* which were known to Leewenhoeck, but have been fully examined only by Purkinje, Deutsch, Miescher, and Müller, are oblong oval bodies, flattened, and pointed at each end, situate between two *lamellæ,* so that their long diameter preserves an oblique direction to the lamella. They are observed in bone which has been deprived of its earthy matter by acid, like minute specks of a brown colour, transparent in the middle and bounded by a distinct opaque line. Their size varies. From them proceed many dark-coloured striæ, so that they present the appearance of ovoidal bodies with small fibrils or roots proceeding from them. Their long diameter is from .0048 to .0072 ; and their transverse diameter from .0017 to .0030 of one line.

These bodies are formed in the primary or ossifying cartilage; around them ossification takes place; and it appears that their presence is of great importance to the original formation of the bone.

When these *corpuscula* are examined, by a powerful microscope, with refracted light, they appear like black oblong specks, with the dark *striæ* proceeding from their surface in all directions, but most abundantly from their lateral regions. When they are examined by reflected light, they appear like bluish-white specks of a milky colour, with the *striæ* of the same colour proceeding from them.

What the nature of these corpuscula may be, has been a source of much inquiry. When laminæ of bones finely polished are boiled in potass, and thereby deprived of their translucency, the calcareous matter of the part formerly translucent adheres, exactly as if the structure of the animal matter had been in no way changed. In all the intermediate spaces the substance of the corpuscula appears finely granulated; and the white grains equal nearly the size of the diameter of the radiating canals of these bodies.

Müller thinks it merely probable that these *corpuscula* may be a sort of secreting organs to deposit osseous matter ; and he therefore is disposed, though not very confidently, to term them *organa chalikophora*, or earth-bearing organs. He allows, however, that it is impossible on this subject to speak with certainty.

Miescher states the following conclusions: 1*st*, The spongy or cancellated tissue is nothing but enlarged *canaliculi*. 2*d*, The medullary canal, as to formation and signification, must be regarded as the union of such *canaliculi*. 3*d*, The canals, therefore, surrounded by concentric lamellæ, and containing marrow, furnished with abundant blood-vessels, are the primary form of the osseous tissues completed by growth.*

In these results there is nothing new. Indeed, the only new fact in the whole is the existence of the *corpuscula*. The idea of *lamellæ* is not new. Their existence was maintained by Gagliardi, Havers, Reichel, Blumenbach, and Soëmmering; and it may be doubted if the opinion be well founded.

As to the *corpuscula*, they are stated to exist in the primary or ossifying cartilage or callus; and it is very probable that they in some manner contribute to the formation of bone, as it is eventually observed to exist.

Though bone has been submitted to analysis by many eminent chemists, the results hitherto obtained cannot be said to be quite satisfactory. The most complete is that of Berzelius, who, in 100 parts of bone from the thigh of an adult, gives the following proportions: of gelatine, 32.17; blood-vessels, 1.13; phosphate of lime, 51.04; carbonate of lime, 11.30; fluate of lime, 2.00; phosphate of magnesia, 1.16; hydrochlorate of soda and water, 120.

These results by no means agree with those obtained by Fourcroy and Vauquelin, who found neither fluoric acid nor phosphate of magnesia, but discovered oxides of iron and manganese, silica, and alumina, in bone. The statement of Berzelius regarding the presence of fluate of lime has, on the other hand, been confirmed by Dr George Wilson, who found it in recent bones of the human body, and in those of various mammalia, and in fossil bones. Sulphate of lime, which was found in the experiments of Hatchett, was shown by Berzelius to be formed during calcination.

It is, however, obvious that a little more than a third part of bone consists of animal matter, which appears to be either entirely gelatine, or a modification of that principle; and that the remainder, nearly equal to two-thirds, consists of earthy matter, which is chiefly phosphoric acid combined with lime. From the experiments of Dr Rees it results that $\frac{3}{5}$ths are earthy matter; and $\frac{2}{5}$ths are

* De Inflammatione Ossium, eorumque Anatome Generale. Exercitatio Anatomico Pathologica. Auctore Friderico Miescher, Med. et Chirurgiæ Doct., cum Tabulis

animal matter.   s the ca   onic aci   sa   to   ime
also not a result of the decomposition of the animal matter?   The
other saline substances are not peculiar to bone, but being common
to it and the other animal tissues, and even the fluids, may be supposed, without much injustice, to be derived from the blood left in
the bone at the moment of death.

The cylindrical bones of the extremities contain more earthy
matter than those of the trunk; the bones of the upper extremity
contain more earthy matter than the corresponding bones of the
lower extremity; and the bones of the head contain considerably
more earthy matter than the bones of the trunk.*

It is most difficult to say what is the nature of the animal matter
of bones.   At one time it was presumed to be cartilage; but this
appears to be a mere assumption, derived from the superficial resemblance which it bears to this substance.   It does not appear to
be mere gelatine; for though this principle is obtained in quantity
from bone, and bones are economically used in manufacturing glue,
they do not furnish the same proportion of jelly as tendon, nor are
they so useful in making soups, as was once paradoxically and absurdly enough maintained by some chemists.   It is probable that
the gelatine, as we have already stated, is under a peculiar modification, or combined with some principle which is not well understood.   Is there no albumen in this animal matter?   The sulphur
formed during calcination seems to show that there is.   There is
no fat in bones; and in the experiments in which this substance has
been found, it is evident that it was merely marrow which had been
mingled with the bones employed, or which had not been removed.

Though bones were arranged by the ancients among the bloodless organic substances, they receive a considerable proportion of
this fluid, and injection shows them to be highly vascular.   In early
life, especially, these vessels are numerous; and even in the grown
adult, when death takes place by strangulation or by drowning, the
bones are found to be naturally well injected.   In old age the
vessels are less numerous, but they are larger.   From the capillary
vessels distributed through their substance, bones derive the pale
blue or light pink colour by which the healthy bone is characterized.
When this tint becomes intense, it indicates inflammation or some
morbid state of the vessels of the bone.   When it is lost, and the
bone assumes a white or yellow colour, the part so changed is dead.

Anatomists distinguish three orders of vessels which enter the
substance of bones; the first, those which penetrate the bodies of

---

* On the Proportions of Animal and Earthy Matter, &c.   By G. O. Rees, M. D.
Medico-Chirurgical Transactions, Vol. XXI. p. 406.   London, 1838.

long bones to the medullary cavity, (*arteriæ nutritiæ, arteriæ medullares* ;) the second, those which go to the cellular structure of the bone; and the third, those which go to the compact or dense matter of the bone. This view is only partially correct. The large vessels termed nutritious certainly proceed chiefly to the cavity of the bone, and are distributed in the medullary membrane. These, however, are not the only vessels which proceed to this part of the bone. *First,* I have often traced several large vessels, entering not by the middle, but the ends of the long bones, into the loose cancellated texture, and actually distributed on the *medulla* in this part of the bone. In dried bones also the canals of these vessels may be demonstrated extending from the surface to the body of the bone. *Secondly,* the nutritious vessels are not constant; and when they are wanting, those of the ends of the bone, or of the *cancelli,* are much larger and more numerous than in ordinary circumstances. The communication between these and the branches of the nutritious vessels, which is admitted by Bichat, may be easily demonstrated. The third order of vessels are those which may be termed *periosteal,* in so far as they consist of an infinite number of minute capillaries, some red, some colourless, proceeding from the periosteum to the bone, and contributing to maintain the connection between the two. The short bones and the flat bones, which are destitute of nutritious arteries, receive blood from the two latter orders, but principally from the periosteal vessels. In the skull these vessels are often highly injected in apoplectic subjects, and in persons killed by drowning or strangulation.

The veins of bones are peculiar in their arrangement. The nutritious artery is accompanied by a social vein; the articular and periosteal vessels are said to be destitute of corresponding venous vessels. According to Dupuytren, however, minute venous capillaries arise from the substance of the osseous tissue, precisely as in other tissues, and, uniting in the same manner, form twigs, branches, and trunks, which finally terminate in the neighbouring veins.

Lymphatics are not found in the substance of bones. Bichat, however, thinks analogically, that nutrition implies exhalation and absorption ; but it is manifest that this does not demonstrate the existence of true lymphatics. Nerves in like manner have not been traced into this substance.*

To complete the anatomical history of bone, it is requisite to examine shortly the marrow. The interior of the long bones con-

* On these points see Scarpa, *de Anatome et Pathologia Ossium Comment.* p. 38, &c. ; and Howship, Med. Chir. Tr. Vol. VIII. p. 66.

tains a notable quantity of fat, oleaginous matter, which has been long known under the name of *marrow* (μυελος ὁςιτης, *medulla ;*) and a similar substance, though in much smaller quantity, is found in the loose cancellated tissue of the flat and short bones. It is in the first situation only that it is possible to examine the anatomical cha-racters of this substance. It is sufficiently similar to fat or animal oil in other parts of the body to lead us to refer it at present to that head. In other respects, its chemical qualities have not been much examined; but an analysis by Berzelius shows that it consists chiefly of an oily matter, not unlike butter in general properties. The filaments, blood-vessels, albumen, gelatine, and osmazome found by this chemist in marrow, are to be regarded as derived from the filamentous tissue in which the medullary particles are deposited, and by no means to be arranged with it. They did not exceed 4 parts in the 100. The medullary membrane, which has been con-sidered as an internal periosteum, is but imperfectly known. There can be no doubt, however, of its existence, which is easily demon-strated by opening either transversely or longitudinally the medul-lary canal of a long bone, and boiling it for about two hours. The marrow then, as is well known to cooks, drops out; and it will be found on examination to be deposited in the interstices of a fila-mentons net-work of animal matter, which is not unlike very fine filamentous or cellular tissue, which may be traced not only into the lattice-work of the extremities, but into the longitudinal canals of the cylindrical bones. It is traversed by blood-vessels, which are observed to bleed during amputation. No nerves have been found in it. The medullary membrane, in short, may be regarded as an extensive net-work of very minute capillaries united by deli-cate filamentous tissue. From these capillaries the marrow is de-posited as a secretion.—(Mascagni, Howship.)

The development or progressive formation of the osseous system has given rise to many interesting researches by Kerckringius, Vater,* Baster,† Duhamel,‡ Nesbitt,§ Haller,‖ Dethleef,¶ Reichel, Albinus,** David, Troja, Scarpa, John Hunter,†† Senff,‡‡Howship,§§

* De Osteogenia Naturali et Præternaturali. Haller, Disput. Anat. Vol. VI. p. 227.
† De Osteogenia. Haller, Disp. Anat. Vol. VII.
‡ Mém. de l'Academie Royale, 1741–42, &c.
§ Human Osteogeny, &c. By Ro. Nesbitt, M. D. Lond. 1736.
‖ Opèra Minora, Tom. II. XXXIII. p. 460.
¶ Dissert. Ossium Calli generationem exhibens. Goett. 1753.
** Annot. Anat. et Eikones Os. Foet. Hum. Lug. Bat. 1753.
†† Medical and Chirurgical Transactions, Vol. II.
‡‡ Nonnulla de Incremento Ossium, &c. Halle, 1781.
§§ Medico-Chirurgical Transactions, Vol. VI. p. 263.

Meckel,[*] Medici, Serres, Lebel, Schultze, Beclard, and Dutrochet; and it is a proof of the difficult and complicated nature of the subject, that it still continues to give rise to fresh investigation. The inquiry naturally resolves itself into two parts,—the history of the process of ossification, as it takes place originally in the fœtus and infant, and the history of its progress as a process of repair when bones are divided, broken, or otherwise destroyed or removed.

From the first formation of the embryo to the termination of fœtal existence and thenceforth to the completion of growth, the bones undergo changes, in which various stages may be distinguished. In the first weeks of fœtal existence it is impossible to recognize anything like bone; and the points in which the bones are afterwards to be developed consist of a soft homogeneous mass of animal matter, which has been designated under the general name of mucus. Sometime between the fifth and the seventh week, in the situation of the extremities, may be recognized dark opaque spots, which are firmer and more solid than the surrounding animal matter. About the eighth week, the extremities may be seen to consist of their component parts, in the centre of each of which is a cylindrical piece of bony matter. Dark solid specks are also seen in the spine, corresponding to the bodies of the vertebræ; and even the rudiments of spinous processes are observed in the shape of minute dark points. In the hands and feet rings of bones are seen in the site of the metacarpal and metatarsal bones. All the joints consist of a semi-consistent jelly-like matter liberally supplied by blood-vessels. At ten weeks the cylinders and rings are increased in length, and are observed to approach the jelly-like extremities, which are acquiring the consistence of cartilage, and when divided present irregular cavities. At the same time the parts forming the head are highly vascular; and between the membranes are deposited minute points of bony matter, proceeding in rays from a centre, which, however, is thinner and more transparent than the margin or circumferenc e—(Howship.)

Between thirteen weeks and four months the cavities in the jelly-like cartilaginous matter receives injection. The membranes of the head are highly vascular, transmitting their vessels through the intervals of the osseous rays, which are occupied abundantly by stiff, glairy, colourless mucilaginous fluid.

In the seventh month, the bony cylinder of the thigh-bone and its epiphyses contain canals perceptible to the microscope. In the

[*] Journal Complementaire, Tome II. p. 211.

head, the bones are proceeding to completion; the pericranium and dura mater are highly vascular; and a quantity of reddish semi-transparent jelly between the scalp and the skull, which contained numerous minute vessels, Mr Howship regards as the loose cellular state of the fœtal pericranium. This is, however, doubtful. The cylindrical bones have at this period no medullary cavity, but present in their interior a loose bony texture.

Between the seventh and eighth months, in a fœtus ten inches long, I find the humerus consisting of a cylinder of bone placed between two brownish firm, jelly-like masses, which correspond to the epiphyses, enclosed by periosteum, which adheres loosely by means of filamentous and vascular productions. The radius is a thin bony rod, also between two jelly-like epiphyses. The ulna is still thinner, more slender and flexible, and even compressible. The interosseous ligament is a continuous duplicature of the periosteum. The metacarpal bones are much as before, only larger. The hands and fingers are complete; but the phalanges consist of minute semi-hard grains, enclosed in periosteum, which forms a general sac to them, and to the intermediate connecting parts. The middle and unguinal phalanges can scarcely be called osseous. The *femur*, like the *humerus*, is an osseous cylinder between two jelly-like epiphyses, enveloped in loosely adhering periosteum. The *tibia* and *fibula* like the *radius* and *ulna*. The metatarsal bones are cylindrical pieces, firm, but not very hard. The first phalanx of the toes is complete; the other two, though the toes are fully formed, are much of the consistence of cartilage. The carpal and tarsal bones are in the state of the epiphyses, but of a gray colour.

In this state of the osseous system, the periosteum, which is continuous, and appears to make one membrane with the capsular ligaments and the deep-seated portions of the fascia, adheres to the bone chiefly by arteries and filamentous productions; and so loose is this connection, that a probe may be inserted beneath it, and carried round or inwards, unless where these connections are situate. Another point where the periosteum adheres firmly is at muscular insertions. Thus it adheres to the *humerus* most firmly at the insertion of the deltoid, and to the *femur* at that of the *glutæus;* and at these parts the bone is already rough.

In the vertebral column the bodies of the vertebræ and the spinous plates are formed; and minute specks are beginning in the site of the transverse processes.

In the skull, the parietal bones are well-formed shells of bone, though very deficient at the mesial plane, the anterior margin, and the upper anterior angle. The pericranium is distinctly membranous and vascular; and the red jelly-like fluid noticed by Mr Howship is exterior to this membrane.

At the period of birth, the cylindrical bones contain tubular canals filled with a colourless glairy fluid, and terminating in the surface of ossification. As the bones previous to this period are homogeneous, and contain no distinct medullary cavity, but present in their interior a soft or loose bony texture, it is reasonable to suppose that the development of the longitudinal canals is connected with the formation of the medullary cavity. At birth in the *femur* may be distinguished a medullary cavity beginning to be formed, about half a line broad, but still very imperfect.

After birth the two processes of the formation of tubular canals and medullary cavity go on simultaneously; and at the same rate nearly the outer part of the cylindrical bones acquires a more dense and compact appearance. The epiphyses, also, which are in the shape of grayish jelly-like masses, begin to present grains and points of bone. Preliminary to this, Mr Howship represents them; while still cartilaginous, as penetrated by canals or tubes, which gradually disappear as ossification proceeds. The carpal and tarsal bones appear to observe the same course in the process of ossification.

In the bones of the skull, however, a different law is observed. The osseous matter is originally deposited in linear tracts or fibres, radiating or diverging from certain points termed points of ossification. Each bone is completed in one shell without *diploe* or distinguishable table. Afterwards, when they are completed laterally, or in the radiating direction, the cancellated arrangement of the *diploe* begins to take place, apparently in the same manner, in which the medullary cavity and compact parts of the long bones are formed.

It has been generally supposed that the formation of cartilage is a preliminary step to that of bone. This, however, seems to be a mistake arising from the circumstance, that cartilage is often observed to be converted in the living body into bone. Neither in the long nor in the flat bones is anything like cartilage at any time observed. The epiphyses, indeed, present something of the consistence of cartilage, but it has neither the firmness nor the elasticity of that substance. It is a concrete jelly, afterwards to be penetrated by calcareous matter. The flat bones are from the first osseous; and though their margins are soft and flexible, in consequence of their recent formation and moist state, they have still a distinct osseous appearance and arrangement, and bear no resemblance to cartilage. In short, true bone seems never at any period of its growth to be cartilaginous.

The period at which ossification may be said to be completed varies doubtless in different individuals. It may be said to be indicated by the completion of the medullary canal, by the ossification of the *epiphyses*, and their perfect union with the osseous cylinder, (*diaphysis.*) The first circumstance is always indefinite. The two latter, though more fixed, are still liable to great variation. The epiphyses are rarely united before the age of 14 or 15; and they may continue detached till the 20th or 21st year. I preserved the greater part of the skeleton of a man, who was known to be about 28, and in whose bones the epiphyses were imperfectly united, and many had dropped off. In general, however, they begin to unite, or to be *knit*, as is said, between the 15th and 20th years.

Little doubt can be entertained that the main agents of original ossification are the periosteum and the periosteal arteries. The proofs of this inference are manifest. The formation of bone has never been ascribed but to the vessels of two agents,—the periosteum and the medullary membrane. That the latter cannot be concerned in the production of bone in the fœtus must be inferred from the fact, that at that period it cannot be said to have existence. To the periosteum, therefore, and its vessels must be ascribed the process of fœtal ossification. Of this a cumulative proof may be found in the circumstance, that the periosteum adheres more firmly at the ends than the middle of the bones; and that the pericranium and *dura mater*, which perform the part of periosteum to the bones of the skull, are visibly concerned in the formation and successive enlargement of these bones. But though the periosteal vessels are the main agents of ossification originally, there is reason to believe that the medullary vessels contribute to its growth and nutrition after it is formed. This may be inferred from the phenomena of fractures, of diseases of the bones, and of those experiments in which the medullary membrane is injured. The periosteum, however, does not act by ossification of its inner layers, as Du Hamel, misled by a false analogy between the growth of trees and bones, laboured to establish. This leads naturally to the examination of the phenomena of ossification as a process of repair. This, however, is introduced more properly under the next section.

The teeth, as a variety of bone, demand attention. Every tooth consists of two hard parts; one external, white, uniform, somewhat like ivory, the other internal, similar to the compact structure of bone.

The first, which is named enamel, is seen only at the crown of the tooth, the upper and outer part of which consists of this substance. It is white, very close in texture, perfectly uniform and homogeneous, yet presenting a fibrous arrangement. Extending across the summit of the tooth in the manner of an incrustation, it is thick above, and diminishes gradually to the root, where it disappears. This fact is demonstrated by macerating a tooth in dilute nitric acid, when the bony root becomes yellow, while the crown remains white.

The enamel is not injectible, and is therefore believed to be inorganic. It is also filled and broken without being reproduced; nor does it present any of the usual properties which distinguished organized bodies. The piercing sensation which is communicated through the tooth from the impression of acids seems to depend on the mere chemical operation, and not on the physiological effect. Upon the whole, the enamel is to be viewed as the result of a process of secretion or deposition, but as inorganic entirely.

The bony part of the tooth is the root and that internal part which is covered on the sides and above by the enamel. It consists of close-grained bony matter, as dense as the compact walls of the long bones, or the petrous portion of the temporal bone. The fibres which are said to be seen in it are exactly of the same nature as those in bone.

In the interior of the bony part of each tooth is a cavity which descends into the root, and communicates at its extremity with the outer surface by openings corresponding with the number of branches into which the root is divided. This cavity, which is larger in young or newly formed teeth, and small in those which are old, contains a delicate vascular membrane, which has been named the pulp of the tooth. It is best seen by breaking a recent tooth by a smart blow with a hammer, when the soft pulpy membrane may be picked out of the fragments by the forceps. It then appears to be a membranous web with two surfaces, an exterior adhering to the bony surface of the dental cavity by minute vessels;

the other interior, free, and, so far as can be determined of a body so minute, resembling a close sac.

The development and growth of the teeth is a process of much interest.

At what time the first rudiments of teeth appear seems not to be determined with accuracy. In the fœtus, between the seventh and eighth month, I can merely distinguish in the centre of the vascular membrane of the alveolar cavity a minute firm body like a seed. I have, however, seen the crowns of teeth formed in fœtuses, which I have reason to believe had not attained the seventh month. But whatever may be the exact period, the process is nearly as follows.

As the bones of the upper and lower jaw are in the process of formation between the third and fifth months,* cavities at their lower and upper margins are gradually formed by the growth of the osseous plates, which afterwards form the *alveoli*. As these cavities are formed, they are lined by a large, soft, membranous, vascular sac, which, in the manner of a serous membrane, consists of two divisions, one lining the *alveolus*, the other folded within that, and forming a closed cavity. In the inside of this cavity the process of dentition commences some time between the fifth and seventh month, by the deposition of matter from the vessels at the lowest point of the alveolar division of the sac. This matter is to constitute the crown of the tooth, which is invariably formed first. After the deposition of the first portions, these are pushed upwards by the addition of successive layers below them, and necessarily carry the inflected part of the sac before them. As this process of deposition advances, the tooth gradually fills the sac, and rises till it reaches the level of the alveolar margins. If a tooth be examined *in situ*, near the period of birth, it is found to consist of the crown, with portions of enamel descending on every side, and forming a cavity in which a cluster of blood-vessels, proceeding from the sac, is lodged.

After the enamel has been deposited the bone begins to be formed; and as this process advances, the tooth is still forcibly thrust upwards by the addition of matter to its root. When the latter is well completed, the vessels become smaller and less abundant; until, when the tooth is perfect, they shrink to a mere membrane, which lines the cavity of the tooth, and still maintains its

* Fourth and Fifth, Bichat, p. 93, Tome iii.

original connection with the alveolar membrane, by the minute vascular production which enters the orifice or orifices of the root. Physiological authors have thought it important to mark the period at which the teeth appear at the gums; and in general this takes place about the sixth or seventh month after birth. This mode of viewing the process of dentition, however, gives rise to numberless mistakes on the period of teething. The process, as we see, commences in the early period of fœtal existence ; and the time at which they appear above the gums varies according to the progress made in the womb. In some the process is rapid ; in others it is tardy ; and even the fabulous stories of Richard III. and Louis XIV. may be understood physiologically, without the aid of the marvellous. Generally speaking, the crown is completed at the period of birth; and, according as the formation of the root advances with rapidity or slowly, dentition is early or late.

What is here described is the process of the formation of the first or temporary set of teeth, which consist, it is well known, of 20. In that of the second set the same course is observed. In the same manner is observed a row of follicular sacs, though not exactly in the original *alveoli* ; in the same manner deposition begins at the bottom of the free surface of the sac by the formation of the crown ; and in the same manner the crown is forcibly raised by the successive accretion of new matter to its base. The moment this process commences, a new train of phenomena takes place with the primary teeth. The follicular sacs of the new or permanent teeth are liberally supplied with vessels for the purpose of nutrition ; and as these blood-vessels increase in size, those of the temporary teeth diminish ; and the supply of blood being thus cut off, the latter undergo a sort of natural death. The roots which, as being last formed, are not unfrequently incomplete, now undergo a process of absorption ; and the tooth drops out in consequence of the destruction of its nutritious vessels. Some authors have ascribed this expulsion to pressure, exercised by the new tooth. They forget, however, that before the new tooth can exert any pressure, it must be in some degree formed; and to this a vascular system is indispensable.

The increased number of the teeth when permanent, the enlargement of the jaws, and the consequent expansion of the face, though interesting, are foreign to the present inquiry.

Another part of the osseous system requiring notice are the sesamoid bones. These derive their name, it is well known, from their minuteness, (σησαμη, a grain,) most of them, excepting the knee-pan, being of the size of a grain or pea. They are confined to the extremities, and are situate chiefly in positions in which they give points of support to the tendons of the flexor muscles. (Tendons of the *gemelli, tibialis posticus, peronæus largus,* &c.) The peeu-liarity of these bones is, that they are formed invariably in the sub-stance of fibrous organs, as tendons in the case of the knee-pan and the sesamoid bones of the *gemelli, tibialis posticus,* and *peronæus l. ;* or ligaments in the case of those situate between the metacarpo-pha-langeal and metatarso-phalangeal articulations. With this pecu-liarity their mode of ossification corresponds. At first albuminous or fibro-albuminous, in process of time they are penetrated by cal-careous matter, and present an osseous texture, which, however, is much less firm than that of genuine bones. The period at which this deposition commences and is completed varies in different indi-viduals; and hence, scarcely in any two persons of the same age is the number of sesamoid bones the same. Though the patella may be ossified at the 20th year, the minute sesamoid bones are some-times not formed before the 30th or even the 40th. In the patella, when ossified, we find a medullary organ. But it is uncertain whether the others acquire this mark of osseous character. These bones resemble the epiphyses in uniting, when divided, by fibro-albuminous matter.

SECTION II.

Osteitis ; Inflammatio.—Though all practical authors admit that bones may be inflamed either spontaneously, or in consequence of injury, yet it is remarkable that none have communicated any precise idea of this process; and while they admit it as a patholo-gical fact, they have too often lost sight of it in one or more of the changes to which it gives rise. To Mr Howship we are in-debted for the first attempt to determine with precision the anato-mical characters and pathological nature of this process.

It may at first sight seem doubtful whether genuine bone is sus-ceptible of such a process as inflammation. For though a bone constituted as already described is doubtless an organized substance, and therefore liable to the actions of organized bodies, yet whether a particle of completed bone, as in the compact parts of the cylin-drical bones, becomes itself the seat of inflammation, may seem

3

questionable. The morbid process, however, to which the actual bony particles may not be competent, the membranous covering and the vascular filamentous penetrating web, are unquestionably powerful agents in effecting. In short, while bone as a secretion is almost passive in its morbid relations, we observe it obeying the slightest influence of the periosteum and its vessels on the one hand, and those of its medullary system on the other.

Having premised these remarks, it is to be observed that inflammation occurring in bone may assume various forms.

1. *Adhesive Inflammation.*—Of these the simplest is that which takes place in the process of union after fractures,—*the healthy ossific inflammation* of Mr Hunter, a variety of the adhesive. In this three distinct stages are enumerated. In the first, effusion of blood from the periosteal vessels into its substance, and from the medullary vessels into the fracture, is after coagulation followed by effusion of a colourless viscid fluid, which also coagulates into a jelly. (J. Hunter, Bichat, Howship, &c.) In the second, the soft parts, and especially the periosteum, become hot, red, swollen, and, in short, are in a state of inflammation. (Du Hamel, Howship, &c.) If at this time the fracture be examined, the periosteal and medullary arteries at the line of fracture are large, numerous, and are seen emitting vessels into the coagulated blood and lymph effused beneath the periosteum, and from the broken ends, and converting them into organized masses, sometimes distinct like granulations, sometimes irregularly continuous. This substance, which is of a reddish-gray colour, and of the consistence of firm jelly, is what is named *callus*. The third stage may be distinguished by the appearance of osseous points which now begin to be deposited from the new vessels, which penetrate from the periosteum and medullary filaments to the *callus*. As the arterial action advances, these osseous points extend from the broken surface and coalesce. The exterior swelling at the same time diminishes and disappears; the periosteum falls to its natural size and its ordinary rate of vascularity; the medullary canal is restored in greater or less perfection; and the broken portion of bone after some time recovers the same organization and firmness nearly which it originally possessed. Instead of the longitudinal canals which are found in compact healthy bone, however, the renewed part presents a series of irregular cavities, varying in size and direction, and which contain a vascular, filamentous, medullary web. (Howship.) According to

Mr. John Bell it remains for years more vascular than the contiguous bone.* According to Howship it possesses a larger proportion of animal matter.†

In some instances of fracture union is not accomplished in this perfect manner; but is effected merely by a fibro-albuminous cicatrix, which unites the fragments loosely. This is observed especially in fractures of the neck of the thigh-bone, (Bell, Desault, Cooper, Howship;) of the knee-pan, (Camper, Callisen;) of the *olecranon*, and other parts consisting of loose cancellated structure. Upon the reasons of this physiologists are not agreed. By some it is ascribed to defect of periosteum, as in the neck of the thigh-bone (A. C. Hutchinson;) by others it is attributed to inefficient nutrition in the part broken off, which is then certainly less freely supplied by blood-vessels. (J. Bell, Sir A. Cooper.)

Further, in fractures in which there is much contusion and comminution, and especially where it is complicated by a communicating wound of the soft parts, reunion is rarely complete. The suppurative inflammation which then succeeds precludes the adhesive and ossific, and generally renders the latter imperfect or entirely abortive. In such circumstances more or less of the bone dies, and is thrown off in dead splinters. In some instances even necrosis may be produced, as is exemplified in compound fractures produced by gunshot.

Even in simple fracture may occur a variety of incomplete union. In some subjects, in whom the fragments have been badly applied, in whom they have been often moved, or in whom the vessels are inadequate to assume the ossific action, though blood and lymph are effused from the periosteum and medullary vessels, and undergo coagulation, adhesion is only partial and imperfect. It is not penetrated by vessels so as to become organized; or those vessels are rent asunder by repeated motions. Under such circumstances, the intermediate substance, instead of acquiring solidity, and becoming penetrated by bone, is partly absorbed; while the broken ends are converted into a secreting surface, which discharges se-

* Principles of Surgery, Vol. I. p. 507. Disc. 12. " Having cut off the limb of a soldier whose limb had been broken in America twelve years before, I found upon injecting the bone, that while the bone itself received the red colour of the injection pretty freely, the callus, which goes in a zig-zag form, joining together the several ends and points of a very oblique fracture, was very singularly red."

† Experiments and Observations, &c. By J. Howship. Med. Chir. Trans. Vol. IX. p. 143.

rous, purulent or sero-purulent fluid in small quantity. This forms what is termed *false joint.*

In the pregnant, or persons labouring under scurvy, and in those affected with the constitutional symptoms of syphilis, fracture is not united by bony union.

2. *Diastasis.*—Next to fracture may be placed detachment or disunion of the epiphyses, (*diductio epiphysium.*) In young subjects, while the epiphyses are still imperfectly united to the *diaphysis,* this may occur, in consequence of forcible stretching, or injury of the bone. In this manner it is noticed by Palfyn, Reichel,* Wilmer,† and others. Reichel saw it in the humerus, and Wilmer in the tibia. I have seen it in the humerus and in the femur, in which chiefly it occurs. Sometimes it may be traced to injudicious efforts by bone-setters in pulling a thigh-bone supposed to be dislocated. It is liable to be confounded with fracture of the neck of the thigh-bone. If not disturbed, the injury is repaired by union either in the ordinary manner, or with more or less extensive ossification of the neighbouring parts, causing generally stiff-joint. Consecutive disunion of an epiphysis may happen in *mollities ossium* and in *spina ventosa.* (Trioen, Reichel.)

The variety of disunion now mentioned is generally confined to the epiphysis of one bone. A more general disunion, however, occurring in most of the epiphyses of the skeleton, may take place in scurvy. This was remarked especially in the scorbutic epidemic of Paris 1743, and has since been occasionally seen. (Lind.) Inspection shows that the bones are penetrated by bloody extravasation, —that the vessels are relaxed and atonized,—and that nutritious deposition is suspended. This scorbutic diduction, which depends on a disease affecting the whole system, may be removed by the same means which remove that morbid condition. Too often, however, it takes place in that stage of the disease in which recovery is impossible.

3. I have above stated that it may be justly questioned whether bone itself undergoes the organic process of inflammation. Most of the facts hitherto collected, when well investigated, favour the inference, that the inflammatory conditions of bone are to be referred to inflammation taking place either in the periosteum; or the tomentose medullary web; or, finally, in the articular synovial

* M. Georgii Ch. Reichel, de Epiphysium ab Ossium Diaphysi Diductione. Sandifort Thesaur. Vol. I. p. 1.
† Cases and Remarks, &c. Lond. 1779. P. 228.

membrane or cartilage; and most of the morbid states observed by authors in bone may be traced to some variety or degree of inflammation in one or more of these textures. ·

a. When the periosteum becomes inflamed, one of several effects may follow.

α. It may induce effusion of coagulable lymph into its substance, or between that and the bone,—constituting simple node, and the tumour termed *gumma.**

β. By a modification of this action it may effuse lymph, which afterwards becomes ossified,—constituting the *ossific node* of Hunter and Howship, or simply, osseous node, (*periostosis.*) This appears in the form of loose bony masses, plates, or scales, on the surface of such cylindrical bones as the *tibia* and *ulna*, which are, nevertheless, quite natural. In some instances this osseous node appears to consist in ossification of the inner part of a circular area of inflamed periosteum. In both cases, instead of the regular arranged longitudinal canals, the new osseous deposition presents irregular cavities, varying in size and direction.* This, together with great vascularity, constitutes the anatomical character of such deposits. In one skull under 7 in my collection, periosteal inflammation has produced on the parietal bone a circular area the size of a shilling, of minute spherical or spheroidal eminences, surrounded by a smooth whitish ring, and that enclosed by a darker coloured ring. The circular area, with rough eminences, marks the space from which the periosteum was detached. It is thicker and less translucent than the rest of the bone. The white ring indicates the tract where the pericranium was inflamed, but not detached.

γ. If the inflammation be acute, as in that from injury, it may produce ulcerative absorption of the subjacent bone, which then presents a denuded, rough, reddish surface, progressively increasing in extent and depth. This occurs particularly in young subjects. I have seen it in the bones of the skull destroy both tables, and expose the *dura mater ;* and the fact shows that the tendency to suppurative inflammation in the bones of the young is great. Of this the following case is a good example.

A young girl of 10 or 11 years of age received on the head a blow from a stone, which divided the scalp down to the bone, but without causing fracture or depression. The wound

* Chirurgical Observations and Cases. By William Bromfield, Surgeon to Her Majesty and to St George's Hospital. Vol. II. Chap. i. p. 14. London, 1772.

† Howship in Medico-Chirurg. Trans. Vol. VIII. pp. 90, and 105, 106.

bled freely and was dressed in the ordinary way. A few days after the parents requested the advice of an able surgeon, who, finding the wound swelled, hot, and painful, with scanty discharge, recommended the application of an emollient poultice, and the use of low diet with laxative medicine. In the course of a few days, suppuration took place to a great extent, yet without any appearance of the wound healing or adhering. The patient also complained of pain in the head, especially girding frontal headach; the appetite was gone; the pulse was quick, above 120; she looked pale and unwell; and occasionally felt shivering sensations.

At this stage, about 15 or 16 days after the infliction of the wound, the surgeon requested me to see the child. The following was the state of matters. The lips of the wound were red, large, and gaping; much matter was proceeding from it; and it was the seat of very distinct pulsation, synchronous with that of the arteries; while, when the child cried, or breathed strongly, or coughed, matter issued copiously from the wound. When this matter was removed by the use of dry charpée, it was then distinctly seen that an aperture had been completely formed through the bone into the *dura mater;* that the brain and its membranes were exposed at the bottom of the wound, showing the two motions of the brain. The wound was in the right parietal bone near the coronal suture.

The question was, what was to be done? I recommended that a little blood should be drawn from the arm; that the poultices should be given up; that the wound should be kept clean and cool by occasional ablution with cold water; that a light dressing consisting of lint dipped in cold water, or a solution of sulphate of zinc, should be applied over the surface of the wound; and that the patient should be kept quiet, and on moderate unstimulating diet.

This plan was immediately adopted. In a few days the headach had subsided, the discharge was greatly diminished, the pulsating and heaving motion of the wound was no longer observed; new bony matter was deposited, and closed the aperture in the parietal bone; and in about 10 days more the wound was entirely healed.

In this case, as there was ulceration of bone and loss of its substance, there must have been deposition and new formation of it. The process I regard as peculiar to the young.

It takes place also in the tibia, in the sternum, and other superficial bones. In a more chronic form I have seen it cut through both nasal bones by insensible ulcerative absorption. This process corresponds with the *insensible exfoliation* or *decomposition* of Tenon;

F f

the *absorption* produced by tumours, aneurisms, and other compressing agents; (Louis, Wilmer;) and the peculiar absorption described by Mr Russell.*

δ. A similar process, by causing suppurative destruction or even death of the periosteum, may kill the subjacent bone (*nekrosis,*) which then becomes white, yellow, or black, and presents a denuded but uniform surface, bounded at certain points by an irregular rough line; (crena.) This line, which denotes the establishment of ulceration on the confines of the living bone, becomes more complete and deeper, till the dead portion is loosened and removed. This process is denominated *exfoliation,* and the part so removed is said to be *exfoliated.*† By Weidmann, who justly remarks that these terms are too limited, the process is designated by the general name of *separation ;* while the part separated is distinguished by the epithet *ramentum.* Though it takes place chiefly in the bones of the skull and in the front of the tibia, it may occur in the lower jaw,‡ in those of the pelvis,§ in the femur, and wherever the structure is close and compact. In this manner the odontoid process of the *epistrophe* (*vertebra dentata*) has been known to be removed.‖ In bones containing much cancellated structure, for instance the *vertebræ, sternum,* the carpal and tarsal bones, this suppurative destruction and death of the periosteum produces not death and exfoliation, but *caries* or ulceration, (τεϱηδων), with death of minute particles of bone, (*separatio insensibilis.*)

ε. Certain forms of periosteal inflammation give rise simultaneously to osseous deposition and ulceration or caries. Thus nodose inflammation of the tibia and fibula may terminate in ulcers of the periosteum, and produce irregular deposition on the surface of these bones, which appear thick, but without the usual aspect of healthy bone, present irregularly shaped masses of structure, partly like honey-comb cells and partitions, partly like confused network. The course of phenomena here is first chronic thickening and induration of the periosteum, with deposition of bone beneath it;

---

* Edinburgh Medico-Chirurgical Transactions, Vol. I. p. 74.

† Memoires sur l'Exfoliation des Os, par M. Tenon, dans Mém. de l'Academie R. des Sciences, 1758. P. 661, &c., and 1760. See, among others, good cases in Howship's Practical Observations, Case 107, pp. 404, and 113, p. 434.

‡ Exfoliations of the lower jaw from disease or injury of the alveolar processes are common. The hasty and reckless use of the tooth-key I have known produce not a few examples of exfoliation of both jaw-bones.

§ In Mr J. Bell's case of Gluteal Aneurism exfoliation from the ilium and sacrum took place. Principles, Vol. I. p. 423.

‖ Mr James Syme's Case in Med. and Surg. Journal, Vol. XXV. p. 311.

then ulceration of the periosteum ; and lastly, ulceration or caries in the new bony matter, which appears to continue to be deposited irregularly. This, which is the *carious ulcer (ulcus cariosum,)* of practical authors, may be seen in the legs of those who have been affected by the constitutional symptoms of syphilis, and who have undergone for its cure repeated courses of mercury.* In the cases in which I have seen it, it gave rise to extreme local pain and great constitutional disorder, requiring amputation ; and one case terminated fatally. Occurring in the bones of the cranium, which it occasionally does, it is one of the forms of the disease described by the older authors under the fantastic appellation of the garland of Venus ; (*Corona Veneris.*)

ζ. *Exostosis Periostei. Osteo-sarcoma.* That the periosteum may be concerned in extensive but morbid secretion of osseous matter, giving rise to that form of tumour which has been termed by some *exostosis,* and by others *osteo-sarcoma,* has been already noticed. (P. 424.) The periosteum becoming thickened and morbidly vascular and painful, assumes additional energy in the deposition of bony matter over a certain space. But the bone so deposited is never arranged in the manner of healthy bone. Sometimes it is in the form of a large shapeless prominence deposited on the outer surface of the original bone. This, which was remarked by Pouteau,† Houstet,‡ Herissant,§ Flajani,‖ and Monteggia, has been verified by Howship. Sometimes it occurs in one point of the bone in the form of a spheroidal tumour, in which the osseous matter is arranged in the form of long needle-like fibres, radiating from one or more points, not unlike radiated zeolite. In other instances it occurs in the form of amorphous masses of bone, much like pieces of calcareous sinter. (Houstet.) In others again, a central granular mass is surrounded by acicular bony fibres.

Of these growths the interior structure varies. They are never masses of solid bone ; but the bony matter is so arranged that it leaves spaces or intervals filled in some instances with soft flesh-coloured spongy matter ; (the *fungous exostosis* of Sir A. Cooper ;)

* Of this kind appear to be the tibia and fibula delineated by Roberg. See his Dissert. in Haller Disp. Chirurg. Tom. IV. p. 561.
† Œuvres Posthumes, Tom. III.
‡ Mém. de l'Acad. de Chir. Tom. III. p. 130.
§ Mém. de l'Acad. Roy. des Sciences. 1758, p. 676.
‖ Collezione d'Osservaz. e Rifless. Tom. II.

in others with cartilage; (J. Bell, A. Cooper,) (the *cartilaginous exostosis*;) in others with colloid or jelly-like matter, (J. Bell;) in others with semifluid blood-like matter, (Houstet;) and in some instances they have been known to contain hydatids, (Keate, &c.) In all cases the periosteum is thickened; the tumour is penetrated by numerous large vessels; and the bone in which the exostosis is formed is more or less thinned and destroyed by absorption. (Houstet, J. Bell, Palletta,* Sir A. Cooper.)

Though periosteal exostosis may take place in any bone of the skeleton, it most frequently appears on the inner side of the thigh-bone above the internal condyle, or upon the shaft, which it may enclose completely, (Houstet;) next upon the *tibia*, which, with the *fibula*, it may encompass more or less perfectly; next upon the humerus, (J. Bell and Cooper;) next in the bones of the pelvis, (Cheston and Sandifort;) and finally, on such bones as the lower jaw, the temporal, and other bones of the cranium. It is most likely to take place at muscular or tendinous insertions.†

In these forms of osseous deposition the vitality of the new deposit is small. Its organization is indistinct and imperfect; and in no long time it proceeds, apparently by pressure, to destroy the struc-ture of the adjoining bone, which then becomes rough, yellowish, or even black, and undergoes absorption. The bony mass at the same time is changed interiorly, presenting cavities containing ge-latinous or sanious fluid. The adjoining soft parts are generally destroyed by pressure; and when they give way are wasted by bad; but not cancerous ulceration. The bone thus exposed is generally black, rough, and carious. Though no exact analysis of these os-seous tumours has yet been made, it is known that they consist of phosphate of lime with animal matter.

The bony tumours occurring in the carpal, metacarpal, and pha-langeal bones, as described by Severinus, Mery, and Mr John Bell, I am inclined to refer to the head of exostosis depending on disease of the medullary membrane.

b. The medullary filamentous web is perhaps still more impor-tant than the periosteum in its morbid influence on bone. It is, in the first place, liable to inflammation; and, according as this takes place in the medullary web of the cylindrical bones, or in that of their epiphyses, or of the short irregular bones, different effects re-sult.

* Exercitationes Pathologicæ, Cap. ix. Art. iii. p. 112-115.
† On Exostosis, by Sir A. Cooper in Surgical Essays, Part i. London, 1818, p. 155.

α. Nekrosis. The term *nekrosis* means the process or state of dying or mortification in general ; but it is restricted by pathologists and surgeons to designate death taking place in bone. This may be accomplished in various ways, and may be the result of the operation of various agents. A compound comminuted fracture, a gun-shot which breaks and shatters a bone, or any other considerable degree of violence, may be followed by death of the portions most directly injured, and even those less immediately injured. It is observed also in the course of diseases and accidents that when any one of the compact bones is denuded of its periosteum, the part so denuded is very liable to become dead and to be then separated as a lifeless part. In some instances it has been observed that the agency of fire applied to the human body accidentally or intentionally has caused, by denuding the bone, the same result. Thus the actual cautery applied to the scalp has caused death of the external table; and I have seen a portion of the same external table destroyed, and made to exfoliate in an epileptic patient who in one of his fits had fallen into the fire.

A peculiar sort of nekrosis of the bones of the face, especially the superior jaw, has been made known by one of the manufactures of modern times. It is observed, that persons engaged in lucifer-match manufactories are liable to be attacked with pain and swelling of the face; and eventually it is observed, that the soft parts about the nostrils suppurate, and portions of dead bone are discharged evidently from the upper jaw. The process is chronic, tedious, and exhausting; and sometimes the face is greatly deformed. This disease is ascribed to the agency of phosphorus in vapour, which is believed in this manner to produce death of the bones of the upper jaw.

All these are modes in which nekrosis or death of bone may be produced.

The term is nevertheless most commonly applied to designate death in any of the cylindrical bones, in which the disease is seen in its greatest perfection ; and, as it is sometimes under certain circumstances attended with attempts to form new bone to supply the place of the dead bone, the term has been often understood to embrace the latter process as well as the former. The formation of new bone, nevertheless, does not take place always ; and that must be regarded as a distinct part of the process.

Nekrosis may come on in different modes. Often it is sponta-

neons in origin, and its appearance cannot be traced to any external cause. In other cases it is observed to appear some time after
a blow, or other injury, in which the bone has suffered considerable
concussion.

The disease may make its appearance in two forms; either as a
chronic malady, which is most usual ; or as one of great acuteness,
with intense symptoms of general and local disorder.

When it approaches as a chronic disease, the individual has pains
in the leg, or thigh, or arm of the part to be affected, which is referred to the bone; the pain is aggravated by walking and all motion; and there is in the limb a sense of weight with weakness,
which makes the patient afraid lest anything is to injure it. After
some time swelling takes place all over the limb. Occasionally
attacks come on like rose affecting the limb; and either soon or
after several of these attacks matter is formed; and upon being
discharged spontaneously or by art, the bone is found bare, in more
or less extent, and sometimes rough and parts of it loose.

In another class of cases the patient suffers deep-seated gnawing
pain, referred to one part of the bone, which is aggravated and
extended over the whole bone on attempting to walk or otherwise
persisting in using the limb. The patient is also lame and in general little able to walk. The limb is swelled; over the bone much
thickening and swelling are felt; generally pain on pressure is felt;
and the surface is unusually hot. At length, from some very slight
and inadequate cause, as endeavouring to stand on the limb, or in
the course of walking, if that has not been abandoned, the patient
is seized with sudden and immediate loss of power in the limb, and
he falls down helpless and motionless. When the bone is examined, it is found that fracture has taken place.

In some rare cases this fracture unites after a considerable time
in the usual way, with much effusion of callus and deposition of
bone. In a much larger proportion of cases suppuration takes
place ; matter finds its way to the surface ; and when by an opening
by art or spontaneously, it is allowed to escape, the bone is found
to be extensively stripped of periosteum, to be rough and irregular,
and without any attempts at union. This suppurative process advances, enfeebling the patient, who pines away in hectic fever, and
in no long time dies.

The state of the bone is then remarkable. No attempt at union
is observed ; the broken ends of the bone are white, rough, and
lifeless, and for a considerable space deprived of periosteum. The

medullary canal contains purulent matter; on the removal of which the *cancelli* are observed also to be white and rough, while a little farther away from the fragments the medullary web is vascular, swelled, and discharging purulent matter. In general, beyond the white portion of bone, a rough depressed line is observed between the living and dead parts, the former having in general the periosteum attached, and which is thickened, vascular, and evidently in a state of inflammation.

The acute form of the disease is greatly more violent in phenomena and more rapid in progress. All at once a limb or a portion of it, for instance the leg or thigh, is attacked with general swelling, diffused over the whole limb, great and intense pain both superficial and deep, while the surface is hot and tense, of a dull red colour, or sometimes very faintly red; and the patient, besides a feeling of great weight in the limb, is entirely deprived of all powers of moving it. The constitutional disorder is great. Generally there are rigors succeeded by heats; the pulse is quick, full, and strong; pain is felt in the head; the tongue is furred and dry; the patient distressed with thirst, restlessness, and anxiety, and is in certain cases delirious; the complexion is brownish-red as in *phlebitis;* the eyes are glaring; and the expression is a mixture of wildness and great suffering. This general disorder is in certain cases so intense, and causes so great a shock to the system, that the patient expires in the course of three or four days; and before the local disorder has lasted sufficiently long to produce suppuration.

If the patient, however, survive this period, the swelling invariably proceeds, until suppuration takes place in one or more parts. In the course of one or two days more, matter points in one, two, or three places simultaneously or successively; and when this is allowed to find issue either by art or spontaneously, it is ascertained that inflammation has existed over the whole bone and the soft coverings, and that this has proceeded most extensively to suppuration. The skin and adipose membrane are by this detached from the *fasciæ;* the *fasciæ* are detached from the muscles; the muscles from each other; and the whole soft parts are more or less detached from the periosteum, which, again, is either shreddy and killed, or is detached in parts from the subjacent bone, which is in these points rough, white, and evidently either deprived of vitality or very much injured in texture. When the bone is cut open longitudinally, the medullary membrane is swelled and very vascular; loaded with blood and serum, and presenting in various points drops of purulent matter.

The veins of the limb are inflamed; and their coats are thickened and sometimes obliterated. The arteries are denuded, brittle, and present traces of having partaken in the general inflammatory orgasm.

This form of *nekrosis* appears very similar to an attack of diffuse inflammation of the adipose and filamentous tissue; and I have occasionally entertained doubts whether it ought not to be regarded as such primarily, or as general inflammation of the soft parts affecting eventually and necessarily the bone. It also presents some resemblance to inflammation of the blood-vessels, and especially of the veins. The point is practically of little moment. The bone is killed; whether primarily or secondarily appears of little consequence, unless we could thereby discover some means by which an action so destructive might be stayed in its progress.

An important question presents itself; to determine what is the anatomico-pathological cause of nekrosis; which is the texture concerned in its production; whether it be always one and the same texture, or whether, in different cases and different forms of the disease, different textures are concerned. This question it seems difficult to determine. All that is already known tends to show that nekrosis may be the effect of previous disease of the periosteum, previous disease in the medullary membrane or in both, or of the whole of the soft parts investing the bone. The rest may be understood from what follows.

Nekrosis interna.—That the medullary web of the cylindrical bones is liable to inflammation is a well established point. The tendency of this is not so well understood. It may proceed either to suppuration, forming a collection of matter within the cavity of the bone; or by producing effusion within the interstices of the medullary web it may, by causing induration and swelling, induce expansion of the walls of the diaphysis; or by destroying the medullary membrane, it may kill the bone from within outwards.

That inflammation of the medullary web causes swelling and effusion into its interstices may be regarded as established by the phenomena of fractures, simple and compound, and especially by those experiments in which this texture is expressly injured. When it proceeds without being resolved, it may cause a uniform expansion of the bone, which very often precedes the extinction of its vitality.

Thus in most of the instances of the incipient stage of nekrosis, a local enlargement, or rather dilatation of the bone, takes place, while the bone, though its texture is softened, is still alive. This is the process which Scarpa distinguishes under the name of *expansion*, and in which he imagines the reticular structure to be relaxed or unfolded. The fact is well established, but the explanation is gratuitous. It is doubtless the early stage of the process which terminates in nekrosis.

Suppuration in the cavity of the long bones, which was seen by Cheselden, (p. 40), Gooch, (Vol. II. p. 357,) Hey, (p. 26 and 32,) and others, is generally a process so severe as to cause death by constitutional irritation. If it fails to effect this, it first distends and softens the bone, and then kills it from within outwards, inducing *nekrosis.* This may affect either part or the whole of the diaphysis, which is then separated from the periosteum and epiphysis, which is rarely killed. In process of time the dead portion or portions (*ramenta,*) become enclosed more or less completely by a thick shapeless cylinder of new bone, with or without openings in its sides, and which is placed between the epiphyses and covered by the periosteum, which is much thickened. If death take place at this period, the bone thus formed is found to contain the original shaft, loose and dead. If life be still prolonged, the old bone generally piecemeal is gradually brought to the surface through the openings in the new osseous case and expelled. The fragments thus discharged, which are of a dirty, yellow, drab, or black colour, and somewhat corroded or worm-eaten at the ends and margins, are named *sequestra* by Troja,* David,† and other French surgeons; and *ramenta* by Weidmann. The channels or openings through which they are expelled, which are temporary deficiencies in the new bone, are termed *cloacæ.*‡

The above is a brief description of the process of nekrosis with regeneration, as it occurs in the cylindrical bones. Its effects were known long before its mechanism was understood. The fact of portions of the cylindrical bones of the extremities being removed or expelled without impairing the motion of the limb, and of one

* De Novorum ossium regeneratione exp. Paris, 1775.

† Observations sur une Maladie connue sous le nom de Necrose. Paris, 1782.

‡ J. Petr. Weidmann, M. D., &c. De Necrosi Ossium. Francofurti ad Mœnum. 1793. Folio.

bone being found within another was remarked Duverney, Ruysch,[*] a Meek'ren,[†] Cheselden and others of the older anatomists and surgeons; and even Portal speaks of the circumstance of one bone rattling within another as a curious and unexplained phenomenon.[‡] Next to the case given by Cheselden, Laing[§] in 1737, and Johnston[||] in 1742, described cases of removal of the *tibia* and regeneration of the bone. Trioen[¶] and Amyand[**] describe the same facts under the name and as examples of *spina ventosa*; and Mackenzie,[††] William Hunter,[‡‡] Ludwig,[§§] Bromfield,[||||] and others describe the disease with the process of regeneration under various names, as detachment of the *epiphyses*, caries, loss of a bone, or reproduction, destruction of the *diaphyses*, according as any one part of the process was most prominent, without appearing to be aware of its true nature. Ludwig, indeed, appears to have been the first, or among the first, who investigated carefully the nature of the change. He published in 1772 two cases of the disease; one in the *tibia*, with recovery; and another in the femur, in which the patient had died, and in which he described the appearances found in the bone. In the latter case a considerable dead fragment of the *os femoris* had come away in the fifteenth year of the patient, six years after the commencement of the disease, followed by about 30 fragments varying in size. This patient survived to her 25th year;

* Thesaur. Anatom. VIII. Fig. 2, 3, 4.

† Jobi a Meek'ren Chirurgi Amstelodamensis Observationes Medico-Chirurgicae. Amstelodami, 1682. Cap. LXIX. p. 328. Part of the *humerus*.

‡ Anatomie Medicale, Tome I. p. 32.

§ The larger space of the Tibia taken out, and afterwards supplied by Callus. By Mr David Laing, Surgeon at Jedburgh. Edin. Med. Essays, Vol. I. Art. XXIII. p. 238. Edin. 1737.

|| A History of the Tibia taken out and regenerated. By Mr William Johnston, Surgeon in Dumfries. Ed. Med. Essays and Obs. Vol. V. Art. XL. p. 452. Edin. 1742.

¶ Cornelii Trioen, Med. Doc. Observationum Medico-Chirurgicorum Fasciculus. Lugduni Batav. 1743, 4to. p. 105.

** Some Observations on the *Spina Ventosa*. By the late Claudius Amyand, Esq., F. R. S., &c. Phil. Transactions, Vol. XLIV. Part I. for 1746. London, 1748, p. 193.

†† A Remarkable Separation of part of the Thigh Bone. By Dr Mackenzie, read 14th July 1760. Med. Observations and Inquiries, Vol. II. London, 1762, p. 299.

‡‡ An Account of a Diseased Tibia, as a Supplement to the last article. By William Hunter, M. D. Ibid. p. 303.

§§ Tractatio de Diaphysibus ossium cylindricorum laesis exfoliatione separatis et callo subnato restitutis. Ludwig Adversaria Medico Practica, Vol. III. Part I. Lipsiae, 1772, p. 45, Art. II.

|||| Chirurgical Observations and Cases. By William Bromfield, Surgeon to her Majesty and to St George's Hospital, Vol. II. p. 18, and Plate I. This represents what is called, "a very remarkable carious bone from the Museum of Dr Frank Nicholls," p. 342. It is a nekrosed *os humeri*. London, 1773.

and after death the shaft or diaphysis of the *os femoris* was found very thick, rough, irregular, and with a large hole and cavity passing into the interior of the bone. He is the first author who speaks of reproduction of the bone.

Louis appears to have first applied the epithet *nekrosis;* but Chopart and David were the first who directed the attention of surgeons to the process of regeneration ; and about the same time Troja and David, and afterwards Blumenbach, Koeler, Macdonald, and Desault, investigated the manner in which this is effected.

Meanwhile Andrew Bonn, who published in 1785 an account of the diseased bones contained in the museum of Hovius, gave six examples of the disease, sometimes without, sometimes with attempts at reproduction of bone. In the cases in which reproduction took place, the usual phenomena of great and extensive deposition of bone round the site of the old bone, with much irregularity of figure and thickness, perforations in the remains of them, on the body of the new osseous matter, and fragments of mortified bone, ulcerated, and showing traces of having been subjected to maceration in purulent matter. His general conclusion deserves attention. "By these various instances," says Bonn, "from Plate XV. to Plate XXIII. it is proved, that by a uniform law of nature, a bone diseased and mortified is separated from the living bone, by a notch, [*crena,*] or ulcerated depression, and by the successive growth of membranous matter which is eventually converted into bone."*

Two circumstances in the history of nekrosis merit attention ; *first*, the cause of the death of the bone ; and, *second*, the agent of its reproduction. I have already stated inflammation of the medullary web to be the cause of the former ; and this I conceive to be proved not only by the phenomena of the disease, but more directly by the experiments of Troja, David, and Macdonald, who have performed experiments of the same description. From these experiments it may be inferred, that suppurative destruction or death of the medullary web is necessarily followed by death of the surrounding bone.

The same experiments, with the relative situation of the new bone, unequivocally prove that the periosteum and its vessels are the agents of reproduction. Whether by accident or spontaneously the medullary web is destroyed, if the periosteum be uninjured, it becomes thick, swollen, and highly vascular ; bony matter in the fluid form

* Andreæ Bonn Descriptio Thesauri Ossium Morbosorum Hoviani. Lipsiæ, 1784. Tabulæ, 1785, 1789.

is then deposited with more or less regularity from its interior surface; and after this has acquired a due degree of thickness, the
vascularity and swelling of the periosteum gradually diminish, till
the membrane is restored to its natural state.   When, on the contrary, the periosteum is injured or destroyed, regeneration is imperfect or altogether deficient.   (Weidmann.)   In some instances
also, in which necrosis affects one portion only of the internal surface of a cylindrical bone, reproduction appears not to be effected.
The outer part of the bone then becomes soft, and at length
carious, and forms apertures (*foramina grandia*, Troja), (*cloacæ*,
Weidmann,) similar to those in new osseous cases, through which a
sequestrum is discharged.   (Weidmann, p. 31.)

In short, the doctrine of those who have maintained that the
periosteum is the chief agent of reproduction, is that the old bone,
or that which was first diseased and then mortified, has no concern
in the formation of the new bone.   It may be the periosteal vessels,
or various vessels of the soft parts in general, they argue; but it
cannot be the vessels of the bone, properly so called.

This doctrine, though supported by the observations and experiments of a number of able observers, has nevertheless been strongly
controverted, first by Ludwig and Palletta, and afterwards by
Scarpa and Richerand.

Ludwig appears to have early maintained that the new soft mass,
by which the loss of bone was to be supplied, grew or sprouted
from the sound bone;* and Palletta, from the facts of a case which
he observed with great care in the year 1790, arrived at the conclusion, that the growth of the new bone proceeds not from the periosteum, which was in this case destroyed, but from the substance
of the bone itself.   In the case now adverted to, nekrosis of the
left *tibia* was induced in the following manner.   A man of 50 was admitted into the hospital, on the 24th December 1789, for an ulcer
of the leg, which progressively denuded the whole tibia, so that the
posterior surface of the bone only was left covered by soft parts.
A trihedral portion of the front of the *tibia*, five Paris inches
long, became dead, and was ejected.   After this, new flesh sprung
from the surface thus exposed, and formed, according to the account, a firm bony support, such, that after the lapse of eight
months and a few days, the man could support his person on the
limb. He was gradually recovering strength until September 1796,
when he was destroyed by an attack of rose.

* Adversaria Medico-Practica, Vol. III. Pars I. p. 62. Lipsiæ 1772.

The recently repaired bone was of a very blood-red colour, spongy, crowded everywhere by certain smooth nodes, and slightly bent to the outer or fibular side. It was a white, almost cartilaginous substance, yet sufficiently strong, which Palletta thinks must have become firmer in time. The periosteum was not thicker than natural. It could be drawn from the recent bone, and appeared merely laid over it. The bony matter proceeded from both extremities of the *tibia* to mutual contact. Yet the meeting portions did not coalesce, but were united as it were by intermediate cartilage.*

Scarpa, who adopts this doctrine, maintains, that what is commonly regarded as new bone, is the old *cortex* or compact tissue expanded and relaxed; that this, by a great effort of nature, is everywhere enlarged and becomes spongy; that growing inwardly it repairs the loss of the marrow, and swelling outwardly increases the walls of the bony tube; that hence the old bone is enclosed, as it were, in a sheath, which, though at first spongy, soft, and flexible, becomes hard by the gradual reception of earthy particles, and at length becomes entirely like the old bone.

Scarpa, in short, first assumes or maintains in the living textures a vital property which he calls the *expanding faculty.* He then maintains on the strength of cases of nekrosis and various experiments, that no reproduction of bone takes place except from callus produced from ossific fluid, not secreted from the periosteum or the cellular tissue in the medullary membrane, but elaborated by the intimate structure of the bone, and which is effused sometimes between the ends of the broken or excised bone, sometimes exudes from the external surface of bones, and being hardened in both situations, assumes the bony organic character.†

It must be admitted that the hypothesis of Troja and Weidmann labours under certain difficulties; and in exposing these difficulties and the objections to which they give rise, Scarpa has been more successful than in establishing his own hypothesis, which is exposed also to difficulties perhaps still more insur-

* Exercitationes Pathologicæ, Auctore Joanne Baptista Palletta. Mediolani, 1820. 4to, p. 28.

† De Anatome et Pathologia Ossium, Auctore Antonio Scarpa. Turin, 1827, p. 82- 87-96.

Verum idcirco, et unicum organon elaborationis, et secretionis succi ossifici est os ipsum; neque aliunde quam ex universa ossea compage, sive *laxa* ea sit et *reticulata,* sive *dura* et *compacta,* liquor ille glutinosus plasticus, fila trahens, extillat, qui cum in centro fracturæ, tum in marginibus, tum in extima fracti ossis superficie effusus, cogetur in exiguas rubras carunculas, dein in majora carni similia tubercula, demum in carti- laginem, postremo in os commutatur et *calli* nomine venit, p. 104, 105.

mountable than those belonging to the hypothesis of Weidmann. It is impossible here to consider all the facts adduced and the whole train of the reasoning employed by the professor of Pavia. It is sufficient to observe, that, independent of the violent and gratuitous nature of the assumption of the expanding faculty, which he ascribes to bone, there is some inconsistency in saying, that the old cortex is expanded, and becoming spongy, and advancing inwards, forms medullary membrane, and swelling outwardly increases the walls of the bony tube; and that thus the old bone is inclosed within a sheath. In this representation the old bone is made at once to inclose and to be inclosed.

Another objection is still found in the following fact. In all the instances in which considerable or large *sequestra* have come away, how does it happen that these *sequestra* resemble so closely the shafts or portions of the shafts of old bones as they do? Excepting in the circumstance of their broken, irregular, ulcerated extremities, and the carious and worm-eaten appearance of the surface, they present all the characters of an old or dead portion of a cylindrical bone. It is to be observed, that from the moment the bone becomes dead from whatever cause, whether external injury or inflammation of its medullary membrane, instead of being capable either of undergoing this expanding process, or in any way contributing to the formation of new bony substance, it is a lifeless, inert mass, and acts as a mechanical irritant, exciting and maintaining, for the purpose of its own expulsion, an excessive suppurative inflammation, which instead of promoting and facilitating the formation of new bone, is the main cause above all others, which retards, impedes, and renders impossible the necessary secretion for that purpose. It is a well-established fact, that as long as the old bone or any of its fragments are in the affected limb, the deposition of new bone is so much retarded and often rendered impracticable. Conversely, it is only when these sources of irritation and wasting suppuration are withdrawn, that new bone begins and proceeds to be regularly and steadily deposited. The irritative actions are excessive, and prevent the effusion of lymph and liquid *callus* and their consolidation.

A third argument, which may be advanced against the doctrine of Scarpa, is the following. In all the cases of nekrosis with reproduction, the newly formed bony mass appears to be so certainly the result of the operations of tissues exterior to the bone, that it is impossible to understand, how the old bone can have any share in the process of new deposition. The reproduced bone is always a large, thick, shapeless mass, sometimes imperfect, that is with breaches or gaps in its bony walls, irregular on the surface, and in every well authenticated case three or four times the diameter of the old bone. It is in contact with, if not closely invested by inflamed and thickened periosteum, all the vessels of which and the surrounding tissues are engaged in conveying blood and lymph to the scene of effusion and deposition. Lastly, it is in some parts soft, loose, and spongy, in others firm and solid, the former being the most recently formed, the latter the last deposited portions.

Scarpa appears to have adopted the idea of the formation of bone in nekrosis from the phenomena of fractures, in which certainly the vessels of the bony fragments are instrumental in the secretion and modulation of liquid *callus*. It may be admitted, that in a certain class of cases of what may be called fragmentary or limited nekrosis, taking place chiefly in compound fractures and gunshot wounds, the living fragments of bone may present materials for the formation of new bony matter. But this is a very different process from that which takes place in nekrosis of an entire bony shaft, in which the bone is already dead, in the midst of living parts, and consequently cannot be supposed to be the agent of living actions.

Notwithstanding these objections, the hypothesis of Scarpa has been espoused more or less strongly by various authors, anatomical and surgical, who have also apparently confined their views to the phenomena of bones comminuted by gunshot wounds or compound fractures, for instance, Leveillé, Richerand, Jourdan, and a few others. Richerand in particular, regards the theory of Troja and David as erroneous in this respect, that it represents as a uniform law, a phenomenon which takes place in a small number of cases only. By others again, as Boyer, Ribes, and Beclard, attempts have been made to reconcile the two hypotheses. The attempt seems hopeless and impracticable, unless in the circumstances already specified, in which portions of living bone are really left to perform the duty assigned. In cases of extensive nekrosis of a cylindrical bone, it seems a contradiction in terms to say that the dead bone can reproduce a living one.

In 1836, Mr Gulliver examined various points connected with this subject. He doubts the possibility of absorption of the *sequestrum*, and for this he has probably good reason. He undertakes to prove that tissues, at least bones, being dead, possess the power amidst living tissues of attaching, as it were, from the blood particles similar to themselves; and in this he appears to confirm certain of the views of Scarpa.*

Lastly, several observations by Dr Watson Wemyss favour the inference, that the living parts of the old bone do not contribute to the formation of the new one; and that in *nekrosis,* the periosteum is the agent of ossific reproduction.†

Regeneration is most frequent in the *diaphyses* of the cylindrical bones. Many cases of reproduction of the *humerus,* the femur, and especially the *tibia,* are on record. Of the ulna three only are mentioned, and of the radius only one, of the clavicle one, and of the scapula one. Of the lower jaw, regeneration, either partial or total, has been recorded by various observers.

The flat bones of the skull are very rarely regenerated; and perhaps it would be difficult to produce an authentic and unequivocal example, unless that given by Weidmann (pl. xii.) be admitted. Mr Russell, however, states that he has seen instances of apertures of the cranial bones being supplied by solid matter which, to his observation, possessed all the qualities of solid bone. This nevertheless resembles more the reproduction after fracture than that after nekrosis.

The short or cuboid bones appear never to be reproduced.

β. *Spina Ventosa.*—Inflammation of the medullary web of the epiphyses and the cuboid or short bones produces very different effects; and seems occasionally and in certain circumstances to be the cause of the disease so vaguely spoken of under the name of *Spina Ventosa.*

The history of this disease is curious, and deserves attention from the erroneous notions that have at different periods prevailed on its correct pathology.

The name *Spina Ventosa,* or flatulent, or wind thorn (Der Winddorn), was employed by the Arabian surgeons of the tenth century to designate certain painful affections of the bones, which were probably not always of the same kind, and which, there is strong reason to believe, did not depend on the same pathological cause. By Rhazes, who is believed first to have described the disease, it is represented to consist in swelling, erosion, and corruption of the bone, from the presence of hot humours corroding and perforating its substance.‡ Similar is the view given by Avicenna, who represents the cause of

---

* On Necrosis. Medico-Chirurgical Transactions, Vol. XXI. p. 1. London, 1838.

† Edinburgh Medical and Surgical Journal, Vol. LXIII. p. 302. Edinburgh, 1845.

‡ Joannis Freind, M. D., Opera Omnia Medica. Londini, 1733. Folio. Historia Medicinæ. Pars Secunda, p. 487.

spina ventosa to be sharp humours penetrating to the bone and cor‑ roding it; and the approach of the disease to be indicated by pain in the joints, yet the matter of the disease to be seated in the bone. These ideas, which are derived entirely from external symptoms, were adopted by the surgeons of the 16th and 17th centuries, with‑ out question whether they were accordant with fact or not. Such were the doctrines of Joannes de Vigo in 1513, and of Pandolphi‑ nus a century later.

Peter de Argellata, indeed, near the close of the fifteenth cen‑ tury, gave a more definite notion of the distemper by saying, that it consisted in matter collected within the substance of a bone, either from weakness of assimilative power or weakness of the member, and there causing abscess, on opening which by incision the whole substance of the bone is found corrupted.*

About the beginning of the 17th century, it appears to have been not unusual among anatomists and surgeons to apply the term *spina ventosa* to caries of the smaller spongy bones. Scultetus tells us, that while he was at Padua, studying medicine and practising surgery, he saw a young nobleman, who had been for several months labouring under œdematous swelling of the left hand, which ter‑ minated in ulcerated openings. The patient was then submitted to Spigelius, at that time professor of anatomy; and he, finding, on introducing a probe, the bones bare, rough, and corrupted, imme‑ diately said that the disease was *spina ventosa*. As Spigelius died in 1625, in his 47th year, this must have been about 1620.

Pandolphinus, who was a surgeon at Fermi, published in 1614 a treatise on the disease, which was by Mercklin, about 60 years after, thought worthy of a learned and elaborate commentary.† The commentary is now more valuable than the text.

Marcus Aurelius Severinus adopted (1629) partly the notions of de Argellata, partly those of Pandolphinus, and modified the doc‑ trine by views of his own. While he teaches that *spina ventosa* consists in abscess within the substance of the bone, he adds that it takes place chiefly if not solely in children, and is mostly found in the joints and ends of bones, and in bones of spongy cancellated

* Petri de Argellata Chirurgia. Venetiis, 1480. Lib. V. Tract. xxii. Cap. 2.

† "Ventositas spinæ est ossis corruptio cum partis tumore ac intemperie, ab humore corrumpente procedens." Josephi Pandolphini a Monte Martiano Medici ac Philo‑ sophi Tractatus de Ventositatis Spinæ saevissimo Morbo. Revisus, correctus et anno‑ tationibus novisque tum proprii tum alienis observationibus, illustratus a D. Georgio Abrahamo Mercklino jun. Med. Noribergæ. Noribergæ, 1674, 12mo. Cap. III.

texture. To me he appears to have considered carious and strumous disease of the small joints, especially in the wrist and fingers and in the tarsal and metatarsal bones, as *spina ventosa ;* and the latter he maintains to be an erroneous and improper name.* He regards it as produced in the manner of the cold or congestive inflammation.

The great evil of all essays and writings in those days was confounding the remote, efficient, and proximate or pathological causes together, and rendering all their doctrines more or less obscure by mingling ideas on the generation or formation of a disease with its actual nature. This is the case not only with Pandolphinus and Severinus, but with Peter de Marchettis, who has left a short essay on the subject. (1665.) Amidst these notions, however, it is easy to see that he regards the pathological characters of the disease as consisting in denudation, roughness, and caries of the bones of the wrist or metacarpus, the tarsus or metatarsus, and sometimes of the ends of the radius or ulna, the tibia or fibula. (1665). He also maintains that the bone is first affected, and then the periosteum.†

If any doubt could be entertained as to the locality of the disease assigned by de Marchettis, it would be dissipated by this circumstance, that he tells his reader, that after the first indications of the disease is pungent, acute, lancinating pain, without swelling, the matter of the disease then raises the affected joint into a swelling, at first soft, loose, and indolent, of the same colour with the skin ; and afterwards becoming hard ; and when the probe is introduced, the bone is felt corrupted or carious. It is clear that he, like Spigelius and Severinus, describes here the inflammation of the articular ends of bones taking place in strumous persons. This affection, he further states, he observed mostly in persons of both sexes about the 25th year.

A doctrine similar, though in a more decided shape, was about the same time taught by Paul Ammann, professor at Leipsic. According to him, *spina ventosa* is a corruption, abscess, or sphacelism in a bone, not only round joints, but also about other parts, affecting the substance of bones earlier than the periosteum, equally common in adults as in children,—arising from inflammation, sometimes with great pain, sometimes with dull pain, with change of co·

. * De Recondita Abscessuum Natura. Lib. V. De Paedarthrocace, c. III. IV. V. VI. XI., p. 103.

† Petri de Marchettis Patavini et Observat. Medico-Chirurg. Sylloge. Amstelodami, 1665, p. 195, 196, 197.

lour in the bone, sometimes with hardness, sometimes with softening of the bone, and always with a thin sanious discharge.*

Next in this series may be placed the doctrines of Mercklin, as
given in his commentary on the treatise of Pandolphinus. This
author collects the opinions and observations of all his predecessors
and contemporaries; and, though it be not easy to discover his own
views, yet, upon the whole, it may be said that he leans most to
those of Ammann. He regards the disease as arising from inflammation in the substance of bones, which he thinks may cause either
abscess with caries or sphacelus; and that this inflammation may
affect any portion of bones or any order of bones; and may arise either
from scurvy, the venereal poison, or the presence of morbid fluids.†

The nearest approach to the true pathology of this malady was
probably made by Freind, who placed the primary action in the
marrow, which becoming diseased and enlarged, separates the outer
lamellæ, and distends the periosteum with pain and swelling.‡ We
still require, nevertheless, the collateral illustration of actual cases
and dissections.

Cheselden observed, in 1713, that matter was liable to be formed
within the large medullary cavities of the cylindrical bones; and
that this increasing and wanting vent, partly by corroding and
rendering the bone carious and partly by pressure, tears asunder
the strongest bone in the human body; and of this he mentions an
example, in which all the internal hard part of the bone containing
the medulla was separated from the rest, and being drawn out
through the place where the external caries made a vent, the patient received a perfect cure.§ This was manifestly a case of nekrosis. In his OSTEOGRAPHIA, published in 1733, containing several views of diseased bones, especially from the effects of mercury,
he gives, in his 49th plate, the view of a *sequestrum* of the *os humeri*
which had been removed from the arm of a girl of 13; and in his
55th plate, another figure of an *os humeri*, both reproduced, and
with the *sequestrum* or fragment of the old bone.§ These he mentions without seeming to consider them as making examples of
spina ventosa.

* Pauli Ammann Diss. de Spina Ventosa. Lipsiæ, 1674. 4to. Cap. ii.
† Josephi Pandolphini Tractatus, &c. Cap. v. 3, p. 198, *et passim*. Noribergæ, 1674.
‡ Joannis Freind, M. D., Opera Omnia Medica. Historia Medicinæ. Pars Secunda, p. 487. Folio. London, 1733.
§ Osteographia. By William Cheselden. London, 1733. Folio. And Anatomy of the Human Body, 12th edition. London, 1784. P. 40.

In 1742 and 1743, Cornelius Trioen, a physician-surgeon at Leyden, published a series of medico-chirurgical cases, containing also observations on *spina ventosa*. This he distinguishes into three forms; *spina ventosa, spina venenosa*, and *spina mitior*. After stating as a general definition that *spina ventosa* consists in expansion or distension of the bony substance, and a sort of separation of the smooth or compact tissue of the bone and its *tubuli* from the substance, that is the cancellated tissue of the bone, by which the bone and the incumbent soft parts are enlarged much beyond their wonted diameter; he adds, that the first is that in which the texture of the bone is not penetrated with purulent matter or other fluids, and that the threatened rupture of the bone is anticipated by death; while the bony substance may be inflated like a large globe. Of this he gives one instance in which the lower extremity of the femur is certainly expanded in this fashion into a large irregularly globular tumour (p. 106, 108,) yet without the presence of ichor, purulent matter, or offensive smell, and in which the patient was destroyed by repeated hemorrhage. It must be allowed that the figure given of this case resembles much that kind of disease to which several surgeons in recent times have applied the name of *Spina ventosa*.

The second form of the disease admitted by Trioen corresponds, it appears to me, with caries as it shows itself in the short or irregular bones of spongy cancellated tissue; for instance the bones of the carpus and metacarpus, and the tarsus and metatarsus, and the vertebrae. These he allows to be attended with swelling, small, livid, deep ulcers, admitting the probe to rough, denuded, often softened bones, and as occurring mostly in young persons of delicate constitution, corresponding to the *Paedarthrocace* of Severinus; (p. 111.)

The third form of the disease, which he terms *spina mitior*, corresponds, if we judge from the example of it adduced, with *nekrosis*. He describes it as affecting the middle or hard substance of bones, and after inducing swelling, causing the separation of the compact substance like plates, with discharge of matter, yet without fœtor. Of this he gives three examples taking place in the tibia, in each of which the fragments of dead bone were separated and expelled, with recovery of the patient. (P. 115, 118.)*

It appears, therefore, that Trioen knew and described under the

* Cornelii Trioen Medicinæ Doctoris Observationum Medico Chirurgicarum Fasciculus. Lugduni Batavorum, 1743. 4to.

same name of *spina ventosa* three forms of disease of the bones; the first enlargement and expansion of the extremities of the long bones, the second caries or chronic strumous inflammation of the short irregular bones, and the third nekrosis, as it appears in the cylindrical bones.

In 1746, there was read to the Royal Society by the late Claudius Amyand, Sergeant-Surgeon to the King, a paper containing observations on *spina ventosa*, and giving in illustration two instances of *nekrosis*, one in the *os humeri* of a man of 22, another in the same bone of a man of 26. Mr Amyand begins by observing, that " what practitioners generally understand by the *spina ventosa* is a caries in the bone from the extravasation of some sharp juices within it relaxing the tone of the fibres, and swelling and increasing its bulk beyond the natural bounds." He farther allows that in certain cases the cariosity is encrusted and covered with an exostosis, that is, with bony matter; that when the bone swells, the nutritious fluid is deposited outside, and forms *callus* ; that in certain cases, in the first stage of the disease, purulent matter lodged within the substance or cavities of the bone, causes some exfoliation or detachment of it; and that, in the last stage of the disease, the bone is perforated with holes, tubulous cavities, and fistulous openings; and that it is highly probable that a suppurated phlegmon in the marrow was the original cause of the *spina ventosa* in the two cases recorded.

From these facts it appears that Mr Amyand describes as *spina ventosa* the disease now known by the name of *nekrosis ;* that he rightly inferred that this disease, *nekrosis*, arises from inflammation of the medullary membrane of cylindrical bones; that he was aware that new bony matter was formed outside the old or original, but diseased bone; and that the original or diseased bone was exfoliated and detached.*

In 1751, the Treatise on the Diseases of Bones, by M. Du Verney, appeared. Though this surgeon noticed various cases of *necrosis*, yet he does not mention *spina ventosa.* The editor, however, in his preface, mentions shortly that inflammation of the *medulla* produces pain, heat, throbbing, swelling, abscess, caries of a bad character, and even *spina ventosa*, if the cause be internal; and that the corruption of the *medulla* without external wound, or that which is produced by an internal cause, is called *spina ventosa*, in consequence of the corrosion and destruction of the bone attended

* Some Observations on the Spina Ventosa ; by the late Claudius Amyand, Esq. F. R. S. Sergeant-Surgeon to his Majesty. Phil. Trans. 1746, Vol. XLIV. p. I. p. 193. London, 1748.

with pungent pain and swelling.* There is good reason to think·
that the author has in view some of the multiplied effects of secondary syphilis or mercurial disease.

It appears, indeed, for a long time, to have been a common prae-
tice to regard as *spina ventosa* many of these affections of the bones,
which arise either from the operation of the syphilitic poison, or the
hurtful effects of mercurial medicines; and I think it certain, that
many of the painful affections of bones, dependent on one or other
of these causes, were regarded as instances of *spina ventosa*. Such
appear to have been the ideas of the first Monro, Cheselden, and,
at a later period, Schlichting, who states that he observed the *spina
ventosa* to be very like the venereal disease, and to corrupt the humours and vessels of the body.† Cheston, (1766,) who was desirous
chiefly to distinguish.the disease from white swelling, after referring to Avicenna and Mercklin, concludes with them that it begins
originally within the bone, which is more or less enlarged. It is
evident, however, that he had not formed any very clear or distinct
idea of the nature of the malady.‡

Warner places it (1756, 1784) in the marrow and vessels of the
bone,§ (p. 322); and Bromfield, we have seen, (1773) regards it
as abscess of the marrow, without appearing to be aware of the relation between this and *nekrosis*‖. (P. 20-22).

It is not wonderful, therefore, that Augustin, who published in
1797 a learned treatise on the subject, complains of the confused
ideas and contradictory views given on this disease. He had endeavoured, after studying the preparations in the museums at Berlin, Halle, and Goettingen, to form a distinct and precise notion of
the disease; and he has certainly added to our knowledge. Yet
it cannot be said that his distinctions are so clear and precise as
might have been expected. At that time it appears that several
teachers called every internal caries by the name of *spina ventosa ;*
others confounded it with every sort of swelling in bones.

Spina ventosa Augustin represents to consist in internal inflam-

---

* Traite des Maladies des Os. Par M. Du Verney, M. D. &c.   Paris, 1751, Tom.
I. Preface. VII.

† Philosophical Transactions. London, 1742. No. 466.

‡ Pathological Observations and Inquiries on Surgery from the Dissection of Morbid Bodies.   By Richard Browne Cheston, Surgeon to the Gloucester Infirmary.
Gloucester, 1766, 4to. p. 117.

§ Cases in Surgery, with Introductions, Operations, and Remarks.   By Joseph
Warner, F. R. S., Senior Surgeon to Guy's Hospital. London, 1760 and 1784.

‖ Chirurgical Observations and Cases. By William Bromfield, Surgeon to Her Majesty, &c.   London, 1773.   Vol. II. pp. 20 and 22.

mation of a bone with swelling, universal in a small bone, partial in a large one, causing the greatest pain, terminating successively in swelling of the soft parts, not unfrequently in fistulous ulcers, and caries, by all which the affected bone is converted into a large, irregular, and tuberous mass of hard or highly corrupted structure. From caries he distinguishes it by the presence of swelling or enlargement, and by the absence of ulceration; and from *exostosis* and *hyperostosis* by the parietes of the bone being separated and destroyed.[*]

Among the four figures given by Augustin to elucidate the character and nature of the disorder, it appears that, with great irregularity and spiny roughness of the bones affected, and enlargement, there is deposition of bone in irregular forms and masses. It is in these an abnormal nutrition or misnutrition in the bony texture. In one, (fig. 3,) a tibia, there is enlargement and separation of the walls of the bone, and irregular exostotic deposits; and in another, (fig. 4,) the lower third of the *os femoris* is enlarged into a great irregular mass, very irregular on its surface, and with manifest indications of new bony deposit.[†]

These views, nevertheless, appear to have been overlooked by Petit, Bordenave, Portal, and others, who, regarding it as a variety of *exostosis* occurring in the scrofulous, and complicated with suppuration in the substance of the bone, by a wish to simplify, have rendered the subject more complex. Scarpa, especially in his Commentaries, maintains that *spina ventosa* differs in degree only from exostosis and *osteo-sarcoma*.[‡] The opinion of Bichat is not very distinct.[§] That of Monteggia and Palletta[||] is much more explicit. The former represents it as commencing in the marrow, which inflames slowly, swells and wastes, or passes into a slow suppuration, distending the parietes of the bone all round, and then bursting its compact shell, giving vent to the medullary sanies, and causing the inflammation and suppuration of the soft parts, at the bottom of which the bone is found bare and carious, or covered with fungous granulations, but with one or more orifices penetrating into the medullary cavity.[¶]

[*] De Spina Ventosa Ossium. Scripsit Fridericus Ludovicus Augustin, Med. et Chirurgiæ Doctor. Halae, 1797, 4to. Accedunt Icones IV. § 4, § 5, § 7, § 34.
[†] De Spina Ventosa Ossium, § 27, § 28, § 29.
[‡] De Anatome et Pathologia Ossium, p. 76 and 78. Ticini, 1827, 4to.
[§] Anatomie Generale, Tome III. p. 112.
[||] Exercitationes Patholog. Mediolani, 1820, p. 120.
[¶] Istituzione Chirurgiche, Vol. II. 645, p. 275.

This view errs only in placing the disease in the marrow, which, as an inorganic secretion, is incapable of orgasm, healthy or morbid. The true agent of the process is the vascular medullary web, especially of the *epiphysis*, of such bones as the vertebræ, the carpal and tarsal bones, and the phalanges. The cancellated arrangement of the osseous matter and of its medullary web in these bones explains the progress and phenomena of the disorder.

Palletta adopts the distinctions of Trioen; and admits, in true *spina ventosa*, expansion of the bony walls. *Spina mitior* he allows to be the same as *nekrosis.*

Though various modern surgeons have directed their attention to this subject, it is still surrounded with confusion and uncertainty. Some allow that the disease does not affect the *epiphyses*, but the shafts of the bones, and admit, however, the expanding process. Dupuytren, who was aware of the confusion in the application of the term, has not, however, done much to remove it. From the few cases which he records under this head, it appears that the disease affects the head of the *humerus* by enlargement and expansion of the osseous walls, and the phalanges and metacarpal bones in the same manner.   He admits that the disease is seated in the cavity of the bone; that in certain cases there is a deposit of cancerous matter which distends the bone; that it is an affection of the medullary membrane ; and that there is secreted a new substance, fungous, gelatiniform, gray, yellow, lardaceous, sometimes gypseous and serous.*

It is clear, from the account now given, that this eminent surgeon had formed on the intimate nature of this disease no distinct or precise ideas ; and he has left the subject in as great confusion as when he found it.   The subject is certainly unsettled from the contradictory and inaccurate manner in which the term has been employed.

From the facts here adduced, the following conclusions may be established.

1*st*. It appears that the early writers on *spina ventosa* had no distinct or precise notions on its characters and nature, and that most of them, like Vigo, de Argellata, Pandolphinus, and Severinus, regarded as *spina ventosa*, caries of the articular ends of bones, chiefly dependent on chronic inflammation of the medullary membrane.

* Lecons Orales de Clinique Chirurgicale.   Tome Deuxieme, Article XII. p. 268—
275. Paris, 1839.

2*d.* It appears that several surgeons during the 18th century, as Trioen, Amyand, and Bromfield, when the knowledge of morbid processes was deriving advantage from anatomical enquiry, regarded as instances of *spina ventosa*, cases which were examples of *nekrosis.*

3*d.* It appears that, up to the present time, very great confusion and inaccuracy prevails as to the exact import of the term *spina ventosa*, which with one set of observers means an ordinary though morbid affection of bone, and with others is employed to designate a malignant or heterologous disease of bone.

And 4*th.* It appears, nevertheless, that all agree in considering enlargement of the bone and expansion of its bony walls as a uniform result.

If we look to specimens in collections, we find that the opinions of surgeons are by no means the same, and present much discordance. Thus we find, in one pathological museum, marked as *spina ventosa*, a greatly enlarged end of a long bone, the bony wall extruded, and a large irregular cavity formed internally. In other instances, we find placed under the head of *spina ventosa* instances of enlargement of the metacarpal bones and phalanges. In others, again, we find bones with great enlargements, and covered with numerous rough spines and *spiculæ*, considered as *spina ventosa.* In short, every disease of bone not previously referred to a definite place, is accounted by different individuals *spina ventosa.*

From the specimens which I have examined, I think that enlargement of the bone and expansion of its osseous walls must be admitted as one character. Two points, however, remain to be determined, which is the agent of this enlargement ; and are the new deposits analogous or heterologous ? In general I think that they are analogous, that its products are those of inflammatory action of a peculiar kind, or at most of misnutrition. They do not, in legitimate *spina ventosa*, appear to be scirrhous or cancerous. The fungous granulations appear to be the product of the medullary web in these particular circumstances.

That this is the seat of its action is to be inferred first from the phenomena of the disease ; and secondly, from its effects, as seen in diseased bones. *Spina ventosa* never occurs in a bone with distinct medullary canal, unless at the epiphyses, where the structure is cancellated. When it takes place in these situations, it first induces enlargement of the epiphyses, with extreme pain deep in the bone. Soon after the periosteum becomes thick and swelled ; and in no long time sanious matter is found beneath it issuing from the *can-*

celli, which are then softened, partially destroyed, and excavated. If in this state such a bone be examined, the broken cancelli are filled with a reddish, soft, spongy vascular mass, producing flabby granulations *passim*, and secreting bloody sanious fluid.   The compact shell is partly destroyed by irregular ulceration, and partly extruded by the distending force of the swelled medullary web. The diseased epiphysis then presents a large irregular anfractuous cavern filled with soft spongy substance, which is either the web itself, or the new products which its inflammation has generated.* In this manner it is frequent in the upper end of the tibia, or the lower end of the femur, or in the extremities of the radius or ulna.

With deference, therefore, to the observation and assiduity of Mr Howship, I cannot agree with this author, that *spina ventosa* is an enlargement affecting the cylindrical bones, unless with the limitation above stated. . The only cylindrical bones in which its occurrence may give colour to this opinion are the phalanges.   These, however, have no distinct medullary cavity, and resemble in all respects the epiphyses and the short irregular bones in general.   In these the disease occurs in children and young persons.   It occurs also in the lower jaw, and occasionally in the vertebræ.

γ. *Enostosis.   Medullary Exostosis.*—To this head I do not refer the examples quoted by Houstet from Ruysch, Cheselden, and Daubenton, and which I conceive belong to necrosis.   There are nevertheless instances of cylindrical bones having an accretion of bony or osteo-colloid matter deposited in their interior, to such an extent as at once to enlarge much the dimensions of the bone, and obliterate the medullary cavity.   Examples of this are recorded by Cheselden,† Mery,‡ Tripier, Houstet,§ and J. Bell; and Sir A. Cooper describes the disease·at length under the name *exostosis* of the medullary membrane.   According to the observation of this experienced surgeon, the disease occurs in two forms, the *fungous* and the cartilaginous.   Both originate from the medullary web; both produce enlargement, expansion, softening, and separation of the osseous walls; and both ultimately terminate in ulcerative absorption of the affected bone.   In certain circumstances, however, they differ from each other.   The fungous exostosis consists of lo-

* See Observations on the Morbid Appearances and Structure of Bones, &c.   By John Howship, Esq. Med. Chir. Tr. Vol. x. p. 176, and several fine delineations of the disease.   •

† Osteographia, p. 53.

‡ Mém. de l'Academie des Sciences, 1706, p. 245.

§ Mém. de l'Acad. Roy. Chirurgie, Tome iii. p. 130.

1

bulated masses of soft, spongy, vascular substance like fat, brain, or clotted blood, which emits malignant *fungi*, and discharges blood-coloured serum. After some time it not only distends, separates, and destroys the bone, but it undergoes an alternate process of sloughing and hemorrhage. Though, in compliance with the views of Sir A. Cooper, I placed it under this head, it is scarcely entitled to the character of *enostosis* or *exostosis*, but is manifestly of the nature of the éncephaloid tumour. The cartilaginous, or genuine enostosis, consists of masses of firm chondrodesmoid structure, whitish-red or gray, producing by its enlargement progressive separation and destruction of the bone, but not possessing the fungating or malignant tendency.*

M. A. Severinus, Mery, and Mr J. Bell have described a variety of monstrous enlargement of the bones of the hand, which I think is to be viewed as belonging to the head of enostosis. Though they are termed tumours of the phalanges, it is impossible to doubt, from perusing the authentic description of Mery especially, that the disease consisted of inordinate enlargement of the ends or articular heads of the phalanges.† This enlargement was confined to the ends of the metacarpal and middle row. The shell of the bones was extenuated, and in some parts broken. The interior structure consisted of irregular bony masses, fibrous and cellular, or cavernous, containing reddish semifluid jelly. The contiguous articulations were ankylosed. These changes depend doubtless on morbid action of the medullary web. Any change in the structure of the bone and periosteum in such circumstances is secondary. A similar case is given by Scarpa, (Tab. 6.)

δ. *Pædarthrokake. Osteo-arthritis. Joint-ill of Children.*—This name was applied by Pandolphinus, Marcus Aurelius Severinus, Mercklin, and various other authors of the 17th century, to designate a disease which they conceived to be the same with *spina ventosa*. From the facts already adduced on this head, it is clear that they committed a great mistake, and that they confounded two diseases which are essentially different. It is evident that the disease which they most frequently saw, was that in which the articular ends of the bones, more especially the small bones of the extremities, become affected with caries, in consequence of previous disease of the synovial membrane, or chronic inflammation of the medullary mem-

* Surgical Essays by Sir A. Cooper. Part i. Pp. 165–173.
† Mémoires de l'Acad. des Sciences, 1720, p. 583. See also J. Bell's Principles Surgery, Vol. iii. pp. 73 and 80.

brane of the *epiphyses.* The last circumstance, nevertheless, is of small moment. The main fact to be attended to is, that the articular ends of the small bones of the extremities are liable to become denuded of their membranous coverings, to be rough and softened on their surface, to be swelled, and discharge a bloody, serous matter, and that no tendency to eject the diseased portion in mass is exhibited; while minute atoms of the bone are removed by ulceration and carried away in the discharges.

This disease may originate either in the synovial membrane of the articulation, and proceed thence to the subjacent cancellated tissue of the bone, or, beginning in the medullary membrane of the cancellated tissue, it proceeds outwards to the synovial membrane, which is affected with secondary inflammation and ulceration.

This sort of disorder may affect any articulation in the whole body. But those, in which it is most usually observed, are the articular surfaces of the carpal and tarsal bones, the articular ends of the metacarpal and metatarsal bones, and those of the phalanges of the fingers and toes. A considerable number of examples of the disease in the bones of the wrist, metacarpus, and fingers, I have seen in young females; and I think, that in them it is more frequent than in males.

The first indication of the approach and presence of the disease is swelling, generally of a puffy character, over the joint attacked. Pain is also felt; and the surface is in general hot and red. The disease, however, whether originating in the medullary tissue or in the synovial membrane, proceeds so rapidly and insidiously, that often the whole articular end of one bone, if not both of those of the articulation, is stripped of its covering, rough, and irregular, before the true nature of the malady is suspected.

The *cancelli* thus attacked are softened and reddened; and the part immediately affected is manifestly enlarged. In cases where opportunities of inspecting the bones have been afforded, they are found denuded of synovial membrane, cartilage, and periosteum. Their exposed surface is rendered irregular by numerous holes or cavities varying in size; and from which is seen issuing a reddish or brown-coloured sero-purulent matter, with which also the *cancelli* or lattice-work of the bone is filled.

The whole of this destruction is occasioned most commonly by inflammation of the cancellated medullary membrane, in some instances by that of the synovial membrane. Yet, notwithstanding the nature of the parts affected, recoveries are occasionally observed to take place. Adhesive inflammation comes on; lymph is effused; a stop is put to the disorganizing action; and new ossific matter being formed, sometimes with the preservation of the articulation, sometimes with ankylosis, partial or complete, the disease altogether disappears.

The disease is liable to affect the *vertebræ*, and often does affect them. There, however, it is much less likely to subside. In short, as it most frequently attacks bones which have cancellated tissue, as the short bones and the vertebræ, so it in them causes most havoc, and is least likely to undergo this spontaneous cure.

This disease affects mostly and preferably young persons. It begins to appear about the 6th or 7th year; and may take place at any time between that and the 21st year. After the latter period it is much less common, but may take place, especially in females. I have seen it, nevertheless, in some rare cases, affecting the bones of the feet in men above 40 and 50.

c. The third source of disease in the osseous texture are the articular synovial ·membranes and cartilages. Inflammation of the first soon passes to the second, in which it causes erosion or ulcerative absorption. From the cartilage this may proceed progressively to the epiphyses, the upper surface of which is sooner or later excavated into numerous holes or caverns of various size and shape. This process, which I refer to the vessels passing from the cartilage to the medullary web of the epiphyses, is accompanied with deep-seated aching pain, particularly distressing during the night. It is very common in that form of disease of the joints which arises from inflammation of the synovial membrane and cartilages; and several instances are recorded by authors.* It occurs in the hip-joint and knee-joint especially, and is one of the preliminary steps to ankylosis. I have seen this take place in the knee-joint, and have ascertained the point by dissection.

This also is one of the modes in which the vertebræ become carious. Chronic inflammation affects the synovial membrane and cartilages of an oblique process, and passing into the bone produces ulceration and carious excavations. This process not unfrequently causes in the incumbent and contiguous textures, irritative suppuration constituting an extensive abscess, which, according to circumstances, may take the anterior, the posterior, or the inferior di-

---

* See Cheston, who delineates two examples of it, and is at some pains to distinguish it from *spina ventosa*.

rection. As the original seat of the disease is generally the lower dorsal or upper lumbar vertebræ, the disease is termed *lumbar abscess.** It may appear either in the lumbar region, at the margin of the rectum, or in the groin. Several vertebræ are found excavated or destroyed by caries. As in the other articulations, however, this disease may terminate in irregular osseous union of several vertebræ, forming a species of ankylosis.

The forms of disease now enumerated are chiefly varieties or effects of the inflammatory process. Those which yet demand attention, though dependent in like manner on some abnormal action of the periosteal or medullary vessels, are nevertheless so peculiar, that it is impossible to refer them to the same general head.

d. Cartilaginous union of the ribs and other bones. In September 1828 I met with a singular instance of malformation in the ribs of a child, to which I have not yet heard of any example entirely similar.

In the body of a boy, two years and four months old, I was struck by the shape of the anterior surface of the chest. On each side, instead of the usual convex swell of the ribs, there was a remarkable depression extending from the third to the seventh rib inclusive, commencing about two inches from the sternum, and extending in breadth along the chest from one inch and a half to two inches. This depression consisted in each of these ribs presenting a defect of conformation from their posterior convexity to the junctions with the cartilages. At the former point each rib was suddenly bent from its normal curvature to an angular or sharp turn, as if it had been broken, and thence proceeded flat, and in some sense straight, to the cartilage, its union with which was marked by a depression and a large and evident knob or tuberosity not unlike an articulation. The deformity thus produced was so distinct, that any one would have readily pronounced it the result of a fracture. But to this idea, the circumstance of its extending through so many ribs, and being found with the same uniformity on both sides, formed an objection of some weight. To obtain some light on the matter, I removed several of the ribs, and made of these longitudinal and transverse sections. By this means the following facts were ascertained.

The bony portion of the third, fourth, fifth, sixth, and seventh ribs, underwent at the posterior-lateral convexity a sudden change

* Camper, Demonst. Anat. lib. ii. cap. 1. art 6. Cheston's Pathological Inquiries and Observations, Case iv. p. 128, and v. p. 130. Howship, Morbid Anatomy, chap. vii. p. 365.

of direction, so that the second or straight portion formed with the first or curved a sharp turn sufficient to constitute exactly a right angle. Longitudinal and transverse sections of these ribs showed that no breach of continuity had taken place, and, therefore, that this turn was not the result of fracture. It presented a uniform, firm surface, ash-gray in colour, and traversed, as usual, by minute red lines, yet without manifest trace of interrupted continuity. From this rectangular bend the substance of the bone was of the usual appearance, but looser and more cancellated as it approached the sternal extremity, which was large, soft, and very sectile. It was also forced inward from the cartilage, so as to form the remarkable depression observed on the exterior of the chest, while the cartilage itself projected in the shape of a large round tubercle or eminence. Nothing like false joint was observed either at the point of curvature or at the cartilages.*

These appearances were observed in the third, fourth, fifth, sixth, and seventh ribs; in the four last most distinctly; in the third and eighth faintly, but still sufficiently well to contribute to the general aspect of deformity on the exterior of the chest. All the ribs were soft and flexible, and spongy and sectile; and I cannot convey the idea of this condition more distinctly than by simply stating the fact, that in removing several of the ribs and making sections, I did not use the saw, but simply cut them both transversely and longitudinally. As has been already stated, they were in all respects the same on both sides of the chest.

Connected with this was a peculiarity in the bones of the skull not dissimilar. Before dividing the scalp there was observed a deep longitudinal furrow in the situation of the sagittal suture between the two parietal bones; and another transverse one extending, though less deep, on each side along the coronal suture, between the posterior margin of the frontal bone and the anterior edge of the parietal bones. Not only was the fontanelle incomplete for about two inches; but no attempt had been made, or was likely to be made, to unite the two parietal bones with each other, and these with the frontal, by the ordinary process of dove-tail ossification. The longitudinal furrow in the situation of the sagittal suture was so large as to leave an inch at least between the parietal bones; and along this space these bones were united by firm fibro-ligamentous structure. The coronal suture on each side down to the temporal bone

---

* Edinburgh Medical and Surgical Journal, Vol. XXXII. Plate I. Edinburgh, 1829.

was so much divided in like manner, that the transverse furrow thus formed easily admitted the introduction of the tip of the finger ; and the frontal and parietal bones were also united by firm fibro-ligamentous tissue. When this was inspected attentively, it appeared to consist of pericranium and *dura mater* firmly adhering, and without the smallest trace of intermediate bone. This was shown, indeed, by the state of the fontanelle, at which the pericranium adhered so firmly to the *dura mater*, that it was impossible to separate them otherwise than by the knife. This double membrane was quite fibro-cartilaginous, and was so tensely stretched between the bones, that while it was bound down in the centre to the *dura mater*, it was raised to the margins of the bones on each side of the depressed channel or *sulcus.* Much the same substance surrounded the whole parietal bones, though with less separation of the lambdoidal and temporo-parietal sutures, and with more traces of ossification. Yet so imperfect was this process, that I removed both parietal bones by strong scissors ; and without using the saw, inspected the whole brain completely. The other peculiarities will be understood by a short sketch of the appearance of the right parietal bone.

The bone is very thin, and, in the situation of the parietal protuberance, translucent. The anterior or frontal margin presents no serrated appearance; but becoming quickly attenuated, terminates in fibro-ligamentous structure, which was leaden gray coloured, opaque, and very tough, but which has dried very hard and brittle, and is translucent and traversed by red vascular lines. At the upper mesial extremity of this margin, the bone, instead of presenting the usual rectangular process, is very deficient, and terminates in a portion of fibro-ligamentous membrane, at least eight lines broad. The inner or mesial margin, which forms the sagittal suture, which is equally void of serrated edge, is completed by the same sort of texture; but the posterior margin, corresponding to the occipital anterior of the bone, is firmer, and presents in some parts points of ossification ; and one of these is what would afterwards have constituted a Wormian bone. The inferior margin, where it corresponds to the temporal bone, is separated from that bone by a thin portion of the same membranous substance, about two lines broad, but without trace of bony matter. The bone was soft and sectile, as indeed were the bones of the skull in general ; and as a proof of this, the instrument has divided the scaly portion of the temporal bone, and left it attached by ligamentous matter to the parietal.

Though the sudden rectangular turn or change of direction had at first sight the appearance of a fracture which had been afterwards consolidated, yet there was no reason to think, from the history and circumstances of the case, that this injury was the cause of the malformation. The peculiar bad configuration of these ribs had existed from the moment of birth, and appeared to have attracted little attention from the relatives. It was found, as already stated, on both sides of the chest; and it was impossible, in making sections of several of the ribs, to discover any of those marks, by which the existence of a previous fracture is recognized.

The state of the cranial sutures is less uncommon than that of the ribs. For I believe it may be regarded as a variety of that malformation which has been distinguished by some authors as *opening* of the sutures. Portal especially, in speaking of the occurrence of this phenomena in young subjects, remarks, that though rare, it is occasionally observed to the age of two or three years; but adds, that at a more advanced age it is uncommon to find the sutures separated, in consequence of the operations of an internal cause.[*]

This child had been destroyed by *bronchitis*. But all the other internal organs were sound.

On the cause of this deficiency in the bones of the chest and head it is difficult to offer even a conjecture. It was the opinion of several relatives of the mother, that the peculiar misshaping of the chest had been caused by tight lacing and excessive compression during pregnancy. To the operation of this cause being adequate, the chief objection is the fact, that it is difficult to imagine any degree of compression of this kind, which would not rather have caused the death of the child.[†]

In 1828 M. Dupuytren published in the *Repertoire Generale d'Anatomie*, with four illustrative cases, an account of a malformation or deformity in the bones of the chest, not dissimilar. This he represents to consist in a depression more or less considerable of the bones of the chest, in proportional prominence of the sternum, of the belly anteriorly, and of the vertebral column posteriorly. In infants affected by this deformity, the sternum projects forward like the keel of a vessel; the spinal column rises like the back of an ass; and the ribs are not only flattened but depressed towards the

[*] Anatomie Medicale, Tome i. p. 96.

[†] Account of an Instance of Malformation in some of the Bones of the Skeleton. By David Craigie, M. D. Edinburgh Medical and Surgical Journal, Vol. XXXII. p. 51. Edinburgh, 1829.

chest, nearly as if at the period, when they were soft, flexible, and capable of taking all shapes and curvatures, they had been com-pressed from one side to the other, as is done in killing pigeons, by placing the fingers beneath the wings and compressing the sides of the chest. This deformity is so considerable in some children that it is possible to embrace both sides of the chest with the fingers of the same hand. The transverse diameter of the chest is dimi-nished from one-fourth to one-third, or even one-half, while the antero-posterior and vertical diameters are in a similar rate increased.

This change in the natural figure and dimensions of the bony walls of the chest exerts great and hurtful effects on the functions of the contained organs. Respiration is habitually short and oppress-ed, with inexpressible anxiety and anguish, and threatening suffo-cation; the infant cannot suck; afterwards speech is short, inter-rupted, and panting. The motions of the heart are oppressed, con-strained, and irregular. Sleep is disturbed, noisy, and accompanied with great labour in breathing; while the sufferers lie with the mouth open. Their repose is often interrupted by frightful dreams.

Of the anatomical state of the bones M. Dupuytren says, that M. Breschet only recognized some retardation in the development of the skeleton, disjunction of the bones of the *cranium* at a period at which these bones should normally have been united, persistence of the *epiphyses*, or swelling of the extremities of the cylindrical bones, sundry torsions of their *diaphyses*, and little consistence in their tissue, so that they were sectile rather than fragile, and re-sembled bones softened by immersion in weak nitric acid. Denti-tion was retarded; the teeth of the first or second dentition altered the crown eroded, partly destroyed, and furrowed on their anterior surface.

The most remarkable circumstance in the internal and soft or-gans observed by Dupuytren in this sort of deformity, is the swel-ling of the tonsils, with which it is almost invariably attended. These glands are often so much enlarged as seriously to impede respiration, and require to be partly or wholly resected.*

The lungs are depressed towards the vertebral column; and ge-nerally bear on their surface the impression of the ribs. The

---

* Memoire sur la Depression Laterale des Parois de la Poitrine. Par M. le Baron Dupuytren. Repertoire Generale d'Anatomie et de Physiologie, Tome Vquieme, p. 110. Paris, 1828.

Leçons Orales de Clinique Chirurgicale, &c. Tome Imier. Deuxieme edition. Paris, 1829. Article ix. p. 182.

children are sometimes affected with pulmonary catarrh, and emphysema of the lungs.

This disease may prove fatal during the first days or weeks of existence; and if it do not, it gradually wears down the sufferers by certain steps to extreme emaciation and debility, terminating in death.

Though I have mentioned these two instances of deformity of the bones together, and though in several respects they strongly resemble each other, yet I am not sure that they are exactly alike. It is remarkable that M. Dupuytren says nothing of any cartilaginous union of the ribs at the point of depression,—a circumstance which, if present, could scarcely have escaped the notice of M. Breschet.

On the other hand, in the case detailed by myself, though the child had died of a bronchitic attack, the tonsils were not larger than usual. Again, I see daily young persons with tonsils more or less enlarged, some so much that I know the presence and degree of the enlargement by hearing them speak; yet in these I see no deformity of the walls of the thorax.

I think it, nevertheless, highly probable that both affections, whether they are to be regarded as alike or different, depend on, or are connected with the same general cause; some peculiar state of the osseous system, by which its ossification at the normal rate is retarded.

It is necessary to say, that this congenital depression of the thoracic walls must not be confounded with a depression which also takes place in infants and children, in connection with chronic pneumonia, pleurisy, empyema, tubercles, and other affections of the lungs. The depression here adverted to is the effect of the great and incessant efforts made to dilate and compress the lungs, in the laboured actions of respiration induced by morbid states of the lungs.

5. *Rickets.* *Rachitis.*—This disease, of which no distinct trace is found in the writings of the ancients, or in those of the authors of the middle ages, was first described by Glisson as appearing in England in the course of the 17th century. Though still frequent in these islands, it is not peculiar to them; and it is by no means unknown in other countries of Europe. In the time of Petit it was common in France. At present it appears to be occasionally seen in Belgium and Holland. Notwithstanding the fact above mentioned, the disease is not to be regarded as new. Its occurrence in infancy only was the cause of its escaping observa-

tion. Its influence, however, in leaving more or less deformity of the skeleton must have at all times attracted notice. Deformed dwarfs have been known in all ages. The *gibbi*, the *vari*, and the *valgi* of the Romans must have been more or less rachitic in infancy. From this cause the deformity of Thersites might have originated. It is also to be remarked, that Fabricius Hildanus delineates the serpentine lateral curvature of the spine in a girl of 8, whose bones were soft as wax,* which could be produced by no other cause save rickety softness.

When the disease first attracted notice, and the chemical constitution of bone was understood, it was believed that rickets consisted merely in the late deposition of phosphate of lime. Of this theory the defect is its simplicity. Though the earthy matter is doubtless very deficient, this is not the sole change in the rachitic skeleton. The bone is light, spongy, and cellular. The close or compact structure is said to disappear. The truth is, that it is not yet formed. The interior of the bone is homogeneous like that of a fœtal bone, without distinct medullary cavity, without cancellated structure, and without compact bone; but presenting the loose cellular or areolar arrangement observed at that period of life. The interstitial cells are filled with brownish jelly-like substance,† which appears to be a secretion from the medullary arteries. The bone is soft, of the consistence of cartilage, and is easily cut by the knife. Its colour is some shade of red, but varies from light pink or brown to an orange or fawn-coloured tint. This it derives from its vessels, which are numerous, large, and loaded with dark-coloured blood deficient in fibrin. The periosteum is generally thickened, and occasionally detached. (Cheselden, Bichat, Bonn.) In short, the rachitic bone is the fœtal bone in internal structure, but destitute of its proportion of calcareous matter.

One of the peculiarities of the rachitic condition of the osseous system is, that though the bones present the characters now enumerated during its continuance, they afterwards acquire equal or even greater firmness and density than sound bones, by the deposition of calcareous matter. While this takes place, the distinction between the cancellated and compact structure begins to be established, and the formation of medullary canal is also begun.

---

* Cent. 6, Obs. 75.

† Morel in Jour. de Med. Paris, 1757, Vol. VII. p. 432 ; Portal sur la Nature du Rachitisme, 2de Partie, Art. iii. p. 246 ; Tacconi in Comm. Bonon ; and Stanley in Med. Chir. Tr. Vol. VII. p. 407.

When this process once commences, it proceeds much as in healthy bone. In one respect, however, its completion is peculiar. Instead of the compact matter of the bone being equally distributed on each side of the medullary canal, as in sound bones, it is more abundant at the internal than the external side of the incurvated bone. Thus if the femur, as generally happens, is incurvated outwards, the greatest deposition of compact bone is at the internal wall. This deposition may be so considerable in bones which are much bent, as to obliterate entirely the medullary canal.* The restored ra-cbitic bone is said to contain more earthy matter than healthy bone.

6. *Mollities Ossium ;—Malakosteon ;—Osteo-malacia ;—Osteo-sarcosis.*—To the ancients this peculiar state of the osseous system appears to have been as little known as rickets. Omitting the un-certain traces of its existence, which are found in the writings of Ebn-Sina, and several of his European commentators, the first dis-tinct record of the malady was given in 1665 by Banda, who, in 1650, observed for ten years the progress of the disease in the case of a citizen of Sedan ;† and in 1688 by Gabriel, who found all the long bones of a lady soft, flexible, and converted into a reddish flesh-like substance, void of fibres.‡ Still more distinct cases were published by Saviard in 1691,§ and by Courtial and Lambert in 1700.‖ About the same time Valsalva met with an instance, which, however, was published only in 1760 by Morgagni.¶ Previous to this, however, had been published a case by Mr S. Be-van in 1742 ;** that of the woman Supiot, the details of whose his-tory were given in France by M. Morand, and in England by Mr Bromfield ;†† the case of Mary Hayes by Pringle and Gooch ;‡‡

* Observations on the condition of the Bones in Rickets, &c. By Edward Stanley, Esq. &c. Med. Chirurg. Tr. Vol. VII. p. 404.

† Traité des Maladies des Os. Par M. Du Verney. Paris, 1751. Tome I. Pre-face v. p. 136.

‡ Eph. Nat. Cur. Dec. 3, An. 2, Obs. 3. This is the case noticed by Gagliardi the following year, 1689, which Scarpa also mentions as the first. The Professor of Pavia seems not to be aware that the case did not belong originally to Gagliardi but to Ga-briel. The earliest case, however, appears to have been that of Peter Siga of Sedan.

§ Nouveau Recueil, &c. Obs. 62, p. 274. 1702.

‖ Histoire de l'Acad. R. des Sciences, 1700, Obs. 2. et Relation de la Maladie de Bernarde d'Armagnac, &c. This young woman, a native of Thoulouse, died in the Hospital of St Jacques de la Grave on the 19th November 1699.

¶ Epist. lviii. 4.   ** Phil. Tr. Vol. xlii. p. 488.

†† Histoire de la Maladie Singulière, &c. Par M. Morand Fils, 1752. Mém. de l'Acad. 1753. The particulars of this case are published also in the Philos. Transact. for 1753–1754, Vol. xlviii. where she is called Queriot, and in Bromfield's Chirurgical Observations and Cases, Vol. ii.

‡‡ Phil. Tr. 1753, Vol. xlviii. p. 297.

and that of E. Winckler by Ludwig.* Since that time cases have
been published by Mr H. Thomson†, Acrel,‡ Renard,§ and Howship.‖

From these and similar cases it results, that in this disease
the bones gradually lose their firmness and consistence, become
soft, flexible, and may even be broken. The change is remarked
first in the cylindrical bones, and though it extends to the others,
it there continues to be most conspicuous. It consists in the bone
becoming soft, sectile, reddish, and something like a mass of flesh.
When any part remains unchanged, it is in the shape of thin scales
or crusts at the outer part of the *diaphysis,* or occasional bony
plates like portions of egg-shell intermixed. The cancellated structure of the epiphysis entirely disappears, and in its place is found
a soft homogeneous reddish mass. The situation of the marrow is
occupied by a red, thick, semifluid matter like clotted blood, mixed
with grease or suet. The flat bones of the skull are generally
equally soft, flesh-like, and sectile. The cancellated structure of
the *diploe* is equally destroyed, and its place is occupied by a uniform soft reddish substance, from sections of which bloody serum
exudes. The periosteum is sometimes thickened, but is often unchanged.

The cause of this change is quite unknown. The most ingenious and probable conjecture regarding it is that by Howship, who,
from the necroscopic appearances of a well-described case, infers
that it is the effect of a morbid action of the capillary arteries upon
the medullary membrane within the bone; and that the disappearance of the latter is the effect of absorption exercised by the morbid
secretion.¶

7. *Friability. Fragility.* In the disease now described the bones
may be broken by the weight of the person, or slight action of the
muscles; and perhaps most cases of spontaneous fracture are referable either to incipient *osteo-sarkosis,* to *nekrosis,* or to *spina ventosa.* One instance of this I certainly traced to incipient nekrosis.
Others, perhaps, are more equivocal. Is the animal matter absorbed?

8. *Interstitial absorption.*—Under this name Mr B. Bell Jun. de-

* Haller Disp. Med.-Pract. Tom. vi. p. 327, Lips. 1757.

† Med. Obs. and Inquiries, Vol. v. p. 259.

‡ Dissertatio, &c.   Upsalæ, 1788.

§ Ramollissement Remarkable, &c.   Mayence, 1804.

‖ Medico-Chir. Tr. Ed. Vol. ii. p. 136.

¶ Case of *Mollities ossium,* &c. Med.-Chirurg. Tr. Edin. Vol. ii. p. 136.

scribes a peculiar sinking or condensation of the cancellated texture of the neck of the thigh-bone, occurring chiefly in aged subjects.* The affected part of the bone is highly vascular. In the only instance of this in my possession, the head of the bone has lost its spherical shape, and is flattened down upon the neck not unlike the *pileus* of a mushroom. The most internal part of its cartilaginous covering presents a series of holes passing into the *cancelli*. The neck is about one-third of its usual length, so that the head of the bone is lower than the great trochanter. This change must have been effected by the medullary vessels of the head and neck of the bone.

9. *Angiectasis.*—The arterial system of bones is liable to a peculiar abnormal development, in which they become much enlarged, and forming a cyst in the substance of the bone, gradually effect its absorption. Cases of this description I have already stated were observed by Pearson and Scarpa. Similar cases have occurred to M. Lallemand and M. Breschet.†

10. *Eburneoid, or Ivory-like Induration.*—This, which consists in bone acquiring extraordinary hardness, density, and closeness, is occasionally seen in bony tumours, or exostosis, in bones which have been fractured, and sometimes in those of the skull, without evident morbid condition. In the case of Petit, however, an osseous tumour as large as a melon, and of the ivory aspect and consistence, was developed in the temporal bone.‡

A species of eburneoid or porcelain degeneration is liable to attack the articular extremities of bones after synovial rheumatism. An effusion of sero-albuminous fluid first takes place; and when this undergoes coagulation, it is found to contain some earthy matter, which some have said is lithate of soda, and others carbonate of lime. After some time, by the motion of the articular surfaces, this deposit undergoes a degree of polish; and the more the articular surfaces are moved, the smoothness increases, communicating the aspect of ground-ivory, or porcelain. In some instances, also, the cartilages are worn or removed by absorption, as the effect of the same disease; and their place is in some degree supplied by this eburneoid or porcelain-like deposit. The subject shall be noticed under the head of the synovial membranes.

---

* Essay on Interstitial Absorption of the thigh-bone, Ed. 1824.

† Repertoire Gen. de Breschet, T. ii. part 2d. Paris, 1826.

‡ Maladies des Os, Tome ii. p. 292.

11. *Osteo-sarkoma.*—Though this is mentioned as a distinct variety of morbid change, it is probably of the same nature as exostosis. In this light it is viewed by Scarpa and Boyer. Upon the whole, though I cannot agree with the former in accounting it of the same nature as *spina ventosa*, I think the examples of osteo-sarkoma may be referred to the cartilaginous variety either of periosteal or. medullary exostosis.

12. *Encysted Tumours. a. Osteo-steatoma.*—The formation of steatomatous tumours in the substance or at the surface of bones, has been noticed by Kulm,* Hundtermark,† Herrmann,‡ Pott,§ Murray,‖ Sandifort,¶ Reil,** Von Siebold,†† and above all, by Palletta‡‡ and Weidmann.§§ The tumour is generally encysted; and though it is represented by J. Bell as originating in the medullary tissue, it seems occasionally to arise from the periosteum. Its contents are not invariably, as its name seems to indicate, of an adipose nature. They vary from gelatinous, oleaginous, and meliceritious, to atheromatous and sebaceous, irregularly intermixed with *spiculæ* and *lamellæ* of bone. Their progressive enlargement causes by pressure and absorption destruction of the contiguous bone. This is the process which by Palletta is termed *ossivorous.*

b. Hæmatoma ; (Blood-cyst.)—Of all the examples of this disease (*abscessus sanguineus,*) collected by Palletta, one only I find originated in the substance of a bone,—the tibia in its upper epiphysis, which was consumed by carious absorption. (Case 22.) In several, however, the tumour, though originating in the adjoining tissues, had produced by progressive encroachment the same effect.

c. Fungus Hæmatodes.—This is the same as the fungous medullary exostosis above noticed. Whether it originates in this manner, or from the contiguous textures, it produces the same erosive destruction of the bones. An instance of this originating in the peritonæum I saw destroy the bones of the pelvis, and reduce the upper half of the right *os femoris* to a thin net-work of bone, which broke asunder a few days before death.

13. *Scirrho-Carcinoma.*—Though this seems never to originate

* Haller, Disp. Med.-Chir. Vol. V. p. 653.
† Haller, Disput. Med.-Pract. Tome VI. p. 349.
‡ Diss. Inaug. J. G. Herrmanni de Osteo-steatomate, Lipsiæ, 1767.
§ Phil. Trans. No. 459.   ‖ Dissert. de Osteo-steatomate, Upsalæ, 1780.
¶ Mus. Anat. I. 161.   ** Archiv. III. B. 453.
†† Sammlung Chirurg. Beobacht. u. s. w. II. B. p. 310 and 412.
‡‡ Exercitat. Patholog. p. 111.   §§ De Steatomatibus, Moguntiae, 1817.

in the osseous texture, it often spreads to it from the contiguous one. Thus most surgeons have seen cancer of the lip or scirrhus of the parotid affect the lower jaw; cancer of the female breast erode the ribs; cancer of the penis affect the *ossa pubis;* and cancer of the eye or eyelids, in both sexes, affect the frontal, malar, or superior maxillary bones.

14. Tubercular destruction may occur in bones; but it most frequently originates in the periosteum or adjoining tissues, and passes thence to the enclosed bone, in which it produces the usual destructive erosion. (Palletta.)

15. Hydatids of the social form were seen in the tibia by Cullerier.[*]

16. In early life the growth of the osseous system may be suspended or interrupted, so that the parts of the skeleton are incomplete. This deficiency generally takes place on the mesial plane, at the line where the bones of each side are approaching to unite with each other. It is most common in the spinous processes of the vertebræ, in the bones of the head, and those of the upper jaw and palate. In the spine it is generally connected with the abnormal effusion of fluid from the membranes of the chord, or the chord itself, when it constitutes *spina bifida* or cleft spine. The same deficiency I have seen in the frontal and nasal bones; and in hare-lip it is by no means uncommon in those of the palate and superior jaw.

17. Before concluding this chapter, a few words may be said on the morbid states incident to the teeth.

The enamel is liable to be worn down by the mutual attrition of the teeth of the upper and lower jaw. This detrition, which has been particularly described by Prochaska,[†] is most conspicuous in the crowns of those of the lower jaw, which in some subjects are so much worn down as to expose the central osseous pith of the tooth. Though effected chiefly by attrition, it is much facilitated by the use of acid substances, and by those states of the stomach and alimentary canal which favour the formation of acid. Another form of the same destruction may take place in the corresponding sides of two teeth which are too closely implanted together. The mutual pressure exercised during the process of mastication appears to be the first cause of this. After it is once established, it destroys

---

[*] Cruveilhier, Anat. Pathol. Vol. I. p. 230.

[†] Observationes Anatomicae de Decremento Dentium Corporis Humani. Apud Operum Minorum. Partem IIdam, p. 355, &c. Viennae, 1800.

first the enamel, and then the bone of the tooth, causing caries in the latter, which become blue or black, and is gradually excavated into a hole.

The most frequent cause of disease of the teeth, however, is inflammation of their internal pulp. This, which is attended by intense pain, by progressively destroying the membrane, impairs the nutrition of the tooth, which becomes carious in the bony pith, while the enamel cracks, and is cast off in the form of concave scales or crusts. The bony part thus exposed proceeds still more rapidly to destruction. It becomes excavated, breaks down, and at length is expelled in fragments.

Inflammation of the membrane of the alveolar cavities also, by injuring the connecting vessels, may cause carious destruction of the teeth. But it is generally combined with more or less affection of the pulp. In the rachitic its destruction causes the development of the teeth to be checked, rendering the individual toothless.

CHAPTER V.

GRISTLE, CARTILAGE, *Cartilago,— Tissu Cartilagineux.*

SECTION I.

THE cartilaginous system or tissue is found at least in three different situations of the human body ; 1*st*, on the articular extremities'of the movable bones ; 2*d*, in the connecting surfaces or margins of immovable bones ; 3*d*, in the parietes of certain cavities, the motions or uses of which require bodies of this elastic substance.

The organization of gristle is obscure and indistinct. On examination by the microscope, its structure is said to be uniform and homogeneous, like firm jelly, without fibres, plates, or cells. William Hunter, however, represents the articular cartilages as consisting of longitudinal and transverse fibres.* Herissant represents those of the ribs as composed of minute fibres mutually aggregated into bundles connected by short slips, and twisted in a spiral or serpentine direction.† By Lassone, the articular cartilages are

---

* Phil. Transact. Vol. XLIII. No. 470.
† Mem. de l'Acad. Roy. 1748. P. 355.

said to consist of a multitude of minute threads mutually connected and placed as right angles to the plane of the bone, but so as to radiate from the centre to the circumference.* The general fact of fibrous structure is confirmed by Bichat, who says, that with a little attention it is possible to recognize longitudinal fibres, which are intersected by others in an oblique or transverse direction, but without determinate order. In its purest form no blood-vessels are seen in it, nor can they be demonstrated even by the finest injections. In the margins of those pieces of gristle, however, which are attached to the extremities of growing bones, blood-vessels of considerable size may often be seen, even without the aid of injection. In young subjects a net-work of arteries and veins, which is described by Hunter under the name of *circulus articuli vasculosus*, may be demonstrated all round the margin of the cartilage at the line between the epiphysis and it. They terminate so abruptly, however, that they cannot be traced into the substance of the latter. The most certain proofs, however, of the organic structure of this substance are the serous exudation which appears in the course of a few seconds on the cut surface of a piece of cartilage after a clean division by the knife; and that it becomes yellow during jaundice, and derives colour from substances found in the blood. Neither absorbents nor nerves have been found in it. The cellular texture said by Bichat to form the mould for the proper cartilaginous matter appears to be imaginary.

The articular cartilages adhere to the epiphyses by one surface, which consists of short perpendicular fibres placed parallel to each other, and forming a structure like the pile of velvet. This is easily demonstrated by maceration first in nitric acid and then in water. The free or smooth surface is covered by a thin fold of synovial membrane, which comes off in pieces during maceration. The existence of this, though recently denied by Gordon, was admitted by William Hunter, and may be demonstrated either by boiling, maceration, or the phenomena of inflammation, under which it is sensibly thickened. All other cartilages are enveloped, unless where they are attached to bones, by a fibrous membrane, which has been therefore named *perichondrium.* The existence of this may be demonstrated by dissection, and also by boiling, which makes it peel off in crisped flakes.

The chemical properties of cartilage have not been accurately

---

* Mem. de l'Acad. Roy. 1752. P. 255.

examined. Boiling shows that it contains gelatine; but as a good deal of the matter is undissolved, it must be concluded also that it is under some modification, or united with some other principle, perhaps albumen. Immersion in nitric acid or boiling fluids induces crispation; and it dries hard and semitransparent, like horn.

SECTION II.

Cartilage is subject to inflammation, which in the chronic form passes into ulceration or erosion,—an affection common in the articular cartilages of the thigh-bone and tibia.

In this state cartilage becomes reddish or vascular, and flaccid, or soft and spongy, with a lardaceous appearance and distinct fibrous arrangement. It swells and acquires a size double or even four times larger than natural. In this state it does not become yellow, nor is dissolved by boiling. This is most common in the hip-joint. (Bichat.)

When inflammation continues some time, it produces erosion. The first trace of this consists in minute reddish perforations appearing at the synovial surface of the cartilage, and gradually extending and becoming deeper. At first they are circular; but as these perforations by extension coalesce, irregular abraded patches are produced, which at length become so deep as to expose the denuded bone. When this takes place, as the process advances, irregular excavations are hollowed in the epiphyses, which then present the state described at p. 477. This form of caries, which resembles in some respects *spina ventosa*, is, I conceive, the one to which Severinus alludes, and to which he wishes to restrict the epithet of *paedarthrokake*. I have seen it in adults, however; and it is most frequent in the knee-joint, in which I have seen it remove every trace of cartilage. In this process Hunter represents the transverse fibres as giving way first; but this distinction is too refined. The disease may terminate in bony *ankylosis*. It occurs also in the hip-joint and in the elbow-joint.

In the cartilages of the larynx inflammation takes place either primarily or by extension from the perichondrium or the mucous membrane of the throat. When it takes place primarily, it is represented by Mr Porter as preceded by ossification. When it takes place secondarily, it may occasionally be traced to ordinary inflammation from exposure to cold, the poison of syphilis, or the unfavourable operation of mercury. In either case it produces a bad species of ulceration, with mortification of the cartilages, which are sometimes coughed up as dead sloughs. This constitutes one of the worst forms of laryngeal consumption, (*phthisis laryngea.**)

In strumous subjects the cartilages of the nose are subject to a species of enlargement or thickening, accompanied with increased vascularity, and terminating in unfavourable ulceration. In some instances, tyromatous deposition in the tubercular form takes place, and renders the nostrils tumid, irregularly knobbed and painful. This, which also tends to very bad ulceration, is one of the forms of the disease described under the general name of *Noli me tangere.* That it originates in the cartilages I have observed more than once; and its ravages are seldom stopped till they are completely destroyed, leaving much deformity.

It has been supposed that cartilage does not readily granulate. But this must be a mistake, unless in regard to the laryngeal and tracheal cartilages; for when bones are removed from articular cavities, granulations have been known to rise from the cartilaginous surface; and there is no doubt that wounds of cartilaginous tissue are frequently united by granulation. All that fact and observation permit to be said is, that often they do not readily granulate.

Cartilage is also liable to ossification, as is seen in those of the larynx and of the ribs. In these the osseous matter is disseminated in irregular points and patches. In diseases of the hip-joint, the cartilages of the thigh-bone and acetabulum become not only bony, but may be converted into a substance similar to ivory. (Bichat.)

When textures, originally cartilaginous, have thus become penetrated by bony or calcareous matter, they manifestly lose part of their vital properties. They are much less capable than formerly of resisting the approaches of disease. They are more liable to inflammation. And they are prone to become affected by mortification or nekrosis exactly as bone; and in this condition they cause as much irritative suppuration as dead bone. This disorder is observed principally on the cartilages of the larynx.

A new formation of cartilage is frequently found in various tissues, but especially in the serous and synovial membranes, to which it is not uncommon to find cartilaginous bodies attached. Cartilaginous texture is also found in those sarcomatous tumours which eventually pass into insanable ulceration.

* Observations on the Surgical Pathology of the Larynx and Trachea, &c. By W. H. Porter, A. M., &c. Dublin and London, 1826.

CHAPTER VI.

FIBRO-CARTILAGE,— *Cartilago Fibrosa,*—*Tissue Fibro-Cartila-gineux,*— *Chondro-Desmoid Texture.*

SECTION I.

INTERMEDIATE between the cartilaginous and the fibrous tissues, Bichat ranks that of the fibro-cartilages, which comprehends three subdivisions. 1*st*, The membranous fibro-cartilages, as those of the ears, nose, windpipe, eyelids, &c.; 2*d*, The inter-articular fibro-cartilages, as those found in the temporo-maxillary and femoro-tibial articulations, the intervertebral substances, and the cartilaginous bodies uniting the bones of the pelvis; 3*d*, Certain portions of the periosteum, in which, when a tendinous sheath is formed, the peculiar nature of the fibrous system disappears, and is succeeded by a substance belonging to the order of fibro-cartilages.

Beclard follows Meckel in rejecting the first of these subdivisions, the individuals of which are quite similar to ordinary cartilage. Like it, they do not present the distinct fibrous structure, but are covered by perichondrium, the fibres of which have evidently caused them to be regarded as fibro-cartilages. On this principle Beclard gives the following view of the fibro-cartilages.

1*st*, Fibro-cartilages free at both surfaces; those in the form of *menisci*, which are placed between the articular surfaces of two bones; (*fibro cartilagines inter-articulares.*) These are seen in the temporo-maxillary, sterno-clavicular, and femoro-tibial articulations, and occasionally in the acromio-clavicular and the ulno-carpal joints. These ligaments are attached either by their margins or their extremities, and are enveloped in a thin fold of synovial membrane. 2*d*, Fibro-cartilages attached by one surface. Of this description are those employed as pulleys or grooves for the easy motion of tendons; for instance the chondro-desmoid eminences attached to the margin of the glenoid cavity for the long head of the *biceps*, and at the sinuosity of the ischium for the tendons of the *obturatores*. 3*d*, Fibro-cartilages, which establish a connection between bones susceptible of little individual motion, as the intervertebral bodies; or which unite bones intended to remain fixed, unless under very peculiar circumstances, as those which form the junction of the pelvic bones. (*Symphysis pubis, sacro-iliac synchondrosis.*) The peculiarities of these substances consist in their partaking in different proportions of the nature of cartilage and white fibrous tissue, and, consequently, in possessing the toughness and resistance of the latter with the flexibility and elasticity of the former. The structure of the fibro-cartilaginous tissue is easily seen in the intervertebral bodies, or in the cartilages uniting the pelvic bones. In the former, white concentric layers, consisting of circular fibres placed in juxta-position, constitute the outer part; while the interior contains a semifluid jelly. The concentric fibrous layers are cartilage in a fibrous shape. In the latter situation, the fibrous structure is equally distinct; while the cartilaginous consistence shows the connection with that organic substance. A similar arrangement is remarked in the interarticular cartilage of the temporomaxillary articulation, and in the semilunar cartilages of the knee-joint. In all, the fibrous is said to predominate over the cartilaginous structure. Their physical properties are distensibility with elasticity. Though they are at all times subjected to considerable pressure, they speedily recover their former size. Their chemical composition appears to be entirely unknown.

Section II.

There is little doubt that the fibro-cartilages are liable to inflammation, either originally commencing in their own substance, or communicated to them from contiguous parts, especially synovial membrane, with which many of them are invested. Suppuration of that which forms the *symphysis pubis* was seen by a friend of Hunter,* and by Ludovici, in the person of a puerperal female. This was the effect of excessive stretching during labour. In other instances they are torn asunder, so as to cause diastasis without suppuration. In one instance, separation of this kind appears to have been congenital. Palletta and Brodie have described a variety of vertebral disease which always commences with, and sometimes consists in erosion of the intervertebral cartilages; and most surgeons have seen the semilunar cartilages of the knee-joint inflamed and eroded. The intervertebral fibro-cartilages have been found softened, swollen, and distended with fluid. Ossification is not uncommon, and in those of the sacro-iliac and pubal junctions

---

* Med. Obs. and Inquiries, Vol. II.

(*symphyses*), is remarked in adults, or those advanced in life so frequently, that it cannot be regarded as disease. In the vertebræ it is also observed, though less frequently. It has been seen most generally in the dorsal and lumbar vertebræ, which are thus indissolubly ankylosed.

The *accidental*, or new development of the chondro-desmoid tissue, is not uncommon; and its appearance constitutes the anatomical character of the most usual form of scirrho-carcinoma. In this state irregular or amorphous masses of fibro-cartilage are developed in isolated points of the organs; and by their coalescence progressively invade or destroy the original texture of the part. In some instances, a mass of cartilage is traversed irregularly by intersecting white or yellow fibrous bands. In others, irregular nodules of cartilage are separated by ligamentous partitions. This deposition, which ever manifests a tendency to fatal disorganization, is most frequent in the female breast, in the womb, in the lacrymal and parotid glands, and in the intestinal canal of both sexes. In its progress to ulceration, cavities are formed containing brownish jelly-like fluid; and as it approaches the surface, fungous growths and hemorrhage are frequent.

BOOK IV.

MEMBRANOUS, ENCLOSING, OR INVESTING TISSUES.

THE organic substances, which have been already described, consist either of those which are ramified or distributed extensively through the animal body, or of those which are confined to definite situations. Those which are now to be examined, are extended continuously over considerable spaces, and tissues or organs very different sometimes from each other. They are *envelopes* or *mem-branes*, and consist of skin, mucous membrane, serous membrane, synovial membrane, and compound membrane.

CHAPTER I.

SECTION I.

SKIN, *Cutis*, *Pellis.*—CUTANEOUS TISSUE.—DERMAL TISSUE.—*La Peau, Tissu Dermoide.*—DIE HAUT; DAS FELL. FELL, old English. WITH ITS APPENDAGES, SCARF-SKIN OR CUTICLE, NAIL, HAIR. EPIDERMIS; CUTICULA. UNGUES. PILL.—*Tissu Epidermoide et Tissu Pileux.*

SKIN has been said to consist of three parts, true skin, (*cutis vera*,) mucous net, (*rete mucosum*,) and scarf-skin, or cuticle. Haller, Camper, and Blumenbach are inclined to deny the existence of the mucous net in the skin of the white, and to admit it in that of the negro only; and, in point of fact, indeed, its existence has been demonstrated in the negro race only, and inferred by analogy to exist in the white. " When a blister has been applied to the skin of a negro," says Cruikshank, " if it has not been very stimulating, in twelve hours after, a thin transparent grayish membrane is raised, under which we find a fluid. This membrane is the cuticle or scarf-skin. When this with the fluid is removed, the surface under these appears black; but if the blister had been very stimulating, another membrane, in which this black colour resides, would also have been raised with the cuticle. This is *rete mucosum*, which is itself double, consisting of another gray transparent membrane, and of a black web very much resembling the *pigmentum nigrum* of the eye. When this membrane is removed, the surface of the true skin, as has been hitherto believed, comes in view, and is white like that of a European. The *rete mucosum* gives the colour to the skin; is black in the negro; white, brown, or yellowish in the European."*

Cruikshank distinguished the membranes spread over the surface of the true skin into five, each of which he conceived are cuticles or secretions from the outer surface of the skin, undergoing transformation into cuticles.

The first and most external of these is the cuticle or *epidermis*, properly so named, that is the completed covering investing the whole, and which is semitransparent. This is constantly rubbed off or falling off in scales; and its place is as constantly supplied by layers arising from and secreted by the next covering.

This is the *rete mucosum*, which according to Cruikshank is double, consisting of an outer or consistent layer, and an inner or softer, and which is secreted by the vascular surface of the true skin. These two with the cuticle proper form three coverings.

The next or fourth is more equivocal in existence. It is a vascular membrane spread over the outer surface of the true skin, which becomes most distinct in various cutaneous inflammations, as small-pox, measles, and scarlet fever. In this the small-pox pustules are situate; and certainly it seems to form the layer in which these pustules are first developed.

Lastly, when a piece of skin has been macerated, and this fourth vascular membrane is removed, it is possible to observe a fifth resting immediately on the surface of the true skin.

These distinctions seem rather minute. The cuticle is probably one membrane only secreted by the *rete mucosum* as it is required ; the external layers being hard and firm, the inner soft and pulpy.

The *rete mucosum* is evidently a secretion from the outer vascular surface of the skin.

With regard to the other two they seem to be the external surface

---

* Experiments on the Insensible Perspiration of the Human Body, showing its affinity to Respiration. By William Cruikshank. London, 1795, p. 3 and 4.

of the true skin itself.' It was, however, the opinion of, Cruikshank, that these membranes are not created, but only demonstrated or rendered distinct by eruptive diseases in consequence of the large quantity of blood impelled into the skin.

Bichat denies the existence of a mucous coating or varnish (*corpus mucosum*,) such as Malpighi describes it, and regards the vascnlar surface of the corion as the only mucous net. ·

According to Chaussier, the skin consists of two parts only, the *derma* (δερμα) *cutis vera* or corion, and the epidermis, cuticle, or scarf-skin ; the first embracing the organic elements of this, tissue ; the second being an inorganic substance prepared by the organic, and deposited on its surface. This opinion is adopted by Gordon, according to whom the skin consists of two substances placed above each other like layers or plates (*laminæ*,) the inner of which is the true skin, the outer the cuticle or scarf-skin. Beclard, on the contrary, thinks that a peculiar matter, which occasions the colour by which the several races are distinguished, is found between the outer surface of the corion and the cuticle ; and that no fair race is destitute of it except the *albino*, the peculiar appearance of whom he ascribes to the absence of the mucous net of the skin.

According to M. Gaultier, the mucous body of the negro skin consists of four parts ; 1*st*, a series of minute vascular bundles, to which M. Gaultier applies the name of *gemmulæ sanguineæ*, and which are really the termination of vessels ramified on the papillæ; 2*d*, the deep whitish layer, consisting of white vessels, and indicated in an oblique section of the negro skin, by a white line between the surface of the corion and a darker undulating line ; 3*d*, the coloured layer, named by M. Gaultier *gemmulæ*—the true colouring matter of the skin,—indicated by the undulating line already noticed ; 4*th*, the superficial white layer, consisting of serous vessels as the first, indicated by a white line between the dark undulating line and the cuticle.

The vascular eminences, (*gemmulæ sanguineæ*) of M. Gaultier, are the termination of the cutaneous papillæ; and this induces M. Dutrochet to give the following view of the constituent parts of the cutaneous tissue. 1*st*, the derma, or corion, the true skin of the ancient anatomists; 2*d*, the papillæ, or minute elevations of this membrane; 3*d*, the epidermal membrane of the papillæ, which is the deep whitish layer of M. Gaultier ; 4*th*, a coloured layer, the proper colouring matter of the skin ; 5*th*, a horny layer, which corresponds to the superficial whitish layer of Gaultier ; and, 6*th*, the epidermis, or cuticle.

The *corion* of the human skin, (*pellis, corium, derma, cutis vera*) seems to consist chiefly of very small dense fibres, not unlike those of the proper arterial coat closely interwoven with each other, and more firmly compacted the nearer they are to its outer or cuticular surface. The inner surface of the corion is of a gray colour ; and in almost all parts of the body presents a number of depressions varying in size from one-twelfth to one-tenth of an inch, and consequently forming spaces or intervals between them. These depressions, which correspond to eminences in the subjacent adipose tissue, have been termed *areolæ*. They are wanting in the corion of the back of the hand and foot only.

The outer or cuticular surface of the corion is quite smooth, of a pale or flesh-red tinge, and is much more vascular than its inner surface. It presents, further, a number of minute conical eminences (*papillæ,*) which, according to the recent observations of Gaultier,[*] and Dutrochet,[†] are liberally supplied with blood-vessels (*gemmulæ sanguineæ,*) and are the most vascular part of this membrane. In the ordinary state of circulation and temperature during life these eminences are on a level with the surrounding *corion ;* but when the surface is chilled, this membrane shrinks, while the papillæ either continue unchanged, or shrink less proportionally, and give rise to the appearance described under the name of *goose skin ;* (*cutis anserina.*) This surface was said by the older anatomists to present numerous openings, orifices, or pores ; but according to Gordon, if we trust to mere observation, no openings of this kind can be recognized, either by the eye or the microscope, except those of the sebaceous follicles. The hairs, indeed, are found to issue from holes in the corion, but they fill them up completely.

In certain situations, for instance at the entrance of the external auditory hole, at the tip of the nose, on the margins of the eyelids, in the arm-pits, at the nipple, at the skin of the pubes, round the anus, and the female pudendum, are placed minute orifices, from which exudes an oleaginous fluid, which is quickly indurated. These openings lead into small sacs or cavities called follicles, (*folliculi,*)

---

[*] Recherches sur l'org. de la peau, &c. Paris, 1809 and 1811.

[†] Observations sur la structure, &c. Journal de Phys. Mai 1819, and Observations sur la structure de la peau, Jour. Compl. Vol. V.

or sebaceous glands, (*glandulæ sebaceæ.*) Of these sacs the structure is simple. They appear to consist simply of hollow surfaces secreting an oleaginous fluid, which is progressively propelled to the orifice, where it soon undergoes that partial inspissation which gives it the sebaceous or suet-like aspect and consistence. In the negro races the secretion exhales a peculiar strong odour ; and in the fair or red-haired European races the odour is also strong.

The corion is liberally supplied with blood-vessels, nerves, and absorbents. After a successful injection, its outer surface appears to consist of a uniform net-work of minute vessels, subdivided to an infinite degree of delicacy, and containing during life blood coloured and colourless. It can scarcely be doubted that this vascular network (*rete vasculosum*) is the only texture corresponding to the *reticular body* of the older anatomists.

It is well known that this membrane when boiled sufficiently long is converted into a viscid glutinous liquor, which consists chiefly of gelatin, (Chaptal, Seguin, Hatchett, Vauquelin, &c.) and that glue is obtained in great quantity from it for the purposes of art. As, however, in these operations a portion of matter is left undissolved, and as glue is completely soluble in water, while skin resists it for an indefinite time, it may be concluded, that though the chief constituent of the corion is gelatin, it is under some peculiar modification not perfectly understood. The union of this organized gelatin with the vegetable principle denominated *tannin* forms leather, which is quite insoluble in water.

Cuticle or scarf-skin, (*epidermis, cuticula*), is a semitransparent, or rather translucent layer of thin light-coloured matter, extended continuously over the outer surface of the corion. Its thickness varies, being thinnest on those parts least exposed to pressure and friction, but thickest in the palms and soles. It is destitute of blood-vessels, nerves, and absorbents ; and there is reason to believe, from observing the phenomena and process of its reproduction, that it is originally secreted in the form of a semifluid viscid matter by the outer surface of the corion ; and that, as it is successively worn or removed by attrition, it is in like manner repaired by a constant process of secretion or deposition. This semifluid viscid matter, which, in point of fact, is found between the outer surface of the corion and the firm cuticle, appears to be the substance mentioned by Malpighi, and so often spoken of as the mucous body or net ; (*corpus mucosum.*) It is certainly quite inorganic ; and it is impossible to explain its production otherwise than by ascribing it to the outer or vascular surface of the corion.

Cuticle is rendered yellow, and finally dissolved by immersion in nitric acid. It is also dissolved by sulphuric acid, in the form of a deep brown pulp. These, and some other experiments performed by Hatchett, appear to show that it consists chiefly of albuminous matter somehow modified.

This description shows, that, if strict observation be trusted, the mucous net has no existence, at least in the European. In the Negro, Caffre, and Malay, however, a black membrane is said to be interposed between the corion and cuticle, and to be the cause of the dark complexion of these races. On this subject I refer to the description given by Cruikshank,* which is the best, the Essay of M. Gaultier already quoted, and the observations of Beclard. What is found in the skin of the mixed or half cast races, *i. e.* the offspring of an African and European, or of a mulatto and European? and how is the transition between this colouring layer and its insensible diminution effected?

Nail is a substance very familiarly known. On its nature and structure we find many conjectures, but few or no facts in the writings of anatomists; and almost all that has been written is the result of analogical inference, rather than of direct observation. It is known that the nails drop off with the scarf-skin in the dead body; that they are destroyed or diseased by causes which act on the outer surface of the corion, and produce disease of the cuticle; and that, if forcibly torn out, the surface of the corion to which they were attached, bleeds profusely and inflames. In other respects they are quite inorganic; but these facts appear to warrant the conclusion, that the root of the nail is connected with the organic substance of the corion, and that the whole substance is the result of a process of secretion quite similar to that by which the cuticle is formed.

According to the experiments of Hatchett, they consist of a substance which possesses the properties of coagulated albumen, with a very small trace of phosphate of lime.

The *root* of a hair is not only that part which is contained in the bulb, but the portion which is lodged in the skin. The *middle part* and the *point* are those which project beyond the surface of the skin. The *bulb* is a small sac fixed in the inner surface of the corion, in

. * Experiments, &c. p. 31.

the contiguous filamentous tissue, and receiving the extremity or root of the hair implanted in it.

Every hair is cylindrical, tapering regularly from the root to the point, and solid, but containing its proper colouring matter in its substance. The colour varies, but the root is always whitish and transparent, and softer than the rest; the fixed or adhering part of the root is almost fluid. When hair is decolorized, it becomes transparent and brittle, and presents a peculiar silvery-white colour; and as hairs of this kind are few or abundant, it gives the aspect of gray, hoary, or white-hair.

The bulb, though visible in a hair plucked out by the root, is too small in human hair to be minutely examined; and Chirac, Gaultier, and Gordon, have therefore described its structure and appearances from the bulbs of the whiskers of large animals, the seal for example, in which it is much more distinct. According to researches of this kind, every bulb forms a sort of sac or follicle, which consists of two tunics, an inner one, tender, vascular, and embracing closely the root of the hair; and an outer, which is firmer and less vascular, and surrounds the inner one, while it adheres to the filamentous tissue and the inner surface of the corion. When the hair issues from the bulb, it passes through an appropriate canal of the corion, which is always more or less oblique, but which, as has been already said, it fills completely; and it afterwards passes in a similar manner through the scarf-skin. Nervous filaments have been traced into the bulbs of the whiskers of the seal by Rudolphi and the younger Andral. The bulb or follicle, in short, is inorganic, and forms by secretion the inorganic hair.

The structure of hair itself appears to be either so simple, or so incapable of being further elucidated, that anatomists have not given any facts of consequence regarding it. Its outer surface is believed to be covered with imbricated scales, because in moving a single hair between the finger and thumb, it follows one direction only.

Hair is believed to be utterly inorganic, though the phenomena of its growth, decoloration, and especially of the disease termed Polish plait, (*plica Polonica*,) have led various authors to regard it as possessed of some degree of vitality. These phenomena, however, may be explained by the occurrence of disease in the bulbs or generating follicles. Hair is insoluble in boiling water, but Vauquelin succeeded in dissolving it by the aid of Papin's digester. From the experiments of this chemist, and those of Hatchett, it may be inferred that hair consists of an animal matter, which appears to be a modification of albumen, a colouring oil, and some saline substances.*

SECTION II.

The cutaneous texture and appendages are liable to many forms of disease. Most of them, however, may be referred to some form of the inflammatory process, or to changes in texture either original or acquired.

I. *Inflammation* assumes in this texture a great variety of forms, which it is the province of pathological anatomy to distinguish accurately. This was first attempted by Cullen, whose *phlegmon* and *erythema* were intended to designate two forms of cutaneous inflammation, according as the vessels of the internal or external surface are the seat of morbid action. The distinction, though judicious, was overlooked; and those who confided in his practical instructions, without attending to the correctness of his pathology or the fidelity of his descriptions, transferred the seat of phlegmon from the skin, in which it was placed by Cullen, to the cellular tissue, where it has since remained. This error was abetted by J. Hunter and C. Smyth, whose distinctions of inflammation, according to the tissues in which it occurs, place rose in the skin, and *phlegmon* in the cellular membrane. These views were generally adopted till the appearance of Bichat, who attempted, after the example of Cullen, to distinguish cutaneous diseases according to their seat in the cutaneous tissue.† As this is obviously the most rational method, and, though not much followed by practical authors, has received the approbation of such observers as Meckel and Beclard, it is best calculated for the order to be observed in the present treatise.

Cutaneous inflammation, though it eventually affect the substance, which, however, is not frequently, may be conveniently distinguished in the following manner. *First*, it may be seated in the exterior or cuticular surface of the corion; *secondly*, it may affect the *papillæ* or minute elevations of the corion; *thirdly*, it may affect the substance of the corion; *fourthly*, it may occur at the inner or attached surface of this membrane; *fifthly*, it may affect the sebaceous follicles ; and *sixthly*, it may be connected with

* Annales de Chimie, 1806. Tome LVIII., and Philosoph. Trans. 1800, Vol. XC, p. 327, *et seq.*

† Anatomie Generale, Tome IV. p. 721.

l

the sacs and bulbs of the hairs. If these circumstances be adopted as the basis of general division, subordinate characters may be derived from the mode in which the inflammatory process advances, and from the effects which it produces, in the following order.

§ 1. *Diffuse or spreading inflammation.*—I. Cutaneous inflammations seated in the outer or cuticular surface of the corion, (*cutis vera, derma,*) and generally spreading along it.

Measles,	Rubeola.
Morbillose eruption,	Morbilli.
Rash fever, scarlet fever,	Scarlatina.
Nettle-rash,	Urticaria.
Rose-rash,	Roseola.
Common rash,	Erythema.

§ 2. *Effusive inflammation.*—II. Cutaneous inflammation seated in the outer surface of the corion, producing a fluid which elevates and detaches the cuticle.

Rose, St Anthony's fire,	Erysipelas.
Bleb fever, bullose fever,	Pemphigus, febris bullosa.
Simple blebs,	Pompholyx.

§ 3. *Punctuate papular inflammation.*—III. Cutaneous inflammations commencing in circumscribed or definite points of the corion, producing minute eminences.

Gum, gown, red gum, tooth gum,	Strophulus.
Sun-rash, prickly heat,	Lichen.
Itchy rash,	Prurigo.

§ 4. *Punctuate desquamating inflammation.*—IV. Cutaneous inflammations of the outer surface of the corion, more or less circumscribed, affecting its secreting power, and producing exfoliation of the cuticle.

Scaly leprosy,	Lepra.
Scaly tetter,	Psoriasis.
Dandriff,	Pityriasis.
Fish-skin disease,	Ichthyosis.

§ 5. *Punctuate vesicular inflammation.*—V. Cutaneous inflammations originally affecting the outer surface of the corion, circumscribed, definite, or punctuate, producing effusion of fluid first pellucid, afterwards slightly opaque, with elevation of cuticle, with or without further affection of the corial tissue.

Miliary rash,	Miliaria.
Shingles, vesicular ringworm, or fret,	Herpes.
Heat spots, or red-fret,	Eczema.
Limpet shell vesicle and scab,	Rupia.
Cow-pox vesicle,	Vaccinia.
Chicken-pox,	Varicella.

§ 6. *Punctuate phlegmonous or pustular inflammation.*—VI. Cutaneous inflammations originally affecting the outer surface and vascular layer of the corion, afterwards its substance, sometimes the sacs and bulbs of the hairs, and producing purulent matter more or less distinct.

Small-pox,	Variola.
Plague,	Pestis.
Malignant pustule, Persian fire,	Anthrakion.
Itch,	Scabies.
Moist or running tetter,	Impetigo.
Scall or pustular ringworm,	Porrigo.
Great pox,	Ecthyma.

§ 7. *Punctuate chronic phlegmonous inflammation.*—VII. Cutaneous inflammations originating in the substance of the corion, or in the sebaceous follicles, sometimes at the bulbs of the hair, and terminating in partial or imperfect suppuration, with formation of scales, crusts, &c. and more or less destruction of the sebaceous follicles, the piliparous sacs, or of the corial tissue.

Boil,	Phyma, Furunculus.
Carbuncle,	Anthrax ; Carbunculus.
Whelk,	Acne.
Scalp or chin whelk,	Sycosis.
Soft tubercle,	Molluscum.
Canker,	Lupus, noli me tangere.
White scall,	Vitiligo.
Yaws,	Framboesia, rubula.
Sivvens,	Sibbenia.

§ 8. *Punctuate phlegmono-tubercular inflammation, chronic.*—VIII. Cutaneous inflammations, chronic, attended with general affection of the fibro-mucous tissues.

Arctoic leprosy, Radesyge,	Lepra Norwegica.
Lombard evil, Pellagra,	Pellagra.
Scherlievo, Falcadina,	Lepra Pedemontana.
Asturian itch or scab, Mal di Rosa,	Lepra Asturiensis.
Crim evil, Krimmische krankheit,	Lepra Taurica.
Arabian leprosy,	Elephantiasis.
Wart,	Verruca.

§ 1. *Cutaneous inflammations seated in the outer or cuticular surface of the corion, and generally spreading along it.*—Inflammation of the outer surface of the corion may be diffuse and continuous, as in scarlet fever, diffuse and interrupted, as in common rash (*erythema,*) nettle-rash, and rose-rash, or diffuse and of determinate figure, as in measles and *morbilli.* The redness with which superficial cutaneous inflammation is attended varies. Though it disappears on pressure, it returns immediately. In scarlet fever, though its tint is indicated by the name, it often has a shade of brown ; in *erythema,* or simple rash, it is rarely so vivid as in other forms of cutaneous inflammation ; in rose it has a tinge of yellow. In measles it assumes the shape of crescentic or lunular patches. In simple rash it terminates gradually in the sound skin ; but in one variety of this rash, (*erythema marginatum,*) and in rose, it is marked by a distinctly circumscribed edge, or is said to be *marginate.* The swelling of superficial cutaneous inflammation is rather a general distension than obvious elevation. When it is obvious to the eye, or felt by the finger, and is at the same time confined to definite red patches, these are named wheals. A familiar instance of this occurs in the effect produced by the bite of several insects, the blow of a whip, or the stinging of nettles. Spontaneously it is seen in the disease named nettle rash. In rose, elevation, extensive and

3

continuous, conterminous with the redness, and like it bounded by a distinctly circumscribed edge, is uniformly observed.

Superficial cutaneous inflammation being seated in the extensive vascular net-work, (*rete vasculosum, reseau vasculaire,*) of the corion, always destroys to a greater or less extent its scarf-skin, which comes away in small portions or scales, sometimes in larger pieces, while a new but thinner and more transparent scarf-skin is formed. The process by which these changes are effected is termed desquamation, and is observed in measles, scarlet fever, nettle-rash, rose-rash, common rash, and rose when it does not proceed to the formation of blebs. As the process thus defined forms a good mode of distinguishing its varieties when seated in the outer or cuticular corial surface, I adopt it on the present occasion.

According to the definition above given, it comprehends the following diseases:—Measles, rash-fever or scarlet fever, nettle-rash, rose-rash, common rash.

This must be regarded as the simplest form of cutaneous inflammation. It may indeed be doubted whether it can justly be termed inflammation; for though the capillaries of the cuticular surface of the corion are unnaturally distended with blood, and the usual functions of secretion and perspiration are suspended, it does not induce those consequences which succeed the inflammatory process in other tissues, or even in the same tissue, in a state of unequivocal inflammation. It may, however, be remarked, that, in other respects, the phenomena of the disorders referred to this head afford fair examples of inflammatory action. The skin is permanently red, either continuously or in patches, or in spots of definite figure, diffusely swelled, and unusually warm, or rather hot and dry. Its sensations are also deranged; for the parts are either painful, smarting, or itching, as in nettle-rash, rose-rash, and common rash, or the skin is generally tense and sore, as in measles and scarlet fever. In each of these diseases, also, the capillaries of the outer or cuticular surface of the corion are inordinately distended with blood, which appears to move very slowly, or stand entirely motionless in them. The skin of a person cut off during the progress of measles or scarlet fever is marked by innumerable minute vessels disposed in various modes, arborescent, asteroid, reticular, &c.; and, in some instances, minute specks of blood are effused on the corion or into its substance. In scarlet fever, confined chiefly to the skin, the outer surface of the corion of the face, neck, and trunk, is particularly injected; and towards the close of the disease, this capillary injection is brownish or purple. The injection of the mucous surfaces shall be noticed afterwards. In nettle-rash, this injection is in circumscribed patches, and accompanied with elevation, but disappears greatly after death. In erythematous inflammation I have observed the cuticular surface of the corion of a scarlet red, and soft velvety texture, and distinctly traversed by numerous minute arborescent and asteroid patches, which, however, become much paler in a few days.

§ 2. *Cutaneous inflámmations situate chiefly in the outer surface of the corion, producing sero-albuminous fluid, which elevates the scarf skin into pushes, blebs, or blisters,* (Bullæ, Phlyctænæ,) *commencing in certain parts of the corion, but spreading continuously.*

The outer surface of the corion may be inflamed in such a manner as not to terminate in desquamation or resolution, but to pour forth a sero-albuminous yellowish fluid, which detaches the cuticle and elevates it in the form of a bleb or blister. This is very well seen in the instance of scalding by boiling fluids, on the application of the blistering fly, (*Meloe vesicatorius,*) or even in some cases of friction to parts naturally tender. In each of these cases, in a short time large watery elevations or bladders appear. The same process takes place spontaneously in rose, in common blebs, and in the bullose or bleb fever. The form of these blebs is not determinate; nor even are they always uniform in appearance. The action by which they are produced, though more violent in degree, is not different in kind from ordinary cutaneous inflammation. It is attended, nevertheless, with more swelling of the corion, more exquisite burning heat, and more searing or scalding pain, than the other forms of superficial cutaneous inflammation. The fluid secreted by this process is sero-albuminous. When the raised cuticle is divided a yellowish transparent watery fluid escapes; and when the cuticle is detached so as to expose the inflamed spot, the inflamed skin is found covered by a quantity of soft, cellular, gelatinous matter, of a yellow-white colour, somewhat tough, and similar to coagulable lymph. This substance is traversed by firm linear partitions, not uniform in number or direction, but forming interstices from which serous fluid, the same as that which escaped first, is discharged. The coagulable matter, which is albuminous, at the same time contracts; and forming a covering to the corion, while the latter begins to secrete a new cuticle, is at length thrown off in the form of opaque patches. In the liquid secreted by the corion during the application of a blister, and that contained within the vesications produced by scalding, the same facts may be recognized. That obtained from the vesication of a blister separates spontaneously into coagulable and fluid portions; and the addition to the latter of the smallest portion of nitrate of silver is followed by a copious formation of opake albuminous matter. These facts show that the new secretion, though discharged fluid, afterwards separates into a serous and an albuminous portion, and is an imperfect or modified coagulable lymph; that both are the product of the inflammatory process; and that the latter is analogous to that producing albuminous exudation from serous membranes. This analogy has not escaped Bichat, who remarks, that vesications do not occur in the latter, solely because they want epidermis. To this head belongs the inflammation of cutaneous whitloe.

§ 3. *Cutaneous inflammation commencing in circumscribed or definite points of the outer surface of the corion, and producing minute eminences or pimples* (papulæ,) *which disappear gradually or terminate in scurf, or minute exfoliations of the cuticle.*

When cutaneous inflammation appears in the form of innumerable minute points, which, without spreading or coalescing, remain in general distinct, it differs in nature from that which has been already considered as the spreading or diffuse inflammation. The simplest form under which this is observed to occur, is that which consists of the minute pointed elevations named pimples (*papulæ,*) which may be described as small conical eminences, surrounded by a red circle, and sometimes attended with superficial redness of the neighbouring skin, but without definite figure. They are slow in progress, do not proceed to suppuration, and after remaining an uncertain time, subside gradually, occasioning a branny or scurfy exfoliation of the scarf-skin, with which they are covered.

These seem to have been the circumstances which induced Dr Willan to consider pimples as arising from inflammation of the *papillæ* or conical eminences of the corion. I cannot say that personal observation has enabled me to determine, whether this is at all times truly the case or not; and I therefore will not positively deny the accuracy of the opinion. On this point, however, I remark,—that I have seen and daily see instances of *strophulus* in which the papular eruption can neither in form nor distribution be traced to the cutaneous papillæ; that the eruption of *lichen* in adults appears in situations in which the papillæ are few, as regularly and abundantly as in those in which they are numerous; and that we meet with local examples of papular eruption in which it is difficult to suppose the disease to be an affection of the papillæ of one region of the skin only. For these reasons it may be justly doubted whether in all instances papular eruptions consist in inflammation of the papillæ.

Of the anatomical characters of pimples, little is accurately known. They are not diseases necessarily fatal; and when death takes place during their presence, their distinctive characters are either much changed, or entirely gone before the anatomist can inspect them. In some instances of strophulus in infants cut off by other diseases, I have seen the corion rough and slightly raised in irregular spots, which were the seat of closely-set pimples during life.

§ 4. *Cutaneous inflammation of the outer surface of the corion, more or less circumscribed, affecting its secreting power, and thus producing first, exfoliation of the scarf-skin, afterwards vitiated scarf-skin.*

Though the scarf-skin (*cuticula, epidermis,*) and nails are incapable of injection, and are therefore believed to be inorganic, the former is remarked to be more sensible, when thin and semitransparent, than when thick and opaque, which it may be in certain regions. It is also observed, that when it is removed by a blister, or the effect of a scald, the surface of the corion, when it ceases to discharge the sero-albuminous fluid already noticed, becomes covered by a thin pellicle of transparent membrane, so delicate, that it affords very little defence to the subjacent skin. This same transparent pellicle is observed in the skinning or cicatrization, as it is named, of cutaneous wounds. If, under these circumstances, the formation of this pellicle be observed, it will be found that it is deposited from the outer or cuticular surface of the corion, like a secreted substance in a viscid or semifluid state, and afterwards becoming hard, dry, and semitransparent. When the first and thinnest pellicle is formed, the outer surface of the corion, which in the healthy state never suspends its secreting function, continues to deposit more of the semifluid, viscid matter, which in like manner, but more slowly, becomes firm; and as successive depositions continue to be formed beneath that last secreted, the cuticle in its perfect state consists of successive layers of matter secreted from the outer surface of the corion. It is not to be imagined, nevertheless, that they can be distinguished from each other. The secret-ing or depositing power of the corion is a process which is inecs-sant and uninterrupted; and after the first secreted portions become firm, others subjacent undergo in like manner incessant deposition and induration.

While this process of repair is going on at the surface of the corion, a process of wearing or destruction is with the same rapidity in the healthy state going on at the outer or exposed surface of the cuticle. A piece of black or blue cloth rubbed gently over the skin becomes quickly whitened by minute portions of scarf-skin, which are thus detached from the firmer and more recent portions. A black silk stocking drawn on the leg for a very short time, even when the skin has been carefully washed with soap and water, comes off covered with numerous thin white amorphous scales, which are found to be minute portions of decayed cuticle, ready to be thrown off by the first slight friction. In like manner, the friction of dress, of washing, rubbing, &c. tends to remove the exposed portions of cuticle. These several facts show that this membrane is a sub-stance secreted from the outer surface of the corion; that its pro-duction is a successive and incessant process; and that it undergoes a constant wearing or detrition. As numerous facts show that it is an albuminous substance much indurated (Hatchett,) so it would appear that when this induration becomes extreme, as takes place in the exterior portions, their connection with the recent and softer portions is destroyed, and detachment is the result. Such is the course of phenomena in the healthy state.

When the outer surface of the corion becomes inflamed or other-wise disordered, its secretion is no longer performed with the same perfection or regularity. The effect of this is seen in the vitiated state of the scarf-skin, which is no longer the uniform, continuous, firm, semitransparent membrane observed in health, but becomes broken, thickened, opaque, and divided into numerous scales. Of the various modes in which this secretion may be deranged, and of the varieties in cuticular disease to which it may give rise, too little is known to speak with precision of their individual forms. But it may be con-sidered as certain, that every morbid state of the outer surface of the corion gives rise to certain unnatural conditions of the cuticle, and that every abnormal state of the cuticle depends originally on a mor-bid state of the cuticular or secreting surface of the corion. In general, this morbid state consists in some degree of inflammation, or at least it is attended with some degree of this process, though in the chronic form. In some instances, this chronic inflammation is obviously the immediate cause of the derangement of secretion; but in other instances, the disordered secretion continues after the inflammation subsides. The former is observed in the Greek leprosy (*Lepra*,) and the scaly tetter, (*Psoriasis*,) in both of which the formation of the morbid opaque scales is preceded and attended by a red inflamed state of the corion taking place in minute spots. It is less obvious in dandriff, (*Pityriasis*,) in which the surface of the corion, though dry, harsh, and rough, is not particularly red or vascular, and which, therefore, appears to exemplify the latter statement. The fish-skin eruption (*Ichthyosis*,) is in general so chronic, that it is difficult to say, whether it is or is not attended with any degree of the inflammatory process; but when its commencement can be traced, it is generally possible to recognize marks of inflammation of the outer surface of the corion.

: § 5. *Cutaneous inflammation originally affecting the outer surface of the corion, circumscribed, definite, or punctuate, producing effusion of fluid, first pellucid, afterwards slightly opaque, with elevation of cuticle, with or without further affection of the corial tissue.*

Inflammation may be developed in many minute points of the corion simultaneously, and, continuing limited to these points without spreading, may terminate in each in the formation of a pellucid fluid, afterwards becoming more or less opaque. These may either be confined to the outer surface of the corion, without affecting its substance, or beginning originally at the surface, may thence affect its substance.

a. The individual points appear first like a common rash, with general redness of the skin, sometimes like pimples or minute elevations, with a good deal of redness surrounding them. After some hours, a white pearly point appears at their summits, while the surrounding redness diminishes in breadth, so as to form a mere circle or hoop (*areola*,) which, if minutely examined, is found to consist of a zone of vessels, circumscribing the inflammatory process, and forming in their centre the fluid which gives the elevation the white appearance. After 12, 20, or 30 hours more, according to circumstances, the white pearly appearance extends, assumes a tint of yellow, and is depressed on the summit, indicating the advancement of the process of circumscribed inflammation. In the course of two or three days, there is detached a thin crust or scab, which consists of the cuticle of the part with the dried fluid adhering to it. Minute elevations of this description have been termed vesicles (*vesiculæ*), and the contained fluid *lymph* by Dr Willan. The fluid thus distinguished is not the same as the coagulable lymph of J. Hunter. It is nevertheless sero-albuminous, and appears to be quite similar to that which is secreted in the first stage of suppuration. The process, by which it is secreted, is confined to the vascular surface of the corion, and is not attended by ulceration of that surface in millet rash, shingles (*herpes*), and the red-fret or mercurial eruption (*eczema.*) In chicken-pox it is sometimes attended by ulceration of the corial surface, sometimes not.

b. In the other two forms of vesicular inflammation, though the process commences at the surface of the corion, it finally affects the substance of that membrane.

c. In the limpet-shell vesicle (*rupia*), inflammation of the punctuate or circumscribed character commences in one or more points of the outer surface of the corion, and causes the secretion of a thin clear fluid, which first elevates the cuticle into a broad flat vesicle, and soon becoming opaque, oozes through the broken cuticle, and is hardened into thin, superficial, but in general laminated scabs. These vesicles are surrounded by a red, hard, and painful margin or base, indicating slow inflammation of the corial tissue.

The progress of this form of cutaneous inflammation demonstrates clearly and satisfactorily the gradual transition of the morbid action from the surface to the substance of the corion. The inflammation confined at first to a small spot by the usual zone or areola, causes merely sero-albuminous secretion and consequent elevation of the cuticle. If at this time the cuticle be removed accidentally or intentionally, the subjacent surface of the corion is intensely red, soft, or velvety and pulpy, elevated, and extremely tender, while the surrounding ring or hoop of skin is hard, and equally elevated and red. From the softened inner portion the secretion of sero-albuminous fluid, generally of a reddish tint, continues; and the surface itself begins to become rough, and to lose its velvet aspect. This indicates incipient ulceration, which proceeds to affect the substance of the corion, until it is either much or wholly destroyed, generally in the form of an inverted cone; while the place of the destroyed skin is supplied by the sero-albuminous secretion, which hardens as it is formed, and seems thus to sink deeper and deeper into the skin. In the meanwhile, the surrounding portion of the skin is much indurated and inflamed, and seems to form a hard ring in the skin; and the whole process is attended with extreme pain, searing heat, and constitutional distress. These phenomena are most distinctly seen in the *rupia prominens* and *r. escharotica*, and in a variety of the eruption, which I have witnessed in the persons of those who have been affected with the constitutional symptoms of syphilis, and who have for this been subjected to repeated courses of mercury; (*rupia cachectica*.)

This is an example of inflammation with destruction of parts, either by ulcerative absorption, or by phagedenic ulceration.

d. Cow-pox (*vaccinia*,) whether in the teat of the cow, or the skin of the human subject, consists in local inflammation of the outer surface of the corion, which, by causing the secretion of a thin semitransparent fluid, elevates the cuticle into a vesicle. At the same time, the surrounding skin is red, sore and hard (*areola;*) and the inflammatory process denoted by these signs causes suppuration of the corion, with some destruction of its substance, or what is termed ulceration.

If the thin fluid secreted by the vaccine vesicle either in the teat of the cow, or in the skin of the human subject, be taken before it has become opaque or puriform, and applied to the surface of the human corion exposed by scratching, slight incision, or suitable abrasion of the cuticle, it is followed by local inflammation of the same characters as those of the original sore or vesicle, from which the morbid fluid is taken. The vaccine inflammation is naturally divided into two stages.

1. About the second or third day, or from fifty to seventy hours, after insertion of the fluid, the point of skin becomes red and slightly raised. This redness and elevation continue to increase, till the cuticle is gradually elevated about the fifth or sixth day into a flat pearl-coloured spot or vesicle, which is found to derive its appearance from the secretion of thin semitransparent fluid, formed during the inflammatory process of the corion. The figure of this spot or vesicle varies according to the manner in which the vaccine fluid has been applied to the part. If it is by a longitudinal incision or scratch, as is commonly done, the shape of the vesicle is oval; if it has been by longitudinal and transverse ones of nearly equal size, or by simple puncture, then it is more or less regularly circular; and if the scratches have been numerous and irregular in direction, or if the fluid has been applied irregularly, the shape of the vesicle is also irregular. From its first appearance

its upper surface is uneven, the margin being more elevated than the centre, and shining, firm, and distended, so as to project slightly beyond the plane of its base, or unaffected cuticle. This appearance it presents till the eighth day, when the surface is observed on the ninth to be even ; and in some instances the centre may be higher than the margin. At this time, when the vesicle is supposed to be fully formed, it is found to consist of many minute communicating cells, in which the fluid is contained. This cellular disposition is characteristic of the vaccine vesicle ; for it is found to occur under every variety of circumstances when the origin of the vesicle is genuine, and its progress uninterrupted.

2. The circumstance now remarked may be regarded as denoting the termination of the first and the commencement of the second stage. About the same time, the skin round the vesicle becomes hard, tense, and red, so as to form a ring or hoop, from one to two lines broad all round, and from a quarter of an inch to two inches in diameter, according to the size of the vesicle. This hard red hoop, which has been named *areola*, marks an augment or increase of inflammation in the substance of the corion, which continues with pain, tension, and hardness, in some instances with obvious swelling of the contiguous parts, till the end of the tenth or the beginning of the eleventh day. At the same time the fluid of the vesicle becomes opaque and thick like purulent matter, rendering the centre yellowish, and depriving it of its pearly distended aspect. On the eleventh and twelfth days, as the marginal redness fades, the surface of the vesicle becomes brown in the centre, and less clear on the margin; the cuticle begins to be separated; and the fluid of the vesicle gradually thickens into a hard round scab or crust of a reddish or yellow brown colour, which afterwards becomes black, dry, and shrivelled, and is loosened, and drops off about the twentieth day after the time when the vaccine fluid was first applied. It leaves a permanent uniform scar, distinguished by minute pits or depressions corresponding to the number of cells of which the vesicle consisted.

During the progress of the local inflammation some disorder of the constitution takes place generally about the seventh or eighth day, in the form of loss of appetite or sickness, slight thirst and heat, and dryness of the skin. The pulse is almost never affected. The vaccine vesicle may also produce sundry cutaneous inflammations, very transitory, and of a secondary nature. Of these the vaccine rose-rash (*roseola vaccina*) is the most important and frequent.

It must not be understood that vaccine fluid when applied to the human body ever produces a general eruptive disease like itself over the person. This, indeed, was believed to be the case at first by Jenner, Pearson, Woodville, and perhaps some others. But more correct knowledge of the history of the disease shows, that its action is confined in the human body to the identical spots, to which it is applied; that these, and these only, become the seat of genuine vaccine inflammation ; and, that whatever eruptions or other morbid changes in the skin succeed, or have been said to succeed, the communication of cow-pox to the human body, are not the result of its genuine or proper action. It is strictly and truly a local morbid process.

The history above given of the progress and characters of the vaccine vesicle, shows clearly that the application of the vaccine fluid, under proper conditions, is succeeded by a local inflammation of the corion, which observes a definite progress, divisible into two stages. In the first of these stages, which may be termed the *primary* or *immediate*, the inflammatory process is confined with great accuracy to the cuticular surface of the corion, and, diffusing itself very uniformly from the point of insertion at equal distances in every direction, terminates in effusion of lymph or sero-albuminous fluid, and elevation of the cuticle. During the first stage, which lasts about seven or eight days, the minute cells are formed. They appear to consist in separate points of inflammation, at which the corial vessels discharge, as in other examples of the inflammatory process, sero-albuminous fluid, which is soon coagulated in a definite form. The coagulated portions form the partitions of the cells, within which the fluid part is contained. The appearance of the red ring, (*areola*), which takes place about the eighth day, indicates the commencement of the *secondary* inflammation. This consists in the action being propagated to the substance of the corion, which is effected to some depth in the formation of puriform or purulent matter, and in destruction of part of its tissue. The subsequent phenomena and effects are easily understood.

It is a remarkable property of cow-pock inflammation, that it modifies considerably not only the variolous inflammation, but that produced by itself. The second application of the vaccine lymph in a person who has previously undergone this disease, produces a smaller vesicle of the same characters, but less intensely marked. If the application be made while the first is still in progress, and before its *areola* has appeared, it produces a vesicle which runs its course more rapidly than the original one, and terminates nearly at the same time with it. This constitutes the *test-pock* or vesicle of Mr Bryce. (*Vaccinella.*)

e. Of chicken-pox as a cutaneous inflammation sometimes affecting the corial substance, I have already merely spoken. Like instances of the punctuate inflammation, though it commences at the surface of the corion with sero-albuminous secretion, it very often proceeds to suppuration, and occasionally affects the corial tissue. This is seen in the lenticular and more distinctly in the conoidal chicken-pox, in which the suppurated points are marked by depressions. The cutaneous punctuate inflammation of chicken-pox may be considered as the link which connects the vesicular and the pustular eruptions.

The facts now adduced show that it is impossible to draw a distinct line between the vesicle and the pustule, as was attempted by Willan and Bateman. Looking only at the pathological process by which they are developed and advance to maturity, it is more natural to consider them as differing in degree only, and as gliding by imperceptible shades into each other, than as always capable of being accurately distinguished. What is a vesicle when first observed, may assume the appearance of a pustule on the following day ; and the thin sero-albuminous fluid, by which they have been supposed to be distinguished, may be converted into purulent matter before the termination of the disease. As the terms, nevertheless, are useful as precise distinctions in nomenclature and description, and as they occasionally may be traced to a pathological difference, I retain them in the present observations.

§ 6. *Cutaneous inflammation originally affecting the outer surface and vascular layer of the corion, afterwards its substance, sometimes the sacs and bulbs of the hair, and producing purulent matter more or less perfect.*

Inflammation of the minute circumscribed kind, though commencing originally on the surface, may speedily affect the substance of the corion, and in its progress may produce more or less loss of substance, with formation of purulent matter. The objects thus formed are named *pustules,* and are to be viewed as instances of genuine phlegmonous or rather purulent inflammation of the skin. Practical authors enumerate four forms under which this species of cutaneous inflammation may take place:—1st, the *psydracium;* 2d, the *achor ;* 3d, the *favus ;* and, 4th, the *phlyzacium.* To this number I add the *phlyctidium.*

1. The *psydracium* may be viewed as the connecting link between the vesicle and pustule. It is small, often irregularly circumscribed, producing but slight elevation of the cuticle, and terminating in a laminated scab. It is attended with little or no redness of the surrounding skin (*areola*), does not affect the corion deeply, and rarely, almost never, leaves a hollow scar. Several of them often appear together, and becoming confluent after discharging the scanty puriform matter which they furnish, pour out a thin watery fluid, which on drying forms an irregular incrustation.

2. The *achor* differs not much from the psydracium. It appears in the form of a minute pointed elevation, of a yellow colour, and succeeded by a thin brown or yellowish scab. It contains straw-coloured matter of the appearance and consistence of strained honey; it is surrounded with little inflammatory redness, and seems to affect the corion as little as the psydracium. In ordinary circumstances it leaves no scar.

3. The *favus* may be esteemed the next degree of inflammation of this tissue. It is larger and flatter than the last-mentioned pustule, not pointed, and contains a more viscid matter than the *achor*. It is surrounded by a slight-red, irregular, marginal ring, indicating a more considerable affection of the corial tissue. It is succeeded by a yellow, semitransparent, and sometimes cellular scab, like honey-comb.

4. A form of pustule referable neither to these nor to that which is to follow, I must here mention,—the *phlyctidium* or genuine small-pox pustule. It consists in a circular or annular spot of inflammation of the corion, encircled by a red ring or zone, which is observed to consist of the outer corial surface highly vascular and elevated. Within this suppuration takes place. Though the *phlyctidium* is observed spontaneously in the distinct small-pox, it is also produced artificially by friction of tartar-emetic ointment.

5. The *phlyzacium* is the most perfect example of the most violent degree of this form of cutaneous inflammation. It is described as a large pustule, raised on a hard circular base, of a lively red colour, and succeeded by a thick, hard, dark-coloured scab. It is generally slow in progress, and, commencing at once on the surface and in the substance of the corion, is attended with considerable surrounding inflammation ; and the suppurative process which follows is always accompanied with more or less destruction of the corial tissue. It often leaves a hollow scar. The surrounding

3

redness, hardness, and elevation ; the slow progress and sometimes tedious suppuration ; and lastly, the loss of corial substance, are the circumstances which indicate the peculiar seat of this form of cutaneous inflammation.

Into the pathological characters of the individual pustular inflammations, the limits of this treatise do not permit me to enter. On one or two of them, however, I shall offer a few remarks, which may tend to illustrate the general nature of cutaneous pustular inflammation. I begin with small-pox as one of the most interesting.

a. From Dominico Cottugni we learn that it was the opinion of Astruc, that the poisonous matter of small-pox (*venenum variolarum*) affects particularly and exclusively the mucous body (*corpus mucosum*), which Malpighi describes between the skin and cuticle, and that it was the property of this poison to induce in it the peculiar variolous inflammation. This opinion appears to Cottugni to be correct, because it is confirmed by dissections made by him of the incipient and complete small pox pustule. These dissections, Cottugni states, showed the incipient pustule to consist of the raised cuticle without affection of the substance of the corion ; that this elevation of the cuticle was occasioned by the intermediate mucous body (*corpus mucosum*) being expanded like jelly, without separation of parts or intervening cavity ; and that such separation and cavity could be perceived only when the pustule was completed. Variolous pustules, he then asserts, are of two kinds, the *umbilicate* or *depressed*, and the *vesicular* or *crystalline*. The umbilicate are those, the apex of which is, from the very beginning, flattened or truncated, and which are rather lenticular than conical, as most pustules, except the variolous, are. This shape they retain until in the course of inflammation they grow to their full size, which may equal or exceed that of a lentil either on the eighth or ninth days, or on the tenth and eleventh. The cause of this depressed figure is the navel (*umbilicus*) in the centre of the pock, which is at first like an indistinct point, but afterwards, as the pock grows, becomes more elevated, with a flatter figure. From this central point or *navel* he represents all the actions of the pock, inflammation, suppuration, and drying or scabbing to proceed. For while it, as a seat of the poison, remains fixed, the surrounding part, not of skin, but of mucous body, is raised into an inflammatory ring or mound, which prevents the morbid action from spreading. In the conflu-

ent small-pox this provision is not observed. No outer swelled or
red ring is observed, and the mucous body of Malpighi is not in
such circumstances affected with the just and laudable action of the
disease. These results he ascribes to the spongy structure of the
Malpighian membrane, which swells and secretes a lymphy fluid.
In the crystalline small-pox, the fluid of which is almost pellucid,
he asserts that the mucous body, instead of being converted into
good matter, is filled with a caustic eroding humour, which seldom
fails to leave deep scars.*

Though these crystalline pocks are nearly allied to his second
kind, the vesicular, they must not be entirely confounded with them.
They are utterly destitute of depression from their origin, are quite
similar to minute blisters, and he conceives them to be generated
in a similar manner, that is, by the inflammatory action operating
like a scald, and detaching very rapidly from the mucous body the
cuticle, so as to form vesicles or vesicular pustules. The purple-
like pocks he explains in a similar manner. They are merely vesicular elevations of the cuticle, containing at first a watery fluid,
but mixed afterwards with blood or bloody fluid exuding from the
mucous body or vessels of the skin. They are generally mixed
with petechial spots, the origin of which depends on the same
cause.

In short, the doctrine of Cottugni is explicitly the following.
The natural and ordinary character of the small-pock is to produce in the mucous body (vascular web) of the skin a pit or depressed point, which is soon surrounded with an elevated circle, indicating inflammation of the corial surface. As this inflammatory
process proceeds from the central pit or navel to the circumference,
the elevated ring of mucous or vascular web is gradually converted into purulent matter, which necessarily renders the summit of
the pock flatter and more extensive, while its centre remains depressed. The formation of purulent matter is indicated, he says,
by the appearance of a whitish ring (*albidus annulus*,) which is at
first at the vertex, but extends successively to the base of the pock.
In this course, he says, it does not affect the corion (*cutis*) if the
pocks be good; for before it reaches this membrane the purulent
matter occupying the circumference of the pock either by bursting
it escapes, or by the itching which it causes at length gets an out-

* Dominici Cottunnii Regii Anatomes Professoris de Sedibus Variolarum Syntagma. Vienna, 1771. lxxx. paragr.

let. Meanwhile the site of the pit or navel (*umbilicus,*) which was previously sunk and hollow, not only attains the uniform convexity of the rest of the pustule, which renders it spherical instead of lenticular, but is raised into a top or apex, which first allows the contained matter to escape. This hardening forms a crust which covers the pustule during the subsequent process of drying (*persiccatio,*) which now commences; when this is completed the crust or scab drops off, leaving the skin uninjured.

This is, according to Cottugni, the natural and most perfect process of variolous suppuration, from which all others are more or less deviations. Thus the umbilicate pocks may degenerate into the gangrenous, corruptive, crystalline, and warty; the vesicular deviate into the purple-like pox only.

The most doubtful point of this account of the variolous inflammation, is that which relates to the disease being entirely confined to the mucous body of Malpighi. The existence of this membrane is very doubtful, and if it cannot be demonstrated, the opinion of small-pox being confined to it is obviously inconclusive. If the term *outer surface or vascular layer of the corion* be substituted for mucous body, the whole description may be regarded as not far from the truth. The depressed pit or *navel* of which Cottugni speaks, corresponds with the central slough of John Hunter, to which I shall advert in its proper place. At present, the process of variolous inflammation, if divested of hypothetical language and opinions, may be stated in the following terms.

The small-pox eruption consists of circumscribed points of inflammation developed simultaneously in many spots of the corion. These inflamed spots (*phlyctidia*), always commence at the cutieular or outer surface, and in general penetrate to a depth which is greater or less in different circumstances. After no long time, each *phlyctidium* is surrounded with a hard red circle somewhat raised, which may be conceived to indicate the process of cutaneous inflammation. Hunter would say, and perhaps did say, that this inflammation is of the adhesive kind, and arises from lymph effused into that part of the corion which is red, hard, and swelled. I believe it cannot be in every instance shown that this hard swelling depends on effusion of lymph; and it may be doubted whether it arises from such effusion in the case of small-pox. *First*, hardness and swelling take place at a period of the eruption so early, that it appears unreasonable to ascribe them to effused lymph; *Secondly,* hardness and swelling accompany every example of circumscribed or definite inflammation; *Thirdly*, it is not easy to understand in what particular part the lymph could be effused, for the corion does not contain cells or cavities like the filamentous tissue, but the outer surface consists of a smooth dense membrane, abounding in minute blood-vessels; *Fourthly*, it is as easy and more natural to think that if effusion took place, it would do so into these minute vessels. In point of fact, the capillaries of the corion of the pustular redness and hardness are numerous and distended; and I believe that the truest conclusion is, that the redness, hardness, and swelling of each pock, consist in the unusual distension of the corial capillaries with blood.

Pustular inflammation of the skin naturally terminates in suppuration, which may be either with or without destruction of the corial tissue. In the variolous *phlyctidia*, when distinct, destruction of the skin is rare, but may occur. There is reason to infer that it takes place in consequence of a true process of ulceration.

According to the observation of John Hunter, there is another mode in which destruction of the corion, and a permanent scar may be effected. "The most certain character," that is the most certain pathological character, " of the small-pox," says this writer, " is the formation of a slough, or a part becoming dead by the variolous inflammation, a circumstance which hitherto, I believe, has not been taken notice of. This was very evident in the arms of those who were inoculated in the old way, where the wounds were considerable, and were dressed every day; which mode of treatment kept them from scabbing, by which means this process was easily observed; but in the present method of inoculation it is hardly observable. The sore being allowed to scab, the slough and scab unite and drop off together. The same indistinctness attends the eruptions on the skin; and in those patients who die of, or die while in the disease, where we have an opportunity of examining them while the part is distinct, this slough is very evident. This slough is the cause of the pit after all is cicatrized; for it is a real loss of substance of the surface of the *cutis*, and in proportion to this slough is the remaining depression."

" The chicken-pox comes the nearest in external appearance to the small-pox; but it does not commonly produce a slough. As there is generally no loss of substance in this case, there can be no pit. But it sometimes happens, although but rarely, that there is

·a pit in consequence of a chicken pock; then ulceration has taken place on the surface of the *cutis*, a common thing in sores."[*]

The circumstance of a slough at the bottom of each pock or inflamed point has been particularly insisted on by Joseph Adams, a most zealous admirer of the pathology of Hunter, and an active commentator on his principles. "We have before seen," says Adams, "that the peculiar property of some morbid poisons is to produce death in a part, whether the inflammation be violent or not. Of this kind is the small-pox, every individual pustule of which is found with a slough at the bottom, which may be removed with ease, after time has been allowed for its separation by suppuration. The progress of the small-pox is therefore to form a number of sloughs under the skin, (on the cuticular or outer surface of the corion,) and the danger depends on the number formed, and the violence which the constitution suffers from the first shock of that *stimulus* which excites it into this process. If the *stimulus* of the small-pox virus is moderate, its local action follows by adhesive inflammation and slough; after which, the parts and constitution have sustained the first shock, and the subsequent process of suppuration, to separate the slough, is accomplished with so much ease, that the constitution is rarely sensible of any general inconvenience. But the face having sustained the first shock, the actions on that part began with the greatest rapidity, and continue so throughout their whole progress; in consequence of which the pus has a higher tinge, and the progress of skinning beginning as soon as the slough begins to separate, this irregularity produces an inequality in the surface of the pustule. On the contrary, the actions being slower in other parts, the pustules acquire the property of common sloughs, and granulation follows suppuration for the restoration of the lost part."[†]

According to the observations of Cruikshank, this white slough is not situate in the corion, but in a vascular membrane exterior to it, and immediately beneath the cuticle. This anatomist macerated in water for a week several portions of small-pox skin, which he had previously injected, and kept for some time in spirits. "The spirits with which they had been impregnated made them resist the effects of this water longer. Cuticle and *rete mucosum* were already turned down; and upon the eighth or ninth day I found I could separate a vascular membrane from the *cutis*, in which were also situated the

---

[*] Philosoph. Transactions, Vol. LXX. p. 133. Mr Hunter's account of a woman who had small-pox during pregnancy.

[†] Morbid Poisons, p. 364.

injected small-pox pustules. These last consisted of circles of long floating *villi* at the circumference, but of a white uninjected substance in the centre. This central part Mr Hunter had previously said was a slough formed by the irritation˙of the variolous matter."[*] He subsequently comes to the conclusion, that on the surface of the skin (corion) lie five membranes, the outermost of which is cuticle, the next two-fold is *rete mucosum*, and the fourth is the first vascular membrane in which the small-pox pustules are chiefly seated.

From these facts and observations, as well as those which it has occurred to myself to make, the following conclusions may be drawn.

The *phlyctidium* or pustule of small-pox consists of a cutaneous inflammation, which may produce;—

1*st*, Secretion of puriform fluid without permanent injury or destruction of the corion. In lenticular chicken-pox, and distinct small-pox, there is no doubt that though suppuration takes place from the cuticular surface of the corion, it is not necessarily connected with destruction or ulceration of that membrane.

2*d*, Suppurative ulceration of the corion. In conoidal chicken-pox, in some instances of distinct small-pox, and in many instances of small-pox partially or wholly confluent, each pock proceeds to ulceration of the corion. It does not appear that the pock slough described by Hunter is present in every case. It is admitted by Adams to be wanting in the vesicular small-pox, which appear after cow-pox, and in some other occasions.

3*d*, Death of numerous spots of the corion constituting sloughs. In some cases of distinct small-pox this has been observed; but it is most frequent in the confluent eruption. It then appears in the form of a white circular patch lying at the bottom of each pock.

4*th*, Along with sloughs at individual points, an extensive spreading redness of the skin rapidly terminating in sloughs of irregular shape and limits not unfrequently occurs in certain bad forms of variolous eruption.

b. Oriental plague I place among the examples of pustular cutaneous inflammation, because the carbuncle to which its poison gives rise, is, I conceive, an instance of punctuate inflammation of the corion. I am aware that Willan, and˙ after him Bateman, placed this disease among the order of tubercular eruptions. But this they have done, I am satisfied, without due consideration either of the characters of the pestilential carbuncle, or of those which they assign to the order of tubercles.

* Experiments, &c. p. 41.

From careful comparison of the most authentic accounts of pestilential carbuncle, it commences as an inflamed spot in the corial surface and substance. The inflammation of the surface speedily induces sero-albuminous secretion and detachment of the cuticle, which is elevated in the form of a bluish irregular blister; while beyond this the skin is of a fiery-red colour, hard, and the seat of searing pain. The simultaneous inflammation of the corial substance speedily kills that membrane, which is then felt in the form of a hard black mass, surrounded by living but highly inflamed skin. This dead portion is afterwards, if the patient survive, detached in the form of a mortified slough. The carbuncle of oriental plague seems not to be quite similar to the ordinary carbuncle seen in this country.

c. Of the disease termed *malignant pustule* by the French, and Milzbrand, and Black-Pocks by the German authors, (*Anthrakion;* Nar al-Parsi; *Persian fire,*) we can scarcely speak from experience in this country, in which, so far as I am aware, the disease is unknown. From the description given by Enaux and Chaussier, Vicq-D'Azyr, Pinel, Ozanam, Rausch, Hoffmann,* and Regnier,† it appears to consist in inflammation of the outer surface of the corion, speedily depriving that membrane of its vitality. It may commence in one of two modes; *First,* as a hard, red, burning, not elevated point, speedily causing bluish or reddish-blue fluid secretion, elevating the cuticle into a purple or pale-blue blister, (*phlyctæna ;*) *Secondly*, as a hard, knotty substance slightly elevated into a doughy swelling, and causing detachment of the cuticle by similar effusion. In both cases the affected corion undergoes mortification, partial or general, and is then detached as a foreign body. In some respects this resembles the ordinary carbuncle of this country. But it differs particularly in this, that the malignant pustule (*anthrakion,*) is ascribed by the best authorities to contagion, and very often is traced to epizootic contagion, or pestilence occurring among the lower animals. Its presence depends on the local application of a morbid animal poison.

d. The great pock, (*ecthyma,*) consists in an eruption of red, hard, sore pustules, (*phlyzacia,*) distinct, seldom numerous, without primary fever, and not contagious. In the three species of ordinary

---

* Der Milzbrand, oder Contagiose Carfunkel der Menschen. Von Johann Friedrich Hoffmann, Oberwundarzt in Bernb irg. Stuttgart, 1827. 8.

† De la Pustule Maligne, ou Nouvelle Exposé des Phenomenes observés pendant son cours, Par J. B. Regnier de Semur, Cote-d'or, D. M., &c. Paris, 1829. 8.

(*E. vulgare*), infantile (*E. infantum*), and dingy pock (*E. luridum*), the pustules are round or oval hard masses fixed in the substance of the skin, which is red, hard, and swelled, and terminating first in elevation and desquamation of the cuticle, and then in imperfect softening, discharging a serous and generally blood-coloured fluid, which concretes into a foul dark-brown or reddish scab, which at length drops off, leaving the subjacent skin reddish, and marked by a depressed scar, indicating the affection of the corial substance.

It seems probable that these ecthymatous pustules may occasionally be seated in the sebaceous follicles. If so they ought to be arranged under the following head.

§ 7. *Cutaneous inflammations originating in the substance of the corion, sometimes at the bulbs of the hair, sometimes in the cutaneous follicles, terminating in partial or imperfect suppuration, with formations of scales, crusts, and occasionally sloughs, and more or less destruction of the corial tissue.*

The pathological reader may perceive that the last disease, which came under consideration, forms a preparatory step to those of the present order. The hard phlyzacious pustules, by which it is distinguished, denote a more complete affection of the corial substance than is known to take place in any previous cutaneous inflammation; while the slow, crude, and imperfect solution which they undergo, and the discharge of blood-coloured rather than purulent fluid, indicate a variety of the inflammatory process different from those already examined, and approaching to those now to follow. The transition, therefore, if not insensible, is at least natural, to a tribe of diseases of which the general character is inflammation of the corion, which, modified in various ways, gives rise to the varieties of disease referred to this kind. The principal modifying circumstances may be referred either to duration, to circumscription, to difference in kind, or to the integral elements of the skin affected.

1. The influence of duration is observed in the comparative difference of progress of the common boil, which is rapid, and that of the whelk (*acne*), canker (*lupus*), and yaws (*framboesia*), which are slow and tedious. 2. The influence of circumscription or diffusion is evinced in those inflammations which are confined to a spot, and those which spread to some extent. In the whelk and boil the inflammatory process is restricted to one point; in carbuncle, on the other hand, it affects a great extent of the corion through its entire thickness. 3. Whether the inflammation of the corial substance be different in one disease from what it is in another, there are few means

of ascertaining. Though various facts seem to indicate something of this nature, too little is known to justify positive conclusions.

a. The boil or bile (Die Beule; *Furunculus;* le Clou; il Ciccione;) may be adduced as an instance of acute inflammation of the corion confined to a certain spot. Pearson. admits that its seat is the skin; but, by afterwards saying that it may occur in any part which abounds in cellular membrane, leaves the alternative either that skin contains this substance abundantly, or that boils may occur in many other tissues. Boyer, by placing its seat in the cellular tissue, confounds it with phlegmon. The opinion of Bichat differs from either, but partakes of both. This anatomist represents the corion to be penetrated by a great quantity of cellular tissue, which fills its *areolæ*, and is the exclusive and proper seat of the boil. The truth of this opinion depends on the idea attached to the term *cellular tissue.* If by this be meant the loose fatty matter with its intersecting threads, on which the inner surface of the corion rests, the opinion is erroneous; for this is the proper subcutaneous cellular tissue. To this, doubtless, the inflammatory action of boil may descend; but the phenomena and termination of the disease show, that it consists at first of circumscribed inflammation of the corial substance, soon but slightly affecting the subjacent cellular tissue. The circumstances which indicate the corion, or its follicles, as the seat of furuncular inflammation are,—the defined knotty tumour with which the complaint begins, the minute pustule to which it gives rise, and the imperfect and tardy suppuration with formation of sloughs, and the perforated appearance of the skin.

In various instances the presence of boils seems to depend on a peculiar affection, either of the sebaceous follicles, or of the pil'parous sacs. A sebaceous follicle becomes inflamed, and is affected by mortification. It then requires to be ejected as a dead substance; and, to accomplish the object, suppuration is excited all round. This is a frequent cause of cutaneous boil. The core, as it is called by surgeons, is the mortified sebaceous follicle.

Of the same nature and tendency is inflammation of a hair-sac or bulb. When this takes place, it is much disposed to cause death in the sac or bulb, or both. Or one hair-sac or bulb may be at once smitten with death, and then it equally acts as a foreign body; and, to accomplish its ejectment, suppuration is excited. The frequency, with which boils are observed to originate round hairs, is familiar to many observers.

It is further to be remarked, that the boil of the sebaceous folliele is often induced by full or rather gross living, by the transition from moderation to some degree of excess; and sometimes boils are critical, as in diseases of the lungs, and in some of those of the alimentary canal.

b. Of the same nature are the inflammatory tumours termed Epinyctis and Terminthus mentioned by all authors almost from Celsus to Wiseman.

c. Though in this place I notice carbuncle as an example of spreading inflammation of the substance of the corion, yet the question of its precise seat is not free from ambiguity. Hunter believed it to begin in the skin, and going deeper to affect principally the cellular membrane, in which it caused mortification; and with this Pearson agrees. Boyer places it in the integuments and subcutaneous cellular tissue; while Monteggia, who repeats the fact that it destroys a considerable portion of the teguments and cellular substance down to the muscles, seem to regard it as a peculiar action affecting several tissues simultaneously and successively.

The statement of Hunter I was at one time disposed to regard as exhibiting a just view of the pathology of carbuncle, and to think that Willan laboured under a mistake in referring the seat of carbuncle to the skin. From observing the progress of several carbuncles from their origin to their termination, and from cutting them open more than once and examining their morbid relations as carefully as it is possible to do in the living body, I am satisfied that the opinion of Hunter is not correct, and that that of Willan is not altogether wrong. In several carbuncles which I have observed from the beginning, the inflammatory action commenced in the skin in the form of a hard knotty pustule; a circumstance which corresponds with the admission of Hunter. If cut open at this time, which may be done not only with safety, but with benefit, the corion is found to be thicker than natural, much redder, and more vascular; and these marks of inflammation pervade not only the substance of the corion to a considerable extent, but the subcutaneous cellular membrane in a slighter degree. This inflammation of the cellular membrane spreads indeed along with that of the skin; but it also kills this tissue almost immediately, or at least speedily gives it the usual appearance of mortified matter. At the same time, the inflammation of the corion extending quickly, kills at least its exterior surface; and Hunter is inaccurate in saying that the skin does not die, but gives way by ulceration. Death of the corion is an early effect of carbuncular inflammation; and though it does not preclude the formation of ulcerated openings, it may take place without them. According to my own observation, death takes place most generally in patches of the corion, which may afterwards burst as it were by distension; ulceration takes place at points which have not been killed, and in general at the union of the dead and living skin.

There is no ground for believing that the subcutaneous cellular membrane is killed by the confinement of matter in its cells, as Hunter imagines. The ordinary mode in which this appears to take place is by the spreading inflammation of the corion, extending along its lower surface, and producing death, as it appears to do in diffuse inflammation, in which it spreads and does not readily cause suppuration.

Upon the whole, it may be concluded that the corion is the primary seat of disease in carbuncle, and that the affection of the cellular membrane, with which it is uniformly accompanied, is the effect of inflammation of the corial tissue spreading to the adipose membrane.

4. *Diseases affecting chiefly the sebaceous follicles.*—These, which are *acne, sykosis,* and *molluscum,* show the influence of texture or the elements of the skin affected.

The whelk (*acne; ionthos; varus, vari,* Celsus;) consists of minute portions of corion, round, oval, or spheroidal, hard, circumscribed, and elevated. Of the four sorts enumerated by Bateman, three only, the simple (*A. simplex*), the inveterate (*A. indurata*), and the crimson (*A. rosacea*), can be considered as examples of inflammation of the substance of the corion; and even these are affections of the cutaneous follicles.

d. *Acne simplex* and *Acne indurata* are manifestly affections seated in the sebaceous follicles of the skin, and appear to consist partly in changed secretion in the surface of these minute glands, partly in chronic inflammation of the substance of the glands.

They may appear either on the face or on the person. Their character is that of small tumours or tubercles, mostly ovoidal, situate in the follicles, the orifices of which are swelled and closed. They are chronic in duration and slow in progress; and often, when they begin to appear, they continue to distress the patient for years. Their appearance is believed to be connected with some deranged state of the alimentary function.

When this eruption appears on the person, it is chiefly the posterior surface of the trunk which the pustules occupy. They then appear in the form of oblong ovoidal tubercles, with the long diameter corresponding to the axis of the body. There also they are slow in progress. It is possible by a glass, sometimes by the eye, to recognize the orifice of the follicle closed; and the follicle swelled and enlarged all round. In general these swellings undergo slow and partial suppuration; and in some severe cases, the follicle is mortified and ejected by suppuration, like a part deprived of life. ·

Both the simple and indurated whelk may produce ulcerative destruction of the true skin, and leave a smooth depressed scar; and I have seen them by extending to the roots of the hairs render the skin entirely depilous.

The black whelk (*Acne punctata*), doubtless arises from disease and obstruction of the mucous follicles, or sebaceous glands.

Demodex Folliculorum.   Follicular worm.—A singular circumstance relating to the sebaceous follicles of the face and their diseases, is the fact that they become the residence of a peculiar species of parasitical animal or worm, not dissimilar in appearance to the grub of a common fly. The existence of this animal in the sebaceous follicles of the face was first discovered in 1842 by Dr Simon of Berlin;[*] and since that time it has been repeatedly seen by observers in this city, and is fully described by Mr Owen.

The animal belongs to the lowest organized forms of the order Arachnida; and like the parasitic Cymothoe and Bopyrus of the Crustaceous class, makes a transition from the *Annelides* to the higher *Articulata*.   In length the animal, which has been named the *Demodex folliculorum,* ranges from one-fiftieth to one-hundredth part of one inch.   The head and mouth are confluent with the abdomen.   The thoracic appendages, eight in number, as in the Articulata, are simple and rudimental, and are terminated by three short *setæ*.   The integument of the abdomen is minutely annulated.   The mouth is suctorial and proboscidiform.   The entozoon occupies the hair follicles and the sebaceous follicles.[†]

e. The crimson whelk (*A. rosacea, gutta rosea ;* dartre pustuleuse couperose of Alibert), is an affection rather complicated; and I doubt whether it is justly classed with those now mentioned. It is doubtless an affection of the corial substance; but it commences

---

[*] Muller's Archiv fur Physiologie. Berlin, 1842. P. 218.

[†] Lectures on the Comparative Anatomy and Physiology of the Invertebrate Animals. By Richard Owen, Esq. &c. London, 1843.

with redness and slight diffuse swelling of the skin of the nose and cheeks, not unlike that of *erythema marginatum*. This is followed _by the appearance of two or three small seedy particles very hard, but red and tending to suppurate, which they at length do partially at their summits, while the base remains hard, red, and firm. As the red appearance of the skin spreads, the roughness increases; fresh particles of the same seedy consistence arise and undergo the same course; and some coalescing form broad tubercular blotches of a crimson or livid colour, and irregular notched surface. The skin is not, however, in this state. at all times permanently red. I have seen this affection in patches on the cheeks and nose so light coloured, that in the morning it could not be recognized; but in the latter part of the day, after taking wine, and becoming warm, they assumed an intense red inclining to crimson. In the advanced stage, when numerous tubercles appear, and the surface is generally rough and red, the skin swells diffusely and becomes doughy, and is traversed by tortuous purple veins; the nose is enlarged; the nostrils become distended, their surface notched into lobular masses; the red hard bodies of the cheeks become large and coherent; and the whole countenance is converted into a crimson tumid mass, in which the original features are prodigiously deformed. These whelks do not often undergo suppuration, but are constantly casting the cuticle in the form of peelings, or scales, or crusts. When suppuration occurs it is liable to terminate in bad and intractable sores.

f. The chin and scalp whelk, (*Sykosis; Mentagra;* dartre pustuleuse mentagre,) consists in chronic pustular inflammation of the substance of the corion at the bulbs or conduits of the hairs, and probably of various sebaceous follicles besides.*

g. On the subject of *molluscum contagiosum* much information has been recently communicated by the researches of Dr Robert Paterson, Dr Reid, and Dr A. Thomson.

According to the observations of Dr Paterson the appearance of the bodies commences in the shape of minute pearly granulations, which increasing in size, become more of the natural colour of the skin. When as large as a vetch, on their apices appears an opening emitting a whitish milky fluid. Their size varies from a pinhead to that of a hazel-nut; and their progress in attaining the largest size, though varying, is slow.

* Celsi, Lib. vi. 3.

The structure of the small bodies is that of numerous cells se-creting the milky fluid, which under the microscope is entirely com-posed of nucleated cells oblong or ovoidal in shape. These are about one-thousandth part of one inch in diameter.*

From the position which the tubercles of contagious *molluscum* occupy in the face, it seems certain that they are seated in the fol-licles. They are generally found round the lips, or on the chin, near the nose, and in those situations in which the follicles are mostly placed.

h. The chronic soft tubercle (*molluscum diuturnum*), is a rare disease; and I have seen only one example of it in the person of a man of 40, in whom these bodies were disseminated over the cu-taneous surface of the face and scalp, the trunk, the upper extre-mities, the nates and thighs. Of two of the larger tumours which were removed from the *palpebræ*, the greater part was composed of firm, tough, whitish gray matter of the consistence of condensed cellular texture, penetrated through its whole extent by numerous minute blood-vessels, but exhibiting in no other respect traces of or-ganization. This substance, when macerated in water, was resolved into gelatinous, flocculent filaments, easily lacerable, and present-ing no definite structure. Imbedded in this, and removable most easily by maceration, were several small bodies not larger than a pin-head like fat in appearance, of a regularly spheroidal shape, of a lemon-yellow colour, and specifically lighter than water. The matter of these bodies was unctuous. It communicated an oily stain to paper; it liquefied and became transparent at a temperature not exceeding 97° Fahrenheit, so that, when attached to the body, it must have been fluid; it was insoluble in alcohol, ether, and water, but formed in the volatile oil of turpentine a colourless solution. When this was exposed to the temperature of the spirit-lamp, the greatest part of the volatile oil was evaporated, leaving a transpa-rent, colourless, but viscid and semifluid substance, communicating to paper a stain becoming less deep, but not wholly removable by exposure to a high temperature. These results favour the idea that the matter of these bodies is oleaginous; but I was unable to observe any action of *aqua potassæ* or *aqua ammoniæ*, after repeated

---

* Cases and Observations on the *Molluscum Contagiosum* of Bateman, with an Ac-count of the Minute Structure of the Tumours. By Robert Paterson, M. D. Edin-burgh Medical and Surgical Journal, Vol. LVI. p. 279. Edinburgh, 1841.

† Du Molluscum Recherches Critiques sur les formes, la nature, et le traitement des Affections Cutanées de ce nom. Par Maximilian-Maurice Jacobovics, Docteur Me-decin de la Faculté de Pesth. Paris, 1840, 8vo.

trials, both at the ordinary temperature of the atmosphere, and when liquefied by a gentle heat. By the sulphuric acid it is hardened and blackened; by the nitric acid its yellow colour is rendered more intense.*

Whether the presence of these yellow adipocirous bodies is uniform in the *molluscum* I have had no subsequent means of ascertaining. If they are, it may be reasonably conjectured, that their formation depends on some morbid or vitiated state of the sebaceous follicles. I have indeed no doubt that in the case referred to the small tumours consisted in lesion of the cutaneous follicles.

i. Under the head of canker, *lupus*, (*noli me tangere*, wolf of Wiseman and others, *dartre rongeante*, Pinel and Alibert,) may be noticed a disease consisting in hard elevated tubercles set in the corion, from which they appear to grow. The name of *noli me tangere* is applied by Wiseman to a " small round acuminated tubercle" without much pain, unless when " touched, rubbed, or otherwise exasperated by topics." Though most frequent on the face, it may occur on other parts. One of these, of a bluish colour, and looking like a *vein*, appears from the description to have been of the nature of erectile tissue.

One example of bluish spherical tubercle I have seen in the person of a woman of about 65 years of age, otherwise healthy. It was situate on the side of the nose near the middle of the nasal bone. It appeared first in the form of a small red prominence less than a pea, but gradually shot up from the skin, so as in the course of twenty months or two years from its commencement, to project at least one-third of an inch from the surrounding skin. It was then round or spherical, smooth, and even shining, and of a blue or light purple colour, which, on close examination, was derived from numerous minute vessels. It was connected to the skin by a neck, the base being narrower than the summit, but did not adhere to the bone. What was the ultimate fate of this person I did not learn; but no doubt can be entertained that if life were continued a sufficient time, the tubercle would terminate in destructive fungating ulceration.

I have seen also many cases of ragged ulceration of the countenance, and one or two in the incipient state before it spread to

* A good painting of the subject of this case was made by my late friend, Staff-Surgeon Schetky, and by him deposited in the pathological collection of Chatham Hospital.

any extent. One mode in which this disease appears to commence is by the formation of a patch of hard red skin, slightly but diffusely swelled, and which is the seat of a hot, gnawing, smarting sensation. Though smooth on the surface, it is found by examination to be irregular, or very soon becomes so by the formation of small hard round bodies, (pustulo-tubercular), which after some time begin to be acuminated, and cast the cuticle in thin peelings. Occasionally they give rise to thin watery vesicles of no determinate shape, which either burst the cuticle and discharge their fluid, or appear to cause an insensible dewy oozing all over the surface. The most usual seat of this form of cutaneous inflammation is the side of the nose, one of the *alae*, or a small portion of the cheek. After subsisting in this form for some time, it may disappear spontaneously, the skin becoming of its natural colour, soft and without pain. More frequently, however, the cuticle continues to be cast off in peelings; vesicles and pustules continue to be formed; and one or other more red and painful than the rest is at length covered by a scab, which dropping off discloses a small sore with a smooth ungranulating surface, and a scanty, thin, bloody-coloured, puriform discharge, which generally forms a fresh crust or scab. This either spreads without showing any disposition to heal, or coalesces more or less completely with other sores which are generated in the same mode, and undergo the same process. . After proceeding in this manner for weeks or months, a tendency to heal is manifested in some parts, while others continue to spread. The parts which heal are irregularly seamed and scarred. This form of disease appears to correspond with what Wiseman describes under the name of *Herpes Exedens*.

k. Another form of local pustulo-tubercular disease I have seen take place on the skin of the face, generally on the forehead, in the form of round hardish bodies, with flat summits, to the number of eight, ten, or twelve, disposed in a circular arrangement. The surface of the skin was red, glossy, and occasionally casting cuticular scales and shreds. These bodies were stated to be the seat of an uneasy sensation of heat rather than of pain. They had not advanced to ulceration. Upon removal by the knife, they became pale, white, and considerably shrunk. Internally they consisted of gray coloured substance, interspersed with a few blood-vessels, not hard, so much as doughy, tough, and fibro-cartilaginous. They did not, nevertheless, present the characters of carcinoma, but seemed to consist in an inflammatory induration of the corial tissue.

On the anatomical characters of the white scall (*vitiligo*), I possess no accurate information. I have often suspected that the appearances referred to this disease are in truth the effects of others more known.

1. (Yaws) (*frambœsia*), consist in chronic inflammation of the corion taking place in circumscribed spots, attended partly with death of a portion of the corial substance, partly with growth of granular fungi,—the result of a peculiar morbid poison.

On the nature and characters of this disease much misconception has prevailed, chiefly from the erroneous notions to which its station, in the arrangement of Cullen, gave birth. These were first corrected in 1791 by Dr Jonathan Anderson Ludford, who showed that yaws is a true cutaneous inflammation, which, though more chronic, yet, like small-pox and other acute cutaneous eruptions, is preceded by febrile motions, and observes regular periods of accession, height, and decline.[*] The general accuracy of these facts has been confirmed by the testimony of Dr William Wright,[†] Dr Winterbottom,[‡] Dr Joseph Adams,[§] and Dr James Thomson,[‖] who observed the phenomena of the disease in negroes or Europeans in the West Indies or elsewhere. Dr Dancer, who admits that they seldom make their appearance without previous indisposition, alone doubts the propriety of comparing them with small-pox and other eruptions.[¶]

It cannot be doubted, that the appearance of yaws is invariably preceded by more or less indisposition,—as languor, pains of the limbs like those of rheumatism, chillness or shivering succeeded by general heat and uneasiness, amounting in most cases to fever, and always more severe and distinct in children than in adults. The first trace of eruption is a white mealy scurf covering the whole cutaneous surface. A few days after small firm pimples may be

* Tentamen Med. Inaug. de Frambœsia et Jon. Ludford Ed. 1791.

† Apud Adams on Morbid Poisons.

‡ Account of the Native Africans, &c. by T. M. Winterbottom, M.D. London, 1803, Vol. II. c. viii.

§ Observations on Morbid Poisons, &c. by Jos. Adams, M.D. 2d Edit. Lond. 1807, chap. xvi.

‖ Observations and Experiments, &c. Med. and Surg. Journal, Vol. XV. 321, and XVII. 31.

¶ The Medical Assistant, &c. by Thomas Dancer, M.D. Kingston, 1801, chap. ix. p. 201. 2d Edition. St Jago de la Vega, 1809. P. 226.

seen on the forehead, face, neck, groin, and round the anus.
These increase for six or ten days, when their tops are covered by a
crust; and an opaque whitish fluid, which is ill formed matter, may
be recognized.   Thus converted into pustules, they gradually enlarge, still covered by crusts, which are loose and irregular, until
they attain the size of a sixpence or even of a shilling,—the largest
being in general those which appeared first.   If in this state the
crust be removed, it exposes a foul sloughy sore, or, according to
Adams, a rough whitish surface consisting partly of slough, partly
of living animal matter.   The pustules may also burst spontaneously, and discharge thick viscid matter, which hardens into a foul
crust or scab on the surface.   In the large pustules from this surface at length shoots up a red granulated excrescence composed of
minute lobes, not unlike a wild rasp or mulberry, which is the
proper yaw, and gives the disease its peculiar appearance and character.   Its size varies according to that of the pustule from which
it rises, from a pea to that of a mulberry of considerable dimensions.   Its colour also varies according to that of the general health
of the subject.   In the healthy and robust it is red like a piece of
flesh and prominent; in the weakly and puny it is pale and white
like a piece of cauliflower, not elevated, and bleeds on the slightest
touch.   The yaw-fungus has little sensibility, and does not smart
when capsicum-juice is applied, never suppurates perfectly, but
discharges a sordid glutinous fluid, which dries into a scab round
the edges of the excrescence and covers its upper part, if much
elevated, with white sloughs.   This glutinous fluid is the proper
yawey matter, and communicates the disease by inoculation.

   The time at which the fungous granulation rises is irregular.
Thomson met with it so early as one month and so late as three
after the first appearance of the eruption; and he concludes that
its formation cannot be taken as a mark of the second stage of the
disease, as was thought by Adams.*   Each pustule, as it attains a
certain size, undergoes the same process.   After remaining some
time, the yaw gradually contracts, diminishes in height, and, as the
pustule heals, is finally covered by skin.   It leaves in general no
mark except in those places in which inflammation has been violent,
when a scar similar to that of cow-pock, but broader and more superficial, is left.

   This description shows not only that yaws are an inflammatory

* Morbid Poisons, p. 201.

disease of the skin, but that they are not, strictly speaking, an example of tubercular disease of that membrane, as in the arrangement of Willan is erroneously represented. The phenomena show that they consist in an inflammatory process of the corion, commencing in minute points, and gradually spreading in extent and penetrating in depth, till it generates a peculiar morbid product, which, after undergoing certain changes, is at length spontaneously removed, and allows the sore to heal. Thomson justly remarks, that the disease is first papular, then pustular, and afterwards consists of yaw, though the latter is not constant, as the ulcer may heal without this substance, when it must be accounted pustular. At no period does it appear to be tubercular; for the yawey growth, to which alone this term can be applied, is rather an effect of the pustular or chronic corial inflammation modified by the proper yawey action. It may, in short, be inferred, that when the yawey action is sufficient without being excessive, it generates the proper fungous growths, under which the corion is either not materially injured or is regenerated; if the action be too violent, this growth is either destroyed or prevented from appearing; and in either case the corion is irreparably injured.

m. Sivvens, though a disease affecting not only the skin, but the fibro-mucous membranes, is entitled to notice in this place, as causing cutaneous inflammation not dissimilar to that of yaws. Like most inflammations depending on the action of a morbid poison, when it affects the constitution it induces inflammation of the corion in the shape of pustules terminating in bad ulceration and sloughs, —of furuncular tubercles and ulcers,—and of pustular sores affording the raspberry granulating fungus. *

§ 8. *Cutaneous inflammations, chronic, affecting at once the surface and the substance of the corion, and attended with general affection of the fibro-mucous tissues.*

Of the disorders which I refer to this head, several are so similar, that they are probably to be viewed as varieties of the same morbid action. Of this kind are the Radesyge, Spedalsked, Liktraa or northern leprosy, the Pellagra or Lombard evil, the Scherlievo of the same place in Italy, the Mal di Rosa of Asturia, and a cuta-

* Gilchrist in Essays and Observations, Phys. and Lit. Vol. III. Art. xi. Ed. 1771. Diss. Inaug. de Syphilitide Insontium, &c. Auct. A. Freer. Ed. 1776. Cases in Surgery, &c. By James Hill, Surgeon. Ed. 1772. Observations on Morbid Poisons, &c. By Joseph Adams, M. D. London, 1807, Chap. xv. 2d Ed.

neons disorder prevalent in Crim Tartary. In whatever points these disorders differ, all of them agree in being preceded by distinct febrile commotion, in consisting of inflammation affecting the corion in definite points, and in causing at the same time more or less inflammation, punctuate or diffuse, of the mucous and fibromucous membranes of the nasal cavities, the throat, the Eustachian tube, and tympanal cavity.

In these diseases the affection of the corion is neither pustular nor tubercular, but consists in inflammation of its substance occurring in many minute points, and causing first an appearance like papulæ, or sometimes only an extensive diffuse redness and roughness of the skin ; then desquamation of the cuticle ; then pustulotubercular or minute hard eminences seldom suppurating completely, but sometimes causing, partly by sloughing, partly by ulceration of the corion, deep foul sores, destroying the corial texture and the bulbs of the hair. This is particularly the case in the Radesyge, the form of disorder prevalent in Iceland, the Scandinavian peninsula, the Feroe Islands, and the peninsula of Jutland. In those prevalent in Italy, Asturia, and Crim Tartary, ulceration of the corion appears to be less frequent.

The limits of this treatise do not permit me to enter at large into the history of these diseases, which are not to be viewed as merely cutaneous affections ; and I shall simply refer to the best sources for further information.*

* For Radesyge, Dissert. Inaug. de morbo cutaneo luem veneream consecutivam simulante, auctore C. F. Ahlander. Upsaliæ, 1806.

Diss. Inaug. sistens obs. in exanthema arct. vulgo Radesyge, auctore Isaaco Vought. Grypheæ, 1811.

. Geographische Nosologie von Fried. Schnurrer, M. D. p. 440.

Morbus quem Radesyge vocant, &c. Commentatio Auctore Fred. Holst, M. D. Christianiæ, 1817.

Ueber die Aussatzartige Krankheit Holsteins, &c. Von Ludwig Aug. Struve, M. D. 1820.

Die Radesyge Oder das Scandinavische Syphiloid. Aus Scandinavischen Quellen dargestellt. Von Dr Ludwig Hünefeld, Professor zu Greifswalde. Leipzig, 1828. 8vo.

Erkenntniss und Cur des Sogenannten Dithsmarsischen Krankheit. Von Dr E. A. L. Hübener, Pract. Aertze en Heide. Altona, 1835.

For Pellagra, S. Const. Titii orat. de Pellagræ Pathologia. Viteberg. 1792.

De Pellagra Obs. quas collegit Caietano. Strambio, 1784-89, Mediol.

Franc. Frapolli. Mediol. Animadvers. in Morbum vulgo Pellagra, Med. 1771.

N. X. Jansen de Pellagra, Lug. 1787. Frank Delect. Tom. IX. p. 325.

Holland in Medico-Chirurgical Transactions, Vol. VII.

For Mal de Rosa, Thierry Observations de Physique et Medecine, Tom. II. Chap. vi.

To this head also may be referred some of the cutaneous eruptions which occur either among the secondary symptoms of syphilis, or in the persons of those who, for this disease, have been subjected to one or more courses of mercurial medicines. Though these eruptions may appear sometimes in the form of *papulæ*, sometimes as a variety of *rupia*, and sometimes as *ecthyma*, they are also not unfrequently of the chronic pustulo-tubercular nature, originally taking place in the corion, and causing more or less ulceration of that membrane. Their connection with inflammation of the mucous and fibro-mucous membranes is well known.

Upon elephantiasis so much accurate information has been collected by Dr Adams, Mr Lawrence, and Dr Lee, that little difficulty can be experienced in settling its characters as a morbid state of the skin. The case described so well by the last of these observers, I had repeated opportunities of seeing; and the appearance of the skin could leave no doubt of the disease affecting the substance of the corion. The exact nature of this affection is perhaps less easily determined. By calling it a tubercular eruption, after the manner of Dr Bateman, little exact information is communicated. Bichat states that he has seen the corion manifestly disorganized in elephantiasis,* but says nothing of the anatomical characters of this disorganization. Pinel, Beclard, and Meckel, are equally silent on this subject. In short, though we have good descriptions of the external visible appearances of Arabian leprosy, an accurate description of its anatomical characters is still a desideratum.

Wart and corn are believed to depend on morbid accumulation of cuticle. The former, however, is vascular at its basis; and it may therefore be inferred that its production depends on morbid action of the surface of the corion at the particular point at which it appears.

II. § 1. *Dermatæmia, Dermatorrhagia.*—Hemorrhage of the skin appears under two forms; either that of a bloody or blood-coloured fluid oozing from certain regions, or of blood effused in the form of purple specks, spots, patches, or livid stripes on the surface of the corion below the scarf-skin. The former discharge is rare, and takes place chiefly as a supplementary evacuation to some natural one accidentally suppressed, as the menstrual discharge in

For Scherlievo, Annali Universali de Medecina.
For Crim Tartary Disease, the Travels of Falk, Gueldenstadt, and Pallas.
* Anat. Generale, Tome IV. p. 688.

females.   The latter is of a different nature, and is both the effect and proof of a morbid state of the system.

Restricted in this manner, hemorrhage from the corion may take place in two modes; either when the corion only is affected, or when it is affected in common with many other membranes. The first case constitutes the simple purple disease (*purpura simplex*) of authors; of the second we have examples in the hemorrhagic purples (*purpura hemorrhagica*) or land-scurvy, and in the genuine sea-scurvy, (*scorbutus.*)

The anatomical characters of the disease consist in bright red or crimson spots, becoming in a day or two purple or livid, afterwards brown, and when about to disappear, assuming a yellow tint. They are occasionally attended with long livid stripes (*vibices, molopes*), or patches (*ecchymomata ;*) and in some instances the cuticle is raised into vesicles or large purple blebs, (*phlyctænæ,*) containing bloody or purple serous fluid.   These spots consist of blood or bloody fluid, effused on the outer surface of the corion, which is soft or pulpy, velvety, and reddish, from injection of its vessels.

§ 2. *Angiectasis.*—Anastomotic aneurism is frequent in the corion, and has been observed by J. Bell, Freer, Travers, and Wardrop. Though congenital, it must not be confounded with the *nævus maternus* or birth-spot (*l'envie,*) which appears to consist in a peculiar original malformation of the corion.   A similar congenital defect is the white-spot (*leucosis, leucæthiopia,*) which consists in the absence of the polished vascular surface of the corion.   Occasionally it takes place during life, and in minute spots is observed to follow diseases in which the cuticular surface of the corion has been destroyed by ulceration.

III. *Tumours.*—§ 1. *Meliheris ;* Cutaneous or Follicular Wen. The only encysted tumour which takes place in the skin consists in the immoderate enlargement of one or more of its mucous follicles, in consequence of obstruction of the excretory duct. When from any cause this takes place, the sebaceous matter, which in the healthy state is propelled to the surface and removed, accumulates in the interior of the follicle, which is thus inordinately distended, till by removing the obstruction the orifice is opened and the inspissated matter eliminated.   It almost invariably again accumulates, unless care be taken to keep the excretory duct pervious,—an object which is most easily and certainly attained by frequent ablution.   This mode of explaining the origin of the cutaneous folliculated tumour

3

was understood by Morgagni,[*] Haller, Plenck,[†] and Monteggia,[‡] and has been recently revived by Sir Astley Cooper.[§]

~§ 2. *Keloid or Cheloid Tumour;* (*Kelis*[||] *Cheloidea.*)—This name has been applied by M. Alibert to a peculiar tumour of the skin, which bears a resemblance to the scar or discoloured, irregular, and puckered *cicatrix* of a burn, or any sore which has healed in similar circumstances. In shape it is oval or cylindrical, generally elevated above the level of the skin. The colour is of various shades of red, sometimes deep-red, wine-red, or pink-coloured, and sometimes only flesh-red. The surface is irregular, that is, elevated into eminences, with intermediate depressions; and often it is seamed or scarred. In general, it is a little firmer than the surrounding skin; but in some cases it presents a sort of velvet-like or spongy softness, which allows it to be pressed. From the margins of the tumour occasionally proceed processes like the feet of an animal ; and this circumstance, with its irregular appearance in general, has been supposed to be the reason, why it is occasionally called the cheloid or crab-like tumour.

The keloid tumour may consist of one, two, or three portions, the lateral margins of which are deeply implanted in the skin. The surface is hard and in general resisting, communicating a sensation quite different from that of the sound skin. It is void of pulsation, and in this respect differs from cutaneous *nævus*.

The origin of this disease, and the causes on which its formation depends, are not well known. It is rarely congenital. When it first appears, it is small, but is liable to enlarge in extent. It proceeds, however, very slowly ; and months or years may elapse be-

* Adversaria Anatomica.

† " Sedes meliceridis," says Plenck, " in glandula subcutanea esse videtur. Quicquid ergo porum excretorium glandulæ subcutaneæ obdurat, contentum succum inspissat, vel ejus absorptionem impedit, meliceridem producere valet." Systema Tumorum, Cl. vii. p. 153. Viennæ, 1767.

‡ Istituzione Chirurgiche, Volume ii.   § Surgical Essays, Part 2.

|| It is quite uncertain whether this term should be written *Cheloid* or *Keloid*. M. Alibert, to whose neological talents we are indebted for the term, gives the following synonymes. *Kelos ; Cheloide ; Cancroide ; Tubercules durs ; Cancelli ; Cancroma ; Cancre blanc ; Le Crabe.* If the name be derived from the supposed resemblance to the crab, then the orthography is *Cheloid.* On the other hand, the term *Kelis, Macula,* a spot, was used by various ancient authors to signify a foul scar or ulcerated mark ; and as one of the characters of the keloid tumour is, that its surface and margins sometimes resemble the *cicatrix* of a burn, this may be with most propriety regarded. as the term from which the denomination for this cutaneous affection should be taken.

fore much change in its size or appearance can be detected. In some instances its formation has been preceded by a burn or some ulcerative process of the skin ; in some by an attack of small-pox ; in other instances, it is said, by the syphilitic poison affecting the skin. Most commonly it occupies the sternal region ; but it has been observed on the face and neck.

As to the nature of *Kelis*, though some have regarded it as allied to cancer, this seems by no means well established. The tumour has been observed to remain a long time on the body, without showing any tendency to pass into cancerous ulceration.

§ 3. *Scirrho-carcinoma* of the skin is not uncommon. Though it may occur in any part of the cutaneous covering, it commences most frequently in situations where the corion is delicate and thinly covered. The skin of the face, especially of the eyelids, prolabium, and nose, is á frequent seat of this disorder ; and next to these, perhaps, are to be placed the nipple of the female and the penis of the male, the corion of which are liable to be affected by this morbid structure. The scrotum is very often the seat of that peculiar carcinomatous destruction occurring in the persons of chimney sweepers. In all these cases the structure is much the same.

It may appear either in the shape of tubercular cancer, or in that of reticular cancer. In the former case small hard tubercles appear to be formed either in the substance of the corion, or in the cutaneous follicles. These coalesce and become elevated, forming a patch of skin, red, hard, irregular, hot, and the seat of stinging pain. After some time, scales are formed on the surface ; and along with or after these slight softening takes place. The scales and crusts are ejected ; and in general there is left a hollow, ulcerating, non-granulating surface, secreting serous fluid, and gradually increasing in depth and extent. Commonly two or three tubercles, simultaneously or successively, are the seat of this process, so that the part presents several hollow ulcers, with hard, elevated edges beginning to be everted or already everted.

When the disease assumes the reticular shape it generally affects a considerable portion of skin with hard, scirrhiform swelling, irregular in surface, and tending, after some time, to the formation of an ulcerated surface, with sanious discharge, and hard, elevated, everted edges. The internal structure of reticular scirrhus in the skin is similar to that structure in other tissues.

In the situation of the corion is seen á tough firm substance of fibro-cartilaginous structure, the fibrous bands being generally arranged in a waving direction. In the most distinct example of the disease which I examined personally—a case of scirrho-carcinomatous degeneration of the whole skin of the penis, these fibrous bands were disposed transversely to the long direction of the part, and appeared to consist of a fibro-cartilaginous long band folded repeatedly on itself.

IV. *Reproduction.*—The reparation of the corion when destroyed has been maintained by many authors. Notwithstanding their assertions, however, this membrane is never, after its substance has been injured, restored to its original state. The breach is filled up by firm cellular tissue, the upper surface of which never acquires the organization of the outer surface of the corion. It is nevertheless capable of furnishing cuticle by which this new corion is covered. These facts may be verified in the cicatrization of burns and other injuries in which the corion has been destroyed.[*]

V. *Parasitical Animals.*—By these the skins both of animals and the human race are liable to be infested. One of these proper to the human race, (*Demodex Folliculorum*) has been already noticed when speaking of acne. Besides these there are others more easily recognized, especially the several species of *Pediculi;* the *Ped. Capitis;* the *Ped. Corporis;* and the *Ped. Pubis,* or *Morpiones.* These are well known, and require no notice here. Of one parasitical animal, however, the existence has been so much contested for two centuries, that it was alternately admitted and denied, until, by the aid of the microscope, its existence and nature were placed in 1833 beyond the reach of doubt. I refer to the itch insect, (the *Sarkoptes scabiei*). A rapid notice of the discovery and recognition of this animal is all that can be admitted in these pages.

For several centuries the inhabitants of the south of Europe recognized the existence of an insect in itch, and were in the habit of extracting and destroying it. In the 12th century it is mentioned by Abenzohr; and in the 15th and 16th centuries more or less fully by Ingrassias, Gabucinus, and Laurence Joubert, each of whom agreed in ascribing to the movements and ravages of this animal beneath or within the skin the fierce itching of scabies.

---

[*] Ottonis Huhn Commentatio de Regeneratione, &c. 1787. P. 23, &c. Andreæ J. G. Murray, Commentatio de Redintegratione, 1787. P. 50. A Dissertation on the Process of Nature in the filling up of cavities, &c. By James Moore, Member &c. London, 1789. Sect. ii. p. 54, &c.

These facts, which were known to the industrious Thomas Mouffet, are confirmed in 1634 by the testimony of his own observation ;* and about the same time, Hauptmann and Hafenreuffer noticed the existence of the insect. The fact, nevertheless, appears by many to have been received with scepticism or positively denied; and even in 1683, when Bonomo addressed to Redi a letter on the existence of the insect of the itch, it was supposed, to be one of those examples of credulity which foreign naturalists occasionally exhibit.† Bonomo, nevertheless, had described the animal from nature; and in 1703 his description was communicated to the Royal Society, by Mead,‡ and afterwards by Baker and Schiebe, in such a manner that showed that the latter two had ascertained the existence of the animal, and examined it by the microscope.

The authority of Bonomo prevailed with various foreign naturalists ; and Linnaeus, who admitted the existence of the insect as a species of *Acarus* or mite, adopted the description of the Italian naturalist.‖ · Bonomo, however, had committed an error in considering the itch insect as similar to the common mite ; and this was rectified by De Geer, who in 1778 both established the existence of the

---

* " Syrones have no certain form ; only they are round. Our eye can scarcely discern them ; they are so small that Epicurus said it was not made of atoms, but was an atom itself. It dwells so under the skin, that when it makes its mines, it will cause a great itching, especially in the hands and other parts affected with them, and held to the fire. If you pull it out with a needle, and lay it on your nail, you shall see it move in the sun, that helps its motion : crack it with the other nail, it will crack with a noise ; and a watery venom comes forth ; it is of a white colour, except the head; if you look nearer, it is blackish, or from black it is something reddish. It is a wonder how so small a creature that creeps with no feet, as it were, can make such long furrows under the skin. This we must observe, by the way, that these syrones do not dwell in the pimples themselves, but hard by. For it is their property not to remove far from the watery humour, collected in the little bladder or pimple, and where that is wasted, or dried up, they all die shortly after." Insectorum sive Minimorum Animalium Theatrum, olim ab Wottono Gesnero, et Pennio inchoatum. Folio. London, 1634. The Theatre of Insects or Lesser Living Creatures. By Thomas Mouffet, Doctor in Physick. London, 1658. Folio, Chapter xxiv. p. 1094 of Topsel.

† G. C. Bonomo Osservazioni intorno a pellicelli del corpo umano. Florenza, 1683.

G. C. Bonomo Obs. circa humani corporis teredinem. Ephem Nat. Cur. Dec. II. Ann. X. App. p. 33.

‡ An Abstract of part of a Letter from Dr Bonomo to Signor Redi, containing some Observations concerning the Worms of Human Bodies. By Richard Mead, M. D. Phil. Trans. for 1703, No. 283, p. 1296. Vol. XXIII. London, 1704.

‖ Linnæus Exanthemata Viva. Amœnitatis Academicæ, V. n. 82, et VIII. p. 73 and 283.

animal, and specified the differential characters between it and the vegetable mite.* In 1786 and afterwards in 1791, Wichmann, a physician at Hanover, published a work on the itch insect†; and his descriptions were verified by Goeze.

From the testimony of these observers it might have been expected that the existence of the itch insect was recognized as established. English dermatologists were, however, sceptical; and they were supported on the continent by the authority of Sagar, Baldinger, Jonas‡, Volkmann,§ Hartmann,‖ Weise, Alexander, and Mieg; and this feeling was increased by Joseph Adams, who, while he showed that a particular kind of insect(ouçao) burrows in the skin in the natives of Madeira, maintained that, as this was not the itch insect, no animal of that kind existed. This scepticism, both among English and French physicians, was much increased by the proceedings of M. Gales, a pupil of Alibert, who, in 1812, presented as the genuine itch *entozoon,* figures and bodies of the common cheese mite.

At length, however, in 1831, M. Raspail having discovered in the itch pustules of the horse, an insect similar to that delineated by De Geer, was satisfied that it was possible to discover a similar parasite in the itch eruption of the human race. It was, however, still the entomologists of the south of Europe who were to determine this as an unquestioned fact. M. Renucci, a student of medicine from Corsica, surprised to find the existence of the insect questioned, showed it to several observers, among others to M. Raspail; and it is solely to the labours of the latter that we are indebted for a correct description of this long doubted and doubtful animal.¶

The itch insect is white at first sight, but with some reddish-brown points on its circumference. It may be seen without a

---

* De Geer Memoires pour servir a l'histoire des Insectes. Stockholm, 1778. 4to, T. VII. p. 92, Pl. 5.

† Jo. Ernest Wichmann Ætiologie von der Kräze. Hanover, 1786.

‡ Jonas Dissert. Dubia circa Ætiologiam Wichmannianam Scabiei. Halae, 1787.

§ Volkmann Diss. sistens quæstiones medicas super Wichmanni Ætiologia Scabiei. Francofurti ad Viadr, 1787.

‖ Hartmann Dissert. Quæstiones super Wichmanni ætiologia Scabiei. Fr., 1789.

¶ Bulletin General de Therapeutique, Septembre 1834.
Raspail Memoire Comparatif sur l'histoire naturelle de l'insecte de la Gale. Fig. 8vo. Paris, 1834.

magnifying glass moving on a coloured surface, especially if dark. It is about $\frac{39}{10000}$ parts of one inch in diameter. With one glass, the feet may be numbered, the mouth distinguished, and all the other details of outline recognized. The head and fore feet are capable of being concealed under the body by incurvation downwards; and in this attitude these five members seem withdrawn within coverings. The posterior portion of the body placed in the same position presents eight *setæ* or hairs, gradually decreasing in size, till they approach the vent. Four of them belong to the hind feet; and of the other four, two are inserted on each side of the vent.

When examined lengthwise by the microscope, the animal appears flattened; and in the transparent places it presents parallel curved striæ, which give it the appearance of the shell of a fish viewed by the same magnifying power. These *striæ* cover the whole surface of the body of the insect, forming a large cellular network, the *cellulæ* of which are linear and hollow, the interstitial partitions relieved and prominent. This network strongly resists cutting instruments, so that it is difficult to kill the insect with the point of a needle while extracting it.

When placed on the back, so as to examine the anterior or inferior surface, the organization of this insect appears greatly more complicated. The head and the four anterior feet are implanted in an equal number of cases, not dissimilar to incomplete *elytræ*. The head is simple and curved downwards by the snout or proboscis, or sucker. Placed in acetic acid, two transparent vesicles come into view, which might be taken for eyes. The articulations of the legs require long observation to be quite visible. Each of these articulations is covered by hairs, of which those only on the sides are visible. The last joint is covered with short prickles, and armed beneath with a stiff hair, which is terminated beneath by a flexible cavity capable of producing a vacuum, like the soft glutinous pads of certain animals much higher in the scale, such as the tree-frog. To these pads, which enable the animal to fix itself in any position, M. Raspail applies the denomination of *ambulacra*.

There are four posterior legs, which are smaller and shorter, and less easily distinguished than the anterior legs. They are so small and slender that by De Geer they were mistaken for hairs or *setæ*. They have the same organization and the same locomotive apparatus as the anterior legs, excepting the part called by Raspail *ambulacrum*,

3

instead of which are very long hairs. The anterior or abdominal surface of the insect is striated as well as its dorsal surface.

. ⸺This insect is not an *acarus*, as imagined by Linnæus and other entomologists. In consequence of the differential characters, it has been referred by Raspail to a separate genus under the name of *Sarkoptes*, or *Flesh-roaster*, (Σαρξ, *caro*; Οπταω, *torreo*.)

It has now been seen by so many observers, both in France and this country, that there is no chance that its existence can again be questioned. It works its way beneath the cuticle by making burrows or paths in the vascular layer of the skin.

The nails, like the cuticle, may be diseased in consequence of a morbid state of the corial surface and vessels by which they are nourished. In one or two instances of strumous children, I have seen them fissured into several longitudinal portions, much thickened, and indurated like horn, and incurvated. In others of the fingers of the same individuals, they were small and imperfectly developed; and in some their place was supplied by a small portion of thick horny cuticle. Similar changes are sometimes induced by disease or by injury.

Of the hairs, the most extraordinary morbid state is the Polish plait (*plica Polonica;*) so named from being endemial in Poland, Lithuania, Hungary, and Transylvania, from the source of the Vistula to the Carpathian mountains. It occurs also in Prussia, Russia, Switzerland, and in some parts of the Low Countries. It is impossible to doubt that this abnormal condition of the hairs depends on disease taking place in their bulbs or nutritious sacs. This is proved by the state of the skin from which the diseased hair grows, and by the unctuous, viscid, and blood-coloured fluid which the hairs in this state contain. We nevertheless possess no very precise information on the nature of this diseased state of the capillary bulbs; and in the absence of exact facts I abstain from offering conjectures.

The piliparous sacs lose their energy under certain morbid states of the system; for instance, fever, pulmonary consumption, and the constitutional symptoms of lues. The hairs then drop out; and if at this time the bulbs be examined, the sacs are found to contain, according to Bichat, at least in persons who have passed through fever, the rudiment of new hairs. The shedding of the hairs, which takes place in the decline of life, and the period of which varies remarkably in different individuals, Bichat represents as depending on a total death of the piliparous sacs.

Accidental and abnormal developement of hairs is not uncommon. In the skin this appears in the shape of hairy moles and similar congenital marks.* Their occurrence in the stomach, intestines, and bladder, as noticed by a variety of authors, is also to be regarded as abnormal. Lastly, the accidental developement of hairs is observed in encysted tumours, especially those of the ovaries, in which masses or balls of hair mixed with fat, oleaginous, or adipocirous matter, have been frequently found.† On the mode in which these hairs are formed nothing satisfactory is known.‡

CHAPTER II.

Section I.

MUCOUS MEMBRANE, VILLOUS MEMBRANE.—*Membrana mucosa, M. mucipara, M. villosa,*—Tissu Muqueux, Bichat.

The organic tissue or membrane, to which the name of *mucous* or *villous* has been applied, consists of two great divisions, the gastro-pulmonary, and genito-urinary.

A. The first or gastro-pulmonary mucous surface comprehends that membranous surface which commences at the various orifices of the face, at which it is contiguous with the skin; and is continued through the lacrymal and nasal passages, and even the Eustachian tube, by the larynx on the one hand to the windpipe and bronchial membrane, and by the œsophagus on the other through the entire tract of the alimentary canal, at the opposite extremity of which, it is again identified with the skin.

B. The distribution of the second division, or the genito-urinary mucous membrane, is slightly varied according to the differences of sex. In the male it is connected with the skin at the orifice of the urethra, from which it proceeds inwards toward the bladder;

---

* Haller, Elementa Physiologiæ, Lib. XII. Sect 1. § XVII.
† Bichat, Tom. IV. p. 828.
‡ Meckel, Journ. Compl. T. IV. and Bricheteau, Journ. Compl. T. XV.

sending previously small prolongations through ducts on each side of the *veru montanum*, from which it is believed to be continued through the *vasa deferentia*, to the *vasa efferentia* of the testicle. Continued over the inner surface of the urinary bladder, it is prolonged through the ureters to the pelvis and infundibula of the kidney. In the female, besides passing in this direction, it ascends into the womb, and passes through the Fallopian or uterine tubes, at the upper extremity of which it terminates in an abrupt opening into the sac of the peritonæum,—the only instance in the whole body in which a mucous and serous surface communicate freely and directly.

These two orders of membranous tissue have each two surfaces, an attached or adherent, and a free one. The adherent surface is attached, 1*st*, to muscles, as in the tongue ; most of the mouth and fauces, œsophagus, and whole alimentary canal, and the bladder ; 2*d*, to fibrous membranes, as in the nasal cavities and part of the larynx, in which it is attached to periosteum or perichondrium, the palate, ureter, and pelvis of the kidney ; 3*d*, to fibro-cartilages, as in the windpipe, (*trachea*,) and bronchial tubes.

The free surface is not uniform or similar throughout. The appearance of the pituitary or Schneiderian membrane is different from that of the stomach or intestines ; the surface of the tongue and mouth is different from that of the trachea ; and the free surface of the urethra is unlike that of the bladder. These variations depend on difference of structure, and are connected with a difference in properties ; yet anatomists have improperly applied to the whole what was peculiar to certain parts only, and have thus created a system, in which some truth is blended with much misrepresentation.

Mucous membrane consists, like skin, of a *corion* or *derma*, and an *epidermis* or *cuticle*.

The mucous corion is a firm dense gray substance, which forms the ground-work of the membrane in most regions of the body, but which is evidently represented by the fibrous system, *e. g.* the periosteum or perichondrium, in some other situations. It is most distinctly seen in the mouth and throat, and in various parts of the alimentary canal. In the first situation it is more vascular, less gray and dense than in the intestinal mucous membrane.

It possesses two surfaces, an inner, adherent to the submucous filamentous tissue, and an outer or proper mucous surface. In the stomach, the mucous corion is in the form of a soft but firm membranous substance, about one-sixth or one-eighth of one line thick, tough, of a dun-gray or fawn colour, (intermediate between Sienna-yellow and ochre-yellow, Syme,) slightly translucent, and sinking in water. The attached or inner surface is flocculent and tomentose, and a shade lighter than the outer, which presents a sort of shag or velvet, consisting of very minute piles. This, when examined by a good lens at oblique light, appears to consist of an infinite number of very minute roundish bodies closely set, but separated by equally minute linear pits, and occasionally circular depressions. In the ileum it presents much the same characters; but the minute bodies of its shaggy surface are still larger and more distinct, and may be seen by the naked eye. In the windpipe, again, it is rather thinner and lighter coloured; and while its outer surface presents numerous minute pores, it is much smoother than in the alimentary canal, and entirely destitute of those minute bodies seen in the latter. It nowhere presents any appearance of fibres.

The mucous corion rests on a layer of filamentous tissue, pretty firm and dense, and of a bluish white colour,—a character by which it is easily distinguished from the soft fawn-coloured mucous membrane. This submucous filamentous tissue is what is erroneously termed the nervous coat by Ruysch, Albinus, and some of the older anatomists. In certain parts the mucous corion is covered by a thin membrane, which has been named the epidermis or cuticle.

It is exceedingly difficult to demonstrate this membrane distinctly. It is very thin, quite transparent, and is perhaps most easily shown by boiling or scalding a portion of mucous membrane, and then peeling off with care the outer pellicle. This experiment succeeds best in the mucous membrane of the mouth and palate, in which, therefore, the existence of mucous epidermis cannot be doubted. In cases of death by swallowing boiling water, the epidermis is raised in the form of vesications on the base of the tongue, on the epiglottis, and even sometimes at the arytenoid membrane; and I have seen the epidermis of the epiglottis forming vesications in consequence of the deglutition of sulphuric acid. The observations of Wepfer, Haller, and Nicholls, and especially of Bleuland,* are sufficient to prove its existence in the œsophagus. Bichat admits that, though it can be demonstrated at the cutaneous junctions of

---

* Jani Bleuland, M. D. Observationes Anatomico-Medicæ de sana et morbosa œsophagi structura. Lug. Bat. 1785.

the mucous surfaces, it can no longer be shown to exist in the stomach, intestines, bladder, &c.   Beclard renders this conclusion precise, by showing experimentally that mucous epidermis cannot be traced in the œsophagus beyond the cardia ; in the genito-urinary system beyond the neck of the womb, and that of the bladder.

 The termination of the epidermis at the lower end or cardiac junction of the œsophagus is very remarkable.   It is seen by the eye, but more clearly by the aid of a good glass.   It is observed to form or send out long triangular processes, the base connected with the œsophageal epidermis, the apices free, leaving also between them triangular spaces.   The length of these processes varies from one-third of an inch to half an inch and two-thirds of an inch. Their number is also variable, and sometimes in the same subject they differ in size.   They are rendered very distinct by immersing the œsophagus in boiling water, which renders them opake, or in nitric acid, which imparts to them an orange-yellow tinge, leaving the intermediate and adjoining mucous corion little changed.

In the *uterus* it is quite easy to see that the epidermis does not advance beyond the upper extremity of the *vagina*.   The uterine mucous membrane presents no appearance of *epidermis*.

The structure of mucous membrane varies in every situation and in every organ; and as the mucous membrane of the alimentary canal has been most frequently examined, on that, accordingly, the greatest amount of information has been communicated.

This division of the mucous system presents most distinctly and in greatest perfection three sets of objects, the true structure of which it is believed highly important to understand aright.

These are the tubulo-cellular structure of the stomach, the *villi*, and the muciparous follicles or glands.

The mucous membrane of the stomach, which first deserves attention, is not villous, properly speaking, so much as cellular.   Hewson had early observed, that at the upper part of the stomach, the villous coat appears in a miscroscope like a honey-comb, or like the second stomach of ruminating animals in miniature, that is, full of small cells which have thin membranous partitions.   Towards the pylorus these partitions are lengthened so as to approach to the shape of the *villi* in the *jejunum*.

These cells Sir E. Home represents as found in the form of a honey-comb in the upper end of the stomach, and to be of greatest depth in this region, though seen over the whole cardiac portion, but so faintly that a high magnifying power is required to render them visible. In the pyloric portion the same cellular appearance continues; but here and there are small clusters, the sides of which rise above the surface, giving the appearance of foliated membranes.

These cells are, according to Dr Boyd, about $\frac{1}{80}$th of one inch in diameter near the *cardia*. Not half an inch from the *cardia*, however, these large cells give place to small regular cells which characterize the whole internal surface of the organ. When the mucous membrane is extended, they appear regular both in shape and size, varying from $\frac{1}{200}$th to $\frac{1}{300}$th part of one inch in diameter, being smaller in the young than in the adult. Near the *pylorus*, again, they are enlarged, being about $\frac{1}{100}$th of one inch in diameter. The floor of each cell appears perforated by numerous circular openings, as if a number of tubes opened on it; and on making a vertical section of the mucous membrane, it is seen to be composed of *striæ* or fibres running perpendicularly from the free surface of the membrane to the cellular coat beneath.

These *striæ* or fibres are known to be small tubes lying parallel to each other. These tubes are longest, and are most distinctly seen near the *pylorus*, and indeed all over the organ. At the cardia they are short, little more than simple rings, lying close to each other. They are about $\frac{1}{600}$th part of one inch in diameter, appear to have no immediate connection with the cells into which they generally open, and are supposed to be subservient to a different function.[*] There is strong reason to believe, nevertheless, that these tubes are concerned in some mode in the secretion of gastric fluid.

In the human stomach, glands or follicles are found mostly at the pylorus. In other regions they are, in the state of health, not very distinct. Indeed, the gastric follicles of the human stomach are always in the healthy state indistinct. A kind of minute gland-like bodies nevertheless is sometimes perceptible along the small arch.

The next peculiarity which it is important to notice is the existence of minute piles or villosities in the gastro-enteric division. These bodies are best seen by detaching, inverting, and inflating a portion of ileum. When this is immersed in pure water, the observer may perceive, by means of its refracting power, an infinite

---

[*] Essay on the Structure of the Mucous Membrane of the Human Stomach, by Sprott Boyd, M. D. Edinburgh Medical and Surgical Journal, Vol. XLVI. p. 382. Edinburgh, 1836.

number of minute prolongations, which are made to wave or move gently amidst the fluid; but even a very powerful magnifying glass does not render them so distinct, as to determine whether they are round or flattened, whether they are solid or hollow, or whether they are obtuse or acuminated. The shape and structure of these villosities are indeed imperfectly known.

These piles, (*villi*, die zotten,) though seen by many anatomists, were first examined in 1721 by Helvetius, who represents them as cylindrical prominences in quadrupeds, but conical in the human subject.* Their intimate structure, however, Lieberkuhn undertook first by microscopical observation to demonstrate. According to this observer, each *villus* receives a minute branch of a lacteal, arterial branches, a vein, and a nerve; and in each the lacteal branch is expanded into a minute sac or bladder (*ampullula, vesicula,*) like an egg, the capacity of which he estimates at $\frac{1}{2}$th of a cubic line, and in the apex of which may be seen by the microscope a minute opening.† Upon this sac the arterial branches are ramified to great delicacy, and terminate in minute veins, which then unite into one trunk; while its inner surface he represents as spongy and cellular. The space between the *villi*, which do not touch each other, he further represents to be occupied by the open orifices of follicles, so numerous that he counted eighty of them, where were eighteen villi; and both, he asserts, are covered by a thin but tenacious membrane similar to epidermis.

Hewson, while he admits in each villus the ramification of minute arteries and veins, denies the saccular expansion, and infers that the lacteals are ramified in the same manner as the blood-vessels, and that the whole constitute a broad flat body,‡ the spongy appearance of which he ascribes to the mutual ramification of the latter. With this in general Cruikshank agrees;§ while Sheldon, who found the villi not only round and cylindrical as Hewson, but bulbous as Lieberkuhn, and even sabre-shaped, rather confirms the statements of that anatomist.‖ Mascagni and Soemmering agreeing in the general fact of vascular and lacteal structure, seem to

---

* Mém. de l'Acad. des Sciences. 1721.

† J. N. Lieberkuhn, M. D. &c. Dissertatio Anatomio-Physiologica de Fabrica et Actione villorum Intestinorum Tenuium Hominis. Lugduni Batavorum, 1745. 4to; et cura J. Sheldon. Londini, 1782, § ii. iii. &c.

‡ Experimental Inquiries, part ii. p. 175, chapter xii.

§ The Anatomy of the Absorbing Vessels, &c. p. 58.

‖ The History of the Absorbent System, p. 36 and 37.

represent the shape of the *villus* as that of a mushroom, consisting of a stalk and a *pileus*.

Some of these discordant statements Hedwig attempts with equal ingenuity and industry to reconcile. The difference in shape he refers to differences in the animals examined; and in one class finds them cylindrical, (*e. g.* in man and the horse;) in another conical, (the dog;) in a third club-shaped, (the pheasant;) and in a fourth pointed or pyramidal, (*e. g.* the mouse.) The interior structure he also represents as spongy in all the animals which he examined; and invariably also he found at the apex the orifice of the duct, which, after the example of Lieberkuhn, he conceives constitutes the *ampullula.**

These conclusions are not exactly confirmed by the researches of Rudolphi, who examined the *villi* in man and a considerable number of animals. This anatomist never found the orifice seen by Hedwig, notwithstanding every care taken to perceive it. He maintains that the *villi* are not alike in all parts of the intestinal canal of the same animal, as represented by Hedwig, but may be cylindrical in one part, club-shaped in another, and acuminated in a third. Admitting their vascular structure, which he thinks may be demonstrated, he regards the ampullular expansion as doubtful, and denies its cellular arrangement.†

About the same time Bleuland, who had previously examined the intestinal mucous membrane, after successful injection of its capillaries, undertook to revive the leading circumstances of the description of Lieberkuhn. By examining microscopically well-injected portions of intestine, he shows that the *villi* are composed of a system of very minute arterial and venous capillaries, enclosing a lacteal which constitutes the *ampulla*, and in the interior of which a certain order of these capillaries terminates. He also revives the statement of the absorbing orifice at the extremity of each *villus*.‡ The rest of the observations of this author pertain rather to the distribution of the minute vessels, and shall be more particularly noticed under that head.

The observations of Beclard on these bodies are most perspicu-

* Disquisitio Ampullularum Lieberkuhnii Physico-Microscopica. Lipsiæ, 1797. 4to.

† Einige Beobachtungen über die Darmzotten von D. Karl A. Rudolphi, in Reil. Archiv. iv. b. 1797, p. 63 and 340. Und Anatomische-Physiologische Abhandlungen, Von Karl Asmund Rudolphi, Mit. Acht Kupfertafeln. Berlin, 1802. 8vo. III.

‡ Jani Bleuland, M.D. &c. Vasculorum, in Intestinorum Tenuium Tunicis, &c. Descriptio Iconibus Illustrata. Trajecti ad Rhenum, 1797.

ous. According to this anatomist the intestinal *villi* appear neither conical, nor cylindrical, nor tubular, nor expanded at top, as described by several authors, but in the shape of leaflets or minute plates so closely set that they form an abundant tufted pile. Their shape varies according to the manner in which they are examined, and according to the part. Those of the pyloric half of the stomach and *duodenum* are broader than long, and form minute plates; those of the *jejunum* are long and narrow, constituting piles; at the end of the ileum they become laminar; and in the colon are scarcely prominent. They are semitranslucent; their surface is smooth; and neither openings at their surface, or cavity, or their interior, or vascular structure can be recognized.*

Follicles and Crypts.—In most mucous membranes are found minute, oval, or spheroidal bodies, slightly elevated, and presenting an orifice leading to a blind or shut cavity. As they are believed to secrete a fluid analogous to or identical with mucus, they are named mucous glands; and from their shape and situation they are also denominated follicles (*folliculi*) and *cryptæ*. Though found in all the mucous membranes in more or less abundance, they have been most frequently examined in those of the alimentary canal, where they were first accurately described by Peyer and Brunner. (*Glandulæ Peyerianæ.*†) In this situation they are situate in the substance of the mucous corion. Their structure, so far as it can be examined, is simple. The orifice leads into a saccular cavity, the surface of which is smooth and uniform, and appears to secrete the fluid which oozes from them. This membranous sac appears to be lodged in a reddish-coloured, dense, abnormal matter, which is probably filamentous tissue enveloping minute blood-vessels; but of the minute structure of which nothing is accurately known. In the state of health these bodies are so minute that it is very difficult to recognize them. I have seen them, nevertheless, in the tracheo-bronchial membrane by the eye and by a lens. When the membranes are inflamed they become larger and more distinct. In the bladder, the womb, the gall-bladder, and the seminal vesicles, they are not distinctly seen, and cannot be satisfactorily demonstrated. It is unnecessary, however, to follow the ex-

---

* Anatomie Generale, chap. iii. sect. 2de, p. 253.

† Joannis Conradi Peyeri Parerga Anatomica et Medica Septem, Ratione ac Experientia parentibus concepta et edita. Genevæ, 1681. Parergon Secundum, p. 79. De Glandulis Intestinalium, 1681. Brunner de Glandulis Duodeni. Francof. 1715.

ample of Bichat in trusting to analogy to prove their existence; for they are not necessary to the secretion of mucous fluid, as he seems to imagine. Those in the urethra, first well described by William Cowper, are distinct examples of follicles in the genito-urinary surface.* The sinuosities (*lacunæ*), first accurately described, if not discovered by Morgagni,† though not exactly the same in conformation and structure, seem to be very slightly different.

The importance of the muciparous follicles in influencing both the functions and the morbid states of the alimentary mucous membrane, renders it necessary to consider with some detail the situation, structure, and anatomical peculiarities of these bodies.

These do not occur at all parts of the alimentary mucous membrane; but are distributed in different modes in different regions of the membrane.

In the *œsophagus* they are not numerous, but are observed like small bodies about the size of flattened pin-heads in various parts of the membrane, and at irregular intervals from each other. With a good glass may be recognized a minute aperture or pore, which proceeds from the centre of the gland and acts as a sort of excreting duct.

At the *cardia* these bodies become more numerous and are more closely set, so that they form a sort of ring round the cardiac orifice.

In the stomach they are rather numerous along the course of the small arch. But they are observed at uncertain intervals in various other regions of the stomach. At the pylorus also they are abundant, and in that region also they may be more easily recognized than in any other part of the organ.

The duodenum is rather peculiar as to its glandular apparatus. The whole duodenal mucous membrane is provided with numerous minute glandular bodies, which are more closely set than in any other part of the alimentary canal, and give its surface an appearance rough and irregular, and a firmer consistence than elsewhere. These bodies nevertheless are not so distinctly observed in man as in certain animals, for instance the horse, ox, stag, dog, and wolf. These glandular or follicular bodies are believed to be seated mostly in the submucous cellular tissue.

The upper part of the *jejunum* does not present many glandular bodies, and indeed is most commonly without them for several feet.

* * Two new Glands near the Prostate Gland, with their Excretory Ducts. By Mr William Cowper. Phil. Transactions, No. 258, p. 364.

† Adversaria Anatomica, IV. 8, 9, &c.

But the lower part of the small intestine, and what is named *ileum*, is provided with two sets of follicles, one solitary (*gl. solitariæ*), or consisting of single isolated follicles, the other aggregated or associated (*glandulæ agminatæ*,) so as to form a patch, plexus, or cluster.

The solitary glands begin to appear about four or five feet above the lower end of the *ileum*. They are not always very distinct or visible. When they are, they are disseminated like minute grains through the mucous corion at irregular intervals. They are often, nevertheless, less conspicuous at the lower end of the *ileum* than a little higher up.

The aggregated glands begin to appear in the *ileum* about from four to six feet from its lower end. From the point where they commence showing themselves, they are invariably disposed along the antimesenteric side of the bowel, or that which is opposite to the mesenteric attachment. They appear in the form of patches, sometimes affecting the circular shape, sometimes irregular, most frequently elliptical, with 'the long diameter corresponding to the axis of the bowel. In size they vary according to the number of integral follicles of which each patch consists. High up in the ileum they are often small, that is, not larger than a silver four-penny piece. But lower down they become larger and affect more decidedly the elliptical figure. They are also closer to each other toward the lower portion of the bowel than at its upper part.

These elliptical patches consist of a great number of follicles or crypts placed contiguous to each other. The number varies from perhaps 20 or 30 to 50, 60, or more. Each isolated component follicle is a small body with a pore or orifice issuing from its centre; and each follicle consists, so far as can be at present determined, of a peculiar sort of dense matter, which I think is merely a species of close filamento-cellular tissue, through which are distributed many minute arteries and veins.

In colour, these patches are usually of a darker tint than the surrounding mucous membrane, mostly of a leaden gray, or slate-blue shade; and when viewed by transmitted light, they are like a dark or opake patch on the more translucent intestine. This, I think, depends on the greater aggregation of their constituent tissue.

Most usually they are, in the natural state, on a level with the surface of the adjoining portion of intestine. They are not very rough or irregular; but by the eye, or a good glass, it is possible to observe considerable irregularity in surface.

All these characters become exaggerated under the influence of disease. They then become elevated, rough, irregular on the surface, and their opacity is increased.

At the lower extremity of the *ileum*, where it enters the *cæcum*, the whole membrane is often occupied with a large and extensive patch of agminated glands, most extensive in the long direction of the bowel, without definite shape, or rather the whole of the lower part of the *ileum*, for the space of from three to four inches, consists of a surface of agminated glands.

The agminated glands, and also the solitary follicles of the *ileum*, are generally larger and more distinct *caeteris paribus* in infancy, than in adult life. In the bodies of infants, they are almost invariably easily seen and demonstrated. In the bodies of young subjects between 14 and 20 or 25, they are still visible, sometimes very distinctly. In general, however, after this period, they are greatly less distinct, and sometimes they cannot be recognized at all. In old age they cease to be observed.

In the colon, the mucous follicles are still different both in shape and disposition.

They appear in the form of small round oblate-spheroidal or orbicular bodies, with circular outline about one line in diameter, not unlike millet-seeds, with a central pore or aperture. These bodies are always isolated, and they are placed at the distance of from half an inch to one inch from each other. They are arranged all round the mucous surface of the bowel, and are not, as is observed as to the aggregated glands of the ileum, confined to one side of the bowel only. In different subjects they are presented with different degrees of distinctness. In some they are scarcely visible; in others they are conspicuous. In dropsical subjects they are usually very distinct, probably from their tissue being infiltrated with serum. Their structure appears to consist of minute colourless vessels ramified in filamento-cellular tissue, and with a central pore or excretory duct. They are placed immediately beneath or in the mucous corion, which over their surface is thin, and descends through the pore into the interior of the gland.

At the lower extremity of the colon, or rather the rectum, there are placed several follicles, often of considerable size. Their structure is in all respects similar to that of those of the colon.

On the minute structure of these follicles, all that is accurately known is the following. If we examine an isolated follicle, it presents the most simple form of glandular arrangement. The intestinal mucous membrane is continued through the minute pore, which is situate at the apex of the follicle downward for about $\frac{1}{100}$th part of one line, forming a blind-sac, or cavity of a sac, and constituting in this manner a crypt or recess. The surface of this short passage is moistened by a fluid which is secreted from it. On this surface are ramified an infinite number of minute arteries and veins, which constitute the vascular system of the follicle. Beneath the mucous membrane of the crypt is situate a close but fine filamentous tissue, which surrounds the arteries and veins now mentioned. This filamentous tissue is gradually connected with that of the contiguous intestine. The existence of excretory ducts on the cryptic membrane has not been demonstrated. It is most probable that upon the free surface of this the arteries open.

The close filamentous tissue now mentioned as forming the parenchyma of the follicle, it is difficult to demonstrate in the healthy state. Some describe as silvery white, others as slightly yellow. When the follicles are affected by inflammation, it becomes thick, hard, and swelled, and it is then more distinctly seen. It then also becomes reddish, or yellow, or orange-coloured.

What the structure of the isolated follicle is, such is that of the aggregated follicles, which, indeed, are merely many isolated follicles adjoining to each other, or united so as to form a patch, (agmen) (glandulæ agminatæ). Each agminated gland has its pore, its crypt, its cryptic membrane, its blood-vessels, and its cellular tissue.

These glands have been denominated muciparous, and are supposed to secrete mucus. The fluid which issues from them appears to be thinner and more liquid than mucus. It may, however, undergo changes after its secretion.

In certain regions of the mucous membranes, more especially at their connections with the skin, are found minute conical eminences denominated papillæ. They are distinctly seen in the mucous membrane of the tongue, where they vary in size and shape, and in the body named clitoris. They are elevations belonging to the mucous corion, and they are liberally supplied by blood-vessels, the veins of which present an erectile arrangement, and with minute nervous filaments. Of the intimate structure of these bodies, however, little more is known. They are covered by a true epidermis.

In the stomach, duodenum, and ileum, this membrane is collected into folds or plaits, which have received in the former situation the name of *rugæ* or wrinkles, and in the latter the name of *plicæ* or folds, and *valvulæ conniventes* or winking valves. In the vagina also are transverse *rugæ*, which in like manner are folds or dupli_catures of its mucous membrane. Those of the œsophagus are longitudinal, and have been described by Bleuland. In the tracheo-bronchial membrane, and in the membranous and spongy portions of the urethra, we find them in the shape of minute plates or wrinkles in the long direction of their respective tubes, but rarely of much length. These folds or plaits are quite peculiar to the mucous membranes; and the object of them appears to be to increase the extent of surface, and to allow the membrane to undergo consider_able occasional distension.

In certain points, where a communication is observed between the general mucous surface and the cavities or recesses of particu_lar regions, anatomists have not demonstrated a mucous membrane, but have inferred its existence as a continuation of the general surface. In the tympanal cavity to which the Eustachian tube leads, the existence of a mucous or fibro-mucous membrane is rather presumed from analogy than proved by actual observation. We know that, where the biliary and pancreatic ducts enter the duodenum, and for a considerable space towards the liver, the interior appearance is that of a fine mucous surface provided with *lacunæ* and villosities; but it is impossible to say at what point of the hepatic duct, or of the smaller canals of which it is formed, the mucous membrane terminates.

The tracheal membrane, when traced to the bronchial divisions, presents no arrangement, either of *papillæ*, piles, or villosities; and nothing is perceived except a smooth uniform surface, of a colour between gray, dun, and red or purple, which is moistened with a viscid semitransparent fluid, and which is as like the peritonæum as the intestinal mucous membrane.

In the ultimate divisions of the bronchial tubes, the mucous mem_brane follows the anatomical arrangement of these tubes to their extremities. It was at one time imagined, that these tubes terminat_ed in enlarged or dilated chambers, which were termed by Malpighi *ampullulæ*, and by others air-cells and vesicles; and it was further believed, especially by Willis and Senac, that various vesicles or ultimate chambers placed at the terminal ends of bronchial tubes communicated with each other in the substance of the lungs. These cells, indeed, Willis represents as clustered together like grapes. It is certain that this is not established by observation.

When a bronchial tube is traced to its further extremity, it terminates not in an enlarged chamber or cell, but merely in a blind sac or cavity; and this sac does not communicate with others. The bronchial tubes, in short, though divided to great minuteness in the substance of the lungs, preserve their character of tubes gradually tapering and diminishing, but do not form ampullulæ, or vesicles or cells properly so named.

It is nevertheless convenient to retain the name of cells or vesicles, understanding thereby merely the terminal ends of the bronchial tubes.

Lastly, the situation where the existence of the mucous system, though believed, is most uncertain, is in the interior of the *vasa deferentia*, and where they take their origin from the *vasa efferentia* of the *testis*. Regarding the organization of these tubes no sensible evidence can be obtained, and whatever is stated concerning it is the result of analogical inference.

Though these membranes have been designated by the general name of *mucous*, it is not to be understood that the action of their surface is in every situation the same. It is not easy to limit the signification of the term *mucus ;* for it appears that this fluid varies in the nasal passages, in the tracheal and bronchial membrane, in the œsophagus, stomach, and intestines, and in the urinary bladder and ureters. But it may be stated as a certain fact, that many parts of the two mucous surfaces never in the healthy state secrete any modification of this animal matter ; and in others the membrane is almost always moistened by a different fluid. The mucous or villous membrane of the eyelids is never in the healthy state occupied with mucus, but is uniformly moistened with the tears ; the membrane of the mouth and throat is moistened with saliva only ; the urethra presents a peculiar viscid fluid, which seems to exude from many minute vessels opening along its surface, as in the *lacunæ*, but which is widely different from mucus. All those parts, in short, which are not in perpetual, but only occasional, contact with foreign or secreted substances, seem to present no mucus in the healthy state ; whereas the surfaces of the stomach, intestines, gall-bladder, and urinary bladder, are constantly covered with a quantity, more or less considerable, of this animal secretion.

. The chemical properties of mucous membranes are completely ˎ
unknown. The analysis of the fluid secreted by them has been
executed by Fourcroy, Berzelius, and others, but is foreign to the
subject of this work.

The mucous membranes are most liberally supplied with blood
by vessels which are both large and numerous. This is proved not
only by the phenomena of injections, but by the red colour of which
many of their divisions are the seat. This coloration, as well as
the injectibility, is not indeed uniform ; for in certain regions mucous surfaces are pale or light blue ; in others their redness is considerable.

Thus, in those regions in which the mucous membranes coalesce
with the periosteum, forming fibro-mucous membranes, e. g. in the
facial sinuses, the tympanal cavity and the mastoid cells, the colour
is pale-blue, or approaching to light-lilac. In the bladder, in the
large intestines, in the excretory ducts, in general, though pale,
this colouring becomes more vivid. In the pulmonic mucous membrane it is a slate-blue, verging to pale pink. In the stomach, duodenum, small intestines, and the vagina, it becomes still more
marked. In the uterus it varies according to the period or the intervals of menstruation.

If these vessels be examined in the gastro-enteric mucous membrane, in which they are probably most numerous, they are found
to consist of an extensive net-work of capillaries divided to an infinite degree of minuteness, mutually intersecting and spreading
over the upper or outer surface of the mucous corion. This vascular net-work, though demonstrated by Ruysch, Albinus, Haller,
and Bichat, has been very beautifully represented in the delineations of Bleuland, who thinks he has traced their minute ramifications into the *villi*, as above stated. These minute vessels are derived from larger ones, which creep through the submucous cellular tissue, and which are observed to penetrate the mucous corion
to be finally distributed at its exterior surface. The substance of
this membrane itself appears to receive few or no vessels. It is
well known, that the vessels which supply the mucous surfaces, enter
between the folds of the serous membranes, at which they are in the
form of considerable trunks. Having penetrated between the folds
of these membranes, they divide in the subserous cellular tissue
into branches, the size of which is considerable ; and here they form
those numerous anastomotic communications which constitute the

arches so distinctly seen in the ileum. From the convexity of these arches in general, are sent off the small vessels, which are then fitted, after passing through the muscular layer and the submucous tissue, to enter the mucous corion.

The capillary terminations, then, of these arteries, and their corresponding veins, constitute the physical cause of the coloration of the mucous membranes. This coloration, however, is not at all times of the same intensity in the same membrane, and varies chiefly according to the state of the organ which the membrane covers. The coloration of the gastro-enteric mucous membrane undergoes, even within the limits of health, many variations. Thus, according to the absence or presence of such foreign substances as are taken at meals, the mucous membrane is pale, or presents various shades of redness. At the period of menstruation the uterine mucous membrane becomes red and injected. Pressure on any of the venous vessels renders the mucous membrane blue, purple, or livid, as is seen in *prolapsus*, and more distinctly in *asphyxia*, in which all the mucous membranes assume a livid tint. (Bichat.) The varieties of red colour observed in the gastric mucous membrane by Dr Yellowly are to be ascribed partly to the latter cause, partly to the vascular redness which the presence of foreign bodies occasions.*

Where death is the result of *asphyxia*, rapid or slow, the gastric and intestinal mucous membranes are often much loaded with blood. In death from disease of the heart, when the fatal event is preceded by great anguish, I have often seen the gastric mucous membrane of a deep red colour, and occasionally livid and approaching to black. The dependant portions of the intestinal convolutions are, under the same circumstances, much loaded with blood, mostly in veins. These appearances must not be confounded with inflammation. They merely imitate that process, and are pseudo-inflammatory.

The pulmonary division of this membrane is of an ash-gray or dun colour, inclining to pale-blue or light-red. These colours vary, nevertheless, according to the facility or the difficulty with which the blood moves through the pulmonary capillary system. It is also freely supplied with blood-vessels derived chiefly from the bronchial arteries. These vessels, after accompanying the bron-

---

* Observations on the vascular appearance in the Human Stomach, which is frequently mistaken for inflammation of that organ. By John Yellowly, M. D. &c. Medico-Chirurg. Trans. Vol. IV. p. 371.

chial tubes and their successive subdivisions, divide into minute branches which penetrate the mucous corion, which here is white, dense, and fibrous, and after anastomosing with the capillaries of the pulmonary artery and veins, form a minute delicate net-work on the outer surface of the pulmonary mucous membrane. According to Reisseissen, to whom we are indebted for a careful examination of these vessels, a successful injection of them from the bronchial arteries, renders the whole mucous membrane of the *bronchi* entirely red to the unassisted eye.[*]

The termination of arteries at the mucous surfaces has at all times occupied the attention of anatomists and physiologists; but it is unfortunately not a matter of sensible demonstration. The thin serous or sero-mucous fluid with which they are at all times moistened, has led every author almost, and among the rest Haller and Bichat, to infer the existence of arteries with open mouths, or what are termed exhalant vessels. If this be entirely denied, the pathologist, as well as the physiological enquirer, is deprived of a convenient source of explaining many vital phenomena. It has been admitted, nevertheless, more on analogical than direct proofs. The injections of Bleuland are the only experiments after those of Kawe Boerhaave, which, so far as I am acquainted, tend to confirm the conclusion.[†] These experiments, nevertheless, require to be repeated and extended.

That lymphatics are distributed to mucous membranes is a point well established. Cruikshank saw the lymphatics proceeding from the pulmonic mucous membrane loaded with blood in persons and animals dying of hæmoptoe. Their existence in the gastro-enteritic mucous membrane has been long established.

The mucous surfaces are also freely supplied by nervous twigs and filaments, derived in general from the nerves of automatic life. It is a mistaken view, nevertheless, to ascribe to these filaments the sensibility and other properties of the mucous surfaces. These mucous membranes possess intrinsically certain vital properties independently of the nervous filaments with which they are supplied; and the principal use of these filaments appears to be to regulate these properties, especially that of secretion.

* Franz Daniel Reisseissen, ueber die Bau der Lungen, u. s. w. Berlin, 1822.
† Experimentum Anatomicum, quo Arteriolarum Lymphaticarum existentia probabiliter adstruitur, &c. a Jano Bleuland, M. D. Lug. Bat. 1784. Item ; Jani Bleuland, M. D., &c., Vasculorum Intestinorum tenuium Tunicis subtilioris Anatomes Opera Detegendorum Descriptio Iconibus illustrata. Trajecti, 1797.

The progressive development of mucous membrane, and especially of its *villi*, has been studied by Meckel in the intestinal tube. This anatomist states, that in the beginning of the third month he first recognized them distinctly in the form of long plaits, (Längenfalten) thickly set on the inner surface of the intestine, and scarcely indented on their free edge. The number and depth of these folds, and their indentations, are gradually increased, till in the end of the fourth month, sometimes sooner, in place of the simple long plaits, the observer may distinguish an irregular multitude of minute elevations, which become proportionally larger at a later period of fœtal existence. He therefore infers that the *villi* are formed by the gradual indentation and decomposition (Zerfällung) of simple longitudinal plaits.*

The connection between the mucous membranes and the skin, I have elsewhere stated, was first well demonstrated by Bonn, who traces their mutual approximation and reciprocal transition into each other, and represents the former as an interior production of the latter enveloping the internal as the skin incloses the external organs.† This view has been adopted by Meckel and Beclard, to whom I refer for the proofs of its accuracy. I cannot conclude the subject, however, without observing that one of the most conclusive arguments in its favour is derived from the circumstances of the development of the intestinal canal during the first months of uterine life. The history of this curious process, which has been so happily investigated by Wolff and Oken‡, and so well traced by Meckel, shows that at this period the gastro-enteric mucous membrane, which is previously formed by the vitellar membrane of the ovum, and the *allantois* or vesical membrane, which afterwards forms the genito-urinary mucous surface, are in direct communication on the median line, and afterwards at the navel with the skin or exterior integument.§ The detailed history of this process belongs, however, rather to special than to general anatomy ; and I notice it here as the strongest proof which occurs to me of the connection between the skin and the mucous membranes, and as an

---

* Deutches Archiv für die Physiologie von J. F. Meckel, 3ter Band. Halle und Berlin, 1817. P. 68.

† Specimen Anatomico-Medicum Inaug. &c. Continuationibus Membranarum, &c. &c. In Sandifort Thes. Vol. II. p. 265. Rotterod. 1769.

‡ Jenaische Zeitung, S. 207–208.

§ Deutches Archiv für die Physiologie, Dritter B. Halle und Berlin, 1817:

anatomical fact which furnishes the solution of some curious congenital malformations, and of various morbid processes, which affect simultaneously, successively, or occasionally, both orders. of membranes.

SECTION II.

The morbid states of the mucous membranes are numerous and important, and constitute a large proportion of the diseases which daily come under the notice of the physician. Generally speaking, these morbid states may be referred to the following heads, inflammation and its effects, sero-albuminous effusion, suppuration and ulceration, hemorrhage, induration and thickening producing contraction or stricture, new growths, and malformation.

I. The inflammatory process in this tissue gives rise to a considerable number of diseases which long usage has distinguished according to the region, the mucous membrane of which is diseased. These affections, which agree in general characters, and vary only in certain points depending on situation and local peculiarity, may be conveniently arranged according as they take place; A. in the cephalic or facial mucous membrane; B. in the tracheo-bronchial mucous membrane; C. in the gastro-enteric membrane; and D. in the genito-urinary mucous membrane.

A. Cephalic division.	Eyelids and eye,	Ophthalmia.	
	Nasal duct,	Epiphora.	
	Nasal passages,	Coryza.	Ozæna.
	Tympanal cavity,	Tympania.	Otorrhœa.
B. Tracheo-bronchial division.	Throat,		
	Larynx,	Laryngia.	Cynanche laryngaea.
	Trachea,	Tracheitis.	Croup ; catarrh.
	Bronchial membrane,	Bronchia.	Bronchitis ; catarrh.
C. Alimentary division.	Œsophagus,	Œsophagia.	Inflammation of œsophagus.
	Stomach,	Gasteria.	Dyspeptic symptoms.
	Ileum,	Enteria.	Diarrhœa
	Colon,	Colonia.	Dysenteria.
D. Genito-Urinary division.	Ureter,	Ureteria.	
	Bladder,	Cystidia.	Catarrhus vesicæ.
	Urethra.	Urethria.	Gonorrhœa, Blennorrhagia.
	Womb and vagina,	Metria.	Leucorrhœa, &c.

In these several divisions of the mucous surfaces the anatomical characters of inflammation are much the same. The process takes place under two varieties, the spreading or diffuse, which extends over the surface of the membrane; and the punctuate or circumscribed, which affects many points at the same time. The membrane becomes red, injected, traversed by minute red points and vessels, sometimes arborescent or asteroid, sometimes punctular or in minute points, occasionally in linear streaks, and not unfrequently in red patches; the surface becomes swelled and villous or pulpy; and the proper secretions of the part are altered into sero-albuminous fluid, puriform mucus, or actual purulent matter. In situations in which there is epidermis, as in the mouth and gullet, this is elevated into minute vesicles and blisters forming *aphthæ*; or the membrane is cast off in the form of exfoliated patches. In the gastro-enteric membrane the *villi* are removed, and the surface is rendered plane like that of the rectum or bladder. The inflammation may terminate in the formation of ulcers; or in induration and permanent thickening of the mucous tissue by effusion of lymph beneath it, and into its substance. The follicles are at the same time liable to become enlarged and vascular, and occasionally proceed to ulceration; but this is more frequent in the chronic form of the process. The minute peculiarities will be more conveniently noticed under their respective heads.

A. CEPHALIC MUCOUS MEMBRANES.

§ 1. *Ophthalmia serosa et puriformis.*—The ophthalmic mucous membrane (*conjunctiva*) may be become the seat of inflammation, with secretion of sero-albuminous fluid, puriform fluid, or purulent matter. In the former case, in which the natural fluid appears simply to be much augmented, the inflammation is confined chiefly to the ocular conjunctiva, which is reddened and elevated, forming in severe cases round the cornea a prominent ring or excrescence, which appears to start from the eyelids—a state denominated by the ancient surgeons chasm or gaping (*chemosis*), because a small opening corresponding to the cornea is left in the centre of the swelled membrane. This severe form of the disease occasionally terminates in suppuration, ulceration, or sloughing.

Of the second form, two varieties are mentioned, the purulent ophthalmy of infants, and the purulent ophthalmy which affects epidemically large bodies of men in close intercourse with each other. In both cases, the mucous surface of the eye and eyelids is very red, swollen, villous, and pulpy, and puckered into folds by the violent action of the muscles; while the cornea is generally completely concealed by more or less chemosis, and the eyelids are everted. After continuing in this state for eight or ten days discharging much puriform yellow fluid, it may terminate in infants in resolution, but more generally produces specks or opacity of the cornea, ulceration, pustules, or chronic inflammation and thickening of the cornea, rendering that tunic opaque.   In adults, proceeding much in the same manner, its effects are generally more serious.   If it do not at an earlier period of the disease cause opacity, the cornea may be ruptured partially or generally, so as to allow the escape of the humours.   The membranous inflammation becoming in all cases also chronic, the surface of the conjunctiva becomes irregular by numerous minute hardish eminences or granulations; and this granular state of the palpebral *conjunctiva*, though originally an effect, becomes afterwards a cause of further inflammation.

The puriform ophthalmy originating from the gonorrhœal poison, though differing in its cause, is the same in its pathological effects.

β. A pustular form of ophthalmy is sometimes observed.   It consists in the appearance of minute eminences of the sclerotic mucous membrane near the circumference of the cornea.   These bodies, which may be considered either as aphthæ or pustules, are conoidal, and surrounded by a cluster of vessels which run into them either all round in a circular area, or from one side, most commonly the temporal.   When they are situate a line or two from the margin of the cornea, they are broad and flattened.   This disease seldom under proper treatment advances to suppuration or ulceration; and I have seen it disappear in thirty hours after being first seen.   It seems in some instances to consist in a punctuate deposition of lymph, in others to be a peculiar concentration of blood-vessels.   It is not impossible for it, however, to proceed to suppuration and form a minute abscess of the *conjunctiva*.   When these pustular eminences appear in the corneal mucous membrane, they generally pass into ulcers.

In some instances, with abatement of pain, diminution of swelling, and alleviation of other symptoms, the vessels appear much distended and distinct, though tortuous, the membrane is thickened in patches or continuously, and sero-albuminous fluid is deposited in spots or along the course of the vessels.   These appearances mark the transition of the disease into the chronic form.   Their persistence too often leaves the superficial speck (*nebula*), the triangular web, (*pterygium*), or the opaque spot, (*leucoma*.)

§ 2. *Watery eye; Epiphora.*—The mucous membrane of the eye and eyelids communicates with that of the nostrils by the narrow tube termed lacrymal duct.   A minute capillary opening at the

3

nasal extremity of each eyelid, termed *lacrymal* (*punctum lacry-male*), forms the upper or palpebral end of this canal; and its inferior or nasal extremity is a considerable opening in the lower nasal passage, between the lower spongy bone. This canal is lined by a fibro-mucous membrane, the free surface of which is moistened by a thin semitransparent, glairy fluid, not like the mucus of the nasal or tracheal membrane, but merely viscid enough to facilitate the descent of the tears, and to maintain a free communication between the eyelids and nostrils. This membrane may be inflamed in any part of its course, especially at the palpebral extremity; and the swelling attendant on this process in a canal so narrow produces a temporary obstruction to the transmission of the tears,—constituting the simple and acute form of the *watery* eye or *epiphora*. In ordinary circumstances this terminates in resolution, and the canal again becomes pervious in a few days. In more severe cases, however, either in consequence of thickening of the fibro-mucous membrane, or the effusion of albuminous fluid, the obstruction is more permanent; and if not seasonably removed, may induce secondary inflammation of the parietes of the canal, and ulceration and false openings; *(fistulæ.)* In all cases the inflammatory process may affect the subjacent periosteum of the lacrymal, nasal, and superior maxillary bones, and induce caries in one or more of them. With or without this latter complication, the disease constitutes lacrymal *fistula*. In either mode it is sometimes the result of syphilis, and very often where mercury has been given for the treatment of that disease.

Similar disease of the lacrymal duct may take place in consequence of previous chronic inflammation of the eyelids and Meibomian glands.

The mucous membrane of the nasal passages is inflamed in *Coryza*,—an affection forming the preliminary part of catarrh. A secondary *coryza* occurs in nasal polypus; and *ozæna*, which consists in chronic suppurative inflammation of the nasal membrane lining the nasal and covering the spongy bones, is always preceded by similar inflammation. The same process is not unfrequent in the fibro-mucous membrane of the maxillary sinus, in which it generally proceeds to suppuration, forming abscess of that cavity.

§ 3. *Otitis.*—The membrane of the external auditory passage is, strictly speaking, neither skin nor mucous membrane, but a texture intermediate between both. In its morbid relations it is, however, more closely connected with the latter, and is often the seat of inflammation producing a yellow puriform discharge (*otorrhœa*), from the outer surface of the tympanal membrane, and the membrane lining the ear-hole. The membrane is then red, soft, villous, and highly tender. The average duration of this disease is from fifteen days to three weeks, after which the fluid discharged becomes thicker, and in colour, consistence, and odour, resembles caseous matter. The ceruminous glands are disordered during its presence; but as it recedes their secretion becomes abundant.

§ 4. *Tympania.*—Though the membrane of the tympanal cavity and the Eustachian tube presents a smooth uniform surface, moistened by a thin watery fluid possessing little resemblance to mucus, yet, as continuous with the naso-guttural membrane, and as similar to that of the·facial sinuses, it may be placed in pathological properties in this situation. Bichat indeed corrects the error of those anatomists who represent the membrane of the tympanal cavity as periosteum; but in his anxiety to maintain its mucous he overlooks its fibrous character. Its adherent surface cannot be distinguished from the periosteum of the bones to which it adheres. When removed and dried it is thin, crisp, and semitransparent. During the inflammatory process it becomes red, thick, soft, and actually villous; and it secretes first serous, afterwards yellow puriform fluid, which cannot be distinguished from genuine purulent matter, though without ulceration.* In this disease an opening takes place in the membrane, which becomes fungous, or is eventually destroyed; the tympanal bones are discharged; and not unfrequently the inflammatory process spreading into the mastoid cells, fills these cavities with matter more or less viscid. In such circumstances it may affect the periosteal surface and cause caries of the bones, which are then found denuded and rough. Not unfrequently it causes inflammation of the *dura mater*, and cerebral membranes, and the brain itself.

§ 5. *Thrush; Aphthæ.*—The mucous membrane of the mouth and throat is liable to this form of inflammation, which depends on the presence of epidermis in this region. It is then elevated into whitish or ash-coloured vesicles or blisters, sometimes round or oval, sometimes irregular. The contained fluid is separated into two parts, one albuminous, forming the rudiment of new epidermis,

---

* " Le cadavre d'un homme exposé à ces écoulemens pendant sa vie, m'a présenté une épaisseur et une rougeur remarquables de la membrane du tympan, mais sans nulle trace d'erosion." Anat. Generale, Tome III. p. 430.

the other serous, which escapes while the old epidermis is cast in the form of scab or slough.

The mucous membrane of the throat and soft palate is affected by diffuse redness, swelling, and other marks of inflammation during the sore throat of scarlet fever. That of quinsy is more frequently seated in the submucous cellular tissue.

B. TRACHEO-BRONCHIAL MUCOUS MEMBRANE.

b. Inflammation of the tracheo-bronchial membrane may be distinguished as the process is developed; 1*st,* in the larynx; 2*d,* in the windpipe or proper tracheal membrane ; 3*d,* in the bronchial membrane; and, 4*th,* in the small bronchial tubes or pulmonic membrane. Though these inflammations possess certain common characters, each is attended by peculiarities which require attention.

§ 1. *α. Laryngia, Laryngitis. Cynanche Laryngaea. Laryngia acuta.*—Though this disease appears not to have been unknown to Cullen and some previous authors, we are indebted to Dr Baillie, Dr Farre, Dr Percival, Mr Lawrence, and Mr Howship, for a more accurate account of its pathology than we previously possessed.

The proper śeat of *laryngitis,* indeed, its characteristic symptoms and nature, had been overlooked in the attention paid to croup ; and when it was first observed carefully, as in the case of General Washington, it was called Croup in the adult. It is impossible to deny that the disease named *laryngitis* affects children as well as adults; and it may have often been mistaken for croup. From this, however, *laryngitis* differs in the parts which it affects, in the effects which it produces, and, in short, according to my own observation, in its anatomico-pathological nature and characters; and for these reasons I consider the disease separately.

It may be stated as a well-established fact, that the symptoms of this disease arise from inflammation circumscribed to a definite region of the larynx. Though the whole laryngeal membrane, from the *epiglottis* to the tracheal rings, is red and swelled, the particular point at which this morbid action is most injurious is that part of the mucous membrane which covers the arytenoid cartilages, and forms the chink called *glottis.* Though this part of the laryngeal membrane may not be more swelled than any other, a moderate degree of swelling soon diminishes the aperture so much that inspiration is rendered difficult or impossible, and the danger of suffocation becomes urgent. It must nevertheless be observed, that in many instances the margins of the glottis are occupied by an œdematous or puffy swelling, similar to that which occasionally affects the eyelids, prepuce, and female *labia,*—from sero-albuminous infiltration of the submucous filamentous tissue, and the effect of which is to diminish, or in some instances to obliterate, the aperture which regulates the admission of air into the trachea. The redness and swelling of the laryngeal membrane is occasionally more conspicuous at its posterior part than elsewhere; and the epiglottis is sometimes swelled and thickened with injection of its membrane; but whatever variations the disease presents, its effect on the membrane of the glottis is uniform; and this aperture is either much contracted or completely obliterated.

With redness and swelling, the laryngeal membrane is generally occupied by thick viscid mucus, which contributes by adhering to the margins of the glottis to obstruct the aperture. It is most abundant in the recesses called *sacculi,* where it assumes the appearance of purulent fluid. In some rare instances suppuration takes place with breach of surface; and purulent abscesses have been found between the thyroid or arytenoid cartilages, and their investing membrane. Reddening of the tracheal membrane is a complication. Inflammation confined chiefly to the membrane of the epiglottis is described by Sir E. Home;* and this with the arytenoid affection, Dr M. Hall shows, is the effect of the accidental attempt to swallow boiling water.†

Of laryngeal inflammation three terminations may be enumerated; 1*st,* resolution, which takes place some time between the 36th and 60th hour; 2*d,* fatal suffocation, which may take place any time after the 30th hour; and, 3*d,* a chronic state, with redness and thickening of the mucous membrane, sometimes with suppuration or ulceration of some part of the organ, which may be apprehended, if the disease continues without proving fatal for four revolutions of 24 hours.

β. *Laryngia chronica.*—The latter result is most usual after attacks so lenient as not to suffocate, but too severe to be completely resolved. The membrane then continues injected, thickened, and corrugated, rendering the individual hoarse and incapable of laryngeal speech. The duplicatures called superior vocal chords in particular, are irregularly thickened, partly by accumulation of blood within their vessels, partly by effusion of sero-albuminous fluid

---

* Transactions of a Society, Vol. III.   † Medico-Chirurg. Trans. Vol. XI.

into the submucous cellular tissue.   Often the epiglottis becomes
much thickened.   Its investing membrane is always reddened and
rough. After some time ulceration may take place in the epiglottis,
and destroy the top or anterior extremity of it.   This I have observed several times; the round apex of the epiglottis being cut off
as it were transversely by ulceration.   In other instances, it is merely
rendered thick, rigid, and inflexible, so that it no longer, when the
tongue is depressed, covers accurately the upper aperture of the
larynx.

Other appearances are the following.   The lower or true vocal
chords become thickened.   The membrane forming the ventricles of the larynx (*sacculi laryngis,*) is thickened, and occasionally presents minute ulcers of the surface.   The apices of the
arytenoid membranes are red, thickened, and abraded or ulcerated;
and sometimes this ulceration descends to the subjacent cartilages
or their perichondrial covering.   Constantly the perichondrium,
when the disease lasts any time or has recurred several times, is
thickened and rendered rough.

Even when the ulcers of the mucous membrane have been healed,
the membrane itself remains much thickened, rough, and sometimes
irregular by tubercular growths; and the perichondrium of the
cartilages is thick, soft, and easily detached.

In this state the diseased action is liable to spread to the cartilages, rendering them thick, painful, and sometimes producing
ulceration, and occasionally imperfect ossification.

In one or more points ulceration takes place generally in oval
patches, which spread and become deep, affecting the submucous
tissue and the perichondrium.   The ulcers which were previously an
effect, become now a cause of inflammation, and obstinately resisting all tendency to heal, continue to spread with chronic inflammation, and give rise to more or less wasting with hectic fever.   This
constitutes the disease described under the name of laryngeal consumption : (*phthisis laryngaea.*)   (Cayol.)

In some instances suppuration of the submucous filamentous
tissue takes place previous to ulceration of the membrane; and
though, by affecting the perichondrium on the one side, and the
laryngeal mucous membrane on the other, it may cause the same
chronic process as that now described, it is generally a milder and
more sanable disease.

In others it spreads to the cartilages, and by inducing ulceration or death of these bodies, causes an insanable disease speedily fatal. In Mr Dyson's case, in which the epiglottis and upper part of the trachea were ulcerated, the *os hyoides* became carious, and was exfoliated dead.*

Of both acute and chronic *laryngitis*, it is a peculiar character, that death often takes place suddenly, and sometimes when not expected.

The causes of chronic *laryngitis* are the same as those of the acute form ; that is, exposure to cold, previous attacks of the acute form, and extraordinary efforts of the voice in speaking, crying, or shouting. One cause, however, is so peculiar that it deserves mention. It consists in the use of mercury, often in repeated courses. In almost all the cases of chronic *laryngitis* which have come under my observation during the course of twenty-five years, the sufferers had been subjected to one or more full courses of mercurial medicines, and sometimes to several repeated courses. The effect of this was to render all the mucous surfaces prone to irritation and inflammation ; and especially where these surfaces are near the periosteum or perichondrium. The cases are always susceptible of alleviation ; but the symptoms invariably recur, showing the chronic nature of the disorder, and the firm hold which it takes of the larynx.

γ. *Ulceration of the Laryngeal and Tracheal membrane in phthisis.* —In persons cut off by tubercular consumption, minute ulcers of the laryngeal and tracheal membrane are not unfrequent. They vary in size, and are irregular in shape; but in general they appear in the form of angular or oval spots, from which the mucous membrane has been entirely removed. In the larynx of a young woman in my collection, I count five of these eroded spots affecting the oval shape, none of more extent than one square line, and one patch evidently formed by the coalescence of two, as large as the section of a split pea ; and in the tracheal membrane of the same subject, at the bronchial bifurcations, large patches of the same description are visible. In the latter situation, indeed, this destruction is more common and more extensive than in any other point.

The most frequent site of ulcers of the larynx, according to Louis, is the junction of the vocal chords; then the vocal chords themselves ; and lastly, the base of the arytenoid cartilages, the upper part of the larynx and the *sacculi.* In the trachea these ulcers occupy chiefly the posterior part. The bronchial mem-

* Mem. Med. Society, Vol. IV.

brane is, according to the same authority, less frequently ulcerated; but when not so, it is almost invariably reddened.

b. Ulceration of the Tracheal Membrane and Cartilages.—This is not a very frequent lesion, but it is liable to take place. It is seen mostly in the posterior surface of the trachea; and though probably it may take place in several points, yet I have never seen more than one or at most two ulcers, one generally large. No doubt can be entertained that ulcers of this kind are the result of inflammation attacking the mucous membrane of the trachea; but on the early history of these ulcers we possess no correct information. The following details will convey some idea of the appearance and characters of these ulcers.

In one case, taking place in a man of about 48 or 50 years of age, the individual suffered much from constant difficulty of deglutition, a sense of soreness and rawness in the throat, great hoarseness, cough, difficult breathing, and scanty expectoration occasionally streaked with blood. All solids and fluids caused during deglutition much suffering, and a feeling of impending suffocation; and the patient of his own accord requested food of a semifluid character. Even this was swallowed with little less difficulty, and with much of the gasping and suffocating feeling. Soon after death took place.

The laryngeal mucous membrane was red, thickened, and covered with a considerable quantity of thick puriform mucus. This was abundant in the *sacculi* between the superior and inferior vocal chords. The laryngeal mucous membrane presented abrasions and ulcerations. The epiglottis was thickened, reddened, rigid, and ulcerated at its apex. The tracheal membrane was very much reddened, and as if roughened. About one inch and a half below the cricoid cartilage, immediately above the bifurcation of the trachea on the posterior surface, was first one elliptical ulcer, then another smaller, both with the long axis in the long direction of the windpipe. The first ulcer was about three-fourths of one inch or nearly one inch long; the other about one-fourth of an inch long. Both were formed by total destruction of the mucous membrane and part of the sub-mucous tissue; and the base of the ulcer was formed by part of that connecting the windpipe to the œsophagus. The edges of both were ulcerated, irregular, and ragged, and consisted of jagged points; but this was caused by the projection of the extremities of the cartilaginous rings, which were cut right across, and being less destroyed than the connecting mucous membrane, left between them hollow spaces. The cartilages also projected into the interior of the trachea, being no longer held down by the mucous membrane uniting with those of the opposite side.

This man, like many persons under laryngeal disease, had been previously subjected to several courses of mercurial medicines.

In another case I saw an ulcer of the trachea take place under peculiar circumstances.

A female between 40 and 45 years of age was affected with chronic *laryngitis;* and over this was super-induced an acute attack so intense, that immediate suffocation was threatened. For relieving her sufferings and averting the fatal termination, it was deemed necessary to perform the operation of laryngotomy or tracheotomy. This was accordingly done with very beneficial results, the breathing being much relieved, and the urgent symptoms of suffocation in•the meantime removed. The tube was inserted and kept in the wound for about three weeks or longer, being withdrawn only to cleanse the wound, and remove mucus and purulent matter.

About this time it was recommended to the patient to try to breathe without the tube; but she found that this was impracticable. Meanwhile the same course was pursued for about three weeks longer, during which the patient did not appear to be recovering the power of breathing through the larynx. Uneasiness and soreness were felt in the windpipe; and this it was natural to ascribe to the wound. After some days longer of struggling, irritation, distress and agony, the patient suddenly expired.

The laryngeal membrane was red, thickened, rough, and irregular; and when the abundant mucus was removed, minute abrasions were observed. The chords, both superior and inferior, were thickened and swelled. The wound was healthy and granulating, though slowly and irregularly. At the posterior surface of the trachea, about one inch and a-half below the cricoid cartilage, a large elliptical ulcerated destruction of the mucous membrane had taken place. The edges and outlines of this were irregular. The long diameter corresponded to the axis of the trachea. In some parts this ulcer was deep, almost proceeding through to the œsophagus; in others it was more superficial. The ulcerated extremities of the cartilaginous rings were, however, exposed in the same manner, and prominent, as in the case last mentioned; and gave the ulcer the same ragged appearance.

This large ulcer corresponded so accurately to the extremity of the tube, which was kept in the wound, that it seemed impossible to doubt that it had been produced by the constant pressure and irritation of the tube on the posterior surface of the windpipe. I am aware that it may be said, that if the tube were so placed, it was improperly placed ; and not only must have produced irritation in the windpipe, but could not have acted as a tube to convey air into the windpipe and out again in the actions of respiration. It is also possible that some ulcer or ulceration may have existed there previously, and may have been associated, as is often the case, with chronic disease of the larynx. To this it is not necessary to give any other answer than merely stating the facts of the case.

This patient had been subjected to the use of mercury in full courses, more than once; and of this the laryngeal affection was the result.

§ 2. *a.* Croup (*Bronchiasis albuminosa*) may be defined to be inflammation of the tracheo-bronchial mucous membrane, terminating in sero-albuminous exudation. The points deserving attention in the pathology of this disease, are, 1*st*, the fact of.inflammation; 2*d*, the extent of the process ; and, 3*dly*, its effects. The inflamed state of the tracheo-bronchial membrane is established beyond doubt. Home observed that it was redder than natural when the concrete covering is detached; Rumsey recognized manifest traces of inflammation ; in Cheyne's cases the vessels of the membrane were large, distinct, and sometimes numerous, (9th.) The same was seen by Albers, Jurine, and Bretonneau. In short, whether the membranous exudation be present or absent, the tracheobronchial membrane is always more or less red, bloodshot, villous, and swollen ; and puriform fluid oozes from the bronchial tubes.

This inflammation is seated in the tracheo-bronchial membrane solely. It begins immediately below the cricoid cartilage, and extends along the tube into the *bronchi* and bronchial membrane. It is less frequently observed to affect the laryngeal membrane; and when it does so, this is to be viewed as a complication not essential to genuine croup. It may, nevertheless, in extreme cases, affect the pharynx, larynx, and trachea, covering their surface with a false membranous exudation. The disease, from this circumstance, receives the name of *Diphtheritis.*

The effect of this inflammation is to produce from the surface of the membrane a fluid or semifluid secretion, which soon undergoes

o o

coagulation after exposure to the air. In the upper part of the
trachea this substance is firm and in the form of a tubular membrane moulded on the canal; below and in the bronchial divisions
it is less firm ; in the tubes it is completely fluid.* (Home, Cheyne,
Bretonneau.) The nature of this morbid exudation has been a
matter of ambiguity. Home, who remarked that the tubular membrane when complete is tough and thick, might be soaked in water
for days without dissolving, that it does not adhere to the windpipe, as there is always fluid matter beneath it, and that beyond it,
the windpipe, bronchial tubes, and pulmonic vesicles, are covered
by pus or purulent mucus, thought it of the nature of thickened
mucus. In one case Rumsey calls it viscid mucus or phlegm; in
others he likens it to the buffy coat. Field regards it as coagulable
lymph; Cheyne, with some confusion, compares it to the exudation of the inflamed pleura or peritonæum, and accounts it thickened
puriform fluid; while by Pinel and most of the recent authorities,
it is identified with albuminous exudation. According to the investigation of its chemical properties by Schwilgué, Maunoir and
Peschier, and Jurine, it appears to contain albumen in various proportions, and to owe to this principle its tenacity and firmness.
Bretonneau, in particular, endeavours to establish a distinction
between the tracheo-bronchial exudation, the albuminous concretions of serous membranes, and the buffy coat, but without success.†
It may be inferred, therefore, that this substance, without being
either wholly coagulable lymph, or thickened mucus, or dried purulent matter, is a morbid product secreted from the tracheo-bronchial mucous surface, in a semifluid form, and undergoing, in consequence of the presence of albuminous or albumino-gelatinous
matter, coagulation, as it is more freely exposed to air.

Death is produced in this disease chiefly by the albuminous fluid
in the bronchial tubes and vesicles excluding the air from the pulmonary membrane.

β. *Bronchiasis albuminosa adultorum.*   *Polypose inflammation of
the trachea.*—Not very dissimilar is that morbid state of the tracheo-
bronchial membrane, in which a membranous concretion, moulded
on the tube, is, from time to time, brought up by coughing either

---

* " We can even demonstrate," says Cheyne, " the adventitious membrane degene-
rating into the puriform fluid, and again gaining consistence in different parts of the
same membrane."

† Des Inflammations du Tissu Muqueux, et en particulier de la Diphtherite, &c.
Paris, 1826. P. 293.

in fragments or entire. Instances of this disease, which is not common, were first observed by T. Bartholine,[*] N. Tulpius,[†] Ruysch,[‡] Clarke,[§] Lister, Cheselden, Bussiere,[||] Samber,[¶] F. Nicholls,[**] Warren,[††] John Andrew Murray,[‡‡] Callisen,[§§] Baillie, and Laennec.

The mode of their formation is not established without ambiguity. In many instances they are the result of a modification of the inflammatory process. In some, however, in which they are connected with bronchial or pulmonary hemorrhage, they appear to be formed by the coagulation of blood not discharged at the time of hemorrhage.

§ 3. *Bronchial Inflammation, acute, and chronic. Bronchiasis puriformis ; Bronchitis.*—Bronchitis may be distinguished into two varieties, according to the portions of the air-tubes which it affects. The disease may be confined chiefly, if not solely, to the large and middle-sized bronchial tubes, in short, where the mucous membrane lines tubes, properly so called ; or it may either, with or without affection of these, be seated principally in the terminal ends or vesicles where the membrane is more delicate, and the tubes are much smaller. In the former case, the impediment to respiration is much less considerable than in the latter, in which, from their small size, any thickening or new secretion produces most serious and alarming labour in breathing, with great anxiety and distress. The former may be termed tubular *bronchitis*, the latter vesicular *bronchitis*, or bronchitis of the vesicles, or of the small bronchial tubes and terminal ends of the small bronchial tubes.

I am aware that the latter is by some believed to constitute pneumonia or inflammation of the lungs; and, in point of fact, in all cases of pneumonia or inflammation of the substance of the lungs, there is a considerable affection of the terminal ends of the *bronchi ;* and in cases of affection of the vesicles on the other hand, there is sooner or later some affection of the pulmonic tissue. In short, the two diseases pass into each other, and in most cases co-exist.

* Centur. iii. Hist. 98.   † Obs. Lib. ii. Obs. 7.
‡ Epistola Anatomica, VI. p. 9 et 11. Amstelodami, 1659. Op. Om. Tom. II.
§ Phil. Trans. No. 235, p. 779 and 780. Vol. XIX.
|| Ibid. No. 263, p. 545. Vol. XXII.
¶ Ibid. No. 398, p. 262.   ** Ib. No. 419, p. 123.
†† Transactions of College of Physicians, Vol. I. p. 407.
‡‡ Commentatio de Polypis Bronchiorum. Goettingæ, 1773. Opuscula, Vol. I. 1785. VI. p. 255.
§§ Observatio de Concretione Polyposa, Cava, Ramosa, tussi rejecta. Acta Societatis Medicæ Havniensis, Vol. I. Havniæ, 1777. Art. IV. p. 76.

This, however, is no reason for confounding these affections in a work like the present, in which morbid processes are considered in an analytical manner, according to the individual elementary textures which they affect. This analytical method leads to no error; and it enables the pathologist more clearly to understand the characteristic differences of closely allied diseases.

a. Tubular bronchitis. Bronchitis affecting the large and middle-sized air-tubes.—In tubular *bronchitis*, then, the inflammatory disorder is very much confined to the large and middle sized bronchial tubes; and as this disease as a primary affection is not often fatal, and is chiefly so by recurring frequently, or by the morbid action extending to the small tubes and the vesicles, it is not possible to speak accurately of its anatomical characters as an isolated affection. When in these circumstances the membrane is examined, it is found brown-coloured, sometimes dark red, rough, and swelled, with more or less contraction of the area of the bronchial tubes. These tubes are lined by viscid jelly-like mucus, streaked with blood or embrowned. In some instances the mucus is puriform, yet adheres to the membrane.

This form of bronchitis takes place not only in catarrh, but in the course of continued fever, of typhus fever, in measles, in scarlet fever, and in small-pox. It is also an invariable accompaniment of tubercular destruction in consumption, and is frequent in cases of diseased heart, especially hypertrophy and valvular disease.

By frequent recurrence it is liable to produce symptoms of asthma, or to pass into chronic catarrh, with *dyspnœa*, or into dry catarrh. It then gives rise to winter cough.

Tubular *bronchitis* may terminate in health by the gradual sub-sidence of the inflammation; in vesicular *bronchitis* by extending to the vesicular mucous membrane; in thickening of the tubular membrane and contraction of the tube, (*stenochoria bronchorum*,) causing symptoms of asthma, breathlessness, and more or less ebro-nic cough, aggravated especially in the winter, during cold weather, and on the accession of any slight cold; in emphysema of the lungs with breathlessness; in œdema of the lungs; in serous effusion within the *pleura* (*hydropleura; hydrothorax,*) and in general dropsy.

The formidable terminations last mentioned seldom take place until the disease has recurred several times; and as it is always liable to recur after the first attack, it necessarily renders the bronchial tubes less fit for the purpose of admitting air to the vesicles. In the bodies of those destroyed under this advanced stage of the disease the following appearances are recognised.

· 1. Collapse of the lungs, on opening the chest, either imperfect or none; the lungs inelastic, doughy, and gorged with venous blood; sometimes œdematous, sometimes slightly solidified. 2. The *bronchi* and large bronchial tubes containing a considerable quantity of viscid, opaque, tenacious mucus adhering firmly to the membrane; the membrane itself in the *bronchi* and large tubes reddened, rough, in some parts swelled, and of a colour more or less brown. 3. Several of the bronchial tubes present portions in which the area of their canal is more or less, sometimes considerably, contracted, forming a degree of bronchial stricture. 4. Parts of the lungs, especially near their margin, present air in their filamentous tissue, and sometimes bladders of air, forming *emphysema* of the lungs. 5. In some instances a few of the bronchial tubes, especially towards the lower part of the lung, may be dilated to a greater capacity than natural. 6. In certain cases they are narrowed, or altogether closed and obliterated.

b. Vesicular Bronchitis. Inflammatio Vesicularum.—In the second variety, either with or without the affection of the membrane of the large and middle-sized tubes, inflammation attacks the pulmonic or vesicular division of the bronchial mucous membrane.

The pathology of this disease, though understood by Morgagni, De Haen, and Stoll, has been more fully illustrated by the researches of Chevalier, Badham, Abercrombie, Hastings, and Laennec. Dissections of persons cut off in different stages of the disease show that the bronchial membrane is much reddened and injected, villous or pulpy, and thickened or swelled. As the disease proceeds, it discharges viscid puriform mucus, or muco-purulent fluid, which fills the air-cells or vesicles, and prevents the lungs from collapsing when the chest is opened. The tracheal membrane may be reddened or traversed by arborescent red lines; and though the bronchial membrane is in general entire, in some instances small ulcerated breaches are observed in various parts.

In the chronic form, the membrane, though red and villous, is rarely so much swelled as in the acute disease; but minute ulcers or patches of ulceration are more common.

The effect of this process in the bronchial membrane is to augment the quantity and change the quality of the fluid secreted in the natural state. At the commencement of the process, the bluish,

semitransparent, and particled mucus of health is mixed with mucilaginous, semitransparent, and grayish fluid, not unlike white of
egg, which is secreted in considerable quantity.   As the process
advances, it becomes thicker, more viscid and opaque, and sinks in
water; and when fully established, this viscid mucus is either
mingled with, or converted into yellowish opaque fluid, which cannot be distinguished from purulent matter, and which is generally
more or less streaked with blood.   These changes may be effected
without breach of continuity or ulceration of the membrane.   This
fact, which was first established by Dè Haen,* has since been fully
confirmed by Willan,† Badham,‡ George Pearson,§ and Hastings.‖
The process of suppurative secretion is attended with hectic fever
and wasting.

Though ulcers, however, are not essential to chronic inflammation
of the bronchial membrane, they may occur, and are most common
in the lungs of those whose occupation exposes them to inhalation
of irritating mechanical powders.   Such, for example, has dissection shown to be the state of the bronchial membrane in stone-
cutters,¶ glass-grinders, needle-grinders, and leather-dressers.

  c. *Pustular Inflammation.*—On the nature of a form of ulcer considerably different we have less certain information.   In several
cases of bronchial disease, the membrane becomes the seat of numerous minute eminences, which, as they may be traced through the
stages of inflammation, suppuration, and ulceration, may be regarded
as pustules of the pulmonic mucous membrane.   The ulcers thus
formed are in general round or oval, rarely irregular, with margin
slightly raised, and surrounded by a red circle, (*areola,*) more or
less distinct.   The matter expectorated consists of purulent fluid,
streaked with blood, and mingled with a considerable proportion of
dense mucus.   The analogy between this and certain ulcers of the
intestinal mucous membrane is obvious.   It gives rise to wasting
and hectic fever.

  d. *Induration, Consolidation.*—When chronic inflammation subsists long, the inflammatory action extends to the submucous filamentous tissue, which unites the bronchial tubes and vessels to the
serous membrane of the lungs—the parenchymatous or cellular tissue

---

* Rationis Medendi, I. xi. p. 60.   † Reports, 1796, 20th March.
  ‡ Observations on the Inflammatory Affections of the Mucous Membrane of the
Bronchiæ, &c. pp. 48—76.
  § Phil. Trans. 1809, Part ii. p. 315—321.
  ‖ Treatise on Inflammation of the Mucous Membrane, &c.
  ¶ Johnstone of Worcester, Mem. Med. Society.

of the older anatomists.   Of this the first effect is redness, with vascular injection of the submucous tissue (*infarctio.*)   As the morbid state of the blood-vessels continues or increases, sero-albuminous fluid is effused into its interstices; the part loses its natural softness and elasticity; and as the process extends, the lung loses the spongy lightness which depends on permeability of its vesicles.   In a lung in which the chronic inflammation of the submucous tissue has subsisted for some time, the following phenomena are recognized :— 1*st*, On opening the chest and admitting the air, though there are no adhesions, the lung collapses imperfectly or not at all; 2*d*, The pulmonic tissue surrounding a portion of inflamed membrane becomes hard and dense, and floats deep or sinks in water; 3*d*, Deprived of its elasticity and compressibility, it cannot be inflated, does not crepitate, and resembles a portion of solid flesh.   In such circumstances bronchial inflammation is complicated with *pneumonia.*

  *e. Bronchitis from the presence of foreign bodies.—Bronchitis alienorum.—*A variety of chronic bronchial inflammation, important from its close resemblance to consumption, is that occasioned by the presence of foreign bodies which have dropped accidentally into the windpipe.   Of this species of disease many cases are recorded, as having occurred to different observers; and the facts of these cases show at once the influence of the cause alleged in producing chronic, bronchial, and occasionally pulmonary inflammation, closely imitating pulmonary consumption, and the great efforts made by the system in striving to get rid of a source of great and possibly fatal irritation.

  Foreign bodies which drop into the air passages may produce one of two effects.   First, a foreign body dropping into the larynx may, by fixing itself in the ventricles, or in the *rima glottidis*, cause immediate suffocation.   This result will depend on its shape, or its consistence, and its size.   Thus, portions of food masticated, or imperfectly masticated, are occasionally observed to produce suffocation and immediate death.   Or, secondly, a foreign body may drop into the larynx, and by passing entirely through the *rima glottidis*, may get into the windpipe and one of the bronchial tubes, and stopping there, cause great irritation and inflammation of the parts, indicated by frequent, urgent, and distressing cough; fits of difficult breathing; expectoration of dense, puriform mucus, often with blood; and wasting of the flesh and strength of the individual, nearly in the same manner and to the same extent as in pulmonary consumption. It is, indeed, remarkable that, in all the re-corded cases, the symptoms thus produced have borne so close a resemblance to *phthisis*, that they have in most instances been con-sidered as examples of consumptive disease, and by several they are described as such.

The bodies which have in this manner been known to drop into the windpipe are various; beans,* nuts,† walnuts,‡ cherry stones,§ plumb stones,‖ an iron nail,¶ a leaden shot,** teeth, natural and artificial,†† ears of grass,‡‡, fragments of bones, a fragment of nut-meg,§§ pieces of money,‖‖ and similar substances. Of various pointed and well authenticated examples of this accident and its effects, I published in 1834 a collection, with the view of showing the true nature and effects of the lesion and its degree of frequency; and the most instructive mode of presenting the results of this series of cases, I believe to be placing them in the tabular form which is here subjoined. This list I might have enlarged more than I have done. But I believe that the present table gives a sufficient number of well established and accurately detailed facts to enable the reader to form just ideas on the nature of the disorder, and to compare the facts with the inferences deduced.

* Boussier de la Bouchardiere. Journal de Medecine, xlv. p. 267. Guincourt in Journal de Medecine, continué. xii. p. 44.

Allard, Journal de Physique, T. li.

Klein Chirurgische Bemerkungen, p. 168. Vicq D'Azyr Memoires de la Societé de Medecine, Vol. IV. Chir. N. 3, fatal on 6th day.

† Ephemerides Naturæ Curiosorum, Dec. ii. Ann. i. Obs. 144.

‡ Ephemerides Naturæ Curiosorum, Decad. iii. Ann, iii. Obs. 18. Dr Scott's case in Dr Craigie's Memoir.

§ Ephemerides Naturæ Curiosorum, Dec. ii. Ann. x. Obser. 66. Desault Oeuvres Chirurgicales, 2ieme Tome.

‖ Deschamps in Journal de Medecine, continué, ii. p. 555.

¶ Morton Phthisiologia, Lib. iii. cap. vi. p. 143. London, 1689.

Howship's Practical Observations in Medicine and Morbid Anatomy, p. 222.

Dr Craigie's Case. See page 590.

** Birch History of the Royal Society, Tome III. Robert Hooke, Collections. Transactions of a Society, Vol. III. Lond. 1812.

†† Cases in Memoir by Dr Craigie. Edin. Medical and Surgical Journal, Vol. XLII. p. 103. Edin. 1834.

‡‡ Histoire et Memoires de Thoulouse, II., ejected by abscess in the side ; phthisical symptoms ; and Dr Donaldson's case in Edinburgh Medical and Surgical Journal, Vol. XLII. p. 102. Edin. 1834.

§§ Borelli P. Observationes Medico-Physicæ. Cent. IV. Obs. 63.

‖‖ De la Martiniere dans Memoires de l'Academie de la Chirurgie, Tome V. Re-mained five years. Mr Key's Case ; and the Case of Sir I. Brunell by Sir B. Brodie. Medico-Chirurgical Transactions.

Authority.	Sex and age.	Object which dropped into windpipe.	Symptomatic effects.	Length of time it continued there.	Termination.
Stalpart van der Wiel Observationes Medico-Anatomico-Chirurg. L. B. 1687. Obs. 23, p. 97.	A girl aged 9.	A fragment of veal bone.	Constant cough ; expectoration of purulent matter ; haemoptysis ; fever and wasting.	Four months.	Ejection ; recovery.
Morton in Phthisiologia, Lib. ii. cap. vi. p. 143. Am, 1689.	A young man residing in Cirplegate.	Three iron nails.	Cough ; difficult breathing ; pain in breast and side ; cough most urgent ; complete wasting in the course of five weeks; hectic fever ; and death.	Several ms., without symptoms beyond cough.	Death ; no ejection.
Mr Thomas Amt, Edin. Med. Essays, v. Art. lvii. p.613. 1744	D. Hedderwick. 30 years.	A fragment of veal bone.	Cough ; difficult breathing; purulent expectoration; die ; emaciation.	36 to 40 days, probably longer.	Ejection ; recovery.
M. his in Mém. de Ad. de Chir. T.v. p.528. Paris,1774.	An engraver.	A Louis d'or.	Cough, difficult deg, expectoration, and wasting ; with the usual symptoms of phthisis.	5 years.	Death ; no ejection.
M. et Mem. de l' Ad. de Mr., T. V. p. 532.	Soldier of Piedmont Infantry.	Triangular fragment of bone with sharp angles.	Cough in frequent fits ; great ity in breathing; puriform expectoration ; spitting of blood ; pleuritic pains in left side , wasting.	10 months.	Eject. great and violent efforts, dth. 3 days after.
M. Sue in Mem. de l'Acad. de Chirurg. T. v. p. 533.	A girl between 8 and 9.	Fragment of back-bone of pigeon.	Cough very violent ; difficult breathing , expectoration of puriform matter , haemoptysis , pain in larynx and windpipe , phthisis.	15½ years. Partial recovery at 21.	Eject. ; death 18 m. after at 26.
Frid.Lud.Bang.Acta Regiæ Med. Societ. Hav. 1783. Vol.i. p.96.	A soldier.	A fragment of bone as large as a small nut.	Cough , difficult breathing ; muco-purulent expectation ; die and wasting.	Five months.	Ejection ; recovery.
Ibid. p. 23.	An adult female	Fragment of bone.	Cough at first dry, with pain of left chest, then copious purulent and bloody expectoration; wasting.	18 months.	Ejection ; recovery.
J. B. Borsieri Inst. Medicinæ Pract. Vol.iii. cap.xvii.1787–90	Girl, 10 to 12.	First molar tooth.	Cough ; expectoration tinged with blood ; pleuritic pain.	6 to 7 weeks.	Ejection and recovery.
Desault Oëuvres Chirurg. T. ii. p. 258. Paris, 1801.	Male about 30.	Cherry-stone.	Cough ; difficult breathing, and symptoms of laryngeal phthisis.	2 years.	Death ; no ejection.
Mr Holman in London Med. & Surg. Journal, Vol. vii. P. 126.		Fragment of bone ¾ of an inch long.	Cough, expectoration of blood and purulent matter, hectic and wasting.	15 years.	Ejection and recovery.
Pelletan ue Chirurg. T. i. 5ieme Obs. p. 10. Paris, 1810.	A boy aged 12.	A rounded conical pebble.	Cough, violent and continued ; puriform expectoration ; bile, and difficult breathing, with great anguish ; great wasting and debility.	22 days. Ejected after tracheotomy.	Death at end of 8 months.
P an Clinique Chirurg. T. I. Obs. 6, p. 12.	Individual up in years ; male.	Frag. of woollen cloth with long pile, from his sleeping-gown.	Cough ; expectoration of puriform matter ; difficult breathing ; wasting ; phthisical symptoms.	Several months ; received the previous winter.	Eject. after 3 hours' cough, death.

Authority.	Sex and age.	Object which dropped into windpipe.	Symptomatic effects.	Length of time it continued there.	Termination.
Memoirs of Life and Writings of Dr Lettsom, Lond. 1817. Vol. iii. p. 82.	Boy from 9 to 10.	Foil or worked covering of a button.	Cough, hoarseness, expectoration of puriform mucus, night-sweats, and wasting.	7 to 8 months.	Ejection and recovery.
Trans. of a Society, Vol. iii. Dr Mervin Nooth. Lond. 1812.	Dr Mervin Nooth.	A leaden shot, one-eighth of an inch in diameter.	Urgent cough; difficult breathing; expectoration of dense mucus; constant quick pulse; anxiety, and pectoral distress.	Many months.	Ejection; recovery.
Howship's Practical Observations on Surgery and Morbid Anatomy, p. 222. Lond. 1816.	James Butler, 25, carpenter.	An iron nail.	Cough very violent; expectoration of puriform mucus and blood; great wasting, with fever; hemoptysis.	4 months,—15th April–12th August.	Ejection and recovery.
Schroeder van der Kolk Observationes Anatomico Pathologicae. Amstelodami, 1826.	A young female of 26 years.	A small bone.	Incessant harassing cough; pain in breast; anxiety; pulse frequent and hard; emaciation; hectic; and phthisical symptoms.	Not mentioned; but about 12 weeks, upwards.	No ejection; death.
Dr Craigie from Dr Abercrombie and patient's sister.	A lady of middle age.	An artificial tooth with a metal screw.	Harassing cough; laryngeal and tracheal irritation; dense muco-purulent expectoration; quick pulse; pectoral uneasiness; wasting and debility.	2 years and 7 months.	Ejection and temporary recovery.
Dr John Scott, in Dr Craigie's Paper, Edin. Med. and Surg. Journal, Vol. xlii. p. 379.	A boy 4 years of age.	Fragment of a walnut.	Cough; quick pulse, 120–140; night-sweats; muco-purulent expectoration; wasting of flesh, and weakness.	50 days.	Ejection and recovery.
Dr Gilroy, Edin. Med. and Surg. Journal, Vol. xxxv. p. 293.	A lady 40 years of age.	A chicken bone.	Cough; difficult breathing; quick pulse; expectoration of purulent matter; hectic fever.	82 days.	Death; no ejection.
Dr Evanson, Dublin Journal of Medical Science, Vol. V. p. 19.	An infant, 1 year and 1 month old.	A herring bone.	Cough severe and rending; difficult breathing; symptoms of bronchitis of right lung, and croup.	4 days.	Tracheot. probable eject on 8th recovery.
Dr Houston, Dublin Journal of Med. Science, Vol.V. p. 42. 1834.	John Clare, aged 29.	Body and root of second molar tooth of right upper jaw.	Cough; difficult breathing; great uneasiness in chest; expectoration of frothy mucus; symptoms of bronchitis and pneumonia.	11 days.	Death. No ejection:
Dr Donaldson, Edin. Med. and Surg. Journ. Vol. XLII. p. 102.	Miss E. F., 11 years.	An ear of grass.	Cough; pain of chest; fetid expectoration; disorder of stomach; wasting; hectic.	7 weeks.	Ejection; recovery.
Dr Craigie. See p. 590.	Master M. L. aged 5 years.	An iron screw-nail, rather more than half an inch long.	Cough urgent and harassing; expectoration of dense puriform mucus; p. 110–120; hectic; wasting; temporary recovery; another attack, with great wasting.	From 12 to 13 or 14 months, probably 2 years.	Ejection; recovery.

' This tabular statement contains 24 cases, among which eight terminated in death, five of these being cases in which the body was not ejected.

In each of the cases terminating favourably the usual symptoms of chronic, bronchial, and even of pulmonary inflammation were induced; and purulent expectoration with occasional hemoptysis, and hectic and great wasting, threatened certain death. In each, however, after a lapse of weeks, months, or years, the foreign body was rejected by coughing when least expected, and recovery eventually took place. Though this favourable issue prevents the pathologist from ascertaining with certainty the exact nature and extent of the lesion, it is reasonable, from the facts disclosed by inspection of the fatal cases, to infer that the bronchial membrane certainly, and probably the pulmonic tissue, were maintained in a state of chronic inflammation during the presence of the foreign body.

Among the fatal cases are six in which the state of the parts was inspected after death; and from these we learn several instructive facts.

1. In the case given by Morton, the patient, after the first irritative symptoms were over, suffered so little inconvenience, and was apparently so well, that for several months he pursued his business or profession as a whitewasher, and entered into the matrimonial state. On the evening of the day of marriage, however, he was attacked with most acute pain of the breast and side, difficult breathing, and frequent dry cough, so urgent that he could neither lie in bed nor sleep. Fever followed; and, notwithstanding the active and judicious use of approved remedies, the symptoms of pulmonic inflammation and suppuration with hectic were established, and death took place at the end of five weeks.

The three nails were found a little below the division of the *bronchi*, buried, as it were, in a bed of purulent matter, which was also spreading gradually through the lungs. The cavity of the pleura contained about six pints of purulent matter.

2. In the case of the engraver recorded by De la Martiniere and Louis, the left lung was sound. The right lung was almost entirely destroyed by suppuration. The right cavity of the chest was filled with purulent matter; and the Louis d'or was found placed perpendicularly at the upper part of the right lung at the first bifurcation of the *bronchus* on this side.

In this case the piece of money had produced inflammation, first in the large bronchial tubes, where it was fixed, then in the lung, and afterwards in the pleura.*

3. In the case communicated by M. Lenglet to M. De la Martiniere in which a splinter of bone triangular in shape, with sharp angles and cutting edges, one side 9 lines long, had remained 10 months in the bronchial tubes, the right lung was natural, but the left in a state of putrefaction. About four inches below the bifurcation on the left side was a preternatural cavity of the capacity of a large nutmeg; and in this cavity the bone had been lodged.†

4. In the case given by Dr Milroy, in the centre of the right lung was found a large abscess containing about twenty ounces of purulent matter, of reddish-brown colour, and fetid odour. The piece of chicken bone, which was light and porous, weighing only six grains, lay in the upper part of the right *bronchus*, close to the bifurcation of the trachea. This tube (I suppose the right *bronchus*) communicated with the upper part of the abscess.

5. In the case given by Schroeder, the right lung was occupied by several tubercles, among which was a vomica in the middle lobe, filled not with purulent matter but with black gore. The left lung contained everywhere tubercles and several small *vomicœ*, and in the left *bronchus* about one inch from the bifurcation of the trachea was a splinter of bone covered with black viscid mucus. This bone was rough, and its angles had so completely penetrated the bronchial mucous membrane, that it could be moved neither upwards nor downward.

6. In the case given by Dr Houston, the broken tooth was found lying in the right bronchial tube about one inch beyond its commencement, with the fangs directed towards the lung, and the broken surface of the crown towards the larynx. It lay loose and unattached, and when caught between the points of the scissors was readily removed. The broken surface fitted accurately to that of the crown as presented by the patient to Dr Houston.

The right lung adhered to the *pleura costalis* everywhere except behind, where bloody fluid lay between the pleuræ. The adhesions were soft and easily broken; the right pulmonic pleura was livid. The substance of the right lung was dense and indurated through-

* Memoires de l'Academie Royale de Chirurgie, Tome V., p. 528-531. Paris, 1774.

† Ibid. p. 533. Paris, 1774.

out; and lacerable; much loaded with blood and serum. The left pleuræ adhered universally; and the left lung, though less heavy and gorged, was everywhere reddened and ejected.

The mucous membrane from the larynx to the smallest branches of the bronchial tubes in both lungs was swelled, softened, and of a deep red colour; and the bronchial tubes were filled with muco-purulent fluid round the tooth, but without abscess or breach of surface in the vicinity of the spot where it was lodged.

From the facts now adduced, it seems reasonable to establish the following conclusions.

1. Foreign bodies, such as kernels and stones of fruit, nuts, or fragments of them, teeth, natural or artificial, pieces of metal, wood, or fragments of bones, which pass the glottis and drop into the windpipe, if they do not produce immediate suffocation, cause irritation of the windpipe, *bronchi*, and bronchial membrane, indicated by fits of coughing, more or less continued and severe, wheezing, breathlessness, and weight and oppression in the chest.

2. These symptoms of irritation are speedily succeeded by symptoms of inflammation, sometimes acute, sometimes chronic, but always afterwards becoming chronic, indicated by cough, expectoration of dense puriform or purulent mucus, occasionally streaked with blood; weight and anxiety in the chest; quick pulse; and eventually, hectic fever, with wasting.

3. Bodies of the kind now specified drop not constantly but most frequently into the right *bronchus ;* and their presence is followed by inflammation first in the right bronchial tubes and lungs of right side. The right *bronchus* is normally more directly in continuation with the tracheal canal than the left *bronchus.* One or two instances, nevertheless, of foreign bodies falling into the left *bronchus* have occurred.[*]

4. These bodies, there is reason to believe from their size and shape, must be arrested in the large or middle-sized bronchial tubes; and it must be anatomically and physically impossible for them to descend into the small tubes or the pulmonary vesicles.

5. The disease induced by their presence must therefore be, in the first instance, tubular *bronchitis ;* and though the inflammation may afterwards extend to the vesicular membrane, it is chiefly the tubular variety of the disorder throughout.

6. In all the recorded cases, the symptoms, however intense

[*] Schroeder Van Der Kolk.

during the abode of the body in the *bronchi*, and though enduring from the space of from six to seven weeks, as in the cases of Borsieri, Dr Donaldson, and Dr J. Scott, to that of several months, as in the case by Dr Lettsom, that of Dr Nooth, and the case by Mr Howship, or for years, as in those by Desault, Louis, Sue, and Holman, in general rapidly subided as soon as the foreign body was ejected.

7. In two cases only, that by M. Sue, and the one which occurred to myself, did partial and temporary recovery take place, before the ejection of the foreign body.

8. In certain cases in which the mechanical configuration of the body is unfavourable for detachment and expulsion, the bronchitic symptoms are liable to be extended to the lung, in which suppuration is caused, and to the pleura, in which effusion of lymph and purulent matter is induced.

As the case which occurred within my own experience has not yet been published, and as its progress and termination illustrate well the usual characters of cases of this class, I subjoin a short account of it.

Master L. M., an interesting and apparently healthy boy of about five years of age, had suffered occasionally from cough during winter. In April 1843 he had measles, and made a very favourable recovery. Soon after he was attacked by cough of extreme violence.

For these symptoms remedies were judiciously employed by Dr Watson Wemyss. The cough nevertheless proceeded and became daily more urgent and distressing; expectoration, at first scanty, was attended with the excretion of dense puriform mucus, occasionally slightly streaked with blood; fever was added and became constant; and some loss of flesh as well as of strength had taken place.

In May 1843 I was requested to see the boy. I found the respiration from 32 to 36 in the minute, with little or no motion of the upper part of the right side of the chest, and manifest dulness on percussion all over the subclavicular, pectoral, and scapular regions of the right side. Air did not during the motions of inspiration enter the right side of the lungs freely; and seemed to be stopped and thrown back when the attempt to inspire was made. The voice was a little resonant over the right mammary region; and the beats of the heart were heard as strongly, clearly, and distinctly as if the heart was beating under the ear. Occasionally slight wheezing and faint mucous rattles were heard immediately below the right collar bone and through the right scapula; and when the patient coughed, the expiration sound came against the ear at times faintly, at other times with unusual force. The child complained of pain in the right mammary region; stretching sometimes to the shoulder. The pulse was never under 120; the child perspired much during the night, and in the morning violent and alarming fits of coughing came on and continued long.

On the left side of the chest no morbid sounds were recognized. The motions of the chest were rapid and frequent; but air seemed to enter and quit the bronchial tubes of the left side without much impediment, excepting what arose from the rapid motion of that side, and of the diaphragm and abdominal muscles.

Leeches were applied over the right side of the chest several times, according to the strength of the patient, the urgency of the symptoms, and the effects of the discharge. Antimonial medicines had been given; and ipecacuanha wine, with occasional doses of tincture of hyoscyamus were tried. The bowels were kept open by means of calomel and rhubarb, or castor oil; and afterwards small doses of the gray powder, (*hydrargyrus cum creta*) were given. Leeches were applied often, as they seemed to give most relief; and once or twice the surface of the right side of the chest was blistered.

At length after treatment of this kind for the space of between five and six weeks, the cough became less urgent and frequent; the amount of expectorated mucus was diminished; the pulse became less frequent; the night sweats diminished and better sleep was obtained; and appetite returning, the child took food with some relish. The breathing was reduced to between 24 and 26 in the minute; but there was still much dulness over the whole right mammary region, and little motion of that side of the chest was observed, while the beats of the heart were heard as clearly and distinctly as before.

Sufficient amendment was produced, however, and sufficient strength was recovered to justify the cessation of medical treatment, and to enable the patient to proceed to a country situation in July 1843. Here he remained for six weeks, and improved much in health and strength. The cough had left him; the expectoration had ceased; and he had recovered his wonted looks. In this state he remained the early part of the winter of 1843-4. As the season advanced, however, the cough returned in a more violent form; and in the spring of 1844, in March, symptoms of another attack of catarrh appeared.

At first the usual remedial means were employed. But the cough became daily more urgent, rending, and frequent; the muco-purulent expectoration with the night sweats returned; the pulse was never below 120; the flesh was wasting fast; and, in short, the patient was again rapidly returning to his state in May 1843.

At this time the respiration was 36 in the minute, with almost no motion of the right side; the mammary region emitted a dull sound, and was visibly flattened and depressed; the voice was resonant; and the cardiac beats were clearly and distinctly heard all over the mammary region before, and the scapular region behind. Little respiration was audible, and only now and then a slight rattle. About one inch below the right collar-bone, extending downwards about three inches; and from one inch from the sternum to the outer margin of the large pectoral muscle before, little or no natural respiration was heard. The same phenomena were recognized behind. When inspiration was observed, it appeared that the air never penetrated further down than half an inch, or three-fourths of one inch below the right collar-bone, and about the same corresponding point behind. Respiration was performed mostly by the diaphragm.

On the other hand, over the whole of the left side respiration was clear and good; and though there were rattles in several points, they indicated nothing very bad.

I was satisfied at this time, March 1844, that there had been pleurisy with considerable effusion; pneumonia with consolidation; and *bronchitis*, but of what nature it was not easy to say. From the recurrence of the symptoms, it seemed probable that the lungs were tuberculated; and although there was no distinct evidence of any vomica, or excavated part, the sounds heard led me to think that almost no respiration was performed by the upper and middle lobes of the right lung.

Treatment was resumed, very much of the same kind as before, regulating the diet as carefully as possible. The symptoms proceeded, being sometimes more intense, sometimes alleviated, but never disappearing. At length, after a long, violent, and distressing fit of coughing on the morning of the 10th March 1844, the patient coughed up an iron screw nail, about three-fifths or three-fourths of one inch long, with a head with very sharp edges, covered with purulent matter and a little blood, and completely rusted. This was presented to me at my visit; and though the symptoms were still urgent and by no means diminished, I inferred now that there was every prospect that the patient would get rid of his disease.

In this expectation I was not disappointed. At first after the ejection of the screw-nail, the cough seemed to be aggravated; and expectoration did not immediately diminish in quantity. The patient also suffered from abdominal pains, which depended on a small umbilical hernia, which was protruded during the fits of coughing. Eventually, however, the cough abated; the expectoration gradually diminished, and at length ceased; the respiration fell to 26, 24, 20; the pulse came down to 80; the appetite, which had not been in this attack bad, was active; and flesh and strength returned in the course of about four or five weeks.

The surface of the mammary region was still dull; and little respiration was heard; but the chest was moving a little; and the patient appeared to suffer no inconvenience.

In July he again went to a country situation, and residing there for several weeks, returned home strong and free from any apparent complaint.

When the screw nail was coughed up by this child, it became a point of importance to ascertain when and how it had been introduced into the larynx and trachea. On these points, however, all enquiry was unavailing. One thing only was certain, that the nail must have been in the right *bronchus* since April 1843, probably at a date previous to that time. It must, therefore, have continued there at least 13 months, probably nearer 14 or 15 months.

This boy bas sinee that time remained in good health, and free from any bronchial or pectoral ailment. The mammary region is still flatter and more depressed on the right side than on the left, and emits a sound a little dull; but respiration is performed faintly; and it is clear that the lower part of the right lung is tolerably good.

In this case I think, that it is quite impossible to doubt, that the screw nail had been lodged in the right *bronchus*; that its presence there had caused first, inflammation of the whole of the upper bronchial tubes; then inflammation of the substance of the lung in a certain degree; and at the same time pleuritic inflammation. I have no doubt that the whole upper and middle lobes are adhering by their *pleura* to the *pleura costalis*.

P p

Of this case it is a circumstance not the least remarkable, that decided abatement in the symptoms took place in June 1843, and temporary recovery continued during autumn and winter, while the nail was still fixed in the bronchial tubes.

§ 4. *Emphysema of the lungs as a result of bronchitis.*—Though this probably should be placed under the head of diseases of the substance of the lungs, yet it may maintain the anatomical connection more closely by considering it here.

In the early stage, indeed, of *bronchitis*, there is simply a diffuse or spreading inflammation or congestion of the pulmonary mucous membrane; and after it has subsided under proper treatment, that membrane, both where it lines the bronchial tubes and pulmonary vesicles, sooner or later returns to its natural condition; while the calibre of these tubes, and the capacity of the vesicles, is little or not at all lessened. Either, however, after repeated attacks or long continuance of this disease, not only does the inflammatory process extend from the mucous membrane to the submucous or pulmonary filamentous tissue, but by its long endurance it renders the former thick, villous, and brownish-coloured, secreting either much viscid mucus, or mucus more or less tinged with blood, and even occasionally pure blood, and indurates and solidifies the latter by the extravasation of albuminous fluid; while the increased thickness of the membrane, and the swelling of the submucous tissue, encroach so much upon the area of the bronchial tubes and vesicles, as to diminish remarkably the capacity of these cavities.

This swelling, however, of the pulmonary mucous membrane and filamentous tissue, is not general over the whole of the tubes, nor even over the whole of one tube, otherwise it would produce fatal *asphyxia.* But it in general takes place at certain spots in the course of the tubes more remarkably than at others, producing a species of stricture of one or more bronchial tubes in one or both lungs. The effect of this again is various, according to its degree, and according to the component systems and textures of the lung most affected. One of the most frequent effects of the presence of one of these constricted portions, especially if the membrane secretes much viscid mucus, which requires to be frequently coughed up, is to obstruct the passage so much that expiration becomes either inadequate or is interrupted. As respiration consists, therefore, in alternate inspiration and expiration, if air has been either inhaled by this tube, or by some of the communicating ones, it cannot, during ordinary expiration, be easily expelled. The effect is, that the bronchial membrane and pulmonary vesicles are excited by their physiological properties to frequently repeated expiratory efforts; and, as these are inadequate to expel the air from the lungs, the compression of the expiratory muscles necessarily, by forcing the portion of lung into smaller compass, compresses the air already contained in the vesicles beyond the constricted point. The air thus confined, after many repeated expiratory efforts, forces its way, by its own elasticity, through the delicate mucous membrane of the vesicles into the pulmonic filamentous tissue, and, when once there, it continues to spread rapidly in proportion to the obstruction in the bronchial tubes, and the difficulty of producing efficient expiration. It is then that the air contained in these vesicles renders the chest, when struck, preternaturally resonant; while the extreme difficulty of breathing, with the dry sonorous *rhonchus* or sibilism, indicate the laborious struggle which is made in the tubes, contracted by swelling, and obstructed, as they are, by adherent mucus,—to inspire and to expire in an efficient manner.

In this manner, therefore, bronchial inflammation, either by continuance or repeated attacks, tends to produce *emphysema* and its usual phenomena; and there are few cases of emphysematous distension of the pulmonic filamentous tissue which may not be traced to this cause. In the young, when labouring under hooping-cough, in the aged, after frequently repeated attacks of catarrh, and in the middle-aged after the continuance of bronchial inflammation, in a subacute or chronic state, *emphysema* is with equal certainty, and in equal perfection, produced. In the first case, indeed, as the bronchial symptoms subside, the tubes become more pervious, and expiration becomes so much freer and less interrupted, that the air ceases to be urged through the vesicular membrane, and that which had been already impelled into the pulmonic filamentous tissue is at length absorbed. But in the two latter instances, in which the thickening of the membrane either abates little, or continues unchanged, the emphysematous distension continues to increase, until it has attained an extent almost incredible to those unaccustomed to examine cases of chronic bronchial disease.

Emphysema, however, is not the only effect of this state of the bronchial tubes. The impracticability of inspiring and expiring completely in such a state of the lungs, which implies the absence of the most essential condition of respiration, viz. the frequent and incessant change of air in the bronchial tubes and vesicles of the lungs, interferes with the necessary changes in the blood of the pulmonary artery and veins, which, therefore, passes from the former vessel into the latter, much less completely aërated than it would be in the healthy state. In addition to this, as the motion of the blood through the pulmonary artery into the pulmonary veins is always more free, in proportion as the expansion of the lung by inspiration, and its collapse by expiration, is extensive; and as both the obstruction of the bronchial tubes by viscid mucus, and the swelled and congested state of the bronchial membrane and submucous tissue, prevent the branches of the artery and veins from freely expanding themselves; the motion of the blood through this order of vessels begins to be interrupted and retarded, and thus to induce a congested state of the whole pulmonary system, which not only adds to the *dyspnœa* and *orthopnœa* of such patients, but eventually terminates in dropsical effusion into the pulmonic filamentous tissue, within the cavity of the *pleura*, and even into the general cellular membrane. The pulmonic filamentous tissue is in general the first seat of this dropsical infiltration; and it is one of the most common changes recognized in inspecting the lungs of persons cut off by long-continued bronchial inflammation.

: Chronic bronchial inflammation, further, by its influence in impeding respiration and the circulation of the pulmonary artery and veins, has an indirect tendency to induce disease of the heart. In consequence of the difficulty which the blood encounters in passing through the branches of the pulmonary artery, the trunk of that vessel becomes permanently distended; and the right ventricle, being also distended and incessantly excited to new contractions, becomes affected with hypertrophy, sometimes with dilatation, sometimes without; and in other cases it may be merely enlarged with extenuation of its walls. It is, I conceive, in consequence of the union of the two ventricles in the human subject, that this excessive distension and inordinate action, by being first confined to the right ventricle, gives rise to a similar inordinate action in the left ventricle, that the latter is often found in a state of hypertrophy in persons who have long laboured under chronic bronchial disease. The fact of the connection is at least well-established; and hospital practice presents few instances of bronchial disease in which the heart is not affected; and in most of the cases of disease of the heart, the bronchial membrane and pulmonic tissue are previously affected.

§ 5. *Bronchitis from inhalation of particles of sand, dust, and metal.*
—Next to bronchial disease from the presence of foreign bodies, may
be placed that form of the disease which is the result of the inhalation of sand, dust, or metallic particles in minute mechanical division. This has been already mentioned in a general manner. But
it may be proper to advert more particularly to the changes induced in the lungs as presented by the artisans of Sheffield.

These changes are not, indeed, by any means confined to the
bronchi or their branches and membrane. But as the primary cause
is applied first to the membrane of these tubes, it seems reasonable to consider the different lesions thus arising in the present
place.

In the town and vicinity of Sheffield two sorts of grinding of
edged tools are practised; one dry grinding, on a dry stone, the
other wet grinding, on a stone moistened with water. Many articles, as scissors, razors, and penknives, are ground partly on
dry stone, and partly on the wet stone. Others, as forks and
needles, are ground mostly on a dry stone. Table knives are
ground principally on a wet stone. Saws, files, and scythes are
ground entirely on a wet stone.

Dry grinding is most injurious, and tends most directly and effectually to induce bronchial and pulmonary disease, and thereby
to abridge the duration of life among the grinders. The dry
grinders, therefore, are most speedily destroyed. The life of the
wet grinder is often prolonged to a considerable age.

Of 1000 scissor-grinders above 20 years of age, only 20 attain
the age of between 51 and 55 years, only 10 the age of between 61
and 65, and none live beyond the latter age; while of the inhabitants of Sheffield generally, 244 in 1000 are found living at 65 and
above, and in the midland counties, 413 in 1000. Of artisans in
this branch 843 in 1000 die under 45 years of age.

With the fork-grinders it is worse. Among 1000 fork-grinders,
aged above 20 years, not one attains the age of 59; while in Sheffield, among 1000 persons 155 are living at 59. Of these 1000
persons 472 die between 20 and 29 years, 410 between 30 and 39;
and the residual 115 are all gone before the age of 50.

Among 1000 razor-grinders above 20 years of age, 749 die under 41 years of age; the rest mostly between 41 and 60; between
61 and 65 only 5 are living; and after 65 all are gone.

Of the pen-knife grinders not one in 1000 arrives at the age of

60 ; 731 die before the 40th year; and the rest are all destroyed before the 60th year.

· Saw-grinders, file-grinders, and scythe-grinders, who work on the wet stone, are less liable to bronchial disease and are longer lived. The numbers pursuing saw-grinding are not great.   Yet among 78 persons engaged in it in 1843, 9 were between 60 and 65, and one died between 66 and 70, and one at 79.   The number of scythe-grinders is also not great.   In 1843 there were 30; and of these 8 were between 41 and 60 years of age.   Both the saw-grinders and the scythe-grinders are exposed to accidents, sometimes fatal, from the breaking of the stone.

The lesions which produce this great mortality are of a complicated character.   The most common lesions are chronic inflammation with thickening of the bronchial membrane, enlargement or dilatation of the bronchial tubes, emphysema, and expansion of the pulmonic tissue.*

The bronchial glands are enlarged, or converted into a black hard gritty substance, varying in size from half a marble to a large hazel nut.   In dividing these glands, the sound emitted is the same as if the scalpel were dividing a soft stone ; and the section is black and polished, and grates over the edge of the knife.   Such masses are commonly detected in grinders who have belonged to the most destructive branches.†

Similar soft sectile gritty or stony matter is found in almost every part of the lungs, in portions varying from the size of a currant to that of a bean.

Adhesions between the pulmonic and costal *pleuræ* are also frequent.

In some instances the lungs present an appearance as if black currants had been distributed through their whole substance, and accompanied with similar bodies larger in size, but hard and gritty like them.   These currant-like bodies are also observed on the surface of the lungs.   As to their nature Dr Holland gives no opinion. But Dr C. Fox Favell states that frequent examination has convinced him that they consist of the dilated extremities of veins containing some of the solid constituents of the blood.

* Diseases of the Lungs from Mechanical Causes.   By G. Calvert Holland, M. D., p. 12.   London, 1843, 8vo.
† Ibid. p. 41.

Tubercles are also occasionally found with their consequences, vomicæ.

Another state frequently observed is engorgement or infiltration of the lungs with a dark-coloured fluid, which is ascribed by Dr Holland to the inhalation of the fine black dust floating in the atmosphere during the operation of glazing.

On the mode of production of these lesions, or the order of their succession, observers are not agreed. Dr Arnold Knight and Dr Holland consider the tracheo-bronchial membrane to be the original and principal seat of the disease, and the tracheo-bronchial irritation to be the primary morbid action, and to give rise to all the other effects; the dilatation of the *bronchi*, emphysema, the formation of currant-like bodies, tubercles, pulmonary induration, and pleuritic adhesion. Dr Fox Favell, on the other hand, thinks that the pulmonic tissue or parenchyma is the primary and essential seat of the disease, does not regard the mucous membrane as the original seat of the disease, and maintains that the organic changes found in the structure of the lungs constitute the essence of the lesion; in short, that all the changes seen in the lungs of the grinders depend on congestion and inflammation of their parenchymatous structure.[*] Dr Favell, in short, ascribes as much to the position, the labour, and the debauched habits of the grinders, as to the inhalation of the dust or powder. The question is not easily determined. But it may safely be asked, how the wet grinding is so little hurtful, and the dry grinding so rapidly, powerfully, and effectually detrimental to the lungs. It is also to be observed, that it cannot be said to follow, because the pulmonic parenchyma is found much diseased, that the tracheo-bronchial membrane is not the primary seat of mischief. It is known that various affections of the tracheo-bronchial membrane do extend to the lungs; and there is little reason to believe that the grinder's asthma constitutes an exception to the rule,

§ 6. Bronchial inflammation takes place secondarily in hooping-cough, measles, scarlet fever, small-pox, and typhous fever. In measles I have seen the membrane red, injected, villous, and secreting puriform fluid copiously—the usual symptoms of pulmonary consumption having preceded the fatal event. In scarlet fever not only the pulmonic but the facial mucous membrane is inflamed; and

---

* On Grinder's Asthma. By Charles Fox Favell, M. D. &c. Transactions of the Provincial Medical and Surgical Association. New Series. Vol. ii. 1846, p. 143.

in some severe and fatal cases I have traced the capillary injection along the gastro-enteric division, and in the genito-urinary from the neck of the bladder to the pelvis of the kidney. This general affection of the mucous system explains the fatality as well as many of the symptoms of scarlet fever. Inflammation of the tracheo-bronchial membrane is an occasional consequence of inhaling accidentally certain of the noxious gases.

. Redness and punctular injection of the tracheo-bronchial membrane, with more or less secretion of viscid mucus, was seen in hydrophobic subjects by Beddoes, Babington, Oldknow, Rush, Satterley, Brandreth, and Trolliet, the last of whom labours to prove that the rabid poison affects particularly this membrane. Much of this effect is doubtless to be ascribed to the violence of the abnormal motions of the respiratory muscles; and it is still undetermined how far the appearances now mentioned are primary and essential, or secondary and accessary.

§ 7. *Obliteration and Arctation of the Bronchial Tubes.*—From the operation of various causes at present not well understood, the bronchial tubes are liable to be narrowed or contracted, and in certain instances their canal may be entirely closed and obliterated. Arctation or narrowing of the bronchial tubes has been already mentioned as one of the effects of bronchial inflammation, recurring repeatedly, and becoming at length chronic. In cases of this kind, these walls forming the tube are distinctly thickened by effusion either of blood or lymph, or both, into the submucous tissue; and the capacity of the tube is proportionally diminished. In other instances the presence of indurated or hemorrhagic portions of lung round small bronchial tubes produce the same diminution in their normal dimensions

Of obliteration, M. Reynaud, who has studied this lesion, has observed four forms.

In the first kind complete coalescence of the walls of a bronchial tube takes place without foreign matter contained in their interior, and without any cause of external compression.

The simplest and most elementary degree of this obliteration of the bronchi consists in closure or obliteration of the terminal end of one tube or more.

This sort of obliteration, to which may be referred several lesions of the lungs, takes place both generally over a space of lung more or less extensive, and locally in one or more bronchial tubes. In

the former case, the substance of the organ, instead of being vesicular or spongy, becomes solid, compact, and impermeable to the
air.

· A second sort of bronchial obliteration, differing from the preceding one in its seat, is what is observed in bronchial canals of the
fifth or sixth order, consequently very near their termination, and
some lines from the pleura, yet in the interior of the parenchyma of
the lungs. In this variety the obliteration takes place at a part of
the bronchial tube, where the area is still considerable enough to
furnish divisions. But where the lung is divided, the tube is observed suddenly to terminate in a blind sac; and beyond the point
of obliteration, the bronchial tube is seen distinctly continuous, with
a small firm, resisting cord, itself furnishing small ramifications, and
easily detached by slight scraping from the rest of the lung. · The
bronchial tube may thus be traced to the *pleura.*

·A third sort is that in which the obliteration is seated, as in the
second, at a distance nearly equal from the pleura. The chief difference is this, that while the second form can be recognized only by
cautiously and gradually dividing the small bronchial tubes by means
of delicate scissors, the present form is easily discovered by a common
blunt probe, which, when introduced into the principal *bronchus,* is
suddenly stopped, while, if carried into the neighbouring ramifications placed at the same distance, it penetrates more forward. When
the *bronchus* thus obstructed is laid open down to the site of obstruction, it is observed that the obstruction is owing to an obliteration
seated in a large tube, which, though near the surface of the lung,
does not appear with the characters peculiar to dilatation of the
bronchi. The obliterated *bronchus* is continuous with a fibrous
cord; but this is larger than in the preceding case, though its course
to the pleura is not longer.

To the disposition now mentioned is conjoined another referable
to the surface of the lung, and which denotes the presence of the
obliteration. This consists in more or less shrivelling of the pulmonic surface at the point corresponding to the seat of the obliteration. From this it is reasonable to infer that the shrivelling is
in some manner connected with the bronchial obliteration. It is
indeed not difficult to understand how the obliteration of a bronchus,
not remote from the surface of the lung, involving that of the
branches issuing from it, must, by the consequent contraction, produce contraction or shrinking of the pulmonic substance, and

shrivelling more or less considerable of the surface of the organ at the corresponding point.

These shrivelled spots are easily recognized. The pleura is drawn to one or two points in a series of wrinkles, imperfectly radiated; the surface is perceptibly depressed; and, when the part is touched, it is found to be solid, adherent, firm, and inelastic.

The fourth and last sort of obliteration is that which is observed in bronchial tubes larger than those affected in the previous cases, and furnishing tubes to portions of the lung more or less considerable. This sort of obliteration differs from the third in no respect unless in the greater number of bronchial tubes the obliteration of which it involves. It also produces peculiar forms of morbid structure.

This obliteration is observed in the *bronchi* at all points of the bronchial tree, from the branches issuing from the first *bronchus*, to those which may be divided by ordinary scissors. The obliteration is known as in the third case, by the abrupt termination of a large tube in a blind sac, and with ligamentous cords proceeding from it through the lung.

The most common seat of these obliterations is the upper lobe of the lung and especially its apex, a fact of which it is necessary to be aware, in distinguishing these obliterated spots from alleged healed tubercular cavities. They have been found nevertheless in the lower lobe. Reynaud found the lesion twice in this situation.

As to the state of the *bronchi* and their membrane in this lesion, it is variable. Sometimes, I believe very rarely, it is found in what is called perfect integrity, in that portion accessible to air. This is certainly sometimes the case. On the other hand, the membrane may be and often is red, rough, thickened, and covered with viscid opaque mucus. Occasionally the tube is much dilated immediately above the point of obliteration; and though this dilatation may take place in *bronchi* of all sizes and in all points, yet it is most common in those in which obliteration affects large trunks, at a short distance from their origin.

In some instances the adjoining *bronchi* to one which has been obliterated, are all more or less dilated, and instead of forming cones gradually contracting, as in the healthy state, are either cylinders, or present actual dilated and enlarged portions. In these tubes the membrane is generally reddish, rough, and covered with opaque puriform mucus.

The pulmonary parenchyma round an obliterated bronchus may present two morbid states. It may be either consolidated, dense, and firm, as already mentioned, or it may be emphysematous, that is, containing air in the pulmonic cellular tissue, or in the shape of bladders beneath the pleura. In some instances both states are associated. Immediately round the seat of the obliteration the lung is firm and dense, with shrivelling of the pleura and pulmonic surface; and beyond this dense spot again the surface of the lungs is pale, white, crepitating, and emphysematous; and two or more air-bladders are formed beneath the pleura. Lastly, it is not unusual to find the upper lobe presenting shrivelled patches, and the indications of obliterated bronchial tubes; and the middle and lower lobes to be pale, white, crepitating, and more or less extensively emphysematous.

The blood-vessels are not obliterated; except in the minute branches distributed through the indurated portion.

The solid filaments, the relics of the obliterated tubes, are generally of a deep black colour.

The causes of obliteration of the bronchial tubes are not positively ascertained. All that is known is this; that obliteration takes place in persons who had laboured under severe, repeated, or long-continued attacks of bronchial inflammation, usually chronic, and those who had attacks of chronic pneumonia. Reynaud is inclined to ascribe the occurrence of the lesion to diphtheral or albumino-facient inflammation of the *bronchi;* and there is no doubt that the bronchial membrane is liable to this form of inflammation, and that this form of inflammation may produce or terminate in obliteration. He admits also that he has met with cases of acute *pneumonia* with hepatization of the lung, in which the lesion consisted in inflammation, which had in all the small *bronchi* given rise to the formation of false membranes, which filled more or less accurately all their cavities.[*]

From what I have myself seen, I ascribe the lesion either, as already stated, to severe and repeated attacks of chronic *bronchitis,* or to the effects of chronic pneumonia.

A lady presented the usual symptoms of very severe chronic bronchitis; that is, cough, expectoration of muco-purulent matter, with hectic fever, and pulse varying from 110 to 120. There was

---

[*] Memoire sur l'Obliteration des Bronches. Par A. C. Reynaud, D. M., &c. Memoires de l'Academie Royale de Medecine, Tome ivieme. Paris, 1835. 4to. P. 117.

strong resonance of the voice at the upper part of the right side of the chest; and the cardiac and arterial beats were heard most audibly. Yet, though the symptoms continued long, there was no distinct indication of pectoriloquy. The subclavian and pectoral regions also before, and the scapular behind, emitted a dull sound. These symptoms, which were attended with wasting and much loss of strength, after lasting for many weeks, at length subsided; and she seemed to recover completely. The dull sound on percussion continued, however; and little respiratory murmur was audible in the upper region of the right *demithorax* either before or behind. The air, indeed, seemed not to enter the bronchial tubes of the right lung above at all; and only a little respiration was audible along the back close to the spine, and in the lower region of the chest. She died about two years after of a different disease, and inspection presented the following appearances.

The whole of the upper lobe of the right lung and part of its middle lobe was firm and solid, and inelastic like a mass of solid flesh. The pleura adhered behind, and partly on the sides, and a little anteriorly. On dividing this portion of solidified lung, the bronchial tubes were found to be closed, except at the apex and near the spine, where they were still pervious for the space of not more than half an inch. The pulmonic substance itself was firm, of a light red colour, but totally uncrepitating, and did not admit the air from the tubes. It sunk in water like a stone. On tracing the tubes, they seemed to be compressed together into ligaments or cords, quite solid and impervious; but it was not easy to say whether they had been filled with matter effused from within their canals or exterior to them.

It seems also impossible to doubt that when pneumonia proceeds to abscess or *vomica*, it in like manner entails obliteration of the bronchial tubes; and, if the patient be not destroyed by the disease, various tubes are found obliterated.

Obliteration is also observed in those cases in which tubercular masses are broke down and expelled by expectoration, whether any attempt to close the vomica and heal it is made or not.

Lastly, in the form of pneumonia denominated lobular, or where there appears to be inflammation of the terminal ends of the *bronchi*, obliteration at these ends is very common, in consequence of effusion of albuminous matter from the mucous membrane of their terminal extremities. This effusion or deposit, however, is probably either the same with the tubercular deposit, or very similar to it in the mode and situation in which it takes place.

§ 8. *Dilatation and Hypertrophy of Bronchi.*—In certain circumstances of chronic bronchial disease the *bronchi* become greatly enlarged, and their walls are thickened, with thickening of the membrane. The diameter of the tubes may be increased in this state to half an inch. Of this lesion Dr Carsewell gives an excellent representation in his Fourth Division, first engraving ;* and an instance is described by Mr Watt of Manchester as having been exhibited at the Pathological Society of that place.†

§ 9. *Dilatation of the Bronchial Tubes.*—Of one species of dilatation I have already partially spoken, as taking place along with obstruction and obliteration of these canals. There is yet to be noticed another, which, according to my own observation, takes place either solely or principally in connection with aneurismal enlargement and dilatation of the aorta or *innominata*. Of this I have seen several examples ; and from these, especially one published,‡ I give the following characters of the lesion.

The lesion is seated in the right lung, the lobes of which are generally solidified and inelastic, of a reddish-brown colour, and loaded with blood. The middle lobe and the lower one are generally more completely and extensively solidified than the superior lobe ; and the affection appears often to commence in the lower lobe, and thence proceed to the middle and upper lobes.

The great change, however, is in the bronchial tubes, which in all the three lobes are greatly enlarged, losing their conical figure, and being converted either into large cylindrical canals, or tubes with wide dilated spaces in their course. Bronchial tubes, which in their natural state are not larger than crow-quills, become, especially in the lower and middle lobe, of the diameter of half an inch. Besides this, at various points in their course they undergo still greater dilatation, so as to form cavities communicating apparently with the bronchial tubes, and thereby with each other, but which, when carefully examined, are seen to be unusually enlarged portions of the bronchial tubes themselves.‡

* Illustrations of the Elementary Forms of Disease. By Robert Carsewell, M. D. Folio. London, 1838. Hypertrophy, Plate 1.

† London Medical Gazette, Vol. xxxix. p. 596. No. 1009. April 2, 1847.

‡ Report on the Cases treated during the Course of Clinical Lectures delivered at the Royal Infirmary in the Session 1832-1833. By David Craigie, M. D., &c. Edinburgh Medical and Surgical Journal, Vol. xli. January 1834. P. 106. Case of Janet Waits.

The bronchial tubes in this state are filled with thick opaque puriform or purulent matter, on the removal of which the membrane is seen to be reddened, softened, and thickened.

In some instances the dilatation, though sufficiently distinct, does not proceed to the extreme degree already noticed. The bronchial tubes of the middle and lower lobes are merely rendered cylindrical like goose-quills, and filled with a sort of viscid albuminous puriform matter. The lung is also solidified, and, losing its elasticity, does not crepitate; and, when divided, puriform matter issues copiously from the cut bronchial tubes.

This form of dilatation I have seen only in cases of aneurismal tumours of the aorta and *innominata*. It appears to be caused principally by the compression exerted on the superior bronchial tubes by the aneurismal swelling. In the cases in which I have observed the lesion, the aneurismal tumour invariably compressed much the bronchial tubes of the upper lobe, near the mediastinum, so as to flatten them and contract their area, and prevent the free discharge of the matter secreted by their mucous membrane. The matter retained appeared to be one of the causes of the great dilatation produced in the small tubes of the middle and lower lobes.

At the same time it must be observed, that this same compression causes general inflammation of all the bronchial tubes on which it is exerted, and even inflammation of the pulmonic tissue with the usual morbid products.

In one case the tumour was as large as a good sized pippin, two inches and a-half in diameter, and compressed the right *bronchus* and its divisions and the mesial or internal margin of the lung. In another case the tumour was about the same size, though more ovoidal, and it equally compressed the right *bronchus* and its branches.

That this dilatation of the bronchial tubes proceeds from the cause now specified, must be inferred, I think, from the fact, that in the cases in which it is observed, it is generally in proportion to the size, situation, and compressing powers of the aneurismal tumour, and that the lesion is confined to the bronchial tubes of the right lung, not affecting those of the left lung at all.

I have no doubt, nevertheless, that were the tumour to be situate in that part and side of the aorta in which it could compress the left lung, the same state of the bronchial tubes of that organ would be produced.

In general this state of the bronchial tubes and lung can be known during life. The voice is hoarse, and like that of a person in croup. The cough is peculiarly hoarse and sonorous, as if issuing through a brazen tube. The difficulty of breathing is very great, and often amounts to orthopnœa ; and mucous rattling is heard in the middle and lower part of the right lung only, while at the upper region respiration is performed with a harsh croaking sound.

C. THE GASTRO-ENTERIC MUCOUS MEMBRANE.

In the gastro-enteric mucous surface inflammation may take place either generally or partially ; and it affects either the villous membrane or its follicular apparatus or both.

§ 1. *Œsophagus.*—In the œsophageal mucous membrane inflammation seldom appears, unless as part of the same process affecting the stomach and bowels more or less generally. This is particularly the case in inflammation of the gastric mucous membrane, with which a similar state of the œsophageal is almost invariably connected. The surface is red, injected, and more or less villous, and thickened ; and the œsophageal epidermis is occasionally elevated into apthæ or blebs, leaving, when these are removed, an excoriated or abraded surface. In the chronic form it may affect the mucous glands, and produce ulceration. Irregular patches of the latter I have seen in subjects in whom the colic membrane was extensively covered by ulcers. The cases described by Dr F. Simmons and Dr Gartshore appear to have affected the submucous tissue.

§ 2. *a.* The gastric mucous membrane may be inflamed generally or partially. When a limited portion of the villous membrane is inflamed the disease is seldom violent. The mucous membrane of the inflamed part shows an unusual number of minute vessels, but is rarely much crowded. In some instances, however, it is red or scarlet, with vessels disposed in arborescent, punctular, or striated fashion ; and not unfrequently spots or patches of extravasated blood are recognized. At the same time, the substance of the mucous coat is thicker than natural, of pulpy softness, and when attempted to be detached, is readily lacerated.

The gastric mucous membrane is liable, nevertheless, to a more general inflammatory process, in which its surface presents a light rose-coloured blush diffused all over, and secretes mucous or mucopurulent fluid copiously. The mucous membrane is also pulpy and softened, but not remarkably thickened. This state of the gastric membrane, though occurring spontaneously, may be produced by repletion or improper articles of food, and by several of the acrid poisonous substances. Of this form of *gasteria* a good delineation is given by Dr Armstrong in the second plate of his first Fasciculus.

b. Gasteria psilotica ; Psilosis.—In the persons of those who have long pined under various chronic diseases, the gastric mucous membrane is liable to a form of disease in which some part of it becomes pale white, bluish, rose-coloured, or gray, continuously or in long narrow stripes, or irregular patches more or less thickly set. The spaces so coloured are simply depressed beneath the level of the adjoining membrane, not ulcerated, soft and thin, and converted into a glairy semitransparent pulp. According to M. Louis, to whom the pathologist is indebted for the correct description of this change, when in narrow stripes, it is distributed nearly uniformly over the whole surface of the stomach; when continuous, it occupies the large extremity of the organ, is rarely confined to the great *cul de sac,* and in some instances appears at once at the cardiac and pyloric orifices. The vessels of the submucous tissue, which is generally sound, are large, distinct, and empty.* From the few instances in which I have seen this change myself, I should say that it consists in removal of the *villi* by some process analogous to inflammatory absorption. It is certain that in the affected patches these processes are greatly less distinct, and often totally gone. I may add that this is one at least of the forms of the change which John Hunter describes as *digestion* of the stomach;† and also one of these described by Dr Yellowly,‡ the greater part of which, it is to be observed, occurred in persons cut off by pulmonary consumption. To this head probably are to be referred such cases as that recorded by Mr Douglas, who found the villous coat obliterated except near the pylorus, and the muscular absorbed.§ The theory of its production is further exceedingly obscure; and I abstain from conjecture.

In similar subjects, but more especially in the phthisical, the gastric membrane is liable to become occupied by minute roundish eminences, not unlike granulations separated by superficial furrows,

* Mémoires ou Recherches Anatomico-Pathologiques. Paris, 1826.
† Observations on certain parts of the Animal Economy, p. 226, 231.
‡ Medico-Chir. Trans. Vol. iv. p. 271, 5 out of 20.
§ Mem. Med. Soc. vol. iv. p. 395.

with occasional points of ulceration round or oblong form, from one to several lines in diameter. The colour of the membrane is at the same time reddish, or reddish gray, always thickened, and generally softened, and covered with much viscid mucous. This granular state of the mucous membrane is most frequent in the large curvature, and the parts adjoining to the anterior and posterior surfaces, at the pyloric extremity, the small curvature, and the great *cul de sac*, the whole extent of which, however, is rarely affected.* The granular eminences appear to be swellings of the mucous glands, which are most abundant in the situations in which it is seen.

    c. *Gasteria Diuturna, Gasteria ulcerans, Gasteria Helkosis.*— Chronic inflammation of the gastric mucous membrane is much more frequent than is imagined. The process is in general confined to one or two small spots, which are slightly red, often brown or reddish brown, rough, villous, and firmer than natural. Of these appearances the most constant is the rough villous aspect and firm consistence, which are at once recognized by drawing the finger over the part. The inflammation does not spread, but gradually penetrates to the submucous filamentous tissue which is exposed, and terminates in the formation of an ulcer or ulcers of the mucous membrane.

    The most usual appearance of these ulcers is that of depressed breaches in the continuity of the mucous membrane, with a rough, brown-coloured surface, variable in size, but generally small, affecting an irregularly round or oval shape, sometimes angular, and with edges smooth, but sharp and accurately marked. This character, which is that of a piece of the membrane completely cut or scooped out, is certainly derived from the peculiar properties of the mucous corion, which seems in ulceration to undergo a gradual process of absorption. When the first minute perceptible point of ulceration is formed, the edges are destroyed or absorbed in the same gradual manner, and thus the ulcer is enlarged. The edges are in general some shade of crimson or reddish brown, owing to injected capillaries of the corion; but in other instances the colour does not differ from that of the adjoining surface.

    Many of the examples of this lesion have been described as instances of rupture or perforation of the stomach; and hence it is not easy to ascertain the exact state of the villous membrane in the

* Louis, Recherches Anatomico-Pathologiques sur la Phthisie. Paris, 1825.

incipient stage of the disease. It is nevertheless impossible to doubt that these ulcers, whether in the state of ulcers, or appearing afterwards as perforations, must originate in inflammation which probably attacks one point and is circumscribed to that, while it is slow in progress and chronic in character.

Instances of this lesion have now become numerous. Cases have been recorded by Morgagni,[*] Dr Carmichael Smyth,[†] Gerard,[‡] Dr Baillie,[§] Dr Crampton,[||] Mr Travers,[¶] Laennec,[**] Dr Abercrombie,[††] Dr Elliotson,[‡‡] M. Duparque,[§§] M. Uebersaal,[||||] M. Goeppert,[¶¶] and Cruveilhier.

From these cases, and seven which have been observed and inspected by myself,[***] I conceive the following general conclusions. regarding the nature and character of this lesion may be established.

It is, in the *first* place, remarkable that the majority of these cases of ulcerative destruction of the mucous membrane of the stomach are situate either in the small arch of the stomach, or very near the small arch. In the case by Dr Carmichael Smyth, it was in the anterior part towards the *cardia*. In the first case by Gerard, it was in the small arch, one inch from the pylorus. In his fifteenth case also, a circular hole was found at the right and anterior side of the small curvature. It is unnecessary to refer to all his cases, because he does not distinguish between simple inflammatory ulceration and that which is the effect of tubercular destruction and cancer. In the case by Dr Baillie, it was near the small curvature on its posterior side, about two inches from the cardia. In the case by Dr Crampton, it was at the union of the cardiac and pyloric portions. In the instance of the late M. Beclard, the anatomist, who had laboured under symptoms leading to

---

* De Sed. et Caus. Epist. xxix. 14.   I am doubtful whether this case be not the result of tubercular ulceration.

† Medical Communications, Vol. ii. p. 467.

‡ Des Perforations Spontanées de l'Estomac. Par M. Alexandre Gerard, D. M., &c. Paris, 1805.

§ Morbid Anatomy, Chap. vii.   Lond. 1825 ; and Miscellaneous papers and Dissections, p. 199.

|| Medico-Chirurgical Transactions, Vol. viii. p. 228.

¶ Ibid. Vol. viii. p. 271.

**. Revue Medicale, Mars 1824.

†† Edin. Med. and Surgical Journal, Vol. xxi. p. 3.

‡‡ Medico-Chirurg. Trans. Vol. xiii. p. 26.

§§ Archives Generales, Vol. xxvi. p. 123.

|||| Ibid. Vol. xxvi.

¶¶ Rust's Magazin, 1830. F. 32. 3. C.

*** Edin. Med. and Surg. Journal, Vol. xliv. p. 262. Edinburgh, 1835.

the suspicion of chronic inflammation in the gastric mucous membrane, and in whom these symptoms had subsided under appropriate treatment, after death from disorder of the brain, a cicatrized ulcer was found in the small arch of the stomach the size of a sixpence, about four lines from the *cardia*.*

In the cases by Ubersaal, Goeppert, and four of the seven seen by myself, the ulceration was situate in the small curvature. In two, indeed, of the first three cases described by me, the ulceration of the villous membrane was bisected by the line of the small arch.

In other three cases examined by me, the ulcers were situate in the anterior region of the stomach, about midway between the small and great arch. In one case, that of a young female of 23, there were in this situation two ulcers, one rather larger than a sixpenny piece, one less than a fourpenny piece. The largest had given way; and the rupture was followed by escape of the contents of the stomach, and fatal *peritonitis* in the course of a few hours. The patient was in her usual health at seven in the evening, and she was found lifeless, yet not cold, in bed next morning.

In another case, which took place also in a young woman of about 22, the ulcer was situate in the anterior part of the stomach, but nearer to the pylorus.

In the sixth case, which took place in a boy of 11 years, who had been labouring under granular disease of the kidney, and dropsical symptoms, extensive peritoneal inflammation, with copious effusion of lymph, had taken place over the intestines. But it was not certain whether this had been caused by perforation or not. There was no distinct evidence of escape of the contents of the stomach, which contained a good deal of blood coagulated and semifluid, which must have escaped from some vessel or vessels opened in the margins of the ulcer.

Secondly, Whatever part of the organ they occupy, the different tissues are always destroyed in unequal degrees; — the villous membrane being most extensively destroyed, the filamentous and muscular less so, and the peritoneal least. Indeed, it is by no means certain that the peritoneal is destroyed by ulceration, as it seems rather to give way after the other tissues have been removed from it and cease to support it, than to undergo loss of substance itself.

Thirdly, Though the ulcers now mentioned resemble ulcers in other parts of the body, they have nevertheless a very peculiar

* Billard de la Membrane Muqueuse. Paris, 1825. P. 558.

character. The mucous membrane is always exactly destroyed to certain well-marked limits; and the edges which are formed by the mucous membrane are in all cases sharp, manifest, and well defined. They appear as if some time previously a part had been cut or punched out from the villous membrane with a sharp instrument, and the edges had healed, so as to present a uniform smooth boundary round the excavation which had been made.

Fourthly, It is always possible to distinguish at one part of the ulcer, viz. round its edges, whether perforation has taken place or not, the submucous filamentous tissue and the muscular coat, much less extensively destroyed than the villous membrane. From this it may be inferred, that the process had first attacked the villous membrane, and, after destroying that, had proceeded to the filamentons and muscular. In some instances, only a portion of the villous coat is destroyed, and the bottom of the ulcer is then formed by the filamentous and muscular layers, yet comparatively uninjured. In other instances, however, all the tissues are destroyed down to the peritoneum, in which perforation takes place.

In the *fifth* place, the villous membrane forming the edges of the ulcer is often quite free from redness, vascularity, or thickening, and is always completely without either tubercular deposition, irregularity, or hardness, such as might be expected in scirrhus. The surrounding structure of the stomach is in appearance healthy and unchanged. Sometimes, however, the margins are a little thickened, firm, and sharp, and more or less opaque; and the surrounding mucous membrane is for some space thickened and of a deep fawn-colour ;—changes which depend on effusion of lymph and the afflux of blood to the neighbourhood of the ulcer. It must be admitted, in short, that the destruction of the villous membrane of the stomach must have been the effect of inflammation, originating most probably in the villous membrane, and giving rise to the ulcerative destruction when the membrane was no longer able to resist the intensity of the action. This is evidently inflammation of the substance of the membrane, circumscribed in character and chronic in duration. Is there any reason to suppose that it was the result of inflammation of the submucous filamentous tissue? or do these ulcers originate in affection of the glands of the stomach?

In the *sixth* place, in all these cases it is a common character, that there is at the close of the disease, inflammation of the peritoneal membrane, with effusion of lymph, in proportion as the ulcerative process affects the *peritoneum*.

In the *seventh* place, perforation or rupture, though the natural termination of these cases, is nevertheless not necessary to the disease. Death may take place by mere *peritonitis*, without effusion of the contents of the stomach into the abdominal cavity. In this case, the adjoining organs are generally applied accurately over the part of the stomach where the ulcer is situate, and by the adhesion effected by the inflammatory exudation, perforation and escape of the contents are prevented. No escape took place in four of the six cases inspected by me. Under such circumstances, therefore, peritoneal inflammation is rarely general or extensive. When perforation takes place, of course the inflammation is very general and intense. This result, however, depends much on the position of the ulcer or ulcers. When they are situate on the anterior part of the stomach, at some distance from the small arch, at which no contiguous organs are applied over the stomach, perforation and escape of the contents of the stomach are very liable to ensue.

In the *eighth* place, it deserves to be particularly noticed, that this disease is greatly more common in females, and especially young females, than in males. Among the six cases seen by myself three took place in young females; in those that I have seen examined by professional friends they were mostly in females. The disease seems not unfrequent among female domestic servants.

The symptoms produced by this disease are not well marked. In all the cases almost which have been recorded, though the patients have not been in perfect health, yet they have been free from any symptom calculated to excite apprehension, and they have been in general suddenly and unexpectedly surprised by death.

In the cases which came under my own observation, the individuals had for a considerable time laboured under obscure and imperfectly marked dyspeptic symptoms, with loss of flesh, and increasing languor and weakness. In two of them profuse hemorrhage had taken place from the stomach at different times,—circumstances which were afterwards explained by the position of the ulcer on the line of the coronary artery. A similar source of hæmatemesis was recognized in the case given by M. Goeppert, as occurring in the person of a young man who had suffered from *anorexia* and tension at the pit of the stomach, but without being aggravated by pressure.

Pain is by no means a constant symptom. In the case given by

Dr C. Smyth, the patient had occasional but not severe pain at the stomach. In that by Dr Baillie, the patient had violent occasional pain in the *scrobiculus cordis*, with vomiting, most liable to ensue after meals. In most of the other cases, the sense of pain was either trifling or not uniform. But in all there appears to have been a sense of dull gnawing or aching, either constant or pretty frequent. In one of the cases seen by myself, though the patient always complained of pain, it was referred to a point deep in the epigastric region, towards the spine,—a peculiarity which I think was due to irritation of the extremities of the nervous filaments sent along the small arch.

The pulse is not much affected in this disease.

The circumstances now remarked, however, apply only to the early stage of the complaint, while it is still confined to the villous membrane, or at most does not touch the peritoneum. When the ulcerative action penetrates through the gastric tissues and begins to affect this membrane, it produces also slight and limited *peritonitis*, which, if there be other organs applied on the part, tends to protract the life of the patient, and retard for a little the approach of the fatal event. With this peritoneal inflammation, the pulse becomes quick and sharp, and the patient complains of more or less pain in the epigastric and umbilical regions. But when the ulcerative destruction has reached the peritoneum, the life of the patient hangs by a thread. The most casual occurrence, as a fit of sneezing, coughing, eructation, or vomiting, or, even without these, the distension of the stomach by drink or by air extricated from flatulent food, may produce perforation, and cause the escape of gaseous and fluid contents into the cavity of the abdomen, and general peritoneal inflammation very speedily fatal.

It is, therefore, too often only at the close of this disease that the practitioner can even conjecture its true nature.

In every case, however, in which obstinate dyspeptic complaints are accompanied with a gnawing sensation, more or less constant, referred to the region of the stomach, or occasional acute pain, with loss of flesh, weakness and languor, and with the frequent rejection of *ingesta*, the presence of chronic inflammation and ulceration may be suspected. This conjecture will be converted into certainty, when, after a course of such symptoms, the patient is suddenly and unexpectedly attacked with feelings of faintness and sinking, acute pain generally radiating from the epigastrium or navel, all over the belly, pale, shrunk features, small rapid pulse, followed by rapid breathing and cold extremities; and dissolution may then be certainly apprehended.

This species of gastric inflammation and ulceration has been confounded by several authors with cancerous destruction. From this, however, it is to be distinguished by the absence of any considerable thickening or induration in the vicinity of the ulcer, or in any other part of the stomach, by its presenting less intense gastric symptoms, and by its taking place either principally in young persons, especially young females, or in persons of all ages; while cancer is rather the disease of declining years.

Ulceration affecting the mucous follicles of the stomach is somewhat different. The surface of the swelled follicle begins to be perforated by innumerable minute reddish points, which gradually coalesce, and when this is completed, a reddish brown ragged surface is formed.

Ulceration often proceeds, it has been seen, by successive destruction of the submucous, muscular, and peritonæal coats to perforation, which consists in the occurrence of a ragged opening, through which the contents of the organ escape, and give rise to secondary peritonæal inflammation, which is invariably fatal. This accident, examples of which are recorded by Morgagni, Lieutaud, Carmichael Smyth,[*] Gerard,[†] Crampton,[‡] Travers,[§] Louis, and Dr Abercrombie, may take place at any part of the stomach, but appears to be most frequent in the space between the great and small arches, but nearer to the former. In some rare instances, in which adhesion is formed between an adjoining organ and the edges of the aperture, the contents of the stomach are prevented from escaping, and life may be continued till the progress of ulceration destroys a part where this temporary barrier cannot have place.

The most important point to be known is, that these ulcers may be cicatrized. Independent of the uncertain cases recorded by Atkinson and Reil, we have an authentic and unequivocal example in the person of the late M. Beclard. This able anatomist laboured at one period of his life under obstinate symptoms of gastric disease, the nature of which, though uncertain, seemed to partake of chronic inflammation. The symptoms did not give way without

* Med. Commun. Vol. ii. p. 467.
† Des Perforations Spontanées de l'Estomac. Paris, 1803.
‡ Trans. of the Association, Vol. i.   § Med. Chir. Trans. Vol. vii.

frequent local blood-letting, counter-irritation, and the most rigid regimen. After death, there was found in the small curvature, about 4 lines from the *cardia*, a cicatrized ulcer, the size of a 20 sols piece, with a depressed surface, the middle of which was traversed by a solid cellular band, on each side of which were two *lacunæ* formed by peritonæum. The margins were neither red nor swollen; and the rest of the stomach was sound.*

   d. Solution of the gastric tunics enfeebled by inflammation.—Besides the ulcerative perforation now mentioned, another variety has been described by Jaeger of Wirtemberg, Zeller of Tubingen, Cruveilhier of Paris, and Dr John Gairdner of this place, as occurring in the stomach and bowels of infants generally at the breast. From the elaborate examination of this subject by the latter author, it appears that these perforations are probably not the result of previous ulceration, but are effected by some solvent power of the fluids after death ; that, nevertheless, the parts so eroded and perforated appear to undergo a previous change of structure, in consequence of which they are less able to resist the solvent power. †

   Before I conclude this subject, I may remark, that in some instances the mucous follicles appear to become enlarged in consequence of chronic inflammation, without affection of the gastric membrane. A very good instance of this change is recorded by Haller, who found in the pyloric end of the stomach of a woman of 64, ten or twelve hemispherical bodies like *papillæ*, with black or perforated summits, and cavities full of purulent matter. Though the size of these bodies was variable, the diameter of some was three lines, in others a full inch.‡

   e. A particular cause of gastric mucous ulceration has been supposed to exist in certain substances belonging to the class of corrosive poisons. That in many instances these substances induce inflammation, ulceration, and erosion of the gastric tissues, cannot be denied ; and this is true, particularly of the concentrated mineral acids, as is shown in the cases and experiments of Tartra, Orfila, and Brodie, the cases and experiments recorded by Roupelle,§ and the instances, now rather numerous, in which sulphuric

---

* De la Membrane Muqueuse Gastro-Intestinale, &c. p. 558.   Par C. Billard.

† Medico-Chirurgical Transactions of Edinburgh, Vol. i. p. 311.

‡ Opuscula Pathologica Observat. xxvii.

§ Illustrations of the Effects of Morbid Poisons.   By George Leith Roupell, M. D. The Plates from Original Drawings.   By Andrew Melville M'Whinnie, M. R. C. L. Part I. and II.   London, 1833.   Folio.

acid has been swallowed accidentally, or used for the purpose of self-destruction.

Though it is true, however, that these substances produce in many instances inflammation, and in several corrosion, it is not established that they in all cases cause ulceration.   It is very doubtful even if arsenic itself, to which this property has been often ascribed, ever induces ulceration; for in a large proportion of cases in which particles of the solid oxide have been found in the stomach, no ulceration has been recognized.   The reason of this I conceive to be, that death is effected by the severity of the general operation of the agent, before there is time for ulceration.

From the instances of deglutition of sulphuric and nitric acid which have fallen under my own observation, and from the records of other cases, the following conclusions may, I think, be established.

1st, The first effect of sulphuric acid is evinced in its transit over the membrane of the mouth, throat, and œsophagus.   It there indurates, crispates, and raises into vesications the mucous epidermis, and giving it a brownish colour and greater firmness.   Nitric acid produces the same effects, imparting, however, a citron yellow colour to the epidermis.   Both acids render the terminal boundaries of the epidermis at the cardia much more distinctly visible than in the natural state.

Both sulphuric and nitric acid produce at the epiglottis and upper part of the larynx so much detachment of the mucous epidermis with inflammation generally, as to give rise to symptoms of *laryngitis* and *œdema glottidis*, much as after the accidental swallowing of boiling water.   Even during life the symptoms of gasping and spasmodic depression-of the lower jaw are as well marked as in cases of spontaneous *laryngitis*, and in most instances they are more intense.

In the stomach the effects vary as the organ is empty or contains articles of food.

If it contain articles of food, these are generally blackened, hardened, and charred, as it were, by the contact of the acid.   If the organ be empty, or contain little food, the parts touched by the acid appear like portions blackened, indurated, and charred. The blood in the vessels is coagulated and blackened; and the vessels appear as if they had been filled by a dark-coloured injection which has speedily become solid.   The blackened and indurated patches vary in size and shape.   They may be small, but most commonly they are large, as large, that is, as a crown piece or a half-crown piece. Their edges are distinctly circumscribed.*

In cases in which sulphuric acid is swallowed and death follows speedily, the acid is not only absorbed by the blood but transudes through the tissues; and the peritoneal covering presents a distinct acid reaction. The acid in like manner acts on the concave surface and anterior edge of the liver, rendering it hard and friable; on the transverse arch of the colon, contracting that bowel and rendering its tissues hard and thick; on the *duodenum*, contracting its calibre and rendering the coats firm and thick; and acting in a similar manner on the adjoining folds of *jejunum* and *ileum*.

It occasionally happens that a portion of the stomach is dissolved and corroded, forming a ragged irregular opening; and the contents escape into the abdominal cavity. This happened to a woman who had committed double suicide. She had swallowed oil of vitriol, apparently without its having been known. She then cut her throat with a knife. She was supposed to have died of the effects of the wound in the throat; and certainly vessels enow were divided to cause the loss of much blood; and blood was found, as is often the case in examples of cut throat, in the bronchial tubes. But besides this, there was in the large arch of the stomach a large ragged irregular-shaped and dissolved opening, which presented all round the usual charring and induration caused by sulphuric acid.†

When the mineral acids do not immediately kill, they cause inflammation of the parts touched. The œsophageal epidermis is cast off, and the whole surface of that tube suppurates and secretes lymph and granulates. The mucous membrane of the stomach in like manner suppurates, or sloughs and suppurates, secreting lymph and granulation. Under this process the patient's life may be protracted from five or six weeks to two months, with great suffering, distress, and wasting. But death at length takes place, and the parts are found in the state now described.

The effects of nitric acid on the stomach are very similar to those

* Account of a Case of Suicidal Poisoning by means of Concentrated Sulphuric Acid, with notices of other cases. By David Craigie, M. D. &c. Edinburgh Medical and Surgical Journal, Vol. liii. p. 406. Edinburgh, 1840.

† Cases of Poisoning by Arsenic, Sulphuric Acid, and Muriate of Mercury. By Alexander Watson, F. R. C. S. E. Ibid. Vol. liii. p. 401.

of sulphuric acid. But the citron yellow coloration of the gastric tissues is here also conspicuous.

The vapour of nitric acid also operates on the organs of respiration.

Hydrochloric acid is less frequently employed, either accidentally or intentionally, apparently than sulphuric acid. But its effects are very similar. Crispation and detachment of the œsophageal epidermis; charring of the interior of the stomach; blackening and coagulation of the blood in the blood-vessels; corrosion of the gastric tissue; and a dark mottled appearance of the neighbouring viscera; are all lesions which have been observed after deglutition of this acid. The bile is rendered of a bright grass green wherever the acid comes in contact with it.*

The duration of life after deglutition of the concentrated mineral acids, varies according to circumstances from four or five hours to twenty-five or thirty hours.

The further examination of this point, however, belongs to toxicology.

f. In many cases of canine madness the œsophageal and gastric membrane has been found reddened and covered with viscid mucus; (Morgagni, Baillie, Babington, Ferriar, Marcet, Powel, Pinckard, &c.) and several authors have here been inclined to ascribe the symptoms of that disease to œsophageal and gastric inflammation. Admitting, however, that appearances of this kind are sufficient to constitute spreading or diffuse inflammation of the mucous surface, it does not follow that this is the cause of the hydrophobic symptoms. The œsophageal and gastric redness is not constant; and its presence and degree, which are secondary, depend rather on the violent spasmodic motions of the muscles of deglutition and the diaphragm, than on positive or primary inflammation.

The affection of the gastric mucous membrane occurring in fever, as remarked by Roederer and Wagler, Sarcone, Pinel, and others, shall be noticed afterwards.

§ 3. The *duodenum* is liable to morbid lesions similar to those affecting the stomach. Chronic inflammation appears to be the most common affection in that part of the alimentary canal. Under its influence the duodenal mucous membrane becomes firm, rigid, and a little thickened. Its glandular apparatus also is liable to be hy-

* Case of Poisoning by Muriatic Acid. London Medical Gazette, 1839, No. 15.

pertrophied, rendering the inner surface of the tube irregular and hard.

Chronic inflammation is liable to attack this organ in the circumscribed form; that is, affecting a small spot and proceeding to ulceration of the mucous membrane, and destruction of the whole tissues;—producing perforation of a part of the organ not adherent. The effects are quite similar to those of ulceration and perforation of the stomach.

Chronic thickening of the duodenum is liable to take place at any part of the bowel; in some cases in consequence of inflammation and congestion, in others in consequence of deposition of new matter. If the thickening take place near the point where the common duct enters the bowel, it causes jaundice often of a most obstinate character. It is still worse where the deposit is tubercular or scirrhous. In one case of this kind, the jaundiced colour of the surface was not only very deep, but continued obstinately to the last. It was found after death that the mucous membrane of the *duodenum* was the seat of a deposition of tubercles near and all round the orifice of the common duct; and that these had thickened the tissues of the bowel to so great a degree as to obstruct entirely the orifice of the duct. The surface of this deposition was beginning to be ulcerated, being irregular and abraded; and, had life been prolonged, the morbid process would doubtless have destroyed the tissue of the bowel and caused perforation.

Any other deposit is liable to produce the same results.

§ 4. *Enteria.*—Inflammation of the iliac mucous membrane is greatly more frequent than it has been represented by authors. Whatever be the influence of authority to the contrary, it may be shown that the frequent fluid alvine discharges, to which physicians give the name of *diarrhœa*, are in the greater number of cases to be referred to inflammation of the mucous surface of the intestines, spreading over a considerable extent, and rarely penetrating to the submucous filamentous tissue.

Though it was originally maintained by Glisson on the evidence of dissection, that in diarrhœa the intestinal mucous membrane is inflamed, and a similar idea was entertained by Baglivi and other Italian physicians, the facts on which this opinion rests, appear to have been overlooked, amidst the zeal and ingenuity with which the hypothesis of *inordinate motion* (*motus abnormis*) of the school of Hoffmann and Cullen was defended. Next to the instance recorded by Morgagni in his own person and others mentioned in his 31st epistle, in the Reports of Ludovic Bang for 1782 and 1787, may be found distinct traces of the opinion that intestinal inflammation gives rise to diarrhœa.* Much about the same time, (1798,) Carmichael Smyth conjectured, " that in diarrhœas, from catching cold, the villous or interior coat of the stomach and intestines is sometimes slightly inflamed."† This conjecture was afterwards confirmed by the researches of Baillie,‡ Pinel,§ Hildenbrand,‖ Broussais,¶ Petit and Serres,** Abercrombie, Andral, Latham,†† and lastly Billard. The proofs collected by these authors it is unnecessary to examine minutely. They establish indisputably the inference, that the red or rose tint of mere injection of the mucous membrane is adequate to produce all the symptoms of diarrhœa passing into dysentery. The state of the intestinal membrane, as discovered by necroscopy, may vary according to the extent of the disease, the kind of the inflammatory process, and the parts of the intestinal membrane affected.

Inflammation of the intestinal mucous membrane, to be rightly understood, should be studied both in the villous membrane proper, (*Enteria ; Enteritis mucosa ;*) and in the intestinal follicles, isolated and agminated ; (*Adenitis ; Adeno-enteria.*)

a. In the villous membrane proper, the process is known by redness and vascularity, increased secretion of viscid jelly-like mucus, which is often very adherent, and sometimes tinged with blood, sometimes with a proportion of albumen, so as to form false membrane, and generally some thickening and roughening of the membrane. This is commonly a diffuse or spreading form of inflammation, and in characters acute.

b. *Adenitis ; Adeno-enteria.* Follicular inflammation. *Dothinenteritis.*—The intestinal follicles are subject to at least two forms of in-

* Selecta Diarii Nosocomii Regii Hafniensis, Auctore Frederico Ludovica Bang. Vol. i. p. 47, Vol. ii. and 233, 314, 360, 361.

† Medical Communications, Vol. ii. p. 210.

‡ " It does not always happen," says Baillie, " when a person has died from fatal purging, that there are ulcers in the intestines. In two cases which I have opened of persons who died from this complaint, the small intestines were inflamed, so as to present the appearance of distinct vessels, the small branches of arteries curling most beautifully at the outer surface of the intestine filled with florid blood, and the *villous coat being slightly red.*"—Dissections, &c. p. 218.

§ Medecine Clinique et Nosographie Philosophique, Tom. ii.

‖ Ratio Medendi in Instit. Clinico.   ¶ Phlegmasies Chroniques.

** Traité de la Fievre Entero-Mesenterique. 8vo. Paris, 1813.

†† An Account of the Disease lately prevalent at the General Penitentiary. By P. M. Latham, M. D. &c. Lond. 1825.

flammatory enlargement. In one the mucous membrane is mostly affected. It swells up, becomes dry at first, then is covered with viscid thick mucus adherent to it, while the pore of the follicle is more or less obstructed in consequence of the swelling. When this continues long, it is liable to induce abrasion of the mucous membrane or even ulceration. Yet this does not appear often to take place in this sort of affection of the follicles. The swelling may subside, and the follicle or follicles recover their previous appearance and qualities.

In the second form, in which the fine cellular tissue is most affected, it is very different. The tissue is raised and swelled out, becomes firm, tough, and often assumes a buff or yellow colour, which shows that it is dying or dead. In short this follicular cellular tissue is very easily killed, and then forms a slough below the mucous membrane. The latter, however, being deprived of its support and nutrition, likewise dies, is cast off as a superficial slough, while below there is one more deep. This also is cast off, and a deep ulcer is left, which is almost invariably very difficult to be healed, and which often does not heal, but, by weakening the bowel, causes perforation of the peritoneal coat.

These are forms of inflammation comparatively chronic, that is, lasting from three to six weeks.

1. The simplest form is that in which the mucous surface is light reddish, or rose-coloured over a large extent,—an appearance which depends on superficial injection of the villous membrane. The *villi* are red, and more or less gorged with blood. This state, besides producing copious mucous or sero-gelatinous discharges, is very often the pathological cause of intestinal hemorrhage. In some instances it is shaded from a light rose to blood-colour or wine-coloured crimson.

2. The intestinal membrane may be marked by redness disposed in various forms, arborescent, asteroid, or punctular, or in slender linear streaks. These appearances may occur independent of inflammation, as an effect of transudation, or stagnation during the last hours of existence or after death, and should therefore be distinguished from the same forms of redness in connection with the inflammatory process, when they indicate a slight or incipient form of it.

3. A common form is in red or brown patches, irregular in size and shape, with sensible elevation above the surrounding membrane, forming a sort of puffy swelling, the surface of which is rough and irregular, and, though not hard, void of its natural feel.

Though these patches, which are in the follicles isolated and agminated, may occur in any part of the small or large intestine, they are most common at the termination of the ileum, in which they are seated in the agminated patches of glands, and the beginning of the colon, where they are in isolated follicles. From petechial and ecchymotic blotches, with which they are liable to be confounded, they may be distinguished by the blood being observed in pieces of intestine held up to the light to be still contained within vessels. (Latham.) These red patches are exceedingly prone to proceed to ulceration, which takes place in one or more points near their centre, and by extension and coalition produce in no long time a breach in the continuity of the mucous corion equal in size to the original patch. This is the form of disease described first by Prost, then by MM. Petit and Serres under the name Entero-mesenteric fever, and which, there is reason to believe, is occasionally epidemic in Paris.* Of the same nature is the disease which was prevalent in the Millbank Penitentiary during 1822 and 1823. According to the description of Dr Latham, the patches, which most frequently were circular, and not exceeding the diameter of a pea, were dispersed at intervals through the whole tract of the intestines. These were evidently in the isolated follicles. When larger and more irregular, they appear to have been the result of the coalescence of several small patches; and were most likely in the agminated glands. The transition to ulceration in this instance consisted in the reddened mucous membrane becoming elevated, rough, and unequal to the touch, and in erosion taking place at several points.†

4. A considerable extent of the membrane may be diffusely red or reddish brown, or with a general rose-coloured ground may present red or brown patches of a more intense tint. The membrane is at the same time soft, friable, pulpy, and often thickened; the mucous glands are enlarged and reddish; and the membrane is covered more or less extensively by thick, semi-opaque viscid mucus of a reddish or wine-coloured tint. This form of the disease is also said to proceed to ulceration. When it does so, the process takes place not only in spots and patches of the mucous membrane, but in the follicles, which are converted into a number of oval reddish-brown ulcers.

5. Part of the intestinal mucous membrane may present numerous vesicular or pustular elevations, not unlike thrush vesicles

* Traité de la Fièvre Entero-mesenterique, p. 13. Paris, 1813.
† An Account of the Disease, &c. p. 48.

(*aphthæ*), which may terminate in the formation of abraded spots or minute ulcers.   Excoriation and abrasion is mentioned by various authors; but I think none of them distinguish between this and ulceration, of which I regard it as the incipient stage.   Abrasion consists, properly speaking, in the removal of epidermis; but as the existence of this in the gastro-enteric membrane is problematical, it may be doubted whether there is other abrasion than what I now admit.   These abraded spots or minute ulcers appear to me to be the apices of the isolated follicles proceeding to ulceration.

6. In certain forms of intestinal inflammation, the morbid process appears in the shape of spheroidal or conoidal circumscribed eminences, which are red, fungous, and irregular, and form conspicuous prominences of the mucous membrane. These bodies, which thus resemble pustules, and are surrounded by a red hoop (*areola*), consist in inflammation of the isolated mucous follicles of Peyer, as represented by MM. Bretonneau and Trousseau, and many subsequent observers.   They are often much elevated above the adjoining mucous membrane, not unlike broad circular mushrooms, and are then sometimes named *fungi*.   There is no doubt, nevertheless, that they consist, as above described, of the thickened follicular cellular tissue, with morbid secretions in the apex, and they are tinged with the colouring matter of the excrement.   According to the former of these observers especially, this follicular inflammation, passing occasionally to ulceration, is a most frequent form of intestinal disease not only primary, but occurring in the course of fevers.   Its most constant and frequent locality is the 3, 6, or 10 last inches of the ileum, where the agminated patches are largest, and a long space of the *ileum* consists of agminated follicles without interruption; and when it affects the colon it is near the ileo-cœcal valve, being on both sides of this point much more confluent than at greater distances.   This form of intestinal inflammation M. Bretonneau denominates *dothinenteria* (δοθινη *pustula*, and εντερον *intestinum*.)*

Any one of these forms of morbid condition may produce all the phenomena of diarrhœa or even dysentery.   The most uniform and remarkable effect, however, is after the first discharges of feculent matter to cause abundant excretion of viscid mucous matter, which, though fluid when discharged, undergoes a species of coagulation

* Archives Generales, Tome x. 1826. P. 67 and 169.

not unlike jelly. This may be easily recognized, even when mixed with feculent matter. It is free from the peculiar offensive odour of the latter; and it appears to contain a proportion of albuminous or gelatinous matter, or both.

Ulceration of the mucous follicles is very common after the disease in any of the above forms has subsisted long. This was seen in those of the duodenum by Brunner, in those of the ileum by Leeat, Prost, Petit, and Serres, Bretonneau, and Trousseau, Billard, and Dr Bright. This form of ulceration is invariably more complicated and more difficult of cure than simple ulceration of the villous membrane. The latter, indeed, without affection of the follicles, is so rare that its existence may be questioned.

To render the history of inflammation of the intestinal mucous membrane and its follicles complete, I feel it necessary to take a general view of the disorder, as it takes place at different periods of life and in different circumstances; and though in this view I shall not disregard the observations and descriptions of others, yet I deduce it principally from the results of personal observation continued over a long period of years.

1. Chronic inflammation may attack the mucous follicles of the *ileum* at six weeks after birth, at three months, at six or eight months, or at twelve months, or two years after birth. After the latter period it is less frequent, but may take place under circumstances presently to be mentioned. The earliest period at which I have observed the disease after birth was six weeks. And in the case to which I allude, it must be observed, that the disease had been present for three or four weeks; so that it may be allowed that it commences as early as two or three weeks after birth.

The aggregated patches, which are generally more distinct in the infant than in the adult, are elevated, with rough prominent edges, rough surfaces, so uneven with elevations and depressions that they have been supposed to be ulcerated, and they have been in this condition by some supposed to be in a state of ulceration. When, however, the surface is carefully cleansed by water, it is seen that it is merely irregular, rugose, here prominent and elevated, there depressed; and, in short, swelled or in a state of inflammatory congestion.

The reason of this irregularity is that the inflammatory congestion and injection affects mostly the follicular cellular tissue, which then rising up, where it most easily does so, causes the elevations;

while the intermediate points, at which it does not readily rise, form the hollows and depressions.

This state of the ileal follicles may last for weeks, coming and going, or appearing and subsiding alternately. It may take place in consequence of improper food, but seems also to occur spontaneously or at least without evident cause. It is common in infants fed by the hand or other unnatural modes; and is often induced at the period of weaning, if care be not taken to effect that change gradually. When it has been once commenced it is liable to recur.

Follicular irritation and enlargement, if not proceeding to much thickening and to ulceration of the surface, may subside, and leave the membrane in a healthy state. Children who have it are liable to diarrhœa in fits, or are said to have irritable bowels; but as the follicles return to their natural condition, this symptom disappears.

When it continues long or recurs frequently, and gives rise to frequent, habitual, or violent diarrhœa, the follicles are thickened; and on the apices of several of them small ulcers are formed. But even without ulceration it may prove fatal by the extent over which it is diffused, the over-action and irritation of the intestines, and the violence of the general symptoms, with its wasting effects on the function of nutrition. It is usually observed in cases thus terminating, that numerous invaginations have taken place in the bowel, each invagination being formed over the site of an enlarged aggregated patch. Infants and young children with this disorder are sometimes cut off suddenly, most usually with symptoms of crowing inspiration; and spasmodic contraction of the thumbs, fingers, and toes. In other cases symptoms of *enteritis* or *peritonitis* with obstinate constipation often take place; and then ulceration is found to have extended to the submucous cellular tissue and the peritonæum.

2. Follicular inflammation may take place at a subsequent period, that is, at periods after infancy, and between the third and fifteenth year, or even at later periods.

Though this disease may come on in various modes at the time of life now referred to, the most usual, at least between three and seven or eight years, is the following.

The patient is unwell, languid, with hot skin, especially at night; -the tongue a little furred; the pulse quicker than usual (90, 100, 110); and the appetite impaired, with thirst. Sleep is disturbed .and unrefreshing; the patient starts and is alarmed; and awakes in the morning generally more fatigued and exhausted than at night. Yet there are no very conspicuous or prominent symptoms which denote derangement or disorder of a particular texture or region. This state of matters may proceed for 8, 10, or 12 days. The bowels are then observed to be irregular; sometimes constipated; more frequently slightly loose. In a few cases uneasiness is observed or felt in the umbilical or the right iliac region, or in both. The umbilical region may be somewhat distended; and beneath the fingers air is felt moving in that region, or in the right iliac. Feverishness continues, and is usually aggravated in the latter part of the day and at or during night. At length pain is felt in the belly, generally about the right iliac region or the umbilical; and this may increase to symptoms of enteritis or peritonitis. Diarrhœa stops; vomiting takes place; and the bowels are obstinately bound, while the abdomen is swelled, painful, and tympanitic.

The disease usually under these circumstances terminates fatally; and the intestinal mucous membrane and follicles are found in the following state.

Much viscid mucus adheres to the villous membrane, and more especially to the aggregated patches. When this is removed, the patches are observed elevated, roughened, and indurated in various degrees. In some the elevation is moderate; in others it is great and perceptible, giving them the aspect of pustular eminences, or rendering them like buttons on the villous membrane. Usually this considerable elevation depends on thickening and death of the follicular cellular tissue, which is hard, friable, and of a buff or yellow colour. In certain points the mucous membrane is cast off, disclosing small ulcers; the base of which is sometimes the yellow thick dead tissue already mentioned, sometimes the muscular and peritoneal coat. These ulcers evidently take place in individual follicles; but by two or more coalescing, two or more small ulcers may be converted into one large one. The adjoining intestinal membrane is occasionally but not always thickened; and sometimes vessels are seen traversing it to the patch or patches most thickened. The mesenteric ganglions opposite are enlarged in various degrees and to different extent. At some points a whole cluster of glands enlarged is presented; at others, two or three are enlarged but separate.

· In extreme cases albuminous exudation covers the peritoneum corresponding to the patches or the ulcers; and the peritoneum has in certain cases given way previous to death, allowing the partial escape of the contents of the bowel, and followed by effusion of sero-albuminous fluid from the internal or free surface of the peritonæum.

3. In certain cases the isolated follicles are the seat of chronic inflammation, either alone or along with the aggregated follicle. In either case they present the appearance of pustules a little elevated, or fungous-looking flat tubercular bodies. These isolated follicles pass through the changes already mentioned in proceeding to ulceration. In the form of pustules they have been repeatedly mistaken for variolous pustules; and hence it has been said, that they are small-pox in the intestinal mucous membrane.

A peculiar sort of broad elevated button-like appearance is occasionally seen in the intestinal mucous membrane in this disorder. The individual bodies are about two lines broad, sometimes three, irregularly circular, with flat tops. They are evidently raised above the level of the surrounding mucous membrane, and sometimes their margins project over the latter. The tops are fungous-looking and rough, and of a fawn or dirty yellow colour; and it seems as if the whole follicular mucous membrane had become thickened and hypertrophied. This is the result of a more chronic affection than the one already described. Occasionally these fungous-looking bodies are seated in the isolated follicles; and sometimes in the agminated follicles.

4. The disease now described may take place, as already stated, as a mere intestinal affection. Often, however, it is either connected with fever, or it is an effect of the operation of the febrific poison. In children and young persons it is often connected with the fever described as intestinal remittent fever. In adults it takes place along with fever which has been by several observers described as typhous fever. But when it was manifest that typhous fever, in the great majority of cases, took place, and continues to take place, without affection of the intestinal follicles, the fever in which this follicular disease was said to take place was denominated typhoid fever.

The truth is, that the disease takes place in a fever which may present, according to its treatment, typhoid symptoms during the second septenary period, or rather towards the close of that period. But the fever, in which it most commonly takes place, is a remittent fever, with evening or afternoon exacerbations; and the persons most usually affected are children from 5 to 10, or young persons in general under the 30th year of age. The disease is much more common in certain localities than in others. In Paris it seems

4

frequent, but affects mostly persons coming from the provinces. In London it is also not uncommon. In Manchester I have seen it affecting the Irish labourers. In Edinburgh it is not very common; and a physician treating from 200 to 300 patients in the course of the year my see not above three or·four cases, and only one of these fatal. In certain seasons it is more common than in others. Thus several cases took place in the winter of 1842–1843; and a few cases took place in the end of 1845 and beginning of 1846. At the close of the latter year it was again appearing.

In Edinburgh it is seen in railway labourers, and persons engaged in similar out-door labour.

In Glasgow it is more frequent than in Edinburgh, and is seen mostly among the Irish.

It appears to me not to be contagious, but to affect spontaneously, or in consequence of causes, not easily determined, the persons attacked. From the testimony of various foreign observers, as Frenzel, Ebel, Grossheim, Stannius,* Chomel,† Lesser,‡ and Cramer,§ it appears to depend either on telluric miasma, or on some atmospheric conditions.

c. *Perforation.*—Though any part of the small intestine from the *duodenum* to the *cæcum* may be the seat of ulcers, they are most numerous and largest in the lower part of the ileum. In this part of the tube the ulcerative process may advance so far as to affect the submucous tissue, the muscular layer, and the subserous tissue, upon which the peritonæum generally gives way, and laceration or perforation takes place. That the peritonæum is removed by absorption, or rather gives way when no longer supported by the collateral tissues, may be inferred from the fact observed by M. Louis, to whom we are indebted for the best and fullest account of this accident;—that the margin of the ulcers in which perforation takes place is sharp and clean; that the mucous and submucous tissue are destroyed nearly to the same extent; and that the muscular is less, and the peritonæum scarcely at all destroyed.

The effect of perforation is, as in the case of the stomach, 1*st*,

* Edinburgh Medical and Surgical Journal, Vol. xlviii. p. 145.

† Leçons de Clinique Medicale, faites a L'Hotel Dieu de Paris. Par le Professeur A. F. Chomel. Paris, 1834 : and Edinburgh Medical and Surgical Journal, Vol. xlix. p. 492, and l. p. 175.

‡ Die Entzundung und Verschwarung der Schleimhaut des Verdauungs Kanales als selbstandige Krankheit, dargestellt von Ferdinand Lesser. Berlin, 1830. 8vo. Mit Kupfertafeln.

§ Der Abdominal Typhus. Monographische Skizze. Von Dr F. Cramer. Cassel, 1840. 8vo. ss. 128.

escape of the intestinal contents to a greater or less extent; 2d, the development of peritoneal inflammation, with albuminous deposition on the peritonæum. The period which elapses between the commencement of ulceration and the completion of erosion varies in different cases. According to the observations of Louis, already quoted, it may be inferred that in a space varying from 12 to 25 days, the ulcer or ulcers may effect destruction of the intestinal tunics. The occurrence of the final laceration of the peritoneal coat may be conjectured by the patient experiencing all at once in the belly intense tearing pain, aggravated by pressure, speedily followed by shrinking of the features, vomiting, &c. which, continuing with almost incessant severity from 20 to 54 hours, denote intense peritoneal inflammation terminating in death. In one case, which, however, must be regarded as an exception, life was continued for seven days after the appearance of symptoms of perforation.

d. *Enteria mollescens.*—Under this head may be placed a change observed by Louis in the ileum of many persons cut off by phthisis and other chronic diseases. It consists in the mucous membrane becoming exceedingly soft, almost like mucus or jelly, sometimes thicker than natural, and sometimes redder. In the instances in which I have observed this change in phthisical subjects, the intestinal *villi* were less distinct than natural. But whether this arose from removal of these bodies or from the pulpy swelling of the mucous corion, or from absolute disorganization, I have not been able to determine. It is rarely continuous, and occurs chiefly in large patches, which occupy, however, the whole circumference of the bowel.

§ 5. *Chronic ulceration.*—To this head I refer a form of disease of which I have seen several instances in children labouring under symptoms of mesenteric wasting ; (*tabes.*) I have no doubt that it commences in inflammation of the mucous membrane, or rather of the agminated follicles; but as it was found in the cases to which I allude in the form of ulcerated patches, I prefer, for the sake of obvious and easy distinction, to designate it as above. In the best marked instance in which I have seen it, and the preparation of which is before me, it occurred in the form of three large bands near the lower end of the ileum, extending transversely round the entire circumference of the bowel. The broadest of these bands is about two inches, the narrowest about eight lines. Over the whole of these spaces is the mucous membrane completely removed by the ulcerative process, leaving an irregular surface, partly granulating, partly ulcerated in the mucous tissue. The margins are sharp, clean, and accurately cut, almost as if they had been divided by a knife, and slightly turned up, so as to leave an excavated furrow beneath the mucous membrane which forms the margins. The colour of the bottom of these ulcerated patches, when recent, was reddish brown, and the contiguous mucous membrane was red, verging to pale rose colour and peach blossom. This, however, has disappeared, and at present it is much the same tint as the healthy part of the mucous surface. The mucous membrane is a good deal thickened and rather firmer than in the sound part of the tube. At each of these ulcerated bands the submucous and subserous filamentous tissue is thickened, but indurated and contracted, so as to diminish considerably the calibre of the canal. In the first patch, which is about twelve inches from the ileo-cæcal valve, this thickening consists of a firm knot like a bean, at the mesenteric side of the bowel, and the intestine is contracted to about half its usual capacity. In the second, about five inches from the ileocæcal valve, this indurated knot at the mesenteric attachment of the bowel is equally well marked, and has had, if possible, greater influence in contracting and diminishing the canal of the bowel. The ulcerated surface is very irregular by soft spongy eminences, separated by means of linear furrows. The third occupies the end of the ileum and beginning of the colon, and has entirely destroyed, with the mucous membrane of both bowels, the ileo-cæcal valve. The destroyed part here presents a surface consisting in very minute round granules; and in the beginning of the colon are one or two large irregular granulations. The same inflammatory induration of the submucous and subserous filamentous tissue has here operated in diminishing the capacity of the bowel; and, indeed, previous to being cut open, it seemed almost impervious. The inflammatory process here had produced peritoneal inflammation, and false membrane connecting the *ileum*, *caput cæcum*, and part of the colon together. The vermiform process is unaffected. Opposite to each were enlarged mesenteric glands, and especially at the last mentioned one was a cluster of large knotty masses.

Though I describe the ultimate effects of this destructive process, I have no doubt, from what I have seen of other cases in earlier stages, that it is the result of chronic inflammation of the intestinal mucous membrane, originating in the agminated follicles, at the lower end of the *ileum,* and from them spreading to the adjoining mucous membrane.   I had an opportunity of observing the progress of the disease for more than two years, during which the case was more or less under my care; and during that period it was possible to recognise occasional attacks of inflammation.   The other symptoms were occasional pain of the belly, never severe, unless at the period of the above attacks, and diarrhœa alternating with constipation, afterwards incessant and uncontrollable diarrhœa, wasting, and hectic fever;—in short, all the symptoms imputed to mesenteric decline; (*tabes mesenterica.*)   This process, therefore, or chronic inflammation of the intestinal mucous follicles and membrane, with or without ulceration, I regard as one of the pathological causes of mesenteric *tabes.*   The enlargement of the glands, in which this disòrder has been very generally believed since the time of Wharton, Baglivi, and Richard Russell to consist, is merely secondary, and is a consecutive effect of the irritation exercised at the organic extremities of the lymphatics and lacteals.   This view of the relation between enlarged mesenteric glands and intestinal inflammation, though already stated by Broussais, has not, however, been established by that author on authentic proofs.   Enlargement of these glands is indeed, I have elsewhere said, a common effect of irritation at the organic extremities of their lymphatics.

§ 6. *Typhlitis, Perityphlitis.*—The *cæcum* or blind bowel (*typhlon enteron*) is often the seat of a peculiar disease, which, from slow and almost imperceptible commencements, produces so much havoc as to terminate the life of the individual.

This disease consists in inflammation and suppuration of the cellular tissue connecting the *cæcum* to the *quadratus lumborum* and other parts, or in inflammation and·ulceration of the mucous membrane of the cæcum, and often of the vermiform process, and which, advancing by very gradual and insidious steps, destroys the mucous membrane, affects the submucous cellular tissue and peritoneal coat, and either causes inflammation of the latter with adhesion to the muscular parietes of the abdomen, or perforation and fatal *peritonitis.*   The exact mode in which this disease commences is not always perfectly known.   But from the dissection of those who have perished by it, we may infer that the following description makes a near approach to the facts.

At first the glands or follicles of the *cæcum* become enlarged and thickened and elevated by inflammation. Then the summits of these covered by the remains of purulent matter and adherent mucus are separated; and below are disclosed ulcerated surfaces to the same extent as the glands of follicles originally affected. This process extends and deepens, until the submucous tissue and the peritoneum are affected. Lymph is effused over the surface of the latter; and this for some time either prevents the bowel from being perforated, or it unites the peritoneal coat of the cæcum with the muscular peritoneum and the abdominal muscles. At the same time the mucous membrane of the vermiform process is affected by inflammation of its follicles and subsequent ulceration; so that when the body is inspected after death, this appendage presents numerous ulcers along its internal surface.

When the inflammatory action has caused the agglutination of the cæcal peritonæum to the muscular peritonæum and abdominal muscles, the morbid process is not thereby stopped. Very commonly it is extended progressively to the cellular tissue outside the peritonæum, thence to the muscles in the right iliac region, and it may even produce an external abscess in these muscles, the opening of which on the surface will depend on the time during which life is prolonged.

In one case of this kind, which I inspected in the body of a young female of 11 or 12, the cæcum itself was greatly distended; the extra-cæcal peritoneum was partly adherent to the muscular, and partly destroyed by ulceration; the round or convex part of the bowel was perforated with 6 or 7 ragged apertures, various in size and shape; matter was found all round it and between them, and also externally to the muscular peritoneum, and between the fibres and layers of the abdominal muscles; and the skin, though not destroyed, was undermined. When the disease had reached this point death had taken place. But had life been prolonged a few days more, an opening in the skin of the right iliac region would have taken place; and a fistulous, cavernous abscess passing through the abdominal muscles and into the cæcum must have ensued. In this case also the colon was small, contracted, and almost empty, its size being more like that of the *ileum* than the colon, while the *ileum* was distended by feculent contents to about three or four times its usual size, and presented at first sight the appearance of the colon. This fact deserves, as we shall see, especial attention.

Another mode in which this disease shows itself is the following.

After the disease in the mucous membrane of the cæcum has subsisted for some time, with or without ulceration of the cæcum, it is followed by inflammation taking place in the cellular tissue at the posterior part of the cæcum. The latter bowel, it must be remembered, is tied down and fixed by cellular tissue to the right iliac *fossa* immediately before the lumbar and *iliacus internus* muscles. The inflammation passes to this cellular tissue; and in it causes effusion of lymph and purulent matter, forming a sort of abscess round and behind the cæcum. In the right iliac region there is then recognized a tumour compressible and doughy, and giving a sense of deep-seated matter; painful when pressed at certain points, and tending, as in the last case, to advance to the surface. The disease then shows itself under the form of abscess of the right iliac region.

In this state after matter has been formed one of two results may take place. Either the inflammatory action continuing and the suppurative action advancing, a communication by ulceration may be opened into the cæcum, and through this the matter contained in the tumour passes gradually but speedily into the colon, and is thus discharged into the bowels. Then, if adhesive inflammation and lymphy deposit take place, the tumour is emptied of its contents and recovery is accomplished, the inflammation and suppuration being confined to the immediate neighbourhood and attachments of the cæcum.

Secondly, it may happen that either with or without the opening into the cæcum the agglutinative or adhesive inflammation is imperfect and inert. Lymph is not effused in sufficient quantity to stop the spreading of the suppuration. Matter is effused or infiltrated into the cellular tissue all round and downwards over the surface of the *iliacus internus* muscle; and after great ravages are committed, it appears forming an outlet at the margin of the anus. This is an unfavourable result, because the matter in advancing to the surface is attended with much destruction of parts; and because the progressive advancement of the disease denotes a deficiency of healthy agglutinative and reparative action.

In the third place, the suppurative process may advance to the surface, causing superficial abscess in the right iliac region and ulcerative openings to discharge the purulent contents of the deep-seated abscess. This appears to be not very common; but it occurs in a certain number of cases. It is not very favourable.

Although I began the account of this affection by representing it to originate in previous disease of the *cæcum* and vermiform appendage, yet there occur cases in which the latter circumstance is not always manifest. If the first movements of diseased action have taken place in the cæcum, it has been externally; and hence they have advanced to affect the bowel secondarily. This mode of procedure may best be illustrated by the following case.

A young female, in the rank and occupation of a servant, was sent from Leith to the Royal Infirmary with symptoms believed to indicate the presence of continued fever. The skin was hot, and though not dry, was imperfectly transpiring; the tongue was covered with a whitish gray pasty fur; there was some thirst; the expression of the countenance was languid and feeble, though the face was flushed; the pulse was between 86 and 90, rising to 100; and the strength was impaired. The abdomen was a little distended and slightly painful; yet pressure was borne tolerably well. The sound emitted was clear and natural. But in the right iliac region, where some fulness was manifest, the sound emitted was dull; and considerable pain was felt on pressing or handling this region. This painful sensation also extended backwards to the loins; but was more complained of on the right than on the left side. In the right iliac region also, but most towards the side of the region and its posterior aspect, there was recognized a more firm and resisting yet compressible and doughy state of the parts than natural. Pain was aggravated by coughing.

Some blood was drawn from the arm; twelve leeches were applied over the right iliac region; and laxative medicine was given.

Next day the patient said she felt relieved and more easy. But the state of parts in the right iliac region was not improved; the abdomen was rather more distended, with some tympanitic resonance; the pulse was above 100, not full but hard; the skin was dry; the urine scanty and sedimentous; and the bowels had been moved scantily and imperfectly; the fur on the tongue was much as before.

Twelve leeches were ordered on the right iliac region, to be followed by warm fomentations and a poultice; and an enema was directed to be administered.

Next morning the patient became suddenly very feeble and died.

Inspection disclosed the following appearances.

A portion of bowel between 3½ and 4 feet long, which turned out to be the lower part of the ileum, was greatly distended chiefly with air; of a dark brown-red colour, and with its peritoneal coat covered and penetrated by an infinite number of red vessels. This piece of intestine formed in this state several turns or convolutions; and a considerable portion of it had been pushed over to the right side. The ileum above this was distended but less reddened. When cut open the contents were much as usual, but with more air. The mucous membrane was greatly reddened, friable, rough, and easily detached. The substance of the bowel was vascular and reddened. But of the follicles there was neither elevation nor ulceration. The ileo-cæcal valve was reddened. The interior of the cæcum was also reddened and softened; but no ulceration had taken place. The *appendix vermiformis* presented a few enlarged follicles along its interior. The ascending arch of the colon was comparatively empty; and the rest of the bowel was pretty natural, and void of any thing except thin feculent matter and mucus. The mucous membrane of the colon was not unnatural.

External to the cæcum, on the lateral and posterior aspects of that bowel, were deposits of purulent matter and loose lymph, extending upwards and backwards for a good space. This purulent matter occupied the place of the perityphlic cellular tissue; was not contained within a distinct or well-formed cyst, but appeared to be loosely infiltrated into the space around the cæcum. No perforation of the cæcum had taken place. But all round the cellular tissue was reddened, softened, loaded with bloody serum and specks of purulent matter; and the parts were ash-coloured and offensive smelling, as if proceeding to mortification.

In this case the cause of death was twofold. First, the general inflammation of the lower portion of the *ileum* (*enteritis*; *ileitis*), caused apparently by obstruction and distension of the whole bowel, in consequence of the pressure created by the inflammatory abscess round the *cæcum*; and secondly, this suppurative inflammation of the perityphlic cellular tissue itself, which, though operating chiefly as a cause of pressure on the *cæcum* and obstruction to the peristaltic motion of the bowel, yet did further mischief by the peculiar effects of a bad suppuration on the system at large.

In this case also, there is every reason to believe that the primary morbid action was seated in the perityphlic cellular tissue; and that the inflammation and suppuration there established had acted on the *cæcum* by compressing it, and thus obstructing the descent of the contents of the *ileum*, had caused over-distension of the latter and general inflammation much as a strangulated hernia. Indeed, the appearance of the *ileum* was quite similar to that presented by intestines above a point of strangulated bowel.

The termination of this disease is, nevertheless, not necessarily or inevitably fatal. If the tumor in the right iliac region be recognized before suppuration has taken place, resolution may be accomplished under the use of local and general blood-letting, with very gentle aperients. Several patients in this state I have treated and seen get perfectly well; and there is always more chance of complete recovery if the treatment be commenced in this stage, than if it be delayed until suppuration has occurred. After this event the favourable termination, though less likely, may be effected in the mode already mentioned.

Though all the causes of this disorder may not be perfectly understood, yet several are sufficiently obvious and intelligible. In the first place, the peculiar situation and fixed attachment of the *cæcum* must be regarded as an important disposing cause. That bowel being attached by its whole posterior surface, by means of filamentous tissue, to the muscles of the right lumbar region, and with its blind sac or receptacle below the level of the ileo-cæcal aperture, and in a dependent position, is liable to become distended with excrementitial matter, which the bowel itself cannot easily expel and raise against gravity. Then the vermiform process itself, by its dependent position, may encounter difficulty in evacuating its contents.

Secondly, all articles taken with food, or otherwise swallowed and not easily carried along the bowels, are here, from the position of the *cæcum*, more readily detained. The stones of the drupaceous fruits, seeds, pieces of money or metal, fragments of bones, marbles, and similar substances, are liable to be here stopped, and by their presence to cause irritation. In fatal cases the *cæcum* sometimes contains hardened fæces, concretions; and in one case I found fragments of glass.

Kaltschmidt records the case of an artisan of 25, who, about one month after swallowing many walnuts and medlars, was attacked with symptoms of *ileus*, which, after lasting for 15 days, terminated in death. On inspecting the body Kaltschmidt found the whole tract of the bowels presenting marks of inflammation, and the *ileum* at its lower end near the valve of Bauhin perforated in three parts, and contorted or twisted so as to form three separate cavities filled with indurated feculent matter. The destruction was so complete that the *ileum* seemed detached from the *cæcum*, and adhered by a few shreds only. Feculent matter had escaped into the abdominal cavity near the lacerated portion of *ileum* ; and in this was found about half an ounce of the stones of the medlars eaten, and about as much in the fæces within the *ileum*.[*]

Similar instances of the stoppage of stones of the drupaceous fruits, bones, pieces of money, and similar foreign bodies, are recorded by Younge, Amyand, Fielding, Stoll, and other authors. In certain instances intestinal concretions are formed either spontaneously or around bodies of the kind now mentioned. In either case the stoppage of such bodies in the *cæcum* is at once probable, and likely to produce irritation and inflammation of that portion of the intestinal tube.

These must be regarded as disposing causes.

As to age, it seems to take place most frequently in persons between 20 and 30.

As to sex, MM. Husson and Dance say that it is more frequently seen in males than in females.[†] My own experience, nevertheless, leads to the opposite conclusion. I have seen the disease in a greater number of females than males; I have found it more unmanageable in females than in males; I have never seen a fatal case in a man, but several in females. I infer that the class of females in whom it is most frequent is that of domestic servants and seamstresses.

As to the influence of articles of food, it has been said that the use of oatmeal, which favours the formation of intestinal concretions, is also liable to be followed by this disease. Yet it does not appear that the disease is less frequent in France and England, where wheaten bread is used, than in Scotland, where oatmeal is used as part of food. It appears to me also very questionable, whether among those who in Scotland use oatmeal much as food, it is more frequent than among those who use it little or not at all.

Constipation is probably favourable to its formation; and whatever tends to impede or interrupt the periodical evacuation of the bowels must tend to produce this as it does other disorders.[‡]

---

[*] Caroli Fred Kaltschmidt de ileo a scrupulis Pyrorum Mespilaceorum eroso perforato. Jenæ, 1mo Oct. 1747. Haller, Disput. Medico-Pract. iii. p. 510.

[†] Memoire sur quelques engorgemens inflammatoires qui se development dans la fosse iliaque Droite. Repertoire d'Anatomie, &c. T. iv. p. 74. Paris, 1827.

[‡] Ferrall in Edin. Med. and Surg. Journal, Vol. xxxvi. p. 1. Edin. 1831. And Dr Burne in Medico-Chirurgical Transact. xx. p. 200, and xxii.

§ 7. *Colonia. Dysentery. Colonitis.*—The opinion that dysentery depends on inflammation of the bowels is very ancient; but the authority of Cullen succeeded for a time in throwing doubt and obscurity on a doctrine, in favour of which various positive and unequivocal facts have since been collected. The state of the intestines in this disease has been described by Pringle, Baker, Donald Monro, Hunter, and Baillie, Cheyne, and O'Brien; and their accounts, with some trifling exceptions, in general correspond. In four dissections made by Pringle in the Flanders campaign of 1744, the villous coat of the colon was red or vascular, and abraded or ulcerated; the lower end of the colon, and generally the *rectum*, was in a state termed mortification; the ligamentous bands are said to be relaxed, half corrupted, or entirely obliterated; and the colon, sometimes the ileum and stomach, much distended by air.* In the inspections recorded by Baker of the London epidemic of 1762, the villous membrane of the rectum, colon, cæcum, and occasionally part of the ileum, was more or less reddened, velvety-granular, and occupied by numerous minute bodies like small-pox pustules, but harder and solid when divided, and fungous eminences. These hard pustules and fungous eminences were manifestly seated in the isolated follicles. In one case four or five perforations had taken place in the transverse arch of the colon.† In persons cut off by old dysentery, Monro represents the villous membrane of the rectum and colon as inflamed, with livid spots in the arch of the latter; and in one seized by violent pains of the bowels two days before death the ileum was reddened.‡ From a subsequent account by the same author, it appears that the colic mucous membrane as high as the valve, was occupied by livid or black spots of various size, occasioned by black blood in the submucous filamentous tissue; and that in the centre of each spot there was more or less erosion of the villous membrane. Though no black spots or erosions were seen in the mucous membrane of the ileum, in one or two minute red spots, and slight traces of inflammation were recognized.§ The general accuracy of these statements is briefly confirmed by F. L. Bang in

---

* Observations on the Diseases of the Army, by Sir John Pringle, M. D. London, 1768. Chap. 6.

† De Catarrho et de Dysenteria Londinensi epidemicis utrisque, anno 1762, Libellus. Auct. G. Baker, Coll. R. &c. Lond. 1764.

‡ An account of the Diseases, &c. By Donald Monro, M. D. Lond. 1764.

§ Essays and Observations, Physical and Literary, Vol. iii. article 25.

the following terms. " Perlustrata interna facie intestini cæci atque coli, vidimus tunicam villosam alibi adhærentem, et alibi derasam, ibidemque tunicam vasculosam lividam quasi sanguine plenam, mesenterium rubescens vasis distinctis plenissimum."*

Dr John Hunter, on the contrary, who states that he never saw abrasion or mortification of the villous coat, is inclined to think, that in the dissections mentioned by Pringle, the black colour arising from extravasated blood was mistaken for gangrene. Though it is impossible to doubt that this mistake has been often committed in describing the necroscopic changes of the gastro-enteric membrane, it must not be forgotten that inflammation occasionally terminates in mortification, and that instances of this are not unusual in the tropical form of the disease especially. The general fact of inflammation is further confirmed by Maximilian Stoll, who describes the cæcum, colon, especially its transverse arch, and rectum, in persons cut off by acute dysentery, as swelled, thickened, hard, and fleshy, of a leaden or dull red colour, the mucous membrane of a foul or dingy red tint with blood, or of a deep rank green tinge removable neither by water nor the sponge,—an appearance indicating the commencement of elementary decomposition.†

Occasionally dysentery prevails during summer and autumn in this country; and both in previous seasons and in the summer of 1843, we had opportunities of observing its effects on the intestinal coats. In several cases which I examined, the following were the appearances.

The whole tract of the colon was thick, massive, and heavy, totally different from the usual membranous appearance of that bowel. This thickness was partly in the mucous membrane and partly in the submucous cellular tissue. The mucous membrane was thick, of a reddish colour, firm, and more solid than in the normal state, which was shown by the peculiar mode in which it was cut. Its surface was covered with much viscid, thick adherent mucus, which was indeed partly albuminous. The section showed that it was thickened, apparently from effusion of lymph into its interstitial tissue, or from the great congestion of the vessels; the colour was also of a deeper fawn red here than natural. The calibre of the bowel was much contracted, the size and capacity of the colon being not so large as that of the *ileum*.

* Selecta Diarii Nosocomii Hafniensis, Tom. ii. 1786. P. 223.
† Ratio Medendi, Partis iii. Vol. iii. Sectionis 4.

When the mucous membrane was cleared of adherent mucus, numerous patches, variable in size from that of a pea to that of a sixpenny piece, or even larger, and irregular in figure, appeared covered with a coating of albuminous mucus tinged with the colouring matter of the bile and excrement. When these coverings were removed, they disclosed surfaces destroyed by irregular ulceration of the mucous membrane.

These ulcers had originated in the follicles of the colon, which had become softened at the commencement of the attack, and had then proceeded to sloughing and ulceration. The state now described extended along the whole colon, but was most remarkable in the transverse arch and sigmoid flexure.

In some other cases the disease was confined to the lower part of the sigmoid flexure and to the rectum. The mucous membrane had become thickened, and similar patches of ulceration, very irregular in shape, had been formed, covered in like manner by lymph tinged with the colouring matter of the bile and excrement. The coats of the bowel were in like manner thickened and indurated, and the area of the bowel was contracted.

The necroscopic appearances of tropical dysentery have been described more or less fully by Sir W. Farquhar, Sir George Ballingall, Mr Bampfield, Mr Annesley, whose several testimonies tend to establish the general conclusion, that this disease consists in inflammation of the colic mucous membrane, spreading in general, not always or necessarily, with ulceration, but advancing to this process when not suitably or promptly opposed, and occasionally ending in death of portions of the mucous membrane. Of this inflammation the peculiarities are, 1st, that it is confined with considerable accuracy to the colon or large intestine, and the ileum being but rarely affected, and only at its lower or colic extremity; 2d, that this inflammatory action spreads continuously from the ileocoecal valve along the mucous membrane of the *cæcum*, right branch of the colon, transverse arch and sigmoid flexure, at various rates, and with various effects, but at all times with that of producing frequent copious discharges of mucous, muco-purulent, and blood-coloured stools; 3d, that this process may continue for some time without producing ulceration of the mucous corion, or inflammation of the submucous tissue; that these phenomena may take place, nevertheless, in certain circumstances, at an early period; and that in others they occur towards the conclusion of the disease;

and 4*th*, that though this inflammatory process in general commences with disorder of the circulation, and increased number of the cardiac pulse, it may commence without this, and almost always goes on when once established, without the pulse being much quickened, till the inflammatory process either affects the submucous tissue, or, which is nearly the same thing, begins to effect mortification of the mucous tissue.

The formation of numerous ulcers in the tract of the colon may be said to indicate the chronic form of the disorder. This, from the statements of Ballingall, Bampfield, and Annesley, appears to be more common in the tropical variety of the disorder than in that observed in more temperate climates. The same change, however, was seen by Morgagni, Lieutaud, Baillie, Cooke, and others, in the dysenteric affections of the latter description. In one instance of a man of 65, who had for several weeks laboured under chronic purging, and whose body I inspected for my friend Mr Caird, I found the colic mucous membrane occupied by numerous ulcers, irregular in shape, and varying in size from the area of a split pea to that of a sixpence, and even of a shilling. The lower end of the ileum presented a few small patches of ulceration scarcely penetrating the mucous corion. In the cæcum, on the other hand, they were deeper, and had not only penetrated this membrane, but were destroying the submucous tissue. In the ascending portion and transverse arch they had effected equal destruction, and in one or two the peritonæum only was left. The bottom or surface of these ulcers varied according to the stage of destruction. In the least advanced, in which the mucous tissue was not entirely destroyed, the surface of the ulcer was a sort of pale-red or gray-brown colour. When the surface was formed by exposed submucous tissue it was more ashen-coloured, but with red streaks depending on blood-vessels. The muscular layer gave it a red or brown tint; and where the peritonæum was exposed, it was thickened, reddened, and in general coated by a layer of lymph on its free surface. The edges of these ulcers, if formed of mucous tissue, were generally well-marked, sometimes thickened, and occasionally slightly turned upwards from destruction of the submucous filamentous layer. Seldom were they red; and their most prevailing tint was light or ash-coloured brown. The colic mucous membrane was generally traversed by blood-vessels at variable distances from each other. The *villi* were obliterated and indistinct. The valvular folds also were destroyed, and the cellular arrangement of the bowel could no longer be recognized.

It is not unimportant to know that these ulcers of the intestinal mucous membrane may, under certain circumstances, undergo a process of reparation. The steps of this process, which was origi-nally observed by Dr Donald Monro, have been well described by Petit and Serres in their account of the entero-mesenteric disease of Paris, and by Dr Latham in that of the epidemic of Millbank Penitentiary. From the observations of these authors it results, that the first step towards repair consists in the loose margin of ul-cerated mucous membrane becoming fastened down to the muscu-lar layer or the peritoneal coat respectively, by deposition of lymph all round. This lymphy deposition forms an elevated prominent ring, inclosing a depressed space corresponding to the centre of the sore, and which about the same time acquires a reticular appearance from intersecting filaments of lymph, among which may be seen minute red vessels. As the process advances, these filaments, by acquiring solidity and strength, seem to draw the mucous membrane forming the edges to the centre of the ulcer, while the elevated ring becomes flattened. At length, the lymphy deposition being covered by a thin pellicle newly formed completes the cicatrix. When the ulcerated spots are examined in this state, the ragged edges of mucous membrane are found to be mutually approximated; and the peritonæum at the same time to be puckered or drawn to-gether, appearing as if a small portion of the intestine had been taken by the forceps and tied by a ligature. This shows that the process of repair consists not in the mucous corion being reproduced, but in the opposite margins of its breach making as it were an effort to approach by means of the lymphy exudation from the peritonæum, which was thus necessarily contracted.

§ 8. *Pustulo-tubercular eminences. Probable Tubercular deposit in the isolated Follicles.*—I am not aware that the circum-stances on which the formation of hard pustules or tubercles of the colic mucous membrane depends, have been investigated or determined. Is this membrane liable to a peculiar pustular or pustulo-tubercular inflammation? That they do not occur in all forms of colic inflammation is proved by the fact, that they were not seen in the camp dysentery of 1743, and but rarely in the tro-pical dysentery of the east, while they were observed in every case of the London dysentery. Dr John Hunter, who saw them in all the dysenteric inspections which he performed in Jamaica, describes them as true *pustules*, though they contain no purulent matter, and represents them as seated beneath the villous coat or in the sub-mucous tissue. Each pustule, though at first small, round, and reddish, not more than the one-tenth of an inch in diameter, gra-dually enlarges till it attains the diameter of one-fourth of an inch, becoming at the same time paler. In this stage a minute crack or fissure appears at the top, and gradually enlarges, when the con-tents of the pustule are found to be cheese-like substance. As the opening enlarges, the edges become prominent, the base grows rough, and matter sometimes tinged with blood oozes from it. This is the progress of one pustule or tubercle; but they are ge-nerally in clusters, and may coalesce and form an unequal ulcer-ated surface with a hard thickened base.*

It is impossible to doubt that these pustulo-tubercular bodies are the isolated follicles either in a state of chronic inflammation and enlargement, or infiltrated with tubercular matter, or degenerated in consequence of the long continuance of chronic inflammation. In general there are three forms under which this state presents itself. One is when the subfollicular cellular tissue becomes thick-ened, enlarged, and indurated. Another is when this tissue is infil-trated with tubercular matter. This takes place in dysentery in those of strumous habit, and in the phthisical. A third is when the follicular membrane is degenerated and converted into a hard warty sort of matter, which usually splits or is fissured on the apex. In either of these three cases the follicles are prone to undergo a spe-cies of bad and almost insanable ulceration, causing chronic diar-rhœa with great weakness and wasting.

Of much the same nature are the granulations of the intestinal mucous membrane, described in the persons of the phthisical by Louis. According to this observer, these granulations are of two sorts, the *semicartilaginous* and the *tubercular*. The former, which in the cases inspected were most frequent and most numerous, were distributed equally round the bowel; and though dispersed occa-sionally through its whole length with intervals of two or three square inches, they were generally largest and most numerous to-wards the cæcum. They were not seen in the colon. Generally after attaining the size of a pea, the mucous membrane at top be-

* Observations on the Diseases of the Army in Jamaica, &c. By John Hunter, M. D., F. R. S., &c. Lond. 1784. Chap. 4, Sect. 2, p. 230, 231.

came thick, soft, and gave way; and the destructive process thus begun advanced, forming an ulcer with hard, white, opaque edges. The tubercular granulations, which were less frequent, were never seen ıı ar the duodenum, and, always most numerous near the cœcum, occupied indiscriminately any point of the bowel. They terminated by softening in minute ulcers. It does not appear that the ulcers thus formed are ever cicatrized.*

When cicatrization either of the simple or the tubercular ulcer does not take place, or takes place imperfectly, yet without causing immediate death, it gives rise to the symptoms denominated *lientery* (λειεντεϱια, slippery bowels); and its natural termination is dropsy, abdominal and general.

By these ulcers the colon is occasionally perforated with the same effects as other parts of the canal. Haller records an instance in which an ulcer of the transverse arch, by gradual absorption, perforated the coats of the stomach ;† and Lowdell mentions one in which an ulcer of the sigmoid flexure effected an opening into the urinary bladder.‡

§ 9. *Inflammatory induration.   Skleroma.*—Another effect of inflammation common to the gastro-enteric mucous membrane with others is more or less permanent thickening of its substance, or that of the submucous tissue, inducing contraction of the capacity of the canal.   This takes place in the œsophagus, in the cystic and common bile ducʻs, and in the intestines, small and great.   In the œsophagus it constitutes one of the most manageable forms of stricture of that tube, in so far as the swelling, under proper management, occasionally disappears.   (Grashuis, Bleuland, Monro, Howship.)   Its most usual seat is in the neighbourhood of the cricoid cartilage, and occasionally at the *car ıiu*.   A good example of the former is delineated by Dr Armstrong.   In the common biliary duct I have seen this inflammatory thickening give rise to jaundice; and I suspect this, and not spasm of the tube, is the most frequent cause of biliary obstruction.   In the ileum this contraction is perhaps less frequent than in the colon.   Yet in the case above-mentioned the diameter of the bowel was very much diminished, chiefly by inflammation of the submucous and subserous filamentous tissue; and Dr Charles Combe records an interesting example of thickening of the lower end of the ileum, in which the capacity of the bowel was di-

* Recherches Anatomico-Pathologiques sur la Phthisie.   Paris, 1825.
† Opuscula Patholog.
‡ Mem. Med. Society.

minished to the size of a turkey's quill.* In the colon this inflammatory induration is more frequent. It takes place chiefly in the
sigmoid flexure, and in the connection with the rectum. Of the
former instances are recorded by Haase, Christian Wincker, Lau-
bius, Portal, and Baillie, and delineated by Mr Annesley; and indeed it is no uncommon consequence of tropical dysentery. Of its
occurrence in the latter situation, Willan records an excellent example; and I may add, that I have seen several cases of it in persons who have returned to this country after severe or long-continued dysentery.

. § 10. *Membranous Exfoliation.*—In some rare instances more or
less of the intestinal mucous membrane has become completely dead,
and been discharged like a foreign body. Of this mode of exfoliation
of the mucous membrane of the ileum, occasionally with the muscular
and peritoneal tunics, good examples are recorded by Monro second
from Cullen,† Mr William Dougall,‡ Dr T. Sanden,§ and Mr John
Bower.‖ Dr Baillie records a case in which a large portion of the
colic membrane was voided ;¶ and Mr J. M. Bowman mentions one
in which a portion of the colon and cæcum with attached mesocolon
are said to have been discharged.** This subject has been most fully
examined by Dr William Thomson ; and to his Memoir I refer the
reader.††

An effect of inflammation of the gastro-enteric membrane, as
well as the tracheo-bronchial, is albuminous or sero-albuminous
exudation. This was observed by M. Bretonneau in the œsophagus; by Baillie, Andral, Howship, Godman, and Villermé in the
stomach; and by a considerable number of authors, in the colon.
In all cases the formation of these membranous substances has been
preceded and accompanied by marks of inflammatory action. In
the cases of M. Bretonneau they were connected with tracheal and
œsophageal inflammation.‡‡ In that of Howship it was the consequence of swallowing boiling water ;§§ in the cases of Andral

* Transact. Coll. Phys. Vol. iv. p. 16.
† Essays, Physical and Literary, Vol. ii. p. 395.
‡ Medical Comment. Vol. ix. p. 278.
§ Annals of Med. Vol. vi. p. 296.   ‖ Ib. Vol. vii. p. 346.
¶ Transactions of a Society, &c. Vol. ii. p. 144.
** Med. and Surg. Journal, Vol. ix. p. 492.
†† Abstract of Cases in which a Portion of the Cylinder of the Intestinal Canal,
comprising all its coats, has been discharged by stool. Edin. Med. and Surg. Journ.
xliv. p. 296. Edin. 1835.
‡‡ Des Phlegmasies des Membranes Muqueuses.
§§ Practical Remarks on Indigestion, &c. London, 1825.

it occurred in connection with fever;* and in those of Godman†
and Villermé‡ it was connected with chronic inflammation of the
gastric mucous membrane.   In the intestinal canal it is invariably
the consequence of some degree of inflammatory action.

§ 11. *Febrile Gastro-enteria.*—Gastro-enteric inflammation has been
considered above chiefly as a primary and idiopathic disorder.   It
is, however, not unfrequently observed as a concurrent symptom
or effect of many disorders reputed primarily febrile.   This was
observed long ago in ague and remittent fevers by Baglivi, Sarcone, Roederer, and Wagler, Stoll, Selle, and others; and more
recently by Pinel, Broussais, Petit, and Serres, Andral, Bretonneau, and Trousseau.   In continued fever it has also been seen by
Andral, Bretonneau, and Trousseau, Louis, and Chomel, and by
Cheyne, Reid, O'Brien, and Dr Bright in this country; and it has
been more or less fully described in different parts of Germany by
Killiches, Frenzel, Grossheim, Ebel, Stannius, Kramer, and Lesser.

From the facts collected by these observers it results, that the
action of fever has a peculiar tendency to affect the mucous surfaces in general, and especially the tracheo-bronchial and gastro-
enteric membranes.   In the former it may produce the anatomical
characters of unequivocal bronchial inflammation, proceeding not
unfrequently to the first stage of peripneumony.   Of the latter it
affects more or less intensely different regions.   In some it affects the
gastric, in others the duodenal, in others the ileal or cæcal, and in a
few the colic mucous membrane.   In most instances the membrane is
reddened and vascular, thickened, and occasionally softened.   (Andral.)   In many it assumes the form of red or brown patches, with
or without ulceration.   In many the mucous membrane is occupied by white conical elevations half a line or a line high, as broad
as a lentil at base, but with depressed summits like the pustules of
small-pox.   These are rare in the jejunum and colon, but are frequent in the two lower fifths of the ileum.   (Andral.)   In the colon this punctuate inflammation appears in the form of broad conical bodies, elevated, with pointed tops, of a cherry-red colour, and
injection of the surrounding membrane.   In a large proportion of
cases, according to Bretonneau and Trousseau, the mucous follicles

* Clinique Medicale, &c. Paris, 1823.
† The Philadelphia Journal, 1825.
‡ Archives Generales, Tome xiv. 1827. P. 614.

are enlarged, reddened, softened, and not unfrequently the seat of ulcers. Upon this statement, however, some doubt is thrown by Andral, who maintains, that, though these bodies are highly vascular, and pour forth an augmented secretion when the mucous membrane is inflamed, yet their affording the commencement of intestinal ulcers is not an invariable circumstance.

I have already endeavoured to explain the circumstances under which follicular inflammation is most likely to take place in fever. It does not seem to be necessarily connected with typhous fever; and, therefore, the fever with which it is seen in connection has been denominated typhoid fever.   But it appears to be rather a remittent disorder, to be endemic in certain regions and localities, and epidemic in certain seasons.

Though the frequency of ulceration of the lower extremity of the ileum is proportional to the number of follicles, ulceration is exceedingly rare in the duodenum, in which they are more numerous, larger, and more apparent than in any other part of the gastro-enteric membrane.   From the observations of Dr Bright, nevertheless, and the facts collected by Frenzel, Stannius, Chomel, Cruveilhier, and Lesser, no doubt can be entertained of the fact, that inflammation and sloughing of the mucous follicles is a frequent cause of ulcers.

The comparative frequency of ulcers in different regions of the gastro-enteric surface during fever may be understood from the following table, in which Andral gives the result of 71 necroscopic inspections.

	Cases.			Cases.
Ulcers of the Stomach in .	10	Cæcum,	.	15
Duodenum, .	1	Ascending colon,	.	4
Jejunum, ·	9	Transverse arch,	.	11
Lower part of the		Descending colon,		3
ileum, .	38	Rectum, .	.	1

According to this statement, which is on the whole accurate, ulcers are most frequent in the lower end of the ileum, nearly in the proportion of one-half of the cases, next to this in the cæcum in about one-fifth of the cases, then in the transverse arch, in the stomach, and in the jejunum.   In the ascending and descending colon, they are not very common, and in the duodenum and rectum extremely rare.   Their progress and effects are the same as when taking place idiopathically.

In some instances of fever, Andral remarked that portions of the

intestinal mucous corion appeared to be suddenly struck by mortification, forming a species of mucous carbuncle, (*anthrakion*,) and
like that requiring to be thrown off by a long process of ulceration.
The eschars thus discharged left ulcers extensive and irregular.
On this point I refer to what has been said above on the sloughs
of the muciparous follicles.

§ 12. *Variolous inflammation.*—It has been an opinion not uncommon, that the variolous poison produces in the mucous surfaces,
and especially along the tract of the gastro-enteric mucous membrane, pustules, similar to those of the skin; and sundry instances
of *papillæ*, pustules, and similar bodies in the stomach or intestines,
recorded by Lieutaud, have been supposed to give countenance to
this idea.   Upon this point, however, facts are something discordant.

1. In Mr Heaviside's museum is a preparation demonstrating
the appearance of numerous genuine pustules of the mucous membrane of the pharynx, and half way down the œsophagus.*   In
one subject, in like manner, Wrisberg counted 14 distinct pustules
on the palatine arch, on the posterior and inferior part of the *velum*
more than 12, and many in the neighbourhood of the *epiglottis*,
and in the upper part of the pharynx, but observed general redness only in the rest of the œsophagus.   In another subject he observed on the mucous surface of the larynx and trachea a crop of
singular warty eminences, varying in size from a lentil to a grain
of hemp seed, round or oblong in shape.   These bodies Wrisberg
states he took care to distinguish from inflamed mucous follicles.†
Sir Gilbert Blane, to the same effect, records an instance of fatal
confluent small pox, in which the whole mucous surface of the œsophagus, stomach, duodenum, and intestines, to the rectum, was
found beset with small round ulcerated spots.   These were most
crowded in the duodenum, and in the colon.   They were dark-
coloured in the centre like cutaneous pustules.   In the same subject, the mucous membrane of the *trachea* and *bronchia* was occupied with similar ulcerated spots.‡

2. Notwithstanding these facts, however, which are accurately
stated, it is not absolutely certain that genuine *phlyctidia* have even

---

* Howship, Observations, p. 253.

† Henrici Augusti Wrisbergii, D. M., &c.   Commentationum, Medici, Physiolog.
&c. Argumenti. Vol. i. Gottingæ, 1800. P. 52, &c.

‡ Some Facts and Observations, &c. by Gilbert Blane, M.D.   Transactions of a
Society, Vol. iii. p. 425.

been seen in the stomach or intestinal membrane. The papillæ and pustule-like eruptions which are supposed by some to be of this nature are evidently enlargements of the mucous follicles.

. 3. The variolous poison certainly produces inflammation of the gastro-enteric mucous membrane; but this consists in diffuse redness and injection, or red-brown patches, or both, generally with some affection of the mucous follicles.* In several instances of fatal confluent small-pox, I have seen the gastric mucous membrane deep red, much loaded with vessels, and patches of extravasated blood, and similar appearances with bloody mucus in various parts of the ileum. In the same subjects, the tracheo-bronchial membrane was of a deep-brown colour, and highly vascular.

It is, indeed, always the tracheo-bronchial membrane that is most affected in small-pox. But, excepting at the epiglottis and larynx, it presents no variolous pustules. The larynx, indeed, usually presents the appearance of mere redness, roughness, and swelling. In one case of fatal confluent small-pox, in which the patient was destroyed before the eruption came completely out, I found the whole mucous membrane of the trachea and the large *bronchi* covered by a thin filmy membrane like silver paper, and the membrane of the small tubes much reddened. In other cases in which the patients died with the eruption out, the whole tracheo-bronchial membrane was red, rough, covered with viscid mucus; and the small bronchial tubes effused large quantities of frothy sero-mucous fluid.

These phenomena explain the severity and fatality of this disease.

. § 13. *Tubercular Disease of the Ileum and Ileal Follicles.*—Before concluding this division, I think it right to mention here a peculiar disorder of the *ileum ;* though I am not certain whether it ought to be referred to the mucous membrane, the *peritonæum,* or the whole intestinal tunics. To illustrate the nature of the lesion I give the particulars of an instance of the disease extremely well marked.

A young woman,† of twenty years, had laboured for some time under symptoms of disease of the abdomen ; and at length the ab-

---

* " The pharynx and œsophagus were certainly much inflamed, as was the stomach, and more or less the whole of the intestines ; but after the most diligent search, no trace whatever of the pustular action was found either in the pharynx, œsophagus, stomach, or intestines." Howship, Observations. See also *Cotunnii syntagma,* &c. xliii. xlix.

† Under the care of Dr Paterson of Leith.

domen, which was swelled and painful at certain parts, became distended, and gave evident proofs of the presence of fluid. Dr Paterson, under whose care the patient was, tried for some time all means of producing the absorption of this fluid, and otherwise removing the disease on which it depended. Little or no effect, however, was produced, either by aperients, diuretics, or local applications. Dr Paterson requested me to see her, to consider the propriety of relieving the distension and other sufferings of the patient, by the operation of parakentesis. At this time the abdomen was greatly enlarged, especially towards the infra-umbilical region, where it emitted a dull sound, and gave distinct evidence of fluctuation. When the patient was placed in the supine position, there was something peculiar in the abdomen, as if the intestinal folds were more consistent than natural, and adhered in certain points. When pressure was applied slowly and carried steadily downwards, so as to urge the intestines towards the spine and posterior region of the abdomen, the patient gave manifest indications of pain. She also described her feelings as if something were tied round the bowels. It was clear, nevertheless, that there was no adhesion between the abdominal parietes and the intestinal peritonæum ; for there the abdominal fluid was interposed.

After careful consideration of the case, it was agreed, that, as no medicinal agent had hitherto made any decided impression on the abdominal swelling or the contained fluid, it was desirable to empty the abdomen by operation, and then try the effect of remedies.

The operation was accordingly performed, and about nineteen or twenty pints of serous and sero-purulent fluid withdrawn. The operation was well borne ; and the patient was replaced in bed.

The wound healed in a few days, and the patient seemed to recover from the immediate effects of the operation. But in the course of a few days vomiting came on and death ensued.

Inspection disclosed the following appearances.

In the lumbar and iliac fossæ and in the pelvis there was some sero-purulent fluid, with a few albuminous flakes. A little accumulation had taken place since the operation.

The omentum was drawn up and shrivelled, though thickened.

All the folds of the *ileum*, which came into view, adhered to each other intimately by albuminous exudation, so that not one portion of the *ileum* could be said to be in its natural free position. Even some of the lower parts of the *jejunum* adhered in this manner. The tunics of the *ileum* were thickened, indurated, and in certain parts where the adhesions were most firm and intimate, they were of cartilaginous consistence.

The *ileum* was cut open longitudinally, and the true state of the disease was then seen.

At intervals of from six to eight or nine inches the mucous membrane of the *ileum* presented large irregular ulcerated openings, penetrating directly through all the coats to the *peritonæum*, then from the *peritonæum* of the corresponding adherent portion of *ileum*, through the coats of that portion to the mucous membrane. By these openings direct passages had been formed from one portion of bowel through the coats into the attached portion.

These openings were in shape mostly elliptical or oval, with the long diameter corresponding to the axis of the bowel. Their edges were ragged and irregular; and while the intestinal tissues around them were thickened and cartilaginous, the capacity of the bowel was much diminished.

In size the openings varied from half-an-inch to one inch or one inch and a-half in the long diameter. Their breadth was from half-an-inch to three-fourths.

The number of these openings was considerable. There were at least 20, and probably more.

On examining the lines of adhesion by which they were connected, tubercular matter was visible both at the peritoneal and mucous surface, and in several parts of the peritonæum small tubercular bodies, white and opaque, were deposited. It was not easy to say whether these bodies had commenced at the peritoneal or at the mucous surface. They were in general covered by *peritonæum*, and they were as distinct at the mucous surface as at the serous.

A case similar to this is given by Dr George Gregory.*

An important inquiry suggested by cases of this class is to determine where the ulceration originates; whether at the mucous or at the peritoneal surface of the bowel. The point is not one of very easy determination.

It seems, on the one hand, most natural to think that the ulceration began at the mucous surface. To me these ulcerated openings appear to be in the site of the agminated patches of Peyer. These patches were, I infer, originally penetrated or infiltrated with tubercular matter. They had then proceeded to softening and ulceration, destroying of course the mucous and other tissues slowly

---

' * Observations on the Scrofulous Inflammation of the Peritonæum, &c. Med. Chir. Trans, xi. p. 258.

and progressively. When this destroying action arrived at the *peritonæum*, it caused first adhesion of that, or rather adhesive inflammation, connecting it to the *peritonæum* of the corresponding portion of *ileum*, and then proceeded by the same ulcerative action to destroy the tunics of that portion of bowel, though in the opposite direction; that is, first, *peritonæum*, then cellular and muscular tissue, then cellular and mucous membrane.

This view of the course of the disorder is, nevertheless, not without difficulty. It supposes the process of tubercular deposition and ulceration to advance first from the mucous to the peritonæal surface of a portion of *ileum*, and then from the peritonæal to the mucous surface; or that the process was advancing simultaneously from the mucous membranes of two applied portions of *ileum* to the peritonæal until they met in the latter point.

Notwithstanding these difficulties, this view appears more probable, than that the disease had commenced in the *peritonæum*, and thence proceeded to affect the other intestinal tissues to the mucous membrane. The ulcerated openings also corresponded in figure and size with the patches of agminated glands.

Dr George Gregory takes the opposite view; and his case I therefore refer to the head of lesions of the *peritonæum*.

D.—THE GENITO-URINARY MUCOUS MEMBRANE.

§ 1. The genito-urinary mucous membrane in both sexes is the seat of sundry forms of the inflammatory process.

The urethral membrane, though forming a part of this surface, possesses, nevertheless, certain anatomical and sensible peculiarities. Smooth, and even polished, moistened by a thin transparent fluid, it is formed into the sinuosities named *lacunæ*, which, like the follicles of other membranes, secrete a fluid of a peculiar odour, which, united with that of the general membrane, serves to lubricate the surface. Examined from its opening to its cystic extremity, it presents divisions which may be enumerated in the following order, the spongy, the bulbous, the membranous, and the prostatic or vesical portions, according to the parts of the canal to which the membrane is attached. This membrane may be the seat of inflammation of two sorts;—one circumscribed and unsuppurative, the other spreading, and accompanied with secretion of puriform or purulent matter, more or less abundant.

a. *Urethria simplex.*—Common inflammation of the urethra consists in redness, swelling, and pain of a certain part of the .canal, which thus is rendered very narrow, or even may undergo temporary and partial obliteration.   This affection is attended with painful tension of part or the whole of the penis, suppression of urine, sometimes priapism, and consitutional disturbance proceeding at once from local irritation, and the distress occasioned by difficulty of voiding the urine, or by its total suppression.   This form of urethral inflammation should be distinguished from stricture, with which it is too often confounded.   Instead of spreading along the membrane, it has a tendency to pass to the submucous tissue, and thicken it.   It is probable that it may occur in any part of the canal; but its most ordinary site is the membranous portion.   If properly treated, it terminates in resolution with a gleety discharge, in effusion of lymph or suppuration, not unfrequently with fistulous openings.

b. *Urethria puriformis; Gonorrhœa; Medorrhœa.*—That the fluid of gonorrhœa is of inflammatory origin is proved by the swelling of the urethral orifice, the pain and tenderness of the canal, and the sore or scalding sensation (*ardor urinæ*) occasioned by the transit of the urine over it.   At an early period of the art, when pathological knowledge was defective or erroneous, this discharge from the urethra was believed to consist of seminal fluid, and to issue from the organs by which that fluid is secreted.   Afterwards, when medical practitioners understood the nature of the discharge as distinct from seminal fluid, it was believed to be purulent matter issuing from ulcers in the canal.   This opinion, which, indeed, was more rational, was nevertheless completely disproved, first by Morgagni,[*] and afterwards by John Hunter,[†] who showed by dissection of persons whose death had occurred while they were labouring under urethral discharge, that though minute ulcers may occasionally be found in the canal, they are totally unconnected with the discharge, which in the greater number of cases is secreted by the urethral membrane in a state of inflammation.   According to the most accurate observations several regions of the urethral mucous membrane may without ulceration or erosion furnish puriform secretion.

The first of these is the hollow named navicular *fossa*, about 1, 1½, or 2 inches from the orifice, or the anterior end of the spongy

---

[*] Adversaria Anatom. Epistola xliv. 1, 2.

[†] Treatise on the Venereal Disease, Part ii. Chap. 1.

portion of the membrane. This region abounds with the *canaliculi*, to which Morgagni traced the secretion; and in the dissections of John Hunter it was uniformly found redder, and more vascular or blood-shot than usual, and the *lacunæ* often filled with matter. *Secondly*, in cases in which the inflammation is more extensive, the membranous part of the canal, Cowper's glands and their ducts, are involved in the morbid process. This, however, is exceedingly rare, according to Littre, Morgagni, and Baillie. The first, after inspecting forty cases of urethral inflammation, found in one case only the glands of Cowper morbid. Morgagni met with one or two instances only; and John Hunter remarks, that if the matter of clap were secreted and deposited either beyond or in the bulb, it would be incessantly ejected by the muscles, as occurs in regard to the urine and seminal fluid. In cases yet more extensive, the prostatic part of the urethra has been known to be inflamed; and in very violent forms of clap, the inflammation has been found to extend to the bladder itself. It thus appears that no portion of the canal, from its orifice to the neck of the bladder, is exempt from inflammation; and every part of the membrane between these two points has been found more or less reddened, slightly villous, vascular, and more or less swelled, so as to diminish sensibly the calibre of the canal. It is observed by Dr Baillie, that the inflammation may pass from the mucous to the submucous membrane, and the surrounding tissue of the spongy body, which thus becomes larger and harder, in consequence of loaded vessels and effused lymph, than in the natural state. It is not improbable that this morbid state of the spongy body, by irritating the *ischio-cavernosi* muscles, and exciting them to action, gives rise to the painful affection denominated *chordée*.

The glands of Cowper have been seen indurated and like tubercles, in consequence of inflammation; occasionally their ducts are rendered impervious, and in some instances ulcers take place. And in some instances the effect of this process is to obliterate both the longitudinal folds and the *canaliculi* of Morgagni. Ulceration, to which Morgagni himself had recourse, is not requisite to explain this occurrence, which may be affected by inflammatory thickening of their membrane. When the inflammation terminates in effusion of lymph into the submucous tissue, the swelling induces that contraction of the canal which constitutes stricture.

§ 2. *Cystidia. Cystirrhœa.*—The cystic mucous membrane, like the urethral, is liable to inflammation either over its whole extent or at a single spot. The part most frequently affected is the neck of the bladder and the space termed cystic triangle (*la trigone vesicale*); a circumstance which has been ascribed to one of two causes. The first is, that the neck is most usually affected by mechanical obstructions to the passage of the urine, and is therefore most likely to be the first seat of the irritation which connects injury and inflammatory action. The other is, that its contiguity to the urethra renders it liable to be first affected by inflammation of that canal when disposed to spread, or when, in consequence of bad treatment, chronicity, or other causes, urethral becomes an exciting cause of cystic inflammation.

From either of these causes, inflammation may be developed in the cystic mucous surface near the neck of the bladder, and may thence be propagated over a considerable extent of the membrane, which then becomes marked by red points, villous, highly vascular, and diffusely swelled, with occasional spots of extravasated blood. In general, the character of this inflammation is to spread; and in ordinary cases it does so without affecting the submucous or other tissues. Instances, however, occur, in which it passes successively to the submucous filamentous tissue, to the muscular, and thence to the peritoneal coat. In the spreading form the inflammation is attended with secretion of thick mucous or puriform fluid, which falls to the bottom of the urine.

It may terminate in resolution, in suppuration, in destruction of the coats or ulceration; or lastly, it may pass into the chronic state. The manner in which the two first terminations are effected, is in every respect similar to these processes, as they take place in other mucous surfaces.

The third, or ulceration of the mucous and other tissues of the bladder, is not uncommon, and may occur under two forms. In the first, which is most common, it may be superficial, and remove the whole mucous membrane so as to expose the muscular layer as if it had been neatly dissected. In the second, which is more usual, the ulcerative process advances in minute patches from the mucous to the submucous and muscular tissues, and in some instances to the subserous and peritoneal membrane. This process differs from the other in this respect, that lymph is irregularly deposited, that there is considerable swelling, and sometimes a true abscess is formed. More frequently, however, small portions of the mucous

3

membrane are detached in isolated points by ulceration ; and though the subjacent tissues are exposed, there is no regular cavity or abscess, but merely an ulcerated depression, which secretes purulent matter. (Walter.) In more severe cases, in which the suppurative or ulcerative process penetrates the different coats, communications are formed between the bladder and the neighbouring parts. The most ordinary of these modes of communication are the general peritoneal cavities, or the rectum, in both sexes, and the vagina in the female. In the first case, besides other symptoms, the urine gives rise to fatal peritoneal inflammation ; in the second and third, its escape by unnatural passages induces much local irritation and general distress, and eventually may terminate in death. Sloughing of the cystic mucous membrane has been known to occur, but is not common.

b. *Cystidia Diuturna.*—The termination of *cystidia* in the ebronic form is most frequent in those who have laboured under repeated attacks of acute cystic inflammation ; those who have had urethral or prostatic inflammation, or other disease of these parts ; those having urethral stricture ; those liable to sabulous or lithic concretions, or wherever there is a permanent cause of irritation. It is hence common in persons whose health is impaired, or who are advanced in life. The cystic membrane becomes not only reddish, but brown, villous, flocculent, and considerably thickened. In some instances it become granular and unusually hard. This change was repeatedly seen by Hoffmann, Morgagni,* Lieutaud, Portal, and others ; and it is important to remark, that it never continues long without causing inordinate thickening of the muscnlar layer, and occasionally irregular contraction of its constituent fibres, so as to form *sacculi*, or cavities in the walls of the organ. In most instances it secretes puriform mucus, (Hoffmann, Chopart,) but without destruction of the mucous membrane. The former author relates an instance in which the usual effects took place, while, upon inspection, the cystic tissues were found thickened and condensed, and the vessels of the mucous membrane large, numerous, and loaded, yet without trace of ulceration. This disorder is said to have been the cause of death to Voltaire, Buffon, D'Alembert, and Spallanzani.† On the other hand, the mucous membrane may be entirely removed, as in the acute form, by a process of ulceration

* Epist. xlii.

† Brera Storia della Malattia di P. Spallanzani.

or sloughing. In the case of Professor Barthez of Montpellier, recorded by M. Double,* the cavity of the organ, which contained a mulberry calculus nine lines in diameter, was diminished and filled with purulent matter; its walls were black and sphacelated; of mucous membrane not a trace was left, and the muscular coat was thickened.† From a similar action results the villous, fungating, and granular state of the bladder observed by Ruysch, Walter, Baillie, and others.‡

The anatomical characters, in short, of this disease in its exquisite form are the following. The walls of the organ, especially its muscular coat, are thickened, hardened, and as if hypertrophied; and the muscular thickening, as well as the cellular, may be considerable, that is to say, approaching to half an inch. The cavity of the organ is much contracted, sometimes not larger than the capacity of a small egg. The mucous membrane is very commonly reddened and vascular all over or in patches; in some instances it is partially removed by ulceration; and in some instances it is entirely removed, as if it had been dissected away from the muscular coat. This I have several times seen; and in general the exposed surface was covered with patches of calcareous matter, which was either ammoniaco-magnesian phosphate, phosphate of lime, or carbonate of lime.

The effects of this process is to alter considerably the ordinary secretion of the cystic mucous membrane. The cystic mucus in the healthy state is a thin fluid, easily miscible with the urine, and so trifling in quantity, at least in the urine discharged, that it is rarely observed. What is called *cloudy* urine generally contains a little more of this mucous matter than usual. In the inflamed state it appears in the form of thick, opaque, viscid fluid, which falls to the bottom of the vessel, and in very severe cases it is puriform, or purulent fluid, opaque and milky, but not ropy, and is occasionally reddish or streaked with blood. To account for the origin of this morbid secretion, Fanton conceived that follicles or mucous glands of the cystic membrane became inflamed, and increased their natural action.§ The existence of such bodies in this membrane is nevertheless questionable; and it is unnecessary to look for any

* Hist. Anatom. Med. Obs. 1224, 1266, 1270, 1272, 1274.
† Journal Generale de Medecine. Nov. 1806.
‡ F. A. Walter, Einige Krankheiten der Nieren und Harnblase untersucht u. s. w. Berlin, 1800. P. 31.
§ Dissert. Anatom. 1745.

other tissue save the mucous surface to explain the origin of the discharge.

The truth is, that, as soon as the mucous membrane of the bladder begins to secrete puriform matter, this alters much the chemical properties of the urine. Ammonia is secreted; or rather the urea is decomposed and converted into ammonia or carbonate of ammonia; and either the urine contains ammoniaco-magnesian phosphates, or some other ammoniacal salt.

The other effects of this disease are weight, uneasiness, and sometimes tension in the hypogastric region; heat in voiding the urine; uneasy parched condition of the skin of the legs and feet, with burning of the soles; thirst, quick pulse, impaired appetite, and general wasting. The constitutional disturbance and wasting generally prove fatal directly, or by inducing some fatal disease.

Membranous substances have been observed to be discharged from the bladder by Willis, Ruysch, Boerhaave, and Morgagni. According to the account of the inspections, these are stated to be portions of the mucous membrane of the bladder. Though I feel difficulty in denying the testimony of observers so competent, I feel equal difficulty in admitting this exfoliation, which is indeed analogous to the exfoliations of the intestinal mucous membrane. It is equally possible, and not altogether improbable, that these membranous substances were albuminous concretions from the inflamed cystic membrane.

§ 3. The utero-vaginal mucous membrane of the female is not less important as a seat of morbid action.

The labio-vaginal mucous membrane is often the seat of gonorrhœal inflammation, which seems-to produce in it much the same effects as in the male urethra. In severe cases the *nymphæ* swell so much that they make, with the external *labia*, one shapeless mass. The vaginal membrane I have seen the seat of a thick yellow puriform discharge, which was positively asserted to be unconnected with gonorrhœal infection. This, however, requires further confirmation. In all cases the membrane becomes so much swelled that the *rugæ* are to a certain extent obliterated. The *lacunæ* are stated to be the chief source of the discharge when thick and puriform.

The uterine mucous membrane is liable to various forms of the inflammatory process, most of which, however, may be referred to three heads,—the spreading sero-mucous or puriform, the limited or suppurative, and the albuminous.

Of the spreading inflammation there are two varieties, one with transparent mucous discharge, the other with opaque or white mucous discharge.

In the first case, in which a transparent, gelatinous, imperfectly coagulable fluid issues from the vagina, the uterine mucous membrane is in a state of chronic congestion, and the organ itself becomes ·slightly enlarged. This discharge, which issues from the mucous surface of the womb, and, according to Leake, from the same vessels which are subservient to menstruation, constitutes a large proportion of the cases regarded as *fluor albus*. It takes place as a symptom of prolapse of the womb, bladder, or vagina, of inversion of the womb, of cancer, polypus, and even warty growths of the organ.*

In the second form, though the disease may affect the mucous surface in general, its more particular seat is the cervix of the womb and its mucous glands. It was observed originally by Morgagni,† and afterwards by Leake, that in certain forms of *fluor albus* incident to young females of 8 or 10 years old, the discharge proceeds from the mucous glands of the womb. By observing pain and tenderness uniformly in this part, Mr C. M. Clarke confirms the accuracy of this observation. It causes to issue from the vagina an opaque perfectly white fluid, resembling a mixture of starch and water made in the cold, or thin cream, easily washed from the finger, and diffusible in water, which it renders turbid, sometimes tenacious, like melted glue.

3. When the mucous membrane of the womb or vagina is inflamed, it may secrete puriform or purulent fluid, which is not unfrequently retained within the cavity of the organ. Collections of purulent matter in the former have been recorded by Lieutaud,‡ Portal,§ Dr Clarke,‖ and others. Of these collections the peculiarity is that they are not discharged as they are formed,—a circumstance which is in general to be ascribed to obstruction of the uterine orifice by lymph. This, it is to be remarked, is accidental,

---

* Observations on those Diseases of Females which are attended by Discharges, &c. &c., by Charles Mansfield Clarke. Part i. Lond. 1814, and Part ii. Lond. 1821.

† Epist. xlvii. 14, 15, 18.   ‡ Hist. Anatom. Med.

§ Anatomie Medicale, Tom. v. p. 519.

‖ Transactions of a Society, Vol. iii. p. 560.

and does not establish an essential or specific difference between such purulent collections and those discharges which take place from the orifice of the organ. It is nevertheless to be remarked, that these collections partake in a more conspicuous degree of the characters of genuine active inflammation of the uterine mucous surface.

Puriform inflammation of the utero-vaginal mucous membrane is to be distinguished from abscess of the *labia*, or *nymphæ*, from suppuration of the submucous vaginal tissue, which I have seen take place under circumstances that might lead them to be confounded with each other, from gonorrhœal inflammation, from corroding ulcer of the mouth of the womb, and from cancer of the womb or of the rectum.

The second general form of uterine mucous inflammation is that in which the product of the process is an albuminous membranous concretion. Morgagni records a good instance of redness of the uterine mucous membrane, part of which was at the same time lined by a preternatural membranous substance. It has been further long known, that many females discharge periodically shreds and portions of membranous matter of various size and shape, and some so large that they form almost complete moulds of the inner uterine surface. These facts, which were observed by William Hunter, Leake, Denman, and Hulme, are well known to acoucheurs and those conversant with the management of female disorders. It may be stated as a well established fact, that these membranous productions are analogous to those, which I have above shown, are secreted by other mucous surfaces; and that their formation is connected with an inflammatory state of the uterine mucous membrane. Independent of the fact, that their formation is attended with pain of the uterine region and disturbed function, in some favourable instances in which inspection has taken place, the transition from fluid to solid state has been traced, and the congested state of the uterine vessels demonstrated. In sundry instances, nevertheless, these membranous productions are formed by that action of the vessels which constitutes menstruation, and they are formed chiefly at the menstrual periods. In all cases, their formation implies a state of the uterus incompatible with impregnation; and sterility is the accompaniment of this disease.

§ 4. *Adhesive inflammation of the Vaginal Mucous Membrane.*—It has been observed by Baillie, that the vagina is liable to a violent form of inflammation, which, by producing effusion of lymph, causes mutual adhesion of the sides of the canal.* By Howship, this is ascribed to excoriation between the *labia*, causing at an early age effusion of lymph, so as to resemble *aphthæ;* and he mentions an instance in a child of two months, in which lymph had been secreted, and had become vascular, leaving a minute aperture for the urine at the inferior angle of the vagina.† If these two forms of inflammation be different, the latter is probably of the same nature as that now to be mentioned.

§ 5. *Sloughing inflammation of mucous surfaces.*—To this head I refer two varieties of disease met with, particularly at the communication of the two great mucous surfaces with the skin.

The first. is the disease originally described by Hoffmann and Van Swieten under the name of *cancrum oris*, the water canker of Dr Robert Hamilton of Lynn Regis,‡ and more recently by Dr M. Hall,§ Dr Thomas Cumming,‖ and various subsequent observers. In this disease the mucous membrane of the mouth, cheek, or gums, becomes hot, swelled, of a dark-red colour, and eventually black, hard, and dead. The mortified portion begins then to be thrown off; but in the meantime the original inflammatory process advances; and combined with that necessary for ejecting the sloughs, is accompanied with extreme pain, and much constitutional disturbance. Though this disorder has been thought to originate in the skin, in which it appears when presented to the practitioner, it may always be traced to the mucous membrane of the mouth; a fact which is properly verified by the observation of Dr Cumming.¶

The second variety of this disease is seen in the pudendum of young girls, in whom the labial or valvular membrane is liable to a species of diffuse inflammation, which almost invariably terminates in mortification of the mucous corion, which is then cast in the form of slough. According to the observations of Mr Kinder Wood, to whom we are indebted for the most distinct account of this disorder yet published, the labial mucous membrane becomes of a dark red colour, swelled, and covered by numerous watery vesicles or *aphthæ*, the cuticle of which dropping off discloses deep

* Morbid Anatomy, Chap. xxii. p. 415.
† Practical Observations, &c. Chap. vi. p. 360.
‡ *Apud* On the Marsh Remittent Fever, &c. London, 1801.
§ Edin. Medical and Surgical Journal, Vol. xv.
‖ Dublin Hospital Reports, Vol. iv. p. 330.
¶ Ibid. p. 335.

foul ulcers, surrounded with much redness, and secreting thin offensive matter. Similar aphthæ also appear on the skin of the *mons veneris, perinæum*, and adjoining parts.* Though the disease is often fatal by the severity of the constitutional disorder, in some instances, after the sloughs are cast, effusion of lymph and granulation may take place, and, unless much care is taken in dressing, great part of the vaginal orifice and the labia are united permanently, leaving only a small orifice for the escape of the urine. In this manner the vagina is not unfrequently closed so as to simulate congenital imperforation. It appears from the account of Mr Wood, that this inflammation is confined chiefly to the *labia*, the *nymphæ*, the *clitoris*, and *hymen ;* and it does not seem to affect the vagina.

In a medico-legal point of view it is important to distinguish this disease from the effects of violation, with which it has been confounded.

III. HÆMORRHAGE.—In the mucous membranes hemorrhage is frequent ; and though none of them can be said to be exempt from it, it is most common in the Schneiderian or nasal membrane, in the pulmonic, intestinal, and uterine mucous surfaces. In the hemorrhagic form of land-scurvy, (*purpura hæmorrhagica*), with the bloody spots on the outer surface of the corion of simple *purpura*, are combined spots and hemorrhage from almost all the mucous surfaces. Of the hemorrhages of the mucous membranes the following table may be given:—

Nasal passages,	*Epistaxis.*	
Mouth,	*Stomacace,*	
Bronchial membrane,	*Hæmoptysis,*	*Pneumonorrhagia.*
Stomach,	*Hæmatemesis,*	*Gastrorrhagia.*
Ileum and colon,	*Melæna ; Dysentery,*	*Enterorrhagia.*
Rectum,	*Hæmorrhois,*	*Proctorrhagia.*
Bladder,	*Hæmaturia,*	*Cystirrhagia.*
Urethra,		*Urethrorrhagia.*
Womb,		*Menorrhagia.*

In these several regions of the mucous surfaces, the pathology of hemorrhage, which has been already partially considered, is much the same. The discharge of blood or bloody fluid from any of the mucous membranes is not so much a disease of itself as one of the effects of some degree or variety of the inflammatory process. Thus blood is discharged from the bronchial membrane during bronchial inflammation ; from the gastric mucous membrane dur-

* History of a very fatal affection of the pudenda of female children, by Kinder Wood, Esq. Med.-Chir. Trans. Vol. vii. p. 85, &c.

ing vascular congestion of the stomach; from the intestinal during
the congestion of dysentery; and from that of the rectum during
the vascular state attendant on *hemorrhois*. In these circumstances,
the blood, whether pure or mingled, as it often is with mucous, muco-purulent or puriform fluid, oozes from the mucous membranes
without destruction of tissue, or rupture of vessels, or, in the language of the physiologist, is exhaled. "I have often opened," says
Bichat, "persons who have died during hemorrhage, and have examined the bronchial, gastric, intestinal, and uterine surfaces, yet
have not perceived the slightest trace of erosion, notwithstanding
the precaution of washing them with care, allowing them to mace-
rate, and afterwards submitting them to examination by means of
a lens."*   In this manner, therefore, are to be explained those
slight hemorrhages which take place in pulmonary catarrh (*hæmoptoe*), about the termination of peripneumony, and in young females
after the accidental suppression of the menstrual discharge.

From these the more copious and irresistible hemorrhages from
mucous surfaces differ chiefly in a previous serious lesion of the mucous or submucous tissue.   This lesion consists in vascular injection more or less extensive of the mucous corion, and injection occasionally very complete, and amounting to extravasation, of the
submucous tissue, which is thus rendered red-brown, hard, and
void of its natural elasticity.   Of the former instances are seen in
the gastro-enteric mucous membrane during *hæmatemesis*, *melæna*,
and bloody flux; and the latter may be observed in the lungs during *hæmoptysis*, and in the rectum in *hæmorrhois*.   These principles are so well established by numerous facts, that it is unnecessary to strengthen them by any elaborate induction.   I shall merely adduce the phenomena of a few of the hemorrhagic diseases in
illustration of the general doctrine that hemorrhage is an exhalation from parts, the capillaries of which are previously inordinately
distended.

§ 1. *The Gastro-enteric Membrane.   Hæmatemesis and Melæna.*
—On the pathology of this disorder, so much misunderstood by the
ancients, it is unnecessary to dwell.   Correct views were first given
by Hoffmann, who, from the fact of finding in dead bodies the mesenteric vessels and those of the ileum much distended with black
blood, and the stomach filled with the same, taught that the bloody
discharge, whether from the upper or the lower end of the canal,
proceeds not immediately from the vessels of the stomach, or from

* Anatomie Generale, Tome i. p. 563, 565.

blood extravasated into its cavity, but also from the vessels of the small intestines, especially those of the ileum.* This inference is confirmed by several dissections of Valsalva and Morgagni,† who in hæmatemesis and intestinal hemorrhage found the gastro-enteric mucous membrane always entire, and its vessels more or less injected.

From an extensive collection of cases, Portal derives conclusions still more distinct. This anatomist shows, 1*st*, that the black matter discharged by vomit and by stool, or by vomiting only, is gennine blood, which is seen to ooze after death from the blood-vessels of the stomach and intestines; 2*d*, that this oozing or transudation takes place from the gastric, duodenal, and mesenteric arterial extremities into the cavity of the stomach or intestines, separately or at once, more frequently into the stomach only, in consequence of certain arterial branches receiving more blood than the corresponding veins return ; and, 3*dly*, though compression of the branches of the portal vein may cause this extravasation, the blood is not effused from the *vasa brevia*, in which it flows in an opposite direction.‡

Similar are the views of Abernethy, who states that in the bodies of several persons who died under attacks of this disease, he found " the villous coat of the alimentary canal *highly inflamed, swollen, and pulpy.* Bloody specks were observed in various parts ; and sphacelation had actually taken place in one instance. The liver was healthy in some cases and diseased in others." He concludes, therefore, that the diseases termed *hæmatemesis* and *melæna* arise from " violent disorder, and consequent diseased secretion of the internal coat of the bowels ; and that the blood discharged does not flow from any single vessel, but from the various points of the diseased surface."§ From the same source originates the cocoa-coloured fluid observed by Baillie in fatal cases of *hæmatemesis.*‖

It may therefore be inferred, that the blood discharged in this disease issues from the loaded capillary vessels of the gastric, duodenal, and ileal mucous membrane without breach of surface ; and as it is anatomically impossible to distinguish these vessels into ar-

---

* Medicinæ Rationalis Systematicæ, pars ii. sect. i. chap. iii. § 17.

† Epist. xxix. 10 ; xxxi. 23 ; xxxvi. 11.

‡ Mémoires sur la Nature et le Traitement de Plusieurs Maladies, Par Antoine Portal, Tom. ii. Paris, 1800. P. 108.

§ On the Constitutional Origin and Treatment, &c. p. 30. London, 1811.

‖ Lectures and Observations on Medicine.

3

teries and veins, the dispute whether the blood issues from the one or other order is frivolous. The blood may acquire its dark colour from two causes; 1*st*, admixture with the gastric juice in the stomach and duodenum; and 2*d*, from the action of the carbonic acid, sulphuretted hydrogen, and other substances of acid properties contained in the intestinal canal.

§ 2. *Hæmoptysis; Pneumonorrhagia; Pulmonary Hemorrhage; Pulmonary Apoplexy.*—For the first accurate description of the anatomical characters of pulmonary hemorrhage, we are indebted to the researches of the elaborate Stark, who ascertained the following facts. The air vesicles in some parts of the lungs are filled with blood or bloody serum; the parts do not collapse on opening the chest, but are firm, dark or light red in colour, and can neither be compressed nor distended by the usual inflation. When cut into, thick blood or bloody matter issues from the cut surfaces; and portions of the diseased parts, after being macerated in water, still sink as before maceration. He further showed, by blowing air into the blood-vessels and air-tubes of the sound and diseased portions respectively, that in the latter air passes from the branches of the pulmonary artery and veins into the bronchial tubes; in other words, that the capillary vessels of the lungs communicate freely with the bronchial tubes and air-cells.[*]

The general accuracy of this description has since been verified by the researches of Laennec, who has indeed rendered the pathological anatomy of this disease more precise than formerly. From these, it results that a portion of the pulmonic tissue becomes uniformly hard, of a dark red colour, and impermeable to air. The indurated spot is always partial, from one to four cubic inches in extent, circumscribed with sound or pale-coloured lung, and looks not unlike a clot of venous blood; circumstances by which it is to be distinguished from pneumonic induration, which terminates gradually in sound lung.[†] These changes, which consist in extreme injection of the pulmonic capillaries, and in effusion of blood into the submucous filamentous tissue, and into the pulmonic vesicles, are confined, however, chiefly to the severe forms of pulmonary he_morrhage. They are the effects of previous injection of the capil_laries, which is to be considered as the uniform cause of hemor_rhage.

[*] The Works of the late William Stark, M. D. &c. London, 1788, p. 34.
[†] Traité de l'Auscultation Mediate, &c.

Much the same changes are observed in the rectum and its submucous tissue in hemorrhoidal disease. This is proved by the testimony of Latta,* Benjamin Bell,† Callisen,‡ Monteggia,§ Delpech,‖ Chaussier, Larroque, and Calvert.¶ This disorder is to be distinguished from varix of the veins of the bowels.

I conclude this subject with a few remarks on hemorrhage from the uterine mucous membrane in the state of impregnation. It is generally supposed that hemorrhage taking place at this period is the effect of abortion; and Denman and some other authors employ a good deal of not very intelligible argument to prove the proposition. It may, however, be demonstrated, that hemorrhage, or, to speak more to the fact, the abnormal state of the uterine capillaries, which leads to hemorrhage, is the *cause* of abortion; and that almost no instance of abortion takes place without previous hemorrhagic distension of the uterine or utero-placental capillaries. By Denman himself it is remarked, that "when abortion is about to happen, there is usually between this (the *decidua reflexa*) and the outer membrane of the *ovum*, an effusion of blood, which often insinuates itself through the cellular membrane of the placenta, and between the membranes, giving externally to the whole *ovum* a tumid and unequal appearance, not unlike a lump of coagulated blood, for which it has been frequently mistaken, and then it is popularly called a false conception."** I have had occasion to observe the phenomena of several abortions with some care; and in every one I have traced them to some degree of hemorrhage taking place from the uterine or utero-placental vessels. The blood which Denman remarks is found insinuated through the cellular membrane of the placenta is derived from the vessels of that body. It is not, therefore, the premature effort of the *uterus* to contract that constitutes abortion; but the inordinate distension of its vessels, which terminates in hemorrhage, and the occurrence of which then excites the uterus to premature contraction. The vessels of the uterus and placenta, naturally full of blood, may, from a variety of causes operating on the mother, become unusually distended,

* A Practical System of Surgery, Vol. ii. Chap. iv. p. 34.
† A System of Surgery, Vol. vi., 7. Edit. Chap. xxiv. p. 324.
‡ Systema Chirurgiæ Hodierniæ, Vol. ii. Edit. 4to. p. 126.
§ Instituzione Chirurgiche, Vol. viii. Chap. xv. 389.
‖ Precis Elementaire, &c. Tome iiime, Sect. viii. Chap. 1, § ii. p. 262.
¶ A Practical Treatise on Hemorrhoids, &c. London, 1824. P. 23, 24.
** Principles of Midwifery, Vol. ii. p. 280.

and discharge blood as in other hemorrhagic injections. This exudation taking place either at the uterine surface, or in the substance of the placenta, or in both at once, speedily detaches the placenta from the womb; the usual supply of blood is interrupted; and the fœtus perishes in consequence. In this sense only can the remark of Leake be well-founded. " Whatever may be the cause of abortion, the effect is produced by a separation of the after-burden from the womb, and consequently, the child, being deprived of nourishment, must soon perish and be expelled."* The difficulty here refers to the remote causes, which may be different in different cases. The pathological cause is invariably the same.

Febrile gastro-enteric hemorrhage.—That the black or coffee-ground vomit, (*vomito prieto*,) and dark-coloured, tar-like, or molasses-like stools, which take place in bad remittents, malignant agues, and yellow fever, consist in hemorrhage from gastro-enteric mucous membrane, is established by the researches of Physick, Dr John Hunter, Bancroft, Jackson, and many other authors. In all cases in which subjects dead of these diseases, under these symptoms, have been inspected, the same kind of coffee-ground matter has been found in the stomach and intestines, but without breach of the mucous surface. The matter, however, has been traced almost in its formation, in the circumstance of dark blood oozing insensibly from the capillaries of the mucous membrane. Its colour is necessarily rendered more intense by the fluids of the gastro-enteric surface. This peculiar exudation may be regarded as the result of disorganization of the mucous capillaries, in consequence of previous congestion during the febrile action. Not confined, however, to the gastro-enteric mucous surface, it occurs in the tracheo-bronchial and genito-urinary. It is observed also occasionally in other tissues from the same cause. In short, febrile action either consists in, or is the cause of capillary disorganization in most of the textures.

The process of hemorrhagic injection, like that of inflammation, may terminate in suppuration, with or without breach of surface, in induration, and thickening, dependent on chronic inflammation.

IV. INFLAMMATORY STRICTURE.—To thickening as an effect of the inflammatory process, I have already had frequent occasion to allude. This takes place to a small extent in the mucous corion, and to a much greater degree in the submucous filamentous tissue,

* Vol. i, p. 149.

in which it depends partly on the increased number of vessels, partly on the effusion of lymph, which causes the mutual cohesion of its component filaments. When this is considerable, and takes place in a membrane lining a canal, it contracts its capacity, and forms what is named stricture; (*constrictio*); (*arctatio.*) Though this may occur in any part of the mucous system, it is most common in the lacrymal canal, the Eustachian tube, the œsophagus, near its upper or lower extremity, the rectum or lower part of the colon, and in the male urethra. The constriction, in such circumstances, depends not unfrequently on the presence of some remaining degree of inflammation; and if this subside, the constriction may also partially diminish.* To its entire disappearance, however, the absorption of the effused lymph is essentially necessary; and in all probability this is never completely effected. In the intestinal canal especially, this induration may be so great that the tissue of the tube becomes hard and firm like parchment or cartilage, and at the same time much thicker than natural. The calibre of the canal then becomes so much contracted that nothing passes through it; and life is terminated, partly by inanition and deficient nutrition, partly by irritation. I have already alluded to partial contractions recorded by various authors, from Haase, Wincker, and Laubins, to Dr Combe and Willan. The most perfect example of total contraction with which I am acquainted is recorded by M. Tartra in his Essay on Poisoning by Nitric Acid. In an individual who died three months after swallowing this poison, the alimentary canal was reduced to so small volume, that it might have been held in the hollow of the hand. Its coats were shrivelled, crisp, and indurated; and its calibre through its whole length did not exceed that of a common quill.† Under such circumstances, all the intestinal tissues suffer successively and simultaneously the effects of the inflammatory process; and the contraction is augmented by the violent and excessive stimulus which it applies to the muscular layer.

That a similar change takes place in the mucous and submucous tissues of the bladder is shown by the observations of Guarinonius, Bonetus, Camerarius, Targioni, Morgagni,‡ Dr Barry,§ Dr Gil-

---

* Home. Howship, Practical Observations, p. 254.

† Essai sur l'empoissonnement, &c.

‡ Epist. iv. 13, 19. x. i3. xxii. 4. xxxix. 33. xl, 22. xli. 13. xlii. 20, 33, 34. xliii. 24. xliv. 15. xlviii. 32. xlix. 18.

§ Edinburgh Med. Essays, Vol. i. p. 266.

christ,* Dessault,† Baillie,‡ Fr. Aug. Walter,§ Charles Bell,‖ Forster,¶ and other authors, who found the mucous coat thickened and indurated like cartilage, and the cavity much contracted. It is at the same time generally sacculated.

Another form of inflammatory thickening, causing diminished area of mucous canals, is that which takes place in chronic enlargement of the mucous glands. The best example of this is observed in the enlargement of the mucous follicles of the cardia, which is no uncommon cause of stricture of the cardiac orifice of the œsophagus. This inflammation is very difficult of resolution, and too often terminates in ulceration of the membrane and the glands.

4. *Adhesion.*—It was asserted by Bichat and others, that mucous membrane does not effuse lymph or contract adhesions. The accuracy of this conclusion, which evidently arose from opinions too generalized on the properties of this tissue, the nature of lymph, and the final causes or rather purposes of morbid action, is questionable, and the inference requires limitation. Independent of the well known experiment of John Hunter, who, by the use of a very irritating injection, produced a secretion of coagulable lymph in the vagina of an ass;—I have already shown that each of the mucous surfaces, under certain states and forms of inflammatory action, may effuse a fluid containing a large proportion of albumen, and which, neither in chemical properties nor pathological relations, can be distinguished from the albuminous exudation of serous membranes. The question of adhesion, however, depends not so much upon the fact of albuminous exudation as upon the anatomical disposition of the cavity or canal, whether it be sufficiently small to favour the mutual approximation of opposite and corresponding surfaces. Thus in the gastro-intestinal membrane, which is in general capacious and distended, either incessantly or frequently with foreign bodies, mutual approximation is too imperfect to admit of adhesion. Yet by some observers this is asserted to have happened. In situations, on the contrary, in which mucous surfaces line narrow tubes, as the lacrymal duct, the Eustachian tube, the urethra, and perhaps the Fallopian tubes, obliteration of the canal by adhesion of its sides is more frequent. It is certain

---

* Essays, Physical and Literary, Vol. iii.   † Journal de Chirurgie.
‡ Engravings, &c. 7th Fascicul. pl. I. fig. 2d.
§ Einige Krankheiten der Nieren und Harnblase, u. s. w. p. 31.   Tafel. ix.
‖ Engravings, &c.   ¶ Med.-Chir. Trans. Vol. i. art. 9.

that the surgeon has not unfrequently occasion to observe corresponding points of narrow canals, as the urethra, adhering apparently by concretion of its sides.* I have had occasion to advert above to a mode in which the vaginal mucous membrane may contract adhesions, and present the similitude of congenital imperforation. The assertion of Bichat regarding the inaptitude of mucous surfaces to adhere requires, therefore, some limitation. Certain facts lead me to infer that one of the conditions necessary to the albuminous exudation and the subsequent concretion of mutual surfaces consists in the destruction of the mucous epidermis by abrasion or ulceration, and the subsequent formation of granulations, which in the course of healing unite the opposite edges of the canal.

V. INDURATION AND THICKENING; CARTILAGINOUS TRANSFORMATION OF MUCOUS MEMBRANE AND CANALS. CHONDROSIS. HYPERTROPHY.—It is not easy to say to what head the change here adverted to should be referred. For it is not by any means easy to determine its exact nature; or even whether it be an affection of the mucous membrane solely, or of the muscular structure, or of both taken together. My chief reason for referring it to the present head is because there is a very considerable affection of the mucous membrane, at its free surface.

The lesion consists in the conversion of a portion of mucous membrane and its subjacent tissue, generally muscular or fibrous, into a thick, hard, cartilaginous substance, sometimes with contraction of the canal, sometimes with dilatation. The mucous surface is irregular, honey-combed as it were, and rough, with numerous intersecting ridges, firm and generally of a whitish gray colour.

It is liable to affect the mucous membrane of the œsophagus, and forms there one species of stricture; the mucous membrane of the *rectum*, where it also forms a species of stricture; and the mucous membrane of the colon, where in like manner it generally causes arctation of the calibre of the canal.

The region, however, in which this lesion is most distinctly seen, and proceeds to its greatest extent, is that of the ureters and bladder. The former canals become thick to the diameter of half an inch and more, their coats are hard, firm, of cartilaginous consistence, and a gray-white colour; the internal of mucous surface is rough and

* Smith Ward, Mem. Med. Society, Vol. iii. p. 536. Maclure, Med. and Surg. Journal.

honey-comb like, with innumerable intersecting lines; and the canal of the ureters may be either natural, contracted, or dilated. The bladder is always much contracted. Its coats are thickened either to the extent of that of the ureters or more; from half an inch to three quarters. The thickening is seated both in the mucous membrane and in the muscular coat, but often more in the former than in the latter. The surface is, like that of the ureteric membrane, irregular and honeycomb-like. The substance of the mucous coat is as firm as cartilage; and the same transformation appears to affect the muscular coat. Occasionally the bladder is sacculated.

The causes and exact nature of this change are not well known. It seems like a species of hypertrophy; and from this, nevertheless, it differs. The instances which have fallen under my own notice occurred in persons under 35. But I daresay that it may appear in old age.

VI. MORBID GROWTHS.—§ 1. *Polypus.*—Under this name various morbid growths are mentioned by authors. It is represented as a disease peculiar to the mucous tissue, and is generally observed to take place in those regions at which it is not very remote from the skin. It occurs particularly in the nose, throat, Eustachian tube, the external earhole, and in the neck of the womb. In the stomach and bladder it is less frequent, and it very rarely occurs in the intestinal tube. It appears under one of three forms.

1. It may take place in the form of a soft ash-gray or bluish production, glistening on the surface, translucent, spongy, and compressible, and attached to the membrane by one or more narrow necks, which render it pendulous. This, which is what is termed by practical authors the *benign polypus*, is proper to the mucous tissue, of which it appears often to be merely a relaxed production or growth. It is much under the influence of atmospheric pressure, increasing in size, and causing much uneasiness while the weather is moist and the mercurial column is low. In clear dry weather, on the contrary, and when the height of the barometer indicates vigorous atmospheric pressure, it shrinks and contracts so much that the patient seems to forget its existence. This form of polypus is frequent in the nasal mucous membrane, in which it causes much uneasiness during its distended state. It may grow also from the fibro-mucous membrane of the frontal, sphenoidal, and maxillary sinuses.* ·When removed it presents, with a few blood-vessels, a

* G. F. Gruner de Polypis in cavo Navium obviis.

flocculent tomentose structure, which is well seen by immersion in water, in which it generally floats. It occurs also in the throat; and *polypi* of the same description I have removed from the external auditory hole. Ruysch observed them growing in the maxillary sinus, and proceeding through the passage below the spongy bone into the nostril,—a fact which I find verified by an observation of M. Giles.* The same sort of tumour is occasionally found in the vagina ; and it is a remarkable proof of the general tendency to the formation of these productions, that in some individuals I have seen them occur at the same time in the nasal and vaginal mucous membrane. The formation of this variety of polypus is ascribed by Morgagni to abnormal development of the mucous glands;† a theory in which he is followed by Plenck.‡ This, however, is too exclusive, and is not applicable to all cases.

2. The name of polypus is also given to a firm fleshy incompressible mass, oval, spheroidal or pyriform, opaque, dark red or purple in colour, sometimes with narrow, sometimes with broad and multifid basis. This form of polypus, which is not influenced by the weather, is observed to occur in the pharyngeal or œsophageal mucous membrane, (Monro), in that of the stomach, (Morgagni,§ Monro,‖ Granville ;¶) in the intestines, in the colon, and rectum, (Rhodius, Fanton, Portal, Monro.) In the case of M. Paulo, recorded by Portal, two fleshy concretions as large as the fist were voided during life ; and after death, which was preceded by hectic and wasting, in the ascending and transverse colon were found four polypous tumours, each as large as a nut, and two smaller ones attached to the mucous membrane.** A good example of polypus of the rectum is recorded by Dr Monro, *tertius*.†† In the bladder they are mentioned by Warner, Baillie, and Walter. Instances of uterine polypus, (*cercosis*, Plenck,) are recorded by Mauriceau, Lamotte, Morgagni, Lieutaud, Levret, Sabatier, Baudelocque, Denman, and Clarke. From these it results, that though polypus occasionally originates from the mucous membrane of the *fundus*, it more frequently grows from the inside of the neck, or from the *os tincæ* itself. Upon the nature or the mode of development of this variety of polypus nothing satisfactory is known. It appears to

---

* Phil. Trans. No. 226, p. 472.   † Epist. xvi. 36.

‡ "Causa polypi proxima est papillæ pituitariæ excrescentia seu vegetatio morbosa." Systema Tumorum, Classis iii. p. 173.

§ Epist. xiv. 17, 18.   ‖ Morbid Anatomy, p. 189, pl. vi.

¶ Med. Rep. Aug. 1817.   ** Anatomie Medicale, Tome v. p. 213.

†† Morbid Anatomy of the Gullet, p. 192.

consist in deposition of matter entirely new, either in the mucous corion, or in the submucous filamentous tissue. The tumour is almost invariably covered by a thin pellicle similar to mucous membrane, but much more vascular. It appears, on the whole, to be much of the nature of vascular sarcoma occurring in other textures. It is generally vascular, often traversed by varicose veins, is liable to frequent hemorrhage, and occasionally degenerates into destructive ulceration. It ought not, however, to be confounded with cancer.

3. The name of polypus is also given to a broad, sometimes flat, hard tumour, taking place in the nasal mucous membrane, and peculiar apparently to this region. It is generally of a reddish or brown colour, harder even than the fleshy polypus, smooth on the surface, and presenting the appearance of mucous membrane. From several examples of this disease which I have had an opportunity of examining, I infer that it depends on some abnormal development of the fibro-mucous covering of the spongy or nasal bones. It affects not the mucous membrane only, but the subjacent periosteum, and adheres firmly to the bones, fragments of which are not unfrequently rent off in the attempt to extract this polypus. It has a tendency to induce inflammation and caries of the bones, but does not appear to possess much malignant tendency of itself. Upon the whole, this variety, though commonly denominated polypus, is in truth a tumour of the periosteum, partaking of the polypous character.

§ 2. *Tyromatous* deposition, commonly denominated tubercular, is not uncommon in the mucous tissue. It occurs chiefly in the alimentary canal, and in the uterus in the persons of the strumous. Its characters in the former situation are well described by Dr Monro *tertius*,[*] and have been already considered at length under their proper head. In the uterus it has been observed by several.

§ 3. *Scirrho-carcinoma* is a frequent organic change in mucous tissue. It occurs under four forms,—fibro-cartilaginous deposition, tubercular deposition, colloid deposition, and lardaceous degeneration.

a. Though fibro-cartilaginous deposition may affect any of the regions of these surfaces, it is more frequent in certain points than in others. Thus it occurs very often in the œsophagus, in the cardia, in the pyloric end of the stomach, in the sigmoid flexure of the colon, in

---

[*] Morbid Anatomy, p. 217.

the rectum, and in the uterus, occasionally in the larynx and trachea. In the œsophagus and stomach it has been seen by many observers, among others, by Morgagni, Bleuland, Palletta, Baillie, Chardel, Monro, Howship, Armstrong; in the pylorus it has also been seen by many: (Morgagni, Baillie, Pinel, Holmes, Louis, &c.) and the rectum is perhaps the most frequent seat of scirrho-carcinoma of any of the internal parts. In all these situations the anatomical characters of the disease are much the same. In the mucous corion, or at its attached surface, is formed a deposition of white or gray fibro-cartilaginous substance, the fibrous bands running transversely to the direction of the bowel. This deposition is firm, of ligamentous consistence, and undergoes a self-destroying process in the interior. In general, however, the mucous pellicle forming its free surface undergoes ulceration; or contraction of the canal takes place to such an extent as to interfere with the functions of the organ, and terminate life.

b. Tubercular induration is another form in which scirrhus may affect the mucous tissue. A portion becomes occupied by irregular nodulated masses, consisting of hard spheroidal bodies not unlike cartilage, sometimes softer, like flesh interspersed with cartilaginous points. This is observed in the œsophagus (Bonetus, Bleuland, Palletta, Mr David Hay, &c.) in the cardiac and pyloric orifices of the stomach, and in the rectum. In the latter it forms many of the examples of scirrho-contraction of that organ. This affection appears to consist in peculiar chronic induration with degeneration of the mucous follicles, in situations abounding in which it most usually occurs. It is observed to attack very often the neck of the uterus. It is totally distinct from the tyromatous deposition of strumous habits, with which it has been occasionally confounded by some observers. The tyromatous deposition occurs chiefly in the young, and has been seen even in infants. Tubercular induration is a disease of middle age and declining years. For some judicious observations on the development and distinctions of these two varieties of cancer, I refer to the writings of Bayle and Cruveilhier, and a Memoir of Scarpa in his Chirurgical Treatises.*

By several authorities, on the other hand, it is maintained, that the fibro-cartilaginous and tubercular scirrhus are the same in structure and characters, and differ only in the mode in which the scirrhous matter is deposited. This view may be correct. It is

* Opuscoli di Chirurgia di Antonio Scarpa, &c. Vol. i. Pavia, 1825.

perhaps of no great moment. It may be merely observed, that while the fibro-cartilaginous form of scirrhus is common in the external glands, as the mamma, lacrymal gland, salivary glands, and testicle, tubercular scirrhus is usually seen in the skin and in certain parts of the mucous membranes, as the œsophagus, cardia, pylorus, and rectum; and, according to Scarpa, the uterine end of the vagina and the *os uteri* itself.

c. *Reticular, Areolar, Alveolar, and Colloid Cancer.*—A third form in which cancer may attack the mucous surfaces is that which is named reticular and areolar, from its disposition, and colloid or glue-like from its aspect. The general characters of this species of degeneration are a tumour affecting a considerable portion of the stomach, most commonly the anterior and posterior portions of the large arch of the organ; and in some instances the cardiac portion both anteriorly and posteriorly. It does not seem often to commence in the pyloric portion; but it may extend from the cardiac or the middle region of the organ to the *pylorus*. The tumour is firm, of cartilaginous consistence, and when inspected at the mucous surface of the stomach presents the aspect of a solution of isinglass which has become coagulated, with a sort of honey-comb, or reticular surface like network. The colour is generally light-gray or pearl-like. The structure cuts firm.

The morbid structure affects primarily, and principally, it appears to me, the mucous membrane of the stomach; and this areolar or colloid form of cancer is more frequently observed in this organ than in any other, or in any other texture. It consists apparently in the infiltration of this colloid or gelatiniform matter into the interstitial spaces of the mucous membrane. It renders the stomach thick and hard. The thickness varies from one-fourth of an inch to half an inch, and to three quarters. When divided, the morbid structure appears like a hard or tough solution of firm jelly or isinglass, with numerous communicating cells.

In general this deposit is confined to the mucous membrane; and the muscular coat is pale, hard, thicker than natural, with developed fibres, and in a state of hypertrophy. Several authorities, and especially Cruveilhier, state that the muscular coat is also affected by this deposit. But the statement appears not to be confirmed.

It is also said that this deposit affects primarily the cellular tissue of the stomach. Such appears to be the opinion of Breschet, Andral, and Raikem. This appears to be still more doubtful than the previous statement. The deposit, originating in the mucous coat

3

of the stomach, may extend to the cellular. But that it commences in the cellular appears at present to be a questionable statement, which requires the confirmation of further inquiries.

Scarpa, though not aware of the exact character of areolar or colloid cancer, shows, nevertheless, that he had seen every reason, from preparations and specimens of the disease, to infer, that it commences in and affects the mucous membrane.*

In short, areolar, alveolar, or colloid cancer, is to be distinguished from the other forms of this morbid deposit, both by its physical and anatomical characters, by its arrangement, and by the tissues which it affects. In physical aspect it is semihard, elastic, like stiff isinglass solution. In internal structure it is cellular. And lastly, it is, if not exclusively confined to the stomach, much more common in that than in any other organ.

d. A fourth form in which cancerous disease attacks the mucous tissues is that of lardaceous degeneration. In certain regions, indeed, this is so rare that it is never seen. For example, though not very frequent in the gastro-enteric mucous membrane, it has been observed in the œsophagus and rectum. It is not known in the tracheo-bronchial membrane. In the uterus, however, it is very common; and I have seen several instances in which the neck and part of the body of this organ was converted into a ceromatous and apparently inorganic mass. The decomposition of this morbid deposition is peculiar. It terminates not in ulceration, but in a species of softening and pulpy disorganization or liquefaction, rendering the decomposing surface doughy or pasty like soft lard, traversed by marks of erosion similar to those produced by the gnawing of animals.

. § 4. *Warty excrescences* are occasionally found in mucous membranes. They consist of hard eminences often fissured, sometimes sessile with broad base, occasionally peduncular, and occasionally pass into bad ulceration. They are most frequent in the pharyngeal and œsophageal, and in the cystic and uterine membrane.

§ 5. *Fungous growths* or excrescences are mentioned as occasionally found in the mucous tissues; but little accurate information is given regarding them. They are frequent in the bladder

---

* "Scirrhus and cancer of the stomach," he says, "always begins with induration of the internal mucous membrane of the organ, which becomes thick, hard, cartilaginous, then ulcerates ; and from the inner coat the disease is propagated to the other membranes of the stomach, which are converted into scirrhus, and cancerous hardness, with ulceration." Memoria Sullo Scirro et sul Cancro. Opuscoli di Chirurgia di Antonio Scarpa. Vol. i. Pavia 1825. Folio minore.

of the male (Lecat, Sandifort, Baillie, Walter, &c.) and the uterus of the female, but appear to be more rare in other regions. It is probable that these excrescences named fungous, are in truth the products of an advanced stage of some organic change either already noticed or to be noticed. In the uterus, for instance, authors mention the occurrence of reddish tumours not unlike masses of clotted blood, which are manifestly either *molæ, or fungus hæmatodes*, or some of the products of cancerous ulceration. In other instances, as in the bladder, these fungous growths actually issue from the mucous membrane in a morbid state, sometimes the effect of chronic inflammation, or are the result of enlarged prostate. Upon the whole, accurate facts are wanting on this head.

§ 6. Though *hydatids* are enumerated by some authors among the morbid products of mucous surfaces, it is not easy to understand, without violation of certain pathological principles supposed to be well-established, the reason of their development in these situations. Thus, hydatids have been stated to be coughed up from the lungs, to be voided from the intestines, and to have escaped from the uterus. In the case of the lungs, they are formed originally in the pleura or pulmonic tissue, from which they find their way to the bronchial membrane ; or they may escape from the liver through the diaphragm ; (Dr Foart Simmons, Dr Monro.) In the case of the intestines, they are also in all probability formed in the liver or the peritoneum, and thence proceed by ulceration into the intestinal cavity. The uterus, in short, is the only cavity with mucous surface, in which inspection shows that they have been found.[*] Tyson, nevertheless, states that he found them in the bladder.[†]

§ 7. Deposition of bony matter in certain of the mucous surfaces is mentioned by various authorities. Thus Metzger records an instance of ossification of the œsophagus ;[‡] Walter one of bony deposition in the inner surface of the pharynx ;[§] De Haen mentions an osseous degeneration of the stomach ;[||] Short[¶] and others mention similar deposits in the colon and rectum ; and Hody,[**] Lettsom,[††] Baillie, Odier, and Mackie[‡‡] mention examples

---

* Gregorini Dissert. Morgagni, Epist. xlviii. 13, 14. Portal, Anatomie Medicale, Tome v. p. 527, 528. Rudolphi gives the best account of Hydatids affecting the uterus and other organs. Ueber die Hydatiden thierischer Korper, in Anatomisch-Physiologische Abhandlungen. Berlin, 1802. P. 190.

† Phil. Trans. No. 188.
‡ Adversaria Medica, p. 176 and 177.
§ Catalogi Mus. No. 1536.
|| Rat. Med. Tom. iv. cap. i.

¶ Ed. Med. Essays, Vol. iv. 353.
** Phil. Trans. No. 440.
†† Mem. Med. Society, Vol. v.
‡‡ Med. and Phys. Journal.

of the same occurrence in the uterus. The history of the mode of development of this deposition is not exactly known; and it is not quite certain whether the ossification originates invariably in the mucous corion. This indeed appears to have taken place in the instance mentioned by Walter, and in such cases of uterine ossification as that recorded by Dr Caldwell.* In instances of osseous deposition in the alimentary canal, it is justly suspected by Dr Monro to originate in the muscular fibres.

§ 8. Further, in certain regions of the mucous tissue are found morbid growths which are proper to these regions, and to be found in no other part of the mucous membranes. Thus the milt-like tumour described by Dr Monro has been found chiefly in the stomach and bowels; and the fleshy tubercle of William Hunter and Dr Clark, and the cauliflower excrescence of the latter, are found only in the womb.

The former variety of tumour, for an accurate description of which we are indebted to Dr Monro *tertius*, resembles in structure and consistence the milt of fishes, is of a pale red colour, with an irregular surface, and is covered by a thin but vascular membrane, adheres slightly to the organ from which it grows by a number of small vascular processes penetrating the mucous corion, which is unnaturally thick, and presents a honey-comb appearance. The portion of intestine to which such tumour is attached presents marks of vascular injection. The substance of the tumour, though miscible with water, which it renders turbid, is indurated by immersion in alcohol,—a circumstance from which it may be inferred to contain a proportion of albuminous matter. It emits a fetid offensive smell, and communicates the same to the organ from which it grows. It is chiefly a disease of advanced life,—a circumstance by which; with others, it may be distinguished from hæmatoid fungus.

The fleshy or sarcoid tubercle of the uterus, though apparently not unknown to Morgagni, was first observed by William Hunter, and has since been distinctly described by Dr John Clarke, Dr Baillie,† and Sir C. M. Clarke.‡ According to the accounts of these observers, it appears in the form of one or more tumours of hard whitish substance, sometimes as firm as cartilage, projecting from the mucous surface of the organ, but occasionally growing

---

* Med. and Surg. Journ. Vol. ii. 22.

† Morbid Anatomy, chap. xix. p. 374.

‡ Observations on the Diseases of Females, part i. chap. xviii. p. 243.

between the peritonæal coat and muscular layer. In size they vary from that of a pea to masses of several pounds; and in shape, though generally spheroidal, they are sometimes irregular. They cause a copious mucous discharge and much local irritation, but without much affecting the constitution.

The cauliflower excrescence was also first accurately described by Dr John Clarke; * and his description has been since verified by his brother Sir C. Mansfield Clarke. From the observations of these authors, it results that the cauliflower excrescence arises always from some part of the *os uteri*. When first recognised, it forms an irregular prominence, with a broad base and a granulated surface. As the tumour increases in size, the granulated structure of its surface becomes more distinct, and begins to be parted into numerous elongated granules, which give it the appearance of a cauliflower when it begins to run to seed. In most instances these granules are friable and brittle, and break off, if rudely handled, in the form of minute white fragments; and indeed such fragments are occasionally or periodically discharged with the urine and other fluids. Its surface, which is of a bright flesh colour, is covered by a thin delicate membrane, from which oozes abundantly a sero-albuminous fluid, which mats the linen like starch, and occasionally blood flows copiously. In married women who have had children its growth is rapid; in those not exposed to sexual intercourse it is slow. The attempts made to inject this growth have been unsuccessful. The injection escapes from its surface rapidly; and it shrinks so much after death, that it is impossible to recognize anything but a small loose flocculent membranous prolongation of the part to which it is attached. These circumstances, with its hemorrhagic character, lead Sir C. Clarke to regard it as an assemblage of minute arteries similar to the placental structure. It is probably a morbid variety of erectile tissue.†

VII. DISPLACEMENTS.—The mucous membranes, partly in consequence of their loose connection in many instances with subjacent tissues, partly in consequence of inordinate action in the muscular fibres of their proper organs, sometimes in consequence of inflam- •
mation, are liable to various unnatural changes of situation. Thus the eyelids are liable to eversion, the *rectum*, the *vagina*, and the

* Transactions of a Society, Vol. iii. p. 298.
† Observations on those Diseases of Females, &c. Part ii.

uterus to *prolapsus* and *procidentia*, the uterus to inversion, and the intestinal canal to invagination and hernial protrusion.

VIII. MALFORMATIONS.—§ 1. Lastly, *Malformations* are frequently observed in the mucous system; but it is often difficult to distinguish between those which are proper, and those which are common to it with collateral and subjacent tissues. Occasionally, for instance, parts of the mucous system in common with the other constituent tissues of an organ are wanting. Thus part of the alimentary canal may be deficient, and the urinary bladder or the rectum has been known to be wanting. In other instances, part of the mucous tissue of one organ may be so incomplete, that a direct communication with another is established. Thus the *velum* may be fissured and the palate may communicate directly with the nasal passages; the vagina may open into the rectum, the bladder in the hypogastric region, or communicate directly with the rectum; or the urethra may open into the perinæum. The mechanism of malformations of this description is to be explained by the history of the development of the mucous system during the early months of fœtal existence. The researches of Wolff, Oken, J. F. Meckel, and Tiedemann, show that a slight interruption given to the process of development at this period, while the cutaneous and mucous surfaces are in direct continuation upon the mesial plane, is sufficient to continue through life a peculiarity of structure, which belongs only to the embryo during formation.

§ 2. *Congenital Fistulæ of the neck.*—One of the most curious examples of this sort of malformation is furnished by the *fistulæ* of the neck described by Dzondi,* Ascherson,† and Meyer.‡ These fistulæ are in general known by a very minute, almost imperceptible aperture, on the lateral surface of the neck, appearing in the angle formed by the internal head of the sterno-mastoid muscle and the sternal end of the collar-bone, or at the inner margin of that muscle. This is the external aperture. An internal one is not in all cases ob-

* Carolus Henricus Dzondi, Phil.-Doct. et Chir.-Doct. De Fistulis Tracheæ Congenitis, Commentatio Pathologico-Therapeutica. Halæ, 1829. 8vo.

† Ferdinandus Mauritius Ascherson, M. D., De Fistulis Colli Congenitis. Adjecta Fissurarum Branchialium in Mammalibus, Avibusque, Historia Succincta. Berolini, 1832. 4to.

‡ De Fissuris Hominis Mammaliumque Congenitis. Accedit Fissuræ Buccalis Congenitæ cum Fissuræ Tubæ Eustachii et Tympani Complicatæ Descriptio. Auctore Conrado Meyer Tigurino ; Medicinæ utriusque Doctore. Cum quatuor tabulis æneis, Berolini, 1835. Folio.

served.   The course of the *fistula*, which is so small as often to admit only the lacrymal probe of Anel, is in general towards the
pharynx ; and in some cases water may be injected by the *fistula*
into the pharynx.

From the external aperture of these *fistulæ* exudes, from time to
time, a thin white drop of transparent glutinous fluid, not unlike
white of egg, sometimes like purulent matter.   The inner, surface
of these fistulæ is smooth, reddish, and like that of a mucous membrane.

These *fistulæ*, which are congenital, are the remains of the bran-
chial slits of the early intra-uterine period of the fœtus, in consequence of the process of closure of these slits being in some manner
stopped.   They cannot be healed without inconvenience ; in one case
the attempt was followed by apoplectic death ; and there is reason
to believe that they must have been left open for some salutary purpose.

. They are more frequent in females than in males in the ratio of
about eight to three.

They are observed in certain families more commonly than in
others.

§ 3. The sacs of the *ileum* and bladder, called *diverticula*, appear to
depend on deficiency of the muscular layer, in consequence of which
the mucous corion is protruded through the defective space. (Morgagni ; Palletta.)

§ 4. In other instances, deviations from the normal arrangement
consist in unnatural unions of mucous surfaces, rendering the canals
which they line impervious, and constituting varieties of imperfora-
tions.   Thus the pyloric orifice of the stomach has been found
closed,* the rectum imperforate, and the vagina imperforate. These,
in all probability, are to be ascribed to deficiency of mucous membrane, in consequence of which the contiguous parts contract adhesion.

§ 5. In other instances, again, malformations are the result of disease.   Of this description are the enlarged or distended state of the
pulmonic vesicles, produced by several being burst into one large
cavity ; the central contraction of the stomach ; the sacculated state
of the urinary bladder ; the dilatations of the alimentary canal, in
consequence of the lodgement of foreign bodies or concretions ;

---

* Case by Mr Crooks, Edin. Med.-Chirur. Transactions, Vol. ii. p. 589.

4

and those of the gall-bladder or gall ducts, in consequence of the presence of gall-stones. Another variety of the same description of malformation consists in the fistulous openings occasionally effected between the mucous membranes and the cutaneous surface by the process of progressive ulceration. To this head belong the *fistulae* of the stomach, of which many examples, from wounds and similar injuries, as well as spontaneous abscesses, are now recorded; the *fistulae* which result from the ulceration caused by the discharge of gall-stones; artificial anus so frequent after intestinal inflammation, and especially that which attends strangulated hernia; urinary fistulæ, whether taking place from the bladder in the hypogastrium or rectum, or from the urethra; and destruction of the recto-vaginal septum in females, either by laceration or ulceration. These fistulæ are covered by a smooth callous membrane so similar in its properties to mucous texture that John Hunter, Meckel, and some other authors think it not an extravagant or gratuitous hypothesis to regard them as examples of the abnormal development of mucous texture.

CHAPTER III.

SECTION I.

SEROUS MEMBRANE, TRANSPARENT MEMBRANE;—*Membrana pellucida,—M. serosa ;—Tissu Sereux.*

THE pleura and peritonæum are the best examples of the tissue, which has been named *serous*, from the fluid with which it is moistened, and which may be termed *transparent* or *diaphanous* as its distinctive character.

The distribution or mechanical arrangement of these membranes is peculiar, and was not well understood by anatomists till Douglas, in 1730,* by his description of the peritonæum, rendered it clearer

---

* A Description of the *Peritonæum*, and of that part of the Membrana Cellularis which lies on its outside. With an Account of the true situation of all the Abdominal Viscera in respect of these two Membranes. By Dr James Douglas, Physician in ordinary to her Majesty, &c. London, 1730. 4to.

and more intelligible. Since that time the distribution of these membranes, individually and generally, has been elucidated by the labours of Hunter, Carmichael Smyth, and Bichat, with a degree of perspicuity and precision which leaves little to be done by subsequent observers. Notwithstanding this, Valentin Hansen of Triers, a learned student of the University of Berlin, thought it, in 1834, a subject worthy of further inquiry and explanation; and his dissertation must be allowed to be a good memorial of industry and intelligence.*

In this, nevertheless, there are certain peculiarities which may perplex the beginner, and prevent him from obtaining at first a clear idea of the distribution and configuration of the pellucid membranes. Thus they have neither beginning nor termination; they have neither orifice nor egredient canal; and they are not continuous with any other membrane or texture.

§ 1. Every serous membrane consists of a hollow sac everywhere closed, and to the cavity or interior surface of which there is no natural entrance, a circumstance from which they have been denominated *shut sacs*, (*sacci occlusi; sacs sans ouverture.*) In every serous membrane one part is inverted or inflected, or reflected, as is commonly said, within the other, so that the inner surface of the former part is applied with more or less accuracy to the inner or like surface of the latter. This mode of disposition has suggested to anatomists the homely and trite, but not inappropriate comparison of a serous membrane to a nightcap, one-half of which is folded or doubled within the other, so that while one-half of the inner surface is applied to the remaining half, no communication exists between the inner and the outer surface. Every serous membrane, in short, is a single sac, one-half of which is doubled within the other.

In every serous membrane the outer surface of the unreflected portion is applied over the walls of the region which the serous membrane lines, while the outer surface of the inflected portion is applied over the organ or organs contained in that region. From this arrangement it results that each organ covered by serous membrane is not contained in that membrane, but is on its exterior sur-

---

* Peritonæi Humani Anatomia et Physiologia, Dissertatio Inaug. Quam pro summis in Medicina et Chirurgia Honoribus in Universitate Literaria Frederica Guilelma, rite sibi conciliandis, die 21 Junii 1834, publice defendet Auctor Valentinus Hansen Rhenano-Borussus. 4to.

face, and that of every organ so situate, one part at least, viz. that at which its vessels and nerves enter, is always uncovered. Thus the lungs are on the outer surface of the *pleura ;* the heart is on the outside of the *pericardium ;* the stomach, intestines, liver, spleen, and pancreas are on the outside of the *peritonæum ;* and the testicles are on the outside of the *peridydimis.* In the same manner the lungs, though invested by pleura before and behind, at their apex and their base, are uncovered at their roots, or the points where the bronchial tubes and great blood-vessels enter their substance; the heart is uncovered by pericardium at the upper part of the auricular cavities; and the intestinal canal is uncovered along the whole of that longitudinal but tortuous line by which the mesentery is attached, and at which its proper vessels and nerves are transmitted.

To comprehend the arrangement of the pellucid membranes still more distinctly, it is expedient, by an effort of abstraction, to trace the course of any one of them, having previously thrown out of the question the necessary means by which their interior or free surface is exposed. In this mental process, also, it is requisite to remember that there is no initial point save what is arbitrarily made. If, for example, the course of the *pleura* be traced, the membrane presents no natural mark or boundary from which the anatomist is to commence his demonstration; and he must fix artificially on any point which he finds most convenient for the purpose. Commencing with this understanding, from the circumference of the spot termed *root* of the lungs, the membrane may be traced first along the internal surface of the chest formed by the ribs and intercostal muscles, forwards to the sternum, upwards to the first rib and *apex* of the thoracic cavity, and downwards to the diaphragmatic insertions, and over the surface of that muscle, and the outer surface of the pericardium again, to the circumference of the root or connection of the lungs. From this point again it may be traced over the surface and between the lobes of these organs, both of which, as already stated, are thus situate on the outside of the pleura. The course first described is that of the *unreflected* or *exterior* division of the pleura. The second, or that over the organ covered, is the course of the *inflected* or *doubled* portion of the membrane, which is thus necessarily smaller and less extensive than the former.

The arrangement thus sketched, which may be easily shown to

be applicable to all the serous membranes, demonstrates their two-fold character of lining the walls of a cavity and covering the organs contained. From an idea of this property the older anatomists applied to them the epithet of *membranæ succingentes.*

In tracing the course of the serous membranes, the anatomist observes, that they present productions which float with more or less freedom in the cavity formed by the free surface, and which may be generally shown to consist of two folds of the single membrane produced beyond the inclosed organ, but still maintaining the unity of the membrane. Of these prolongations, the most distinct examples are the *epiploon* and the *appendices epiploicæ* of the peritonæum. Less manifest instances are the adipose folds of the pleura near the mediastinum, and the bladder-like appearance at the base of the heart, within the pericardium. The synovial fringes in the interior of the synovial membranes, which belong to a subsequent head, are nevertheless of the same general character. Between the folds of these productions there is invariably more or less adipose substance, which indeed is observed, in some quantity, in various parts of the filamentous tissue on the outer surface of the serous membranes in general.

Every serous membrane I have above represented as a hollow sac everywhere continuous, and the outer surface of which has no communication with the inner. To this character the only exception is the peritonæum in the female, which is perforated at two points, corresponding to the upper extremity or orifice of the Fallopian or oviferous tubes. This has been already mentioned as the only spot at which the mucous and serous surfaces communicate directly with each other.

Every serous membrane may be described as consisting of a very thin, colourless, transparent web or pellicle, through which the tissue of the subjacent organ or parts may be easily recognized; and every serous membrane presents two surfaces, an attached or adherent, and a free or unadherent.

The attached surface, which is also termed its *outer* one, is that by which it is connected to the tissue or organ which it covers; it is somewhat irregular, flocculent or tomentose, and is evidently connected by fine filamentous tissue. The degree of attachment is very variable in different membranes, and in different points of the same membrane. In general serous membranes adhere much less firmly to the walls of cavities than to the surface of the contained organs.

Thus the abdominal peritonæum and the costal pleura are more easily removed than the intestinal peritonæum and the pulmonic pleura. The peritonæum adheres feebly to the bladder, to the liver, and to the pancreas, more intimately to the different regions of the intestinal tube, and seems to be almost identified with the substances of the female organs of generation. From the interior of the capsular pericardium and from the vaginal coat it is almost impossible to detach the serous pellicle. The former, however, I shall have occasion to show, is peculiar in having between the serous surface and the fibrous membrane no filamentous tissue, upon the abundance or deficiency of which the degree of adhesion depends.

The free or unadherent surface, which has been also named *inner*, is very smooth or polished and uniform, moistened with a watery fluid, from which it derives in some degree its shining appearance, and completely destitute of fibres or any other trace of organic structure. From this smooth polished aspect, which is a peculiar attribute of the free surface of serous membrane, all the organs covered by it derive their glistening appearance. Thus the exterior surface of the lungs derives its appearance from the pleura, the heart from the pericardium, the liver and intestinal canal from the peritonæum. A successful injection of size or turpentine, coloured with vermilion, brings into view so many capillary blood-vessels in this membrane, that it might be supposed at first sight to consist entirely of minute arteries and veins. Farther, by proper management, lymphatics may be injected in it with quicksilver to a degree equally minute and delicate. From these experiments, therefore, it may be concluded, that serous membrane is chiefly composed of minute arteries and veins conveying colourless fluids, and of vessels connected with the general trunks of the lymphatic system. Whether it contain anything else but vessels of this kind, or has a proper substance or tissue, remains to be ascertained. Though nerves are often seen passing along their outer or attached surface to the neighbouring tissues, none have hitherto been traced either into the pleura or peritonæum.

By most of the older anatomists, and among others by Haller and William Hunter, serous membrane is considered as of the nature of filamentous tissue or cellular membrane, more or less closely condensed, (*tela cellulosa stipata ;*)* and this view is adopted and

---

* Elem. Physiolog. Lib. iv., sect. i. § i. xvi. Lib. xxii.

maintained by Bordeu,[*] Bichat,[†] Meckel,[‡] and Beclard,[§] the last of whom, however, thinks they partake of ligamentous characters. Macerated they become soft, thick, and pulpy ; and are finally resolved into flocculent filamentous matter. In the course of decomposition in the dead subject they first lose their glistening aspect, then become covered by a foul dirty coating of viscid matter, which appears to exude from their surface; and eventually they are dissolved into shreds. Immersion in boiling water renders them thick, firm, and somewhat crisp. When dried they become thin, clear, and transparent, and, if preserved from humidity or the attacks of animals, may remain long unchanged. The experiments of Hatchett, Fourcroy, and Vauquelin, show that they contain gelatin and a little albumen ; but no precise information on their chemical composition has yet been given.

The principal character of the serous membranes is that of isolating the organs which they cover, and to the structure of which they are foreign or adventitious, and forming shut cavities, in which there is an incessant process of exhalation and absorption. In some instances they evidently contribute to facilitate the mutual motions of contiguous and corresponding parts and surfaces. From their free surfaces is secreted a fluid containing a very small portion of albumen, (Hewson,[||] Bostock,[¶]) which is greatly augmented during the state of disease.

The mode of development of the pellucid membranes is not very well ascertained. The investigations regarding organogenesy by Oken, Meckel, and Tiedemann, to which I have occasion so frequently to allude, disclose facts which induce Meckel to hazard the opinion that some of them are not at all times shut sacs. I have some reason to doubt, however, whether the fact which he adduces for this purpose necessarily implies the open condition of the pericardium and the peritonæum. In the case of the former the development of the heart proceeds from the basis generally, without affecting the integrity of the investing membrane. In the case of the latter there is more reason to believe, that at the navel at least the peritonæum is either open, or is continuous with the vitellar membrane.

[*] Recherches sur le Tissu Muqueux, sect. i. § i.
[†] Anat. Generale, Tome iv. p. 573.   [‡] Handbuch, B. i.
[§] Elemens d'Anat. Gen. p. 228.
[||] Experimental Inquiries, ii. chap. vii.
[¶] Nicholson's Journal, Vol. xiv. p. 147, and Medico-Chirurg. Tr. Vol. iv.

In the fœtus the serous membranes are so thin, that they are much more transparent than in the adult. In small animals also, they are more transparent than in large, and in cold-blooded animals than in the mammiferous. Of some also the disposition varies at different periods. Thus the descent of the testicle,—a process which has been so well explained by Albinus, Haller, Wrisberg, and Langenbeck,—is necessarily attended with a remarkable change in the arrangement of that portion of peritonæum which the gland impels before it.

The above description applies chiefly to the general characters and properties of serous membranes. I have yet, however, to advert to certain forms of this tissue, which, though similar in general characters, present too many peculiarities to be justly identified with them. The first which I notice as least different is the *pericardium*, or capsule of the heart; the second is the arachnoid membrane, which shall be examined with the cerebral envelopes.

§ 2. The capsule of the heart (*pericardium*) consists of two portions or layers, an outer or proper capsular, and an inner or lining division. The outer or proper capsular part of the pericardium possesses the characters of a fibrous membrane, of some density and considerable strength. When properly washed its colour is gray or grayish-white, and it appears to consist of very minute fibrous threads, which are arranged without any definite order. These fibres are most distinct at its lower margin, where it is connected to the circumference of the tendinous part of the diaphragm. In the young subject it is generally thin and translucent; in adult age or advanced life it is thicker and more opaque. This part of the pericardium is a mere investing membrane, which bounds the region containing the heart, but which extends no further. It embraces the origins of the large vessels above, adheres to the margins of the tendinous centre below, and is on each side connected with the pleura.

When the pericardium is slit open, its inner surface has the appearance of a transparent or serous membrane, through which the fibres of the outer or capsular part may be seen, and which has the usual glistening aspect of such membranes. It is difficult, however, to insulate it from the outer layer, unless by boiling, when it may be peeled off in minute shreds.

Like the transparent membranes, this inner layer has neither beginning nor end, neither origin nor termination. After lining

X X

the inner surface of the proper capsule, it may be traced from the angle at which this capsule adheres to the large arteries and veins, over the auricles, and finally, over the outer surface of the ventricles to the apex of the heart.

In this whole course, it preserves the characters of a thin transparent membrane, with a free surface and an attached one. The free surface is perfectly smooth, glistening, and moistened with a watery fluid. The attached surface adheres, on the one hand, to the inner surface of the capsule, and on the other, to the outer surface of the heart, by means of fine filamentous tissue.

. Injection shows that the pericardium consists chiefly of minute arteries and veins. The substance of the capsular part is probably a modification of the white fibrous system; but it requires to be more carefully examined. No nerves have been traced into any part of this membrane, nor is it quite certain that it contains lymphatics.

§ 3. The cerebral membranes are not uniform in nature, and cannot be conveniently referred to any head save that of compound membranes. The *dura mater* is fibrous; the *pia mater* is supposed to be celluloso-vascular; and Bichat has laboured to demonstrate that the arachnoid is a serous membrane,—a view which is adopted by Meckel and Beclard, but rejected by Gordon. By configuration and disposition, I believe it is more easily referable to this than to any other class ; and I therefore introduce its anatomical history in this place.

The brain has been said to be surrounded by three membranous envelopes, the hard membrane (*meninx dura, dura mater*), the web-like membrane (*tunica arachnoidea*), and the soft or thin membrane (*meninx tenuis, pia mater.*) There is perhaps no great or just objection to this arrangement, which has been adopted by almost all writers. But it simplifies the subject, without impairing the truth of what is observed, to refer them to two only ; one of which, the hard membrane (*meninx dura,* μηνιγξ σκληρη, *dura mater*), is common to the brain with the inner surface of the skull; the other, the thin membrane (*meninx tenuis,* μηνιγξ λεπτη, *pia mater*), is proper to the brain only. They may be distinguished, therefore, by the terms *common membrane of the brain* and *proper membrane of the brain.* The arachnoid, again, is a pellucid web common to the two cerebral membranes.

The first of these, the common or hard cerebral membrane (*me-*

ninx dura, dura mater), presents two surfaces, an outer or cranial, and an inner or cerebral. The outer surface is irregular, filamentous, and vascular ; and the substance of which it consists is distinctly fibrous. ⸱ The fibres, however, do not follow any uniform direction, but are interwoven irregularly. Maceration causes this membrane to swell and become separated into fibrous threads. It is well known that it is liberally supplied with blood-vessels, and that it is connected by these to the inner surface of the skull. No nerves or absorbents have been discovered in it. This outer or cranial surface of the *dura mater* is manifestly of the nature of periosteum. Its vessels may be traced into the inner table; it contributes to the formation of the cranial bones in the fœtus; and various facts show that it contributes to their nutrition during life.

The inner or cerebral surface of this membrane is very smooth, uniformly polished, and shining ; and when examined in water, it appears to be formed of a very thin, transparent membrane, through which the cranial or outer surface and the fibrous structure of the hard membrane may easily be recognized. This pellucid inner membrane, which is termed by Baillie the *inner lamina*, I shall afterwards show, is the exterior division of the arachnoid membrane.

The *dura mater* is an extensive membrane, and lines not only the interior surface of the skull, but that of the whole vertebral column. Here indeed it undergoes some modification. The inner surface of each vertebra has a proper periosteum continuous with the periosteum of the outer surface ; and from this issues a quantity of filamentous tissue, which penetrates directly a membranous canal, evidently of fibrous structure, (*theca vertebralis*,) tough and firm, but more delicate than the cranial *dura mater*. The *dura mater* in its course forms sundry prolongations ; for instance, the large crescentic one named the *falx*, the horizontal one termed *tentorium*, and the small crescentic one named *falx minor* or *cerebelli*.

The thin, soft, or immediate and proper cerebral membrane, (*pia mater, meninx tenuis*,) presents in like manner two surfaces, a smooth or cranial, which is exterior, a filamentous or cerebral, which is interior and central.

The outer or smooth surface of the thin membrane, (*pia mater*,) has a glistening appearance ; and if examined attentively it is found to be formed by a very thin transparent membrane, exactly similar to that which forms the cerebral surface of the *dura mater*.

It is possible to recognize through it the subjacent cerebral part of the membrane, its vessels and the appearance of the brain itself. This surface has been named in the ordinary works the web-like membrane, (*tunica arachnoidea*). It is believed to be a separate membrane from the *pia mater ;* but that which forms the inner or cerebral surface of the *dura mater* has a claim equally strong to this distinction.

The inner or cerebral surface of the proper or soft membrane, I have already said, is filamentous, flocculent, and somewhat rough. It indeed presents a surface which sends out many angular processes of animal substance, which is filamentous and loose in appearance, and which evidently, by numerous minute vessels, arteries, and veins, communicates with the convoluted surface of the brain. These processes, which are the *Tomenta* of the ancient anatomists, correspond to the furrows of the convoluted surface in which they are lodged. In detaching the membrane from this part of the brain, numerous vessels are observed to be drawn out of its substance ; and when the membrane is injected these vessels may be seen distinctly filled, and communicating with the gray matter of the convoluted surface. The veins of this membrane may be traced to the sinuses in those large longitudinal vessels which are lodged in folds of the hard membrane.

After suitable injection, it is difficult to perceive any thing but arteries and veins in the proper cerebral membrane. Neither nerves nor absorbents have yet been recognized in it. Bichat considers that it contains a notable quantity of cellular tissue. This, however, is denied by Gordon, who could not recognize such tissue. The difference, however, consists merely in name. The *pia mater*, indeed, possesses no cellular tissue like the subcutaneous, the submucous, or the subserous. If, however, a portion of the arachnoid be peeled from it by careful management of the forceps and blowpipe, there is found a quantity of loose filamentous or flocculent matter, which evidently unites this tissue to the finer web of the former. It is further remarkable that Dr Gordon himself admits that the inner surface (he should have said the outer or attached) of the arachnoid membrane is more or less *thready* or *flocculent*, according to its connection with the *pia mater*, without seeming to be aware that this thready appearance is occasioned by filamentous tissue. Lastly, the existence of this tissue between the *pia mater* and arachnoid is unequivocally demonstrated by the phenomena of serous infiltration.

The distribution and configuration of the *pia mater* is peculiar; and correct knowledge of these is requisite in order to understand its pathological relations. The *pia mater*, or proper membrane of the brain, consists of two parts, an outer, covering the *convoluted* surface of the brain, and an inner or central, entering the cavities formed by the inner, central, or figurate surface, and spread over this surface in the form of what has been termed the vascular or choroid web; (*plexus choroides; tela choroidea.*) The arrangement of the first or exterior division of the cerebral membrane is well known. Its flocculent-vascular, or tomentose surface, is applied closely and immediately to every part of the convoluted surface, both eminences and depressions (*gyri et sulci*); to every part of the foliated surface of the cerebellum in like manner; and finally, though in a more delicate form, to the surface of the spinal chord, transmitting those vessels which enter and issue from the substance of each part.

The continuity of the *pia mater* or exterior division of the proper cerebral membrane, with the choroid plexus or interior division, may be demonstrated in the following manner. *First,* the *pia mater* may be traced behind and below the posterior extremity of the mesolobe or middle band, (σωμα τιλλοειδες, *corpus callosum,* der balken,) where it is continuous with the transverse web called *velum interpositum,* and which may be regarded in this order of examination as the first part of the central division. *Secondly,* from this point, the situation of the *velum interpositum,* it may be traced forwards on both sides of the mesial plane into the lateral ventricles, spread over the surface of the optic *thalamus* and striated eminence in the form of the vascular web called choroid *plexus,* the right half of which communicates with the left by means of a similar slip of vascular membrane lying beneath the vault (*fornix*), and behind the anterior pillars of that body at the spot termed *Foramen Monroianum. Thirdly,* it may be traced over the geniculate bodies or posterior eminences of each thalamus into the posterior-inferior *cornu,* or sinuosity of the lateral ventricle, where it covers the *great hippocampus. Fourthly,* it may be traced at the angle between the *cerebellum* and *medulla oblongata,* or what is named the bottom of the fourth ventricle, where it forms a very minute choroid plexus seldom noticed by anatomists, but not less distinct, and which may be traced up the fourth ventricle to be connected with the *velum interpositum* in the middle ventricle, and with the lateral portions of the hippocampus on each side.

Each choroid plexus, or, to speak more accurately, each of the divisions of the choroid plexus now enumerated, may be shown to be mutually connected, and to form parts of one general membrane, which again constitutes the inner or central division of the great membrane of which the *pia mater* forms the exterior. Each division of the choroid plexus, in like manner, is connected, by means of minute blood-vessels, to the portion of the figurate cerebral surface on which it rests, and it appears to perform the same function of sustaining vessels as the *pia mater* does to the convoluted surface.

The membranous nature and appearance of the choroid plexus may be demonstrated by immersing it in clear water, when, by a little management of the probe and forceps, it may be spread out exactly like the *pia mater*, which it closely resembles. It presents the appearance of a thin semitransparent web, one surface of which is smooth, the other somewhat flocculent, and the substance of which appears with and without a glass to be traversed by numerous minute vessels. The transparent web, which forms the basis or groundwork of this membrane, possesses the characters of very close filamentous tissue; and it may be regarded as a filamento-vascular web. Its smooth surface, which is also the free one, is manifestly a continuation of the arachnoid membrane. Like that it is smooth, polished, thin as the finest silver paper, and it may be raised from the more filamento-vascular basis of the membrane to which it adheres.

I am now, by describing the characters and distribution of this membrane, to show how far it resembles, and how far it is unlike, the perfect serous membrane.

The fine inner lamina from which the cerebral surface of the *dura mater* derives its glistening aspect, I have already stated, is to be regarded as the outer or cranial division of the arachnoid membrane. This is to be proved, first, by its anatomical characters, and, secondly, by its distribution and transit.

The inner or free surface of the *dura mater* presents, it has been already said, all the characters of the free surface of the *pia mater*, except one, the facility with which the thin pellicle, which gives it these characters, can be detached. This, however, is derived from the want of filamentous tissue intermediate between the fibrous layer of the *dura mater* and the pellucid membrane; and the latter is thus so intimately united with the former, that it is difficult, if not impossible, by the ordinary means, to detach them. This, however, is no more a reason for regarding this pellucid pellicle as the same as the *dura mater*, than the intimate adhesion of the capsular pericardium to its fibrous coat, or of the peritonæum to the female ovaries, is for regarding the membranes as part of these organs. Immersion in boiling water and maceration produce on this surface of the *dura mater* the same effects as on the free surface of the *pia mater*. Lastly, the phenomena of morbid processes indicate that these surfaces are in all respects similar; and if the thin pellicle on the free surface of the *pia mater* is entitled to separate existence, that on the free surface of the *dura mater* is equally so.

The continuity of these two divisions, demonstrated by their configuration, affords proofs of the same description. This is most easily accomplished by tracing the *dura mater* from those points at which it adheres to the inner surface of the cranium, to those at which the several nerves issue from that cavity by the cranial holes. If the optic nerves be attentively examined at the spot where they enter the optic *foramina*, the *dura mater*, which covers the bone around these holes, is found to go a very short distance into them, to stop suddenly, and be reflected backwards, in anatomical language, to cover the nervous trunks, and to extend along the *pia mater*. This reflected portion is in truth the arachnoid membrane which lines the *dura mater*, passing from it along the nervous chords to form the free surface of the *pia mater*. In like manner, if the third pair or oculo-muscular, or fifth or tergeminal nerves be examined at the openings at which they perforate the skull, the *dura mater* is found adhering firmly round their several margins to the bone by its outer or attached surface, while its inner free surface turns back on the nervous chords, and is thence continued over the *pia mater*. In short, the continuity of this thin transparent membrane from the *dura mater* to the *pia mater* may be traced at each of the nervous trunks as they issue from the brain through the cranial apertures.

Another proof of a similar description is derived from examining the free or lower margins of the *falx major* and *minor*, and of the horizontal portion of the *dura mater*, (*tentorium cerebelli*). First, at the upper or convex margin of the great *falx*, where the veins pass from the *pia mater* to the longitudinal *sinus*, it is not difficult to trace the arachnoid membrane from the *pia mater* along their coats, to that portion of the *dura mater* which forms the sinus, and conversely, from the falx along the veins to the free surface of the *pia mater.* In the second place, the lower, or concave margin of the falx, is connected at the bottom of the middle fissure between the hemispheres to the *pia mater* on each side by thin transparent filamentous membrane, which is in truth the arachnoid passing from the falciform process of the *dura mater* to the free surface of the *pia mater,* covering the commutual surfaces of the hemispheres; and the same may be seen at the lower margin of the small or cerebellic falciform process. In the third place, at the inner margin of the transverse portion or tentorium, the transparent pellicle of the *dura mater* may be traced passing to the *pia mater* of the brain above, and of the *cerebellum* below. The same arrangement may be demonstrated in the vertebral cavity, in which it further covers the serrated membrane, (*ligamentum denticulatum*). In short, while the *dura mater* is proper to the inner surface of the skull, and the *pia mater* to the surfaces of the brain, the arachnoid membrane is common to both, and invests not only the free surface of the *pia mater,* as is usually stated, but the inner surface of the *dura mater.*

The arachnoid has a still more extended distribution. After covering the free or inner surface of the *pia mater,* it follows the course of that membrane into the central surface of the brain, and covers the upper or unadherent surface of the several divisions of the choroid plexus. This is demonstrated by the same process by which the continuity of the plexus with the *pia mater* is established.

From the foregoing description it results that the arachnoid membrane possesses in arrangement and distribution a great resemblance to the serous membranes. It differs, nevertheless, in its extreme tenuity, in the closeness with which it adheres to the collateral tissues, and, as will afterwards appear, in its slight disposition, to albuminous exudation. It appears to contain in its structure less filamentous tissue than the pure serous membranes.

I have elsewhere, in treating of the development of the brain, had occasion to speak of the cerebral membranes. The *pia mater* in the twofold form now described exists at an early period of the ovum, before the formation of the brain is commenced. It is then recognized in the form of a very vascular membrane, somewhat confused, but still sufficiently distinct to show, that in the centre of each half, the cerebral matter afterwards to constitute the hemispheres is deposited from the vessels of its central or attached surface. At this period the arachnoid pellicle cannot be distinguished. It is only when a considerable part of each hemisphere is formed that the free surface of the *pia mater* can be shown to be covered by arachnoid membrane. This may be stated in general terms to be between the end of the fifth and the middle of the seventh month. The free surface of the *dura mater* begins to be perceptible about the same time.

§ 4. The *tunica albuginea* of the testicle may be here mentioned as a membrane composed of fibrous tissue, embracing the gland, and a very thin pellucid layer outside, without intermediate filamentous tissue,—a peculiarity in which it resembles the female ovary.

SECTION II.

The serous membranes are the seat of a considerable number of morbid processes, which, according as they take place in one membrane or another, give rise to several of those diseases which it is the province of nosology to distinguish and of medicine to treat. Most of these processes may be referred to inflammation or its effects, dropsy, hemorrhage, morbid deposits, and new growths.

I. Inflammation occurs in serous membrane under at least two forms, acute and chronic. The anatomical characters of the process vary according to its acute or chronic character, and according to the physiological peculiarities of the affected membrane. These characters it is perhaps most convenient to examine, as they appear in the pleura, pericardium, and peritonæum, in which they assume their most perfect form.

§ 1. When inflammation commences in a serous or diaphanous membrane, the first change which is observed to take place in it, is diminution or loss of its transparent and glistening appearance.* It becomes opaque, dull, and in some instances dry. This change is very well seen, not only in the pleura, pericardium, and peritonæum, but in the arachnoid membrane, in which it is distinct when

---

* " When inflammation," says Hunter, " takes place in parts that have a degree of transparency, that transparency is lessened. This is probably best seen in membranes, such as those membranes which line cavities or cover bodies in those cavities, such as the *pia mater*, where in a natural state we may observe the blood-vessels to be very distinct."—4to, p. 281.

other traces of the process cannot be recognized. It is from this circumstance that dulness of the arachnoid denotes, with great certainty, serous effusion within the cerebral cavities.

§ 2. At the same time, red vessels may appear either in isolated spots or over a considerable extent. They are generally arborescent or parted into minute ramifications. Sometimes they consist of minute red lines, radiating from a point like stars; and in other instances they form a confused net-work of red vessels, interspersed with bloody points and spots, amounting occasionally to extravasation. These vessels, which, though placed in the substance of the membranes, gradually approach the surface as the process advances, are not newly developed, but appear to be the colourless capillaries of the sound state of the membranes injected with red blood. These changes, which may be regarded as the essence of the first stage of inflammation in serous membranes, are best observed in the pleura, pericardium, and peritonæum. In these they are sometimes so intense and general, as to give the membranes a red mottled appearance, and prevent the observer from distinguishing the subjacent tissue.

§ 3. After existing for some time, varying in different circumstances (from 6 to 20 hours in the *pleura* and *peritonæum*,) these changes are followed by others, which may be regarded as their effects. The first and most important of these is the formation of a new fluid at the free or unadherent surface of the membrane. The nature of this fluid varies according to the stage, and perhaps the kind of inflammation. I shall describe first that which takes place in the commencement of the acute form.

a. The capillary injection of the inflammatory process is scarcely well established when it begins to cause a semitransparent fluid to ooze in small quantity from the affected points of the surface of these membranes. In this state the characters of the fluid can scarcely be determined. In a more advanced stage of the process, when it is abundant, it is a straw-coloured, homogeneous, semitransparent fluid, which, as it is effused, undergoes spontaneous coagulation. This consists in part of the fluid assuming a solid form in the shape of a semifluid jelly-like layer of variable thickness, with a rough honey-comb surface exteriorly, where it is in contact with the membranes, and interiorly with thready filaments mutually interlacing, and more or less consistent. A thin fluid portion at the same time is found in the interstices of these filaments, and oozes from the surface of the coagulated part. These facts are easily demonstrated, by examining the effused matter while still recent, and while the process of coagulation is going on, but not completed. It is then a soft, spongy, translucent matter, of a straw-yellow colour, and pulpy gelatinous consistence. When removed from the membrane its surface is rough and irregular, like honey-comb, and marked by blood spots more or less numerous, which are occasioned by the forcible rupture of the minute vessels of the membrane passing into the new product; while serous fluid trickles from it and falls to the most dependent part of the cavity. When cut or torn in minute pieces, this serous fluid oozes abundantly from the sections; and the observer may then remark the filamentous and cellular disposition of the solid coagulated portions. The filaments varying in size cross each other mutually, so as to form partitions and intermediate cells, but without regular order.

The matter thus effused is what was named by Hunter *coagulating or coagulable lymph*, in consequence of its property of spontaneous coagulation. It is often mentioned among some of the older anatomists as masses of liquid fat found between the serous membranes; and even Dr Cleghorn speaks of it in this manner. Its property of coagulation depends chiefly on the proportion of albumen which it contains. If a mass of coagulable lymph in its recent, straw-coloured, and translucent state, be immersed in alcohol, it instantly becomes shrivelled, indurated, of a white colour, and perfectly opaque; and the same changes result from immersion in dilute acids or in boiling fluids. It also becomes much tougher and firmer. From this circumstance it has been denominated by the foreign authors *albuminous exudation*. Of its soft state, when recently effused, it is of the utmost importance for the physician to be aware, in consequence of the fact which I have now verified several times, that in the pleura it communicates to the ear the same stethoscopic and percussive phenomena which arise from the presence of fluid.

b. After its first coagulation this substance undergoes other changes which are highly important in a pathological relation. As the diaphanous membranes are at all times mutually applied, a very common effect of this effused substance and its coagulation is to connect the corresponding points more or less firmly. The process by which this is accomplished was understood by Hunter and Baillie, and may be stated in the following terms. As the lymph is effused and separated into clot or coagulable part and fluid, the former is observed to be soon penetrated by minute red vessels, which may be demonstrated by injection, and the existence of which is also proved by the fact above-mentioned, that the surface of a piece of detached lymph is marked by numerous blood-spots, occasioned by the rupture of the elongated capillaries of the inflamed membrane. These vessels may be traced from the latter into the extravasated substance, in which they are observed to ramify. Red spots, like effused blood, also appear through the substance of the lymph, and in the course of a few hours these are discovered to be new vessels. As this process, which constitutes the organization of the lymph, advances, the penetrating vessels become more numerous, and the lymph becomes more firmly attached to the inflamed surface of the membrane. At the same time the fluid part of the exudation oozes away and drops down to the most dependent points of the cavity, or, if not abundant, it is absorbed. In the former case it forms the serous or sero-purulent fluid, occasionally found in considerable quantities within the *pleura* and *peritonæum*. Meanwhile the albuminous portion becoming firmer and something opaque, the soft, pulpy, gelatinous, translucent, straw-coloured substance is gradually converted into a firm, white, opaque body, uniting more or less exactly the corresponding surfaces of the membrane. The new vessels of its interior substance at the same time contract, and ultimately convey only colourless fluid. The substance thus rendered organic and the seat of an incessant process of exhalation and absorption, is termed *membrane of adhesion* (*concretio, concrementum,*) or false membrane. The process by which it is formed is termed *union by adhesion,* or simply *adhesion.*

These phenomena are most commonly observed in the *pleura,* *pericardium,* and *peritonæum,* in each of which they are modified according to the local peculiarities of the membrane.

In the pleura it appears in the form of a broad layer, variable in thickness, extending between the convex surface of the pulmonic and the concave surface of the costal pleura; or it may occur in the spaces between the lobes; (interlobular pleurisy of Laennec); or it may be stretched between the pleura of the inferior concave surface of the lung and that of the thoracic or convex surface of the diaphragm. When the lung is affected by tubercles or tubercular excavations, it often occurs in the form of short membranous slips, and very generally as a membranous capsule covering the apex of the lung, and connecting it to the thoracic pleura.

In the pericardium the constant motion of the heart modifies the appearance of the albuminous exudation. As this motion prevents during coagulation the exact apposition of the surfaces of the capsular and cardiac divisions of the membrane, the most prominent parts, or those which least change relation only adhere. This forms the irregular laminated processes mentioned by Baillie as giving the appearance of lace-work ; and if the capsule be separated from the heart in this stage of the process, it gives the result noticed by Laennec, who compares it to the appearance produced by the sudden separation of two pieces of slab united by a thick layer of butter. At a later period this disunion will afford the calf-stomach surface (*caillebottée ; bonnet de veau*),* which may be regarded as the link connecting the organizable state of the deposition with that in which it forms an adherent tissue.

In the peritonæum it takes place chiefly along the line of one portion of ileum with another, and between the prominent points of these and the omentum, or the muscular portion of the membrane. In some instances every fold almost of ileum is connected with some other, and the whole are matted together by long triangular prisms of lymph, generally opaque, of a lemon-yellow colour, and of a pulpy or gelatiniform consistence.

Albuminous exudation or lymph is much less frequently found between the surfaces of the arachnoid membrane. That it is actually secreted by this membrane, however, is well established. Dr Stark records three cases in which coagulated lymph was found between the *dura* and *pia mater*, and round the membranous coverings of the *medulla oblongata* and spinal chord.† One example of this exudation is delineated by Baillie ;‡ and Hooper represents three in which he traces its progress from simple inflammation to organized membrane.§ Instances of albuminous exudation on the surface of the arachnoid are also mentioned by Tacheron, Andral, and Dr Abercrombie.‖ In the body of a woman who died with symptoms of intense coma, I found a thin but distinct albuminous deposit on the free surface of the arachnoid, extending from the

* Laennec, Observ. 1, 2, 3, 4, and Art. ii. Obs. 4.
† The Works of the late William Stark, M. D. Lond. 1788. Part iv. p. 69.
‡ Plate iv. Fascic. x. § Plates i. and ii.
‖ Pathological and Practical Researches, &c. p. 51—56—60.

optic commissure to the posterior margin of the annular protuberance. It was less firm and more translucent than in the pleura
or peritonæum, but presented in other respects the usual properties. This albuminous deposit I have seen take place over the superior and lateral regions of the arachnoid in adults, though it is
much less frequent, spontaneously, than in consequence of external
injury.* Albuminous exudation I have likewise observed in the
arachnoid membrane of the base and lateral regions of the brain in
children who have died with symptoms of meningeal inflammation,
or water in the brain. Similar depositions have been remarked in
various regions of the arachnoid by Parent-Duchatelet, Martinet,
Bayle, and others.

c. Baillie and most other observers notice, besides coagulating lymph
or albuminous exudation, a serous fluid, limpid, yellowish, reddish,
or brownish, according to circumstances. Though this fluid has
been supposed to be derived immediately from the blood, there is
no doubt, that it is the serous or watery portion of the morbid exudation, from the surface and interstices of which it may be seen
trickling. The red or brown tint it derives from blood issuing
from the newly formed capillaries opened by laceration of the lymph
from the membrane. Shreds of lymph are at the same time found
floating in it. This is most generally seen in the pleura and pericardium.

I have already stated that the exudation of inflamed serous membrane owes its coagulability to the presence of albuminous matter ;
and indeed upon the proportion of this ingredient the process of
coagulation depends. In certain instances, in which the inflammatory process is believed to be less genuine and energetic, this principle is so scanty that coagulation is partial and imperfect; and instead of a uniform layer of lymph between the mutual surfaces,
each presents a series of loose shreds and patches, with a considerable quantity of reddish, or whitish, semi-opaque fluid in the dependent part of the cavity. This constitutes the link between the
albuminous and the purulent, sero-purulent, or serous products of
inflammation in these membranes.

§ 4. Examined more minutely we find that the fluid varies in its
proportion of albumen in different membranes, and according to the

* Clinical Report of Edinburgh Royal Infirmary for 1836-1837. Edinburgh Medical and Surgical Journal, Vol. xlvii. p. 305.

form of the inflammatory process. These variations may be referred generally to two heads, puriform and serous secretions.

The varieties of puriform secretion may be classed under the
heads of sero-purulent, puriform, and purulent.

The sero-purulent is often connected with the albuminous, from
which it is separated during the process of coagulation. It consists
chiefly of serous fluid with minute granules of albuminous matter,
which subside to the bottom and leave the supernatant liquor like‘
whey or chalk-water. It always contains flakes of lymph. It takes
place in pleuritic and peritoneal inflammation, acute and chronic,
and is generally found in the dependent part of the cavity, *e. g.* in
the posterior part of the chest, and in the lumbar and hypogastric
fossæ in the peritonæum.

The puriform fluid of serous membranes consists of serous fluid,
with an opaque and thicker matter not coagulable in mass blended
with it more equably than in the last case. The granular matter
is less abundant or entirely wanting; and the opaque milky fluid is
not so easily separable as in the sero-purulent fluid. Though it is
often associated with the albuminous, and contains flakes of lymph,
yet, as little lymph is found on the surface of the membranes, and
as the quantity of the latter is often in the inverse ratio of the quantity of puriform fluid, it may be regarded as less nearly allied to the
pure albuminous inflammation than the sero-purulent. Both are
to be regarded as abortive efforts to effect albuminous exudation.

The puriform secretion occurs in all the serous membranes, but
is most frequent in the peritonæum. It is in particular very common in that form of peritoneal inflammation which occurs in the
persons of women in childbed; and Hunter, who was aware of the
fact, states it as an instance of the combination of the adhesive with
the suppurative inflammation,—a circumstance to which he ascribes
the unfavourable issue of such cases.* It is occasionally the combination, and sometimes the substitution of the suppurative for the
adhesive process. This is amply confirmed by the necroscopic appearances of peritoneal inflammation in puerperal females, in which
every shade of morbid effusion is seen, from albuminous lymph,
with separation of proper serous fluid, to puriform or purulent collection.

* " This mixing of the suppurative with the adhesive, or the hurrying on of the suppurative, I have frequently seen in the abdomen of women who have been attacked
with the peritoneal inflammation after child-birth, and which, from these circumstances
became the cause of their death."—On the Blood, &c.

Genuine purulent fluid, as it is represented by pathological authors,—a white, or cream-coloured, opaque, and homogeneous fluid,
—is another product of inflammation of serous membranes. Though
always combined with more or less albuminous exudation, which is
found in loose irregular patches on the membrane, and in the form
of shreds and flakes in the fluid, it is more uniform in composition
than the puriform, being destitute of the granular matter, and not
separating, when allowed to rest, into thin and solid matter.   It occurs in chronic pleurisy, (*empyema*,) in pericardial inflammation as
an effect of the acute, and in *peritonitis*, acute, subacute, and chronic, especially the puerperal.

It was at one time believed that genuine purulent matter could
not be formed in these membranes, unless as an effect of the preliminary process of ulceration.   Instances of purulent collections
in the chest without ulceration of the pleura, and of purulent matter
in the abdomen without breach in the peritonæum, might have led
pathological writers to the inference, that suppuration may occur
in a serous membrane without ulceration, and that secretion of purulent matter is one of the effects of simple inflammation of serous
tissue.   The truth of this fact, however, appears not to have been
established before the time of William and John Hunter, the last
of whom notices it as a point not previously ascertained.   Speaking of the transition or gradual change from coagulable lymph to
purulent fluid, he infers " that suppuration takes place in serous
surfaces without a breach of solids or dissolution of parts," mentions it as a circumstance " not commonly allowed," and considers
this suppuration as the effect of a more advanced stage of the process than that which gives rise to effusion of lymph, and union by
adhesion.   Of this fact, he informs us, he first became aware in
1749 and 1750, when, in the inspection of a young subject, the
left side of the chest was found to contain a considerable quantity
of purulent matter without breach of the pleura or surface of the
lungs; and, at the same time, it was regarded by Dr Hunter and
Mr Samuel Sharpe as a new fact.*   It has since been often observed both in the pleura and peritonæum; and as such is mentioned by William Hunter,† Baillie, Black, and Willan.   It is, in
truth, seen almost daily by those conversant in morbid anatomy.

* Treatise on Inflammation, &c. p. 379. *Note.*

† " Another kind of *pus* is that which is formed without any apparent breach or
dissolution of the solids, and therefore is only a sort of inspissated *serum*, or an inflam-

The purulent fluid in this case and many others is secreted partly from the surface of the inflamed membrane, partly from the organized layer of lymph, partly from both. In the first case, the puriform or purulent fluid is secreted directly by the capillaries of the inflamed membrane. In the second, it is derived from those of the organized false membranes, which assume the suppurative action. In the third, both sets of vessels are concerned. These facts are demonstrated in instances of chronic pleurisy, and of chronic inflammation of the *peritonæum*.

§ 5. A second effect of inflammation of the diaphanous membranes is effusion or secretion of fluid in the subserous filamentous tissue. When the arachnoid membrane is inflamed the delicate filamentous tissue which connects it to the *pia mater* is almost invariably distended with serous fluid, more or less transparent. This change makes the arachnoid membrane look as if it were raised or detached from the *pia mater* by the interposition of a transparent or slightly opaque gelatinous matter uniformly spread between them. If a puncture or incision, however, be made, a small portion only trickles from it, being that which is exposed to the immediate incision. The fluid of the contiguous parts does not escape,—a circumstance which with inspection shows that it is contained in the interstices formed by the mutual crossing of the filaments of the subserous tissue. In this manner and in the same situation albuminous fluid may be effused, especially at the base of the brain. In pleurisy this effusion is less common, unless the pulmonic tissue is at the same time inflamed,—a peculiarity which appears to depend on the intimate union between the pleura and lungs. It nevertheless takes place and dissects the *pleura* from the substance of the lungs. In inflammation of the pericardium it takes place beneath the. cardiac fold of the membrane, and occasionally assumes the form of minute ah-

matory exudation. We occasionally meet with collections of this kind in all the natural internal cavities of the body. I have seen it in great quantity in the cavity of the abdomen or of the *peritonæum*, in that of the thorax or of the *pleura*, and in the *pericardium*, where there was no visible suppuration, ulceration, or dissolution of the solids, or any part of the surface all round. This kind of *pus* is generally thinner than that of an abscess ; and the containing surface is more or less covered with a glutinous concretion, or slough of the same colour as the fluid, in some parts adhering very loosely, in others so firmly, that it can hardly be rubbed off ; but still the surface covered by these sloughs is without ulceration or loss of substance."—Medical Observations and Inquiries, Vol. ii. p. 61.

Baillie, Morbid Anatomy, *passim.*

Black, Clinical and Pathological Reports. Newry, 1819.

Willan, Reports on the Diseases of London, 1797. P. 186. 8vo Edition.

scesses in the subserous tissue and on the surface of the cardiac fibres. In inflammation of the peritonæum it is more common; and careful inspection may detect effusion below the intestinal, and more distinctly in some instances below the muscular peritonæum. In this situation, indeed, may be found patches and minute deposits of purulent fluid, not only in the ordinary forms of peritonæal inflammation, but in that which takes place in the persons of puerperal women.

§ 6. A third change mentioned as a consequence of inflammation in serous membranes is inordinate thickness and some degree of pulpiness.* On this point there is among pathologists some difference of opinion. The occurrence of thickening is contradicted by Laennec, who denies that inflammation produces thickening of the *pleura*, and contends that observers have been misled by morbid deposits on its surface, or the formation of new membranes. Without doubting the discernment or candour of this pathologist, I must remark, that, as Baillie expressly mentions thickening as a consequence of inflammation in the *pleura, peritonæum*, and mesentery, and as this is confirmed in regard to the *peritonæum* by the testimony of Pemberton† and Black,‡ the question resolves itself into one of individual observation. If, in some instances of acute inflammation of serous surfaces, thickening is not recognized, there are few in which the chronic form of the process affects the pleura, pericardium, and peritonæum, without more or less thickening of the membrane. The appearance of this, indeed, may arise from effusion into the subserous filamentous tissue; but in cases of chronic inflammation the membrane itself appears to be not only thicker, but harder and firmer than natural. Does this change depend on effusion of lymph into its component tissue, or development of vessels which are loaded with various fluids? The thickening to which I allude is mostly at the attached surface; and I think that in that situation it depends on the effusion of lymph into the subserous cellular tissue. In chronic peritonitis I have observed the attached surface of the membrane manifestly loaded with extravasated matter in the interstices of the filamentous tissue. What are the cases in which the serous membranes become pulpy or softer than natural, while they are also thickened? On these points accurate information is still wanting.

On the other hand, it must be allowed, that the conditions usually mentioned as examples of thickening of the serous membranes, are,

---

* Baillie's Morbid Anatomy, p. 54, 127, and 200, in reference to the mesentery.
† On the Abdominal Viscera.   ‡ Clinical and Pathological Reports, &c.

in truth, new deposits on their free surface. A deposit of lymph which has become contracted and indurated, or even cartilaginous, a deposit of tubercular matter, and patches of cartilage are formed on the free surface of the membrane; and though they appear to render it thicker, yet are they adventitious and easy removable by dissection, after which the free surface of the membrane comes into view.

§ 7. The next effect of the inflammatory process in serous membranes is destruction of their tissue by ulceration. Though this may happen in the acute form of the disease, it is not common. But after it has subsisted for some time, one or more points of the membrane begin to be affected by the ulcerative process, which at once spreads superficially, and penetrates its substance. The manner in which this takes place is invariably by the inflammatory process affecting the subserous tissue, and causing their suppuration in a circumscribed point. The serous membrane being no longer supported at this point, gives way sometimes in round irregular patches, sometimes in ragged linear fissures. This process is not equally common in all the serous membranes. It is most usual in the pleura, pulmonic and costal, and in the muscular peritonæum.

By some pathologists, and, if I do not misunderstand him, by Hunter, ulceration is ascribed to pressure exercised by purulent matter; and thus, indeed, this author explains the tendency which collections of matter betray to proceed towards the surface. The pressure of such agents, doubtless, operates as an irritating cause, and may therefore produce what Hunter terms *ulcerative inflammation*. In several examples, however, ulceration may occur as a direct effect of the inflammatory process, without the formation of matter sufficient by pressure to cause destruction of the tissue; and in such circumstances I have in general traced it to previous suppuration of the subserous tissue, as already mentioned. In cases of empyema and chronic peritonitis, especially the puerperal form, in which this ulceration is not unfrequent, both causes may be in operation. But even in the interesting case of peritoneal inflammation given by Hunter to illustrate the nature of what he terms the relaxing process, it is impossible to doubt, that, before the muscular peritonæum was detached in the shreds and fragments in which it was found on inspection, inflammation and suppuration of the subserous filamentous tissue had taken place.* In short, from

* Treatise on the Blood, &c. Part ii. Chap. vi. Sect. vi. p. 461. 4to.

the cases recorded, and from several which I have examined personally, I infer that ulceration of the serous tissue is always preceded by inflammation and suppuration of the subserous; that the attachment of the former being thus destroyed, its vitality is impaired, and its cohesion thereby weakened; and that it gives way rather in the manner of laceration than genuine ulceration.

§ 8. Observation has not yet determined whether gangrene be an effect of inflammation of the serous tissue. That it is occasionally involved in this process I infer from seeing the *pleura* in gangrene of the lungs, and the *peritonæum* in that of the bowels, soft, black, or greenish, shreddy, and lacerable. But it is still uncertain whether primary inflammation of a serous tissue exclusively may terminate in mortification of that membrane. With this process ulceration with bloody effusion or blood-coloured patches must not be confounded. Bichat states, that in numerous bodies which he inspected, he met with gangrene of the *peritonæum* only; and that he never witnessed an instance of this change either in the arachnoid membrane, in the *pleura*, in the *pericardium*, or in the *perididymis*.*

On the surface of the lungs there is occasionally observed a species of gangrene, circumscribed and limited in extent. A patch, dark coloured and dead, of a shape nearly, sometimes exactly circular, is formed at the surface, that is, the pleural surface of the lung. The size of these patches varies from the size of a sixpenny piece or a shilling to a crown piece. The patch is in certain cases observed still adherent, though black and dead. In other instances it has dropped off, leaving a cup-like cavity, pretty exactly circular in outline, regularly hollowed out in the substance of the lung, which is red but otherwise natural and free from appearance of gangrene.

In this lesion, which I have described as circumscribed gangrene of the lungs, the pleura is affected by gangrene; but whether primarily, or only in connection with the substance of the lung, it is impossible to determine. The portions so affected appear exactly as if they had been destroyed by the direct application of the hot iron, or touched by a portion of caustic potass.

This circumscribed form of gangrene of the pleura and surface of the lungs is sometimes associated with diffuse gangrene in the deep-seated parenchyma of the organ.†

* Anat. Generale, Tome iii. p. 517.

† Cases and Observations illustrative of the Nature of Gangrene of the Lungs. By David Craigie, M. D., &c., Edinburgh Medical and Surgical Journal, Vol. lvi. p. 1. Edinburgh, 1841.

§ 9. The second general head of secretions, or those termed *serous*, have been long received as the distinctive character of the disorders named dropsies; (*Hydropes.*)

To the influence of inflammation or capillary injection in causing effusion, extravasation, or secretion of *serum*, I have already in part alluded.   In no texture is this more conspicuous than in the serous or transparent. The mechanism of this process it is perhaps not very easy to explain satisfactorily, unless by referring it to the same principles to which I have already referred, the ordinary albuminous and purulent exudations.   I shall attempt, however, to state as briefly as possible the ascertained facts which tend to establish the general conclusion,—that inordinate accumulation of serous fluid from the free surface of the diaphanous membranes is a frequent result of a process of capillary congestion, or even of inflammation.

I have already stated that the serous membranes in general are understood to be the seat of a process of incessant exhalation and resorption.   This may be regarded as demonstrated in the case of the *pleura, pericardium, peritonæum,* and *perididymis,* by the experiments of Haller, Bichat, and others; and of the arachnoid, the same as presumed from analogy.   The fluid thus secreted, though in the healthy state very scanty, is distinctly albuminous.   This may be regarded as demonstrated by the rude experiments even of Hewson and Bichat.   The difficulty in the healthy state of obtaining a quantity sufficient for analysis led Berzelius to examine that of *hydrocephalus,* which he supposes makes a nearer approach to the normal condition than the others; and of this he found 1000 parts to contain 1.66 of albuminous matter, with salts of potass and soda, and some animal matter combined with lactate of soda.*   This result is confirmed by the researches of Bostock and Marcet, which show that though some muco-extractive matter is present, albumen forms the chief part of the solid contents of the serum of the blood and the fluids of the serous membranes.   Lastly, Marcet, who examined all the dropsical fluids, found that they contain coagulable matter; but that those of the pleura, pericardium, and peritonæum, contain much more than the arachnoid, and that of hydrocele most of all.†

The inordinate augmentation of these fluids varies in degree,

* General Views of the Composition of Animal Fluids. By J. Berzelius, M. D., &c.   Med.-Chir. Transactions, Vol. iii. 251.

† Medico-Chirurg. Trans. Vol. ii. p. 331.

from a few ounces to several pints; and it varies according to the site of the membrane from which it is effused. Thus the fluid secreted by the arachnoid membrane may not amount to above half an ounce, or at most to two or three ounces, which is to be regarded as a great quantity. In some recorded instances it is said rather vaguely to amount to six. The fluid secreted by the pericardium may not be above one ounce, rarely exceeds two or three, and in a few instances only amounts to six, eight, or ten. In the pleura, on the contrary, it may amount to three, four, or five pints or quarts; and in the peritonæum has been known to amount to several gallons.

The quality of this fluid varies. That of the arachnoid is limpid and colourless, like clear water, with a slight saline taste, and contains traces of albumen. In the pericardium it is light coloured and semitransparent. In the pleura it may be straw-yellow and semitransparent, but is more frequently reddish, or brown and something opaque. In the peritonæum it is semitransparent, yellow, or greenish, sometimes with various shades of red or even brownish, like chocolate or coffee. In each of the three last cases it is invariably combined with albuminous matter.

The hypothesis of Cullen, who ascribes this inordinate accumulation to any cause which increases exhalation or diminishes absorption, though plausible, is too general, and does not comprehend all the facts of the case. One of the most uniform and powerful agents in augmenting exhalation from serous surfaces is that state of the capillaries in which they are injected, distended in such a manner as to constitute congestion or even inflammation. The influence of this cause appears to have been first well understood by Cruikshank,* Baillie,† and Parry,‡ nor had escaped the obser-

* " The second species of dropsy is very common, and is that which arises in consequence of previous inflammation of a cavity, and may take place in any habit of body. If an inflammation arise in a cavity, it may terminate in a number of different ways ; one of these is by increased secretion of fluid of surfaces. A man receives a blow on the testicle, inflammation takes place, and the consequence is frequently a hydrocele or dropsy of the *tunica vaginalis.* A child's brain inflames, and this inflammation ends at last in *hydrocephalus,* or collection of water in the brain. Pleurisy frequently terminates in hydrothorax, or collection of water in the chest. I have often taken away forty or sixty pints of water, which had accumulated in the cavity of the abdomen in the few days the peritonæal inflammation had lasted, during the usual species of childbed fever. This is to be considered as the substituting a less dangerous disease for another. Peritoneal inflammation kills often in three days, but acute may last twenty years."—Anatomy of the Absorbing Vessels.

† Morbid Anatomy, p. 57. 4th edit. Lond. 1812.
‡ Collections from the unpublished Medical Writings, &c. p. 205, 207, 208.

vation of Pemberton.[*] Its reality, however, was first investigated and formally maintained by Grapengiesser of Gottingen,[†] by Rush of Philadelphia,[‡] and was subsequently made the subject of much research and inquiry by Wells,[§] Blackall,[||] Crampton,[¶] and Ayre. The results of the inquiries thus instituted may be stated in the following manner.

Though accumulation of fluid in the cavities of serous membranes depends on increased exhalation from the vessels of these membranes, that exhalation is not to be regarded merely as an increased form of the natural action, but is a process of morbid secretion, depending on a state of the blood-vessels, either identical with, or analogous to inflammation. The vessels of the membranes are numerous, enlarged, and in general injected. When they are not so, the stage of injection has passed, and been succeeded by that of exhalation. The presence of albuminous flakes in the effused fluid furnishes proofs of the same description. The membranes are more or less opaque and dull, and covered by shreds and patches of lymph in various spots; and fluid is effused into the subserous tissue. Thus, in several instances of dropsical infiltration, with effusion into the cavity of the pleura, 1 have found that membrane not only vascular, but coloured of a red-brown tint, opaque, void of its glistening aspect, and covered by patches of albuminous exudation. The same is observed in ascites. One of the most decided examples is afforded by the inspection of Sir James Craig, well described by Dr Somerville.[**] The peritonaeum was found covered by lymph in various points, and lymphy flakes were found abundantly in the fluid. On the same point the dissections of Dr Crampton in the Transactions of the Dublin Association afford unequivocal and satisfactory evidence.

In most cases of this class, however, it will afterwards be shown, the kidneys are affected with granular degeneration.

In the case of the cerebral membranes it is not quite so easy to obtain evidence. The arachnoid is averse, if I may use the term,

* Abdominal Viscera, p. 12. " Sometimes a resolution of the inflammation takes place from the throwing out of a fluid, when ascites is produced."

† De Hydrope.

‡ Medical Inquiries and Observations. By B. Rush, M. D. Philad. 1805. Vol. ii. p. 159.

§ Transactions of a Society, Vol. iii. p. 167, 183, and 194.

|| Observations on the Nature and Cure of Dropsies.

¶ Clinical Report on Dropsies. Transactions of Association, Vol. ii.

** Medico-Chir. Tr. Vol. v. p. 340, &c.

to albuminous exudation; and though this occurs occasionally, serous effusion is greatly more frequent. The inflammatory origin of this effusion, however, is proved by several circumstances.

1st, The *pia mater* and choroid *plexus* are more or less, sometimes · highly vascular. The arachnoid is always dry, opaque, dull, and elevated by infiltration into the subjacent tissue. In some instances this infiltrated fluid contains albuminous matter; and in some patches of lymph are deposited on the free surface of the arachnoid membrane. In one of the most distinct cases of this disease which fell under my personal observation, I found the free surface of the cerebral arachnoid adhering to that of the falciform process in the great fissure between the hemispheres by well marked filaments of albuminous exudation.

2d, In the case of violence inflicted on the head, which it is well known has a tendency to induce inflammation, when that inflammation proves fatal, almost invariably we find effusion from the membranes, in some cases to a great extent. In proof of this, I prefer referring to the cases of other observers than to such as I have inspected. In the fatal cases recorded by Pott and Dease the most uniform appearance is water in the ventricles, which evidently proceeds from the choroid plexus, or inner division of the cerebral membrane. In the numerous and well described cases of Schmucher also, this effusion is always one of the changes recorded; and vascularity of the *pia mater*, and dulness of the arachnoid, with subarachnoid infiltration, are frequently remarked. Similar results may be derived from the cases given by Dr Thomson, and from those of Dr Hennen. In short, it may be inferred that traumatic inflammation of the cerebral membranes always induces more ,or less serous effusion. It is scarcely necessary to remark, that this explains a fact observed by most practical physicians, that *hydrocephalus* is very often ascribed to blows or falls on the head, the tendency of which to induce congestion of the vessels cannot be denied.

3d, To the same purpose it may be said, that the effusion resulting from the operation of the process of fever, whether intermittent, remittent, or continuous, demonstrates the influence of vascular congestion in inducing it. Thus in ague, meningeal effusion is not uncommon; in remittent it is frequent; and in continued fever it is perhaps the most usual cause of the fatal termination of the disease. The extensive body of evidence collected on this point of late years by writers on remittent and yellow fever, and on the ordinary continned fever of this country, renders it unnecessary to dwell longer on this point.

In favour of the same inference, the connection so often remarked between dropsy and hemorrhage might be adduced. My limits, however, do not permit me to add more.

II. PECULIARITIES IN INDIVIDUAL INFLAMMATIONS.—The principal pathological facts regarding the process of inflammation in serous membrane have been so fully stated, that it is superfluous to dwell on the individual diseases. I shall merely, after enumerating them, make a few remarks on some peculiarities presented by the chronic forms of these disorders. They may be arranged in the following order, showing their transition into dropsies.

Acute form.	Chronic form.	Dropsical form.
Cerebral envelopes,	*Meningitis ; Arachnitis,*	Hydrencephalus.
Pleura, *Pleuritis,*	*Empyema,*	Hydrothorax.
Pericardium, *Pericarditis,*	*Pyocardia,*	Hydrocardia.
Peritonæum, *Peritonitis,*	Chronic peritonitis,	Ascites.
Perididymis, *Orchitis,*	*Empyocele,*	Hydrocele.

Visceral divisions of the peritonæum.

Gastric peritonæum,	*Gastritis.*
Intestinal peritonæum,	*Enteritis.*
Colic peritonæum,	*Colitis.*
Mesenteric peritonæum,	*Mesenteritis.*
Omentum,	*Epiploitis.*
Cystic peritonæum,	*Cystitis.*
Hepatic peritonæum,	*Hepatitis.*
Splenic peritonæum,	*Lienitis.*
Uterine peritonæum,	*Hysteritis.*

§ 1. Chronic pleurisy (*empyema*) is remarkable for the effects which it produces. *First,* the great accumulation of fluid forces the lung towards the mediastinum and spine, and compresses it into so small bulk that it appears to be destroyed. Inspection shows, however, that it is merely compressed. Its vessels are crushed together ; its bronchial tubes and vesicles closed ; and the whole organ is rendered unfit for respiration. This is the condition mentioned by Broussais under the name of atrophied lung.* *Second,* suppurative destruction may take place in the pulmonic pleura and corresponding part of the lung, and lay open one or more bronchial tubes, causing pulmonary *fistula* and *pneumothorax.* Sero-purulent or purulent fluid is then discharged by coughing in a forcible and continuous stream. Of this kind are many cases of pulmonary abscess reported to be cured.

* Phlegmasies Chroniques, Cases 19, 20, 24, 25, 27, 28, 30.

Thirdly, suppurative destruction may take place in one or more points of the costal pleura, and discharge a considerable quantity of puriform fluid through openings between the ribs, which are occasionally carious.* When these two modes of opening are combined, pneumothorax and emphysema take place.† *Fourthly,* the inordinate accumulation of fluid in the left sac of the pleura may be so great as to thrust the heart to the sternum, and eventually into the side of the chest, in which its pulsations are then felt.‡ This change I have several times witnessed in chronic pleurisy.

§ 2. Chronic peritoneal inflammation is distinguished by three circumstances :—1*st*, Purulent or sero-purulent fluid may be secreted in one or more distinct sacs, formed by the union, and secretion of effused lymph. This, which was early noticed by Morgagni, (Epist. xxxiv. 221,) is verified by J. Hunter,§ and subsequently by Baillie, Black,‖ Mr Cooke, and others.

2*d*, Purulent fluid may be secreted by the whole inflamed membrane, without breach of surface. This proposition I should scarcely have thought requisite, after what has been said above, to state formally, did not the valuable remark of John Hunter, that " the cavity of the abdomen acquires all the properties of an abscess," appear to be forgotten by Dr Black of Newry, who, in recording a case in which the " abdomen contained more than two quarts of thin purulent fluid of a turbid appearance," seems to think it extraordinary that the matter was secreted by inflamed surfaces. In other respects the case is a good confirmation of the general principle now stated. I may add, that in several cases of peritonitis lasting for several weeks, which have come under my own observation, I have seen many folds of small intestine connected by lymphy exudation, and a considerable quantity of genuine purulent fluid

---

* Miscell. Curios. Dec. iii. An. v. Obs. 49.   Mem. Med. Society, Vol. iii. p. 127. Kirkland, Med. Surgery, Vol. ii. p. 178. Withering's Remarks on Dropsy, &c. Works, Vol. ii. p. 304, § 35.

† Treyer, in Annals of Thomann, Vol. i. Dr Duncan, in Trans. Med.-Chir. Society, Edin. Vol. i. and Contributions to Morbid Anatomy, No. iv. Empyema and Hydrothorax, in Med. Surg. Journal, Vol. xxviii. p. 302.

‡ Morgagni, Epist. xx. 6. Barry, p. 405, 406. Abercrombie, in Med.-Chir. Transactions.

§ " Inflammation attacks the external coat of an intestine. The first stage of this inflammation produces adhesions between it and the peritonæum lining the abdominal muscles. If the inflammation does not stop at this stage, an abscess is formed in the middle of these adhesions."—Treatise on the Blood.

‖ Clinical and Pathological Reports, p. 133, 176.

bathing the adherent masses, and filling the hollows of the lumbar, iliac, and hypogastric regions. The omentum is sometimes glued down at its corners to a fold of ileum ; in other instances it is drawn up and shrivelled into a roundish or cylindrical mass.

3d, Ulceration may take place at one or more points of the muscular or intestinal peritonæum, by a process, the mechanism of which has been already explained. The first is most common, and may be so extensive and complete as to destroy the whole membrane on the fore part of the abdomen, and expose the transverse and straight muscles as distinctly as if they were cleanly dissected, and leave the tendons of the lateral muscles in rags, partly gone, partly in the form of slough. At the same time, the intestines are covered with a coat of lymph, which is believed by Hunter to prevent the matter from irritating, and producing ulcerative inflammation of the bowels, and from diffusing itself over the abdominal cavity.* Its chief use is to prevent inflammation of the subserous tissue.

The rarity of the latter, which is well established, is ascribed by Hunter to the indisposition to ulceration manifested by the intestinal peritonæum.† It is the express testimony of Baillie, that he " did not recollect to have seen one instance in which the ulcer had begun on the outer or peritonæal surface of the intestines, and had spread inwards." To show that this termination, though uncommon, is not unknown, I mention, that of 16 cases of chronic peritonæal inflammation reported by Broussais, in one only did perforation of the intestines take place ;‡ and that in the case of Willan above alluded to, the colon was superficially ulcerated in several places.

In the sero-purulent and purulent collections, which are the result of peritoneal inflammation in puerperal females after it has passed the acute stage, a peculiar mode of termination is not unfrequently observed in an opening taking place spontaneously generally at the navel, and allowing the issue of a large quantity of fluid. This opening is effected first by distension, the pressure of the matter separating the *recti*, and enlarging the umbilical aperture afterwards by laceration, while the peritonæum detached from the supporting tissues, and sustained only by the skin, at length gives way, and forms an opening. Examples of this are recorded

---

* On the Blood, &c. Part ii. Chap. vi. Sect. vi. p. 461, and Sect. ix. p. 467.

† " If the disposition for ulceration was equal on every side of the abscess, it must open into the intestine, which is seldom the case, although it sometimes does." P. 236.

‡ Phlegmasies Chroniques, Section ii. Chap. iv. Obs. lv. p. 480.

by Hulme,[*] Leake,[†] Denman,[‡] Mr John Burns,[§] Gordon,[||] Armstrong,[¶] and Hey.[**] Gordon and Denman mention cases in which matter was discharged by the urethra with favourable issue. The fluid of ascites in females has a peculiar exit, by which not unfrequently it escapes, the Fallopian tubes.

§ 3. *Puerperal Peritonitis.*—That in the disease termed puerperal fever, in a certain proportion of cases, peritoneal inflammation of one or other of the forms above-mentioned takes place, is established by the observation of the best authors, and by daily experience. In every case in which the symptoms of the disease appear during life, we find in the peritonæum more or fewer of the marks of the inflammatory process above described. This variety of peritoneal inflammation, nevertheless, is peculiar in commencing almost invariably in some part of the peritonæum investing the organs of reproduction. Thus the first, the most abundant, and the most invariable traces of inflammatory action, are found either in the uterine, or the ovarian peritonæum, or in that of the Fallopian tubes, especially at their fimbriated extremities, and within these tubes, or all three at once.

The most usual appearances which I have remarked in a large proportion of cases, are opaque, dull, and lustreless aspect of the uterine and ovarian peritonæum; blood-spots or vascular injection, especially of the ovarian peritonæum; albuminous exudation of the uterine and ovarian peritonæum often agglutinating the latter to that of the oviferous tubes; and sero-purulent or purulent fluid, with albuminous shreds, in the hypogastric, iliac, and occasionally the lumbar *fossæ*, and purulent or albuminous exudation between the bladder and uterus, and the uterus and rectum.

In a certain proportion of cases, in which the disease is not attended by well-marked symptoms, yet destroys the patient rapidly and certainly, the appearances are not very distinctly presented. The uterine peritonæum is covered with a sort of unctuous looking sero-albuminous fluid, or rather mere coating, which is liable to be entirely overlooked by hasty observers. Yet it is seen all over the anterior and posterior surface of the womb, and along the sides of that organ, as a semifluid glutinous coating. In certain cases the Fallopian tubes and ovaries are covered by the same coating; and

[*] On the Puerperal Fever.   [†] On Child-bed Fever.
[‡] Introduction, &c. Fever.   [§] Elements, &c.
[||] Treatise on the Epidemic Puerperal Fever, 5th and 6th Cases.
[¶] Facts and Observations, p. 158.   [**] On Puerperal Fever.

in one class of cases the principal circumstance is purulent matter within the Fallopian tubes. The difficulty of recognizing this peculiar unctuous looking coating has led several persons to deny the occurrence of peritoneal inflammation in this disease. There is, nevertheless, no doubt of the fact, and it should further be remembered that this appearance takes place in cases of the greatest rapidity, with the most obscure symptoms, and in which the disease is occasionally developed before labour. Some females I have known die with the disease undelivered.

It must be observed, however, that puerperal fever is not a simple but a complicated lesion ; and that it varies in different seasons in the same locality, and in different localities. Thus several forms of the disease, to which the name of puerperal fever is applied, have been ascertained to affect the uterine, ovarian, and abdominal *peritonæum*, the womb, the ovaries, and Fallopian tubes, the uterine veins, the uterine lymphatics, and the substance of the womb itself. These different elementary tissues it may affect either separately or conjointly ; either two or more of them simultaneously or successively.

Of these lesions some degree or form of inflammation of the *peritonaeum* is the most frequent. Among 222 cases inspected by M. Tonnellé, in 193 traces of peritoneal inflammation were observed, consisting in more or less redness of the intestinal or the uterine *peritonaeum*, or of the mesentery or omentum, sometimes with thin albuminous exudation, sometimes with copious exudation of opaque sero-albuminous fluid.

In puerperal females *peritonitis* appears to originate most commonly either in the uterine *peritonæum*, or in that of the ovaries, or in that of the Fallopian tubes, or in the mucous or inner lining of these tubes. It is not easy to say to which of these points it shows the preference. If we trust to the numerical results given by M. Tonnellé, the disease commences most commonly in some point of the uterine *peritonaeum*, and next to that in the ovarian *peritonaeum*.

This observer found among 222 inspections of the bodies of females, destroyed by symptoms of puerperal fever, the following proportions of the lesions now referred to,—

	Cases.
Marks of peritoneal inflammation in .	193
Changes in the womb and its appendages in .	197
Difference in favour of affections of womb, .	4

Cases.

Marks of inflammation of the peritonæum and changes in the womb
or its appendages were variously associated in .   165
———— separated in   .   .
Viz. traces of peritonitis without affection of womb in   28 ⎫
    changes in womb, including those of ovaries and veins,   ⎬ 57
    without affection of peritonæum, in   .   29 ⎭

In a considerable number of cases of this disease which I had occasion to inspect, the peritoneal covering of each ovary was enclosed
in a layer of albuminous exudation.   In this the fimbriated extremities of the oviferous tubes were imbedded ; and in that of one
side in several cases the adhesion was tolerably firm.   The usual
blood-spots indicating organization were distinct.   Between the
uterus and rectum in several cases was an extensive albuminous exudation, forming a cyst containing purulent fluid ; and a smaller one
of the same kind was found between the uterine and vesical peritonæum.   In more severe cases the inflammatory process spreads over
the intestinal peritonæum, and produces its usual effects.

The commencement of this disease in the uterine and ovarian
peritonæum is not wonderful, when the extraordinary distension of
that membrane during the latter months of pregnancy is considered.   Denman remarks that there are not wanting instances in which
it has been˜evidently forming before delivery, or during labour ;
Joseph Clarke states that he saw reason to date the commencement
of several cases from before delivery, and refers to two in which
this conclusion was justified by the speedy extinction of life after
labour, and the appearances on inspection, (44) ; and Hey refers
to two cases, one fatal, in which symptoms appeared previous to delivery.   These inferences I have now had occasion to verify more
than once.   I had occasion in the summer of 1828 to detract in
two days fifty ounces of blood with corresponding antiphlogistic
measures, in order to check incipient symptoms of peritoneal inflammation in a lady during the latter part of pregnancy.

Though peritoneal inflammation in puerperal females, complicated as it often is with inflammation of the ovaries, of the uterine
veins, or of the uterine lymphatics, often terminates fatally, and
that at an early period ; yet in certain cases it does not immediately end in this way, but causes so much destruction of parts, or
gives rise to such morbid products, that the patient, after lingering
for four or six weeks in a state of great feebleness, usually with
hectic fever, is suddenly or slowly cut off.

The morbid products and changes which take place under these circumstances, prove at once the destructive effects of the disease, and the great efforts made by the system to counteract them. Thus in one instance, in which the disease had been proceeding for three weeks, the patient was brought to the hospital with the symptoms still present, though in a milder form. Pain was much abated though not gone; swelling and tension were likewise diminished. But habitual fever was present; and in the hypogastric region, on the left side of the pubes, was a swelling, painful, elastic, pointing, soft, and evidently containing some fluid. In the course of a few days, a spontaneous opening took place, and much purulent matter was discharged, apparently with relief to the symptoms. The discharge continued, however, and the hectic symptoms and wasting did not subside. Notwithstanding all means calculated to abate the discharge and promote adhesion, the former continued, and in the course of about four weeks more the patient expired.

It was then found that around the left ovary and Fallopian tube had been deposited a great quantity of lymph which connected these parts to the muscular peritonæum of the left puho-inguinal region, and formed connections also with the *fundus uteri;* that within this mass of lymph had been contained a quantity of purulent matter ; that the abscess which was found in the left pubic region at admission had communicated with this purulent cyst; that the ulcerated opening which had been formed through this abscess in the left pubal region still communicated with the interior of this cyst; and that the latter extended downwards a little on the left angle and side of the uterus. The left ovary was enlarged, and contained various purulent collections of small size. The left Fallopian tube contained purulent matter. Lymph and purulent matter were deposited, though less abundantly, in the *fundus uteri,* in the angle between the *uterus* and *rectum,* in that between the *uterus* and bladder, and on the right side of the *uterus.*

In a similar case which occurred to Dr Lee the ovary was converted into a large purulent cyst, which had, by coagulable lymph, formed adhesions with the abdominal *parietes,* and discharged its contents through an ulcerated opening.

This mode of involving the ovaries and Fallopian tubes in lymph containing purulent matter and then forming adhesions with other contiguous parts, as the muscular or the pelvic peritonæum, or the *rectum,* is by no means uncommon in that class of cases in which lymph is effused, and the tendency to limit inflammation is strong. This tendency to limitation, in short, by effusion of coagulable lymph, is either connected with the more favourable and less violent form of the disease, or it is an indication that the disease is not so speedily and certainly fatal.

One of the most extraordinary terminations of cases of this kind occurred in a patient under my own care, in the Royal Infirmary of this place. A woman had been previously treated for fever supposed to be typhoid, until the symptoms had proceeded so far as to render the effect of active treatment questionable. Blood, however, was drawn from the arm, and afterwards, by means of the repeated application of leeches, from the right inguinal region, where pain was felt, and dulness was recognized. About the fourth week after she came under my care, a quantity of purulent matter was discharged from the rectum, with some transitory relief to the symptoms. Death, however, took place; and on dissection I found on the right side of the rectum, between that bowel and the uterus, an ulcerated opening from the cavity of the peritonæum, whence the matter had escaped. The right ovary was found covered with purulent lymph ; and the right Fallopian tube was filled with thick purulent matter.

§ 4. *Tabes mesenterica; Marasmus.*—A species of chronic *peritonitis*, giving rise in children to the symptoms of this disease, is described by Dr George Gregory. Its anatomical characters are much the same as in the ordinary instances of peritoneal inflammation ; but it also tends to induce thickening of the peritonæum, secretion of matter termed *scrofulous,* (*tubercular ? tyromatous ?*) and finally ulceration of the peritonæum. In consequence of this ulceration, the mucous and peritoneal surfaces of the bowel communicate directly, so that instead of forming a continuous canal, as in the normal condition, they constitute a mass of tubes communicating freely with each other, and with thickened and ulcerated peritonæum, by numerous openings. From the early symptoms combined with these changes, Dr Gregory considers this disorder as primarily commencing in the peritonæum.* The justice of this view I have already attempted to consider.† I have only to observe, that not only the symptoms, but even the appearances of peritoneal inflammation may be explained, by supposing the ulcerative process to originate in the mucous membrane, and proceed to the pe-

. * Observations on the scrofulous inflammation of the Peritonæum, &c.   Med.-Chir. Transact. Vol. xi. p. 258.

† See page 650, § 13.

ritoneal, in which the effusion of the contents of the tube necessarily produce inflammatory exudation.   For a case illustrating
this mode of progress, I refer to Howship, p. 264.

§ 5. *Meningitis* and *Arachnitis.*—These two affections are generally combined,—in other words, inflammation of the *pia mater* is
generally accompanied with that of the arachnoid membrane.   It
assumes acute, subacute, and chronic forms.

The acute and subacute forms constitute the disease described
by practical authors under the name of *water* of the head, *water* of
the brain, *hydrocephalus,* and *hydrencephalus.*   This inference,
which was originally advanced by Quin, and adopted by Rush and
Garnet, was first verified by Cheyne, and has been since amply confirmed by the inspections of Golis, the inquiries of Dr Blackall, of
Dr Ayre, Dr Abercrombie, the dissections and researches of Parent-Duchatelet, Martinet, and Senff.   The proofs collected by
these authors, it is unnecessary, after the general remarks already
submitted, to detail.   From the account also of the distribution of
the proper cerebral membrane, it is easy to explain the necroscopic
phenomena of hydrocephalic brains.   The natural result of this
distribution is, that when the membrane is inflamed, and its vessels
in consequence secrete watery fluid, while that from the outer division is deposited beneath the arachnoid coat, that of the inner trickles
from the membrane, on the figurate surface of the brain, or in the
ventricles, in which its effects are in proportion to its quantity.   If
small, it produces little change on the parts of the brain.   If copious, it raises the vault, pushes out the walls of the ventricles, enlarges their capacity and dimensions, breaks down the median *septum,* forming a large communicating aperture, and may ultimately
extrude the substance of the organ, and render it so thin as to give
it the appearance of a mere bag, containing a considerable quantity
of water.

In some instances fluid is not found in the ventricles.   The *pia
mater* and *plexus,* however, are highly injected; the arachnoid is
opaque, dull, and dry-looking ; and the subarachnoid tissue is infiltrated.   This demonstrates that the symptoms of the disease depend not on the effusion, but on the previous vascular injection.

In addition to these proofs derived from inspection, that the fluid
proceeds not from the brain but its membranes, it may be added,
that in the fœtal state, previous to the formation of brain, fluid may
be derived from the congested vascular membrane.   The new ac-

z z

tion thus established gives a sudden check to the normal action of the vessels; and as the formation of the brain is thus interrupted, the individual is born anencephalous. The same process taking place in the vertebral portion of the membrane during the early months of fœtal life, causing at once serous effusion, interruption to the growth of the chord, and arresting that of the spinal plates, and their mutual union, constitutes *spina bifida*.

The influence of acute *meningitis* in deranging the mental faculties, though questioned by Bayle, appears to me undoubted, for the following reasons.

1*st*, In several cases of the disease taking place in adults, and in which its nature was confirmed by accurate inspection, I have remarked the same confusion of thought, incapacity of judgment, and incoherence of speech as in the maniacal. In general, in this delirium gay and pleasurable ideas predominate. In the most distinct of these cases, to which I have already alluded, the nature of the disease was unequivocally demonstrated, not only by the fluid of the ventricles, but by the vascularity of the *pia mater* and plexus, subarachnoid infiltration, dulness of the arachnoid, and albuminous exudation from the free surface of that membrane. 2*d*, In several cases of the disease occurring in infants, without proving immediately fatal, I have traced to this cause a degree of idiocy which was supposed to be congenital. This idiocy is in many cases associated with deafness, dumbness, or both, sometimes with squinting, and sometimes with amaurotic blindness. Upon inquiry, it always appeared that the infant had undergone soon after birth an anomalous and little understood disorder, after which, hearing and sight seemed much impaired, and the vivacity of the infantile age was not observed. Inspection at a subsequent period demonstrated the nature of the affection.

Symptomatic meningeal inflammation, or rather congestion, I have formerly said, takes place in fever continued, intermittent, and remittent, after injuries of the head, and occasionally in other diseases.

From the appearances of a considerable number of cases of the ordinary continued fever of this country, which since the beginning of 1817 I have inspected personally, or have seen inspected, I infer that subacute congestion of the cerebral membranes is one of the most frequent phenomena of that disease, and one which very often contributes to its fatal termination. I have elsewhere attempted to show, however, that this is not the cause of fever ; and

4

though the cause of many of its symptoms, especially the confused thought and incoherent speech, that it is one only of an extensive and general morbid state of the capillary system induced by the action of fever. It may nevertheless occasionally amount to inflammation.

With the admission of the facts now stated, further, it must be remembered, that the main cause of the symptoms of headach, delirium, convulsions, and stupor during life, and of the appearances after death, is the circulation in the vessels of the brain of blood not oxygenated, blood containing much carbonaceous matter, and several elements which in the state of health are expelled; blood, in short, poisoned by the operation of fever, of whatever type.

§ 6. *Delirium in the Phthisical not an instance of Metastasis.*— Subacute meningeal inflammation I have seen take place in the phthisical during the last days or weeks of existence. Upon examining the brains of persons of this description who have had delirium for some time before death, the *pia mater* and *choroid plexus* are more or less sometimes highly injected; the arachnoid is dull, opaque, and lustreless; the subarachnoid tissue is infiltrated, especially in the vicinity of the vessels; and serum is effused in the ventricles. In an extreme case of this nature, which occurred under the care of Dr Renton, and in which the patient had *delirium* amounting to *mania* for three weeks previous to death, I found among other lesions, the whole *pia mater* most extensively injected, and its minute vessels of a scarlet-red colour, while the large vessels were filled with dark blood. The scarlet-coloured capillaries were distinct and abundant at the convoluted surface, and in particular at the base of the brain, and in the portion which covers the outer surface of the *hippocampus major*. The arachnoid was dull, opaque, and elevated by subserous infiltration. At the inner margins of the hemisphere, in the neighbourhood of the falx, the arachnoid of the *pia mater* adhered to that of the *dura mater* with albuminous effusion; and pisiform or lenticular eminences like those described by Greding and others were found proceeding from the *pia mater*. The choroid plexus was also injected; and serum to the amount of about one ounce or ten drachms was found in the ventricles. The substance of the convoluted or gray matter of the brain was extensively traversed by reddish vessels, in which the blood was still fluid.

§ 7. *Inflammation of the Choroid Plexus or central Pia Mater.* —This lesion, though rare, is observed occasionally to take place.

The choroid plexus becomes thick, solid, and firm, and is matted into a mass with lymph effused between its folds and interstices. It may then be drawn from the ventricles and their divisions like a thick solid mass. The ventricles, at the same time, contain turbid sero-purulent fluid.

This change commmonly affects both choroid plexuses, in all their divisions.

The external effects by which it is attended are variable and not very distinctive. The patient, besides shivering and being hot and uncomfortable, is feeble, tremulous, and has a sort of paraplegic appearance in the lower extremities, and sometimes of the whole person. The patient has a stupid look, complains little, except of weight of the head, and weakness of vision or blindness. In some instances he is at first affected by ringing in the ears, and is afterwards deaf. At length speech is imperfect; great weakness follows, generally with coma; and after some hours of this, death ensues.

§ 8. *Chronic Meningeal Inflammation. The pathological causes of insanity.*—However general be the opinion, that mental derangement may exist independent of anatomical change in the state of the brain or its coverings, we find in the writings of various authors, and in the results of anatomical inspection, ample proof of four facts; that, though mental derangement may, in first attacks and in cases of short duration, depend on some dynamical change in the circulation of the brain or its membranes, yet when long continued, it is always connected with some change in the organization of these parts; that mental derangement, as commonly observed, is usually connected with a morbid state of the membranes, or the brain, or both; that most abnormal changes give rise, sooner or later, to confusion of thought, incoherent ideas, and insane actions; and that deranged intellect is one only of several symptoms which may occur in consequence. Already, when enumerating the morbid changes incident to the brain, I have alluded occasionally to several of those which may induce insanity. I am now to advert to states of the cerebral membranes, which, there is every reason to believe, are a very uniform cause of that malady.

The elaborate inspections of Greding, to whom I have had occasion formerly to allude, afford the first traces of comprehensive views on the abnormal states of the brain and its coverings, in the persons of the maniacal and epileptico-maniacal insane. According to the researches of this physician, the *pia mater* and arachnoid membrane are rarely sound in those affected with insanity. In

120 cases inspected, though in a few (5) the *pia mater* is stated to be pale, in more (9) it was reddish ; and in a number still greater its vessels were injected with dark blood. The exterior surface was in 29 cases white, thick, and mucous ; sometimes dry and lardaceous, like the buffy coat of inflamed blood, near the vertex, along the mesial margins of the hemispheres. In 29 cases this alteration extended more generally over the membrane. In 9 it was observed over the convex and plane surfaces of the hemispheres ; and in 6 it extended round the *cerebellum* and *medulla oblongata.* The white, thick, opaque appearance Greding ascribes to subarachnoid effusion ; the dry lardaceous to albuminous exudation. In 37 cases he found minute, pisiform, or lenticular eminences, like a mustard-seed, a hemp-seed, or a pea, soft or hard, disseminated over the membrane ; in 27 cases more copious and thickly set ; and in 14 cases accumulated abundantly. These bodies, which are to be distinguished from the *glandules* of Pacchioni, by situation, soft consistence, and milky colour, appear to be a product of the inflammatory process. I have occasionally seen them in subjects in whom the traces of chronic inflammation were distinct.*

Similar changes in the cerebral membranes were recognised by Joseph Wenzel of Mayence,† and Chiarugi of Florence. The latter especially, among 59 necroscopic inspections of insane persons, found in 54 more or less thickening of the membranes, serous infiltration of the subarachnoid tissue, with or without injection of the capillaries, and serous fluid to greater or less amount within the ventricles.‡

Much the same results may be derived from the necroscopic reports of Haslam and Marshall. Of 37 cases of insane persons examined by the former, whatever was the state of the brain, the membranes were unsound in all except one (the 33d) ; and in this "considerable determination of blood to the brain shows that the capillaries of the *pia mater* were inordinately loaded." In 23 of these cases, the *pia mater* was injected and loaded with blood, more or less reddened or disordered in its capillary system. In 24 cases, the arachnoid membrane was opaque ; in some instances of milky

---

* Melancholico-Maniacorum et Epilepticorum quorundam in Ptochotropheo Waldheimensi demortuorum sectiones tradit J. E. Greding, Continuatio 2da. Apud Ludwig Adversaria, Vol. ii. Part iii. p. 449.

† Observations sur le Cervelet et sur les diverses parties du cerveau dans les Epileptiques, par Jos. Wenzel, D. M. &c.   Traduit par M. Breton.   Paris, 1811.

‡ Della Pazzia in genere e in specie, Trattato Medico-Analitico con una centuria d'Osservazioni.   3 Tomi, 8vo.   Firenze, 1793, 1794.

opacity; in several thickened; and in one-half at least with infiltration into the subarachnoid tissue. Of these 24, 13 belong to
the first class in presenting traces of injection of the *pia mater*. In
21 cases, serous fluid varying in amount from two tea-spoonful to
four, six, or eight ounces was found in the ventricles; and of these
also 10 corresponded with the first class in presenting traces of meningeal inflammation more or less intense. The presence of this
fluid in the cerebral cavities, I have already shown, indicates previous vascular congestion of the choroid plexus; and though this
membrane was not in all instances much or evidently affected, yet,
since in several it was vascular, thickened, vesicular, or indurated,
the appearance of fluid in the cavities is as unequivocal a mark of
previous inflammation as if it had been reddened, injected, or penetrated by extravasated blood. The opacity, both macular and
diffuse, Dr Haslam regards as marks of inflammation; and the subarachnoid infiltration is of the same nature. In several cases, (5,
7, 8, 14, 15, 18,) the injection had proceeded to extravasated patches.
In one case, in which the patient died hemiplegic, the right lateral
ventricle was distended with dark-coloured blood which had issued
from the choroid plexus; and in one, in which the patient dropped
down lifeless in a moment, much blood was extravasated between
the cerebral membranes.*

The cases dissected by Dr Marshall about the same time, but
published some years after, furnish similar results. Of 22 cases of
insane persons whose brains were inspected by this anatomist, in 21
serous fluid, varying in amount from 1, 2, or 4, to 12 ounces, was
found in the cerebral cavities; and in 17 of these 21 cases similar
effusion was found in the subarachnoid tissue occasionally to the
extent of elevating the arachnoid membrane in minute vesicles or
cysts, (cases 6, 8, 9, 18, 22.) Though the *pia mater* is said to have
been injected in four cases only, and the arachnoid to have been
opaque in two, it results from the fluid effused into the ventricles
or between the membranes, from the vascularity of the substance
of the brain, and from the facility with which the *pia mater* was detached from the convoluted surface, that the capillaries of the latter membrane were in a morbid state.† It is further to be remarked, that in nine of these cases were the arteries of the brain opaque,

---

* Observations on Madness and Melancholy, &c. by John Haslam, 2d edition.
London, 1809.

† The Morbid Anatomy of the Brain in Mania and Hydrophobia, &c. &c. collected
from the Papers of the late Andrew Marshall, M. D. 1815.

thickened, steatomatous, or ossified,—a condition highly favourable for deranging the capillary circulation of the membranes or the inclosed organ.

These results are important in enumerating the most uniform morbid appearances found in the cerebral membranes of the maniacal. Their chief value, however, consists in the verification which they have since received from the researches of Neumann of Berlin, and Bayle and Calmeil of Paris. From the inquiries of the second of these authors especially, it appears almost established that a state of chronic inflammation of the cerebral membranes is invariably the cause of insanity. My limits do not permit me to detail the whole of the proofs on which this inference is founded; nor is it necessary, after collating the dissections of Greding, Chiarugi, Haslam, and Marshall. A short statement of the principal morbid changes recognized by M. Bayle will be sufficient to show how far the inference is justified by facts.

1*st*, The most constant anatomical character of this state of the cerebral membranes is injection, more or less intense and extensive, of the cellular vascular web of the *pia mater*. The vessels are loaded; the membrane is red or scarlet; and blood trickles from all parts on removing it from the brain. In other instances, its interstices are distended with serous fluid, which gives it a pale gray colour, and increases its volume and thickness. The arachnoid is reddish scarcely once in 16 or 20 cases.

2*d*, The arachnoid becomes opaque and thickened, especially in the convex centre of the hemispheres, at their mesial margin, and on their mutual surface. This thickness, which may be so great as to approach that of the *pleura*, the *pericardium*, the *dura mater*, or macerated parchment, M. Bayle ascribes not to albuminous deposition on its surface, but to development of vessels, and extravasation of matter in its substance.

3*d*, The meningeal injection very generally terminates in serous effusion, either from the free surface of the arachnoid membrane into the subarachnoid tissue, or from the arachnoid of the choroid plexus, constituting effusion into the ventricles.

4*th*, *Albuminous exudation* occurred in $\frac{1}{6}$th of the subjects at the free surface of the arachnoid of the *dura mater*, covering its whole extent, confined to the convexity of one or both hemispheres, to the falx, or to the occipital region,—applied, but not adhering to the cerebral arachnoid.

5th, Adhesions of the two surfaces of the arachnoid occurred no more than 8 or 10 times in 100 instances. They are most common in the great fissure, and once or twice were observed in the ventricles. In one case, in which the disease was complicated, M. Bayle found the two folds of the arachnoid intimately united by the interposition of an albuminous patch.

6th, The membranes adhered to the convoluted surface with unusual firmness, so as to carry away portions of brain in one-half of the cases. This took place in spaces varying in size from a lentile or a bean to a five-franc piece or more. The connection of this change with inflammation is denoted by the vascularity and abnormal thickness of the membranes at the adhering points.

7th, The pisiform granulations of Greding were found in not more than $\frac{1}{10}$th of the subjects; a degree of rarity probably dependent on the circumstance that they are in general a product of long-continued inflammation.

8th, Bloody extravasation in the arachnoid cavity, which belongs to a subsequent head, was found in about $\frac{1}{8}$th of the cases.

From these and similar facts, and from the cases of M. Calmeil, it results that the cerebral membranes, more especially the tomentose and vascular surface of the proper membrane, (*pia mater* and *choroid plexus,*) are liable to assume a peculiar state of chronic inflammation, affecting more or less, sometimes very considerably, the convoluted and central surfaces of the brain. Of this morbid change the first effects are more or less weight, uneasiness, and pain of the head; sometimes partial convulsive motions; sometimes tetanic motions or involuntary contractions, *vertigo,* double vision, spectral *delirium,* and occasionally sudden loss of sensation and motion. In other instances, it induces gradually deficient memory, disordered intellect, and some affection of the muscles of speech. *Finally,* it induces palsy, fatuity, and stupor or coma, terminating fatally.

Palsy occurring under these circumstances in the insane is distinguished by peculiar characters. At first the motions of the tongue are constrained; the efforts to speak are unavailing; articulation is impracticable; and the individual struggles and stammers to express his desires like a person under the influence of intoxication. As this becomes intense he is observed to totter, stagger, or reel in walking, and is aware that he cannot direct the muscles of the limbs to move as he wills. At this time the derangement

3

verges to fatuity. At a more advanced period, not only is speech obliterated or converted into inarticulate muttering, but the patient is unable to maintain himself erect; and whenever he wills to make any motion, neither arms nor legs are obedient to his desires. This morbid action of the cerebral membranes, in short, impairs, but does not annihilate the motions of all the voluntary muscles. It induces a general but incomplete loss of power.

The senses are at the same time impaired but not obliterated. The paralytic madman distinguishes light from darkness; he hears a loud sound made at the ears; and he is sensible of pungent odours. But if the skin be touched with two bodies, the one hot and the other cold, he distinguishes no difference. Taste and general sensation are equally obtuse. In this state death is not remote. The duration of the affection varies according to the slowness or rapidity of the meningo-encephalic disorder, from which the palsy arises. Some paralytic maniacs live eight months, a year, eighteen months, and others continue two or three years, rarely longer. The average duration of life, after the commencement of paralytic symptoms indicates affection of the cerebral surfaces extending to the substance, is about thirteen months.

II. HEMORRHAGE.—Discharges of blood from the serous membranes have not attracted so much attention as those of the mucous surfaces. They are nevertheless not uncommon; and though the inaccessible situation of the serous surfaces has made their hemorrhages be overlooked or confounded with other diseases, they constitute a form of morbid action too important to be omitted. They occur in all the serous membranes, are preceded by injection, and take place by exhalation, and may be arranged in the following order.

Cerebral membranes,	*Meningæmia.*	
Pleura,	*Pleuræmia,*	*Hæmathorax.*
Pericardium,	*Hæmacardia.*	
Peritonæum,	*Hæmenteria.*	
Perididymis,	*Hæmatorchis.*	

§ 1. *Meningæmia.*—The nature of the subject compels me reluctantly to begin with hemorrhage of the tomentose or vascular surface of the *pia mater.* In this variety of meningeal hemorrhage, which has been greatly overlooked, the vessels of the attached surface of the *pia mater* become inordinately injected and effuse blood, which is deposited in the convoluted surface generally, and occasionally in the ventricles. Omitting some obscure accounts of this

affection in the older collections, the first good example is given
by Morgagni from Valsalvi, who found in the body of a man of 58
much coagulated blood between the *pia mater* and the convoluted
surface of the right hemisphere. (Epist ii. 19.)   Two similar cases
Morgagni inspected himself. (Epist. iii. 2 and 4.)

The best instance of this hemorrhage, however, is given by Mr
Howship in his 11th case.   It occurred in a young woman of 22,
who for two years had laboured under rheumatic ailments, and at
length, after paralytic and vertiginous symptoms, died lethargic.
Upon inspection the *pia mater* was found vascular and red; its vessels increased in number and size; and blood was diffusely extravasated all under the *pia mater*.   " The extravasated fluid had
formed superficial coagula, corresponding to the *sulci* between the
convolutions."—" It had taken place very universally, and the effusion seemed to have arisen not only from the capillary arteries
upon the external surface of the *pia mater*, but also from those
processes of the membrane which dip between the convolutions
forming the *tomentum cerebri*.   Several of these deep-seated coagula were divided by the knife in the course of the dissection."*

Slighter examples of partial extravasation on the convoluted
surface I have seen myself, and mentioned many years ago,† when
I did not well understand the source of the hemorrhage.   These
partial extravasations are the cause of the orange-coloured depressed spots often seen on the convoluted surface of the brain.   Dr
Abercrombie records two instances communicated by Dr Hunter
and Dr Barlow, in which the extravasation, he states, was from
the superficial vessels of the brain.‡   He does not specify, however, whether the blood was beneath the *pia mater* or above it.   If
it was above, it belongs to the following head.

The lesion now described is to be regarded as a hemorrhage
taking place spontaneously.   Much more frequently, however, blood
effused between the *pia mater* and surface of the brain is the effect
of blows, violence, and similar injuries.   As such it has already
come under consideration; and I have only to repeat what was
formerly stated, that in a medico-legal point of view the distinction
is most important, and the correct knowledge of it may often affect

* Practical Observations on Surgery and Morbid Anatomy, &c. Lond. 1816. Section ii. Case xiv. See also cases xviii. and xx.

† On the Pathological Anatomy of the Brain and its Membranes, Med. and Surg.
Journal, Vol. xviii. p. 487.

‡ Researches, Pathological and Practical.

,the life of a fellow-creature. In general, therefore, it is to be understood that when blood is effused between the *pia mater* and convoluted surface of the brain, or within the ventricles, it proceeds ,from the membranes, and is most likely to be the result of external .violence. When, on the other hand, the effusion is found within the substance of the brain, in fissures or lacerations, it is the result of disease.

In the hemorrhage of the brains of new-born infants, the blood is also situate between the *pia mater* and brain. To this subject, however, I need not recur.

Hemorrhage from the free surface of the arachnoid membrane is more common. It may take place either from that which lines the *dura mater*, and covers the *pia mater*, when it is found between these two membranes; or from the arachnoid of the choroid plexus, when it is found in the ventricles. Of the former, a good instance is given by Haslam, who found this the cause of sudden death in the person of a maniac. The same change was found by Bayle in about ½th of the cases of persons cut off by symptoms of chronic meningitis. The cases of Drs Hunter and Barlow are already mentioned.

Effusion from the interior or central arachnoid is more frequent; and cases may be found in the writings of most collectors. Of this nature are the following. The case of the chamberlain of the monastery of Rheinau, near Schaffhausen, recorded by Wepfer;[*] several described by Morgagni, *e. g.* the case of Cardinal Sanvitali; and those in the 13th, 15th, 17th, 19th, and 22d sections of his second epistle; the cases of Antonio Tita, Pietro Facciolati, and .the Danish ambassador in his third epistle, and one or two in the sixtieth; the case related by Veratti in the Bologna Memoirs;[†] the case by De Haen, called rupture of the choroid plexus;[‡] the 48th of Rochoux;[§] the 4th, 8th, and 12th cases of Cheyne;[‖] one or two cases by Merat;[¶] and the 20th and 21st cases of Serres.[**]

In all these cases, blood or bloody fluid was found in the ventricles; and since it was not connected, as in the ordinary instances of this with rupture or injury of the cerebral substance, and conse. quently had not penetrated, as I have formerly shown, from the substance of the hemispheres, it is inferred that it must have issued

---

[*] Historia Apoplecticorum.   [†] Comment. Bonon. Tom. ii. Chap. i.
[‡] Rat. Med. Pars iv. cap. v. p. 189.   [§] Recherches sur l'Apoplexie.
[‖] Cases of Apoplexy and Lethargy. Lond. 1812.
[¶] Memoires de la Societé Medicale d'Emulation, Tome vii. p. 61.
[**] Annuaire Medico-Chirurgicale, &c.

from the plexus. There is no reason to suppose that the vessels of this web are ruptured in this form of hemorrhage. The fluid is rarely pure blood, generally sanguinolent; but even if pure, the observations of Bichat, Merat, and Serres, show that it may ooze by exhalation from the plexus. It constitutes the meningeal apoplexy of Serres.*

The causes of this form of hemorrhage are often as obscure as those of hemorrhage in the substance of the brain. Yet in certain cases it is possible to trace a connection between these hemorrhages and the state of the arteries, exactly as in hemorrhage into the substance of the brain. For this reason, it is proper, in order to complete the pathology of cerebral hemorrhage, to advert to the state of the blood-vessels which are conveyed along the membranes of the brain.

§ 2. *Effects of the Steatomatous and Osteo-steatomatous Degene ration of the Cerebral Arteries on the Circulation of the Brain and its Membranes.*—Though to this change as a predisposing cause to softening and hemorrhage I have already adverted, it may not be improper to take in this place a general view of the transformation and its several effects.

The tunics of the arteries of the brain are liable, in advanced life, to become penetrated with steatomatous and osteo-steatomatous matter to an extreme degree and a very general extent. They then become rigid, unyielding, opaque, inelastic, and are no longer capable of conveying the blood as pliant transmissible tubes. Though this change affects most usually the internal carotid and its branches, as the Sylvian artery, the anterior communicating arteries, and the circle of Willis, and next to these the basilar artery, yet it may extend over all the arteries of the brain, great and small. In an extreme and extensive example of the disease in my collection, the whole of the trunks and branches of the internal carotid and basilar arteries have become completely penetrated and transformed by this change, and show its effects in various modes. In some parts the arteries are enlarged in external circumference, without increasing the internal capacity, and often diminishing it, in consequence of the deposition between the middle and inner coats. In all parts, the internal area of the arteries is more or less diminished; in some it is contracted so much, that the canal of the vessel appears

* On Extravasations of Blood into the cavity of the Arachnoid, and on the formation of the False Membrane which sometimes envelopes these extravasations. By Prescott Hewett, Esq. Medico-Chirurgical Trans. vol. xxviii. p. 45. London, 1845.

closed, and indeed may be closed. In some points the vessels be_ come tortuous and serpentine. Transverse sections also show an_ other change. The inner coat is separated from the middle by fis_ sures or chinks, caused apparently by the new deposition between them ; and all over the tunics present specks of steatomatous or osseous matter, sometimes rings of bone, and in short they are con_ verted into inelastic, brittle, and more or less rigid tubes.

The effects of this state of the cerebral arteries on the circulation are considerable, though not permanent. The blood is liable to irregularity in its movement, and sometimes to become entirely stopped. In this state the obstructed motion induces an attack of *cataphora*, or stupor and insensibility, lasting for several hours, or even for one or two days. In other cases it induces a degree of confusion and inability to walk, or keep in the erect position, with drowsiness, yet with the patient being capable of being roused, or spontaneously rousing himself at intervals. After some hours of rest, with the use of adequate means, the patient perfectly recovers, and seems as well in intellect, memory, and observation, as ever. He is liable, nevertheless, to recurrences of these fits of *cataphora*, and in one of them death may take place. Fits of this kind, neverthe- less, I have seen come and go in the same individuals for several years, apparently without affecting the health or the intellect, and with only a degree of impaired memory. These attacks of *cata_ phora* are often mistaken for attacks of apoplexy ; but they are not so, and do not require the same treatment. Often, indeed, the pa_ tient recovers spontaneously after a sound sleep. An awkward position of the head and neck occasionally precedes these attacks.

In other instances, the osteo-steatomatous state of the arteries produces more permanent and more serious disorder. By obstruct- ing the circulation, it induces the state formerly described as atro- phy of the convolutions and brain, often with copious effusion into the subarachnoid tissue and within the ventricles. In other cases, the individual speaks thick and inarticulately, is unsteady in his motions, and, though not paralytic, the limbs totter and shake. There is also more or less loss of memory. Such was the state of the person whose cerebral arteries I have above described as ex- tensively affected by this transformation.

Lastly, from this state of the arteries, evils still more consider- able may result: It has been observed several times to give rise to aneurism without or with rupture and hemorrhage. Thus Mr

E. A. Jennings records in a stout healthy man of 54, an instance of aneurism of the basilar artery suddenly giving way, and causing speedy dissolution by hemorrhage. This aneurism, which was about, the size of a pea, was situate on the basilar artery, immediately. after the union of the two vertebral arteries. From this blood had escaped and spread itself over the *medulla oblongata*.* This person was wont to suffer from pain in the head. Death took place about eight hours after the appearance of the first symptoms.

In the course of inspections at the Royal Infirmary of this place, I have observed three instances of aneurism of the cerebral arteries within the space of about five years. Two of these were situate in the anterior arteries of the brain in the fissure of Sylvius. The arteries in both cases were diseased along their whole course. The aneurismal swelling in one case was about the size of a pea ; in the other it was a little larger. In both cases, rupture had taken place, followed by apoplectic death.

A third case I observed in the basilar artery. The tumour here was regularly spherical, and appeared like a small globular body formed in the course of the artery. The preparation is preserved in the museum of the university. A good example of aneurism in the right vertebral artery is given by Cruveilhier. In this case the swelling was almost exactly globular, and extended equally on each side of the artery, being altogether from five to six lines in diameter. The interior shows clots and steatomatous deposition.†

By some, as Mr Porter, it is maintained that aneurism in this situation must be true aneurism, that is, formed by dilatation of the inner and middle tunics alone, as there is no cellular duct to form an external covering, were the inner tunics lacerated. It is certainly remarkable that these aneurisms of the cerebral arteries present examples of uniform and regular dilatation much more complete, than are observed in the aneurisms of other regions. They are in truth the only aneurisms which afford examples of what Cruveilhier denominates peripheral, that is, spherical aneurisms, embracing the entire periphery of the vessel in which they are formed. Cruveilhier, nevertheless, maintains that the whole three tunics are dilated ; and in supporting this proposition, he necessarily maintains that the cerebral arteries possess a cellular tunic as well as those of other regions.

* * Case of Aneurism of the Basilar Artery suddenly giving way, &c. By E. A. Jennings. Transactions of Provincial Association, Vol. i. p. 270. London, 1833.

† Anatomie Pathologique, Livraison xxviii. Pl. iii. figs. 2, 3, 4.

§ 3. It is further an interesting confirmation of the view above given, that hemorrhage of the same nature may take place from the arachnoid of the membranes of the spinal chord, and give rise to similar symptoms, though modified by the situation of the effusion. Of this variety of arachnoid hemorrhage, an instance is quoted by Sauvages from Duverney, under the title of *asphyxia spinalis;* but the best examples are those recorded by M. Chevalier in the 3d volume of the Medico-Chirurgical Transactions, and that by Sir A. Cooper in his work on Dislocation. In these cases blood, coagulated and fluid, was found in the spinal canal between the membranes, and the vessels of the membranes were inordinately loaded.

§ 4. *Pleuræmia ; hæmathorax.*—On this form of hemorrhage, instances of which are recorded by Morgagni and Lieutaud, which has been well described by Merat and Laennec, it is unnecessary to say more. Merat informs us that this hemorrhage proved fatal to Professor Mahon.*

§ 5. *Hæmacardia,* or hemorrhage from the pericardium, has been not less overlooked than the other bloody discharges of the serous membranes. In the few instances which have been recorded, it has generally been ascribed to laceration or rupture of the auricles, venous sinuses, or organs of the large vessels, allowing the blood contained to escape and distend the pericardium. In the instances to which I now advert, the most minute and diligent search was inadequate to detect either rupture, laceration, or minute orifices by which blood could escape ; and it must therefore be inferred, that it issues from the membrane by the process of exhalation.

Of this singular hemorrhage, four distinct and authentic cases are recorded. In the first, by Dr Alston, three pounds of coagulated blood and bloody serum were taken from the pericardium. When the inner surface of the pericardium, and the external surface of the heart were carefully cleansed by sponges, no aperture of any of the large vessels could be discovered ; " but on pressing the heart bloody serum oozed from many small orifices on its surface, and principally near its basis."† The second case, by Dr Thomson of Worcester, is similar in the quantity and kind of blood effused, and in the impossibility of tracing it to rupture or open vessel.‡ In the third case, by Mr Joseph Hooper, about five pints of fluid blood perfectly free from *coagula,* were found in the pericardium, in which no vestige of rupture could, after the most careful exami-

* Journal de Medecine, Tome ix. p. 132.
† Medical Essays and Observations, Vol. vi. p. 111. Art. lvi.
‡ Medical Observations and Inquiries, Vol. iv. p. 330, Art. xxvi.

nation, be found.* Lastly, in a case by Merat, two ounces of pure blood were found in the pericardium of a man of 53, who had laboured under organic lesion of the heart and consecutive dropsy.†

Baillie, to whom these effusions were known, was aware of the difficulty of explaining them, and conjectures that the blood may have oozed by transudation, or escaped from the extremities of the minute vessels, which he supposes may be inordinately relaxed.‡ The last supposition, it may be remarked, virtually admits exhalation.

It must be observed, nevertheless, that the arteries on the surface of the heart are often diseased in this hemorrhage.

§ 6. *Hæmenteria. Peritonæmia.*—Peritoneal hemorrhage is not uncommon. It occurs under two forms, the sanguinolent and the sanguine. · A valuable instance of this hemorrhage, mentioned by Morgagni,§ is that of Laelio Laelii, a medical student, a native of his own town of Imola, in whose abdomen was found about 1½ pound of fluid blood, with black spots of the peritonæum. . The best examples, however, are those recorded by Merat. In the first, there were three pints of bloody serum in the cavity, with evident marks of peritoneal inflammation. In a second, there were between two and three pints, and the membrane was covered with numerous granulations. It is reasonable to infer that this was tubercular disease of the peritoneum causing hemorrhage. In a third case, in which death took place 47 days after the first symptoms, upon inspection there were found about twenty pints of a fluid, first sanguinolent, then like pure blood, and lastly some clots. The marks of inflammation were so intense as to leave few traces of the original form of the abdominal viscera.‖

§ 7. *Hæmatorchis.*—Of hemorrhage from the vaginal coat, Bichat states that he met with two instances only ; and Merat acknowledges that he has not yet seen any example. On some occasions this hemorrhage lays the foundation of the bloody tumour (*hæmatoma,*) occasionally found in the vaginal coat.

From the facts recorded it results that these hemorrhages, like those of the mucous tissue, are the result of exhalation. Bichat states, that after scrupulous examination of the inner surface of the *pleura, pericardium,* and *peritonæum,* under these hemorrhages, he found the surface entire, and the vessels unbroken. There is every

---

* Memoirs of the Medical Society, Vol. i. p. 238, Art. xviii.
† Memoires de la Societé Medicale d'Emulation, Vol. vii. p. 63.
‡ Morbid Anatomy.   § Epist. xxxv. 2.   Case of Laelio Laelii.
‖ Mémoires de la Societé Medicale d'Emulation, Tom. vii. p. 65.

reason to believe that they are in all cases preceded by congestion of the capillaries; for most of those which are hitherto accurately recorded were connected with marks of inflammation, and some with organic lesion.

I have yet to observe, that the serous membranes are liable to become simultaneously the seat of hemorrhage in land-scurvy and in sea-scurvy. In the former disease, these membranes have been found occupied not only by petechial spots and dark or livid blotches, but with considerable effusion of fluid blood. Of this, the cases of Dr Duncan Junior and Mr William Wood are the best examples. In extreme cases of scurvy the same extravasation takes place.

III. Dropsies.—Of abnormal accumulation of serous fluid within the serous membranes I have nothing to add to what is already said in the chapter on the exhalants. These accumulations may almost invariably be traced to disease of the contained organs, or of other organs, as the heart, liver, kidneys, or tubercular deposit in the membranes.

IV. Air is not unfrequently effused into cavities formed by serous tissue. Besides the form of *pneumothorax*, which results from fistulous opening of the lung, another may take place from laceration or wound of the lung. In the peritonæum it is the result either of inflammation, of gangrene and decomposition of serum, of ulcerative perforation, or of organic disease producing the same effect.

V. Tubercles.—Tubercular deposition of different kinds is frequent in the serous membranes. The exact nature of the deposition, however, is not well defined. The tubercular diseases occurring in serous membranes are of two sorts, the genuine *tyromatous*, or that in which tyromatous matter is deposited, in irregular or amorphous masses in the membrane,—and the *cenchroid* or miliary, in which minute lenticular bodies hard as cartilage, but opaque or semi-transparent, are developed in these membranes.

§ 1. The tyromatous deposition occurs in these membranes, but most frequently in the peritonæum, in which it was originally observed by Morgagni, Lieutaud, and Baillie, afterwards well described by Dr Baron, and Scoutetten, and observed by Dr Moncrieff. They are round bodies, varying in size from a vetch or garden-pea to a bean, not always regular in shape, of caseous consistence, and generally softened in the centre. They cause inflammation of the membrane. In the pleura tubercles are noticed by Morgagni, Lieu-

3 A

taud, and Baillie. To this head, perhaps, we may refer a variety of *tyromatous* tumour of the pleura observed by Mr Howship. It consisted in a great number of bulbous processes variable in shape and size, but, apparently from the description, oblong, spheroidal, and attached by narrow stalks or peduncles. The substance of these bodies, which was semitransparent and very firm, of a dull-yellow colour, partly fluid and partly solid, is ascribed by Mr Howship to effusion of lymph. The opacity and increase of density resulting from immersion in alcohol showed that they contained albuminous matter.*

In the membranes of the brain they seem to be also not uncommon, though their origin from the arachnoid is not quite established.

Tubercles or tyromatous depositions in the tubercular form are often found in the *pia mater*, and especially its cerebral prolongations. They occur not only in the exterior division of the membrane, but in that which penetrates the ventricles; and from this circumstance it often happens that tyromatous bodies, which are found in the cerebral substance, have originated in the membranes. Thus of the figures given by Baillie in the 7th pl. of his 10th fasciculus, two tubercular bodies are found actually attached to the choroid plexus; one found in the lower part of the fourth ventricle; and that represented by Dr Hooper in the same situation (12th pl.) appears to have had the same origin; and those said to be found in the brain were very probably originally formed at the filamentous surface of the *pia mater*, between which and the bodies, in most instances, vascular connections are distinct and immediate.

§ 2. The cenchroid tubercles are very frequent in serous tissue. In the pleura they were seen by Wrisberg, Baillie, Bayle, Laennec, and Andral; in the peritonæum by Scoutetten.

These miliary or cartilaginous tubercles are not unfrequently found to occupy all the serous membranes at once, more especially in the bodies of the lower animals. Thus I have often seen them in the pleura, pericardium, and peritonæum in the sheep; and in a specimen of the Paca dissected by my friend Dr Grant, every serous membrane was thickly set with them. They occur chiefly in men and animals long excluded from air and exercise, In the early stage they do not exercise much influence on the state of these membranes. But at a more advanced period they cause inordinate exhalation, opacity, dulness, and other marks of morbid circulation of the tissue.

* Practical Observations on Surgery and Morbid Anatomy, p. 204.

' In the human body cenchroid tubercles occur in the pleura and *peritonæum* in two forms.

In one, very small bodies like the heads of needles or pins, and generally of a white colour, are disseminated over the whole pleural or peritoneal surface. These are very closely set, and communicate to the membrane a perceptible degree of roughness. After some time they cause, at least in the peritonæum, adhesion of the folds of the *ileum*, so that the whole bowels are united in one general adherent mass. These tubercles are seated in the substance of the peritonæum. They do not appear to increase much in size, but they tend simply to induce chronic inflammation of the membrane and union of its parts by effusion of lymph and adhesion.

They likewise tend to cause the effusion of serous fluid from the surface of the *peritonæum*.

In the second variety, small bodies, a little larger than those last mentioned, are most minutely and extensively disseminated over the *pleura* or *peritonæum*. These resemble gunpowder grains, are generally of a light blue colour, and are always extremely hard. They are less liable to cause adhesive inflammation than the small white tubercles. Yet occasionally the intestinal peritonæum is observed adhering extensively, in consequence of their development in that membrane.

They always derange the circulation and secretion of the membrane; and much serous fluid is accumulated within the cavities in consequence. They may take place in one serous membrane only; but they often take place in the *pleura* and *peritonæum* at once, causing in the former hydrothorax, and in the latter ascites.

They affect in the abdomen, the mesentery and omentum; and the latter is doubled or folded up like an oblong tumour across the abdomen between the stomach and colon.*

In the brain they are mostly seen in the *pia mater* towards the base; and they in that situation resemble neither the first nor the second variety of tubercles; being larger than the former, and less hard than the latter.

They may take place at any region of the *pia mater*. But they are more common at the base of the brain and around the *cerebellum* than in any other situation.

Wherever they are found, they induce chronic hydrocephalic

---

* Report of the Cases treated during the Course of Clinical Lectures delivered at the Royal Infirmary in 1832–1833. By David Craigie, M. D. Edin. Med. and Surg. Journal, xli. 122. Edinburgh, 1834.

effusion, with symptoms of stupor, coma, and sometimes convulsions, which terminate fatally in about six or seven weeks, sometimes earlier.

The opinion of Laennec, that miliary tubercles are the incipient form of the tyromatous tubercle, is, in reference to the serous membranes, destitute of proof. The miliary eminences of these membranes have not yet been shown to pass into the tyromatous.

VI. CHONDROMA.—*Cartilaginous degeneration* is not uncommon in the serous tissue. It appears in the form of patches varying in size and shape, attached to the free surface of the membranes. By some authors this is regarded as a preliminary step to ossification. But this is not established.

New development of cartilage is most commonly seen in the *pleura* and *pericardium* in the form of bluish-white patches, highly polished on the free surface, varying from the size of a fourpenny piece to the diameter of one shilling and more. The margins of these patches is irregular and sometimes indented and sending out other thin patches.

In general the formation of these patches is preceded by inflammation, subacute or chronic, in the course of which the spot is covered by lymph, which afterwards undergoes the cartilaginous transformation. Sometimes the part is puckered and shrivelled, as if previously the pulmonic tissue had been affected by inflammation. In old cases of chronic pleurisy and *emphysema*, it is usual for the false membrane to be converted into a fibrous layer of imperfect cartilage, uniting the two *pleurae*.

Similar patches are observed in the hepatic and splenic *peritonæum*; the spleen may be entirely enclosed in a cartilaginous tunic; and often the peritonæum covering the ovaries is entirely transformed into a firm though not very thick cartilaginous covering.

VII. OSSIFICATION.—In no texture, perhaps, is osseous deposition more frequent than in the serous. It occurs in every one of these membranes without exception. In the arachnoid it is not unfrequently seen in the form of osseous plates at the inner surface of the *dura mater*, and the free surface of the *pia mater*. Often, also, numerous thin scales of bony matter with pearly aspect are observed in the arachnoid of the spinal canal. In the pleura and pericardium it is exceedingly common, instances of it being noticed by most authors, and numerous specimens of it contained in museums. In the pleura it is most common in the costal division, large portions of which are sometimes found converted into broad flat patches of bone. The instances of ossification of the diaphragm are of the same nature. In the pericardium it is probably most frequent in the cardiac division, and constitutes those cases vaguely denominated *ossified hearts.* In the peritonæum it is less frequent; but is remarked in particular portions of this membrane. Thus it is common in the muscular, diaphragmatic, splenic, and uterine peritonæum, less frequent in the hepatic and colic, and scarcely seen in the ileal. These patches, though hard, firm, and apparently solid like bone, never present the organization peculiar to that substance. Their presence is generally connected with traces of inflammation or at least injection of the membrane; and Rayer, in an elaborate essay, attempted to prove that osseous deposition is a result of that process.* Indeed, many circumstances render it highly probable that chronic inflammation of serous tissue causes effusion of lymph, which is eventually converted into osseous matter. One of the most satisfactory proofs of this principle is, that osseous induration of the peritonæum is very common in hernial protrusions of the intestine, in which the membrane is subjected to slow inflammation; and that the vaginal coat of the testiele is often cartilaginous, or even bony in cases of old hydrocele.

VIII. MORBID GROWTHS AND PARASITICAL ANIMALS.—§ 1. *Hygroma.*—The serous cyst is not uncommon in the diaphanous membranes. It appears, however, from various observations, to be most frequent in the attached surface, or in the subserous tissue.

§ 2. *Hydatids, Acephalo-cysts.*—These globular sacs are believed to be almost proper to the serous membranes. It is certain that in these they are more frequently observed than elsewhere. Thus they are found attached to the pleura, to the pericardium, to the peritonæum, and to the vaginal coat; and in some rare cases they have been seen in the choroid plexus. Thus Fischer found the *tænia hydatigena* of Pallas, or the *cysticercus pyriformis* of Zeder, attached to this membrane by a peduncle, and vesicular bodies, supposed to be of the same *genus,* attached to the arachnoid surface of the *dura mater.* The writings of Bonetus, Morgagni, and other collectors, contain frequent examples of pulmonary hydatids, several of which were originally hydatids of the *pleura,* and several of

* Archives Generales, Tom. vii.

the subserous tissue. In the peritonæum they are still more frequent; and Dr Monro *tertius* gives a valuable collection of cases,
in which these bodies were found connected with various regions of
that membrane. Though the *cysticercus* or solitary hydatid is occasionally found, those more usually seen in this membrane are the
cænuri and *echinococci*, or the gregarious form of the animal. Of
this description, I have several times observed good examples. In
the body of a man of about 45, who died with the usual symptoms
of dropsy, two globular cysts, one as large as a child's head, were
found attached to the hepatic peritonæum. In each of these were
contained an immense number of globular cysts containing transparent fluid, about half an inch or eight lines in diameter, and surrounded in like manner by a transparent fluid. Two similar cysts,
each containing many small ones, were found attached to part of
the ileum. These were unequivocal examples of the acephalo-cyst,
which is indeed very commonly developed within and in connection
with the peritonæum. These bodies caused during life irregular
prominent tumours of the belly. Hydatids are also common in the
vaginal coat.

§ 3. *Fungus Hæmatodes* is observed to take place in this tissue.
I have seen it affect the *pleura* in the form of numerous pendulous
and sessile tumours. It is, however, more common in the *peritonæum*, both at its free and at its attached surface. One example,
in which it originated in the hepatic peritonæum, and thence proceeded to affect the greater part of the abdominal cavity, and afterwards presented at the groin, where it destroyed the bones of
the pelvis, and the upper end of the thigh-bone, some years ago
fell under my observation. The tumour had attained an enormous
size, and consisted chiefly of cerebriform matter contained in several cysts, and in some instances softened into a dark-coloured pulpy
semifluid mass.

§ 4. Scirrhous induration is said to take place in serous tissue.
There is no doubt that it often affects this tissue from the contiguous ones, especially the mucous and submucous; but it is not
ascertained, that it originates in the serous membrane. It is not
necessary to confound under this name various indurations, which
seem to be the result of the inflammatory process, or the lardaceous
state observed in the omentum and mesentery in old dysenteries,
which by some have been represented as examples of this morbid
degeneration.

IX. Accidental Development.—No tissue perhaps is so liable to be accidentally repeated as the serous. The cysts already mentioned are generally regarded as examples of this repetition; and, indeed, they possess all the characters of serous tissue. These cysts are found in many parts of the body; but they are most frequently observed in the kidneys, sometimes in connection with granular disease of those glands; and they are very common in the female ovary, in which they often constitute the anatomical character of dropsy of that organ. They are also seen in the testicle of the male. The mode of their development is not well ascertained. The hypothesis of dilatation or expansion by mechanical compression was successfully refuted by Bichat; but the one, which he attempts to establish in its place, has not been generally adopted.

Certain of the minute clustered bodies denominated by Laennec *acephalo-cysts*, and the animal nature of which, though admitted by that author, is denied by Cuvier and Rudolphi, belong to the same head. Their formation is equally little understood.

X. Morbid States of the Fibro-serous Membranes.—Before concluding this chapter, I must notice certain morbid states incident to the fibro-serous membranes.

§ 1. The *dura mater*, as a compound membrane, partaking at once of the structure of periosteum and arachnoid, is liable to affections which bear this twofold character. Its outer or cranial lamina is liable to all the morbid processes incident to periosteum. Its inner or arachnoid, it has been already shown, is liable to those peculiar to this membranous pellicle.

I have already shown that the latter surface of the *dura mater* is occasionally covered by albuminous exudation, the result of the inflammatory process. This same substance is occasionally deposited between its laminæ, and causes thickening and some induration.

§ 2. *Thickening of the Dura Mater.*—This membrane is liable, under the influence of various causes, to become greatly thickened. In several instances I have seen it as thick as ordinary leather, very firm, yet otherwise unchanged in structure. This thickening is always connected with symptoms of chronic inflammation, which may take place either spontaneously or in consequence of external violence on the head. Yet the thickening is usually confined to the *dura mater* of one hemisphere, and that the superior part of the brain; and it terminates gradually in the membrane, presenting its wonted character at the base of the organ. The *dura mater* of the opposite hemisphere is in general natural.

In one spontaneous case, in which I found this thickening, the person during life was so addicted to the use of spirits, that he was rarely sober, or at least quite correct. He was in the practice of speaking aloud to himself in the streets, and had a habit of jerking his head to the side from time to time as he walked. He died at last of symptoms of injury of the back and posteriors from a fall, and with them were mingled symptoms of *delirium tremens*.

Most commonly, nevertheless, this lesion is the result of external violence. In one well-marked case which fell under my own notice, and in which I carefully inspected the parts after death, the first exciting cause was a fall down stairs in a state of intoxication, in which the individual struck the head on the steps. He was carried home in a state of insensibility, and in that he continued for nine days. He then began to show signs of returning consciousness; and began to take food and drink, and live a sort of vegetable existence. This state improved a little. But memory, judgment, and all the mental faculties were entirely gone. The patient recovered consciousness and a degree of sensibility, only to remain a paralytic idiot for life. This state continued between two and three years, when death ensued.

The *dura mater* of the left hemisphere was then found very much thickened. The sub-arachnoid tissue was infiltrated with serous fluid to a very great amount. The convolutions were very much atrophied. About four ounces of serous fluid were contained within the ventricles, the cavities of which were dilated, and the walls extruded.

The *fornix* was softened; the *septum lucidum* entirely destroyed; and in its place was a large elliptical aperture, by which the ventricles communicated freely and directly with each other.

Such are the effects of chronic inflammation continued through a long period before they prove fatal.

§ 3. Tyromatous deposition in round nodules also occurs in this membrane, and has been well represented by Dr Hooper in his 6th and 7th engravings. They possess all the characters of the usual tyromatous matter, and consist of whitish or gray opaque substance of the consistence of cheese, of different degrees of firmness, inclosed in a vascular capsule. Generally they grow from the arachnoid surface of the membrane, but sometimes they seem to arise from its substance.

§ 4. The *dura mater* often becomes the seat of a firm tumour, which, as it grows, produces absorption of the cranial bones. In the excellent collection of cases by M. Louis, we find that it invariably proceeded to bad ulceration; but that death in general took place in consequence of interruption to the functions of the brain.

§ 5. In the testicle I have seen a peculiar disease which I refer to the *albuginea* and its serous covering. The testicle seems much enlarged and irregular; but shortly ulceration takes place, and discloses an extensive mass of dead matter evidently exterior to the gland. The sloughing process alternating with ulceration and granulation proceeds till the whole exterior coat of the testicle is expelled. This process, which occurred in a scrofulous subject, and never showed any tendency to malignant ulceration, I ascribe to death of the fibro-serous covering of the testicle, and perhaps of the gland itself.

XI. FIBROUS AND FIBRO-CARTILAGINOUS TUMOURS.—Cartilaginous and bony matter of different degrees of firmness and perfection are often observed in the cerebral membranes, more especially the *dura mater*. Of this change manifold instances are given by Bonetus, Morgagni, Lieutaud, Sandifort, and other collectors; and they are delineated by Baillie and Hooper. These cases are vaguely mentioned under the general title of ossification of the brain; but few of them are entitled to this character, for all of these originate in the membranes. The only authentic instance apparently of bony matter found in the substance of the brain unconnected with the membranes, is that delineated by Dr Hooper in his 12th engraving. The description, nevertheless, is not sufficiently minute to justify positive assertion.

CHAPTER IV.

SYNOVIAL MEMBRANE.—*Membrana Synovialis.*—*Bursæ Mucosæ.*

SECTION I.

BICHAT enumerates several circumstances in which he conceives that serous and synovial membrane differ from each other. Gordon, who doubts how far the distinctions are well founded as the basis of anatomical arrangement, admits, however, peculiarities which shall afterwards be mentioned.

Synovial membrane resembles serous membrane in so far as it is a thin, transparent substance, having one smooth free surface turned towards certain cavities of the body, and another connected by delicate cellular substance to the sides of these cavities, or to the parts contained in them. But it differs from serous membrane in the following circumstances. 1*st*, It possesses little vascularity in the healthy state; no blood-vessels are almost ever seen in it after death, nor can they be made to receive the finest injection. 2*d*, Its lymphatics are quite incapable of demonstration. 3*d*, Very delicate fibres, like those of cellular substance, or like the finest filaments of tendon, are distinctly seen in it after slight maceration. 4*th*, It is considerably less strong than serous membrane. On these grounds, therefore, synovial membrane is to be anatomically distinguished from serous membrane.

The synovial membrane, as described above, is found not only in each of the moveable articulations, but in those sheaths in which tendons are lodged, and in which they undergo a considerable extent of motion, and in certain situations in the subcutaneous filamentous tissue.

The distribution of the synovial membranes is much the same in all these situations. They are known to line the ligamentous apparatus of each joint, capsular and funicular; and they are also continued over the cartilaginous extremities of the bones of which the articulation consists. This continuation, which was originally maintained by Nesbitt, Bonn, and William Hunter, and was demonstrated by various facts by Bichat, was afterwards questioned by Gordon and Magendie, the former of whom especially thinks it unsusceptible of anatomical proof. The cartilaginous synovial membrane is certainly not so easily demonstrable as the capsular, for the same reason which I have already assigned regarding the difficulty of isolating the arachnoid of the *dura mater*, the capsular pericardium, the ovarian peritonæum, and the serous covering of the *tunica albuginea*,—the want of filamentous tissue.

The presence of synovial membrane in the articular cartilage is nevertheless established by sundry facts. 1*st*, If a portion of articular cartilage be divided obliquely, and examined by a good glass, it is not difficult to recognize at one extremity of the section a thin pellicle, differing widely in aspect, colour, and structure, from the bluish-white appearance of the cartilage. 2*d*, If the free surface of the cartilage be scraped gently, it is possible to detach thin shavings, which are also distinct from cartilage in their appearance. 3*d*, The free surface of the cartilage is totally different from the attached surface, or from a section of its substance, and derives its peculiar smooth polished appearance from a very thin transparent pellicle uniformly spread over it. 4*th*, If articular cartilage be immersed in boiling water, this thin pellicle becomes opaque, while the cartilage is little changed. 5*th*, Immersion in nitric or muriatic acid, which detaches the cartilage from the bone, gives this surface a cracked appearance, which is not seen in the attached surface, and which is probably to be ascribed to irregular contraction of two different animal substances. 6*th*, The existence of this cartilaginous synovial membrane is demonstrated by the morbid process with which the tissue is liable to be affected. Upon the whole, therefore, I believe little doubt can be entertained, that the representation of their course, as given originally by Nesbitt, Bonn, and Hunter, is well founded.

The same views may be applied to the synovial linings of the tendinous sheaths, which are equally to be viewed as shut sacs.

Attached to the free surface of each synovial membrane is a peculiar fringe-like substance, which was long supposed to be an apparatus of glands (glands of Havers) for secreting synovial fluid. It is now known that these fringes are merely puckered folds of synovial membrane, and that, although synovia is abundantly secreted by them, this depends merely on the great extent of surface which their puckered arrangement necessarily presents. This arrangement is easily demonstrated by immersing an articulation containing the fringed processes in clear water, when they are unfolded

and made to float, and show their connections, figure, and terminations. They are analogous to the free processes of serous membranes, and like them are double, and contain adipose matter.

The synovial sheaths (*bursæ mucosæ*) are very numerous, and
are generally found in every tendon which is exposed to frequent
or extensive motion.

Though the fluid prepared by these membranes has been examined by Margueron, Fourcroy, John Davy, Orfila, Berzelius,
John, and other chemists, it cannot be said that very accurate results have been yet given of its chemical composition. It is said
to contain water, albumen, incoagulable matter, regarded as mucilaginous gelatine, a ropy matter, and salts of soda, lime, and some
uric acid.

SECTION II.

The diseases of synovial membrane are important.

§ 1. *Hymenarthritis.*—Inflammation is an occurrence not nnfre-
quent in the synovial tissue, and produces effects in many respects
similar to those which are observed in the serous membranes.
Every example of diseased joint, there is reason to believe, commences with inflammation, acute or chronic, of the synovial membrane.   Of this process the anatomical characters are, injection of
the membrane, which sometimes becomes very red with numerous
vessels, and occasionally traversed by crimson or brown spots and
patches, dulness of its surface, opacity, thickening to a considerable
extent, and some degree of pulpiness.   The effects of the process
are effusion of fluid, sometimes serous, sometimes ichorous or vitiated *synovia*, more especially tinged with blood, occasionally sero-
albuminous fluid, which undergoes partial coagulation, and leaves
the cavity distended with a thin sero-purulent liquid.   In other
instances, complete purulent matter, with curdy or albuminous
flakes, are the result of synovial inflammation.

If it fail to terminate in resolution, the fluid effusion in the synovial sac constitutes the simplest of those multiform affections known
under the name of white swelling ; (*hydarthrus.*)   When this is not
abundant, the fluid part is absorbed, and the coagulable matter
may contract adhesion to the free surface of the membrane.   This
is the origin of that species of *ankylosis*, sometimes general and
complete, sometimes partial and imperfect, in which the articular

synovial membrane is found united by *bridles* or ligaments of false membrane.

When sero-purulent or purulent matter is effused into a synovial cavity, especially where the inflammation fails to be resolved, or passes into the chronic state, ulceration of the capsule and the interligamentous tissue is liable to take place, and the ichorous or sero-purulent fluid is discharged by one or more openings through the skin.

In more advanced and chronic states, the synovial membrane often becomes thick, pulpy, and vascular, granular or villous on its surface, and is at length destroyed by ulceration. In some joints, this process is an immediate effect of inflammation, the synovial covering being gradually perforated in numerous points at which the subjacent cartilage is exposed, and then undergoes erosion. Though this process may occur in any joint, the researches of Sir B. Brodie show that it is most frequent in the knee, in which the destruction it occasions is often very great. A disease of this kind I have several times seen remove every particle of cartilage from the articulating extremities, and expose the cancellated structure of the bone. This process is attended with extreme pain and suffering to the patient, more particularly aggravated during the night. The same process takes place in the elbow-joint, but here it often forms fistulous abscesses of the extra-capsular cellular tissue. In the articular processes of the vertebræ, I have seen it often give rise to disease of these bones, and finally terminate in ankylosis, with destruction of the processes, and considerable lateral curvature of the spine.

Inflammation of the articular synovial sacs affects not only the cartilages and bones, but the ligaments, capsular and funicular. Its transition to these textures, which is easy and direct, induces thickening and induration of the ligament, in consequence of effusion of lymph between its fibres and interstices. After some time the action extends to the extra-articular filamentous tissue, which is then injected by jelly-like fluid, sometimes colourless or pale red, at other times reddish or brown. At the same time, this filamentous tissue acquires a granular character and some induration. These several changes, which give rise to swelling round the joint more or less diffuse, constitute one of the most frequent forms of white-swelling. Suppuration may take place, as in the last instance, followed by fistulous openings.

§ 2. *Velvet-like Degeneration.*—I have already mentioned the granular and villous state of the synovial membrane. It is not easy to say whether the change next to be noticed is a more advanced stage of this state, or is to be viewed as a separate organic affection.

Synovial membrane is liable to a peculiar form of degeneration, in which the membrane becomes thick, soft, and villous, not unlike a piece of coarse velvet. The change is evidently in the organization of the membrane, which is entirely destroyed. The surface is red or brown, and no trace of the original structure is left.

This is one of the most unmanageable forms of diseased joint. It may take place in any joint, but is most common in the knee-joint, the hip-joint, and the elbow-joint.

It appears to be attended with chronic inflammation of the synovial membrane, and may probably be the effect of a peculiar form of that process. It seems, nevertheless, by its characters and tendency, to arrange itself rather with the class of organic changes.

Its approach is generally slow but steady, and it is attended with deep-seated pain in the joint, aggravated by motion. It gives rise to general swelling, often with the effusion of some fluid within the synovial cavity. The cellular tissue outside the capsule also becomes diseased, swelling, and being sometimes affected by secondary inflammation and the formation of abscesses.

This disease takes place principally in those reputed of strumous habit; and its presence causes hectic fever, wasting, and debility.

§ 3. *Thecal Inflammation.*—In the synovial sheaths of tendons, inflammation produces effects not dissimilar. The most marked instance of this process is observed in synovial or thecal whitloe, *paronychia thecalis,* in which inflammation of the synovial membrane, I have elsewhere shown, from the anatomical peculiarities of these sacs, not only causes death of the contained tendon, but, by passing to the periosteum, may induce caries of the phalanges.* In other parts of the body, these sheaths are not very liable to inflame, unless in consequence of external injury. From this cause I have more than once witnessed severe inflammation terminating in effusion of purulent fluid in the synovial sheath, between the tendon of the *glutæus maximus* and the head of the trochanter. After incision, however, it terminated favourably, without appearing to impair the motions of the tendon.

* Observations, Pathological and Practical, on Whitloe. By David Craigie, M. D. Edinburgh Medical and Surgical Journal, Vol. xxix. p. 255. Edinburgh, 1828.

§ 4. *Ganglia.*—A milder form of inflammation is occasionally seen in these sheaths, terminating in effusion of semitransparent, viscid, glairy fluid, like white of egg. This effusion causes an oblong prominent hemispheroidal swelling, tense, elastic, and communicating a sense of fluctuation, which has been long distinguished by the names of *hygroma* and *ganglion,* according to the degree in which it takes place. As I restrict the former appellation to the serous cyst, there is no occasion for using two names to varieties of an affection the same in anatomical characters. Ganglion is subcutaneous or tendinous, according to its situation in the subcutaneous or tendinous synovial sacs.

§ 5. *Arthragra.*—During gout the synovial sacs, both articular and tendinous, are the seat of an inflammatory process which terminates in the secretion of synovial fluid loaded with urate of soda.

§ 6. *The Synovial Membranes in Rheumatism.*—Though rheumatism, as affecting the aponeurotic sheaths and membranes, has already been under consideration, it does not, however, confine its action to these tissues. From them it may either spread by contiguity, as already explained, to the articular capsules and the synovial membranes, or it may affect the latter tissues at once. It is then usually denominated articular rheumatism. This takes place both in the acute, in the subacute, and in the chronic forms of the disease. In the two latter, however, rheumatic action produces effects of a serious and unmanageable character.

The mode of the approach of this affection is in general the following.

Sometimes after a slight attack of fascial rheumatism, in the loins, the back of the neck, or one or more of the joints, sometimes without this preliminary circumstance, one joint is attacked with a feeling of stiffness, fulness, as if there were something within it, and dull obtuse uneasiness. These sensations are relieved while the joint is in motion, but become worse when it is at rest; and, always after resting, the sense of fulness and stiffness is aggravated, until it amounts to difficult mobility of the joint.

. Swelling does not appear at first, but always comes on after some time. The joint is then enlarged, elastic, full, and rounded; the articular angles being lost in the swelling; and when examined it is manifest that a fluid is contained within the synovial membrane.

At the same time, it must be observed, that in articular rheumatism, the seat of swelling may be twofold. It may affect the periarthric or extra-capsular cellular tissue, which is infiltrated with sero-albuminous fluid; or it may cause effusion within the capsule and synovial membrane. The former is the most favourable and least injurious. The latter, if chronic, is always a troublesome and sometimes a hurtful lesion.

As the disease proceeds, the stiffness and swelling increase, impeding greatly the mobility of the joint; preventing it either from being fully extended or easily inflected. Pain is also superadded, especially when the joint is moved; and if the joint be one used in supporting the person, as the knee-joint, the individual can no longer support himself without pain.

Pain, however, is not the worst symptom of this disorder. Stiffness, swelling, immovableness; and consequent lameness, are the usual results.

This disease may affect any joint; but it is most commonly seen in the elbow-joints, the knee-joints, the wrists, and the articulations of the fingers.

The pulse is not accelerated, nor are there always indications of fever. After some time, however, the urine evinces alkaline properties, and may deposit or contain ammoniaco-maguesian phosphate.

As stiffness and swelling increase, there is felt on moving the joint a grating sensation, and a rough grating sound may be heard, as if two rough surfaces were moving on each other. In this condition the disease may continue for months and even years.

Death does not often take place in the early stage, or in the course of this disease. In one case, nevertheless, a female who presented symptoms of it in one knee-joint, which had been lasting for many weeks, if not two months or more, was attacked with symptoms of *delirium tremens* and died. The affected knee-joint, which was semibent, was examined, and the synovial membrane was found of a bright scarlet-red colour, with numerous blood-vessels, a little roughened with deposits of blood and lymph, thickened, and at one part it appeared to be wearing away by a species of absorption. This, however, was not ulceration.

The state of the articular cavity and surfaces in cases of long duration, is the following.

At first when the joint is stiff and slightly swelled, sero-albuminous fluid is moderately effused. Afterwards, as the joint is moved, it is effused more copiously. This fluid contains much urate of soda, which is separated and coats the membrane. According to some it also contains lime, which is deposited as a carbonate on the membrane. But whatever be the matter which it contains, the lymph so deposited renders the surface of the membrane rough; limits and circumscribes the mobility of the joint; and, in consequence of the motion to which it is subjected, it becomes hard and polished like porcelain or ground ivory; and in this state forms a sort of imperfect substitute for the synovial membrane.

Some have asserted that in this disease the synovial membrane is removed by absorption and ulceration, and the cartilages are ulcerated. This may occur in extreme cases. But it is not necessary to the disease or its effects; and the most common result is limited mobility of the joint with the eburneoid deposit or degeneration. It is for this reason that the joint so incrusted has been said by foreign authors to be affected with *usure* or friction wearing.

The margins of the articular surfaces, at the attachment of the membranes, present deposits of earthy matter irregularly nodulated, or tuberculated, which are usually termed *exostoses.* They are commonly swellings consisting of phosphate and carbonate of lime. Occasionally the *periosteum,* near the articular extremities in this disease becomes thickened and penetrated with the same material.

On the tendency of this form of rheumatism to affect internal organs, and thereby to influence the duration of life, different opinions are entertained by different authors. In some instances, individuals have lived long with it; in other instances it has suddenly proved fatal by affecting the brain. In all instances it impairs health, and is an indication of feeble digestion, imperfect assimilation, and an unsound state of the circulating fluid.

The nature of this malady is not well known. Some call it articular, capsular, and synovial rheumatism; others refer it to the head of gout; others again term it rheumatic gout. In extreme cases, it has been known to produce ankylosis of all the joints; and in the Museum of the College of Surgeons of Dublin is preserved the skeleton of a person, who was in this manner transformed into an inflexible body.

On the circumstances acting as causes of this disease, the opinions and testimony of physicians are not less discordant than on its nature. By some it is represented as taking place chiefly in those in whom the brain is overworked, and who are much exposed to causes of mental anxiety. This may be the fact in a certain class of cases. But the disease is observed in those, in whom the brain is little or not at all subjected to exertion; and conversely it does not take place in all persons, in whom the brain is much exerted, or in proportion to that exertion. It is observed as much in the temperate and regular as in those of opposite habits ; indeed it almost never appears in persons who live freely. It is greatly more common in females than in males ; and at Buxton and Bath especially, to which patients affected with it resort, the proportion of females to males varies from 5 to 1 to 5 to 2. On the other hand, however, the disease is generally more severe and obstinate in males than in females. It seems to affect the labouring classes and those engaged in corporeal exertion rather in a greater degree than the sedentary.

This disease, when affecting the joints of the hands and fingers, is liable to produce not only *ankylosis* of the joints, but great deformity. The ends of the bones are enlarged, and irregularly tuberculated and knotty. Some of the phalanges are bent forcibly and immovably into the palm of the hand. Others stand out equally immovably, and do not admit of inflection. Others are twisted and contorted ; so that the hand and fingers are of little use. The whole hand then not unfrequently is so deformed as to resemble the root of the parsnip. This is the disease described by Heberden, and afterwards by Haygarth, under the name of Nodosity of the joints.

§ 7. *Purulent collections within the synovial membranes. Arthropyema after phlebitis.*—Though purulent matter may be collected within any of the synovial membranes, in consequence of common inflammation of these membranes, the species of suppuration or purulent collection to which I here advert, is peculiar in taking place after inflammation of the inner coat of a vein or veins. I have already shown that, though venous inflammation often proves immediately fatal, yet instances occur in which the mere venous inflammation does not terminate in death. In this class of cases other processes take place which must be regarded as the consequences of venous inflammation. To several of these, as purulent collections within the serous membranes and extensive suppurations in the cellular and adipose tissue, I have already adverted. Besides these, however, purulent matter is liable to be formed within the synovial membrane of a joint, and to be followed by all the destructive consequences attending suppuration within such a cavity.

This lesion has been supposed to be confined to females with uterine *phlebitis ;* and in them it is perhaps more frequent than in others. I have seen it, however, take place after inflammation of the brachial veins, succeeding to the operation of venesection ; and give rise to

3

all the exquisite effects of this destroying process. In a patient under my care, in whom this accident was followed by secondary effects, the right shoulder-joint first and the knee-joint afterwards, became affected with pain, heat, swelling, and finally, indications of the presence of fluid. The shoulder-joint got better, under the use of various means. But the knee continued swelled, immovable, with much pain, and giving indications of matter in its interior. Death took place soon after. The interior of the synovial membrane of the knee-joint was filled with purulent matter and coagulable lymph, the latter adhering to the membrane in masses, and connecting the opposing and corresponding parts of the membrane. The purulent matter was thick, opaque, yellow well formed matter. After removing most of it, the synovial membrane was brought into view, much reddened and vascular, especially at the marginal connections to the bones and enclosing capsule, where also it was thickened. Over the head of the *tibia* and the corresponding parts of the femoral condyles, it had begun to be destroyed by ulceration; and in several points the cartilage was exposed. At the attached margins also were irregular tubercular bony masses; but it was doubtful whether these were the effects of the recent disease or of some previous orgasm.

It has been maintained by some, that these purulent collections within the joints after venous inflammation are the results of the transport or conveyance of purulent matter by the veins into the interior of the joint. Such they may be in certain cases. But in the present instance, and in others of the same kind, which I have observed, the collection was preceded and followed by all the usual symptoms and effects of inflammation; and I regard the lesion as an instance of inflammation affecting the synovial membrane of the knee-joint, in consequence of previous inflammation of a venous trunk.

§ 8. Hemorrhage of the synovial membranes is not very common, but has nevertheless been observed. M. Pitet, in particular, saw in the knee-joint a collection of blood, which he thinks was exhaled from the articular synovial membrane.* When this effusion does take place, it is an effect of previous injection of the capillaries of the sac. I have often thought that some of the bloody abscesses met with occasionally in the cellular tissue and in the neighbourhood of tendons, depended on synovial sacs in which hemorrhage had followed chronic inflammation. This probably is the origin of

* Bulletin de la Société de Med. p. 222.

the 17th case of Palletta, in which a bloody tumour, containing pure blood, was found in the left ham.* The incision of these tumours is always followed by extensive and malignant, often fatal inflammation of the interior surface of the cyst.

§ 9. *Tyroma.*—Synovial membrane is said to be liable to tubercular deposition. No doubt can be entertained of the frequency of albuminous deposits; and I believe tubercles have been seen in the coxo-femoral synovial membrane in disease of that joint. This, however, I have not had an opportunity of verifying.

§ 10. *Cartilage.*—In some instances, cartilaginous bodies are observed to adhere by a narrow peduncle to the free surface of the synovial membranes. This, though most frequently observed in the femoro-tibial articulation, is certainly not peculiar to it. These bodies may be either generated by morbid action of the synovial tissue, or may be portions of cartilage or fibro-cartilage broken accidentally from some part of the articular apparatus, and suffered again to contract adhesion to the synovial membrane by the inflammation which their presence induces.

§ 11. *Hematoid fungus,* or cerebriform degeneration, is a disease which often originates in the interior of joints. The circumstances under which this begins render it difficult to ascertain the texture primarily affected. It is, nevertheless, most probable that it is chiefly the synovial membrane in which this tumour commences. In the cases of the disease which have been inspected before much destruction has taken place, the articular extremities of one or both bones have presented large fungous spongy masses of matter like brain, and well supplied with blood-vessels; and it has been impracticable to recognize any trace of synovial membrane or cartilage. The analogy between the serous and synovial sacs in this respect is obvious.

The degeneration may take place in any joint, but affects commonly the shoulder-joint, the hip-joint, and the knee-joint.

§ 12. *Scirrho-carcinoma* appears not to originate in this tissue, but certainly affects it from collateral tissues. Some authors have, indeed, with singular vagueness, spoken of certain forms of white swelling or *fungus articuli,* as being a sort of cancerous disease. This, however, is only one of many errors which originate in the practice of applying a vague general epithet to many different morbid states.

* Exercitationes Pathologicæ, p. 207.

BOOK V.

CHAPTER I.

GLANDULAR TISSUE.   THE GLANDS.   THE GLANDULAR SYSTEM.

GLANDULÆ.   DRÜSEN.

SECTION I.

GENERAL CHARACTER OF GLANDS.

A gland may be defined to be an organ, or organized texture, consisting of blood-vessels and nerves; the blood-vessels very nume- rous, arranged in a particular manner, and communicating with a series of sacculated cavities, vesicles, or hollow tubes; intended for the purpose of receiving or preparing from the blood, or secreting, a substance of peculiar properties, either to be applied to some pur- pose within or without the economy, or to be conveyed entirely out of the system.

According to the terms of this definition, the denomination gland comprehends only the secreting or conglomerate glands, or those organs which are known to secrete some substance, generally liquid, and to deposit the same in cavities communicating with an emissary duct or ducts.

These are by various authors denominated perfect glands.

By imperfect glands the same authors understand organs with apparent glandular structure, but without visible secreting appa- ratus, secreted product, or excretory duct, as the thymus gland in the infant, the thyroid gland, and according to some the spleen.   It is evident that the term imperfect gland is equivalent to that of no gland.

Some anatomists, guided by physiological and in a certain sense transcendental considerations, have proposed to add to the order of glands, the lungs, because they separate or secrete carbonaceous matter from the blood; and many have in this manner classed the lungs with the liver and the kidneys under the head of emunctory or excreting organs.

Others again have proposed to refer to the order of glands the ovaries of the female, because they are analogous to the *testes* of the male ; and they have regarded the *ova* as secreted or excreted products ; and the Fallopian tubes as excretory ducts. This view rests, it must be admitted, upon some analogy both anatomical and physiological. But it is enough to mention it here ; nor do I think it proper, in a work of this kind, to introduce views which may require further confirmation.

Under the glandular system I include the following organs; the lacrymal gland; the salivary glands, viz. the parotid, the sublingual, and the sabmaxillary glands; the liver and the pancreas; the kidneys; the *testes*, the prostate gland, and Cowper's glands in the male; and the *mammae* in the female; the sebaceous follicles of the skin, and the muciparous follicles of the mucous membranes.

On no subject in general anatomy has information been so void of precision and accuracy as on the structure of the glands. By several anatomists the structure has been believed to be the same in all ; and consequently, what was supposed to. be ascertained as to one has been applied indiscriminately to all. Little, indeed, was ascertained ; and few accurate facts were recorded. Sylvius and Steno, Glisson* and Wharton,† were the principal inquirers previous to the time of Malpighi ; and both the two latter did communicate some information. These anatomical results, however, were much influenced by various physiological notions on the nature of secretion ; and as the latter were often erroneous, the former were rarely in all points correct.

Malpighi, in 1661, taught that all glands consisted of an aggregation or collection of minute saccular organs, (*utriculi*), in which the blood-vessels were distributed, and which saccular organs he denominated sometimes small glands, (*glandulæ*), sometimes *acini*. *Acini* in the liver he represents to consist of simple glandules collected in clusters, which glandules are hollow membranous cavities. These *acini* are in shape hexagonal or polyhedral. The glandular bodies in the kidneys, on the other hand, are round or spherical like the ova of fishes ; but these *glandulæ* are in like manner hollow.‡

---

* Francisci Glissonii Anatomia Hepatis. 12mo. Londini, 1654.

† Thomæ Wharton Adenographia, seu Glandularum totius Corporis Descriptio. 8vo. Londini, 1656.

‡ Marcelli Malpighii Exercitationes Anatomicæ de Structura Viscerum ; nominatim, Hepatis, Cerebri Corticis, Renum, Lienis. cum Dissertatione de Polypo Cordis et Epistolis Duabus de Pulmonibus. apud Opera Omnia. Tomum Secundum. Folio. Londini, 1687.

Ruysch was confident that the final structure of all glandular organs consists in *fasciculi* of blood-vessels ramified to an infinite degree of minuteness. He admitted, indeed, in 1722, when eighty-five years of age, that sixty years previously he had taught the existence of *acini* or little glands with membranous cavities, according to the received opinion. Afterwards, however, by much observation in injection, he became convinced, that these *acini* are composed of blood-vessels only, and not of little hollow membranes with an outlet.* He allows, nevertheless, that the liver contains *acini* or *acinuli ;* but repeats his doctrine, that these are not small glands or hollow sacs, but very delicate pulpy vessels.†

Ferrein, in the middle of the 18th century, called in question both of these doctrines. He maintained that the liver and the cortical part of the kidney consist neither of blood-vessels nor of small glands, but of a peculiar substance formed by a wonderful collection of white cylindrical tubes variously folded, which, he contended, he demonstrated manifestly in the kidneys,—which he had seen in the liver and renal capsules, and which he believed he could make known in other glandular organs.‡

Haller has collected under the several heads of the pancreas, the liver, the kidneys, the *testes,* the *mamma,* and other glands, the results of the inquiries of different anatomists to his own time (1777.) In the liver he admits the existence of *acini,* and he adopts the view of Malpighi, representing them to consist of simple hollow glandules collected in clusters ; that these *acini* are hexagonal ; and are not an element but a mass of elements ; or, in short, that they are the lobules of the liver enclosed in cellular tissue.§

Each kidney he represents to consist of several little kidneys (*renculus*) ; each of which, again, consists of cortical or vascular and medullary or striated matter.‖

* Opusculum Anatomicum de Fabrica Glandularum in Corpore Humano, Continens Binas Epistolas, Quarum Prior est H. Boerhaave, super hac re, ad Friedericum Ruyschium; Altera F. Ruyschii ad H. Boerhaave, Qua priori respondetur. Amstelædami, 1721 et 1722. Apud Ruyschii Opera Omnia, Tomum iv. p. 71. Amstelædami, 1733, 4to.

† " Acini ibi (in hepate) manifesti semper sunt agniti a me ; sed ego tantum dixi, quod non sunt folliculi membranacei cavi cum emissario, sed quod sint vascula pulposa tenerrima. Epistola, p. 75.

‡ Observations sur la Structure des Glandes, et part. des Reins, et du Foi. Memoires de l'Academie Royale des Sciences. Paris, a. 1749. Hist. p. 92. Mem. p. 489.

§ Elementa Physiologiæ, Lib. xxvi. Sect. I. § xxvi. xxvii.

‖ Elementa, Lib. xxvi. Sect. I. § vii. and viii.

In 1788 Schumlanski published his dissertation on the structure of the kidney, and thereby directed attention to the arrangement both of the cortical or vascular part of these glands, and to that of the *tubuli Belliniani* or excreting ducts. He did not, however, elucidate much the intimate structure of the organ.*

The facts and statements given by Haller were very generally repeated by Soemmering and other anatomists. Bichat alone rejected many without substituting others in their place, and maintained that whatever could not be sensibly demonstrated was to be regarded as uncertain and undeserving attention.

Various inquirers continued to investigate this department of anatomy, with different degrees of success, during the first third of the 19th century. In 1818 Eysenhardt published his dissertation on the structure of the kidneys, in which, with various errors, he gave correct views of the *corpora Malpighiana.*† In 1819 Doellinger, in a dissertation on secretion, adduced several curious facts regarding the arrangement of arteries in several glands.‡ These were followed by the essays of Rathke and Huschke on the structure of the kidneys, the observations of Weber on the salivary glands, and those of Baer on the liver. The researches of all these inquirers, however, though most valuable, have been in a great degree eclipsed by the elaborate commentary on the glands, published in 1830, by John Muller, first of Bonn and afterwards of Berlin, who has, with great skill and much personal research, elucidated the structure of all the glands in a systematic manner, combining the researches of all his predecessors. Since the date of the monograph of Muller, various facts of considerable value, chiefly microscopical, have been added by subsequent observers.

In the following account I shall study to combine the results obtained by all these inquirers.

Muller distinguishes all the glands of the animal body into nine orders, in the following manner.—

I. GLANDS OF THE FIRST AND MOST SIMPLE ORDER.

1. CRYPTS or CELLS. a. Solitary crypts of the mucous membranes. b. Aggregated, agminated, or agglutinated crypts, as the glands of Peyer in the intestines.

* F. Schumlansky Dissertatio de Structura Renum. 8vo. Argentorati, 1788.

† Carol. Guilelm. Eysenhardt de structura Renum, Observationes microscopicæ cum Tab. aen. 4 Maj. Berolini, 1818.

‡ Was ist Absonderung und wie geschieht sie. Wurzburg, 1819.

2. FOLLICLES or PEDUNCULATED VESICLES. a. Solitary, as those of the skin. b. Associated, as the aggregated follicles in the auricular glands of amphibious animals.

3. ELONGATED BLADDERS, (UTRICULI ELONGATI,) sacs, or CÆCA. This glandular apparatus consists in the eversion of a simple membrane, which is prolonged without contraction or terminal enlargement.

These are either, a. simple *intestinula*, occurring in the mucous membranes, or b. aggregated *intestinula*, like the Meibomian glands of mammalia, and the glands of the stomach of birds.

4. TUBULI or BLIND SACS ; (CÆCA.)

These are either, a. solitary TUBULES, as the secretory organs of several insects ; or b. Aggregated TUBULES, as the glands of the oviducts of the ray and shark, consisting of parallel TUBULI, the œsophageal glands in certain birds, and the pyloric appendages of some fishes.

II. GLANDS OF THE SECOND ORDER. COMPOUND CRYPTS. FOLLICLES. INTESTINULES. COMPOUND TUBULES.

1. COMPOUND CRYPTS, or COMPOUND CELLS, in which several crypts are united.

    a. Berry-like crypts, as in the anal glands of the hyena.

    b. Bladders with cells, (CRYPTÆ LOCULATÆ,) as in the præputial glands of the dormouse.

    c. Tubules with internal cells, as the salivary glands of some insects.

    d. Flower-like crypts, or crypts united as flowers, as in the testicles of insects.

2. COMPOUND FOLLICLES, or COMPOUND PEDUNCULATED VESICLES. Follicles united in various modes.

3. COMPOUND CÆCA. Intestinal *cæca* united in various modes.

4. TUBULI COMPOSITI. Tubules or hollow cylinders united in various modes.

III. GLANDS OF THE THIRD ORDER ; COMPOUND CELLS, FOLLICLES, INTESTINULES. *Compound Tubules* united so as to form one glandular sac.

IV. GLANDS OF THE FOURTH ORDER. GLANDS COMPOSED OF SPONGY CELLULAR TEXTURE, variously arranged ; sometimes in the form of tubules, sometimes of cells, sometimes of glandular cells inclosed within membranous partitions (*septa.*)

V. GLANDS OF THE FIFTH ORDER. LOBULATED GLANDS COMPOSED OF AGGREGATIONS OF SMALL INTESTINAL CÆCA.

1. A gland composed of clusters of small intestinal cæca arranged in lobules, as the pancreas of the tunny.

2. A gland composed of blind branching *intestinula*, arranged like leaves in lobules; for instance, the prostatic glands and Cowper's glands in the hedgehog.

3. A gland composed of branched *intestinula cæca* irregularly arranged.

VI. GLANDS OF THE SIXTH ORDER. BRANCHED EXCRETORY DUCTS INCLOSED FROM THEIR ORIGIN TO THEIR TERMINATION BY ELEMENTARY PARTICLES.

This arrangement, which resembles efflorescence, is not terminal, but is similar to the *protracted efflorescence* of botanical terminology. Of this examples are found in the liver of the *crustacea*, the lacrymal gland of the tortoise, and the lacrymal gland of birds.

VII. GLANDS OF THE SEVENTH ORDER. COMPOUND RAMIFICATION IN A LOBULATED GLAND, WITH TRUNKS OF EXCRETORY DUCTS CONTINUOUS AND ENTIRE AMONG LATERAL BRANCHES AND VESICULAR ENDS OF ULTIMATE DUCTS.

The trunk of the excretory duct, entire and continuous, is not divided into branches, but sends out laterally small branches, which are also continued entire and without interruption by lateral ramification. The result of this arrangement is great, small, and very small lobules; because each trunk with lateral branches makes a large lobe; branches with lateral shoots make small lobes of the second order; and from the twigs, and their attached portions the smallest lobules arise. This origin of the lobules is shown from the history of the development of the embryo.

To this mode of arrangement belong the salivary glands, the pancreas, the *mammæ*, and the lacrymal gland of many MAMMALIA.

VIII. GLANDS OF THE EIGHTH ORDER. COMPOUND RAMIFICATIONS IN GLANDS NOT LOBULATED WITH DIVISION OF TRUNKS INTO IRREGULAR BRANCHES, WITH SHORT OR TERMINAL VESI-

CULAR TWIGS, (as in the pancreas of birds; and in the liver of the embryo of birds and mammalia.)

IX. GLANDS OF THE NINTH ORDER.   CONSISTING OF SHORT TUBULES AND VESSELS, NOT RAMIFIED.

The elements of the glands in this order are tubules long and very long; of equal diameter to their short ends; either straight or serpentine. At the origin they are often furcated; after that simple without giving branches. They appear under six forms.

1. From a lateral excretory duct arise bundles of tubules, as in the kidneys of many fishes, and batrachoid animals, and in the *testes* of fishes. The tubules proceed either parallel towards the opposite margin, as in the kidneys of the petromyzon and frogs, and the *testes* of fishes; or they wind tortuous and serpentine, as in the kidneys of the ray family and serpents.

2. Bundles of parallel tubules everywhere issue from branching excretory ducts. Such are the kidneys of the crocodile and tortoise.

3. An excretory duct divided into very long uniform serpentine vessels; as the seminiferous canals of the higher animals, and the prostate glands of the hedgehog.

4. Tubules forked and fasciculated like rays or wheel-spokes, proceeding from an excretory duct; as in the *testes* of frogs and cuttle-fish.

5. Very long vessels; pinnatifid at apex; closed; rising in bundles from a branched excretory duct; as in the kidneys of birds.

6. Very long vessels rising in bundles, at first bifurcated, then pursuing a serpentine course, without branches. The kidneys of the mammalia and man. The proportion between the ureter and the uriniferous ducts varies in three modes.

 a. The ureter is continued to branches; from these arise bundles of uriniferous ducts arranged in separate lobules, externally serpentine, as is seen in the kidneys of the cetacea.

 b. One single ureter passes into a pelvis and *calyces*, which receive the bundles of the uriniferous ducts. These bundles are evolved in the lobated kidney, externally serpentine; but the lobules are not altogether separated, as in the kidneys of several mammalia.

 c. In the kidneys of the rest, even the superficial lobes of the kidneys disappear.

To explain this numerous list of the different forms of glandular structure, it is necessary first to premise certain general facts illustrating the essential characters of glandular organs, and then to attend to the following statements, in which a summary is given of the result of all the inquiries.

The simplest idea of a gland is to be found in such organs as the pyloric appendages of fishes, the pancreas of certain fishes, as the sturgeon, and the kidneys of several of the fishes.

In the first case, that of the pyloric appendages, (*appendices pyloricæ*), which are well seen in the cod and haddock, a great number of cylindrical canals or tubes with closed ends hanging free in the abdominal cavity, and with open ends communicating with the bowel are attached to the pylorus or duodenum. The number of these canals or tubes varies from 50 to 80, 150, or 200 in different genera. They are membranous, and open, as already stated, into the interior either of the *pylorus* or *duodenum*.

These bodies are understood to perform the function of secreting glands. Their inner surface, which is continuous with the mucous surface of the intestine, is believed to secrete a fluid necessary to the proper performance of digestion and solution of the alimentary mass. Part of the food seems to enter them, and after being subjected to the action of this fluid, to be returned into the intestine ; probably allowing other portions in succession to undergo the same action.

This arrangement may be regarded as presenting that of a tubular gland.

The pancreas or pancreatoid organ of the sturgeon is an organ in external appearance and consistence somewhat different, but in internal arrangement similar.

Externally it is a thick fleshy firm mass, triangular, or pentahedral rather, in shape, with one apex hanging free into the abdominal cavity, and with the base attached to the *duodenum*. The colour of the pancreatoid organ is greenish-black, with pansy purple, interspersed with whitish or whitish-gray spots. Its parietes vary in thickness, according to the size of the animal, from half an inch to one inch or one inch and a half.

This organ is attached to the duodenum near its pyloric end ; and with this its cavities communicate by means of a large orifice placed in a recess opposite to the pyloric opening. This orifice is circular or slightly elliptical, sufficiently large to admit the tip of the finger, and even more in large animals.

This large orifice speedily diverges into several similar orifices ; and, when these are exposed by sections, they are observed to terminate in spherical and spheroidal cavities, in which are similar orifices leading to similar cavities,—all communicating in the same manner with each other. The size and capacity of these cavities varies according to the size of the animal. Thus in a sturgeon six feet long they are in general about one inch or more in diameter. In smaller animals they are not more than half an inch ; and in large individuals they are larger. These dimensions, nevertheless, it is difficult to specify ; as their accuracy depends much on the shape of the cavities, which is not exactly spherical, but only irregularly so.

The pancreatoid organ, therefore, of the sturgeon consists of a series of rounded cavities communicating with each other, and with the *duodenum* by one general large orifice. The whole of these cavities are lined by a membrane quite similar to that which forms the inner lining of the duodenum ; and for a particular description of which I refer to another work.*

The surface of this inner membrane evidently secretes a liquid which is applied to the alimentary mass in a peculiar manner. The liquid does not flow by the outlet into the duodenum. But the alimentary mass, after it has been received from the stomach, is conveyed in successive portions into the communicating cells of the pancreas ; there the secreted liquid is effused on them ; and after they have undergone its proper action they are expelled ; and other portions of the alimentary mass are introduced in order that they may be impregnated with pancreatic fluid in like manner.

In all the specimens of the sturgeon which I have examined, I have always found the pancreatoid cells quite filled with chyme or alimentary pulpy matter, evidently in a more advanced stage of digestion, than that contained in the stomach and pyloric end of the duodenum.

The arrangement is singular in this respect, that the chyme is conveyed into an organ to be subjected to the operation of its secreted product ; and after this, is not conveyed through the organ, for which there is no provision, but is withdrawn from its cells,

* On the Anatomical Peculiarities of the Sturgeon. (*Acipenser Sturio.*) By David Craigie, M. D., &c., Memoirs of the Wernerian Natural History Society. Vol. vi. p. 364. Edin. 1831.

and urged on its onward course through the rest of the intestinal canal. The chyme may nevertheless be said to make the circuit of the pancreatoid chambers.

Notwithstanding this arrangement, the pancreatoid organ is regarded by most anatomists as an example of a gland; and excepting the circumstance of the chyme being conveyed to its interior, instead of its secreted product being conveyed to the chyme, it may be regarded as presenting on the large scale, the structure and internal arrangement, which in other glands is so minute and delicate as to elude observation.

In short, the pancreatoid organ of the sturgeon may be regarded as an aggregation of glandular sacs or cells, communicating with each other, and the interior of which furnishes a liquid secreted from its blood-vessels, which are large and numerous.

There is, however, still one point on which information is wanting. This is, how do the blood-vessels terminate and communicate with this secreting surface? On this point no accurate information has been obtained.

The kidneys, or rather the urinary organs, of the sturgeon in like manner may be taken as organs illustrating what may be regarded as the most simple form of glandular structure.

The urinary organs of the sturgeon consist of two long tubular canals, placed on each side of the intestine with the spiral valve, and resting on the spinal column and its muscles, to which they are attached by cellular membrane. These organs resemble neither the kidneys, nor the ureters, nor the bladder of the MAMMALIA and BIRDS, but combine the characters of all these. Their parietes are thin and membranous, so as to seem like elongated bladders or *utriculi*. Their inner surface, which is red, smooth, and mucous, but not distinctly villous, presents a series of minute orifices not larger than pin heads. These orifices or pores correspond partly to the *infundibula*, partly to the uriniferous tubes of mammiferous animals. The lower extremities of these canals widen; and, suddenly contracting, terminate in one common outlet or vent, which opens on the surface behind that of the intestine at the anal fin.

These urinary organs, which in this manner represent at once kidneys, ureter, and bladder, and even urethra, are membranous *sacculi* or *utriculi*, which in this manner act as glandular surfaces, or secreting and excreting surfaces. The small pores are the outlets of the secreting portion; but around them the parts are so thin and membranous, that they may be justly regarded as the rudimental or essential portions of the kidneys.

Of the mode in which the blood-vessels communicate with these pores and their membranes, nothing is accurately known, except that the vessels ramified to an infinite degree of delicacy and minuteness terminate in the membrane.

Thus it appears that the most simple and elementary form of a gland is a hollow cylinder or tube communicating either directly with the surface of the body, or indirectly by opening on a mucous membrane; that the superior, internal, or upper end of this tube presents the form of a closed sac; that the shut end, nevertheless, communicates in different modes with the vascular system; or that branches and ramifications of the vascular system terminate on this closed end. It further will afterwards appear, that the forms which this arrangement and connection with the vascular system presents, may be very much varied.

Meanwhile, it is necessary to state here the general characters of every form of gland.

I. All glands, however much they may depart from the conformation of secreting vessels, nevertheless follow one common fixed law of formation, and present an uninterrupted series from the most simple unramified follicle, to the most complicated structure.

II. Between the secreting organs of Aspondylous animals and the glands of the higher classes no fixed distinction in truth exists. But simple follicles, and tubuliform secreting organs, and closed *intestinula* are repeated not only in animals of the higher classes, but pass by an unbroken series through the different classes of animals, gradually into conglomerate glands. Thus the *mammæ* of the CETACEA and *Ornithorhyncus*, the simple salivary glands of birds, the prostatic glands of several MAMMALIA, and the pancreas of several fishes are formed after the manner of small *cæca* or closed *intestinula*, as observation shows regarding the secreting organs of the CRUSTACEA and INSECTS.

III. All glands with a system of secreting ducts present internally a very large secreting surface. But the variety of forms in which the secreting surface is increased within small space, is innumerable. There is indeed boundless diversity and profuseness; yet there are in all glands certain common characters. The variety in the *testes* or seminiferous canals in insects is so great, as to resemble the profuseness of the forms presented by the vegetable kingdom. Yet of all glands it is a common character, that from the more full evolution of an excreting duct, they increase, in proportion as the canals terminated by closed ends are increased. The hypothesis of Malpighi, accordingly, on the structure of the glands, makes a nearer approach to the truth than that of other anatomists; and its correctness is confirmed beyond doubt, in all the forms of glands. Malpighi, however, was little acquainted with the elementary forms of glands, which he represented in all cases to be follicles and *acini*.

The objects which Malpighi considered to be follicles in the viscera, were bodies consisting of masses of much smaller particles, in which terminate the final twigs of the efferent ducts. Then, besides follicles, the variety of forms of closed sacs in which the secreting canals terminate is great; for they are either *utriculi*, or elongated tubular-shaped *intestinula*, or pinnatifid and paniculate canals ending in closed sacs, or canals everywhere equal in diameter, very long, serpentine, and not branched. This point, however, in which is placed the force of the hypothesis of Malpighi, is certain, that the small twigs of the efferent and secreting ducts are closed at their blind or shut ends in the cellular tissue of the glands.

This is the case with the *mammæ* of the mammalia, the salivary glands in various classes of animals, the pyloric appendages, and the parenchymatous pancreas of fishes, the biliferous ducts of the liver, the tubuli of the kidney, and the testicles.

IV. *Acini*, considered as glandular grains or hypothetical balls of blood-vessels, from which secreting vessels are supposed to proceed, are fictitious. There is no immediate and continuous passage of blood-vessels into efferent vessels either in *acini* or anywhere else. The system of secreting vessels is peculiar, distinct from the blood-vessels, terminating in closed extremities in all forms of glands.

V. *Acini*, therefore, are merely closed ends of secreting canals, or a branchy group of the same parts, that is vesicles, which may be perfectly filled with mercury, and in some glands inflated. Truly solid granules are seen only in the *testes* of a few fishes, the *testes* of which, without excretory duct, send granules into the abdominal cavity, from which they are conveyed by a proper orifice in the abdomen.

VI. The term *acinos* has been employed in different senses, at different periods, by different authors. The word *akinos, acinus,* and *acinum,* from the Greek αχινος and αχονος, was used by ancient writers to signify a grape-stone, the kernel of a pomegranate, or the grain or stone of any stone-fruit. By Glisson, Wharton, and Malpighi it was adopted to designate certain hypothetical parts of glandular structure, into which they thought that glandular structure might be finally resolved. This Malpighi studied to render more definite by saying, that in the liver *acini* were small elementary bodies, hexahedral or polyhedral, or even spherical in shape externally, but with an inner cavity, and thickish parenchymatous walls. These *acini* are further called, both by Malpighi and Boerhaave, one of his great defenders, *utriculi,* or membranous *sacculi.* These bodies Malpighi represents to be round and hollow in the kidneys.

To this view Malpighi probably, and Boerhaave certainly, was led by analogy between crypts and the ultimate elements of large conglomerate glands.

Ruysch, on the other hand, who admitted the existence of *acini* or *acinuli* in glands, maintained that they presented nothing in common with crypts, because they appear not like hollow membranes, and because they have no emissary canal. He further maintained that these *acini* are composed of the final extremities of blood-vessels, united so as to form globular or spherical bodies,[*] and he altogether denies cavity and emissary tube.

After the time of these anatomists, the word appears to have been used either without definite meaning, or in different senses. At one time and with one set of writers it means a clustered structure; (*structura racemosa*); with another it is used to designate a granular structure, or a substance composed of minute granules.

As, however, many glands contain none of this acinated or granular structure, Muller in a great degree renounces the term; and preferably employs the name of ELEMENTARY PARTICLES OF GLANDS, or ENDS OR ROOTS OF SECRETING DUCTS; because under these names may be included the several denominations of vesicles, *utriculi,* tubules, follicles, cells, and canals, straight and serpentine, of which glands consist.

Weber applies the term *acini* to the shut ends of the excretory

* F. Ruyschii Epistola Anatomica de Structura Glandularum, ad H. Boerhaave, p. 69, 70, Op. Om. Tom. IV.

ducts, which are arranged according to their cellular projection ; and also to the primary lobules or their *apices*.

Henle, like Muller, avoids the use of this term *acini*, by which he thinks Malpighi meant the closed ends of excretory ducts, and which probably were primary lobules.*

The most recent authorities withhold the term for the glandular *vesiculæ*. Further, the solid lobules of the liver, and especially the cells of which they consist, are named *acini*.

VII. The smallest blood-vessels pass not directly into glandular parts and ends of secreting ducts ; but the blood-vessels are distributed to the *parietes* of secreting canals exactly as to any other secreting membrane. They do not enter by open ends into the cells of these canals; but they pass between the elementary particles of the glands, and upon these terminate by delicate networks into the small veins. This passage of blood between the elongated *acini* of the liver from one order of blood-vessels into another, may be distinctly seen in the living larvæ of the triton.

VIII. The system of blood-vessels, therefore, in every glandular organ is confined within certain definite limits, by means of an intermediate reticular connection of minute vessels interposed between the arteries and veins.

IX. Of the connection between lymphatic vessels with the excretory ducts in some glands, which has been already noticed under its proper head, Muller is of opinion that it is not proved by the alleged injection ; and that it is entirely accidental.

X. Every system of secreting ducts, without any continuous communication with blood-vessels, bounded and closed by certain shut ends, is to be viewed as an efflorescence or ramification of the excretory duct; because it is proved, that in the embryo it grows or sprouts, as it were, from an excretory duct, at first unbranched.

XI. The ramifications of the blood-vessels accompany the efflorescence of the secreting canals, and with peripheral reticular vessels wind on the elementary parts, and terminations of the secreting canals. As a follicle or *intestinula* rise from the uniform membrane, and send out repeatedly several *utriculi* and canals, so on the efflorescing canals the vascular network advances, itself rising from the uniform membrane. These facts are shown in the phenomena of the incubated egg.

* Allgemeine Anatomie. Lehre von den Mischungs-und Formbestandtheilen des Menschlichen Korpers. Von J. Henle. Leipzig, 1841. Seite 922.
4

XII. While canals, which always in insects and sometimes in the higher animals are observed free, are progressively increased by the new efflorescence, and mutually approximated, connected by blood-vessels,—from these free canals gradually a species of parenchyma arises.

XIII. The most delicate reticulate blood-vessels are still much smaller than the most slender branches of· the secreting canals, and their terminations in the largest glandular viscera. The elemen. tary parts of glands, therefore, though small, are nevertheless al. ways so capacious that they are enclosed and connected by the smallest reticulated blood-vessels. The cortical uriniferous canals are much larger than the smallest blood-vessels in all classes of animals. In the salivary glands of the mammalia and man, the most delicate blood-vessels are many times smaller than the *acini* of the salivary terminal *vesiculæ*. The same is true of the pancreas. The free ends of the salivary ducts in the hamster differ greatly from the very smallest blood-vessels. The closed ends of the bili. ferous ducts in the embryos of birds, amphibia, and mammalia are. much larger than the smallest blood-vessels.

To show the amount of this relation of majority of the secreting ducts to the blood-vessels, and that of the relation of minority of the blood-vessels to the secreting ducts, Muller gives the respective diameters of these two orders of tubes as determined by himself by the micrometer. From these measurements a few examples are here selected.

	Paris inch.
The smallest capillary blood-vessels, (Weber,) .	0.00025 — 0.00050
The same in kidney, (Muller,) .	0.00037 — 0.00058
The same in human iris, . . .	0.00037 — 0.00057
The same in human ciliary processes,	0.00053
Smallest pulmonary cells in man, (Weber,) .	0.00441 — 0.01333
Cylindriform *intestinula* in the lungs of embryo birds,	0.00474
Elementary vesicles of mammæ of suckling hedgehog, .	0.00712 — 0.00928
Terminal cells in salivary ducts of goose filled with mercury,	0.00260
Terminal cells of salivary ducts of parotid in man filled with mercury, . . .	0.00082
Cells of lacrymal gland of goose filled with mercury, .	0.00327
Cells of pancreas of goose filled with mercury, .	0.00137 — 0.00297
Elements of lacrymal gland of *Testudo mydas* .	0.00194
Cells of Harderian gland of hare filled with mercury,	0.00776
Terminal vesicles of biliferous ducts of snail, (*Helix pomatia*)	0.00565
Free terminal twigs of bile-ducts in embryos of birds, .	0.00172
Intestinula of Wolffian body in embryo of bird, .	0.00377
The same from another embryo, . .	0.00300

	Paris inch.	
Uriniferous ducts of Petromyzon, . .	0.00324	
Uriniferous ducts from kidney of *Torpedo Marmorata*, .	0.00469	
Uriniferous ducts from kidney of owl injected from ureter (under air-pump,) . . .	0.00174	
Cortical uriniferous ducts from kidey of squirrel, .	0.00174	
Serpentine cortical uriniferous ducts from kidney of horse injected from ureter, (under air-pump,) . .	0.00137 — 0.20182	
Medullary uriniferous ducts from kidney of horse injected from ureter, the largest near the papillæ, . .	0.01805	
The same from the central medullary matter, .	0.00489	
The same cortical seen in section of kidney, .	0.00140 — 0.00188	
Corpuscula Malpighiana from human kidney, (Muller,)	0.00700	
The same, (Weber,) . . .	0.00666 — 0.00883	
Seminal canals of young cock, .	0.00528	
—— squirrel, . .	0.01453	
—— hedgehog, .	0.00970	
—— man, . .	0.00470	
Tubuli in anal glands of goose, .	0.00990	
Clustered *tubuli* in Cowper's glands in hedgehog, .	0.01022	
Cells in Meibomian glands in man, (Weber,) .	0.00258 — 0.00633	

XIV. In simple glands, which are composed of intestinules and large follicles, the smallest blood-vessels wind along the walls of these intestinules and follicles, exactly as in any other animal membrane; for instance, the pulmonic mucous membrane. In these walls the transition of arteries into veins by reticular arches takes place in the usual manner. In compound glands, however, the ducts of which are small and very small, as in the kidneys, liver, and testicle, the uriniferous, biliferous, and seminiferous ducts are connected only externally with the most delicate vascn-lar networks, without the vessels winding on the thin walls of these ducts.

XV. The ultimate distribution of the blood-vessels does not always follow the formation of the secreting canals. In the liver of the embryo, indeed, where the paniculate and pinnatifid ends of the biliferous ducts spring from the surface, so as to be seen by the microscope, the blood-vessels, though smaller, imitate a similar distribution; for they run in the middle of a *panicula* or *foliolus*, and with their final smallest capillary twigs descend between the closed ends of the ducts or *acini*. But in glands which are formed of serpentine unbranched ducts, everywhere equal in diameter, the blood-vessels are not serpentine, but with very small branches, creep among the *gyri* or turns of the serpentine ducts.

XVI. That the smallest currents of blood run freely between the *acini* of a compound gland, as the liver, and that the blood is in immediate contact with the *acini,* has been inferred by Gruithuisen, on the faith of microscopical observations on the liver of the frog. This inference Müller thinks unfounded. He allows that at first on investigating the development of the liver and kidneys in the embryo, such appears to be the fact. The blood-interstices of the canals appear without certain trace of parietes of vessels ; and the same appearance is presented by the microscopical examination of the liver in live larvæ of Tritons. But Müller is satisfied from microscopical observations on the kidneys of adults, both after injection and recent, that vestiges of the most minute blood-vessels are formed in the tissue which unites the uriniferous canals. Müller allows, nevertheless, that at first new currents, without proper walls, are formed in an amorphous web; but immediately walls, however thin, as more fixed boundaries to these currents, are formed by increased thickness of the substance round the currents.

XVII. The development of the glands in the embryos of the higher animals takes place in the same manner as the glands in the series of animals generally. That is the most complex glands in the embryo of the higher animals consist at first of excretory ducts alone, similar to the secreting vessels of the lower animals.

XVIII. The intimate structure of the glands presents very many varieties, chiefly with the object of increasing the extent of secreting surface. Yet no species of structure is peculiar to any individual gland. In the most different glands the structure may be the same, as in the cortical substance of the kidney, and in the testicle. Conversely the same gland presents a different structure in different animals. For instance the lacrymal gland in the tortoise consists of fasciculated *utriculi,* forming a *cortex* or rind around the excretory ducts. In birds the same gland is cellulated ; in the mammalia it consists of pedunculated vesicles, with ducts appended in the form of clusters. The minute structure of the liver and testicles in like manner presents great variations. The kidneys alone, in all classes, observe one common model of formation, from uniform canals unbranched, either straight or tortuous, though the disposition and walls of the canals undergo the greatest diversity in different classes.

XIX. The structure of glands increases in complication in the series of animals up to man ; yet this increase in complication is not always in the same ratio. The rule seems to be that in every class

the gland which appears first presents the most simple formation.
Thus the pancreas is the most simple in fishes, the liver in the lower
classes of animals, and the kidneys in fishes and amphibia. And
when any gland appears first in any order of animals, it is formed
either of intestinules or follicles, or tubules.

XX. The substance of the canals in the glandular tissue is either
whitish, or whitish-gray, or whitish-orange, however different be the
colour of the secreted products. There is, therefore, no perfect resemblance between the glandular substance and the secreted product, as has been erroneously stated by several writers.

XXI. The elementary parts of glands, viz. cells, vesicles, *utriculi*, follicles, tubules, &c., always consist of one single tissue. The
excreting duct only consists sometimes of several, sometimes of two
membranes, the inner of which, being usually continuous with the
mucous mèmbrane, is generally of the same nature, while the external passes in the substance of the gland into the proper substance
of the canals. The other external membranes of the excretory
ducts, fibrous, or adventitious cellular, terminate in the beginning
of the gland, are sometimes continued in the fibrous investment of
the gland, as in the poison-gland of serpents. In certain cases the
fibrous investment of a gland transmits processes between the segments and lobules, as in the poison-glands of the *Trigonocephalus*,
in the salivary glands of serpents and Birds, and in the anal glands
of the mole. The gland is then divided into compartments, and
the lobules are contained within *septa* or partitions, though externally it appears, and is erroneously considered to be, uniformly
parenchymatous. More frequently, however, the lobules of a gland
are united by loose cellular tissue and vessels.

XXII. The nerves of glands accompany the arteries and veins
in general regularly, and form slender plexuses over the large
branches; and nowhere do the nerves separate from the blood-vessels; so that they may be regarded as rather foreign to the glandular structure.

XXIII. These ducts, canals, or *intestinula*, are all lined or formed internally or at the free surface by a membrane continuous with
some mucous membrane. This membrane has been called *epithelium* by the revival of a name formerly in use. It consists of cells,
mostly nucleated, mingled with granules irregularly dispersed.
These cells are clear and colourless, but often scattered with small
punctula. The *nucleus* is round or oval, from $\frac{2}{1000}$ to $\frac{3}{1000}$ of a
Paris inch in diameter, more or less flat, generally colourless or

pale-red, like blood-globules. These epithelial cells are believed to be detached from time to time in the form of scales.

SECTION II.

THE STRUCTURE OF INDIVIDUAL GLANDS.

THE previous observations are general. It is requisite now to advert shortly to the structure of individual glands. This structure is best understood by tracing it in the embryo.

§ I.—THE SALIVARY GLANDS.

As an example we may take the parotid.

When the parotid gland is examined in the embryo of the sheep or the ox, it appears that it is developed or formed by a species of progressive ramification from the mucous membrane of the mouth. The excretory duct, in short, which is first formed, is a prolongation of the mucous membrane of the mouth. It appears at an early period in the form of a whitish semitranslucent canal, extending in an arched curvature towards the ear, dividing into several very short branches scarcely smaller than the trunk. These branches terminate in a blind or vesicular close cavity, slightly swelling; and this disposition is retained throughout the whole period of the formation of the gland. This branchy arrangement is well distinguished in the midst of a pellucid jelly-like matter, which was regarded by Rathke as primordial, or the *blastema*. Afterwards this jelly-like matter becomes opaque, and is divided into roundish flattened lobules. These dilated *vesiculæ* or *ampullulæ* form the ultimate granules or elementary parts of the gland.

The arrangement of the twigs and branches is the following. The excretory duct is divided into long whitish canals. From these proceed long lateral branches scarcely smaller than the trunks. Each of these goes to a lobule and sends branches into it; in such manner, however, that the twigs then arising are scarcely smaller than the trunks. These twigs again send out new stalks, which all terminate in large rounded bladders or *vesiculæ*.

All the canals are white, even to the extreme tips of the twigs, and they wind about in the same plane of flattened lobules, presenting under the microscope an interesting object.

It is further to be remembered that this ramification is only lateral, that is from each side or margin of the duct and branches, and not all round or peripheral. It appears that the same lateral ramification, with the same arrangement of lobules, takes place in the lacrymal gland, and in the *mammæ*.

The blood-vessels do not follow these ramifications so much as the *blastema*, or primordial matter, to which they are nutrient canals.

As the *ovum* or embryo grows, this growth of ramification or branching like a plant proceeds; and as this advances in producing shoots and pedunculated vesicles, the *blastema* or primordial matter of the lobules is consumed; the internal ramification towards the margin of the lobules, originally spacious, advances; and branches formerly dispersed in the place of the lobules are accumulated over each other.

The vegetation of the ducts of the submaxillary gland differs a little from that of the parotid, according to Rathke, and approaches that of the pancreas.

§ II.—THE PANCREAS.

The arrangement representing this gland in fishes has already been noticed.

In the MAMMALIA, this organ having passed through different stages in reptiles and birds, presents the following characters.—

In the fœtus of the sheep of four inches, the elementary particles of the pancreas have already consumed almost their whole *blastema*, so that scarcely a trace of the common amorphous primordial substance remains. The elementary particles are everywhere freely prominent. These consist of elongated cylindrical *acini* or bunchy *utriculi*, which are larger than the pedunculated vesicles of the salivary glands, and are so generally conjoined, that they constitute *paniculæ* everywhere scattered on the surface. These cylindrical *acini*, or elementary utriculi, proceed alternately from the middle twig, form elsewhere pinnatifid *paniculæ*, as in the pancreas of birds. In other respects they are all very white, equal, not pedunculated, gently expanding in a shut end. In each set of three, four, or five *paniculæ*, Muller observed prominent shoots; the rest, if there were more, were covered by the neighbouring *paniculæ*. The shoots composing one single *panicula* are unfolded in the same place; and in this respect they manifestly differ in structure from the parotid gland. The intimate union of the *paniculæ* Muller was unable to unravel.

3

' In the Hamster (*Cricetus vulgaris*), the pancreas consists of very small lobules, which are almost entirely separate from each other, and adhere only loosely by the different ducts, forming large lobules. The elementary particles are the same almost as in the salivary glands, but half more slender ; nor does the middle part of the canal appear white as in the salivary glands. Each lobule divided into small *fasciculi*, or clusters, or elementary parts, receives in the middle a blood-vessel, which is distributed in twigs among the smaller *fasciculi*.

- The summary of the structure of the pancreas is the following. In AMPHIBIA, BIRDS, and MAMMALIA, in the fœtal state, there is observed a paniculated vegetation of *acini*, or elongated cylindrical *utriculi* or bladders ;. the cylindrical *acini* in the *paniculæ*, proceed from a middle twig like the nerves of leaves ; and all terminate in free, shut, and slightly swelling ends. In adult birds, the secreting canals begin in cellular roots or very crowded small vesicles.

§ III.—THE LIVER.

In the surface of the liver of the sturgeon, Muller observed with the microscope small pinnatifid paniculæ variously dispersed, so that the *acini* or roots of the biliferous canals were united in the pinnatifid manner. The sprouts were otherwise free, slightly swelled at the tip.

In the toad the formation is the following ;—

The proliferous membrane, after surrounding the yelk by growths in all directions, forms a saccated appendix, pendulous from the keel of the embryo, containing the substance of the yelk. That sac is divided into an external very thin pellucid layer, and an internal vascular layer, one of which belongs to the integuments, and the other to the intestines. The inner sac is soon prolonged towards the vertebral column, into an anterior and posterior *lacinia*, which indicate respectively the anterior and posterior ends of the intestinal canal. When the anterior prolongation issues from the common sac, on the right side, in the continuation of the sac of the yelk, is seen conspicuously a whitish swelling, consisting of globules, with slender peduncles, as it were, attached. Observed casually granules appear, and these are the first vestige of the liver. The sac of the yelk is distinguished by innumerable reticular blood-vessels, in which the blood is observed moving distinctly.

After one or two days, the beginning and end of the intestinal

sac are more elongated; and the circular motion of the blood
most fully evolved in the intestinal sac, is distinguished by innumerable arches of reticulated vessels. A trunk of veins bends to
the right, and seems to proceed under the liver, where it sends several small vessels into the liver. The liver itself, situate in the
anterior prolongation of the intestinal sac, is known 'by its whiten-
ing, elongated, almost pedunculated *acini*. These might be called
vesiculæ, if it could be proved that they are already hollow.

In grown animals, the principal difference is in the greater distinctness with which the vessels and the contained blood are seen.

The substance of the liver is very tender, is turned from tawny
into white, not unlike the substance of the yelk : it consists of
elongated *acini*, variously disposed, similar almost to the elongated
bundles of *acini* in the embryo of birds; only these are in BIRDS
more distinct and freely prominent.

As to the liver of BIRDS, the observations of Baer deserve notice.
He states, that from the swelled vascular layer of the alimentary
canal are developed, in the course of the third day after impregnation, the lungs, the liver, the pancreas, the cæcum, and the urinary
bladder.   All these parts are developed from the closed, not the
open end of the alimentary canal, while the mucous membrane of
that canal is covered with the proportional tubes in the vascular
layer.

The liver appears, about the middle of the fourth day, as two
pyramid-like hollow limbs of the intestinal canal, which enclose the
common venous trunk, and pass with their broad basis into the alimentary canal.   Scarcely have these pyramids clasped the veins,
when they are prolonged into the next containing part of the vascular layer, and are ramified in it, a covering from the vascular
membrane at the same time urging them forward.   The protruded
portions appear, with increasing prolongation and contraction of
the alimentary canal, leaf-like, and closely embracing the veins.
In these leaves appear the tips of the advancing quills, while their
basis is progressively narrowed, and assumes the form of a cylinder.
The ramification appears under the microscope as a branching dark
figure in the inside of each leaf.

As soon as the quill-like prolongations, which form the future
hepatic ducts, begin to take the cylindrical form, there appears among
them a retraction which increases gradually, so that at the end of
the third day they scarcely reach the middle of the substance of
the vascular layer, and externally they form nowhere any projec-

tion. The granular inner layer presents at the apex some ramification; which evidently has the aspect of mucous cavities.

On the fourth day, the vascular layer is still farther removed, and resembles semitransparent jelly; the liver is divided into two flat bodies, which surround like plates the portal vein. In these plates both hepatic ducts undergo further ramification, but at the same time at a greater distance from the bowel, so that most commonly they are united at the bases, and at the end of the fourth day are wont to form one common canal.

After this the progress is similar, only to render the vascular and secreting parts more distinct. On the eighth, ninth, and tenth day, the gall-bladder appears.

In short, the liver is formed in the following manner: by eversion of the internal tunic of the intestinal canal into the vascular layer, whence a double excavated cone arises. These two excavated cones are then ramified internally, though united at the base, the common basis being, as it were, prolonged from the intestinal wall, until the two orifices open in one common orifice.

In the MAMMALIA, the terminations of the biliferous ducts end exactly as in birds, free and in shut extremities; but in their internal union they seem to differ in each, so that in some the elongated *acini* are joined in the pinnatifid manner, in others like leaves, and in others irregularly.

Next to the arrangement, disposition, and form of the secreting ducts comes that of the blood-vessels.

The branches and twigs of the portal vein everywhere rise to the surface of the liver, and follow chiefly the distribution of the biliferous ducts; while the branches of the hepatic artery traverse the surface in a peculiar manner. Of the twigs of the portal vein it is a peculiar character, that they are more conical; while the arterial twigs diminish their diameter very gradually, and are distributed in a sinuous course so irregularly, that it is difficult to distinguish trunks from branches.

The smallest blood-vessels are much more minute than the elongated ends of the biliferous ducts.

The smallest blood-vessels in the embryo of BIRDS, and the *larvæ* of tritons and frogs, are not distributed on the walls of the biliferous ducts; but run in the intervals between their bundles and sprouts.

There is no direct communication between afferent vessels, whether portal or arterial, and revehent vessels. In all cases there is an intermediate network of very minute capillaries, that is, vessels all of the same diameter, and all frequently and freely communicating with each other. It is therefore a mistake to say that a blood-vessel terminates in a biliferous duct. If this be the case, no one has ever seen it, even by the microscope; and the phenomena which are supposed to prove it, are irregular, or the result of certain fallacies.

In 1833, Mr Kiernan published a description of the minute anatomy of the liver. He arrived at the conclusion that each lobule is composed of numerous minute bodies of a yellowish colour, imparted to them by contained bile, and of various forms, connected with each other by vessels. These bodies he regards as the *acini* of Malpighi. Each of these lobules consists of a plexus of biliary ducts, of a venous plexus formed by branches of the portal vein, of a branch of an hepatic vein, and of minute arteries. Nerves and absorbents he did not trace into them. He showed also that the hepatic veins do not communicate with the branches of the portal vein; that the interlobular branches of the latter form one continuous plexus through the whole liver; that the portal veins have no direct communication with each other, but anastomose by means of interlobular branches only; and that the portal vein, accompanied by an artery, resembles an artery in its ramifications.[*]

According to Henle, the microscope shows that the *acini* of the liver are formed in a quite different way from all other glandular lobules. They are heaps of closely-crowded, and everywhere closed nucleated cells, which entirely fill up the meshes or intervals between the blood-vessels.

In a fine section of a hepatic lobule, these nucleated cells are seated without the walls of the blood-vessels, sometimes in irregular heaps; sometimes in irregular short rows close to each other, which, if these transverse divisions be examined, appear like minute blood *intestinula*. The medium diameter of these cells is about $\frac{7}{1000}$ parts of a Paris line; the nucleus is usually round, compressed, somewhat flat, from $\frac{50}{10000}$ to $\frac{35}{10000}$ parts of a Paris line in diameter, with one or two nucleated granules. By the mutual pressure of the cells on each other they become polygonal, tetrahedral, or

* The Anatomy and Physiology of the Liver. By Francis Kiernan, Esq. 4to. London, 1834. Philosophical Transactions of the Royal Society of London for 1833, Part II.

pentahedral. Their colour is yellowish. They contain a quantity of fine punctuated *corpuscula*, which appear to be seated on their walls, and frequently in man and mammiferous animals, small and large fat globules, which are never seen in perfectly sound livers. Not unfrequently there are small cells which inclose the narrow nucleus and large cells with two *nuclei;* and some there are, the cavities of which communicate with each other, or between which certainly no partition is visible. Hallmann found cells without *nuclei ;* that is, non-nucleated cells.

Besides these cells, we see only fat in the intervals of the lobules, fibres in the walls of the strong vessels and biliferous ducts, and cylindrical epithelial cells detached from the last. Henle could not observe on the surface of the lobes or between them any peculiar ligamentous tissue ; and Vogel says that it appears doubtful.[*]

These cells, there is every reason to believe, perform an important part in the formation of bile.

§ IV.—THE KIDNEYS.

The kidneys and testes are referred by Henle to the head of Reticulated or Net-like glands.

The substance of the kidneys in fishes consists of long canals of equal diameter, which arise from branches of the ureter, or parallely in bundles from the lateral ureter, and proceed sometimes straight, sometimes in a sinuous course variously contorted, without being divided into branches, which are not attenuated towards the extremities, but terminate uniformly in short ends.

In reptiles, the *vesiculæ* or bladders of the secreting apparatus, or ends of the uriniferous ducts, arise before the ureter itself is distinctly seen. This seems to show that the development of the kidneys begins from the peripheral vesicles. The stalks of these vesicles are prolonged daily, by which the tubules terminated by vesicular rounded *apices* arise, while the *vesiculæ* themselves are more and more attenuated, until the uriniferous ducts observe the same diameter to their shut end. In short, in this order of animals, the substance of the kidneys consists of equal cylindrical tubules rising from the ureter and ascending to the outer margin of the kidney, where they terminate in short extremities.

---

[*] Allgemeine Anatomie. Lehre von der Mischungs-und Formbestandstheilen des Menschlichen Körpers. Von J. Henle. Leipzig, 1841. 8vo. See also Ueber der Feineren Bau der Leber. Von C. Krause in Hanover. Muller's Archiv, 1845. No. V. seite 524.

In adult serpents, the kidneys consist of many lobules, which are connected in order by the ureter, which passes along the internal margin. The lobules on the flat surface of the kidney are less distinct than those on its convex surface. All the lobules, however, are very closely connected. The lobulated appearance, indeed, is the result of the undulated flexures of the renal mass. When the substance, inflected in the undulated fashion, is confined and con-tracted by the ureter, each lobule consists of a convoluted tract, or of a sort of arch, with a median furrow left. Into these median furrows on the one side enter the bundles of the uriniferous ducts; and on the other the blood-vessels. And as the lobules arise by alternating flexures, the bundles of the uriniferous ducts being on the one margin, and the vascular trunks on the opposite one, the former are mostly distributed on the convex surface, and the latter on the plane surface of the kidneys.

The kidneys of the crocodile are also lobulated; but the lobules are not attached in order to the ureter, as in serpents, but are united into an irregular mass, and receive the ureter internally. All the lobules are contorted, and surround the surface with wind-ing *gyri*. When a kidney is divided transversely on the surface, through the *gyri* of the lobules, the section of the lobule or *gyrus* is pyramidal. This shows that the *gyri* of the lobules project with an external acute border, and are united internally at their bases, where they receive the branches of the ureter. The ureter itself appears to be ramified on the deep substance of the kidney, so that the branches pass everywhere into internal *gyri*, according to the arrangement of the lobules.

In Birds at the first period of development, when, besides the heart and the first rudiment of intestine, the other bowels of the trunk are not yet visible, on each side near the vertebral column appears an elongated body, extending from the site of the heart, almost along the whole keel of the embryo. This body observers first mistook for the kidney. Rathke showed, however, that this body is peculiar to the embryon; that it precedes and prepares for the formation of the testes and ovaries, and then, as the fœtus ad-vances in maturity, it becomes shorter, and at the close of fœtal life vanishes entirely. These bodies, which were first described by Wolff, and therefore received the name of Wolffian bodies (*Corpora Wolffiana*), and by Burdach, were called *spurious kidneys*, consist at first of elongated pedunculated vesicles, which being arranged transversely, issue from one common marginal excretory duct, which are gradually elongated into very small *intestinula cœca* or tubules, also transversely placed.   These tubules, at first straight, are gradually curved, until their course becomes serpentine. · They are, however, at all times separated from each other, and without trace of ramification.

Rathke observed the first rudiment of kidneys on the sixth day, and the ureter in the form of a slender filament on the seventh day ; while the Wolffian bodies are still of considerable size, and have extended the whole length of the keel on the fourth day.*   It is further ascertained, that the Wolffian bodies already present the characteristic structure, namely, transverse tortuous intestinula, when the first traces of kidneys, like a mass of very tender grey substance, appears close to and behind the Wolffian bodies.

It is the opinion of Rathke, that the substance of the kidneys is formed from the Wolffian bodies, because, on the sixth and seventh day of incubation, when these bodies are detached from the keel, the kidneys adhere, not to the keel, but to the Wolffian bodies. The view of Müller is different.   The Wolffian bodies, according to him, however, similar to the kidneys in Batrachoid reptiles, yet differ entirely in texture from the kidneys in other AMPHIBIA and in BIRDS ; the first trace of uriniferous ducts being widely different from the intestinules of the Wolffian bodies.   Muller further never could recognise, after very frequent observation, any internal and organic communication between these organs ; the closed intestinules of the Wolffian bodies being at one part, and at another the uriniferous ducts, arranged in brilliant convolutions, also closed and whitish.   Another circumstance which places this question out of all doubt is, that in Batrachoid AMPHIBIA, the Wolffian bodies, though at first sought in vain, Muller found in the upper part of the abdomen, where, at a great distance from the kidneys, they are provided with their excretory duct, and consist also of minute *cœca*. From these facts Muller infers, that the Wolffian bodies have an intimate connection with the development of the organs of generation, as Rathke first suspected.

The substance of the kidneys, on the other hand, is formed from its own proper blastema or primordial matter, by an innate effort.

When the mass of gray substance, situate at the margin and behind the upper part of the Wolffian body, is examined at its first appearance by the microscope, the surface is distinguished by a ver-

---

* By the *Carina* or keel is meant the vertebral column, or what represents it.

micular eruption and varied appearance of *gyri* or convoluted lines, which are in different parts convex and concave; and these gyri again converge everywhere into the foliated form, like the leaves of the oak, fig tree, or cauliflower, variously arranged with undulated margin. The whole kidney at this period consists of mere leaf-like convoluted *gyri*. These gyri form the uppermost part of the substance; but they are continued inwards, as if they were held together in the deep-seated substance by one common mesentery. When the small masses deep in the middle, undulated at margin, and also beyond the margin, are arranged like leaves, the observer thinks he sees the elementary particles of the renal substance in the prominent lobules of the gyri.

At first the *gyri* of the masses appear everywhere with unequal margin. Soon, however, by the aid of the microscope, there is seen on the tortuous border a vesicular eruption like pearls; that is, in the tender substance of the tortuous border, round corpuscles are contained one after the other; but when these are carefully examined, they are found to be round on the margin only; and below, where the gyri penetrate into the interior substance, these corpuscula also descend, and in their course become smaller, as the pedunculi proceed from the deep seated substance, and are unfolded variously on the tortuous and curled border of the gyri. These pedunculated corpuscles are whiter than the rest of the very tender substance, and are arranged one beside the other in very regular order, held together, as it were, by one common mesentery, which, folded and contracted inwardly, but outwardly unfolded by innumerable gyri and a tortuous margin, produces a remarkable resemblance to the arrangement of leaves and lobules. In the same manner the *pedunculi* meet in various points in the deep-seated substance, and outwardly are unfolded in the undulating fashion, terminating in a vesicular or headed end. These pedunculi, though approximated internally, are not really united, but merely approximated in the contracted membranous substance. This may be regarded as the earliest conformation in most embryos.

The arrangement therefore is, that the appearance of granules takes place first on the margin of the gyri; while the vesicles with peduncles are in the deep-seated substance.

The further development consists in this, that the gyri of the uriniferous ducts increase daily, and the undulated margin is contracted into several contorted lobules, whence a more profuse leaf-like vegetation results, so as to fill the intervals between the gyri; and the leaf-like shape of the lobules is gradually obscured. The kidneys now are parted into several distinct masses united by the ureter.

At length all the uriniferous ducts send out near their ends several lateral knots, from which arise short branches scarcely smaller than the trunk, and terminate in short ends. This causes the pinnatifid shape in the apex of each uriniferous duct. These ducts, pinnatifid at end, are quite separate from each other, and, though arranged in regular order, have no mutual communication.

About the close of fœtal life, the uriniferous ducts, at first white, are now everywhere filled with a secretion which from being tawny becomes bright white, which fills the canals almost to their ends, and is best seen in the first days after hatching; and in the young of large birds shows beautifully the structure of the uriniferous ducts on the surface of the *gyri* and lobules.

The kidneys of the adult bird are not only divided into several masses, but these present a surface composed of innumerable minute lobules. These lobules arise from continuous *gyri* variously arranged; the margins of these *gyri* only project, whence the multiform surface, viewed through the microscope, seems to imitate nearly the *gyri* of the convolutions of the brain.

The kidneys of the bird, after being hatched, require no injection to demonstrate the disposition of the uriniferous ducts. Being naturally filled with white solid urine (urate of ammonia), they may be observed in large birds, especially ravens, by the naked eye, in the first, second, third, and fourth day after hatching. All the uriniferous ducts, to their most remote pinnatifid extremities, are swelled with whitish-yellow matter, their proper secretion, consisting of uric acid.

It is difficult to convey a distinct and correct idea of the arrangement now described without figures. But it may appear to be compared to that produced by a long frill or ruffle of muslin or cambric which is doubled up and folded on itself six, eight, or ten times, with the frilled edges allowed to project, and all within an oval or elliptical space of half an inch or less.

By micrometrical measurement, the terminations of the uriniferous ducts are about ·00174, that is, $\frac{174}{100000}$ of one Paris inch in diameter. This is much larger than the diameter of the blood-vessels. Supposing the diameter of the smallest blood-vessels to

3 D

be 0·00025, or $\frac{25}{100000}$ of one Paris inch, then they are seven times smaller, or the ducts are seven times larger.

In MAMMALIA, the following are the most important facts to be known in the development and structure of the kidneys.

In the embryo of MAMMALIA as well as of BIRDS, Wolffian bodies are observed; and as they are largest in the earliest period of embryal life, they have by Dzondi and others been mistaken for kidneys. They consist, as in birds, of very slender closed *intestinula*. In the younger embryos they are larger than the kidneys, and then chiefly simulate these organs; afterwards they are confounded with the testicles, being lower in situation and of the same size as the kidneys, so that it is difficult to distinguish between the three organs. They differ from the kidneys in MAMMALIA in being covered by an external envelope, on removing which the intestinula protrude, arranged transversely.

The kidneys are rounded. In the sheep they present vessels shooting from the notch or umbilicus (*hilus*) towards the circumference in bundles, which are divaricated in arch-like folds and retorted, yet all terminate in large *vesiculæ* pedunculated and hollowed.

In almost all embryos of MAMMALIA, the kidneys consist of multiplied lobules in which the same arrangement of pedunculated and closed tubes is presented and repeated in various forms. In some animals this multiplied division or lobulated form of the kidney is retained through life. In others, certainly the greater number, the kidney appears in the shape of one general organ; but this is caused merely by its external appearance, or, to speak more accurately, by the arrangement of the cortical matter outside. In the human fœtus the lobulated arrangement is manifest, and is in certain instances continued after birth; but in most instances the kidney appears like one undivided organ.

This difference further is of use in illustrating the anatomy of glandular organs in general. The lobulated or divided state is continued through life in certain animals, as the ox, the bear, the badger, and several of the cetacea, especially the porpoise. In these animals the kidneys consist not of one united mass, but of a number, more or less considerable, of separate bodies, each presenting and repeating the same internal structure.

Thus in the ox the kidney consists of a series of sixteen or seventeen lobules or separate parts, each of which presents the following arrangement from the pelvis or common excretory cavity.

First is a large but short duct or canal lined by a membrane continuous with that of the *pelvis ;* this terminates in a shut or closed cavity called cup, (*calyx*) or funnel (*infundibulum*). Into this cavity projects a small conical eminence, (*papilla*), with an aperture in its apex. From this, urine may be made by pressure to exude ; and when the *papilla* is divided by a longitudinal section, it is observed that one short duct from which the urine issues, is the termination of a great number of small capillary tubes which are disposed longitudinally, yet radiating or converging towards the small papillary duct. These are the uriniferous ducts of Bellini ; (*tubuli Belliniani*).

At these upper or peripheral ends is placed a species of structure which is parenchymatous and granular in aspect but vascular in arrangement, that is, it consists mostly of blood-vessels ramified to an infinite degree of minuteness and delicacy. On the mode in which these vessels are arranged at their terminations, Muller states that the arteries terminate in a very minute and delicate vascular or capillary network, which lies between the closed ends of these tubes, and that from this network again veins arise as in other textures of the body.

The papillary cone, which is about half an inch from base to apex, and rather less than half an inch at base, consists of firm solid matter, the colour of which is white or pale gray. Its exterior structure is formed of numerous tubes uniting and converging from the base to the *papilla* or apex.

Beyond this the substance of the tubular part is of a bright pink colour, less firm, but more distinctly consisting of multiplied tubes placed close to each other, and converging from the base to the segment of the frustum, on which the papillary portion rests.

In the bear and badger, these separate lobules or diminutive kidneys are still more numerous ; but the internal arrangement is quite the same.

In the dolphin and porpoise the same multiplied division is carried to a very great length. The masses called kidneys in these animals consist of an immense number of tetrahedral, trapezoidal, or hexadral small bodies, connected to each other by cellular tissue and blood-vessels not very firmly, and in such manner that they may be easily separated. The number of these *renculi* it is difficult in the CETACEA to fix. I am sure I have numbered more than 200, yet have not exhausted them. Each *renculus* presents the internal tubular or medullary portion, consisting of multiplied tubules placed along over each other, and the external cortical or vascular portion consisting of blood-vessels most minutely ramified,

When in any of these simple or integral kidneys the aperture of the *papilla* is examined, it is found to be continued into a short thickish tube not larger than one line or one line and a-half, which then is divided into two small cylindrical trunks. These again, after a short space, are divided into two others of the same diameter almost, very different from, and much larger than blood-vessels. Thence they advance. dichotomous, cylindrical, straight, or deviating little from the straight direction, and in their course constantly double and multiply themselves to the base of the *papilla*, being conjoined by tender cellular substance. When increased in number, without being diminished in diameter, they are collected into one or two bundles separate from each other by blood-vessels. Each of the bundles enters then its own meatus formed by the vascular plexus of the vault or arch. After this, the small ducts contained in their respective fasciculi, and connected with each other, are no longer dichotomous, but proceed singly in the same direction through the substance of the cortex, whence they diverge laterally, and in a serpentine course, contorted in numerous convolutions, and wandering far from the branches. One single serpentine duct, continued from the straight duct, not inserted into the same, deflected laterally, preserves almost always the same diameter and whiteness.

These uriniferous ducts further are continued into the cortical part of the kidney, a fact first ascertained by Schumlansky, and afterwards by Huschke, by injecting them under the receiver of the air-pump. According to Schumlansky, as the straight ducts or Bellinian tubes advance to the periphery of the kidney they diminish in number, or rather they terminate in serpentine ducts, which, with many windings and convolutions, proceed between the few and diminishing straight ducts onwards to the periphery or extreme edge of the cortical matter. Before the straight ducts reach this point or line, all of them have terminated in serpentine ducts which communicate by multiplied arches, so that at the peripheral edge of the cortical matter no straight ducts exist.

Not essentially different is the account given by Huschke. According to his account, when the tubes reach the utmost limits of the medullary matter of the organ, they proceed progressively, separating from each other, until in the surface of the kidney they

3

begin to wind in serpentine directions, forming arches with each other, and again turn backwards and are insensibly lost, becoming still more minute, yet without entering the Malpighian bodies.

The mention of these objects renders it necessary to explain what they are.

Though Eustachi appears to have maintained the existence of a sort of minute glandular grains in the kidney, Malpighi was the first who spoke of them distinctly and confidently. He states that in all the kidneys examined by him, in quadrupeds, the tortoise, and in man, he observed a cluster of minute glandules by the following means. A black fluid, mixed with spirit of wine, was injected into the renal artery, so as to cause the whole kidney to be swelled and of a black colour externally. Then on stripping off the external membrane, there appeared attached here and there to the dividing arteries small glandules stained of a black colour; and on making a longitudinal section of the kidney, it was possible to observe between the bundles of the urinary vessels, (i. e. the ducts,) and in the spaces thereby formed, the same glands, almost without number, attached to the blood-vessels, distended with the black fluid, like apples suspended to the branches of a tree.* He afterwards adds that these bodies are placed in the utmost region of the kidney in almost countless numbers; that he thinks it likely that they correspond to the urinary vessels of which the mass of the kidneys consists; that as to shape, by reason of their minuteness and remarkable translucency, though they cannot be said to be distinctly circumscribed, yet they appear round like the *ova* of fishes; they are blackened when a dark-coloured fluid is injected into the arteries; and they are placed among the extreme branches of the arteries, which wind round them like tendrils, so that they appear surrounded by the former, with this exception, however, that the portion attached to the arterial branch is black, while the rest retains its own colour.†

In these injections, Malpighi explicitly states, that he never saw the liquor thrown into the artery, though it blackened the nearest portion, get into the urinary ducts, or the round masses which he considered as the glandules of the kidney. This agrees with what is long afterwards maintained by Müller.

The round or globular bodies thus described by Malpighi were

* De Renibus, Caput II. apud Opera Omnia, pag. 60. Folio. Londini, 1686.
† De Renibus, Cap. III. p. 92.

seen afterwards by Winslow, Ferrein, Schumlansky,* Eysenhardt, Husckhe, Müller, Henle, Bowman, Gerlach, Bidder, and in short all those who have studied the minute anatomy of the kidney. They have been denominated from the anatomist who first directed attention to them *Corpora Malpighiana.*

At the same time it must be observed, that, whether from some confusion of ideas, or from presuming that these bodies must be well known, almost all those who have spoken of them have given them different names at different times, so that it is difficult to know whether all understood the same objects. Ruysch, for example, regards these round or globular bodies as balls of the extremities of blood-vessels (*glomeres vasculorum*) convoluted on themselves, and not as glands; nor does he allow that they are surrounded by any membrane. Similar opinions were entertained by Berger and Vieussens, and especially Peyer, who contended decidedly for their being winding and contorted vessels. Schumlansky long afterwards calls them *glandulæ auctorum*, and while he in one passage represents the clustering terminations of the arterial capillaries as the glandules of Malpighi, in another he distinguishes these glandules from the *glomeres* and *glomeruli*, or vascular balls of Ruysch. This anatomist, after injecting kidneys, and examining them, concludes that, though the appearances favour at once the doctrine of Malpighi and that of Ruysch, there are, amidst the blood-vessels of the cortical portion of the kidney, granules or globular, polyhedral or polymorphous bodies, which may be injected from the arteries; yet he doubts whether these are hollow like follicles. He allows that they are connected by cellular tissue; and he says further, that they are the terminations of the serpentine uriniferous ducts.†

According to Müller, the Malpighian bodies are *vesiculæ*, or spherical, or spheroidal bladders, which contain glomeruli or globular clusters of minute blood-vessels, and which may be extracted or removed from the vesicular coverings. He thinks also, that another matter besides these blood-vessels is contained in the *vesi-*

---

* Arteriarum rami dant vieissim ramulos laterales, capillares, brevissimos, magis minus copiosos, quibus tanquam *pedicillis* appenduntur grana, cuique unum, seminum papaveris similia, nunc materie turgida. Totus ramus cum suis pedunculis et moleculis subrotundis lustratus, refert fere ribium racemum. En famosas glandulas MALPIGHII, earumque acinos. D. Alex. Schumlansky De Structura Renum Tractatus Physiologico-Anatomicus. Edente G. C. Wurtz, M. D., &c. Cum II. Tabulis Æneis. Argentorati, 1788. 8vo. § xxix. p. 77.

† D. Alex. Schumlansky, &c. § xxxvii., xxxix., xl., et xlii.

culæ, and that this adheres at one point only. When these *glomeruli* or spherical balls of capillaries are extracted, there are left smooth hollow hemispheres, through the wall of which blood-vessels adjacent appear. This *vesicula* forms the capsule of the Malpighian **bodies.**

The diameter of a Malpighian body, at an average, is about $\frac{7}{1000}$ of one Paris inch. The blood-vessels vary in diameter from $\frac{37}{10000}$ to $\frac{58}{10000}$ of one Paris inch. Consequently, the former are from thirteen to eighteen times larger than the latter.

Huschke allows that the Malpighian bodies are filled from the arteries, and are attached to these vessels; in short, that they are, as Ruysch maintained, glomeruli of blood-vessels.

Upon the whole, the Malpighian bodies may be described as globular or ovoidal vesicles, situate amidst or appended to the minute capillary divisions of the arteries, which are curled round them as tendrils of the vine or hop-plant. When the kidney is macerated in water, the Malpighian bodies may also be separately distinguished, lying in all directions between the serpentine uriniferous ducts. There they resemble vesicles, according to Müller; and, while they are attached to the arteries, there is no communication between them and the urinary ducts.*

The accuracy of this last statement is partly controverted by Mr Bowman, who has examined these bodies with much care. He found them to be a rounded mass of minute vessels invested by a cyst of similar appearance to the basement membrane of the tubes. He ascertained also that the investing capsule is the basement membrane of the uriniferous tubes expanded over the tuft of blood-vessels.

It appears further that the terminal twigs of the artery correspond in number with the Malpighian bodies. Arrived at them, the twig perforates the capsule, and dilating suddenly breaks up into two, three, four, or even eight branches, which diverge in all directions like petals from the stalk of a flower, and usually run, in a more or less tortuous manner, subdividing again once or twice as they advance, over the surface of the ball, they are about to form. The vessels resulting from these subdivisions are very small, and consist of one simple, homogeneous, transparent membrane. They plunge into its interior at different points, and after further

* De Glandularum Secernentium Structura Penitiori. Commentatio Anatomica. Scripsit Joannes Mueller. Lipsiae, 1830. Folio.

convolutions reunite in one single small vessel, varying in size, being generally smaller, but in some situations larger, than the terminal twig of the artery. This vessel emerges between two of the primary divisions of the terminal twig of the artery, perforating the capsule close to that vessel, and, like it, adhering to this membrane in its transition. It then enters the capillary plexus which surrounds the tortuous uriniferous tubes.

The tuft of vessels thus formed is a compact ball, the parts of which are held together by their mutual interlacement; there being no other tissue, according to Mr Bowman, forming the capsule except blood-vessels. It is lobulated, at least in certain animals, as man and the horse.

The basement membrane of the uriniferous tube, expanded over the Malpighian body so as to form its capsule, is a simple, homogeneous, and perfectly transparent membrane, in which no structure can be recognized. It is perforated, as before stated, by the afferent and efferent vessels, and not reflected over them. They are united to it at the point of transit. Opposite to this point is the orifice of the tube, the cavity of which is continuous with that of the capsule, generally by a contracted neck. This continuity Mr Bowman observed in mammalia, birds, reptiles, and fishes. When a thin section of a Malpighian body parallel to the neck of the tube is made, the capsule is observed to pass off into the basement membrane of the tube, as the body of a Florence flask into its neck. The basement membrane of the tube is lined by a nucleated epithelium of fine-granular opaque aspect; while the neck of the tube and its orifice are abruptly covered with a layer of cells much more transparent, and clothed with vibratile *cilia*. Within the capsule these cilia cease; and the epithelium beyond is very delicate and translucent. The cavity existing in the natural state between the epithelium and the tuft, is filled with fluid in which the vessels are bathed, and which is continually impelled onwards by the movement of the cilia.

The tubules on quitting the Malpighian bodies become greatly contorted; and this, Mr Bowman infers, is their constant disposition. The tortuous tubes unite again and again in twos, and in their course centrad become straight, forming the pyramids of Ferrein, and the medullary cones of Malpighi. Among these convolutions the Malpighian bodies are imbedded, and are in contact on all sides with the surrounding tubes.

The blood leaving the Malpighian bodies is conveyed by their efferent vessels to the capillary plexus surrounding the uriniferous tubes. The vessels of this plexus lie in the interstices of the tubes, anastomosing everywhere freely, and forming one continuous network lying outside the tubes, in contact with the basement membrane. This capillary plexus is interposed between the efferent vessels of the Malpighian bodies and the veins.

The efferent vessels of the Malpighian bodies never inosculate with each other, each being an isolated channel between its Malpighian tuft and the plexus surrounding the tubes. They are formed by the union of the capillary vessels of the tuft, and, after a course variable in length, they open into the plexus. They vary in size. In general they are smaller than the terminal twig of the artery, and scarce larger than the vessels of the plexus into which they empty their contents. They are larger in large Malpighian tufts.

From the plexus now mentioned, the veins arise and form the set of venous plexus, situate in the nipple-shaped extremities of the cones, round the orifices of the tubes, and pursuing a retrograde course to empty their contents into veins situate at the base of the cones. Another set of venous radiculæ are dispersed through the cortical part of the kidney, and each receives blood on all sides from the plexus surrounding the convoluted tubes.

From the account now given of the arrangement of the vessels connected with the Malpighian bodies, Mr Bowman infers that in the kidney there are *two perfectly distinct systems of capillary vessels*, through both of which the blood in its course from the arteries into the veins passes. The first is that system of vessels proceeding immediately from the arteries, and inserted into the dilated extremities of the uriniferous tubes, (the Malpighian bodies,) the Malpighian capillary system ; the second that enveloping the convolutions of the tubes, and communicating directly with the veins. The efferent vessels of the Malpighian bodies, which convey the blood between these two systems, Mr Bowman regards as performing to the kidney the same function which the portal veins perform to the liver, and these he accordingly regards as collected in the *portal system* of the kidney. The only difference is the absence of one general single portal trunk.

In short, Mr Bowman thinks that he has established the following facts.

1*st*, That each Malpighian body consists of the dilated extremity

of a uriniferous tube, with a small mass of blood-vessels inserted
into it.

2d, That the Malpighian bodies may be easily injected from the
arteries, and that the capillaries surrounding the uriniferous tubes
may be injected though less easily.   When the tubes are injected,
it is by extravasation from the Malpighian tufts.

3d, By the veins, the capillaries surrounding the tubes may be
injected; but neither the Malpighian bodies, nor the arteries, nor,
without extravasation, the tubes.   The main cause of this impediment
to injection and the movement of fluids from the veins into the arteries is the position and small size of the efferent vessels of the
Malpighian bodies, which stand in the way of any fluids being
transmitted to the Malpighian vessels.

4th, The Malpighian bodies cannot be injected from the tubes,
neither can the plexus surrounding the tubes or the veins be injected without extravasation.

5th, There is only one Malpighian body to each serpentine tube.

6th, The epithelium of the tube, when it enters the expanded portion which forms the Malpighian body, becomes transparent, and is
covered with vibrating cilia.*   Within the capsule, however, of the
Malpighian body, the *cilia* cease.

The accuracy of several of the representations of Mr Bowman
has been doubted, and more or less decidedly controverted by
Huschke, Reichert, Gerlach, and Bidder.   Reichert states, that
whatever means be adopted, by making minute sections of recent
kidneys, and using high magnifying powers, he never was able to
observe any transition of the uriniferous ducts into the capsule of
the Malpighian bodies.†

On the other hand, some confirmation of the correctness of this
part of Mr Bowman's representation is furnished by the structure
of the kidney in the Myxinoid fishes by Muller.   In these animals,
which present the simplest type of renal structure, this connection
is undoubted.

Gerlach made trials of the same kind as those by Reichert, yet
without tracing any connection between the uriniferous tubes and

* On the Structure and Use of the Malpighian Bodies of the Kidney, with Observations on the Circulation through that Gland.   By W. Bowman, F.R.S., &c.   Read
February 17, 1842. Philosophical Transactions of the Royal Society of London for
1842.   London, 1843.   Part i. p. 57.

† Bericht über die Fortschritte der Microscopischen Anatomie in dem Jahre 1842.
Von Reichert, Prof. in Dorpat. in Muller's Archiv, Jahrgang 1843.

the capsule. He further denies that the uriniferous ducts terminate in shut ends in the capsule. These ducts or tubules form collars, and what has been taken for shut ends of ducts, are nothing but the capsules, which communicate with the same by means of a short neck, which is evidently thinner than the uriniferous duct. The capsule is not a blind termination of a uriniferous duct, but a retraction or introversion,—a *diverticulum* of the same structureless membrane which forms the uriniferous tubes.

Gerlach admits that the account given by Mr Bowman of the perforation of the capsule by the arteries is correct.

As to the point at which the capsule is perforated by the afferent and efferent vessels, Gerlach thinks that the statement of Mr Bowman is too exclusive, when he represents this point to be always opposite to the opening of the uriniferous tube into the capsule. He gives a figure, (fig. 12,) which shows that the point, at which the afferent and efferent vessels perforate the capsule does not always correspond to the point of communication between the uriniferous ducts and the capsule.

The point in Mr Bowman's statements, which has been most strongly controverted both by Reicher and Huschke, is that as to the free entrance of the Malpighian capillary net-work into the cavity of the capsule; and both justly remark that such an assumption is at variance with all experience hitherto collected on the laws of histological organization; there being no example yet known of vessels lying immediately in the cavity of a secreting tissue. In truth, the representation of Mr Bowman, that the water of the urine is separated from the blood flowing in the Malpighian capillary vessels by simple transudation alone, while the peculiar constituents of the urine are separated through cells at the inner surface of the uriniferous ducts, Gerlach regards as in every respect a rash statement, and to be corroborated by no other fact. On the other hand, all investigations on glands prove, that in the process of secretion, cells are the essential element; and in the present state of science, it is impossible to think of secretion without cells.

He further adds, that when the Malpighian capillary net-work is closely examined, after the capsule has been entirely detached from it, we see it in its whole extent covered by a thick layer of nucleated cells, which are continued from the inner wall of the capsule upon the Malpighian vessels; and the latter lies introverted within a layer of cells, like the intestine within the peritonæum. The Malpighian capillary net-work further possesses the essential element of secretion, in which the blood undergoes those chemical changes, which the metabolic force of the gland-cells imparts to the secreted product. The secretion in the Malpighian vessels differs from the usual secretions, only in so far as between vessels and secreting cells there is no structureless membrane; which last, however, appears not to be an essential condition to the process of secretion.

On the existence of ciliary motions at the point of transition of the uriniferous tubes to the capsule, evidence is contradictory. Huschke and Reichert could observe no ciliary motion in the places indicated by Mr Bowman; and the latter denies even any layer of cells at the inner surface of the capsule. On the other hand, Bischoff is convinced of the presence of *cilia* in the kidneys of the frog. Valentin observed ciliary motions not only in the spots indicated by Mr Bowman, but even within the capsule; and Pappenheim gave a verbal communication on the same fact. The result of the inquiries of Gerlach is as follows. In mammalia he could never, unless he examined perfectly recent kidneys, observe ciliary motions either at the *cervix* or in the capsule. On the other hand, he found the inner wall of the capsule lined with a very slender layer of cells, which is seen very distinctly at the edge of the capsule. Between these cells lining the inner wall of the capsule and those which cover the Malpighian net-work, normally there is found a small interval.

In examining the recent kidneys of the frog, on the other hand, Gerlach convinced himself of the presence of ciliary motions not only in the *cervix* or collar, but also in the whole inner surface of the capsule; and he thinks it probable that ciliary motion is a phenomenon not peculiar to the renal capsule of the frog, but generally diffused over the animal kingdom.[*]

The results obtained by Bidder are not less at variance with those given by Mr Bowman.

Bidder states, first, that in no circumstances, and by no means which he could devise, could he obtain any certain evidence of connection of the *glomeruli* with the uriniferous ducts. The vascular bundles were always found below and between the uriniferous ducts, without interior relation to themselves, either uncovered or sur-

* Beiträge zur Strukturlehre der Niere von Dr Joseph Gerlach, prakt. Aerzte in Mainz. Archiv fur Anatomie, Physiologie, und Wissenschaftliche Medicin, von Dr Johannes Müller. 1845, No. IV. Seite 378.

rounded by the capsule seen by Müller. Never is there seen on the *glomerulus* an unequivocal trace of an appended canal, and never at the inner surface of the capsule, or any where else in the uriniferous ducts, ciliary epithelium. From these facts, Bidder thinks it results, that the representations by Mr Bowman contain one fact which is incorrect. This is, that as stated by Gerlach, the circumstance of vessels being exposed uncovered is quite at variance with all hitherto known as to the laws of organization. He finds, however, from examining the kidneys of the water salamander, that while the representation of phenomena, as seen by Mr Bowman, is essentially correct, the explanation of these phenomena requires in many parts to be rectified.

For the investigation in question, the anterior part of the kidney of the male triton, (*Triton tæniatus*,) is particularly well adapted, because it is by nature expanded in such manner, that for microscopical examination no further artificial preparation is required. Indeed, if one of the leaf-like masses of serpentine canals, of which the part of the kidney specified consists, is simply cut out and placed under the microscope, this is all that is requisite in order to exhibit completely, without exception, the whole of the texture under consideration. Bidder further found that any attempt to improve such a preparation by artificial means, as pulling and tearing with needles, to expand fully the convoluted ducts, usually obliterates the characteristic texture, removes the connection of the *glomeruli* with the uriniferous ducts, destroys the flask-like dilated terminations of the latter, removes the aspect of ciliary epithelium, and otherwise renders the part unfit for examination, so as to give correct results.

In the fact now stated lies the explanation of the negative results always obtained from examining the kidneys of the frog, because the microscope cannot be employed until fine sections of the renal substance have been spread out by mechanical means. He allows, also, that as these parts are not so easily found in the frog, it is no small proof of the perseverance of Mr Bowman, and the solidity of his inquiries, that notwithstanding these unfavourable circumstances in the higher animals, he has been able correctly to give the essential circumstances of the renal structure. In the serpent family and in lizards, the connection of the *glomeruli* with the uriniferous tubes is seen with comparative ease. But never in the higher animals did Bidder find, notwithstanding numerous trials, any fact which could suggest or establish the direct connection of these parts of the kidneys.

In the triton, on the other hand, there are observed in the parts of the kidney specified, at pretty regular distances from each other, shut terminations of the uriniferous tubes, which become dilated in the flask-like shape, and make themselves distinguished from the cylindrical tubes by greater transparency. Before the transition into these dilated parts, the uriniferous tube appears to be sometimes contracted ; yet this is by no means uniform. Normally only one uriniferous tube passes into this sort of dilated portion ; sometimes, however, two uriniferous tubes are connected with the same dilated portion, by which the objection of an illusion taking place thereby is completely set aside, viz. that by pressure the contents of one canal may be forced, without impediment, through the dilated portion into the second canal, and impelled onwards in it. In such circumstances also, the designation may be, instead of a closed termination of the uriniferous tube, rather a general dilatation in the course of such a tube.

Of the presence of an *epithelium* with actively vibrating *cilia*, immediately before the transition of the uriniferous tube into the flask-shaped expansion, and in the *cervix* or collar of the latter, as also in a considerable space of the inner wall of the same, Bidder states that he has completely convinced himself. The representation of Mr Bowman, that the vibratory epithelium layer of the uriniferous canals is prolonged. into the expanded portion, progressively diminishing in thickness, he finds to be quite correct ; but he observes, that not in every instance can we expect, even in the triton, to be able to recognise this circumstance with the desired certainty. He had inspected many preparations before he was able for the first time to be satisfied of the accuracy of the observation of Mr Bowman. The third part, or even the half of the circumference of the flask-shaped expansion presents this ciliated epithelium. If the same appears sometimes to be still more expanded, this depends only on the circumstance, that higher up detached ciliated cells are thrust deeper into the cavity.

On the other hand, the statement which Mr Bowman makes in denying any epithelium to the rest of the walls of the cavity, Bidder finds to be inaccurate. He finds here a simple thin plate-formed epithelium, which appears in pretty regular polygonal forms ; and if this do not appear equally evident in every case, the deficiency appears to depend on this circumstance, that from the contiguous uriniferous tubes entire epithelium cells or their fragments are thrust by the pressure of the covering glass plates into the cavity, and the correct view in the same is destroyed. The original transparency of these cells is frequently lost before the eyes of the observer; and there is thus sufficient opportunity to observe immediately the cause here specified.

Opposite the entrance-spot of the uriniferous tube into that expansion, or on one side of the latter when it is connected with two tubes, the Malpighian vascular tuft enters the uriniferous tube, and advances to a greater or less depth in the expanded portion itself; so that sometimes it fills the half of the cavity, sometimes it occupies a much smaller part of it. As to the statement that the *glomerulus* perforates the wall of the uriniferous tube, lies uncovered and free in this cavity, and is immersed in the fluid of the same, it must be indeed admitted, that the microscopical image on superficial examination appears frequently to agree with this; but that this is nothing but an illusive appearance any one, by more careful examination of all the circumstances taking place, may be convinced in the most positive manner. For, when the preparation has not lost its original translucency by the causes mentioned, it is at once easy to observe, sometimes directly, a partition separating the cavity of the expanded uriniferous tube from the vascular bundle. This partition appears like a fine arch-shaped border denoted by one single line, the convexity of which is directed towards the cavity, and the concavity towards the vascular bundle, which is usually most difficult to be distinguished on the most prominent points of the vascular network, and is most manifest in the distributions on the delicate interstices of the same, the periphery of which is in uninterrupted connection with the proper tunic or basement membrane of the uriniferous tubes. But even if this partition did not present itself to the eye with the desired distinctness, which from its delicacy cannot be wonderful, several convincing circumstances indicate its presence.

1*st*, The already mentioned entrance of the epithelial fragments in the expanded portions; for, while the latter thereby lose their translucency, that of the Malpighian bodies is little or not at all impaired, and remain clear and transparent, while the residual blood globules or their *nuclei* are from the first not in any way diminished in transparency.

2*d*, The phenomena of compression of the preparation prove the existence of such a partition. The fluid granular content of the expanded portions is thus impelled hither and thither without any entrance of the same ever being effected between network of the vascular bundle, and any mutual yielding of the last; and by such pressure the *glomerulus* itself, yet always only in one mass, and not in individual vascular clusters. This proves unequivocally the presence of a medium, by which the network of the vascular mass is held together; and that this connecting bond must be a membrane enclosing the whole vascular bundle, and cannot be a cement holding one of the separate networks to another, is shown by this circumstance, that after drawing the glomerulus from the uriniferous tubes, the vascular convolutions drop from each other, and present at the circumference of the mass disproportionately larger furrows than in the natural disposition of these parts.

Lastly, by continued pressure the glomerulus is forced back from the uriniferous tubes, nay, may be expelled from them entirely; and in such circumstances it may be again evidently perceived, that the whole flask-shaped expansion is surrounded by one uninterrupted outline, on the outside of which the *glomerulus* is placed.

Assuredly the uncovered disposition of the *glomerulus* in the cavity of the uriniferous tube would be contradicted, were it possible to prove that the plate-formed *epithelium*, which, as observed, covers part of the cavity, covers also the vascular mass. Though he allows that he cannot prove this unequivocally, yet he maintains that the rectification here suggested is probable. This he does in the following manner.

The relation of the *glomerulus* to the expanded portion of the uriniferous canal appears to him most properly to be referable to the series of those formations which it is usual to designate as introversions; by which nothing is stated as to their origin, but merely a certain form and kind of position of organic structures within each other is meant. In the case here treated, of such introversions, the same appears to take place at the thinnest and feeblest point of the wall of the shut end of the uriniferous tube. This is proved by the fact, that when, in consequence of strong pressure, the expanded portion bursts, this bursting regularly happens at the point where the proper tunic (basement membrane) of the uriniferous duct coalesces with the *glomerulus*. The outline of the partition mentioned appears also unequally feebler than at the other points of the circumference of the expanded portion. But this undoubtedly has great influence, that the ligamentous substance which lies on the outside of the uriniferous tubes and strengthens their walls, passes in uninterrupted succession, usually upon the vessels going to the *glomerulus*, but never enters the *glomerulus* itself, so that the vascular net-work of the same is actually held together only by the enclosing slender proper tunic of the uriniferous ducts.

In Mr Bowman's representation of the renal texture, a misconception has accordingly happened by this, that the capsule of the *glomerulus* and the expanded portion of the uriniferous duct are fully identified, while both are to be easily distinguished, though, as belonging to one and the same organic part, they pass insensibly into each other. In the agreement in the anatomical basement of the *tunica propria* of the uriniferous ducts and the capsule of the *glomerulus*, it is intelligible, that if the *glomerulus* and uriniferous ducts are separate from each other, in the first no trace of the early connection may be found, while the only available means thereto, viz. the position relation of both, are removed. So it is intelligible, how the *glomerulus*, after artificial spreading out sections of kidney and detachment from the uriniferous ducts, sometimes lies free, sometimes appears surrounded by a capsule. Because this capsule is not the covering belonging originally to the *glomerulus*, but only touches at the nèighbouring connecting tissue, which, after separating the *glomerulus* from the uriniferous ducts, sometimes surrounds the same. Hence proceeds the statement made under these circumstances, that the *glomerulus* lies free within its capsule. Indeed there is here between the vascular packet, the net-work of which is more expanded, and the connecting tissue accidentally lying on the same, a free space ; while the natural capsule of the *glomerulus*, that is, the introverted part of the uriniferous duct, lies close to the same.

The term capsule of the *glomerulus* has also been applied, on the one hand, to the flask-shaped dilated uriniferous duct itself, because it is supposed that the *glomerulus* lies free in the same ; and, on the other hand, the connecting substance surrounding the *glomerulus* after preparation of sections of renal tissue might be viewed as the natural capsule ; in both cases the true capsule would be misunderstood.[*]

* Ueber die Malpighischen Körper der Niere ; von F. Bidder in Dorpat. Archiv fur Anatomie, Physiologie, und Wissenschaftlichen Medicin. Von Dr Johannes Muller. 1845. Heft V. Seite 508.

Lastly, A. Kölliker of Zurich maintains with Mr Bowman not only the connection of the renal ducts with the capsule of the Malpighian bodies, but also at the entrance of the capsule and the contiguous portions of the renal ducts, or in the neck and orifice of the uriniferous tube, the existence of a ciliated epithelium with vigorous acting *cilia*.

According to this observer, whose observations were made on the kidneys of the embryo lizard, uriniferous ducts, measuring from $\frac{2}{100}$ to $\frac{4}{100}$ in diameter, consist of two layers. The outer is formed of a slender structureless membrane, which is easily distinguished by the addition of water, and is altogether a repetition of the outer coat of the renal ducts. The inner is a stratified epithelium, from $\cdot\frac{6}{1000}$ to $\frac{0}{1000}$ parts of one inch thick. The cells of which it consists are roundish, flat, $\frac{85}{10000}$ of one inch thick, $\frac{6}{1000}$ broad, with *nuclei* in two, three, or more layers arranged over each other. The inner layer is remarkable for distinctly developed ciliary processes, from $\frac{6}{10000}$ to $\frac{8}{1000}$ of one inch long, which, by their vigorous action, attract the attention of the most superficial observer, and furnish an interesting sight in transverse sections of the canal. The ciliated epithelium, so far as Kölliker saw, covers the whole length of the canal ; but it is wanting in the common excretory duct of the gland, and in the ends of the canals. These are the Malpighian bodies, the existence of which, in the primordial renal matter, has been established by Rathke's observations on the development of the viper. Every Malpighian body which has a diameter of from $\frac{4}{100}$ to $\frac{8}{100}$ of one inch, is a bladder or *vesicula*, which is placed immediately at the end of the renal duct, and is in free communication with the same. The structureless membrane of the ducts is peculiar to it; so also is the epithelium, only more slender, and is formed of one single layer, and is void of *cilia*. Within the Malpighian body is a cluster of capillary vessels, which enter and emerge at the origin of opposite sides of the canal, and, as it appears, are separated from the cavity of the renal duct or tubule by a layer of cells.*

. M. Kölliker further thinks that it may be owing to the mode of preparing the parts, that Reichert and Bidder did not observe the ciliary motions. If these parts are copiously sprinkled with water,

---

* It does not very clearly appear, from this mode of expression, whether M. Kölliker describes this partition from his own observation or from that of Bidder, by whom I have shown this partition was discovered.

the nucleated cells swell so much, that it is impossible to distinguish the nucleus and contents; and they appear only as pale, apparently homogeneous transparent globules. This renders the ciliated movements indistinct, or annihilates them. But, at all events, M. Kölliker has more frequently seen them in preparations moistened with serum, albumen, or frogs' urine, than in those sprinkled with water; and he has found them most certainly in preparations entirely unmoistened.

In one point only he thinks Mr Bowman's statements not quite correct, viz. regarding the epithelium of the Malpighian bodies. He observed within the capsule a complete epithelium; but the *cilia* be traced no further than the entrance of the capsule. He has satisfied himself, by preparations made with the greatest care, that within the capsule of the Malpighian bodies there is normally no free cavity.*

Such is an abstract of the present state of information on the microscopical anatomy of the kidney and the Malpighian bodies. It will be seen, that, notwithstanding the skill and dexterity of the observers, the facts are contradictory and not easily reconciled. I have nevertheless given them for various reasons; *first,* to show the great difficulty of the subject; *secondly,* to prove what is admitted by Henle, that microscopical anatomy is still in a transition and imperfect state; and also, *thirdly,* to enable readers to form some idea of the minute structure of the glands. Though the kidney is in some respects peculiar in its minute structure, yet it agrees with other glandular organs in certain general and leading characters; and the exposition of these, however incomplete, may serve to communicate an idea of the peculiar characters of glandular structure in general.

Before quitting the subject, however, it is proper to observe that one, if not two of the points on which Reichert, Gerlach, and Bidder differ from Mr Bowman, depend on optical illusions only; that he has described correctly what he saw by the microscope; but that, from some cause not easily understood, he has not given the explanations of the phenomena which they conceive to be correct.

On the uses of the Malpighian bodies we have no positive correct information. All is supposition and conjecture; and those who have most studied these bodies, have been least willing to speak with

* Ueber Flimmerbewegungen in den Primordial Nieren ; von A. Kölliker, Archiv fur Anatomie, Physiologie, und Wissenschaftliche Medicin. Heft V. S. 518. 1845.

confidence. The fact that they are placed among the serpentine renal ducts, and that they are furnished with a peculiar arrangement of capillary arteries, may favour the inference that they are in some way connected with the secretion of urine. If the fact contended for by Mr Bowman, that the Malpighian bodies are connected with the serpentine ducts, were established, this inference would be rendered almost certain. This communication, however, is denied by Müller and others; and Müller accordingly maintains that the Malpighian bodies have no concern in the secretion of urine.

Mr Bowman, on the other hand, who thinks he has shown that each Malpighian body is situate at the remote or superior extremity of a uriniferous tube, and that the tufts of vessels are a distinct system of capillaries inserted into the interior of the tube, infers that, as the arrangement of the vessels in the Malpighian tufts is evidently designed to retard the motion of blood through them, the insertion of the tuft in the extremity of the tube indicates that this retardation is connected with the secreting process. He concludes, therefore, that it is highly probable that the use of the Malpighian tufts is to affuse water abundantly and uniformly over the urine as it is secreted, so as to ensure the perfect solution of all its constituents. Along with this, he thinks that these bodies, by contributing to remove aqueous matter from the blood, act as a self-adjusting valve or sluice to the circulation. The use of the Malpighian bodies, in short, according to Mr Bowman, is to separate from the blood the watery portion, according to the necessities of the system.

I have only to add, in order to complete the description of the renal serpentine ducts, that while they advance through the cortical portion of the kidney to its periphery, they are not always, properly speaking, serpentine.

In the horse, for instance, in which they are so large that they may be perceived by the eye, at least after injection, without the microscope, they do not run in the serpentine and tortuous course, which they observe in man and most other animals. They are continued from the straight ducts, very slightly bending or undulating, but still almost straight, for at least one inch or one inch and a-half. As they approach the surface of the cortical portion, these undulating flexures increase, and at the very surface they are completely converted into serpentine or tortuous tubes.

In the squirrel also, the serpentine ducts are large, and united by little cellular tissue. In that animal they are seen without injection, by the microscope. The Bellinian ducts advance straight through the medullary cones, and then passing into the cortical matter, become bent. They appear a little larger than the medullary ducts upon entering the cortical portion.

§ V.—THE TESTIS.

In the INSECT tribes and ARTICULATE animals, the *testes* assume an endless variety of forms. All, indeed, consist of tubules mostly simple; but these are arranged in so great a variety of forms, that it is extremely difficult to give a short, and at the same time accurate view of these forms.

In FISHES, the organs corresponding to *Testes* appear to be constructed in two different modes. 1. For the most part, the *testes* are composed of multiplied seminiferous canals or ducts. 2. Less frequently the *testes* are entirely solid, and are composed of globules without internal canals, and without deferent duct; the substance of which passes from the external surface into the cavity of the abdomen, from which it is conveyed outwards by one single orifice, exactly as the ova. The best examples of these structures are seen in the eel and *petromyzon*. In such animals the *ova* and the *testes*, or matter composing the testes, are so similar, that they are often confounded.

In the herring and shad the structure is the following. From the efferent duct, running by the side or margin of the milt (*Testis*), the largest tubules proceed close to each other, approaching to the lobes attached to the common duct. But the further division is effected, not only by ramification, but also by numberless reticular anastomoses, so that almost the whole substance of the *testis* or milt consists, in the month of May, of anastomoses of large ducts filled with seminal fluid, which are distinctly seen by the naked eye. From the reticulated *ansæ*, however, proceed also other branching canals, variously separated, which terminate here and there in free but closed ends. Towards the outer margin and at the opposite side of the lobes, the branchy divisions are most abundant, while the anastomoses are less frequent; so that the margin itself is almost composed of straight twig-like tubules, which, little diminished, terminate in the extreme margin and at the surface with closed ends. The internal branches are dispersed in various directions; all the external and marginal ones proceed in a straight course to the surface, so that on the surface of one side of

the testis, the closed ends of the tubules project like rounded corpuscula. The disposition of the tubules is mostly known from the
white seminal matter contained, which renders it more distinct than
the other grey matter. The most singular is the conformation of the male genitals in
the rays and sharks. The glandular organs are of two sorts; one,
corresponding to what has been hitherto described. as testes, consisting of globules, and not of seminal ducts; the other generally
regarded as the epididymis, composed of serpentine canals, yet not
at all joined with the globulose testes. On this account Müller
thinks that these bodies are not epididymides, but peculiar glands.

In man the essential part of the testis consists of tubuli seminiferi, or very minute tubules, which are very numerous, and radiate
from all parts of the circumference of the organ to the centre, or
mediastinum testis, making numberless convolutions, which progressively diminish as they approach the rete testis. Two or more
of the tubuli being collected together, and invested by a common
cellular tunic, form a lobule of a conical shape, with its apex terminating in the corpus Highmorianum. The lobules thus formed
are not entirely distinct, but communicate with neighbouring lobules, the process investing them being incomplete. Krause estimates their number between 404 and 484.

The tubuli of which they are composed are of a white colour,
and uniform in size; but their calibre varies in different subjects,
and in different periods of life, and different states of the system.
They are larger in young adults, and when distended with semen,
than in aged persons, and when the gland is in a state of rest.
From a table of measurements made by Mr Gulliver, and published in the proceedings of the Zoological Society, their diameter appears to have varied from the 1-112th to the 1-77th part of an
English inch, and from the 1-160th to the 1-100th part of an inch
in adults; and in children and infants, from the 1-400th to the
1-230th part of an English inch. Observers, however, vary as to
the diameter of these tubuli. The average diameter of the uninjected canal is estimated by Müller at 1-18th of a line, = 1-180th
of an inch, and by Lauth, 1-185th of an inch. Krause found the
tubuli when filled with semen to measure about one-twelfth of one
line, = 1-120th of an inch, and in old men and youths about 1-16th
of a line, or 1-160th part of an inch.

As to their number and their length little seems ascertained.

Monro estimated the number of seminiferous tubes at 300; while Lauth made their average number 840. The latter author estimated the mean length of all the ducts united at 1750 feet. The individual ducts he found to vary in length, the mean being 25 inches. Krause estimated their entire length at 1015 feet.

That the membrane composing the *tubuli* is of a mucous character has been proved by microscopic examination; and it is further continuous with the mucous surface of the genito-urinary system. There is no appearance of interlobular substance. The ducts are connected by a loose network of vessels, and consequently may be easily separated and unravelled. The tubes are usually injected with mercury, and in this state are shown in most anatomical collections. Sir Astley Cooper injected the tubes with size; but of the method which he followed no account is given.

When the *tubuli* are unravelled, they are found to divide and to form numerous anastomotic unions, which increase in frequency as they approach the circumference of the gland. The tubuli thus form one large communicating network, in which it is impossible to isolate completely either one duct or one lobule. In one instance only did Lauth, who discovered these anastomoses of the seminiferous tubuli, find a duct terminating in a blind sac; and this he regards as an exception. Blind sacs have been more frequently found, however, by Krause.

The convolutions of the seminiferous tubes diminish in number as they approach the mediastinum and cease at a distance of from one to two lines, where two or more unite to form one single, straight duct termed *vas rectum*, whith joins the *rete testis* at a right angle. The *vasa recta* are very slender, and easily give way when injected. Their calibre, which is greater than that of the seminal tubes, is estimated by Lauth at 1-108th of an inch. Their number Haller reckoned at 20; but it is believed that they are more numerous.

The *rete testis* is formed of a plexus of seminal tubes, which occupies the *Corpus Highmorianum* or *mediastinum testis*. The *vasa recta*, after penetrating the walls of the *corpus*, terminate in from seven to thirteen vessels, which, running parallel to each other in a waving course, and frequently dividing and anastomosing, form the *rete testis*. The mean diameter of these vessels Lauth found in injected preparations to be 1-72d of an inch.

From the upper part of the *rete* thus formed issue vessels in num-

ber about twelve or fourteen, but sometimes rising to thirty, which
are named *vasa efferentia.* These ducts, which are arranged in conical shape, and hence named *coni vasculosi,* run straight for the
space of one or two lines, forming convolutions which become numerous and close as the vessels recede from the testis. Lauth, es-
timating the average length at 7 inches 4 lines, and their number
at thirteen, makes the united length to be nearly 8 feet. After forming the vascular tubes, already mentioned, they successively join
one single duct, the canal of the epididymis, at irregular intervals,
the intermediate spaces of the duct varying in length from half-an-
inch to 6 inches. These efferent ducts are more slender than the
canal of the epididymis, and frequently give way under the pressure of the column of mercury.

While the vascular cones form a round bulky mass, which has
been named the head, or *globus major,* of the epididymis, the convolutions made by the efferent ducts form the body and tail, to
which also the name of *globus minor* has been applied.

A shut canal or duct, usually attached to the tail of the epididymis, and with a blind appendage or termination, constitutes what
has been named the *vasculum aberrans.* The length of this duct
varies from 1 to 12 or 14 inches, and it is always more or less convoluted. It is not constant; nor is its use perfectly known. Mr
Curling infers that it serves no particular purpose, and that it is a
mere diverticulum, or process similar to those observed in the intestinal canal.

The canal of the epididymis as it approaches the level of that
body becomes larger, and forms then the *vas deferens* or excretory
duct of the testicle. The course, direction, and termination of this
tube are well known.

The spermatic artery or arteries, or those which supply the testis,
arise either from the aorta immediately below the renal artery, or
come off in one trunk, common to it and the renal artery, a mode
of origin connected with the site of the organ in the fœtus, when it
is placed near the kidney on each side of the spinal column. From
the point now specified they descend behind the peritoneum, forming many convolutions and tortuous windings, obliquely across the
psoas muscle and ureter, to which each artery gives branches, and,
entering the inguinal canal by the internal ring, they are joined
with the chord and reach the gland. Their subsequent distribution is described by Sir Astley Cooper in the following manner.

" When the artery reaches from one to three inches from the epididymis it divides into two branches, which descend to the testicle, and its inner side, opposite to that on which the epididymis is placed; one passing on the anterior and upper, the other to the posterior and lower part of the testis. From the anterior branch the vessels of the epididymis arise. First, one passes to its head; secondly, another to its body; and thirdly, one to the tail and the first convolutions of the *vas deferens*, communicating freely with the deferential artery. The spermatic artery, after giving off branches to the epididymis, enters the testis by penetrating the outer layer of the *tunica albuginea ;* and, dividing upon its vascular layer, they form an arch by their junction at the lower part of the testis, from which numerous vessels pass upwards; and then descending, they supply the lobes of the *tubuli seminiferi.* Besides this lower arch there is another passing in the direction of the rete, extremely convoluted in its course, and forming an anastomosis between the principal branches. The testis receives a further supply of blood from another vessel, the artery of the *vas deferens,* or posterior spermatic artery, which arises from one of the vesical arteries, branches of their internal iliac. This artery divides into two sets of branches, one set descending to the *vesicula seminalis* and to the termination of the *vas deferens;* the other ascending upon the *vas deferens,* runs in a serpentine direction upon the coat of that vessel, passing through the whole length of the spermatic chord; and when it reaches the tail of the epididymis, it divides into two sets of branches, one advancing to unite with the spermatic artery to supply the testis and epididymis, the other passing backwards to the *tunica vaginalis* and cremaster."

The spermatic veins issue from the testis in three sets; one from the *rete* and *tubuli;* another from the vascular layer of the *tunica albuginea ;* and a third from the lower extremity of the *vas deferens.* The veins of the testis pass in three courses into the beginning of the spermatic chord. Of these, two quit the back of the testis, one at its anterior and upper part; and a second at its centre, and thereafter from two to three inches are united into one. The other column accompanies the *vas deferens.* The veins of the epididymis, issuing from the head, body, and tail, with some from the *vas deferens,* terminate in the veins of the spermatic chord. The veins, after quitting the testis, become very tortuous, and forming frequent divisions and inosculations, constitute the plexus named *vasa pam-*

piniformia. After entering the pelvis they form one or two veins which terminate on the right side of the *vena cava* inferior, and on the left in the renal vein, though this is liable to some variety. The left spermatic vein passes under the sigmoid flexure of the colon,—a circumstance important to be remembered, in certain morbid states of the gland and its vessels.

Several anatomists represent the spermatic veins to be void of valves ; and to this circumstance ascribe the occurrence of varicocele. Mr Curling states, that he has several times injected these veins with alcohol, and on laying them open, he observed valves in the larger veins, and found the passage of the alcohol arrested by the valves. Valves are not seen near the testis, or in the small veins forming the plexus, nor did Mr Curling observe them within the abdomen.

§ VI.—THE MAMMA.

The MAMMALIA are the only class of vertebrated animals which possess the glands called MAMMÆ or Breasts ; BIRDS, REPTILES, and FISHES, being destitute of these ; and in this order the conformation of these glands appears under two forms.

1. In the higher MAMMALIA and in man the elementary particles of the MAMMÆ, or the ends of the lactiferous tubes, are small vesiculæ, joined to stalks by small branches of lactiferous tubules in the manner of cluster of grapes or berries, and enclosed by a very delicate cellular tissue. These *acini* of vesicles constitute the smallest lobules. Several clustering *acini* united to the twigs of a larger branch form a large tubule or one of the second order ; and when several of these are conjoined they form a tubule of the third order. These lactiferous tubes then uniting form trunks of lactiferous ducts, which, either united open into the nipple, as in the udder of the RUMINANTS, or separately perforate the nipple, as in the human female and various other mammalia.

2. The second form of *mamma* is more rarely met with, and is observed in families of the mammalia, which may be regarded as the lowest in that class ; namely, in the CETACEA, and in the duck-bill (*ornithorhyncus paradoxus*), and probably in the *echidna*. In these animals the structure is reduced to that of a glandular organ, such as first presents itself in the lowest mammalia, or in the most simple form, that is in the shape of closed *intestinula*, collected in one mass.

CHAPTER II.

MORBID STATES OF THE GLANDULAR ORGANS.

THE morbid states of the glandular organs are very numerous and varied; and if we remember how often their function is disordered, to how many morbid changes their secreted products are liable, how many changes may take place in their circulation, independent of changes in their structure, we must allow that there is scarcely a texture in the whole frame which presents so many forms of diseased action as the glands.

. It would lead me into a field too extensive to consider all the varieties of disorder and diseased action to which I have now adverted. It must also be admitted, that the subject is in many respects imperfectly known; and that the consideration of various changes incident to glandular action would lead me into inquiries inconsistent with the nature of the present work. I propose, therefore, to confine the present sketch very much, if not entirely, to the morbid states most frequently taking place in the system of the secreting glands.

SECTION I.

GENERAL OBSERVATIONS ON DISORDERS OF THE SECRETING GLANDS.

THE glands, from being liberally supplied with blood-vessels, are liable to be affected by all the changes which take place in the vascnlar system. The blood, indeed, may be regarded as the first great agent which affects the state of the functions of the secreting glands. All substances taken into the blood are circulated to the glands, and in a degree greater or less affect their secretions. Thus, mercury and its preparations, which have been erroneously supposed to act on the salivary glands only, act at the same time on the pancreas, the liver, and the kidneys. In the same manner also, spirituous liquors or articles containing them are absorbed by the veins, circulated and conveyed to the different glands, and in this manner always cause unnatural excitement and irritation in their vessels and elementary particles. Saline substances also reach the glands and act on them sometimes favourably, sometimes detrimentally.

Glands are liable to inflammation, acute and chronic, and all their usual effects and consequences; to hemorrhage; to induration; to hypertrophy; to atrophy; to interstitial deposits of new matter; to the obstruction of their duets by blood, lymph, and the products of secretion; to various changes in structure in the elementary or ultimate particles; and to several of the heterologous depths.

When glandular organs are affected by inflammation, that process may affect either the component tubes or the delicate filamentous tissue by which these tubes are united; or both at the same time. When the process affects the tubes, if it do not terminate in resolution, that is, if the orgasm, after subsisting for some time, does not subside without giving rise to inflammatory products, it causes effusion of *plasma*, or of blood within the tubes, which are then for the time obliterated. In this case the gland is enlarged and indurated, sometimes irregular, is the seat of dull pain and weight, and secretion is almost impracticable.

In certain favourable cases, in which the *plasma* or blood is effused in small quantity, it does not undergo coagulation; and the tubes may remain more or less pervious; or even, after a time, may recover entirely their permeability. Instances of this undoubtedly take place both in inflammation of the liver and in that of the kidneys.

In other instances, however, in which the effusion is abundant, the gland remains hard and enlarged for a long time, sometimes for life.

When inflammation affects the outside of the tubes and acini, or elementary particles, and the connecting tissue, it more commonly causes the effusion of purulent matter; in one or more distinct cysts or abscesses.

Lastly, inflammation often attacks first and principally the excretory duct and its divisions, and terminates in effusion of matter more or less copious. This either escapes by the general duct; or, if i do not readily escape, or is entirely confined, the duct and all the communicating parts become greatly distended, containing considerable quantities of purulent matter, and their lining membrane covered with a coating of lymph; and in this case the gland appears to contain a number of separate abscesses. If, however, these be carefully examined, it is seen that neither the gland nor the texture of the ducts is destroyed; that the former is enlarged and extenuated by the distension of the ducts; while the apparent abscesses are formed by the latter. This takes place in the kidneys and prostate gland.

Inflammation of strumous character is liable to affect the secreting glands, more especially the female breast, the *testes* and prostate gland of the male, and the kidneys and parotids in both sexes. The effects of this process, which is chronic in duration, and insidious and not well-marked in symptoms, are denoted by the deposit, in general, within the tubules of the glands of semifluid or fluid tyromatous matter, that is to say, an albuminous animal product, which, though it undergoes coagulation, is nevertheless remarkable for showing little or no tendency to become organized.   This substance, found in the shape of putty-like matter, caseous matter, or caseous mixed with calcareous matter, presents few or no bloodvessels, has no independent circulation, and, in short, gives evidence of possessing a very low degree of vitality, or rather nothing of that property at all.   As already stated, it is found in the ducts of the *testes* and prostate gland, in which its presence gives rise to considerable irregular swelling and pain by pressure on adjoining parts ; it is also seen in the *mamma*, where it likewise causes considerable irregular swelling; and it may affect either the serpentine ducts of the kidney, or the calyces of that gland.

Section II.

§ I. THE LACRYMAL AND SALIVARY GLANDS.

These glands are liable to inflammation, acute and chronic ; the latter most usual.

Inflammation of the lacrymal gland is certainly rare, unless as the effect of injury or the extension of inflammation of the conjunctiva into its ducts. Most usually it is chronic. An instance is mentioned by Beer ;* and the disease is described by Reil and Benedict. Hemorrhage takes place from it sometimes as vicarious of menstruation, sometimes without any obvious connection with this cause. Hemorrhage appearing at the eyes in purpura is most probably from the conjunctiva.

* Georg. Jos. Beer Auswahl aus dem Tagebuch eines practrischen Augenarztes, n. 2. Wien, 1800.

The lacrymal gland may be enlarged from strumous disorder to the size of a nut.   It then makes a distinct tumour at the exterior and superior angle of the eye beneath the orbital plates.

Schmidt admitted that inflammation of the lacrymal gland alone can scarcely be said to take place ; because, the disease thus designated is rather inflammation of the entire orbit, that is of the orbital cellular tissue, embracing also the gland.*   This view is adopted by Benedict, who devotes a whole chapter to the description of the disease and its effects.   As described by this author, it is manifestly an acute inflammation of the ophthalmic cellular tissue, with some symptoms indicative of extension to the cerebral membranes.   Thus, not only is there pain in the eyeball and orbit, but pain of the head, delirium, want of sleep, and great suffering. The characteristic symptoms are the sense of something in the orbit above the eye, the feeling of the orbit being too small for the eye, as if the eyeball were thrust out of it ; then swelling of the upper eyelid, proceeding generally to a great degree; and at last the formation of matter, which points in this situation, or immediately beneath it.†   A similar account is given by Weller.

It is manifest that this is the account of general inflammation of the orbital celluloso-adipose tissue; and not of the lacrymal gland alone.   The gland, however, may be affected; but that is only in a slight degree.

This disorder may terminate in one of three modes.   First, under symptoms of complete *phrenitis*, the patient dies ; secondly, it may terminate in abscess of the orbital tissue ; or, thirdly, complete *ophthalmitis* is associated with inflammation of the eyeball, and suppuration of the latter is superadded to abscess of the orbit.

Next to resolution abscess of the orbital tissue is the most favourable result.   Benedict states that when this does not take place, or an opening is neglected, death has been the result, by the transit of the disease to the brain; and on inspecting the parts, the anterior lobe has been found inflamed, and a collection of purulent matter, both on the surface of the cranium, frontal bone, and in the orbit.

When the lacrymal gland is affected by chronic inflammation, the eye is protruded, the optic nerve suffers from pressure, and

* Johann. Adam Schmidt, über die Krankheiten des Thränenorgans, mit 4 Kupfertaf, gr. 8vo.   Wien, 1803.

† Traugott Guilelmi Gustavi Benedict, de Morbis Oculi Humani Inflammatoriis. Lib. xxiii.   Lipsiæ, 1811.   Liber 7imus, § 153, p. 82.

amaurosis follows ;* or the vitreous humor and lens are so much compressed, that sight is greatly impaired.

Even without this compression the sight may be lost.

This is probably owing to the nervous connection between the divisions of the first part of the fifth nerve,—one of which supplies the lacrymal gland,—and the branches of the same nerve, which are distributed to the ciliary processes.

Portal states, that he found it affected with scirrhus, and even proceeding to ulceration in dead bodies; especially in the body of one female who had cancer in both mammæ, and who some time before death had an attack of chronic ophthalmia.

It is often difficult to distinguish between mere induration, the effect of chronic inflammation and scirrhus of the gland. In both the gland is hard and enlarged, and causes a prominent swelling, more or less distinct, at the superior outer angle of the orbit. The eye is pressed downwards ; and more or less ophthalmia affects the palpebral and ocular conjunctiva. At first the secretion of tears is augmented ; but after the disease has continued some time it is diminished ; and the peculiar symptom called *xerophthalmia* or preternatural dryness of the eye is induced.

The disease named cancer of the eyeball often originates either in the lacrymal gland, or in the *caruncula lacrymalis*. Conversely, if scirrhus affect the eyeball, it may spread to the lacrymal gland.

Guerin states that he extirpated a lacrymal gland affected with scirrhus, while the eye appears to have been unaffected. This he did with so great dexterity, that the *rectus externus* muscle was not touched. The gland formed a swelling so considerable, that it covered completely the globe of the eye. The eye, however, was found quite sound behind the tumour of the lacrymal gland. Richerand, who knew no other instance of extirpation of the gland alone, is inclined to believe the case solitary. It is certainly much more common to remove the gland, sound or diseased, in removing the eye, than to remove the diseased gland alone without the eye.

The lacrymal gland has, nevertheless, been repeatedly removed since that time. Thus it was removed by Duval de Rennes,† by Mr Travers,‡ by Mr O'Beirne in 1820,§ by Mr Todd in 1821,‖

* Reil, Memorabilia Clinica. Vol. i. Fascicul. i p. 118.

† J. L. Duval sur quelques Affections Douloureuses de la Face. Paris, 1814. 8vo.

‡ Synopsis of Diseases of the Eye and their Treatment. London, 1820 and 1824, p. 233.

§ On Diseases of the Lacrymal Gland, by Charles H. Todd. Dublin Hospital Reports, Vol. iii. p. 407.

‖ Ibid.

by Daviel in 1829, by Lawrence in 1826 and 1828,* and by M. Jules Cloquet in 1835.†

It is not perfectly certain, whether in all these cases the gland was affected by genuine scirrhus. It is certain that in its site was a hard firm body, generally much swelled, and forcing the eyeball downwards. In each of the cases almost the structure of the gland was different. In two cases, in which Mr Lawrence operated, he allows that the gland in respect of hardness might have been called scirrhus; but he adds, that he saw no reason for suspecting the disease to be malignant. If this latter conclusion be admitted, then it follows that these are examples of simple induration (*skleroma*) of glands. In all these cases, however, the gland is more or less enlarged, sometimes very much so.

In those cases in which the lacrymal gland has been examined after extirpation, it has been observed that the elementary particles or granules were hard and enlarged, chiefly by the effusion of lymph. But the appearances vary in different instances.

Schmidt, and afterwards Beer, describe the formation of true hydatids as occurring in the lacrymal gland. Their pressure causes a tumour at the upper part of the orbit, and some degree of exophthalmia.

Among the salivary glands, the morbid states of the parotid have attracted most attention.

It is known that the parotid and *socia parotidis* are liable to acute inflammation, forming the disease known by the popular name of Mumps and Branks, and also to various chronic disorders. Of the former I need scarcely speak in this place; because, though a disease not unimportant, yet it is rarely the object of attention to the pathological inquirer; and the accounts given in the ordinary treatises contain all the information which it is necessary to possess on the affection‡ and the diseases in conjunction with which it appears either as an effect or a part.

One or two points only require to be here noticed. The swelling which takes place in the parotid region in remittent fever, typhous

---

* A Treatise on the Diseases of the Eye, by William Lawrence, P. R. S. London, 1833. Chapter xxix. sect. i.

† Du Squirrhe de la Glande Lacrymale et de l'Ablation de cette Glande, par G. E. Maslieurat-Lagemard. Archives Generales, iiie. et Nouvelle Serie. T. vii. ou T. lii. Paris, 1840. P. 90.

‡ Elements of Practice of Medicine. Vol. ii. Book ii. Chapter v. § iv. p. 410.

fever, *synochus*, scarlet fever, and similar diseases, appears to be seated rather in the surrounding cellular and adipose tissue than in the parotid gland. It occasionally proceeds to suppuration ; and this I have seen it do, notwithstanding the use of means calculated to obviate this termination. This result is supposed not to be un-favourable ; and many physicians prefer promoting it by the use of stimulating applications. At the same time, it must be observed that suppuration in this region is not always a favourable result. The following case given by Monteggia is in point.

In a man of 60 years a swelling took place, in the course of fever, in the right parotid region. This speedily subsided, and was followed by a similar swelling in the left parotid region, which terminated in abscess. This being evacuated by an incision made below the ear, the opening continued for one month discharging much matter, and a little coming away daily by the ear-bole. The patient, in the meantime, though the original disease was gone, did not recover properly, continued long languishing, and at length, becoming worse, died comatose.

Inspection of the body disclosed the following facts. The whole cellular tissue on the left side of the head was loaded with fluid. The parotid gland, contracted, rigid, and hardish, was marked in various places with red points. From the external site of the in-cision an ulcerated passage or sinus led to the *meatus auditorius*, the eroded cartilage of which was partly seen. The adjoining part of the bony canal, with the root of the zygomatic process, were struck with caries. In the meatus itself were some loose osseous fragments, along with some testaceous remains of some insect dead in this situation. The temporal muscle presented unequivocal traces of previous inflammation ; and beneath it were some drops of pu-rulent matter on the surface of skull. The intermeningeal space, when the skull was opened, effused a large quantity of fluid on the left side, the veins here being, besides, unusually turgid. When the *dura mater* was detached from the inner surface of the skull on this side, there appeared a purulent space half an inch broad on the surface of the petrous process, where the *foramina* of Valsalva lead to cavity of the tympanum.

The purulent matter, nevertheless, did not proceed from that cavity, in which there was no disease. But the suppuration which had taken place between the temporal muscle and the skull, had transmitted many drops into the cavity of the skull by a small aperture conspicuous in the temporal bone, from which then the fluid proceeding backwards by a linear path had dropped into the space mentioned in the petrous portion of the temporal bone.*

This case, however, merely shows, that when extensive suppurations take place in certain situations and in particular constitutions, the matter may find its way into or among important and essential organs.

In almost all these cases of suppuration in the parotid region, the gland does not itself suppurate, but remains as described by Monteggia, shrunk, dry, hard, and apparently atrophied.

§ 2. The parotid gland and its companion are liable to strumous transformation and infiltration, to chronic induration, to hypertrophy, to scirrho-carcinoma, and to melanosis.

In ordinary circumstances enlargement of the parotid is most commonly strumous or dependent on chronic inflammation. In either case, a tumour variable in size is formed at the auriculo-temporal region, a little above the angle of the jaw. When this swelling is of strumous origin, it usually causes secondary inflammation and suppuration of the surrounding cellular tissue and the incumbent skin; one opening or two may take place; and for a considerable time a thin serous or sero-purulent discharge continues. Usually the gland is not itself much or seriously affected beyond the swelling caused by infiltration of its ducts and *acini*. In certain cases, however, the gland or its ducts seem to pass into the ulcerative stage; and a long continued sore with a salivary fistula is the result. In other cases the ulcerative communication appears to be established between Steno's duct only and the surface. Ulcers and fistulæ of this kind were seen by Hildanus;† and Cheselden states, that he saw patients with the gland ulcerated, and causing a constant effusion of saliva, till, he adds, the greatest part of the gland was consumed by the use of red precipitate.‡ It is not easy to imagine the gland, that is the substance of the gland, to be much consumed in this manner or by this agent, without more serious effects. But we may admit that the remedy, by inducing a new and more decided action, and enabling the most healthy

---

* Joannis Baptistae Monteggia Fasciculi Pathologici. Turici Helvetiorum, 1793. 8vo, p. 17.

† One in a young man of 12. Observat. Chirurgic. Centuria V. Obs. lxxx. Op. Omnia, Francofurti ad Moenum, 1646. Folio. P. 471.

‡ The Anatomy of the Human Body. Book iii. Chapter iii. p. 142. London, 1784, the 12th edition.

part of the gland to assume proper action, had effected cicatrization.

Tenon speaks of a tumour of the parotid gland which attains
a large size, yet he says without change in structure. The instance
which he describes took place in a child, on the left cheek of whom
appeared a tumour almost as large as the fist, extending from the
ear to the angle of the lip. This tumour, which had grown gradually from the birth of the child, was soft, white, indolent, moveable, and composed apparently of glandular grains. It appeared
also traversed by large vessels, which formed in various parts of
the skin networks of spiral form or reddish whorls. The child
died not from the tumour, but from a different cause. Tenon found
that the tumour was formed by the parotid gland, which had acquired great size, and exceeded its usual limits. Large arteries
proceeding from the external carotid and external maxillary entered the lower part of the gland.*

This seems to have been an example of simple strumous enlargement, or at most of hypertrophy occurring in the strumous. If
there was no perceptible change in structure, that must be ascribed
to the short duration of the affection ; for the enlarged state of the
arteries shows that they were conveying much blood into the gland ;
and though this seemed only to be giving rise to simple enlargement, it is impossible to doubt, that the characteristic deposition of
strumous disorganization would soon follow.   A case similar is
recorded by Dr Duke.†

The same species of changes may take place in the submaxillary
and sublingual glands, though in these they have probably attracted less attention.   A peculiar cause of enlargement of the submaxillary gland is the irritation of teething, and especially the
presence of carious molar teeth ; and both these and the sublingual
glands may become enlarged from the irritation of the gastro-intestinal mucous membrane in disorders of the alimentary canal.
These disorders cause sour offensive exhalations to arise, indicating
the bad sort of chyle prepared.   The blood is consequently in an
unhealthy state ; and this, again, appears to irritate the glands, and
to excite their vessels to increased and disordered action.

In adults, a common cause of enlargement of the parotid and
the other salivary glands is the use of mercury in strumous habits.
Whether it be that mercury operates always hurtfully in the stru-

* Memoires de l'Academie des Sciences, 1760.
† Provincial Medical and Surgical Journal, No. XXI. Feb. 19, 1842.

mous, or whether it be, that while it is taken, the individuals are incautious, and expose themselves to cold, or commit errors in diet, certain it is, that in the great majority of cases, the first enlargement of the parotid and other salivary glands takes place either during a course of mercury, or soon after it is completed. All these glands are more or less swelled, sometimes very much; and the parotid being placed in a situation so conspicuous, forms a large bulging tumour on one or both sides of the jaw. These tumours are manifestly of the strumous character, and occur principally in strumous subjects. Often they cause suppuration of the surrounding cellular tissue and skin, forming sinuous ulcers, and leaving ugly scars.

§ 3. The sublingual glands are liable to a peculiar enlargement, generally of a chronic character, immediately beneath the tongue, where its pressure on the sublingual veins causes great distension of these vessels. To this appearance a peculiar name, that of *Ranula,* has been applied, from some fancied resemblance to a small frog. The matter causing this tumour varies. Sometimes it is a simple enlargement of the gland. More frequently, however, it arises from one or more concretions in the excretory duct of one or other of these glands.

. § 4. CHRONIC INDURATION is liable to affect either or all of the salivary glands. The change has, however, been most commonly observed in the parotid gland. The gland is enlarged, hard, indolent, resistent; and constrains the motions of the jaw. Sometimes the tumour is irregular on the surface; in other instances it is smooth. As to pain, evidence varies a good deal; for in some instances there is much deep-seated lancinating or darting pain; in others no pain is felt, except that resulting from pressure and distension of the parts.

Almost all these tumours in the site of the parotid, if a little hard, have been comprehended under the general and comprehensive name of scirrhus; and at present it cannot be said that there is any good diagnosis between simple chronic induration and scirrhus, before at least the tumour has been removed and subjected to proper microscopic examination. Boyer himself admits the difficulty of the diagnosis, and allows that many cases of enlargement in this region, which were strumous, were ascribed to scirrhus. I think it scarcely possible to mistake for scirrhus, as he seems to believe was done, mere strumous swellings, whether of the parotid gland or of the lymphatic glands, when taking place in young persons; and the age of the patient, as well as the appearance of the tumour and aspect of the patient, ought to be taken into account. Neither does mobility avail so much as M. Boyer seems to imagine. A mere indurated parotid gland may, from its position, contract very firm adhesions with the contiguous parts.

The circumstance of age, however, must not be taken alone. Sabatier records a case of considerable enlargement in the site of the right parotid, in a person above 60 years. The tumour extended in the vertical direction from the infra-zygomatic fossa to 5 or 6 centimetres below the angle of the jaw; and in the horizontal, from the lobe of the ear to the anterior margin of the temporal muscle. In shape it was irregular. It was free from pain. To this tumour, which Sabatier removed by operation, he applies the name of *Exuberance*. Upon its inner structure he gives no details. But it must have been an instance either of hypertrophy, or some change different from scirrhus.

What, then, is to be said of the cases, now numerous, in which the parotid gland is recorded to have been removed by operation? For a long series of years, surgical authors have been in the habit of speaking familiarly of scirrhus of the parotid gland, and of the removal of the gland for this distemper. It appears, indeed, at one time, if we form a judgment from the frequency of instances of excision, to have been imagined to be a common disease. Thus Heister, Von Siebold, Souscrampes, Orth, Burgras, Hezel, and Alix, all record cases, which, they say, are examples of excision of the parotid gland.

To the question here suggested two answers must be given. First, it appears certain that scirrhus is by no means so frequent as has been supposed; and, secondly, the alleged instances of scirrhus, from which the gland is stated to have been removed, were certainly either strumous indurations and enlargements of other parts, or affections of the gland not scirrhous.

In several instances these operations could not have been performed on the gland, and must have taken place on enlarged lymphatic glands; and, in other respects, it is more than doubtful that the parotid was affected by scirrhus. Richter and John Bell first; and afterwards Murat, Richerand, Boyer, Velpeau, and the majority of well-informed surgeons, maintain that it is impossible to extirpate the gland without tying the carotid.

In the museum of the College of Surgeons of Dublin, are several preparations of tumours removed either from the site or the substance of the parotid. A. *a* 80 is one from the substance of the parotid gland. It is about the size of a turkey's egg; and it was contained in a fibrous cyst, which adhered to the substance of the gland. Its texture is in some parts fibrous and dense; in others it presents patches of gelatinous consistence; and in one, in spots near the surface, these patches are soft and bloody. This had not recurred 12 years after operation. This tumour was not in the parotid, but only touching it.

A. *a* 81 is the section of a tumour, about 3 inches long, lobulated, firm, and pale in colour, which was contained within a cyst, and was imbedded in the parotid gland.

A. *a* 82 is a tumour of the parotid, in an aged female, supposed to be scirrhous. The texture of the gland is involved. This appears to have been removed after death.

A. *a* 83 is a tumour removed by Mr R. Power from the parotid region of a married female, aged 40. The disease had commenced nine years previously, by a hard swelling about the size of a pea, near the left angle of the jaw.

At the time of admission to hospital the tumour was large; occupying the external part of the parotid gland, displacing the lobe of the ear, extending upwards as high as the zygoma, and backwards to the sterno-mastoid muscle. It was hard and resisting to the touch, and in the fixed condition of the jaw, slightly moveable. The tumour was the seat of sharp tingling pain, and caused considerable difficulty in mastication. Other symptoms were pain in the left eye-ball, with dimness in vision and internal squinting; numbness and soreness of the left side of the face; impairment of articulation and of the sense of taste, with atrophy of the left half of the tongue, which, when protruded, was drawn to that side.* The tumour was easily removed by operation.

The tumour consists of two globular masses, unequal in size. The large portion is firm and heavy, presenting on section the compact hard texture of scirrhus with radiating fibrous bands, with slight softening at one or two points. The small tumour con-

---

* This statement is not quite intelligible. If the tongue were drawn to the *left* side, in which the tumour was situate, it shows that the *right* side was paralysed. It ought, according to all that is known, to have been the left side that was paralysed ; and the tongue would then have been drawn to the right side. The mistake may be clerical.

tains softer substance, not unlike medullary matter, which seems deposited in cells, with hard points interspersed, which had not yet lost their original scirrhous character. A portion only of the parotid gland was removed, and that portion is incorporated with the anterior edge of the tumour, and most intimately connected with it. The disease is supposed to have commenced in the lymphatic gland always situate in this position, and to have secondarily affected the parotid gland.*

In 1805, Dr John M'Lellan of Green Castle, Franklin County, Pa., removed from the parotid region, in a female of 50, a tumour large and ulcerated, believed to be affected with carcinoma. He tied the maxillary and temporal arteries.†

The gland, moreover, has been, when affected by *melanosis*, removed entirely by Dr Mott of New York.‡

M. Larrey is stated to have extirpated the parotid gland in a young man of 19 for scirrhus. I have no doubt that this was mere strumous induration.§

In 1842, M. Jobert stated to the Royal Academy of Medicine that an American physician extirpated, in a man of 62, a large tumour in the parotid region, believed to be affected with scirrhus. The carotid artery was in this case tied.‖

In 1842, Dr Wheeler of Dundaff, Susquehanna, removed from the parotid region of a man, age not mentioned, a tumour of considerable size, stated very confidently to be scirrhous in texture, and to affect the whole parotid gland. The external carotid artery was tied.¶

Professor Vanzetti of Karahoff (Russia) removed from the parotid region of a man aged 40, a tumour weighing three pounds and a-half.**

From the facts now recorded, it can by no means be confidently inferred that in all these cases the parotid gland was affected with

---

* Descriptive Catalogue of Preparations of the Museum of the College of Surgeons in Ireland. Vol. ii. Dublin, 1840. P. 537.

† Case of Extirpation of Parotid Gland. American Journal of Medical Sciences, April 1844. No. XIV. New Series, p. 499.

‡ Case of Extirpation of the Parotid Gland, by Valentine Mott, M. D. American Journal of Medical Sciences, Vol. x. p. 17. 1832.

§ Examinateur Medicale, 15th Aug. 1841.

‖ Archives Generales, IIIieme Serie. Tome LX. p. 232. Oct. 1842.

¶ Extirpation of a Scirrhous Parotid Gland. By H. H. Wheeler, M. D. American Journal of Medical Sciences, No. XVIII. April 1845, 520.

** Annales de Chirurgie. Aout 1844.

scirrhus. Two inferences seem to be established by the cases now noticed. The first is, that these tumours are not in all cases seated in the parotid gland. In the majority of cases they do not at first affect the gland, which is involved only secondarily. Most commonly they are seated in lymphatic glands or cellular tissue. The second inference is, that the tumours of the kind now noticed cannot in all cases be regarded as scirrhous. It is quite impossible to admit that the tumour in the young person of 19 was scirrhus; and as to the others, there is no very certain evidence that these tumours are any thing but strumous glands or swellings.

It appears, nevertheless, that these glands are liable to be involved in the morbid changes and growths so frequently observed in this region.

Lastly, it must be allowed that the most frequent change observed in the salivary glands, and perhaps in all glands, is that of induration, (*skleroma*), in consequence of the effusion of plastic matter during chronic and strumous inflammation, either around their component granules or within these granules.

§5. The parotid gland is liable to the formation of other structures besides induration and scirrhus. Mr Pole records, in the person of a woman of 47, an instance in which a tumour began to be formed in the site of the left parotid gland about 11 years previously. This tumour steadily and progressively increased in size, affecting also the submaxillary glands, until it caused death by suffocation, by compressing the trachea, œsophagus, and blood-vessels. After death, when it was removed, it weighed ten pounds and a half; and contained every kind of substance which usually fills steatoma, meliceris, atheroma, lipoma, and even carcinoma, enclosed in cysts.[*]

Similar to this, though observing an inverted order in succession, is the case given by Cheselden, who shortly states, that he was present at the inspection of a woman who was suffocated by a tumour which began in the submaxillary gland, and extended itself from the sternum to the parotid gland in six weeks time, and in nine weeks killed her. It was a true scirrhus, he adds, and weighed twenty-six ounces.[†]

---

[*] A Case of Extraordinary Diseased Enlargement of the Parotid and Submaxillary Glands. By T. Pole, Surgeon. Memoirs of Medical Society, Vol. iii. p. 546. London, 1792.

[†] The Anatomy of the Human Body. London, 1784, p. 143.

It does not impugn much the judgment of this excellent surgeon, if we doubt whether this tumour were a true scirrhus. If it were not malignant, it might have been a mere strumous enlargement. If it were malignant, it was much more likely to be encephaloid disease than scirrhoma.

But even this point it is very difficult to determine. In most cases of tumours affecting the neck, the enlargement consists either in strumous disorder of the lymphatic glands, affecting probably also the salivary glands; or in *encephaloma*, affecting these glands and the cellular tissue.

A woman of about 40, with a tumour on the right side of the neck, extending from the parotid region downwards to the collar bone and larynx, was admitted into the Royal Infirmary. The tumour was lobulated, and consisted of seven or eight spheroidal masses. It might have affected the parotid gland, the site of which it covered; and, as it dipped under the angle of the jaw, it might also have involved the submaxillary. It was, nevertheless, obvious from its lobulated encysted appearance, and the short time which had elapsed since its commencement, that it was probably encephaloid. It was removed with great dexterity and success by an able surgeon; though it was found requisite to enclose in a ligature a portion which descended deep near the articulation of the lower jaw.

The tumour consisted of about 12 or 13 spherical masses, each enclosed in a separate cyst. The matter contained in these cysts was of a whitish-gray colour, of the consistence between fat and granular cheese, and in all respects resembling the encephaloid growth. It was impossible to detect the substance of the parotid gland, which seemed to be involved in this growth, and was otherwise rendered indistinct by the last incisions.

The wound healed up well. But about three months after, the disease returned and destroyed the patient.

This must be regarded as either a case of encephaloma, affecting first the lymphatic glands and cellular tissue of the neck, and afterwards, perhaps, the parotid gland, or as an instance of the tumour called cystic sarcoma.

The salivary glands are liable to the formation of encysted tumours. Sandifort mentions one being found in the parotid gland.

The observations hitherto made are applicable to the submaxillary and sublingual glands, as well as to the parotid. Both the submaxillary and sublingual glands are liable to be affected by inflammation, more frequently chronic than acute. This process causes hard swellings, with more or less pain, in the site of these glands.

§ 6. OCCLUSION OF DUCTS.—More or less obstruction of the excretory ducts is a disorder common to all glands. This may be occasioned either by the ducts being contracted and narrowed by inflammatory thickening or its products, or by some of the products of secretion sticking in the ducts.

The ducts in which changes of this kind are most usually observed are Steno's ducts in the parotid, and Wharton's in the submaxillary and the sublingual ducts. There is no doubt, nevertheless, that the lacrymal excretory ducts are liable to the same inconvenience.

When the duct of Steno is obstructed by any cause of the kind now referred to, a swelling more or less considerable, and more or less firm, is formed in its course, in the cheek ; and unless the obstructing cause is removed, it sometimes produces ulceration of the walls of the duct, and salivary fistula.

The same accident may happen to the duct of Wharton. Of this sort of swelling, Boyer saw an instance. The gland swelled, and the swelling subsided alternately, as the saliva was retained or was allowed to flow into the mouth. By pressing the tumour whenever the pain allowed pressure to be made, the saliva was urged along the duct into the mouth, and the volume of the gland diminished. This condition continued for months. Boyer recommended the patient to make frequent and long-continued use of mallow water in the mouth. The swelling of the walls of the canal subsided ; the saliva resumed its free course ; and the gland no longer swelled.

§ 7. CONCRETIONS.—The most usual causes, however, probably, of obstructions are the presence of concretions in the excretory ducts. This cause is common to all glands; for the secreted product may be prevented from descending along the ducts, either by its own viscidity and morbid consistence, or by some arctation in the ducts.

All excreting ducts are liable to have their channels contracted by thickening of the walls. But independent of this cause, which has been already noticed, the secretions of all glands, though originally and normally fluid, are liable to vary in chemical and mechanical properties, and thereby to favour the formation of various solid masses. Thus concretions are found to affect the lacrymal and salivary glands, as well as the hepatic and renal ducts.

§ 8. LACRYMAL CONCRETIONS. DACRYOLITHA.—Concretions or hard bodies formed in the lacrymal gland, or its ducts, have been noticed and recorded by many authors. Schurig relates from Paullin the fact, that, in a young peasant, along with the tears small stones were discharged, with heat, itching, and pain.[*] Lachmund relates, that in 1661, in a girl of 13, there arose a painful swelling on the left temple, from which, as well as from the angle of the eye, were discharged small stones at intervals for the space of three weeks.[†] Similar cases are mentioned as having occurred to d'Emery,[‡] Schafer,[§] and Plot.[||] An important case is given by Walther. In a healthy young woman, from the left upper eyelid in whom, two years previously a portion of chalky matter had been removed, without leaving any bad effect, there were formed, amidst evident marks of inflammation, recurring from time to time, in the fold between the eye-ball and the lower eye-lid, opposite the external angle of the eye, white angular stones of the size of a pea, which, in the subsequent course of the disease, became more numerous and larger. After some time the left eye was first delivered from the evil. But a similar formation of concretions began in the right eye at the same place. The phenomena progressively diminished, and at length ceased; yet returned after some years in a milder form. At length the patient got quite well.[¶] Guillié mentions that, in a young person of 15, after marks of violent inflammation, with redness and swelling of the eye-lids, the lower fold of the conjunctiva was filled on the 6th day with chalky deposit like fine sand; and on the 9th day there appeared at the outer angle a small conical-shaped body, as thick as a vetch, reddish yellow, and irregular on the surface, which was loosely attached to the conjunctiva, and was easily removed by forceps.[**]

Dr Kersten,[††] who writes an elaborate paper on these concretions,

---

[*] Schurig Lithologia, p. 100.　　　　[†] De Fossilibus, Sect. iii. Cap. 22, p. 72.
[‡] Journal des Sçavans, 1679, 1 May, p. 66–68.
[§] Ephemerid. Cent. iii. iv. Obs clxxvii. p. 421.
[||] Natural History of Oxfordshire. London, 1677. Folio.
[¶] Graefe und Walther's Journal, Band i. Heft i. S. 163.
[**] Bibliotheque Ophthalmologique, Tome i. p. 133.
[††] Ueber Steinerzeugung aus der Thranenflussigheit. Von Dr Kersten in Magdeburg. C. W. Hufeland's Journal der Practischen Heilkunde. Fortgesetzte von Dr Fr. Busse. 1843. iv. u. v. Stuck April u May, xcv. Band 4 u 5 St. S. 26–63.

thinks, that they may be formed in the *caruncula lacrymalis ;* and he believes that they are formed also in the *puncta*, the canal, and sac. This seems very doubtful as a general inference. These concretions appear generally at the outer angle of the orbit; and it is most likely, that they are most commonly formed in the ducts and orifices of the lacrymal gland, or near this situation.

Sandifort, however, found concretions in the lacrymal canal; and Desmarres records the circumstances of a case in which, in a gouty female of 66, he found a lacrymal concretion impacted in the lacrymal sac of the right side. Manifest swelling was formed over the inner angle of the right eye. The patient had suffered for two years from lacrymation, and latterly a discharge of matter from the eye. The lower *punctum* was enlarged to three times its normal size. In the course of the lower lacrymal duct there was a small, prominent, circumscribed, indolent, and colourless swelling. By means of a probe, Desmarres recognized the presence of a solid body. He then introduced a grooved probe, and, dividing the integuments down to the canal, be extracted a hard, yellowish, pea-like body. The wound was healed in 24 days.[*]

On the frequency of the occurrence of concretions in the lacrymal sac evidence is divided. While some authors, as Nicolai and Waldeck, consider the lacrymal sac as the most usual place for the formation of lacrymal concretions, others, viz. Walther, maintain that they are never found in this receptacle. That this is a mistake is evident from cases recorded by Le Dran, Schmucker, Krimer, Cunier, Stievenart, Thibon, and Maunoir.

Cunier, in particular, gives the details of two cases, one in a man, of 58, another in one of 63, in which concretions were found in this situation,[†] and which seem to leave no doubt of the fact.

Lacrymal concretions of the largest size are observed in the nasal duct; because in the cavity of this canal there is most space for their growth and enlargement with least inconvenience. Of this three examples are recorded; two in the observations of Dr Kersten, and one by Horn in Schmucker's Miscellaneous Writings.

It may be observed that though these concretions occur sometimes in young persons, yet in general their subjects are of middle age or up in years, and persons who have suffered from gout and

[*] Annales d'Oculiste. Paris, 1842.

[†] Observations pour servir a l'histoire des Calculs Lacrymales. Bruxelles, 1842.

rheumatic symptoms. In one of the instances given by Cunier, the patient had, six years previously, viz. in 1831, been cut for stone in the bladder by Dupuytren.

Lacrymal concretions have been analyzed at different times by different persons. Fuchs found in the concretions given him by Walther carbonate of lime, forming the largest part of the weight, and traces of phosphate of lime and albumen. The concretions met with by Cunier consisted chiefly, according to Pasquier, of carbonate of lime, with traces of phosphate of lime and muriate of soda; and in one there was some phosphate of magnesia. Lastly, the concretion removed by Desmarres was analysed by Bouchardat and gave the following results;—solid albuminous matter, 25 parts; mucus, 18 parts; carbonate of lime, 48 parts; phosphate of lime and magnesia, 9 parts; with traces of fat and muriate of soda.*

These facts seem to justify the views taken by Walther, Cunier, and Desmarres, that the formation of lacrymal concretions, like that of other concretions, depends on general causes.

Lacrymal concretions are perhaps disposed to be formed more readily from the complexity and tortuosity of the lacrymal passages, and also from their narrowness and liability to inflammatory thickening and obstruction.

Salivary concretions have not quite so frequently been observed as lacrymal concretions. They are nevertheless by no means uncommon.

The most usual situation for salivary concretions to be presented are either beneath the tongue in the ducts of the sublingual glands, or in the duct of Wharton leading from the submaxillary gland.

In the former situation the cases are so numerous, that it is impossible in this place to enumerate the twentieth part of them. I shall merely mention that instances of salivary concretions have been recorded by Lister, Freeman, Scherer, (1737); Bacciocchi, (1749); Hamberger, (1754); Handtwig, (1754); Hartmann, (1762 and 1784); Hellman (apud von Siebold,) Titius, and several others.

Most of these are from the ducts of the sublingual gland. Flajani gives a case of calculus from Steno's duct, which is the least frequent. Since the time of Flajani cases have been recorded by

* Annales d'Oculiste. Paris, 1842.

Müller (1811) and Seguignol. In the cases by Scherer, Acrel, Hellman, in one by Sabatier, and in one by Boyer, the concretions were from the duct of Wharton.

In the first case, these concretions give rise to an irregular swelling beneath the tongue, and form one variety of the disease named *ranula*. The size of this swelling varies according to the size of the stone, and may be from that of a pea to the size of a filbert, or even a walnut. In some rare instances they give rise to inflammation and ulceration, and thus extricate themselves from the position in which they are confined. More frequently, however, they require the aid of operation. In the case given by Sabatier, it appears that the presence of the concretion in the duct of Wharton caused painful swelling of the submaxillary gland, and this seems to have given rise to more suffering and inconvenience than the immediate swelling caused by the tumour. Two concretions were in this case removed by two separate and successive operations.* Boyer tells us that in a similar case in which the submaxillary gland was likewise swelled, he cured the swelling of the gland by extracting an oblong stony concretion, one extremity of which projected a little beyond the orifice of the duct of Wharton.

I may here mention that salivary concretions are occasionally found in the lower animals. Grognier records two cases of this lesion. In one a concretion weighing 6 drachms was found in the Stenonian duct of a mule; in another a concretion weighing 13 drachms was found in the Stenonian duct of an ass.†

The chemical constitution of these concretions has been several times examined. They consist of carbonate and phosphate of lime coated with animal matter, with traces of muriate of soda.

§ 9. RANULA.—Of this disease it would be unnecessary to say any more, were the terms not employed to designate more than one morbid affection. To every tumour, in short, appearing beneath the tongue, the denomination of *ranula* is given. Munnicks, Louis, and after him Boyer, espoused the opinion that the swelling depended on an accumulation of saliva in the duct of Wharton. But the main point was, why did the saliva accumulate?. Boyer was of opinion that this was caused by obstruction at the outlet of the ducts, or obliteration of those outlets. In point of fact, there

* Sabatier, Medecine Operatoire.
† Grognier in Sceance de l'Ecole Veterinaire. Journal de Medecine continué, 1810, Dec. p. 504.

is no doubt that, from various causes, most frequently inflammatory thickening, the duct is narrowed, and its outlet is either obstructed · or temporarily obliterated. Even inflammation of the mucous membrane of the mouth, by causing obliteration of the outlets of the duct, may be followed by such accumulation. In other instances, again, the presence of a calculus within any of the ducts has the same effect.

Ranula is said to appear in the form of a tumour, in some degree transparent, soft, and fluctuating, and in some instances in the form of one quite hard and firm. At first small, it gradually enlarges, projecting into the mouth, and interfering much with mastication, speech, and even deglutition. It is even said that the effect on speech is so considerable, as to make the voice of the patient resemble the croaking of frogs, and that from this circumstance the disease receives its name. This is probably an idle fancy.

SECTION III.

DISEASES OF THE PANCREAS.

THE diseases of the pancreas may be enumerated in the following order. 1. Inflammation and its effects, adhesion, and suppuration; 2. simple induration; 3. chronic induration; 4. hypertrophy; 5. softening; 6. atrophy; 7. concretions in the ducts or duct; 8. chronic ulceration; and 9. the heterologous deposits.

§ I. INFLAMMATION OF THE SWEATBREAD OR PANCREAS.
PANCREATIA, PANCREATITIS.

That the pancreas is liable to inflammation has been admitted by most morbid anatomists; but it has been also ascertained, that it is very difficult, if not impracticable, to recognize the inflamed state of the gland by symptoms during life. Morgagni believed that he found it twice in a state of inflammation, that is, redder and more vascular than usual; and Wedekind and Daniel have since his time mentioned the circumstance as taking place occasionally. Portal states in general terms that, when inflamed, it is redder than natural not only at its external surface, but in its interior substance; and that it had been found in this state in persons who had undergone an attack of continued fever of more or less intensity, with pains in the abdomen, especially at the navel, frequent fits of violent vomiting, in some instances jaundice, and diminished secretion of urine. Baillie was led by experience to regard inflammation as not very liable to attack the pancreas.

The only inference that can be deduced from these several facts, is, that inflammatory action, if it do take place in the pancreas, does not in all cases evince its presence by well-marked or unequivocal symptoms. Does the inflammatory process, it may be asked, leave distinct effects of its presence?

Of the presence of inflammation in this gland several proofs may be adduced. One is redness of the pancreatic substance with vascularity and more or less softness, generally with effusion of bloody serum in the glandular substance and surrounding cellular tissue. Another is either the effusion of albuminous matter in the neighbourhood, or preternatural adhesion to the adjoining organs. A third effect is suppuration or abscess of the gland, sometimes with, more frequently without, pain and other external symptoms. And a fourth consists in different degrees of induration of the gland, usually with pain in the epigastric region, and occasional vomiting.

§ 1. Redness and vascularity are occasionally observed in the pancreas. But they are most frequently the effect of transudation after death, or some similar pseudo-morbid process. In cases in which they are associated either with effusion of plastic exudation, or purulent matter, or induration or softening, they must be allowed to depend on inflammation. This, however, is not common; chiefly because inflammation of the pancreas is not usually an acute disease, and death does not take place in the early stage of the disorder.

One of the best and least equivocal examples of inflammation of the pancreas is given by Mr Lawrence; and as the appearances observed by Mr Lawrence illustrate well the effects of inflammation, it is proper to mention them.

The case occurred in a married lady of 21, partly during pregnancy, and partly after delivery. During the three latter months of pregnancy, the patient suffered unusually from thirst, and drank large quantities of water. She had also suffered much from pain in the epigastric region, particularly over the site of the pancreas. She became pale, anæmic, feeble, and breathless. She made no good recovery after delivery, but presented symptoms of great weakness and exhaustion; and died exactly five weeks after delivery.

Upon inspecting the body, the cellular texture round the pancreas and duodenum, the great and small omentum, the root of the mesentery, the mesocolon, and the *appendices epiploicæ* of the arch of the colon, was loaded with serous fluid, transparent, bright yellow, and of watery consistence, which escaped abundantly from incisions. The pancreas was throughout of a deep dull red colour, which contrasted very remarkably with the bloodless condition of other parts. It was firm to the feeling externally; and when an incision was made into it, the divided lobules felt particularly firm and crisp. The texture was otherwise healthy. The part was left wrapped in a cloth for nearly forty-eight hours after its removal from the body, when the weather was very cold. At the end of this time the hardness was gone, and the gland appeared rather soft.*

From this it results that redness, and vascularity, and slight hardness followed by softening, with infiltration of serous or sero-albuminous fluid, constitute the anatomical characters of pancreatic inflammation. This case also illustrates a principle formerly mentioned as to the effects of inflammation, namely, that the process renders the tissues friable and easily lacerable.

§ 2. Adhesion of the pancreas to the adjoining organs may be the effect either of suppurative or common inflammation. In general, when suppurative inflammation takes place, more or less albuminous deposition is formed, and connects the gland to the adjoining organs, either to prevent the farther progress of the destructive effects of the suppuration, or to prevent the purulent matter from being absorbed by the veins and transported into the circulating system.

§ 3. *Purulent Inflammation of the Pancreas.*—Collections of purulent matter in the pancreas have been observed by many anatomists. Tulpius mentions the case of a young man who, after an intermittent fever, was attacked with pain in the belly and loins, so violent, that he was unable to lie on any side. After death, besides inflammation of the liver, the pancreas was found suppurated.† Thomas Bartholin found, in a man who had previously fever with pains in the back and in the loins, the pancreas altogether destroyed by an enormous abscess full of fœtid greenish

---

* History of a Case in which, on Examination after Death, the Pancreas was found in a state of active Inflammation. By William Lawrence, F. R. S. Medico-Chirurgical Transactions, Vol. xvi. p. 366. London, 1830.

† Obs. Med. Lib. iv. cap. xxxiii. p. 327. Amst. 1652 and 1672.

matter ;* and Blancard records a similar history ;† and Lieutaud mentions instances which had occurred to various observers.‡ Bonz describes in a man of thirty-eight, an abscess in the right extremity of the pancreas, the purulent matter of which implicated the stomach and the liver, and established a communication between the liver and the abdomen.§ Gautier states that, in the body of a woman who had been afflicted with long-continued *cardialgia*, he saw an abscess of the pancreas which opened into the posterior wall of the stomach.‖ Portal states that he found the pancreas in a state of complete suppuration in a person who, after having experienced violent paroxysms of gout in the feet, upon their disappearance had two or three fits of vomiting, followed by syncope and death.¶ Baillie informs us, that he only once met with an abscess in the pancreas in the case of a young man of little beyond the age of twenty, and in whom the gland was enlarged in size, and contained a good deal of thin purulent fluid without peculiar characters, unattended by fixed pain in the region of the gland, but with a good deal of pain in different parts of the belly.**

Dr Haygarth records the case of a gentleman who laboured under jaundice, bilious vomiting, and disordered urinary secretion with epigastric pain and swelling, and at length the discharge of blood and purulent matter from the intestines. After three months death took place. The pancreas was found greatly enlarged, occupying the site of the tumour felt during life in the epigastric region. The common biliary duct was obliterated where the pressure had been greatest. The gall-bladder was full and the cystic duct pervious. The substance of the pancreas was indurated, and when divided it contained a considerable abscess.††

In cases of this nature the suppuration may be either limited and partial, or extensive and destroying the greater part or the whole of the gland. The matter is usually of a gray-white colour,

* Centuria ii. Hist. xxxix. Tom. i. p. 333. Hafniæ, 1654–1657.
† Anatom. Pract. Cent. ii. Obs. lv. p. 271.
‡ Hist. Anatom. Med. Tom. i. Obs. 1046 and 1060.
§ Nov. Acta. N. C. T. viii. p. 51.
‖ J. L. Gautier de Irritabilitatis Notione, Natura, et Morbis. Halæ, 1793, § 13, p. 129.
¶ Anatomie Medicale, Tom. v. p. 352. Paris, 1803.
** Morbid Anatomy in Works by Wardrop, Vol. ii. p. 238 and 240. London, 1825.
†† Two Cases of Inflammation and Enlargement of the Pancreas, &c. Transactions of Association, Vol. II. p. 132. Dublin, 1818.

similar to that of other abscesses; in a few cases it is greenish. It may be either inodorous or exhale a faint mawkish odour like ordinary matter; and it has in a few instances been found extremely fetid. In some cases it consists of thin serous fluid with curdly clots; and it is then conceived to indicate the presence of the strumous diathesis.

The matter of these pancreatic abscesses is often enclosed within a sac or membranous pouch, formed by the cellular tissue either of the pancreas or covering the gland. Portal states that he has seen two pounds of purulent matter contained within the gland. It may open a passage to itself either through the posterior wall of the stomach, through part of the *duodenum*, through the colon into its cavity, or into the general cavity of the *peritonæum*.

Portal allows that suppuration is in many cases the immediate effect of inflammation of the pancreas. It may be admitted that, in all cases where suppuration has taken place, it is the effect of inflammation; and the only circumstance of difference is the question, whether the inflammation is attended with pain and other feelings of uneasiness, or is unattended by these symptoms? Suppuration seems always to be a process occupying a considerable time; and in this point of view it may be said to be chronic. But it appears from the cases recorded, that suppuration or suppurative inflammation is of three kinds at least; the ordinary, the strumous, and the metastatic. In the two former instances, it must be admitted to be preceded by inflammatory action, however obscure that may be, and however indistinct be the symptoms to which the process gives rise.

It is chiefly important to observe that inflammatory suppuration of the pancreas does not give rise to well marked symptoms at first. But after some time, that is, when probably the purulent collection has become considerable, and begun by mechanical pressure and distension to affect the physiological properties of the gland and the contiguous parts, fits of vomiting, more or less violent and continued, especially after taking food, take place; pains of the loins, which have been often mistaken for nephritic or rheumatic pains, and which prevent the patient from lying on his back, ensue; sometimes pains of the belly, like spasmodic pains (Baillie), are observed; after some time the pulse, which at first was unaffected, becomes a little quick,—from 80 to 86; dyspeptic symptoms, as flatulence, *cardialgia*, and *gastrodynia*, are observed, in some instances with occasional diarrhœa ; the patient appears to derive no nutriment from his food ; and he dies tabid.

The name of *metastatic suppurative* inflammation I have applied to denote suppuration of the pancreas occurring under peculiar circumstances, that is, connected with inflammation of veins, usually the hemorrhoidal or spermatic. It was observed long ago, that in the operation of extirpation of a testicle or testicles, and subsequent ligature of the cord to prevent hemorrhage, among other accidents it occasionally happened that a collection of matter was formed within the substance of the pancreas or around the gland, and the same result was observed to take place in the course of various diseases of the testicle or its vessels. Antony Petit, especially, who had witnessed several examples of the suppurative destruction of the pancreas, adduces them as arguments against the propriety of practising the operation of ligature of the cord after castration. Portal also informs us that he found in a man dead after extirpation of a testicle and ligature of the spermatic cord, a large quantity of purulent matter within the cord and round the pancreas.

The explanation of this singular occurrence is to be found in the fact, that in the old method of inclosing the cord within a ligature, the veins were included, and very often became inflamed and underwent the suppurative inflammation. When this took place, the matter formed in the interior of the spermatic veins was transported to various internal organs, sometimes to the kidneys or their vessels, sometimes to the lungs, and sometimes to the pancreas, and there deposited. According to this view, it is scarcely requisite to regard inflammation as the necessary preliminary of this suppurative deposit, and probably the purulent matter found around or within the pancreas is to be considered as transported from the inflamed part of the tied vein to the other parts of the venous system, and among others to the pancreas.

Suppuration of the pancreas has been observed in persons dead of ague, continued fever, fever after the suppression of some habitual evacuation, diarrhœa, hemorrhoids, the *catamenia*, dropsy, marasmus, convulsions, epilepsy, and hysteria. Regarding the four latter conditions, it is proper to observe, that the state called marasmus is undoubtedly the tabid condition with hectic already noticed, as consequent on the purulent collection within the pancreas ; and convulsive symptoms are so often observed to ensue on any of the disorganized states of the thoracic or abdominal viscera, that they are doubtless to be regarded as symptoms rather than preliminary conditions.

§ 4. SCLEROMA OR INDURATING INFLAMMATION OF THE PANCREAS; SCIRRHUS OF RHAN AND MANY OTHER AUTHORS, IMPROPERLY.—The pancreas is subject to slow chronic inflammation, which, without tending to suppuration, renders the gland much harder than natural, without, it is said, otherwise changing its structure. All that is meant by this, I presume, is, that the structure is not sensibly changed; for if minutely examined and compared with the sound pancreas, it will be found to be considerably altered. This chronic inflammation,.though mistaken for scirrhus, and as such described by Tissot, Storck, Morgagni, Haller, Baader, Rahn, Portal, and others, is quite distinct from it, in so far as it does not present the true scirrho-carcinomatous transformation. It appears to be the same change which has been described by Pemberton under the vague name of Disease of the Pancreas.

Instances of preternatural hardness of the pancreas have been noticed by Riolan, Charles Le Poix, De Paw, Harder, Cheselden, Haller, Morgagni, Tissot, Baader, and Rahn; but all have confounded, under the general name of scirrhus, a change which was evidently the effect of inflammation, probably of a chronic character, acting on the glandular tissue. The observations of these authors appear to have been totally overlooked, at least by English physicians. Cheselden had early observed what has often since been confirmed, namely, the effect of the indurated pancreas in compressing the common biliary duct, and thereby causing fatal jaundice.* But from the time of this author downwards, no attempt is made to explain the anatomical characters of these instances of scirrhus or induration. Dr Latham had the merit of directing the attention of the profession in 1806 to the symptoms of the disorder, as distinct from disease of the liver and other abdominal organs.† In 1816, Mr Bedingfield, in speaking of cases of disease of the pancreas, stated, that in a certain class of cases, all attended with dyspeptic symptoms, and often with jaundice, it was found on inspection that the pancreas was always more or less

---

* The Anatomy of the Human Body. By William Cheselden. Twelfth Edition. London, 1784. Book iii. chap. v. p. 166.

† Remarks on Tumours which have occasionally been mistaken for Diseases of the Liver. By J. Latham, M. D., F. R. S., &c. Read 11th Dec 1806. Medical Trans, Vol. iv. p. 47. London, 1813.

hardened, and sometimes increased in size to the extent of six times its natural bulk.* Mr Todd also described, in 1817, an instance of induration and enlargement, or what must now be called hypertrophy of the pancreas, pressing the common gall-duct ;† and Dr Percival and Dr Crampton recorded, in 1818, examples of the disorder attended with unusual compression of the same duct and the symptoms of jaundice.‡

From the dissection recorded by Dr Crampton, it may be inferred that inflammation attacking the pancreas renders that gland harder, and larger or more tumid than usual, and that, either in consequence of this tumefaction, it compresses and obstructs the common gall-duct, or the inflammatory action extending to the surrounding parts produces a morbid effusion, which gives rise to the same result.

Since the time of Dr Crampton, many instances of different degrees of induration of the pancreas, sometimes alone, more commonly along with affections of the duodenum or other abdominal organs, have been recorded by Dr Heineken, Dr Bright, Dr Wilson, Dr Holscher, Dr Ritter, Dr Landsberg, and other observers, all of which tend to show that induration of the pancreas is not a very uncommon disease; and that this induration, though usually denominated scirrhus, is either the effect of inflammation or aecompanics that process.

From the cases recorded by these authors, it results that, though induration may affect any part of the pancreas, or the whole of that gland, yet most usually it is the head of the organ, that is indurated; and at the same time it may be enlarged.

The pancreatic substance is then hard and cuts firm, grating on the knife.

In some cases it is stated to be like cartilage; in others like the boiled udder of the cow. Usually there are adhesions or recent lymph connecting the pancreas to other adjoining parts. The lobulated acinoid structure is not always very manifest. Ritter

* Compendium of Medical Practice.

† History of a Remarkable Case of Enlargement of the Biliary Ducts. By Charles H. Todd, M. R. C. S. Dublin Hospital Reports and Communications, Vol. i. p. 325. Dublin, 1817.

‡ Two Cases of Inflammation and Enlargement of the Pancreas. By Edward Percival, M. B., M. R. I. A., Bath. Read 1st June 1818. Transactions of the Association of the Fellows and Licentiates of King and Queen College of Physicians in Ireland, Vol. ii. p. 128. Dublin, 1818. Additional Cases, by John Crampton, M. D., &c. Ibid. p. 134.

states, that in a case observed by him it was no longer cognizable. In other instances, however, I am satisfied, from what I have myself seen, that these bodies are certainly not less distinct than before. The change, of which they are the seat, is effusion of lymph, which becomes coagulated. This effusion takes place both into their interior, and externally between the *acini* and lobules; and when the exudation becomes consolidated, the whole is converted into a hard, firm cartilage-like mass.

In some instances the head or duodenal end of the pancreas is thus indurated and enlarged, and at the same time the left or splenic end may be hardened, while the middle portion is comparatively healthy and natural in structure.

The *duodenum* is very generally rough, irregular, and compressed; its interior capacity is diminished; and its mucous membrane is vascular.

With this induration of the pancreas, not unfrequently are associated more or less disease in the duodenum, as chronic ulceration,* thickening, and similar changes in the beginning of the jejunum.

The following instance, given by Cruveilhier, from an infant born at full time, shows that the disease may take place in the fœtus. The pancreas presented a lardaceous appearance, like the structure of a scirrhous mamma, without distinction of glandular grains. The antero-posterior diameter was as great as the vertical diameter. The size of the splenic or left end was as great as that of the right or head. The pancreas adhered to the supra-renal capsule and the right kidney.

I think it is hardly possible to doubt that the whole of the cases now referred to are instances of chronic inflammation of the pancreas. It is quite clear that they cannot in all instances be regarded as scirrhus; for several of the cases mentioned are stated to have been instances of bad health, with symptoms of pancreatic disease, from which the patients recovered. Thus Dr Percival gives one case of this kind, in which recovery took place under the employment of local blood-letting, blistering, restrained diet, and the use of aperients. Dr Crampton gives one case, in which recovery was effected under the same measures. Dr Landsberg gives an instance of what he calls *Tabes Pancreatis*, in which, after about rather more than three months, the patient got well under the successive use of mercury, and mercurial and iodine ointment, and the foot-bath of nitro-muriatic acid. In other two cases, to which

* Two of the cases given by Dr Bright.

he applies the name of *Pancreatitis chronica*, recovery took place in like manner, under the use of foot-baths of mineral acid, (apparently the hydrochloric,) which were followed after a short time by critical diarrhœa.*

Another circumstance, showing that these must have been instances of chronic congestion or inflammation, is that most of them took place in persons comparatively young. The patient of Dr Haygarth was middle-aged. In one of the fatal cases of Dr Crampton, the age was 35. In another favourable case it was 32. In Dr Landsberg's first case the age was 42, in the second 30, in the third 22.

The effects of this change of structure are of two kinds; one order in the adjoining organs; another in the function of digestion and the general health.

Those in the contiguous organs are anatomico-pathological, and have been in some degree referred to already. The most common are adhesions with the duodenum, the right kidney, the jejunum, and in some instances with the gall-ducts and gall-bladder.

Next to these come compression of the gall-ducts, and usually jaundice.

The aorta may be compressed; but the *vena cava* and *vena portæ* are most frequently so. The result is ascites.

The *duodenum*, however, is the organ that suffers most in all this mischief. Its calibre is contracted; the inner surface is excited and injected; and its first curvature is so much obstructed, that a sense of painful distension, flatulence, and acid eructations are common and almost constant results.

There seems no doubt that this induration may proceed to ulceration; and in this way ulceration usually takes place at the head of the gland, and finds its way into the duodenum. Though in strict pathological language this ulceration is not properly malignant, yet to all practical purposes it is sufficiently so to be regarded incurable. It almost never heals when it has once begun. It proceeds destroying the gland, very much like chronic ulceration of the stomach. The havoc then found after death has made most of the cases be denominated *scirrhus* of the pancreas.

The effects on the digestive function are very serious. It is

* Einige Bemerkungen über Krankheiten des untern Magenmundes und der Bauchspeicheldrüse. Von Dr Landsberg pract. Arzte zu Munsterberg in Schlesien. C. W. Hufeland's Journal der Practischen Heilkunde. Fortgesetzte von Dr E. Osann. 1840. Siebenter Stuck Juli, (xci. Bnd.)

unfortunate that Rahn, who has given the fullest collection of cases of induration of the pancreas, has not distinguished the disorder from scirrhus, properly so-named, and has even given as instances of the latter, cases in which tumours, more or less extensive, were formed from the mesenteric and meso-colic glands, and had then implicated the pancreas. It hence results, that it is impossible to attach to his history of symptoms that importance which a correct critical semiographical account deserves. It is important to know, however, that he mentions the following as present in most of the cases.

1. Pains between the ensiform cartilage and navel, at one time occupying the middle region of the belly and stretching to the spine, and at another the right or left hypochondriac region. 2. Tumour in the same region, easily palpable by the finger, hard, moveable, causing a sense of weight while the patient stands or walks, most painful above the lumbar vertebræ, with great precordial anxiety, especially after taking food or drink. 3. A sense of burning in the stomach, not temporary but constant, with a painful sense of soreness and heartburn spreading into the œsophagus, with frequent eructation of a watery, tasteless, or acid fluid which resembles saliva. 4. Constipation. 5. *Anorexia*, squeamishness ; and, 6. Eventually vomiting occurring at uncertain intervals, bringing up *ingesta* and ropy phlegm ; and at length, 7. wasting *(tabes)* and hectic fever with all their attendant symptoms.

The chief objections to this history are, that the same series of symptoms is liable to take place in various disorders of the stomach, the duodenum, and the liver ; that the pancreas is sometimes found indurated without any of these symptoms having taken place excepting the pain and occasional vomiting ; and that the circumstance of palpable tumour is often wanting, and when present is not pathognomonic.

The principal symptoms, judging from the cases recorded by the best observers, are deep-seated pain in the region of the stomach, more or less sickness, sometimes vomiting, with emaciation, general languor, fever especially in the night, and in general a yellow or jaundiced colour of the skin. The urine is in general scanty and high-coloured ; and though the bowels are generally confined, and dyspeptic symptoms are common, sometimes diarrhœa takes place and proceeds to a considerable degree, apparently with salutary effect. Wedekind, who observed this symptom, absurdly ascribed it to a milder degree of pancreatic inflammation, or, as Gautier expresses it, to increased irritability of the pancreas. It may, however; be regarded as a law of inflammation of glandular tissue, that, in the early stage, the secretion is diminished or suppressed, and that, if it seem to be augmented in the latter stage, this is rather the effect and the proof of the subsidence of the inflammation and its final disappearance than of increased action.

In one case of this disorder, in which I had an opportunity of inspecting the parts after death, I observed the progress of the disease for months. The patient, a female of about 48, continued ill for seven or eight years, with pain in the epigastric region, and more urgently unwell for about two years, with pain and tenderness in the same part, frequent attacks of sickness and vomiting, occasional diarrhœa, constant headach, a pulse varying from 88 to 96, most usually at 92, rather full, and hot dry skin, though pale, blanched, and at length leucophlegmatic complexion. The pain, which was most felt in the epigastric, and towards the right hypochondriac region, was so urgent, that the slightest and gentlest pressure could not be borne; it was constant, and underwent no remission; was distinctly referred to the region specified by the patient herself; and was always relieved by local bleeding, and occasionally by general blood-letting. The effect of opiates was immediate but temporary, that of counter-irritation by blister or tartar-emetic ointment more permanent. As the disease proceeded, the fits of vomiting became more frequent and urgent, and were accompanied with distressing hiccup; nothing was retained; the patient wasted, and became waxy-coloured and leucophlegmatic; and life was maintained for some time by nutritious enemata with opiates. Though the emaciation was not visibly extreme, yet the pale waxy appearance of the surface and transparency of the skin, showed the imperfect and scanty degree of nutrition. Death took place apparently by exhaustion and inanition.

It was then found that the pancreas was exceedingly hard, almost like a stone, a little enlarged, but not positively altered in structure. It resisted the knife like firm cheese or cartilage. The acini, which were the parts mostly altered, were of a reddish-gray colour, very close in texture, and extremely firm. It seemed rather less vascular than usual. This body was felt during life, and it never could be pressed or handled without causing much pain. The gall-bladder was greatly distended,—a circumstance which

l

showed that the pancreatic induration had compressed the common biliary duct.

In general, when wasting is far advanced, the gland may be felt more or less distinctly by slight pressure on the belly, which is also attended either with pain or tenderness. In earlier stages of the disease the most effectual mode of ascertaining the state of the pancreas is to make the patient lie prone on the belly, getting him supported so as to allow the hand of the physician to examine the abdomen. If in this position the patient be examined carefully, in general it is possible to recognize not only a painful region, but some swelling.

Induration of the pancreas is attended, after some continuance, either with a leucophlegmatic appearance and anasarca, or with dropsy of the belly, which, though not an invariable consequence, may supervene; and in every case of *ascites*, in which the liver does not appear to be indurated or enlarged, or affected with cirrhosis, or the kidneys are known not to be diseased, it may be apprehended that the pancreas is indurated and compressing some of the veins, either the *vena cava* or some of its branches.

In some individuals induration of the pancreas appears to give rise to that anomalous assemblage of symptoms called *hypochondriasis;* and probably in this manner we are to explain the fact mentioned by Baillie, that in one instance there were pain in the hips and a sense of numbness in one thigh or leg. Difficulty and pain in stooping are also not unfrequent symptoms. It must not be omitted that this disease is sometimes one of the lesions found in the bodies of the insane.

These statements are, it must be admitted, not satisfactory ; and their chief use is to show the extreme difficulty of recognizing the presence of this disease during life, at a period sufficiently early to enable us to form a correct and useful diagnosis. This difficulty led Pemberton to conclude, that it is chiefly by negative reasoning that the physician must infer the existence of disease of the pancreas; that is, if in a case in which there is deep-seated pain in the epigastric region, and more or less sickness and emaciation, the patient does not at the same time present the other symptoms denoting the presence of primary disease of the stomach, of the posterior part of the liver, of the gall-bladder or ducts, or of the small intestines, he may infer the evidence of disease, that is chronic inflammation, of the pancreas.

To one symptom, which, if constant, must be important, Dr Bright, in 1832, directed attention. This consists in the discharge of oily or fatty matters from the bowels in certain affections of the pancreas. In three cases in which the pancreas was considerably indurated, and had contracted firm adhesions with the adjoining parts, with ulceration in the duodenum, there were discharged from the bowels, with the usual matters, a quantity of material like melted grease or tallow, and which was ascertained, by chemical examination, to be either adipocire or stearine. Dr Bright has been led, from various facts, to connect this symptom with disease, probably malignant, of that part of the pancreas which is near to the duodenum, and ulceration of the duodenum itself.* There is no doubt that the suspension of the pancreatic secretion must exert great influence on the process of duodenal digestion ; but it has not been proved by subsequent cases that this oily or fatty discharge never takes place without disease of the pancreas.† In other cases the pancreas was merely indurated.

§ 5. HYPERTROPHY.—Enlargement of the pancreas as an effect either of chronic inflammation or of over-nutrition, is often associated with induration ; but may take place with a natural state of the consistence of the gland. When the gland does become enlarged in this manner, it is almost superfluous to say that the lesion causes more or less of a firm, solid, tumid mass in the epigastric region. The bulk which the hypertrophied gland attains varies in different circumstances, chiefly according to the duration of the disorder. Riolan mentions a case in which it was as large as the liver, (Riolani Anthropographia); in a person mentioned by Tissot, its size was three times the natural size, (De Melæna et Morbo Nigro); and in a woman seen by Storck, it is said to have been so large as to weigh thirteen pounds. In the case of a woman of forty years, detailed by Rahn, the gland measured nine inches long and seven broad, and weighed a little above four pounds, and its internal structure was like lard. Westenberg describes a case in which the

---

* Cases and Observations connected with Disease of the Pancreas and Duodenum. By Richard Bright, M. D., &c. Medico-Chirurgical Transactions, Vol. xviii. p. 1. London, 1833.

† Case of Jaundice with Discharge of Fatty Matter from the Bowels, &c. By E. A. Lloyd, Esq. Ibid. p. 57.

On the Discharge of Fatty Matters from the Alimentary Canal and Urinary Passages. By John Elliotson, M. D., &c. Medico-Chirurgical Transactions, Vol. xviii. p. 67. London, 1833.

gland weighed six pounds. The natural weight varies from one ounce and a half to six ounces.

In some instances the hypertrophy is only partial, and it then affects chiefly the right side of the pancreas, which may attain the size of the fist, while the left side is natural. (Rahn, cases 4th, 5th, 6th, 11th, 12th.) A common result, then, is pressure upon and obstruction of the common biliary duct, and consequent distension of the gall-bladder, and, if the obstruction be complete, a jaundiced colour of the surface.

Dr Holscher records an instance, in a man of 48, otherwise stout and healthy, in whom the enlargement, by compressing the *duodenum*, caused contraction or stricture of that bowel, and fatal ileus. The duration of the symptoms of epigastric pain was eight months; but the symptoms of ileus continued not longer than six days. Dissection presented no marks of inflammation. But the pancreas was void of its normal granular condition, soft, succulent, and fleshy; its sections presented neither tubercular matter, nor any formation like scirrhus, or encephaloma; but it was enlarged to the size of a fœtal head of four months; and it had so closed the duodenum for the space of three inches, that the contracted portion did not admit a goose-quill.*

This enlargement appears to be of the same nature as that which is observed to affect other secreting glands, as the mamma, the testicle, and the liver. In general the individual lobes and *acini* may be observed to be perceptibly enlarged; and usually large and numerous blood-vessels are observed entering the gland. The enlargement seems to depend on additional matter deposited in the interstitial spaces of the *acini*, and perhaps into their substance.

The case mentioned by De Haen, in which he represents the pancreas to have degenerated into numerous scirrhous tumours of various size, closely cohering to each other, may belong to this head. Does the change bear any analogy to the early stage of *cirrhosis* of the liver?

In some cases the gland is enlarged and resembles lard or suet. In such circumstances the change probably belongs to encephaloma.

§ 6. MALAKOSIS. SOFTENING.—Softening or diminution of con-

---

* Medizinische, Chirurgische und Ophthalmologische Wahrnehmungen. Von Dr Holscher. Hannoversche Annalen fur die ges. Heilkunde v. Band 2. Heft, 1841.

sistence is observed under certain circumstances to take place in the pancreas. If attended with increase of size, this may be regarded as the effect of inflammation. In other instances, for example, in persons labouring under scurvy, in cachectic persons, and after several eruptive disorders, especially small-pox and scarlet fever, it seems doubtful whether the diminished consistence can be ascribed to inflammatory orgasm. Portal states that he found it much softened without being reddened or swollen, in two children cut off by measles; and in the body of a young man between fifteen and eighteen years, who died on the tenth day of confluent small-pox.

When the pancreas is softened, its texture is loose, soft, easily lacerable, of a yellowish gray or yellowish green colour, and seems permeated by dirty purulent matter.

When the tissue is reduced to a soft, greenish-coloured fœtid pulpy mass, it is believed to constitute gangrene of the pancreas,—a very rare affection. A case is mentioned by Portal.* I have seen the pancreas in this state, of a pale brick-red colour, the *acini* still a little firm, but softened all round their margins, and with purulent matter oozing from the interstices of the gland. It seems difficult, therefore, to say, whether the change described as softening of the pancreas is to be regarded as a species of diffuse suppuration, or as gangrene.

Dr Holscher gives a case, in which a person who had been dyspeptic from his 30th year, began in his 39th to suffer extremely from violent constriction in the region of the transverse arch of the colon, and afterwards from squeamishness, acidity, and sore aphthæ in the mouth and tongue, with great emaciation. In the course of twelve months more, after various oscillations, these symptoms terminated fatally. There was then found, one inch and a-half beyond the *pylorus*, in the duodenum, an ulcer larger than a shilling, with slightly everted edges, surrounded with many blood-vessels, and which had proceeded to perforation about the size of a pea. The pancreas, void of its usual granular structure, seemed partially fleshy, bore some resemblance to the thymus gland of a three months' infant; was softened and very abundant in blood-vessels, which, when divided, effused blood copiously.

In this case the pancreas appears to have been softened, and to

* Anatomie Medicale, Tome v. p. 354.

have lost its characteristic lobulo-granular structure, in consequence
of, 'or along with increased vascular distension.*

§ 7. ATROPHY of the pancreas or diminution of its size, sometimes
with, sometimes without, condensation and induration of its substance, may be regarded as one of the effects of enlargement and
hypertrophy of some one of the other abdominal viscera, for instance the stomach, the liver, spleen, or the right kidney. The pancreas is also in general diminished in size, in chronic inflammation
and ulceration of the intestines. It is not so much an effect of inflammation, as of the opposite state of diminished supply of blood
for nutrition. By some, however, it is regarded as a remote effect
of inflammation, which has either been partially cured, or has proceeded to suppuration, and the matter of which has been discharged.

This is the most convenient place to mention, that the arteries of
the pancreas have been found ossified. This takes place chiefly
when the abdominal aorta and the cœliac and mesenteric arteries
are affected by osteo-steatomatous deposition. The most characteristic case is the following. A shipmaster, aged 59, and who had
been 37 years at sea, had always enjoyed good health. All at
once, however, he began to suffer from headach, *anorexia,* squeamishness, thirst, a sense of burning heat, following the course of the
œsophagus, and constipation. Emaciation speedily followed ; and
at the end of six weeks, death. Upon inspection the pancreas was
found small, shrivelled, dense, of a deep gray colour. Its excretory
duct was obliterated ; and all the arteries, viz. the small branches
of the splenic, the pancreatico-duodenal, and those from the superior mesenteric were ossified.†

It is not improbable that the morbid condition of the arteries was
in this case the cause of the atrophy.

It will be seen from the subsequent head, that the pancreas may
be shrunk and rigid when the ducts are filled with calcareous matter. It would be wrong to consider these two circumstances in the
relation of cause and effect. But we may infer that there are two
conditions or forms of atrophy of this gland ; one in which it is
shrunk, shrivelled, and indurated, and another in which it is small,
yet softened.

---

* Medizinische, Chirurgische und Ophthalmologische Wahrnehmungen. Von Dr
Holscher. Hannoversche Annalen für die Gesammte Heilkunde v. Band ii. Heft 5
Falle. S. 328-369.

† Lancet, Vol. ii. No. 680. 1835-36, 10th September, p. 825.

§ 8. CONCRETIONS.—Concretions are said by Baillie, who had known only one example, to be a rare lesion. Yet they have been observed in the pancreas or its ducts by several. Instances are given by Van der Wiel, Panaroli, Matani, Ten Rhyne, Eller, Sandifort, Portal, Cowley, and lastly by Dr Arthur Wilson and Dr Adam Schupmann. Dr Wilson found the pancreatic ducts in a man of 41, universally filled with compact white earthy matter, which, examined chemically, was found to contain almost pure carbonate of lime on a nucleus of animal matter. The pancreas itself was hard and shrunk, in short atrophied.* Dr Schupmann found in the main duct of the tail of the pancreas, in a man of 57, a concretion one inch and six lines long, weighing three drachms and one scruple. In the lateral ducts were two smaller concretions. These consisted of carbonate of lime, with animal mucus, and traces of phosphoric acid.†

This fact as to chemical constitution corresponds with the result of other analyses.

§ 9. HETEROLOGOUS GROWTHS. a. SCIRRHUS.—Of these the most common in the pancreas, if we can trust the statements of authors, is indubitably scirrhus, or the common fibro-cartilaginous cancer. An immense number of instances under this denomination are recorded by authors. But when we consider these cases, we find no details as to the facts, on which they were referred to that head; and all that we learn is, that either the pancreas is said to be affected with scirrhus, on the testimony of the observer,—or it is stated that the gland is very hard.

It is impossible, therefore, to avail ourselves of the cases recorded by old observers in this matter; and it seems to me doubtful whether we can ascend to a more remote period than the last twelve or thirteen years for evidence as to the pancreas being affected with scirrhus.

From various cases recorded by Mondiere, Holscher, Ritter, Battersby, and other authors, excluding those cases which are doubtful or referable to the head of induration, I think the following inferences may be established.

Scirrhus does not very frequently attack the pancreas primarily. Much more frequently it appears rather to extend from the stomach

---

* An account of a Case of Extensive Disease of the Pancreas. By James Arthu Wilson, M. D., &c. Medico-Chirurgical Transactions, Vol. xxv. p. 42. London, 1842

† C. W. Hufeland's Journal. 1841, April. xcii. Bd.

or *duodenum* to that gland, or it involves that gland in common with other organs. Holscher gives two cases, one of which he calls scirrhus of the pancreas, the other cancerous degeneration of the pancreas. In the former he describes the gland as greatly expanded and developed, and so cartilaginous that it could scarcely be cut by the knife. It retained, nevertheless, its granular structure. This case, therefore, is doubtful. In the second, he states that however much the pancreas may be disposed to scirrhous degeneration, it nevertheless resists the operation of the carcinomatous process in the neighbouring organs; and among 60 cases of cancer of the stomach, in two only did the pancreas partake of the morbid action. One of these was in a man of 80 years, in whose body the pancreas was found little enlarged, but containing, dispersed through its substance, knotty tuberosities, which, when divided, showed a fibro-cartilaginous structure, with intermixture of dull streaks, and several of which had proceeded to softening. The softened portion was like dissolved cheese, and exhaled a peculiarly disagreeable odour. One of these tubercular elevations was opened by an ulcerative process advancing from within, and had elevated bloody edges covered with some thin fetid ichor. It had not proceeded to the formation of fungi. The carcinomatous pancreas had contracted adhesions with the neighbouring organs.[*] This bears much more the character of a heterologous growth, and appears to have been an instance of tubercular scirrhus.

In the case of a married female of 40 years old, and who, after suffering for months under pain in the epigastric region, anxiety, squeamishness, and vomiting, with great emaciation, died, inspection presented the following state of parts;—the stomach normal as far as the indurated portion of the pylorus; but the pancreas indurated, enlarged to twice its proper size; its lobular structure obliterated; the parenchyma hard and solid, yellowish-white in colour; the duct of Wirsung and the hepatic vessels pervious; the former filled with a viscid liquid. The pancreas was morbidly adherent before and behind.[†]

Dr Engel found in the body of a female who died in her 65th year, after vomiting and intestinal discharges of dark-coloured matters with emaciation, besides an ulcer in the stomach and one in the duodenum, immediately beyond the pylorus, which was

[*] Medizinische, Chirurgische und Ophthalmologische Wahrnehmungen. Hannoversche Annalen, v. Band. 2 Heft. 1841.

[†] Scirrhose Verhartung des Pancreas. Von Ritter, Medizinische Zeitung. 1. 1840.

covered by the pancreas, the pancreas as large as a fowl's egg, with an uneven, solid fibrous covering, pale, bloodless, with an irregular fibrous structure, with many eminences larger than peas at the surface, in which was found a jelly-like brain-like matter. The *acini* were completely compressed. Right in the middle of the largest eminences were roundish bands, which might be traced to the pancreatic duct. The latter, normal in diameter, was buried deep in the mass, had thick, rigid, resisting walls like those of arteries; but upon quitting the mass now mentioned became suddenly large, flaccid, and with thin walls.

If these bodies were of medullary structure, as Dr Engel seems to think, then this was rather an example of encephaloid than scirrhous pancreas. He allows that the ulcers in the stomach and duodenum were not cancerous but simple.

The same observer found in the body of a female dead with symptoms of intense jaundice in her 76th year, the pancreas small, very firm and solid; the excretory duct more than a goose quill in calibre, with many prominent valve-like processes in the interior, and filled with a gray coarse frothy fluid; at the head, however, directed outwards, of normal calibre and condition.*

A case given by Dr Battersby is entitled to attention from the correctness of its details. In a widow lady, aged 60, who, after suffering for twelve months from pains regarded as rheumatic, became much emaciated, a tumour about the size of an orange appeared in the epigastric region, and which was the seat of pulsation. In the course of one or two months the tumour subsided; but emaciation proceeded; dropsy followed; and death took place.

The gastro-hepatic epiploon, especially that part in front of the *foramen* of Winslow, was very dense, hard, and thickened; and the vessels and ducts were intimately cemented together. This thickening and hardening affected the cellular tissue surrounding the cardiac orifice of the stomach, which resisted the introduction of the little finger. The stomach was universally connected with the left extremity of the pancreas, which was hard and enlarged, and had lost every trace of its natural structure. Near the centre of this gland was a thin translucent horny cyst, which was slightly prominent, about the size of a walnut, and lay directly over the

* Nachtrag zu den Krankheiten des Pancreas und seines Ausführungsganges; von Dr Joseph Engel. Medizinische Jahrbucher des K. K. Osterreich. Staates. xxxiii. Band oder xxiv. Band N. Folge, 1842.

aorta. Its base was surrounded by a hard cartilaginous scirrhous structure partly projecting into it. The rest of the gland consisted of less solid yet unyielding heavy substance, composed of dense closely interwoven membranous bands.

The pancreatic duct was pervious for about one inch only from the duodenum. The *ductus choledochus* and hepatic ducts were pervious.*

The pancreas is liable to be involved in the heterologous structures of other parts. Thus it may be involved in new heterologous structure, arising either in the interperitoneal cellular tissue, or in the mesenteric glands, or in the pylorus, or in the duodenum. In the 7th case given by Dr Bright the pancreas was involved for a great portion of its space in a new growth which had affected the liver and the whole of the abdominal absorbent glands.† And in a case given by Schupmann, in which cancer affected the pylorus and pancreas, the head of the latter gland was enlarged to three times its usual size, while the gland itself consisted of separate masses mutually connected, longish, from the size of a hazelnut to that of a walnut, and the interior structure of which was hard and gristly-like.‡ No ulceration had yet taken place. But the mesenteric glands had partaken in the disease, and were firmly united to the pancreas.

In all cases of scirrhus affecting the pancreas, the lobulo-granular structure of the gland is either greatly or entirely obliterated. The *acini* are so much changed, that the granular character cannot be recognized. In the place of this there is substituted more or less of the following structure. First, there may be deposited a hard homogeneous matter of whitish gray colour, and as firm as cartilage, which is diffused in amorphous portions varying in size through the gland. These masses are traversed by bluish-white lines of firmer matter, which look like fibrous bands. Secondly, there may be deposited the same substance in the form of tubercles or nodules, varying in size from a small pea to a bean. Both of these forms of new deposit tend to softening.

§ 10. ENCEPHALOID DISEASE.—On this point information is not

---

* Two Cases of Scirrhus of the Pancreas, &c. by Francis Battersby, M. B. Dublin Journal, vol. xxv, p. 219. Dublin, 1844.

† Cases and Observations connected with Disease of the Pancreas and Duodenum, Medico-Chirurg. Transact., vol. xviii. p. 36. London, 1833.

‡ Pförtner und Pancreas-Krebs, von Dr Ad. Schupmann, W. C. Hufeland, Journal der Practischen Heilkunde Sechstes Stuck. Juni 1840.

more precise than on that of common scirrhus. I have already alluded to one case which probably is to be referred to this head ; and hitherto almost all have been considered as belonging to one category. The instances of adipification, or rather lardaceous degeneration, mentioned by Lobstein and Dupuytren, appear to belong to the present head. Bang records in his reports the case of a soldier of 40, in whom, for at least half a year, much pain had been felt in the middle of the abdomen, followed by loss of appetite, constipation, and wasting, and for two months considerable swelling in the left hypochondre. In the course of six weeks more, after great emaciation, death took place ; when, besides much bloody serum contained in the abdomen, the liver was found occupied by white steatomatous tumours, (manifestly encephaloid) ; and the pancreas, which was enlarged to the size of the head of a child, consisted of large glandular tumours, in various parts suppurated and emitting an offensive odour, with extravasated dark putrid blood. This Bang denominates cancer of the pancreas. It appears to have been either *encephaloma* or chronic strumous suppuration.*

It seems doubtful, indeed, if encephaloid disease frequently originates in the pancreas. It often arises in the liver, and thence spreads to the stomach, duodenum, and pancreas ; and it often also arises in the interperitoneal cellular tissue. In this manner I have more than once seen encephaloid tumours developed in the abdomen and affecting successively many different organs. In cases of this description globular masses of whitish semihard matter like granular suet or cheese, varying in size from a walnut to an orange, appear involving and penetrating the mesentery, the intestines, the pancreas, the liver, and not uncommonly the ovaries in the female. It must, nevertheless, be observed, that, amidst these masses of new deposite, it is usually possible to find the substance of several organs less injured than might be expected. Amidst this new structure, the pancreas is in general found, compressed and concealed, but retaining its characteristic granular structure.

Of the changes and combination of changes now mentioned, examples are given in almost all pathological collections. Thus, both in the museum of Mr Langstaff, and in that of St Bartholomew's Hospital, when the pancreas presents medullary or encephaloid tumours, the same are found in the brain, in the kidneys, in the liver, or in the interperitoneal tissue.

* Selecta Diarii Nosocomii Regii Fridericiani Havniensis. Auctore F. Lud. Bang. Hafniae, 1789, ii. p. 409.

. § 11. TYROMA.—Does tubercular structure affect this gland? In some instances it is possible. to recognize in it small bodies with the aspect of tubercles, when the spleen and the peritonæum are affected by these growths. At the same time, that the lesion is not very frequent may be inferred from this fact, that in tubercular disease of the lungs, when the intestines are also much affected, the pancreas is most rarely affected by the same or any similar deposit. It is necessary, however, to distinguish between strumous and scirrhous tubercles. The latter, that is, scirrhus in the tubercular form, are seen occasionally ; the former very seldom.

§ 12. MELANOSIS seems to be more frequent than tubercle in the pancreas ; yet much less so than either *scirrhus* or *encephaloma*. A good example of the deposite is given by Langstaff in the third volume of the Medico-Chirurgical Transactions, and the original of which is preserved in his museum, (now in the College of Surgeons.) In this instance the disease affected the brain, liver, intestines, sternum, and ribs ; and it projected externally in the axilla.

From a similar instance preserved in the museum at St Bartholomew's Hospital, it may be inferred that *melanosis* is often combined with encephaloma.*

SECTION IV.

MORBID STATES OF THE LIVER.

The morbid conditions, to which the liver is liable, may be distinguished into two orders; first, those proper to the liver; and secondly, those affecting the gall-bladder and gall-ducts.

The morbid changes proper to the liver may be enumerated in the following order; Inflammation of different kinds and its effects, such as adhesion, suppuration, induration, and softening; hypertrophy; atrophy; cirrhosis; fatty degeneration; concretions in the ducts; entozoa, or parasitical animals; and the heterologous deposits.

Among those belonging to the gall-bladder and gall-ducts must be placed inflammation of these parts, and their effects; contraction and obstruction of the ducts; biliary concretions and their effects; and entozoa or parasitical animals.

§ 1. INFLAMMATION.—When inflammation attacks the liver, it may affect either the peritoneum, or the hepatic substance, or both.

* A Descriptive Catalogue of the Anatomical Museum of St Bartholomew's Hospital. Published by order of the Governors. Vol. i. Pathological Anatomy. London, 1846. 8vo. Series xx. p. 347.

In the former case the disease constitutes hepatic *peritonitis,* a disorder already noticed generally under the head of the peritoneum: One or two points only deserve particular attention.

1. It is usually supposed that hepatic *peritonitis* is always an acute disease, or rather, that acute inflammation of the liver always affects the peritoneum. This is a mistake. The disease may, like other inflammations of serous tissue, assume either the acute or the chronic form; and it is not easy to say, from what is seen in the inspection of bodies, which is the most frequent.

Hepatic *peritonitis* is a disease not uncommon, especially when the substance of the liver is either congested, indurated, or affected with cirrhosis. In cases of this kind, almost uniformly, the whole convex upper surface of the liver is found adhering to the diaphragm.

Hepatic peritonitis is liable to take place in the concave surface of the gland, when the stomach is inflamed or affected by chronic ulcer. This ulcer, it has been shown, most commonly is seated in the small arch of the stomach; and, if it destroy the gastric tissues down to the peritoneum, *peritonitis* then follows, with effusion of albumen, which may be in various states of consistence, from soft and semifluid up to organized membrane, according to the duration of the disease.

Occasionally inflammation attacks the peritoneum covering the concave surface of the liver, in the site of the capsule of Glisson, and is mostly confined to that region. This is most commonly, nay, very generally, attended with yellowness of the surface. The inflammation extends over the hepatic ducts and vessels in the capsule, and causes more or less constriction of the ducts.

2. Inflammation may attack the hepatic *peritoneum* at the anterior-inferior margin of the right lobe, either along with, or in consequence of, inflammation of the peritoneal coat of the colon, or even the pyloric end of the stomach. The former is the most common. A good specimen of this I had occasion, on the 10th of January 1839, to observe, in inspecting the body of a man destroyed by continued fever. A band of firm false membrane, about two inches broad, and from three to four inches long, extended from the anterior margin of the liver and the fundus of the gall-bladder to the transverse arch of the colon, about one inch to the left of its angle, and connected that bowel firmly to the liver and gall-bladder. Instances even are recorded, in which, in consequence of biliary calculi

6

ulcerating a passage out of the gall-bladder into the intestines, similar adhesions had been previously formed between the peritoneal
coat of that organ and the peritoneal covering of the bowels. Similar inflammation and adhesion take place in India in consequence
of disease of the colon and cæcum.

3. Inflammation of the hepatic *peritoneum* of the inferior surface
of the liver may arise either spontaneously, or from some cause of
irritation in that region, as biliary *calculi* sticking in the gall-ducts,
or inflammation of the *duodenum* or *jejunum*, spreading to the capsule of Glisson. In all these cases the same effects are produced.
The membrane becomes injected, vascular, and rough, and afterwards effuses albuminous exudation, which unites the contiguous
organs by adhesion.

In all the cases now mentioned, hepatic *peritonitis* arises from
some morbific cause applied to or seated in the membrane. But it
may be also the result of another cause seated in the hepatic substance. When the substance of the liver is inflamed, whether it
proceed to suppuration or not, it is a very common consequence for
the peritoneal covering over the inflamed or suppurating portion to
become red, injected, and at length covered on its free surface with
albuminous exudation, which more or less quickly unites the membrane with the organs to which it is applied. It may hence be said
that though hepatic *peritonitis* may often take place without inflammation of the hepatic substance, the latter is almost never inflamed
without being followed or accompanied by hepatic peritoneal inflammation.

§ 2. SCAR-LIKE MARKS ON THE SURFACE OF THE LIVER.—
In examining dead bodies, it is not uncommon to observe on the
surface of the liver marks like the remains of scars or *cicatrices.*
The peritoneum at these marks seems drawn or depressed into the
substance of the liver at one point; and, radiating from this point,
are lines gradually lost in the space of about from half an inch to
three-quarters of an inch. At these parts, the peritoneum adheres
very firmly; and there is often a sort of contraction or drawing together of all the parts.

The cause of these appearances is in all probability inflammation
of the hepatic peritoneum, taking place at a particular point, and
connected with inflammation either of the liver or of the sub-serous
cellular tissue.

§ 3. CARTILAGE-LIKE PATCHES.—The hepatic peritoneum is often
found covered with patches of cartilage-like matter. The con-

vex surface is the most usual seat of this deposition and transformation; and it is most common in females. There are evidently
layers of albuminous effusion, the result of chronic inflammation.

§ 4. TUBERCLES.—The hepatic *peritoneum* is, like other parts of
that membrane, liable to be affected with osseous degeneration;
and it may be occupied with minute hard semitranslucent tubercles, when the peritoneum is affected by these bodies. All these
conditions are liable to be attended with inflammation of the membrane, that is redness, congestion, roughness, and exudation of
coagulating lymph, but which is slow in progress, and in other
respects of a chronic character.

It then usually happens that the hepatic peritoneum adheres
more or less extensively and firmly to the diaphragmatic, the gastric, or the muscular peritoneum. This disorder is most usual when
the abdominal peritoneum generally is affected by tubercles.

It has been formerly mentioned that in one order of tubercles
adhesion is most common; and in another ascites.

§ 1. INFLAMMATION OF THE HEPATIC SUBSTANCE.—Inflammation of the substance of the liver has been generally, since the time
of Cullen at least, believed to be of a chronic nature; and doubtless
the trifling or obscure symptoms which appear in cases, in which
dissection discloses a considerable abscess of the organ, are highly
favourable to this opinion. For, independent of the avowed difficulty of ascertaining the existence of what has been termed chronic
hepatitis during life, almost all authors abound with examples of
abscess of the organ discovered on dissection, yet in which no decisive symptom had led to the suspicion of such an event. The
truth of this I can verify by personal testimony. Various reasons,
however, lead me to doubt whether hepatic inflammation is invariably chronic; and several facts prove that it assumes, under certain circumstances, a sufficiently acute form.

1. In the tropical regions, inflammation of the hepatic substance
is often attended with acute pain, quick pulse, and all the marks
of a violent disease; and unless remedies be seasonably and energetically employed, suppuration takes place in a period sufficiently
short to warrant the opinion of the inflammation being acute,
(Clark, (Med. Com. xiv. p. 322,) Ballingall, Marshall). 2. In tropical countries, also, there are two forms of hepatic inflammation,—
one, acute, rapid, and with well-marked symptoms; the other slow,
long-continued, and with indistinct symptoms. 3. Though, in

temperate climates, this disease is undoubtedly milder, slower, and less violent than in countries where the atmospheric heat is excessive, yet instances are not wanting in which the disease appears with distinct symptoms, runs a rapid course, and terminates in more or less extensive suppuration. It is true that the distinction, according to duration or severity of symptoms, is liable to be vague and undefined; but it is the only one which is pretty obvious, and which may be useful in diagnosis. 4. Lastly, both in temperate and hot climates one form of inflammation of the liver consists in a slow and gradual enlargement of the gland, which appears to depend on chronic congestion, if not inflammation, without tending to suppuration, but mere hardening.

From these facts, it may be inferred that hepatic inflammation is of two kinds, suppurative and unsuppurative; that the former, which is analogous with the phlegmonous inflammation of Cullen, Smyth, and others of the same school, may be acute or chronic, severe in character, and rapid in progress, or moderate in action, and slow in progress; that the latter is always chronic, unless, when, under certain circumstances, it may suddenly pass into the acute form; and that, though all forms of the disease may occur in temperate countries, yet warm or tropical regions are the situations most common for the several forms of hepatic inflammation. I enumerate, according to these principles, the following varieties.

A. Acute suppurative; B. Chronic suppurative; C. Acute congestive or enlarging; D. Chronic congestive or indurating.

A. Of the first the best examples are afforded in the cases of Dr John Clark, occurring in the East Indies, Dr James Clark, occurring in Dominica, those of Sir G. Ballingall, Mr Annesley, and Mr Geddes, in the East Indies, and those of Mr Marshall in the Island of Ceylon.   Its most common symptoms are more or less pain in the right hypochondriac or epigastric region, tenderness in some part of the side, difficulty or pain in lying on the right, sometimes on the left side, sickness, vomiting, heat, thirst, quick strong full pulse, and constipation, with scanty high-coloured urine.   The pain is generally increased on pressure; but, in some instances, there is merely an undefined sense of soreness or of weight, or of gnawing emptiness, deep in the right hypochondriac and towards the epigastric region.   These sensations are generally aggravated by lying on the left side, in some instances by lying on the right side; and occasionally no ease is procured unless when the patient is on his back. It is probable that this variety of complaint depends on the part of the organ most severely affected. The aggravation caused by lying on the left side appears to denote that the left lobe is inflamed; that resulting from lying on the right side denotes inflammation of the right lobe, each being respectively pressed by the weight over a tender and inflamed part; while the ease derived from the supine position indicates a deep-seated inflammation verging towards the upper obtuse margin, and the concave surface of the organ. The sickness, vomiting, and constipation are not constant symptoms; but if present with local pain and quick pulse, denote the disease, with considerable certainty, as extending to the concave surface. The heat, thirst, quick strong pulse, and scanty high-coloured urine are merely connected with the general feverish state of the system. It rarely happens that, in this form of hepatic inflammation, there is sufficient enlargement or hardening of the organ to cause a sensible increase in the bulging of the hypochondriac region. This only occurs towards the latter end of the disease, when it threatens to terminate in suppuration, or to pass into the chronic form. Clark of Dominica considers inability to sneeze as a certain sign of the malady.

The acute hepatic inflammation terminates, 1st, in resolution; 2d, in suppuration; 3d, in induration or chronic inflammation.

Termination by resolution is when the symptoms gradually decline either spontaneously or by the use of suitable remedies, and the patient is restored to health without further complaint. If the resolution be spontaneous, it is generally accompanied by some evacuation, for instance, hemorrhage from the nose or from the intestines, diarrhœa, critical sweating, or a copious sediment in the urine. Saunders states that he has seen a great increase of bronchial secretion attend the resolution of this disease; and perhaps this is an instance of transfer of morbid action.* Termination in suppuration is more common, and is fatal either speedily or more slowly. In the former case the right or left lobe is converted into a large abscess or collection of matter, purulent, sero-purulent, or purulent with masses of flaky lymph. If the whole hepatic tissue be not destroyed in this manner, the inner surface of the abscess is somewhat irregular, having the appearance of an ulcer thickly covered with purulent matter, or flaky lymph. The substance of the organ for about a third of an inch from the ulcerated surface appears unus-

---

* A Treatise on the Structure, &c. p. 208.

ually red, and may be hardened a little, but beyond this the glandular substance is healthy. In some instances the hepatic substance is destroyed or entirely removed at one spot or over a great extent, and the purulent fluid is contained in a sac formed by the peritoneal coat. The quantity of purulent fluid varies from one to seven pounds, the most usual quantity being about two or three pounds. At the same the contiguous hepatic substance is denser, larger, and heavier, and weighs, exclusive of the purulent matter, from one to three pounds more than in the healthy state it would do. This increase in bulk and weight is occasioned partly by blood in its capillary system, partly by new products from the blood, causing swelling or enlargement of the organ.

When a considerable abscess of one or both lobes has formed, death generally takes place very quickly, apparently in consequence of the feebleness and waste of vital power induced by a violent disease. If, however, life is protracted a little, the purulent collection increases in size, and finds its way to the surface of the organ. Ulceration of the peritoneal covering takes place at one or more points, and the contents escape by the openings. An abscess may in this manner be discharged; 1st, into the abdominal cavity; 2d, through the diaphragm into the air-cells and *bronchi ;* 3d, by the adhesive process into some part of the intestinal canal, the stomach, transverse arch of the colon, or even the duodenum ; 4th, by the same process to the outer surface of the body.

1. When the matter escapes into the abdominal cavity, it produces immediate peritoneal inflammation, generally terminating fatally. This termination is most usual when the abscess is seated about the posterior inferior surface, and the acute margin of the gland. This is believed to be a rare termination.*

2. If the collection be seated about the upper surface and right lobe of the organ, the liver, diaphragm, and lungs become united by adhesive inflammation, and the matter passes into the air-cells, from which it is discharged by expectoration with frequent coughing. In fatal cases the hepatic portion of such an abscess presents a wide hollow, to the margin of which the lungs and diaphragm are firmly attached ; the muscular structure of the latter is destroyed to the extent of the ulcerated surface, and the lungs are hardened, and void of crepitation. This termination is generally fatal in a short time. The symptoms become complicated with those of

* Vide Bang Selecta Diarii Havniensis, Tom. ii. p. 65, where a case with dissection is given. A case by Mr Macmillan Jameson in Mem. Med. Society, vol. iii. p. 579.

pulmonary consumption, and the patient is worn out by incessant irritation, difficult breathing, coughing, and hectic emaciation.* Yet, according to Marshall, recoveries from this state have occurred; they are indeed rare, and perhaps occur only when the abscess is small, and the consequent inflammation of the lungs not extensive. (Vide John Clark, pp. 405, 407.)

3. Mr Marshall mentions a case in which the left lobe adhered to the stomach, and part of the contents of an abscess had passed through a large opening into its cavity. Sir G. Ballingall states, that, in many instances, extensive adhesion takes place between the liver and transverse arch of the colon; and though he never met with a case in which an opening was effected, yet he infers that it has taken place, so as to discharge matter and effect a cure. Mr Marshall adheres to the mere fact of no communication ever being formed, and is not aware of a cure having been accomplished. Dr John Clark, however, records a case, which he considers, from the discharge* of purulent matter, to have been of this nature, (p. 416). Two examples of this communication are given by M. Petit.†

4. Among the cases of hepatic abscess related by Valsalva, in one the biliary duct communicated with the abscess by a large orifice, and was considerably dilated. Morgagni infers, that there is no reason to doubt that this duct frequently conveys blood and purulent matter from the substance of the liver into the duodenum; and he mentions that, in one case in which many pounds of purulent fluid were voided at different periods during life, much matter was found after death in the intestines, biliary ducts, and liver, and the ducts were much dilated, the intestinal extremity being large enough to admit the little finger. (xxxvi. 10.) The probability of this mode of outlet in consequence of purulent matter being formed either in the vicinity of the ducts, or in the concave part of the liver, is noticed by Petit, and afterwards by Saunders; but he appears to have been misled by speculative views, and to have inferred that, because adhesion generally attends suppuration and ulceration, it was difficult to explain the mode in which the hepatic abscess made its way into the duodenum, and falls into some philosophical inconsistencies. (See Chap. iv. Sect. i. 7–13.)

5. The passage of an hepatic abscess to the surface of the body

* See cases by E. Barry, Ed. Med. Essays; Dr Ludlow, Mem. Med. Society, vol. iii. p. 145; and Larrey, Expedition en Egypte, p. 191.

† Des Apostemes du Foie, Memoires de l'Academie de Chirurgie, tome ii. p. 61, cases 2 and 8. Paris, 1753.

appears to be uncommon; and its spontaneous opening by ulceration of the integuments almost unknown. Clark of Dominica records several cases in which, by an external incision, he discharged considerable quantities of matter, (1, 2, 3, quarts, half a gallon, a pint, &c.) sometimes so as to effect a permanent cure. Marshall, however, states that no case occurred in the Kandyan country among any of the classes of troops in which it was deemed advisable to make an incision through the abdominal parietes into an hepatic abscess; and in those cases in which bulging of the false ribs appeared to indicate the performance of this measure, it was found on dissection that adhesion was not sufficiently intimate to render it successful. In three cases in which the abscesses were small, the operation was performed with good result.

The termination of acute hepatic inflammation in hardening or chronic disease shall be noticed afterwards.

Acute suppurative inflammation of the liver may be said to be endemial in tropical climates. It is so in the West Indies; in India, but particularly the Coromandel Coast, (John Clark); in the Mysore, especially at Bengalore, (Mouat); and in the whole of the Presidency of Madras; in Ceylon, (Marshall); and on the coast of Africa, (Winterbottom). It may occur, however, in temperate or cold climates. Morgagni mentions examples in Italy, Portal in France, and Bang in Denmark. (See Selecta Diarii, pp. 62, 224, 285, 315). Two cases have fallen under my observation in this country.

It attacks indiscriminately natives and Europeans, but especially the latter, in the East Indies. In Dominica, the negroes were as frequently attacked as the whites. Not unfrequently it succeeds ague or remittent fever, or may be complicated with them. Exposure to cold, moisture, or extreme heat appears equally to favour its production.

B. Chronic suppurative hepatic inflammation differs from the acute in its mode of attack, the degree of severity, and its effects on the substance of the organ. It generally comes on slowly and insidiously, either originally in constitutions previously exhausted by long residence in hot climates, and repeated attacks of acute disease, or it follows remittent fever or ague. The patient is languid, listless, averse to exertion either bodily or mental, and sometimes apprehensive. Yet he does not complain of pain, or that distressing uneasiness which attends the acute disease. The hypochondriac region, on the contrary, may be insensible, or the seat of a gnawing sense of emptiness. At the commencement it is not enlarged or prominent, but becomes so as the disease advances. The pulse, at first slow and natural, becomes afterwards quicker, varying from 90 to 100, and sharpish; the skin is cold, and dry or unctuous; the tongue furred; the complexion sallow, and the look anxious. The appetite is variable, at one time apparently good, at others completely gone, while squeamishness and even vomiting may succeed. The matters discharged are chiefly tough phlegm, with disordered bile and the portions of food eaten. At the same time, the patient is hot, thirsty, and restless. The bowels are generally bound; the stools darker or lighter than natural; afterwards they are loose, frequent, and lienteric. The urine is scanty, depositing a copious red flaky sediment.

But the most distinguishing character of this disease is, that whatever variation these symptoms may present, and however obscure they may be, there is a distinct accession of fever during the night. The pulse may be calm and of natural frequency, the skin may be cool, and the sensations of thirst and hunger may be natural during the day;—in the course of the night the skin becomes hot, the face reddish, the pulse strong and frequent, the mouth dry and parched, and the patient is restless, or enjoys only disturbed slumber; as morning advances slight sweating comes on, with abatement of his sufferings and tolerable sleep. If the disease is not arrested, all the symptoms, and especially those of night fever, become more severe and distressing; the patient tosses about in bed with a dry burning skin, and scalding palms, constant and insatiable thirst, and, in some instances, a severe husky cough; his nights become sleepless, and it is only in the morning, after the urgent complaints are relieved by partial sweating, that he falls into a laboured, interrupted, and unrefreshing slumber. His strength and flesh waste, his appetite decays, and he at length sinks into hectic, which shortly terminates in death.

Dissection shows, instead of an abscess of considerable size, several small distinct collections of purulent matter similar to the small abscesses (*vomicae*) of the lungs. They may be very numerous, and not larger than peas, or fewer in number, and as large as a hen's egg. The whole mass of the liver is altered in colour; it appears as if parboiled, and its texture is firmer than natural, giving when cut the sensation of the knife passing through a soft cartilaginous mass. Very little blood issues from the incision. In some instances the surface of the organ is sprinkled with white spots of various dimensions, or tubercles are interspersed through its substance. These appearances may be conjoined with hydatids; but these are rarely met in the disease as it occurs in India. The bile differs from healthy bile in a slight change of colour or consistence; but it has not been chemically examined. The gall-bladder seldom presents any change of structure, or is merely thickened in its coats.

This form of hepatic inflammation is very common in India, especially in those who have resided long in the country, who have been exposed to the causes of ague and fever, or whose habits have been rather intemperate. It is not unknown, however, in European countries; for Bang describes an instance of it in his Copenhagen Reports, occurring in the month of April 1783, and with symptoms somewhat acute. (Tome i. p. 88, Selecta Diarii Havniensis.) Two instances have come under my own notice in this country.

In various instances of the disease, a single large abscess is formed in the liver without acute symptoms, or with the usual train of chronic complaints. I had occasion in 1827 to examine the body of an aged person who had been labouring for about five or six weeks under symptoms of inflammation of the intestinal mucous membrane, and in whom, besides the usual traces of disease in the colon, I found a large abscess in the right lobe of the liver, containing fully four pounds of purulent matter, mixed with lymphy flakes. To this head Mr Andree's case in the Transactions of the Medical Society appears to belong. " The formation," says Mr Marshall, " of a large abscess in the liver sometimes takes place without much indication of disease, in as far as the feelings of the patient are concerned. So little obvious occasionally are the symptoms which indicate a large accumulation of pus in that organ, that the pointing of the abscess outwards has been mistaken for a superficial collection, and an opening made into it by means of a lancet. The issue of three or four pounds of purulent matter undeceived the operator. (P. 155.) Are such collections to be regarded as the result of chronic inflammation, or of a scrofulous disease of the liver, as they are in other organs? or are they the result of secondary deposition through the medium of the veins, as takes place in certain cases of intestinal ulceration? A peculiar modification of hepatic suppuration is described by Sandifort in the eighth chapter of the second book of his Academical Researches.

C. I have made a distinct head of *acute congestive inflammation*, for the purpose of referring to it an affection of the liver, which is described by Dr Chisholm, as prevailing epidemically in some parts of the West Indies. The disease began with headach, pain at the pit of the stomach, general languor, and a sense of tightness and oppression at the breast, with difficult breathing. The skin was dry, harsh, and cool; the tongue moist and foul, without thirst; the belly natural; the urine freely secreted; and the pulse was soft, about 70 or 80 in the minute, and of natural fulness. In some cases the pulse was quick and hard from the first, the skin hot and dry, and some swelling of the belly, especially at the umbilical region, was remarked. The pain varied in situation, being some time confined to the right hypochondriac and epigastric regions, in other instances extending from these to the shoulder, especially the right, across the belly to the navel, or from the navel through to the spine. It was remarkable, that, when the pain was fixed, it was felt in the left side, under the false ribs.

In about two days the headach increased much, but without giddiness; the pain at the pit of the stomach became more excruciating; and shivering came on, with chilness of the skin to the touch, but an intense burning sensation when pressed strongly. The tongue was covered with a thick moist fur, purplish at the edges; the cheeks, nose, and eyebrows assumed a copper hue, exuding large drops of sweat, while the skin, in general, was covered with an unctuous moisture; the pulse rose from 80 to 120 or 140; dry cough, or rather a sudden catching mode of expiration, with a sense of compression of the lungs, came on; and about the sixth day, all the symptoms increasing, the skin became cold and clammy, the pulse exceedingly quick and small, deglutition became difficult, and coma came on, terminating in death.

On dissection the liver was found greatly enlarged; its surface, especially the convex, was clouded irregularly with red, purple, and tallow-coloured spots; the peritonæum sound and transparent. The hepatic substance was of natural consistence, without any appearance of suppuration, but so much enlarged as to occupy in eight of ten cases not only the right hypochondriac and epigastric region, but the left hypochondre. Its vessels were enlarged, but empty. These appearances seem to arise from an unusual accumulation or congestion of blood in the liver. It appears to be the same described by Marshall at p. 146, and which he regards as a passive engorgement of the vascular system of the gland.

This sort of hepatic inflammation prevails occasionally as an epidemic in Grenada, Dominica, and others of the later settled islands. Although persons of all colours, ages, and of both sexes may be attacked, yet blacks and young people from eight to twenty-five years are most liable.

D. SKLEROMA.—To the fourth head, or that of chronic congestive inflammation, may be referred those examples of liver disease, in which the organ becomes slowly indurated, generally with, sometimes without, enlargement, but always with obscure symptoms of ill health, until the structure of the organ is so generally changed, that it is no longer fit for its functions of receiving the venous circulation, or performing the secretion of bile. The symptoms of this disease are so similar to those of suppurative inflammation, that it is impossible in the present state of knowledge to attempt a complete history. The principal, according to Pemberton, are a sense of weight and dull pain in the right side, weary heaviness of the right arm, and frequently pain at the top of the shoulder. The tongue is usually whitish, the appetite impaired, the countenance sallow, and the bowels slow, and stools clay-coloured. The pulse is about 90, almost invariably intermitting, and there is a sensation of fluttering at the pit of the stomach,—symptoms which Pemberton ascribes to the impeded motion of the arterial and venous blood through the hardened gland. These symptoms, however, it may be remarked, appear only when the disease is far advanced, when the natural structure is much injured.

The organ is harder than natural, and when cut gives a gristly sensation. Its surface is mottled, irregular, and marked with depressions not unlike *cicatrices*. Its substance is also generally paler than natural, sometimes of a wood-brown colour; and sometimes like a recent section of nutmeg in tint; and, if immersed in clear water, appears quite different from the sound state. It is traversed with gray or light-coloured particles, which seem to be infiltrated between the *acini*, or glandular granules. In some instances it is possible to distinguish between the *acini* a bluish-gray firm sort of substance, which is indurated cellular tissue.

Not unlike, perhaps, is the hard state of liver observed in drunkards. Dr Marshall describes them as yellowish, containing little blood, and communicating a gristly sensation, when divided, sometimes loose and granular, at others solid and tenacious, weighing generally five pounds.

Such a state of the liver gives rise to all the symptoms of imperfect digestion and impaired nourishment, and eventually terminates in dropsical effusion within the *peritonæum* (*ascites,*) or uncon-

trollable hemorrhage from the mucous surface of the intestinal
canal. This is the early stage of that change, which is afterwards
to be described as kirrhosis.

This disease may succeed the acute form, or may be developed
slowly and insensibly after ague, remittent fever, or in the persons
of those accustomed to the use of spirituous liquors. It is certainly
a common disease in tropical climates, but is by no means unknown
in more temperate latitudes. It is much seldomer found in females
than in males.

§ 2. ANATOMICO-PATHOLOGICAL CAUSES OF SUPPURATION AND
ABSCESS OF THE LIVER. INFLUENCE OF SUPPURATIVE DISEASE
IN OTHER TISSUES. INFLUENCE OF PHLEBITIS.—Though the
inquiry into the circumstances acting as precedents or antegre-
dients, and esteemed causes of suppuration of the liver, involves
the consideration of causes of inflammation in general, yet the
formation of purulent collections within the substance of the liver,
is attended by circumstances so peculiar, that, in order to render
the pathological history of these collections complete, it is necessary
to consider these circumstances a little in detail. Abscess of the
liver, indeed, is a lesion so frequent, and in a certain number of
cases takes place so steadily and regularly, yet so insidiously, and
often in connection with injuries of the head, that the subject is entitled to particular consideration.

The circumstances usually observed to precede suppurative
inflammation of the liver are; 1st, external violence or injury ;
2d, internal irritation, as from the presence of bones, concretions,
or other objects which may irritate the gland ; 3d, suppurative
inflammation of bones, especially of their veins; 4th, inflammation
of a vein or veins, whether purulent or lymphy ; 5th, the presence
of ulcers in the intestinal or colic mucous membrane, or ulcers in
the stomach, duodenum, gall-bladder, or gall-ducts, or ulcers or
abscesses in the pancreas; 6th, previous congestive states of the
liver ensuing on the operation of excessive solar or atmospherical
heat; and 7th, the operation of the poison or miasma producing
intermittent and remittent fever.

Of all these causes, though it be difficult to appreciate the comparative influence of each, yet little doubt can be entertained that
the most common and the most potential are venous inflammation,
or the presence of purulent matter in certain veins, and ulceration
of the intestines, either small or great.

1. External violence is rarely the cause of hepatic abscess.

More commonly this produces either laceration, with hemorrhage, or it gives rise to inflammation of the hepatic peritoneum, which is then found to have formed adhesive connection with the diaphragm, with the internal surface of the hypochondriac region, or with the stomach, colon, duodenum, or kidney. Lentin records one case from external violence.* Bretin mentions another which he ascribes to this cause.† And two cases are recorded by M. Petit the younger, (Case 3d, the·kick of a horse; Case 4th, a contusion on the epigastric region).‡ Yet it is evidently not frequent. Among sixty cases, collected in tabular form from different sources by Dr Budd, in one only, a case recorded by Andral, could the disease be traced to a blow. In this case were two abscesses on the convex surface; and in all probability they were collections of purulent matter between the hepatic and hypochondriac peritoneum.

2. From the irritation of internal objects the disease is more common. Thus cases are recorded from the presence of biliary concretions.§ In general, the presence of these bodies causes, first, inflammation and ulceration of the gall-bladder and gall-ducts, and then of the hepatic substance. One of the most pointed cases is given by Mr George Mallet, of Bolton-le-Moors. A clergyman who had been ill with general bad health, accompanied with fits of excruciating pain in the epigastric region, died after the course of eight years. Inspection disclosed an ulcerated opening through the coats of the gall-bladder, communicating with an abscess beneath the concave surface of the liver, containing about six ounces of purulent matter. The ulceration was caused by the irritation of a moderately-sized gall-stone which was found near the opening, but still within the gall-bladder. The pancreas contained in a cyst a gall-stone about three-quarters of one inch in diameter, and which must have ulcerated its way into that gland at some period anterior, as no recent traces of inflammation or suppuration were observed.‖

3 and 4. Hepatic abscess after venous inflammation is much more frequent. In 16 cases which fell under the observation of

---

* Beobachtungen Eineger Kranken, p. 94.
† Journal de Medecine, Tom. lxv. p. 546.
‡ Memoires de l'Academie de Chirurgie. Tome ii. p. 59.
§ Ephemerides Naturæ Curios. Dec. I. Ann. I. Obs. 66. Obs. 105.
  Fournier in Journal de Medecine, Tome xlv.
  Lombart in Recueil Periodique de la Societé de Medecine a Paris, No. 32.
‖ Transactions of the Provincial Medical and Surgical Association. Vol. ix.
art. ix. London, 1841.

Louis and Andral, four may be traced to this source. In 15 cases seen by Dr Budd in the Dreadnought hospital ship, only one belongs to this head.

Inflammation of any vein may be followed by the formation of purulent matter in one or more collections in the liver; but the veins, in which inflammation is most generally followed by this result, are the veins of bones, often very minute, and the veins of the intestinal viscera, from the stomach to the rectum.

The influence of inflammation in the veins of bones in producing hepatic abscess appears in different modes. One of the most common is after injuries of the skull.

It had been observed by Paré, Pigray, (1658,) De Marchettis, (1665,) a Meek'ren, (1682,) and other surgeons of the seventeenth century, that after wounds of the head and fractures of the skull, abscess of the liver was an occurrence so common, as always to be apprehended. Various attempts, some odd enough, were made to explain this combination of pathological phenomena, which was too regular to be regarded as accidental. Little regard was given to the modes of explanation, however, till the middle of the following century, when, within the lapse of some years, the subject exercised the ingenuity of Petit, Bertrandi, Andouillé, Pouteau, and other members of the French Academy, and Richter, Bianchi, Morgagni, Cheston, (1766,) and other observers in different countries of Europe.

Previous to the time of Bertrandi, two opinions appear to have been entertained regarding the cause of hepatic suppuration after injuries of the head. Paré, a Meek'ren, and the cotemporaries of the latter merely note the conjunction of the two phenomena, and suppose the suppuration first formed within the brain, and thence absorbed and deposited in the liver. By another party, among whom may be placed Goursaud, it was ascribed to sympathetic affection of the nerves, or the reflux of purulent matter. This author, in a memoir presented to the Academy in 1751, gives two cases, in one of which hepatic abscess followed a wound of the finger, and in another a blow on the *tibia*, and ascribes them generally to nervous influence.*

This phenomenon Bertrandi ascribed to derangement in the motion of the blood in the brain. He supposed that, after every violent concussion of the brain, the blood flows in greater abun-

* Récueil des Pieces qui ont concouru pour la Prix de l'Academie de Chirurgie, Tome iii. Paris, 1759. Sur la Metastase, p. 3.

dance to this organ, and returns in greater quantity by the jugular veins; so that while a large stream is brought downwards by these veins, and a considerable quantity of blood is conveyed by the superior *vena cava* against the inferior, the blood of the latter is made to regurgitate and accordingly pass into the *vena cava hepatica* and its tributaries; and in this manner, more blood than the liver is capable of admitting being thrown on the vessels of that organ, inflammation follows, and terminates in suppuration and gangrene, the former most commonly.*

This theory was favourably received by the French academicians, especially David; and was illustrated and commended by M. Andouillé.†

The justice of this hypothesis was questioned in this country by Cheston, and in France by Pouteau.

Cheston expresses his general belief of the improbability of the disturbance in the circulation assumed by Bertrandi, and has recourse to three suppositions in order to explain the occurrence of hepatic suppurations after injuries of the head. 1*st*, Abscesses may exist in the liver after an injury received on the head, without being derived or occasioned by falling, from the head to that abdominal viscus. 2*d*, Abscess in the liver may be the result of translations of matter from one part to another, as are frequently observed after amputation of the larger limbs. 3*d*, In severe injuries of the head, the functions of the liver are injured by sympathetic irritation of its vessels and neighbouring parts from the diseased state of the brain; and this disorder may cause obstruction, terminating in suppuration.

To these Cheston adds as an accessory circumstance, that, in those accidents in which the brain suffers, as by falls from some height, being thrown violently from a horse, the body must receive a severe shock, which may not only aggravate the injury inflicted on the head, but, from the size and soft pulpy texture of the liver, affect the functions of that viscus in particular, and thereby not a little assist in confirming those obstructions which afterwards could not be terminated but by suppuration.‡

* Sur les Absces du Foie qui se forment a l'occasion des playes de la tete. Par M. Bertrandi. Memoires de l'Academie de Chirurgie, Tome iii. p. 484. Paris, 1757.

† Observations sur les Absces du Foie, par M. Andouillé. Memoires de l'Academie de Chirurgie, Tome iii. p. 506. Paris, 1757.

‡ Pathological Inquiries and Observations in Surgery from the Dissection of Morbid Bodies, &c. By Richard Browne Cheston. Gloucester, 1766. 4to, chapter iii. p. 32—42.

The doctrine of Cheston was long afterwards espoused in a divided form by Desault and Richerand.

According to Pouteau, on the other hand, who maintained that it was not proved that either the quantity or the velocity of the blood in the superior *cava* was increased, the impediment to the circulation takes place in the arteries. Admitting that after a blow on the head the blood is accumulated in the arteries of the brain, this accumulation extends, he maintains, to the carotid and vertebral arteries; and consequently, the blood being resisted in the upper divisions of the arterial system, is accumulated in the abdominal aorta and the rest of the blood-vessels; while the substance of the liver being soft, and its vessels large and numerous, readily gives way to this new orgasm, and becomes affected by inflammation and suppuration.*

Desault rejected both explanations, and confined himself to admitting the fact of a relation unknown, but real, between the brain and the liver, more intimate than between other organs; and the proof of this relation shown by the living body by sickness and vomiting; and in the dead body by the formation of abscesses in the gland.† This explanation, or rather statement, of the two facts was long received in the French schools, apparently in consequence of the high reputation of its author, and his commentator Bichat.

Curtet, a military surgeon at Brussels, appears first, in 1800, to have doubted the sufficiency of all those hypotheses. Regarding these hepatic collections as secondary or consecutive, he looked for some other cause than any hitherto assigned; and this cause, he believed, he found in the absorbing function of the lymphatic system. Goursaud, we have seen, had shown that hepatic suppuration may follow ordinary suppurating wounds of the extremities. Roose, a surgeon at Antwerp, had communicated to the Society of Medicine and Surgery at Brussels, a memoir containing cases of whitloe, in consequence of which abscesses were found in the liver. Rejecting the explanation of this sym-phenomenon given by Roose, but receiving the fact, which he confirms by other two cases, Curtet ascribes the suppuration in the liver to absorption of matter by the lymphatics, and the transport of the same by these vessels to the liver, first, into the thoracic duct, and thence, both by the hepatic artery and portal vein to the gland. He invokes also

* Melanges de Chirurgie par M. Claude Pouteau, D. M. et C. A Lyon, 1760. P. 123 ; et Oeuvres Posthumes de M. Pouteau, Tome ii. Paris, 1783. P. 111.

† Oeuvres Chirurgicales, 2 tomes. Paris, 1801.

3

the aid of various accessory causes; viz. the size of the liver, the softness and vascularity of its structure, and the slowness with which its blood moves through the organ.*

It is impossible to deny, that the single fact of proving suppuration of the liver in other circumstances besides those after injuries of the head, was one great step in the inquiry; and to refer the process to the absorbing powers of the lymphatic vessels was another. It showed at once that hepatic suppuration might take place in the course of suppurative processes in other parts of the body. It is singular, that, in this respect, the memoir of Curtet has been so much neglected.

Dissatisfied with the whole of these accounts of the connection of these two phenomena, Richerand brought forward a different view, first, in 1803, and afterwards in 1815. According to this author, the large size and the weight of the liver are the main cause of its becoming the seat of suppuration in consequence of injuries of the head. The weight of this gland, between three and four pounds, is so considerable, that it exercises on the diaphragm great tension, which causes inconvenience and pain unless counteracted. The liver also, from its size, weight, and the looseness of its tissue, void of fibres or plates, is easily lacerated by slight violence; and, of all the organs, is next to the brain most exposed to the effects of concussions and shocks, as in falls from some height.

In illustration, he gives two cases; and conversely one, in which, after a blow on the head, causing fracture and fatal inflammation of the brain, the liver was quite sound.†

Not satisfied with this evidence, Richerand tried experimentally the effect of throwing dead bodies from a height of eighteen feet above the ground on the pavement below. By precipitating in this manner more than forty dead bodies, he found that the brain and the liver were always more or less injured; that in some cases the latter presented deep lacerations; that heavy bodies presented the most severe injuries; and that while fractures of all kinds and dif-

---

* Observations et Reflexions sur les Depots Consecutifs qui ont lieu au Foie, particulierement a la suite des Lesions traumatiques. Par le Cn. Curtet, officier de Santé a l'Hopital Militaire de Bruxelles, &c. &c. Actes de la Societé de Medecine, Chirurgie, et Pharmacie etablie a Bruxelles, Tome i. 2ieme partie. A Bruxelles, An. 8. 1800. P. 93.

† Nosographie et Therapeutique Chirurgicales. Par M. Le Chevalier Richerand, Prof. d'Operations de Chirurgie, &c. Cinquieme edition, Tome iiiieme, p. 70—75. Paris, 1821.

ferent luxations were observed, no viscus, not even the brain, suffered more than the liver from these violent concussions produced artificially by falls.

It is easy to see that this explanation is the same, in one circumstance, as that given in 1766 by Cheston.

The explanation of Richerand was very generally received, both in France and in various countries of Europe.

That the explanation, nevertheless, was unsatisfactory and inadequate, appears from the fact, that hepatic abscesses are observed in the case of injuries of the head, in which the individual had sustained no fall, and his person had received no shock, except the blow on the skull, and in injuries and especially compound fractures of the extremities.

Though Curtet had, at the end of last century, made a considerable advance in the right line of inquiry on this subject, it was not till near thirty years after, that the explanation, which may be regarded as the correct one, was given. Mr Arnott showed, in a paper read to the Medico-Chirurgical Society in 1828, that, when the phenomena of injuries of the skull or other external parts are followed by suppuration or abscess within the liver, there is every reason to believe that the veins of the former part are inflamed, and that, in consequence of this venous inflammation, secondary deposits take place in the liver. Mr Arnott showed, in short, that secondary deposits take place in this way both in the abdominal and the thoracic viscera, and sometimes in both sets of organs at once. He further showed, that the injury which the head had sustained consisted, in two-thirds of the cases, of fracture or fissure of the skull, in all compound; and though, in one-third, the skull was neither fractured nor fissured, yet with wound of the soft parts, in several, part of the outer table and diploe had been sliced off, while in all the bone was exposed. As inflammation of the osseous substance must, in all these cases, have existed, Mr Arnott infers that this process taking place in the numerous veins ramifying between the two tables of the skull, and in those distributed to the soft parts externally, may be attended with similar consequences to those which follow *phlebitis* in other parts; that is, collections of matter in internal organs.*

Cruveilhier subsequently showed, that injuries affecting bones,

* A Pathological Inquiry into the Secondary Effects of Inflammation of the Veins ; by James Arnott, surgeon. Medico-Chirurgical Transac. Vol. xv. p. i. London, 1829.

causing inflammation of the osseous tissue, and involving the veins of that tissue, are very commonly followed by abscess in the liver. The veins so affected may be so minute as to escape notice ; and hence the errors and misconceptions that have so long prevailed on this subject. The experience of the three days of July 1830, which furnished many cases of gun-shot wounds and injuries of bones, contributed to throw light on this mystery. It was then found, that, in some cases, injuries and fractures of the cranium, in other instances, compound fractures of the bones of the extremities, were followed by purulent collections within the liver ; and always almost was it found, that the veins of the fractured and subsequently inflamed bone were inflamed, and contained purulent matter.

The veins of bones, it must be observed, allow this species of suppuration and deposit within the liver more easily than the veins of other tissues; because, being contained within incompressible canals, they do not collapse, and remaining open, they are more likely to become inflamed than the veins of other textures.

Though inflammation and suppuration in the minute veins of bones may be generally requisite, in order to be followed by secondary purulent collections, yet probably it is not requisite that this inflammation extend far up within the venous trunks arising from these minute veins. Even it may happen, that inflammation and suppuration of the inner venous coat may not be requisite ; and that the veins act as the mere carriers from the inflamed tissue.

It has been from a very remote period observed that suppuration within the liver after injuries of the head is a most insidious affection, and takes place with very imperceptible external indications of its presence ; and most probably this is to be ascribed to the circumstance, either that it is a peculiarly chronic and insidious process, or that it consists merely in the successive transport of purulent matter by the veins from the parts suppurating as the matter is formed. The testimony of Pigray, given in the middle of the seventeenth century, is remarkable; and its accuracy has been confirmed by all subsequent observers. "Wounds of the head," he says, " are of great importance, from the variety of symptoms and accidents which follow them, which it is good to foresee and consider. In certain years, almost all these wounds, both small and great, are mortal ; and this may be ascribed to the constitution of the air, of which it is difficult to form a judgment. I remarked one year in which wounds of the head, almost all, were followed by gangrene of two or three fingers' breadth, with little fever; and nevertheless few died. Several others I have seen, in which no manifest accidents followed; and nevertheless there died, namely, of the smallest wounds, principally those in whom fever began the third day after the infliction of the wound; but in almost all those who so died, we found a purulent abscess in the substance of the liver."*

This insidiousness led Bertrandi to observe, that the writers by whom these instances of hepatic suppuration after injuries of the head are recorded, were unaware of the existence of such collections in the liver before the body was inspected.

Without dwelling longer on this subject, I only add, that it is not impossible that in several cases the operation of trepanning itself, by inducing inflammation of the bone, may have been a cause of hepatic suppuration.

5. Instances of purulent collection or collections within the liver, in consequence either of inflammation of the veins of the intestines, or of these veins opening at purulent surfaces, are often observed. Cruveilhier mentions a case in which a man of 60 had a protruded rectum replaced, after repeated and violent attempts, which caused much pain. He speedily became ill, with the usual symptoms indicating disease of the veins, and on the fifth day expired. Several small abscesses, superficial and deep-seated, were found within the liver. In other instances, the puriform collections were formed after operations on the rectum, where the actual cautery was employed; after the operation for the cure of *fistula ani;* and after that for strangulated hernia, in which a portion of irreducible omentum underwent suppuration.

It is not easy to say whether in these instances suppuration within the veins is always necessary ; or whether the veins merely transport the purulent matter to the liver. Inflammation is seldom found to extend far from the spot; and almost never into the interior of the large veins. It is probable that when hepatic abscess takes place after ulceration of the intestinal canal, it is rather to the transporting power of the veins than to their actual inflammation, that this sym-phenomenon is to be ascribed.

Of twenty-nine instances of this conjunction given by Annesley, in twenty-one, or nearly three-fourths, were these ulcers more or

* Epitome des Preceptes de Medecine et Chirurgie. Par Pierre Pigray. A Rouen, 1658. 12mo. Liv. iv. chap. ix. p. 368.

less extensive in the large intestine; and in other two cases the colon was contracted with stricture, showing the presence of dysentery at some former period. Among fifteen fatal cases which fell under the observation of Dr Budd in the Dreadnought, in eight cases there were ulcers in the large intestines; in one case, two ulcers were observed in the stomach; and in two cases the state of the intestines was not observed; so that in nine among thirteen cases hepatic abscess was conjoined with ulcers in the colon or stomach. Among sixteen cases collected by Andral and Louis, in two cases ulcers in the large intestine and lower end of the ileum are noticed; in one case, ulcers were observed in the lower end of the *ileum* only; in four cases, ulcers were seen in the stomach; and in one case, in the gall-bladder. In one of these cases of ulcer of the stomach, the ulcer was caused by the abscess opening into the stomach; and this case may therefore be excluded. With this deduction, however, there are, among fifteen cases, seven in which the existence of abscess of the liver was preceded by ulceration of some part of that extensive mucous membrane, from which the capillary veins arise and proceed to unite in the *vena portae.*

I have already, in page 863, mentioned that, in 1827, I met with a remarkable example of the conjunction of large hepatic abscess, with extensive ulceration of the colon; and in which the formation of the former was so insidious, that its existence was not suspected during life. It appeared to me at this time that some connection between the two phenomena subsists; and that this connection is not accidental. Of this connection I had little doubt, after reading the Memoir of Mr Arnott, already referred to; and if I had, that doubt must have been removed by the facts given in 1833 by Cruveilhier.*

On the other hand, it is agreed, that, in the case of this symphenomenon, in various instances hepatic suppuration precedes the formation of ulcers of the intestinal canal. This, however, merely shows, that the same general causes which produce hepatic abscess, that is, excessive solar heat, terrestrial miasmata, and full living, may be followed by inflammatory processes in two sets of organs much exposed to the hurtful influence of these physical causes.

It must also be observed, that, for aught that is hitherto known, mere inflammation, or even vascular congestion of the mucous membrane of the alimentary, may, considering the direct relation

* Anatomie Pathologique, Livraison xi. pl. 1, 2, 3. Paris, 1833.

of its venous system with that of the liver, give rise, in the latter organ, to irritation, which might readily terminate in suppuration. Physicians in India, where this union is most commonly seen, ascribe the dysenteric disorder to the passage of irritating bile. Were this always the case, then it ought to be expected that the small intestine should be diseased before the large intestine. This, however, is so far from being the case, that most commonly the colon is first diseased; and, in many cases, the colon alone is ulcerated, while the *ileum* remains sound. The bile, if it irritate, must irritate most the membrane which it touches first; and, before it reaches the colon, its irritative properties ought to be abated, if not extinguished. Yet the effects of this irritation are presented in no degree almost by the small intestine, and in a most remarkable degree by the large intestine. From these facts, it seems natural to infer, that whatever be the cause of ulceration in the colon, it is not irritating bile; that the blood sent from the diseased intestinal mucous membrane irritates through the branches of the portal vein the substance of the liver.

§ 3. SPHAKELUS—GANGRENE OF THE LIVER.—Gangrene of the liver is a rare affection; and we must be cautious in admitting, as examples of the lesion, all the instances given by authors. In the majority of cases, from Morgagni downwards, the descriptions are too vague, and merely represent portions of the liver to be in a state of sphakelus. The lesion nevertheless may take place; first, either by gangrene attacking an abscess of the liver, generally with more or less inflammation of the veins; and, secondly, in consequence of, or in connection with, gangrene of some part of the surface, for instance, the toes or the sacrum, and the gangrenous inflammation passing thence, apparently by the veins, either to the liver or the lungs, or to both simultaneously.

In the former case, a large portion or the whole of the walls of an abscess are soft, flaccid, and filamentous, exhaling an offensive odour, while the adjoining portion of liver is also more or less softened, dark coloured, and lacerated. In the latter case, the lesion appears in the form either of one gangrenous abscess, that is, an abscess with soft, ragged, dark brown fetid-smelling walls; or in the shape of several collections, of the same characters, while the neighbouring veins contain fetid purulent matter.

Gangrene of the liver is occasionally associated also with gangrene of the lungs.

The cause of this lesion is not well understood. Are we to believe that it is an affection originally gangrenous? or are we to believe that the gangrenous termination is an effect of inflammation? To me, it appears to be the result rather of inflammation of peculiar intensity, in persons of a certain kind of constitution, than of a gangrenous form of inflammation. The course of phenomena, or rather of the process, seems, in general, in cases of this nature, to be as follows. *First*, inflammatory action or vascular congestion distends and overloads the vessels of the part, and causes interstitial extravasation of blood, of lymph, and of serum ; *secondly*, by this the tenacity, pliancy, and elasticity of the texture are destroyed ; it becomes friable, lacerable, and easily softened ; its physical properties are altered and impaired ; and its vital properties are enfeebled ; *thirdly*, as this action or inaction continues, the texture of the part is still more completely changed from its normal state ; and at length, on any slight increase in the morbid distension, the parts, already deprived, in a great degree, of their vital properties, give way ; vessels are broken open, and expose their contents ; parts lose their cohesion ; and the process of gangrene, which is a mixture of the mechanical with the weak vital, is established.

On the other hand, gangrenous suppuration of the liver may follow the formation of an external gangrenous sore.

In the collection of pathological drawings made by the late Dr Thomson, is an instance in several respects important. A person attempted to destroy himself, first, by cutting his throat, and afterwards by discharging a pistol at his forehead. Death did not ensue immediately. The wound of the throat mortified; and exfoliation from the frontal bone took place. After death, which took place in about ten days, a large abscess, with ragged, dark-coloured, softened walls, was found in the upper part of the right lobe of the liver.*

In this remarkable case, we observe the illustration of two pathological principles, which I have attempted to establish. *First*, the abscess in the liver was evidently secondary, and consecutive either on the wound in the frontal bone, or on that in the throat, most likely the former. The suppurating process in the medullary membrane of the frontal bone, rendered necessary to eject the dead

---

* A Practical Treatise on Diseases of the Liver and Biliary Passages. By William Thomson, M.D., and the private collection of that gentleman.

bone and heal the living one, gave rise to the formation of matter, which was conveyed by the vessels of the bone by the veins to the liver. *Secondly*, as this purulent collection was then forming within the liver, it was struck with sphakelus, most likely in consequence of the previous mortified and sloughing state of the wound in the throat.

It is necessary to distinguish gangrene of the liver from those changes in colour,—blue, black, dark-green, dark-brown, mottled dark-green and brown, which are so common in this organ. These colours are effects of mere death changes. No change in colour, without an evident change in consistence and demolition of structure, can be received as indicating the presence of gangrene.

It has been supposed that hemorrhage may be the cause of gangrene. It seems rather the effect in the majority of cases.

§ 4. MALAKOSIS.—SOFTENING of the Liver has been observed, in certain circumstances, to take place. The substance of the liver is then soft, friable, easily torn and broken down between the fingers; and, in some instances, the change in cohesion is so great, that the hepatic substance resembles softened spleen. ·

Dr Marshall met in Ceylon with instances of softening of the liver without other remarkable change. In other instances the parenchyma was granular, and broke down between the fingers, while the peritoneal coat came away with unusual facility. He mentions one case in which the liver was softened in such a manner in a patient with dysentery, that the pulpy substance resembled hasty pudding. The liver weighed in this case $7\frac{1}{4}$ pounds—more than double the average. In all such cases the softening is the effect of a species of vascular congestion or orgasm.

Of this lesion, Andral distinguishes two varieties,—one indicated by the red colour of the hepatic substance; the other by a pale or whitish colour. In the former, the substance presented the appearance of softened spleen; in the latter, of a species of gray coloured pap, and with little blood in the tissue. In the former case, the softening appeared to be the effect of inflammation of the peritoneum, general and hepatic. In the latter case, it appeared to be the result of lesion of nutrition; as the gall-bladder contained not bile, but colourless and insipid serum. The latter also appears to be more chronic in its progress and duration than the former.*

§ 5. HEPATIC PHLEBITIS.—Inflammation of the veins of the liver is not very frequent; and when abscesses and purulent collections

---

* Case by M. Snetiwy. Oesterreich. Med. Wochenschrift. 1842. N. 32.

are found within the gland, these are the result either of inflammation of the parenchyma or of the transporting property of the veins, which, however, themselves remain unaffected. Inflammation may nevertheless affect veins either spontaneously or from the irritation of foreign bodies.

M. Lambron records the case of a man of 69 who was attacked with squeamishness, sickness, uneasiness in the right hypochondre, and irregular shiverings. In the course of four days, jaundice appeared slightly, and increased in the subsequent three days. At the end of one week, the shiverings, which had not been very distinct, were present in the evening, generally with hiccup, and imitated the rigors of ague. The symptoms continued with great and increasing weakness; and the patient expired on the 25th day from the appearance of well-marked symptoms.

Inspection revealed the following state of parts. The portal vein was filled with wine-lee matter and purulent matter; in the trunk of the superior mesenteric vein a fish-bone, which, implanted in the head of the pancreas, had entered the anterior wall of this vein from before backwards, and was fixed in the posterior wall of the same vein. This bone was about 3 centimetres, or one inch and a little more than a line long; as thick as a stout pin; yellowish, hard, and resisting; and the extremity was twisted like a cork-screw. The cavity of the mesenteric vein was obliterated by slate-gray false membrane. Below this obliteration the divisions of the superior mesenteric were sound, but contained fibrinous clots of blood. The splenic vein was in size, colour, and consistence normal; but it contained a quantity of wine-lee coloured matter; and the same matter was found in the divisions of the portal vein, while its sinus was filled with purulent matter mixed with blood. The liver presented no metastatic abscess; but its tissue at the level of the portal sinus was very much softened. The sub-hepatic veins were sound.*

The same observer gives the case of a man of 48, who had been ill for eight days with debility, slight fever, and was incoherent at admission. Four days after he had violent and distinct rigors; while it was observed that the size of the spleen was palpably enlarged. The rigors underwent temporary abatement; but

---

* Observations d'Inflammation de Veines du Foie. 1mo, de la Veine-Porte produite par une arete de poisson; 2do, des veines sus-hepatiques, due au voisinage d'un abces metastatique. Par Ernest Lambron. Archives Generales. Juin 1842. Tom. lix. p. 129.

without improving the condition of the patient; and in rather more than three weeks they returned, accompanied with delirium, followed by profuse sweatings and diarrhœa. In ten days more death followed, the whole duration of the illness having been about 73 days.

At the pyloric end of the stomach was an ulcerated cancer, which had destroyed the mucous membrane to the extent of more than a shilling. The liver was in size normal, but yellowish, and as if fatty; and part of it was dotted with red points, which were traced to the inter-lobular veins. Disseminated in the hepatic substance were seven or eight purulent collections, which looked like metastatic abscesses. The largest of these was the size of a hen's egg. One of these abscesses was situate near one of the trunks of the sub-hepatic veins, as they enter the *vena cava*, where that vessel is attached to the base of the lobule of Spigelius. This abscess had caused inflammation in the venous trunk, so that the latter showed, at some lines from its opening into the *vena cava*, an ulceration about eight millimetres ($\frac{5}{10}$ of one inch) in diameter, while matter easily flowed from the abscess into the cavity of the vessel. The portion of the vein between the ulceration and the *vena cava* was quite covered with lymph sufficiently thick to protect the interior of the vein from the entrance of the purulent matter. Above the ulceration the vessel was intensely inflamed; and its area was obliterated by lymph and fibrinous clots. The circulation was thus completely interrupted.*

This disease is generally fatal. Yet I have stated in a former part of this work, (p. 127,) that I have met with a case in which the trunk of the portal vein, together with those of the splenic and superior mesenteric veins, were completely filled and obstructed by a solid coagulum of lymph apparently, or lymph with fibrin of blood.

In this case it is probable that the obstruction or closure of the vein in this manner must have arisen from one of two causes; either inflammation within the vein, or pressure externally. If the former were the cause, then the closure was perhaps

* These cases have since been quoted in a German journal, in order to prove that splenic inflammation and enlargement is the primary cause of intermittent fever, not the effect; and in order to accomplish this, the speculator has added to the report of the first case, that the spleen was strongly developed and distinctly circumscribed, and in the second, that its volume was evidently increased.

one means of averting the immediate fatal termination. In this person further, the right lobe of the liver was so much shrunk and diminished, that the whole organ weighed only about one-fourth of its usual amount; while its shape was greatly altered, being rounded and drawn from the sides and circumference to the centre; so that the whole gland was represented by a small shrunk left lobe. The effect of this lesion, which is one species of atrophy, was obstinate and incurable ascites.

§ 6. HEPATORRHAGIA.—I am quite satisfied that occasionally the biliary ducts and the liver pour out blood, which is discharged into the intestinal canal. I have more than once seen in patients large quantities of blood-coloured bile, and even blood discharged in this manner, which I am satisfied came from the biliary ducts and the *pori biliarii*, in which this liquid had been poured out . abundantly. This is a species of hepatic hæmorrhage.

Another variety, however, of hepatic hæmorrhage takes place, one in which blood is poured into the substance of the liver, which is rent and lacerated, much as is the brain in apoplexy. Sir G. Blane gives, in a boy of eight, a case in which, after eight days of illness, ending fatally, several fissures were found in the left lobe of the liver, and much blood was effused within the abdomen.* M. Andral mentions the case of a person who, without any previous complaint or indication of illness, felt one morning on awaking, pains in the abdomen, and accordingly remained in bed. In the course of a few hours he was found dead. The peritoneal cavity was filled with a large quantity of dark-coloured blood partly coagulated; and several clots were found between the diaphragm and the convex surface of the liver. Near the centre of the right lobe, on the convex surface, was an opening of sufficient size to admit the tip of the little finger, and which was the orifice of a cavity in the hepatic substance as large as a pippin, and filled with blood. A large vessel which had been rent opened on a point in this cavity; and this vessel was found to be a branch of the portal vein. The surrounding parenchyma was healthy.†

Dr Honore presented, in 1834, to the Academy a liver, in which were several cavities containing blood. It was uncertain, however, whether this proceeded from torn vessels or was the effect of exhalation.

M. Louis mentions one case in which, along with an abscess,

* Transactions of a Society, Vol. ii. p. 18. London, 1800.
† Medecine Clinique. Partie Vieme. Livre IIieme. Set. I. chap. iii.

3 K

there was in the liver a cavity as large as a nut, containing blood coagulated in concentric layers. No laceration in any of the blood-vessels was recognized.

Instances of this lesion have been given also by Dr Heyfelder and Dr James Abercrombie. In the former case, which took place in a man of 60, the heart was affected with hypertrophy of the right ventricle, and the rent, which was in the right lobe of the liver, communicated with the laceration in the portal vein.* In the latter, which occurred in a lady of 35, who had been several years in India, the liver presented, at its anterior and upper surface, a large sac, containing two pounds of blood. This sac was the peritoneum. The blood had escaped from a branch of the portal vein. The accident occurred in the eighth month of pregnancy. The liver was softened, lacerable, and pulpy.†

The causes of this lesion and its external effects are equally unknown.

In those affected with scurvy, the liver, as other organs, is liable to present effusions of blood, which, in this case, undergoes imperfect coagulation.

§ 7. TRAUMATIC LACERATION AND HEPATORRHAGIA.—In falls from a considerable height, especially on hard ground, and after death by heavy bodies which have passed over the trunk, laceration and hemorrhage of the liver is by no means uncommon. On the 1st of January 1824, three soldiers, in attempting to get out of Edinburgh Castle, mistook their way in the dark, and fell over the perpendicular side of the rock. They were found dead next morning; and in all the liver was lacerated.

Cases of rent either from violence or falls are given by Morgagni and Dr Pearson;‡ and instances of the same accident from the transit of a carriage or waggon over the trunk or abdomen are given by various authors.

In all these cases, hemorrhage to a greater or less extent takes place; and as the blood flows into the cavity of the peritoneum, if life be not immediately or speedily extinguished, the quantity may be estimated by the degree of swelling which takes place, with the dull sound always emitted on percussion, when blood is contained within the abdominal cavity.

* Memoire sur plusieurs Maladies du Foie. Par Dr Heyfelder. Archives Generales, t. li. p. 468. Paris, 1839.

† London Medical Gazette, September, 1844, Vol. xxxiv. p. 507 and p. 792. One case twice given.

‡ Transactions of College of Physicians, vol. iii. art. xxiv. p. 377. London, 1785.

Death is, in these cases, generally immediate, or at most follows in no long time. A young boy of five or six was crossing the street at the South Bridge, about two o'clock in the day. He was knocked down some way by a carriage passing, and one if not both wheels passed over the trunk before the coachman could stop his horses. The boy was taken up immediately and brought to the Infirmary, where I was at the time. He was quite dead; and it was manifest, from the appearance of the abdomen, which was already enlarged, that blood was copiously escaping into its cavity. When the body was examined next day, it was found that the liver had been much crushed, and had not only been rent across the right lobe, but as if broke down. About four or four pounds and a half of blood in clots and fluid were found in the abdominal cavity.

My limits do not, however, allow me to say more of these cases, nor of the important order of wounds of the liver, for information on which I refer to the writings of military surgeons.

§ 8. HYPERTROPHY.—By hypertrophy is meant increase of the liver in size and weight, without any palpable change in structure. The normal weight of the liver varies at different ages, in the two sexes, and according to the size and stature of the individual. In general, in an adult of between 25 and 35 years of age, and of the height of 5 feet 8 inches, the liver will weigh about three lbs., and from two to six ounces imperial weight, or about 53 ounces. In general, it may be stated that the weight of the liver is between the 29th and 30th part of the weight of the whole person.*

---

* Facts and Inferences relative to the Condition of the Vital Organs and Viscera in general, as to their Nutrition in certain Chronic Diseases. By John Clendinning, M. D., &c. Medico-Chirurgical Transactions, vol. xxi. p. 33. London, 1838.

Mr Marshall gives several important facts regarding the weight of the liver in the troops in Ceylon. Of 55 livers belonging to Europeans that died of fever, 25 were deemed sound. The average weight of these livers was 4 pounds 6 ounces. The extremes were 6 pounds and 3 pounds 7 ounces. 27 appeared unusually soft. The average weight of this division was 4 pounds 15 ounces. The largest weighed 6 pounds 8 ounces ; the smallest 3 pounds 13 ounces. Two were found indurated. One weighed 2 pounds 10 ounces ; the other 10 pounds. Mr Marshall states afterwards, that of two examples of indurated liver, in which the gland cut hard and gritty under the knife, and in both of which the liver was rounded or drawn together like a ball, without any of the usual distinctions into lobes, one weighed 3 pounds, the other 4 pounds. [This is *kirrhosis*.] He adds, that " the livers of European soldiers were found to vary in weight from 2½ pounds to 5 pounds, without any satisfactory trace of pre-existing disease."—Notes on the Medical Topography of the Interior of Ceylon. By Henry Marshall, Surgeon to the Forces. London, 1821. P. 141, and 151 and 152.

These numbers are higher, on the whole, than those which we have been accustomed to observe in this country. I have weighed a great number of livers at the Royal

Above this standard the weight of the liver may rise greatly; for instance, to 6, 8, 9, or even 10 pounds; and its volume is proportionally increased. At the same time, the organ is in a high degree vascular, firmer than natural, and cuts hard under the knife. The intimate structure is generally understood not to be impaired, or in any way changed; and in one sense this is correct. The structure resembles, except in increased firmness and greater vascularity, the usual structure of the liver; yet, when examined carefully and closely, the granular tissue of the organ appears more fleshy than in the normal state, and occasionally portions of the liver are harder than the surrounding texture. In certain periods of the disease, which I supposed must be more advanced, the vascularity of the organ appears diminished; at least less blood escapes from incisions.

. The increase in volume which the liver acquires, when enlarged by hypertrophy, may be very considerable, and with its increase in weight, produces great uneasiness and derangement in some of the thoracic and all the abdominal viscera. The gland is enlarged in all its dimensions, and may press up the right side of the diaphragm and right lung, while it prevents the diaphragm from descending freely. It also thrusts upward the tendinous centre and the heart a little. These effects, nevertheless, vary according to the posture of the patient. Thus, in the horizontal position, the hypertrophied liver is decidedly higher up in the right side of the chest than in the erect. In the latter, while its bulk prevents the free descent of the diaphragm, its weight draws that muscle downward. In the abdomen it may come down as low as the crest of the os ilium, while at the same time it extends beyond the median line into the left hypochondriac region, and makes usually a decided bulging prominence in the right hypochondriac and epigastric regions. From the circumstance of the liver lying transversely below the diaphragm, this bulging is generally more marked above than below, the gland being tied closely to the diaphragm by its ligaments.

The hypertrophied liver usually has contracted preternatural adhesions with the neighbouring organs; the stomach; the transverse

Infirmary, and generally found those supposed to be free from disease to be from 3 pounds to 3 pounds 5 or 6 ounces. Very rarely did they ascend to 4 pounds, unless in conjunction with palpable marks of disease. In females, the weight was usually about 2 pounds 10 ounces to 3 pounds. One fatty liver in a young female dead of consumption I found to weigh 8 pounds and 7 or 8 ounces. The low weight of the liver given by Mr Marshall is less astonishing than the high weight within the limits of healthy structure. These weighty livers were probably hypertrophied.

arch of the colon; the duodenum, or the pancreas, or all these at the same time.

Instances of hypertrophy of the liver have been long observed. They were seen by Morgagni, Bianchi, Bang, Stoll, Portal, Foderé, Baillie, Bailly, and all who have observed the morbid changes incident to this gland. The lesion is at present common in different forms and degrees.

Hypertrophy may be the effect of the third variety of inflammation, the acute, congestive, or enlarging. But more commonly it advances slowly and steadily, until the size of the organ and its projection under the right hypochondriac margin and the epigastric region renders the enlargement no longer doubtful. As it advances, it gives rise to effusion of serous fluid within the abdomen.

Hypertrophy, both in moderate and extreme degrees, arises in this country from the intemperate and long continued use of spirits. One of the most marked instances of the disease which have come under my notice, in which the liver projected fully four inches below the margin of the right hypochondre, arose in this manner. When first seen, it was in the early stage, with symptoms of inflammatory and vascular congestion. Under the use of remedies chiefly depleting, the size of the organ was reduced, and the dropsical effusion within the peritoneum disappeared. But when the patient left the hospital, he returned to his previous habits, and in no long time came back, with the liver as large, heavy, and prominent as before. He soon sunk under the disease. The liver was found to weigh upwards of 10 pounds.

Instances of the disease I have seen come from Norfolk, in some parts of which county it is the effect either of ague or the physical causes of that disease. The change has also been observed in all aguish and marshy districts; in Lincolnshire and some parts of Essex in England; in the department of the Maritime Alps, according to Foderé; in the island of Walcheren and many parts of Holland; in the Maremma in Italy; in the marshy and low coasts of the West India Islands; and in various parts of the East Indies. In these situations, hypertrophy of the liver may either follow one or more attacks of ague, most usually quartan ague, or it may be established slowly and steadily without being preceded by any distinct attack of this disease. In these circumstances, it is clear that the hypertrophied state of the gland arises from a previous long continued vascular orgasm or congestion. This congested state of the liver, however, is always preceded and accompanied with a greatly deranged condition of the vascular system of the stomach, *duodenum*, and whole intestinal canal. In this disease the gall-bladder usually contains thin watery bile ; the surface is more or less tinged yellow ; and the intestinal discharges are light coloured. A state of *anaemia* with ascites follows.

§ 9. ATROPHY.—The term Atrophy of the Liver has been applied to more than one state of that organ ; certainly to two at least. The first is a state of diminished size, with contraction, as it were, of the parenchyma in all directions, from the periphery to the sinus of the vessels, and often mostly in the left lobe, sometimes with persistence of its parenchyma, though diminished in volume, sometimes with the disappearance of the red, vascular, or acinoid tissue of the gland, and the substitution of a whitish dense tissue, which is manifestly the cellular substance of the gland. The second consists in diminished volume also of the organ, but with more or less induration; and a granular or tubercular appearance of the liver; in short, one of the forms of kirrhosis. Thirdly, I have mentioned an instance in which the whole gland, but especially the right lobe, was shrunk and contracted to about one-third, or between that and one-fourth of its usual size, in connection with an obstructed state of the portal vein.

It is not easy to say, in the present state of our knowledge, to which of these states the term Atrophy ought to be confined. One point is clear, that the name includes, according to present usage, several morbid states of the liver, which are in all probability different, and proceed from different causes. It is clear that the contracted state of the liver in *kirrhosis* ought not to be regarded as an instance of atrophy, though part of the hepatic tissue in that disease is atrophied. The shrunk and contracted state of the gland in that affection is secondary and consecutive.

That there are cases in which the glandular matter of the liver is diminished or atrophied must be allowed, from such cases as that given by Andral, part v. livr. ii. chap. iii. section ii. obs. 12.

§ 10. MOSCHATISMUS JECORIS.—In certain circumstances, the liver, when divided, presents on the surface of the sections a mottled or party-coloured aspect of brown-coloured spots, set in a lighter coloured basis, so as to resemble the section of the nutmeg. It is very doubtful whether this appearance indicates any change in structure. The dark-coloured spots appear to be merely sections of granules or lobules which have been largely injected with blood, while the light-coloured basis retains its normal colour. This nutmeg aspect of the liver is connected with certain states of the vascular system of the chest and abdomen, in which some impediment is presented to the circulation of the blood. Thus it takes place in various affections of the heart, hypertrophy, valvular contraction, and similar affections, in which the blood of the *vena cava* does not easily return to the heart, and in which consequently the *vena cava hepatica* is inordinately distended. It may also take place in consequence of some morbid states of the abdominal circulation.

§ 11. JECUR GRANULATUM.—JECUR TUBERCULATUM.—KIRRHOSIS.—It has been already mentioned, that, in consequence of inflammatory congestion, the liver is liable to become hardened, and as if tuberculated or granulated. It may be that this is the early stage of the state which is to be described under this head by the name of Granulated Liver, Tuberculated Liver, and to which Laennec applied the epithet of Kirrhosis. To English observers, it was known partly under the name given by Baillie of Tuberculated liver, and more frequently in its exquisite form under the name of hob-nailed liver.

Kirrhosis appears under two forms, one an early, another a more advanced and perfect.

In the early form of the disease the substance of the liver is firm, doughy, yet not irregular. The surface is coloured with patches of yellow, variable in size. The whole organ is in general somewhat enlarged, and usually weighs between four and five pounds or more. When divided it appears of an orange red colour, or between that and orange brown; sometimes with patches of this colour diffused through the natural colour of the gland; and when a slice is immersed in water it soon imparts to the water a green colour, which is repeated after several immersions. Closely examined, the section shows innumerable small bodies like millet seed or grains of barley, of an orange colour, dispersed through its substance. Such livers are vascular in the red granular portion mostly.

This lesion does not usually prove fatal of itself at this stage; but persons occasionally die with the liver in this state, from disease of the heart, granular disease of the kidneys, fever, or disease of the intestinal canal.

In a more advanced stage the surface of the liver presents at various parts small irregular shaped elevations like the heads of vetches or peas, separated by irregular linear furrows. These elevations may not extend over the whole liver, but occupy at first only one part, viz. generally the convex surface. When the peritoneum is stripped, which is always difficult to be done, it is observed that the elevations are the prominent parts of roundish or irregular-shaped bodies about the size of tares or small peas, and some as large as peas. The colour of these bodies is orange-brown or wood-brown, sometimes a shade lighter than the colour of the sound liver. A section of such presents an aggregation of bodies varying in size, affecting a roundish irregular outline, united or separated by whitish fibrous or filamentous lines. The liver in these parts is decidedly firmer and harder than in the last described case. Other parts of the liver are firm, doughy, and generally of the orange-yellow or orange-brown tint.

The liver in this state may not be larger than usual, and if it be, it is only in a slight degree larger.

Sections of this sort of liver, when macerated in water repeatedly changed, continue long to impart a green colour to the liquid.

In the most complete form of the disease the appearance of the liver is the following. The liver is seldom larger than natural. It either retains its normal size, or it is smaller, and apparently shrunk and contracted. The whole surface of the liver presents the appearance of numerous irregularly round bodies, elevated so as to give the organ an irregular tuberculated or knotty look. These eminences are as large as peas or small beans, a few larger. Their colour externally is of that light brown usually designated wood-brown. They are separated by well-marked linear furrows, which seem all continuous, so that the surface of the liver presents a resemblance to a shoe covered with hobnails. This appearance extends over the whole surface of the liver ; but in general it is most distinct and conspicuous on the convex surface.

The shape of the liver is at the same time in general more or less altered. The convex surface is more decidedly convex; the anterior edge is obtuse, thick, and as it were bent downwards ; all the sharp edges are rounded or obtuse ; and in general, by the bending downwards of the right and left margins, and the anterior margin, the lower surface is more concave than in the natural state. The last character, however, may be wanting; and the lower surface either remaining even, though irregularly granulated, or partaking in the general elevation, the whole gland appears thick, but rounded, and contracted apparently towards the sinus of the vessels.

When sections of a liver in this state are made, these sections present the same appearance of irregularly rounded bodies aggregated together, as is seen at the surface. The colour is in general more of the orange-yellow tint, or that combined with wood-brown. These bodies are united by a species of gray filamentous or ligamentous tissue; and both structures become more distinct on immersion in water, and after boiling.

These bodies, though affecting the globular figure, vary much. Many are ovoidal or spheroidal; many are irregularly angular; not a few are elongated with rounded or angular ends; and some look like the small stony fragments set in porphyry, or a small grained breccia.

In size also they vary. Some are, as already stated, as large as good sized garden peas; and this volume they do not often exceed. Others are smaller, of the magnitude of dried peas; others, again, like tares or vetches; and some not larger than millet seed. All are mixed confusedly together without any order.

The peritoneum may be stripped from these bodies; and they then present the appearance of an aggregation of orange-brown or wood-brown looking bodies, all closely united and packed. This close conjunction is evidently the cause of their variation in size and shape; for it is manifest, that if all were round, they could neither touch each other nor be of the same size; whereas, being different in size, the small bodies are interspersed between the large ones; and the shape of all is modified by the contiguous bodies.

In general, I think in the cases examined by me, the bodies at the surface are both larger and more regularly rounded than those in the substance of the liver.

I have several times macerated sections of kirrhotic liver; and I always found that they required a long time, months at least, to part even with a portion of their greenish colouring matter. In several cases I kept slices of granulated liver, for spaces of from 20 to 24 months, in water periodically changed, before attempting to put them in spirits; and even then, in the course of a few weeks, the spirits were completely coloured green, and required to be changed; and the spirit in which the section so prepared was immersed, was again tinged green. This fact shows the tenacity with which the colouring matter adheres to these granules.

This green colouring matter is precipitated by the addition of hydrochloric acid. A fatty matter is taken up by ether.

From the prominent characters now described, Morgagni applies to this state of the change the name of *jecur granulatum;* Baillie terms it tuberculated liver; many physicians, both in this country and abroad, term it granulated liver; and Laennec applied to it the name of *kirrhosis*, or yellow degeneration of the liver, from the colour which the liver so changed often presents.

Besides the forms now described, the disease in certain instances appears in the form of yellow matter dispersed through the substance of the liver like peas; or presents an appearance similar to the vitellarium of the common fowl.

In some instances small empty cavities are found in the interior of the granulated liver; and in others are small cavities containing a greenish jelly-like liquid of little consistence. This, which appears to have been observed by Portal, is made the ground of another stage of the disease more advanced than the one last mentioned. The distinction I think entirely useless, as the state mentioned is found, though not very often, in the state already described as the third stage.

Laennec, who considered this yellow matter a new formation, characteristic of the lesion, admitted three forms of *kirrhosis*; one in masses, a second in patches, and a third in cysts. This idea of the separate new morbid formation has not been generally recognized; and it is probable that these distinctions, which apply rather to the external form than the essential character of the lesion, are fanciful.

A liver in the exquisite and perfect form of granulation presents in its substance appearances so characteristic, that, though not easily described, they have attracted general attention. The orange-coloured matter has been sometimes described as like sole-leather, when attempted to be cut by the knife; and in other instances the section has been compared to impure bees wax. Both of these statements are either inaccurate or exaggerations. The granulated liver is certainly not so tough and inflexible as sole leather; neither does it present the hard yet friable property of yellow bees wax. It resembles a solid, close, dense, fleshy mass, consisting apparently of numerous small bodies irregularly aggregated together, which, when closely inspected, are of an orange or orange-brown colour.

This disease tends certainly and invariably to the formation of incurable abdominal dropsy. At first the liver is larger than usual; but afterwards it returns to its normal size, though not to the normal shape, or it becomes smaller and shrunk, as already described.   I have seen three persons among about 32 cases die with intestinal hemorrhage.   Becquerel observed this five times in 42 cases.

It is not uncommon for the granulated liver to be affected with superficial or peritoneal inflammation, and thus to contract adhesions to adjoining parts.   In two cases I found the convex surface adhering extensively by false membrane to the diaphragm.   This might have taken place previous to the granular transformation. I have seen the liver also adhering in this state to the stomach, and to the duodenum.

Sometimes the gall-bladder is found thickened, and adhering preternaturally to adjoining parts.

The capsule of Glisson is usually thickened, and appears to have been the seat of chronic inflammation.

The state of the bile varies.   In some cases it appears not perceptibly changed.   In others it is dark-coloured, viscid, ropy.   In a few it is liquid, light-coloured, and manifestly serous.   In these states there appears to be nothing regular.

ATTENDANT LESIONS.—*Kirrhosis* may take place alone, that is, without lesion of other organs, or at most with a morbid state of the alimentary canal and its mucous membrane.   But it is more common for it to be conjoined with lesions of other organs.   The most common morbid accompaniment in this country is granular disease of the kidney ; and I have seen a great number of instances in which the latter lesion was conjoined with *kirrhosis* either in the early or in the advanced stage.   Becquerel, who has studied the lesion particularly in this view, found among 42 cases only 7 which could be said to be simple or unconnected with lesion of other organs.   Among these were 19 in which the granulated state of the liver was complicated or associated with the granular state of the kidney; in 21 kirrhosis was complicated with disease of the heart in different stages, and in two with *pericarditis.*   The most usual cardiac lesion was hypertrophy of the left chambers ; hypertrophy of the right chambers; and changes in the valves of the left chambers in the order now observed.   In 9 cases he found pulmonary emphysema ; and in one case pulmonary tubercles.

In this country the disease is not so frequently associated with well-marked disease of the heart; but in almost all the cases which I have examined, there were traces of chronic bronchitis and emphysema.

Though abdominal dropsy is the constant and invariable effect of this lesion, so much so, that in every case of abdominal dropsy which is unattended by manifest enlargement of the liver, it may be inferred that this gland is in the granulated state, yet the disease may be followed or associated with other lesions which precede the fatal event. Thus it may cause chronic peritonitis; pleurisy, especially the chronic form; less frequently pericardial inflammation; pneumonia occasionally; pulmonary apoplexy; and if not, expectoration tinged with blood.

From the observations of Dr Eichholtz of Konigsberg, I infer that the conjunction of granulated liver with granular kidney is also frequent in Germany.*

The nature and cause of this degeneration has given rise to much inquiry and considerable difference of opinion. We have seen that Laennec imagined that it consisted in the formation of a new morbid product, which was infiltrated into the substance of the liver, which was liable to be formed in the same manner in the parenchyma of other organs, and which appearing at first in an incipient or nascent state, proceeded eventually to softening. It was further the idea of Laennec, that as the kirrhotic bodies were developed, the substance of the liver disappeared and was absorbed.

The correctness of this idea was first questioned by M. Boulland, who denies the fact of a new formation, and maintains that *kirrhosis* consists in what he calls a dissociation of the elements of the liver, viz. the glandular yellow portion and the red vascular portion. In the early stage, he conceives that the vascular network is enlarged and much loaded with blood. In the second stage, this vascular network, which is interposed between the granules of the yellow portion, becomes impermeable, but large; it assumes a colour varying from gray rose to pale green, and allows turbid serum to escape. This idea implies that the granulated state of the liver is owing to congestion.†

Andral ascribes kirrhosis to hypertrophy of the yellow or granular matter of the liver, while the red or vascular matter remains either the same, or may be changed in colour to an olive-green,

* Ueber die Granulirte Leber und Niere, und ihr Verhältnis zur Tuberculösen und Krebsigen Dyscrasie. Von Dr H. Eichholtz zu Konigsberg. Muller's Archiv fur Anatomie und Physiologie. Jahrgang, 1845. Berlin. Seite 320.

† Memoires de la Societe Medicale d'Emulation. Tome ix.

with increase or diminution in its volume; the latter being the cause of the shrivelling.*

Cruveilhier, as well as Andral, denies the formation of a new substance; and considering the appearance and relation of the minute bodies constituting this change, he infers that they are part of the *acini* or glandular granules of the liver in a state of hypertrophy, while, in consequence of these hypertrophied granules, the others are atrophied or wasted.†

In 1837, Dr Carsewell brought forward, on the nature and formation of this disease, an hypothesis which has had in several points several followers. Rejecting the idea of Laennec, that *kirrhosis* depends on the formation of a new tissue, Dr Carsewell regards the change as consisting in atrophy of the lobular, that is the glandular structure of the organ, produced by the presence of a contractile fibrous tissue formed in the capsule of Glisson. ‡ This idea has been more or less decidedly adopted by Mr O'Ferrall, Mr R. W. Smyth,§ and some others; while part of the hypothesis, that relating to the induration of the substance of the capsule of Glisson, corresponds with an hypothesis presently to be mentioned.

In 1839, Dr Hallmann of Berlin announced formally in his dissertation an hypothesis which had been in various modes and quarters occasionally produced. This is, 1st, that in kirrhosis, hypertrophy of the cellular or ligamentous tissue of the liver takes

* Clinique Médicale, Partie Vieme, Liv. IIieme, Section I. Chapitre III. Paris, 1834.

The ideas of M. Andral regarding the granular liver are founded on his notions of its natural anatomical structure. This is perfectly correct were these notions well founded. But either these are not accurate, or they do not accord with the idea of the majority of anatomical observers. He states that in the liver two substances exist naturally, so arranged as to represent the form of a sponge. One more or less white represents the solid part of the sponge, contains large vessels which traverse without ramifying in it, and consequently contains little blood. The other is a red substance, extremely vascular, in appearance cavernous, and is deposited in the *areolæ* of this white substance.

The white substance of which M. Andral here speaks appears to be the interlobular and intergranular cellular tissue. The red substance is indeed vascular, and is contained in its *areolæ;* but besides this, there is an orange or yellow substance, which is the granular or acinoid, and which consists of the ends of gall-ducts throughout the whole gland.

† Anatomie Pathologique, Livraison xii. Paris, 1837.

‡ Illustrations of the Elementary Forms of Disease. By Robert Carsewell, M. D. London. Folio. 1838. Atrophy 2, Plate ii.

§ Dublin Journal, Volume xxv. p. 521_524. Dublin, 1844.

place; 2d, that in this hypertrophy of the hepatic cellular tissue consists the essential character of the pathological change called kirrhosis. These propositions he maintains that he proved, by showing microscopically the increased quantity of cellular tissue which the kirrhotic liver presents; and chemically, by the quantity of gelatin which he obtained by boiling from the kirrhotic liver, and which is to that of the sound liver, by taking like weights, as five to one. He obtained from three ounces of kirrhotic liver 66 grains of dry gelatin, and from the same quantity of healthy liver only 13 grains.

Dr Hallmann further observes that the yellow bodies (granulations, kirrhotic nodules) consist partly of cells filled with more or fewer fat globules, and thereby often expanded beyond their proper volume, and partly of large free fat globules. Their medium diameter is about 106 thousandth parts of one Paris inch. The fat may be forced from them by pressure; but seldom do they show a distinct nucleus. By maceration in solution of caustic alkali, the fat is dissolved. The accumulation of fat within and without the cells is not peculiar to the kirrhotic liver, but is observed in the drunkard's liver, and occasionally in livers reputed sound. The basement tissue which surrounds the yellow granules, consists partly of closely compressed cells, partly of thin compact fibres, which are much more abundant here than in the sound liver. From the several facts now specified, he concludes that the toughness and hardness of the granular liver proceeds from an augmentation of the cellular tissue of the capsule of Glisson, caused by chronic inflammation.*

Imperfect as this hypothesis is, it is supported by Muller of Berlin, who closes some interesting observations on the structure of the liver with the following remarks. "According to my observations, kirrhosis consists principally in hypertrophy of the interlobular ligamentous tissue, at the expense of the glandular or lobular substance of the liver, by which individual lobules and separate masses of lobules are removed and as if extruded from the others in a striking manner. In a remarkable specimen of kirrhosis in the Anatomical Museum, this is so palpable, that it may be seen in the section of the liver by the naked eye. I con-

* Bemerkung uber die Lebercirrhose von Dr E. Hallmann. A Berlin. Muller's Archiv fur Anatomie, Physiologie, un Wissenchaftliche Medicin. Jahrgang. 1843. Berlin. 475.

jecture that kirrhosis depends on local dissimilar hypertrophy of the interlobular or interacinous connecting tissue."*

I mention the hypothesis of Muller in this place, because, though not published till 1843, it appears that it had been taught by the author previously.

Meanwhile Becquerel adduced in April 1840, a view which has always appeared to me more consonant with the facts, and which, in truth, I had myself maintained before the appearance of the essay of that author.

Becquerel maintains that in kirrhosis the only tissue primarily affected is the yellow substance of the liver; that this yellow substance, which he should have called the glandular tissue, is infiltrated with plastic or albumino-fibrous yellow matter, quite similar to the false membranes of the serous tissues; that from this results hypertrophy of the yellow substance of the liver; and that from this hypertrophy arises at first compression, and subsequently atrophy of the greatest part of the red or interlobular substance. He further thinks, that, though it is difficult to speak positively on the cause of the infiltration of this yellow matter in the glandular tissue of the liver, yet most probably it is the result of repeated vascular congestions.†

It is impossible to doubt that this makes the nearest approach to the correct explanation of the phenomena; and as it is that which I have for several years been in the habit of teaching in demonstrations and lectures,‡ I do not hesitate to add a few words in further explanation.

It has been formerly shown, that the hepatic substance consists of three separate elementary tissues; a red, or vascular; an orange or glandular; and a gray or filamentous.

The vascular tissue consists of the capillary or minute vessels of the hepatic artery, portal vein, and the origins of the hepatic veins. This constitutes, in the healthy liver, and especially in early life, the largest proportion of the gland.

Disseminated through this capillary network, which forms the

---

* Uber den Bau der Leber. Anmerkung zur Vorstehenden Abhandlung von Herausgeber. Archiv fur Anatomie. Jahrgang. 1843. Berlin. P. 343.

† Recherches Anatomico-Pathologiques sur la Cirrhose du Foie. Par Alfred Becquerel. Archives Generales de Medecine. Tome lii. Avril 1840. P. 398 et 407.

‡ Report on the Cases treated during the Course of Clinical Lectures delivered at the Royal Infirmary in Session 1832-1833. By David Craigie, M. D. F. R. S. E. &c. Edinburgh Medical and Surgical Journal, Vol. xli. p. 112—118. Edinburgh, 1834.

basis of the gland, is the second tissue, generally of an orange colour, in the form of minute granules or atoms, which consist of the
terminal ends of biliary ducts, or what have been named *acini*. It
is not easy to say whether single acini, or groups and clusters of
acini, thus form these orange-coloured interposed granules. The
question is of little moment. The main fact, which it is important
to know and remember, is that this orange-coloured matter is surrounded by or enclosed in the vascular network, as it were; that
it is the proper granular or secreting part of the liver; and that it
is formed by the superior or terminal ends of the biliary *pori*. This
matter is much less abundant, and occupies much less space of the
gland, though disseminated through its entire substance.

The third substance is white or gray, and consists of filamentous
tissue, which encloses the vessels on the one hand, and the bile-
ducts on the other, throughout the whole gland, connecting all together in one body. This is supposed by some to be a prolongation or process from the capsule of Glisson, and thence to be continued along the vessels through the parenchyma of the gland.
There is no doubt that this hepatic cellular tissue is connected with
the capsule of Glisson, and may be traced from it; but it is of little
moment whether we admit that it is a prolongation of that capsule
or not. This third substance is easily known by the gray or whitish intersecting lines which it forms all through the liver.

Now, of the three elementary tissues thus constituting the liver,
it is the second, viz. the orange-coloured granular substance, which
is primarily affected in kirrhosis. This affection consists in enlargement and induration of the granular bodies, until they attain
the size, shape, and general appearance of kirrhotic granulations
or nodules; in short, are hypertrophied. That this is the fact, I
conceive is proved, first by their appearance in complete states of
kirrhosis; and, secondly, by the other phenomena which have been
mentioned in the general description. The appearance of granulations of different sizes, from pin-heads up to the volume of peas
or hazel-nuts, can be produced only by the growth and enlargement of the original granular bodies of the liver. These bodies
are of different sizes, because necessarily the morbid process commences in some granules, before others are affected; and those in
which it first commences, must be, and are largest. Secondly, these
bodies contain the colouring matter and fatty matter of the bile,
indeed the parts that cannot escape by filtration; and this circum-

stance alone is sufficient to show that the glandular or granular portion of the liver is the part affected by kirrhosis.

It must not be forgotten therefore, that though the hypertrophy affects the whole of the granular or orange-matter of the liver, it affects it unequally; some being more, others less affected.

As to the exact change induced in these bodies, it is most probable that the bile-tubes are first contracted, and eventually obliterated by adhesive inflammation; for little genuine bile ever reaches the hepatic ducts, in the established form of the disease; and in all the largest tubercles, it is reasonable to think that the ducts are either much contracted or completely closed.

The red or vascular portion of the gland is, at the same time, atrophied; and its waste or diminution appears in some instances to proceed to a very great extreme. Baillie observed that the granulated liver contains little blood; a fact which is confirmed by daily observation. The granulated liver cannot be injected to any extent. The small vessels are obliterated evidently by the pressure of the granulated bodies on them.

It is, therefore, not hypertrophy of one set of granules, and atrophy of another, as imagined by Cruveilhier, that is the essential circumstance in kirrhosis, but hypertrophy of the whole of the orange-coloured tissue, and atrophy of the vascular portion.

The reason why it has appeared to many that the granular part could not be hypertrophied, when the whole liver was actually smaller, is the circumstance, that they overlook the anatomical fact, that, in the sound state, the granular portion of the liver makes but a small proportion of the gland, while the vascular portion forms the most considerable; whereas, when hypertrophied as in kirrhosis, the granular portion constitutes almost the whole.

Along with these changes, the interlobular, cellular, or filamentous tissue is hardened, apparently by inflammatory adhesion. This has been assumed to be the cause of the other changes; but it is manifestly merely a concomitant effect. It is always most remarkable in the concave portion of the liver, and much less so in the convex. Conversely the granular degeneration is usually most complete and furthest advanced at the convex surface of the liver, and least so in the neighbourhood of the capsule of Glisson and the sinus.

The remote causes of kirrhosis are not very accurately known; and all the information which has been given on this subject is rather conjectural than positive. During the years 1817 and 1818, when my attention was first directed to the granular or tuberculated liver, I inspected a considerable number of cases, several of the subjects of which I had opportunities of seeing during life. A good proportion of these cases, at least two-thirds, occurred in persons who had been as soldiers in the expedition to Walcheren; and after becoming acquainted with this fact, I inferred that it is one of the states of liver disease induced by miasmatic poison. Subsequent observation, however, satisfied me that this conclusion is too limited. I afterwards met with instances of granular liver in all its stages in persons who had not been in aguish districts. Between 1831 and 1845, I saw cases of the disease arising apparently under every variety of different circumstances; residence in cold countries, residence in hot and tropical climates, in persons who had never been out of Great Britain. At the same time, while a considerable proportion of cases was found in the persons of Irish who had migrated to Scotland, it was not always ascertained that these persons had been in the bog districts of Ireland. The cause which seems most usually and generally to be followed by the development of this degeneration is the habitual use of spirits; and to this cause, both in London and in Edinburgh, great numbers of granulated liver may be traced.

While the influence of this agent is admitted by Becquerel, he adds various other circumstances; gloomy and distressing mental emotions, bad and innutritious food, and residence in damp situations and dwellings.

The influence of sex and age it is not easy to determine. Among 18 cases of simple kirrhosis, Becquerel found 12 to be in males and 6 in females. Among 45 cases of complicated kirrhosis, 28 were in males and 17 in females. Among the cases seen by myself in 1817 and 1818, all occurred in males. Among those seen afterwards, 3 among females were observed to 5 among males.

Among 18 cases noted by Becquerel, 7 took place between the ages of 30 and 40, and 5 between 50 and 60. Among those in which the age was noted by myself, two cases took place in young females of 20, two in females between 35 and 40, one in a man of 35, and other three in men between 35 and 50. The disease, therefore, seems to be most prevalent between 30 and 50, or 30 and 45.

As to exciting pathological causes, Becquerel maintains that disease of the heart is a frequent antecedent, and must be considered as a cause of granular degeneration of the liver. This inference he adopts, because he found 21 instances of kirrhosis among a series of 55 instances of disease of the heart. Granulated liver is doubtless found often associated with disease of the heart; but often also the latter disease is without the former, while the nutmeg state of the liver is present. Again, it is not doubtful that kirrhosis is often associated with vascular congestion and irritation of the stomach, duodenum, and jejunum; and it is almost certain, that the mode in which the habitual use of spirituous drinks operates in causing kirrhosis, is partly owing to this irritation, partly to absorption into the abdominal venous system.

When kirrhosis is associated with renal granulation, it seems less reasonable to ascribe the one of these affections to the presence of the other, than to ascribe both to the same cause. They also appear to be similar forms of degeneration of the glandular tissue in different glands.

It is not doubtful that kirrhosis is quite adequate of itself to cause death. It must nevertheless be allowed, that it is often found associated with other lesions which are usually fatal; for instance, chronic bronchitis, hypertrophy and valvular disease of the heart, and disease of the kidney, occasionally continued fever, and, in a few instances, pulmonary consumption. When fatal without these diseases, it is invariably found terminating in incurable ascites.

It could not be expected that so great a change in the structure of the liver should be without effects on the health and general system. Yet, in the early stage, it rarely produces conspicuous symptoms. Kirrhosis is, indeed, an insidious disease, causing little disturbance until the liver is altogether changed in structure. The liver is seldom so much enlarged in the early stage as to give rise to manifest and palpable swelling; and there is at this time also little or no serous fluid within the abdomen. Pain is not felt, at least not mentioned by patients; and all that can be observed is a feeble and irregular state of the digestive function, denoted by want of appetite, thirst, constipation, a sense of heat at times in the palms of the hands, and general feebleness and languor. Nutrition is manifestly impaired. As the disease advances the liver is enlarged, and continues so for some time. Then it is diminished; and no tumour may be felt in the hypochondriac region.

Bile is evidently not secreted; for the motions are usually paler than in their normal state. Yet jaundice is an occurrence so rare that I have never seen it in a distinct and well-marked form. All that is observed is a peculiar dingy brownish or sallow colour of the face and skin generally, which is so characteristic, that, though not strongly marked, if once or twice seen, it can rarely be mistaken. It has often appeared to me also, that the perspiration of patients with this disease has a peculiar odour. All perspire during the night or towards morning with a peculiar unctuous discharge. The urine contains no bile; but it is scanty, deep-coloured, contains a large proportion of urea, and deposits a sediment of urate of ammonia.

At length fluid is accumulated within the abdomen; and the strength is still more completely impaired.

Death occasionally takes place by coma, the bile not being climinated, and acting as a poison.

Kirrhosis may be complicated with abscess of the liver.[*]

§ 12. STEATOSIS. PIMELOSIS. FATTY DEGENERATION.—Though the liver even in the human body, in its healthy state, contains in its cells some oily matter, which may be obtained from it by various means, yet in ordinary circumstances this is so small, that it has been generally overlooked.

On the other hand this element, if element it be, is liable to be augmented to so great an extent, that it is infiltrated interstitially into the *acini* and around them, and constitutes a peculiar morbid state, to which the name of fatty liver has been applied.

A liver in this state is very generally larger and heavier than in the healthy state, sometimes amounting to double the weight, or 7, 8, or 9 pounds. It may, nevertheless, be not above 4½ or 5 pounds. When large, it may be felt during life in the form of a large, prominent, but smooth tumour, under the margin of the right hypochondre, which it raises, filling the epigastric region, which is rendered prominent and full, and extending somewhat into the left hypochondriac region. All over this space the tumour emits a dull sound on percussion, but feels not unusually hard.

The fatty liver generally covers the stomach and transverse arch of the colon, and descending about three inches below the margin of the hypochondre, and spreading beyond the median line, appears prominent and conspicuous, concealing all the viscera in the epigastric region. The enlargement usually affects the whole gland.

A liver in this state, when first exposed, is of a pale orange, or reddish yellow colour, or yellowish marbled, some parts being deeper and others lighter coloured. These colours are dispersed in patches, various in size, over the liver. The surface is smooth,

---

[*] Case by Dr H. Beer in Oesterreichische Mediz. Wochenschrift. 1843. N. 22.

and something doughy, or compressible-inelastic to feeling; less solid and dense than the natural liver. When divided, the sections are yellowish red, or with the tint of the fat of old oxen mixed with the red colour of the liver. In advanced stages, the colour is still more highly yellow, approaching to gold yellow. The substance is soft, doughy, and sometimes lacerable. These sections leave on the knife a distinct dirty, greasy mark; and even paper applied over the cut surface receives an oily stain, while fresh particles of dirty grease ooze from the surface.

This fatty matter is deposited or infiltrated partly within the *acini* and granules, partly at their exterior; while the *acini* in the advanced stage of the disease, though present, are compressed. Under the microscope, a bit of yellow or orange-coloured fatty liver appears, according to Albers, like a pale-white sponge, which contains individual bladders of clearer colour with viscid fluid, and there are dispersed in various points remote from each other individual dark-brown *punctula*. These he regards as the atrophied acini of the liver. In the portions of the liver retaining their reddish-shaded colour, these *acini* are large, and more in the normal state, while the morbid intermediate tissue is neither so yellow nor so abundant. From this circumstance he infers that the intermediate or cellular tissue is over-nourished and enlarged, or hypertrophied; and that by this hypertrophy of the cellular tissue the *acini* are atrophied.

The fatty state of the liver is said to be commonly confined to that gland alone; while all the other parts of the system are atrophied. It is observed most usually in pulmonary consumption; and has been by some supposed to denote the most advanced stage of this disease. This inference must nevertheless be regarded as erroneous; since, on the one hand, in many cases of advanced consumption, it is not observed; and, on the other, the adipescent liver is observed in persons who have not died of consumption.

Analysis shows that the adipescent liver contains matter which is something a little different from pure animal fat. Andral found that it was almost entirely cholesterine; and, according to Vauquelin, in 100 parts, 45 consist of oil, 19 of parenchyma, and 36 of water.

The size and weight which the adipescent liver may acquire varies from five to eight or nine pounds. In one remarkable case, in which I recognized the disease during life in a young female labouring under consumption, the liver descended fully three inches below the margin of the right hypochondre, approaching close on the crest of the *os ileum*, extended into the epigastric region, which it might be said to fill, and a little into the left hypochondriac region. Its weight was nearly eight pounds.

On the pathological causes of this transformation, nothing is certainly known. Pathological speculations have appealed to the fattened liver of the goose, to show that it is produced by overfeeding and too little corporeal exertion; and unquestionably this may give rise to the transformation. But the change has been observed in the bodies of persons who, if well fed, have not been underworked. Again, it is seen in those who are corpulent, and who are addicted to the use of nutritious food and spirituous and fermented liquors. Its occurrence in consumption is supposed to depend on the obstructed state of the circulation through the lungs, on the diminished power of decarbonization thus induced, and on the greater quantity of blood believed to be sent to the liver, and the greater amount of duty thrown upon that organ.

The liver in its sound state is said always in the adult to show that its acini contain oil and fat globules, which are further said to be most abundant in those who use fat and oleaginous articles of food. It is possible that this may be one of the sources of the adipose infiltration. Another is more evident. The bile certainly is liable by some means to have its elements converted into cholesterine; and it is reasonable to suppose, that, in the transition to this decomposition, its elements may be converted into fat.

Another illustration of this subject I add from comparative anatomy. The livers of all the finny tribes abound in oil to so great extent, that it is one of the products of spontaneous decomposition. It is most likely that the separation and deposition of oil in this organ is connected with the mode of respiration presented by this class. Gills are evidently less favourable to the elimination of much carbonaceous matter than lungs; and while a small part of the carbonaceous matter is separated by the gills, part may also, in union with hydrogen, be separated by the liver.

As this disease is generally associated with others, as pulmonary consumption, its external effects are not well known. Various symptoms indicative of indigestion are said to denote its first formation. But as upon these no reliance can be placed, I do not mention them. It is known in its advanced stage by the swelling

6

in the right hypochondriac and epigastric region, which is uniform, smooth, and emits a dull sound on percussion, while pain is often considerable in the epigastric region.*

§ 13. CONCRETIONS IN THE DUCTS.—Under certain circumstances the ducts of the liver are filled more or less completely with concretions, which appear to be either bile, or that product in a state passing to the formation of biliary concretions. Concretions may be formed in any part of the course of the secreting and excreting apparatus of the liver; 1st, in the upper or terminal ends of the *pori* or small ducts; 2d, in the middle sized ducts which form the hepatic duct; 3d, in the hepatic duct; 4th, in the gall-bladder; 5th, in the cystic duct; and, 6th, in the common duct.

In the first-mentioned situation, these concretions are, so far as is known, less common than in the others. Cruveilhier gives a very good instance of them in the fourth plate, book xii. of his collection.† These concretions appear under the aspect of grains of a deep green colour, irregular in shape and size, disseminated through the sound structure of the gland, the yellow colour of which forms a strong contrast with that of the grass-green colour of these bodies. No information is given as to the chemical nature of these bodies; but from their colour, it may be inferred that they are nearly pure bile. The glandular substance of the liver appears of a deeper yellow colour than natural ; a condition probably to be ascribed to the obstruction in the ducts preventing the bile from descending.

In some livers, especially in those of children, tubercular bodies are occasionally found disseminated in minute grains through the substance of the liver. These grains are deposited in the terminal portions of the ducts ; and it is the opinion of Cruveilhier that they are the result of the formation now mentioned, namely, biliary concretions. The ducts in which these bodies are thus formed are usually dilated into cysts; while the ducts below these dilated portions may be entirely obliterated. It seems not unlikely that this obliteration of these ducts may have been caused by inflammation at some previous period, and that this obliteration may thus

---

* Einiges zur Pathologie und Pathologischen Anatomie der Leber. Von J. F. H. Albers, Professor der Medizin in Bonn. Rust's Magazin fur die Gesammte Heilkunde, 53 Band, 3 Heft, Seite 511. Berlin, 1839.

† Anatomie Pathologique, Livraison xii. Planch 4. Paris, 1828-1833.

be the cause of the formation of the concretions and the cysts in which they are inclosed.

§ 14. AKINOPYESIS. SUPPURATION OF THE ACINI.—These terminal ends are nevertheless subject to inflammation, so as to form an immense number of minute abscesses in the substance of the liver. Cruveilhier gives an instance in a female of 45, who had jaundice with febrile symptoms for 10 days previous to admission to hospital. The symptoms proceeded, notwithstanding the use of remedies ; and at the end of 55 days she died, that is, 65 days after the appearance of the jaundice.

It was then found, besides two pounds of greenish serum in the abdominal cavity, that the liver, though natural in size, was of an olive colour, and adhered intimately to the diaphragm, the duodenum, and the transverse arch of the colon ; that the whole surface of the liver presented a yellowish-white marbling ; that the lower surface presented two small abscesses, which were on the point of bursting into the peritoneal cavity ; and that the substance of the gland, when divided by the knife, brought into view numerous small abscesses, containing purulent mucus thickened, orange-yellow, deep-green, and greenish. These small abscesses had no determinate shape. Some were formed by an enlarged biliary terminal duct ; others by a duct dilated and perforated ; others by several dilated and perforated terminal ducts, communicating mutually so as to form multilocular abscesses. The adjoining substance of the liver was, he states, not sensibly inflamed. Yet these abscesses were in thousands, not throughout uniformly, but mostly in the right lobe of the liver.

The *ductus choledochus*, narrow at its duodenal end, was dilated immediately above, and contained a concretion which imperfectly filled its cavity ; and at this point a slough in the walls of the duct had been formed.

This appears to be an example of inflammation of the terminal ends of the biliary ducts, confined mostly to these bodies, and not extending beyond them. The inflammation Cruveilhier ascribes to irritation, partly from distension of the ducts by the bile not permitted to descend ; and which, there detained, is liable to form miliary hepatic concretions.*

§ 15. ENTOZOA.—a. Parasitical animals have been observed in the liver by many anatomists. In the livers of the lower animals,

---

* Anatomie Pathologique, Livraison xl. Plate 1. 1839.

these entozoa are very frequent; and the fluke, (*Distoma hepaticum*,) especially, is seen often in the bile ducts of the liver. This is a broad, flat, lancet-shaped animal, from one to four lines long, and half a line to one line broad, which generally is found within the hepatic ducts and their branches. This animal has been found in the liver of the ox, the pig, the hare, and in that of man. In the last, however, it is greatly more rare. It was seen by Malpighi, Bauhin, Wepfer, Pallas, Chabert, Bucholz, and Brera.

The presence of these animals causes some enlargement of the hepatic tubes, and consequent irregularity on the surface of the liver. In the lower animals, the walls of the tubes become ossified, and after some time the parasites die.

b. The hydatid, (*acephalocystis*), is by far the most common parasite in the human liver; and while numerous instances of it are recorded, it is of no unfrequent occurrence. The liver, also, is the most common locality of these animals in the human body.

Of the acephalocyst there are two sorts or species; one the manifold acephalocyst, (*acephalocystis socialis ;*) the other the solitary, (*acephalocystis eremita vel solitaria.*)

In the former case numbers of hydatids are found in one or more cysts in the liver. In the latter in general only one or two large hydatids are found.

The acephalocyst appears in the shape of a globular or roundish bladder, or a ,cubical shaped bladder with truncated and rounded corners.

In the manifold or social hydatid, the figure is in general round or globular; but by pressure on each other the figure is often irregular. One large hydatid globule may contain twenty or thirty small-sized hydatids; or fifty or sixty hydatids of the diameter of half an inch or three quarters may be contained within one large cyst.

In size hydatids vary from the volume of a hempseed to that of an orange, or even larger. In the liver their most usual size is that of a middle-sized gooseberry; but of course this must depend on the length of time elapsed from their original development.

These bodies, whether large or small, consist of a thin, semitransparent, or transparent, homogeneous membrane, in which, by the naked eye, it is not possible to trace either fibrillar or vascular arrangement, and which, externally, is smooth and uniform. Internally there are often eminences or inequalities, to which, in all probability, the small hydatids are or were attached. As it is not possible in these spherical bladders to recognize either head or tail, it is from this circumstance that Laennec applied to them the name of acephalocyst.

Of the internal eminences some are irregular, white, more or less extended in surface ; others are spherical, white, opaque, united in greater or smaller number, and showing the transparence of the enveloping cyst in their intervals. The smallest of these bodies have no cavity. The largest have a small cavity, which enlarges as the granulation itself increases. In other instances these granulations are not opaque, but colourless and transparent, like the walls of the acephalocyst itself. Lastly, there are some in which colourless granules present not rounded but varied forms; some elongated, others cuboidal, others flattened. The largest, which approach the globular figure, when punctured, discharge a little serous fluid.

These bodies, indeed, are the prolific gemmules by which the ani-. mals are propagated. The cyst appears to be a general envelope.

The cavity of the acephalocyst as seen in the liver is filled by a liquid, most commonly quite limpid, and which has all the properties of pure or slightly albuminous water.

The acephalocyst, it has been stated, contains others within it. In general one large acephalocyst contains many of smaller size. These again contain others still smaller ; and it has been inferred that in this succession they may proceed to a great extent. This arrangement is probably the strongest proof of their living character; for it appears to show that one hydatid may produce many.

Of the animal nature of these bodies, the best authorities entertain little doubt.*

---

* Neither Rudolphi nor Bremser appear willing to admit as a distinct species of hydatid the cysts described as the acephalocyst. That distinction was first made by Laennec in 1805 and 1814, and afterwards illustrated by Lüdersen and H. Cloquet, and adopted by most of the French authors. Laennec, Rudolphi mentions hastily, giving no opinion of the merits of the distinction. And Bremser states that he lost the notes which he had made in Paris on Laennec's dissertation.

Laennec distinguishes these cysts, regarding them as animals, into three species ; 1st, The acephalocyst with *ova* or true eggs ; A. *pyriformis, simplex, vesicularis, corporibus ovatis praedita intus ;* 2d, The acephalocyst with sprouts or *gemmulae : A. surculigera,* A. *pyriformis, simplex, vesicularis, surculis praedita intus ;* and 3d, The acephalocyst with granules ; *A. granulosa,* A. pyriformis, *simplex, vesicularis, granulis intus praedita.* Thus it appears that these three species differ ;—in the first presenting in its walls small spherical white opaque bodies, little adherent and often hollow in the cen-

The mode in which hydatids are formed in the liver appears to be twofold. *First,* they may be formed in the peritoneum, and are attached to the peritoneal covering of the liver, forming round tumours, attached either to the upper or lower surface of the liver. In this case it is not unusual for Acephalocysts to be attached to the intestinal peritoneum at various points. *Secondly,* the hydatids may be developed within the substance of the liver; and gradually enlarging by the prolific multiplication of their numbers, they may form irregular elevations or tumours of considerable size at the surface of the gland. They are said to be more common in the right lobe, than in the left; but in this there seems to be nothing regular. They may occupy both lobes at once.

Hydatids when thus formed may undergo changes in themselves, or they may induce changes in the surrounding tissue of the liver.

In certain circumstances, the fluid which the membranous cysts contain becomes thick and jelly-like. The hydatids may die, and then the membranous coverings usually become opaque, thick, and indurated, sometimes almost horny. In both cases apparently they induce inflammatory irritation in the substance of the liver, followed by suppuration; and they may in this manner ulcerate their way outward, either into the mucous surface of the alimentary canal, the duodenum, or the transverse arch or ascending portion of the

tre ; the second presenting at its two surfaces small *gemmulae* or buds, very irregular and varied in shape, scarcely visible, and of the size of a hemp seed ; and in the third being covered interiorly with transparent granulations of the size of a millet seed. Though in appearance little different, these three sorts of acephalocyst are never found in the same cyst. (Bulletins de l'Ecole de Medecine, a Paris, an 13.)

Rudolphi had read the dissertation of Lüdersen and formed an opinion of it. Lüdersen had found in the interior of hydatid cysts, as others have done, innumerable vesicular granules, which could not be referred to the head of *Echinococci ;* and these, therefore, after Laennec, he denominates human acephalocysts ; which, Rudolphi adds, perhaps may be admitted. (Henrici Caroli Ludovici Lüdersen Dissertatio de Hydatidibus. Gottingæ, 1808.) But if these hydatids are taken for animals, says Rudolphi, it is a mistake ; for they are void of certain organs, proper motion, and therefore of life. The acephalocyst of the hog Rudolphi refers to the head of Echinococcus. And the same, he adds, is either always or sometimes true of the human acephalocyst. " De acephalocystide humana idem forsan semper aut quandoque valet ; ipse saltem hydatidibus compluribus hepati debitis, ab aegro deorsum dejectis, solicite examinatis, vermiculos sed rarius in iisdem offendi." (Entozoorum sive Vermium Intestinalium Historia Naturalis. Auctore Carolo Asmundo Rudolphi, Vol. I. and II. Amstelædami, 1808 et 1810. Vol. II. part ii. 367.)

De Blainville is of opinion that acephalocysts ought to be arranged neither with the *Taenia hydatigena,* or with the *Coenurus* or *Echinococcus,* but that they should be placed near the Monadariæ in the type of AMORPHOZOA.

colon, or to the surface of the body. When they cause progressive ulceration into any part of the intestinal canal, they are generally discharged through the rectum. Sometimes there is reason to believe, if situate near the upper surface of the liver, they may cause inflammation and ulceration through the diaphragm into the lungs, and be thence expelled by cough and expectoration. Lastly, in several instances, they have come to the surface of the body, and formed a pointing fluctuating tumour, on puncturing which the escape of purulent matter containing the *debris* of hydatids, has shown the true nature of the case. Of this latter termination, various cases are recorded by Heuerman, Rebentisch, Yeats, Sherwin,[*] Placido Portal,[†] and other observers.

c. ECHINOCOCCUS.—Another of this family of parasitical animals, much more rare, is found in the liver. The *Echinococcus* is a vesicular parasite with a pyriform body, globular, or round at head, and with the caudal extremity much narrower, but also rounded. The head is furnished with a circlet or ring, surmounted by a row of hooklets or prominent spikes, slightly incurvated at the extremity,—the whole apparatus forming a sort of diadem or coronet.

Of the occurrence of this animal in the liver only three cases are recorded. One is contained in the Museum of the College of Surgeons, London, and was originally in the possession of John Hunter. The second occurred to Mr Rose of Swaffham, who observed them in the purulent discharge from an abscess in the liver, which be had opened.[‡] In this instance, the *Echinococci* were associated with acephalocysts. The third is recorded by Mr Curling, who found them in a cyst in the left lobe of the liver, in the body of a man aged 71, who had died in the London Hospital of disease of the urinary organs.[§]

As the cyst in this last case, when first opened, presented the usual appearances of the acephalocyst, and the peculiar characters of the inhabitants of the cyst were only ascertained by microscopical examination, it comes to be a question, whether, in many other

* Case of a very large Abscess containing Hydatids connected with the Liver terminating favourably. By H. C. Sherwin. Edin. Med. and Surg. Journal, Vol. xix. p. 223. Edinburgh, 1823.

† Annali Universali di Medicina, Vol. xcvii. 1841.

‡ On the Vesicular Entozoa, and particularly Hydatids. By C. B. Rose, Swaffham, Norfolk. London Medical Gazette, Vol. xiii. p. 204. London, 1834.

§ A case of a rare species of Hydatid (*Echinococcus Hominis*), found in the Human Liver By T. B. Curling, Esq. Medico-Chirurgical Transactions, Vol. xxiii. p. 385. London, 1840.

instances of large cysts like those of the acephalocyst, they may not belong to the same animal.

In this instance the mode of generation is different. In the echinococcus, the young animal is formed between the layers of the parent cyst, and is detached from the external surface of the inner layer.

§ 16. HYGROMA.—It is doubtful whether serous cysts are formed in the liver; and it may be argued that any instances of this kind are to be referred to the head of Hydatids, especially that named the solitary acephalocyst. The circumstance is certainly not common, and not very well authenticated. Cases referable to the head of Cysts are nevertheless recorded by Dr Todd,* and Dr Stocker.† An instance is believed to be given by Dr Hesse, in Horn's Archiv, in which a female of 42, unmarried, was affected, some years after a fall on the right hypochondre, with a fluctuating swelling as large as the head of an infant. This tumour was punctured; and large quantities (five pounds) of serous fluid escaped without any trace of relics of hydatids. The patient did not recover, but died one year after the operation. It was then found that the liver was very much enlarged; and that the right lobe contained a large cyst, which, when divided, allowed to escape twelve pounds of serum, at first watery, then turbid and flocculent.‡

Mr Cæsar Hawkins describes certain encysted tumours as forming on the margin and at the surface of the liver, and occasionally sinking into its substance, and seldom exceeding the size of a filbert, or, at most, a walnut. These tumours contain clear semi-transparent or pellucid liquid, scarcely coagulable by heat, and in which there is found a peculiar animal matter, named by Dr Marcet muco-extractive.§

According to Mr Hawkins, these cysts rarely secrete purulent matter; and when this fluid is formed in them, it is not of a healthy character.

§ 17. HETEROLOGOUS GROWTHS.—A. Of these it has been observed, that occasionally one or other of the encysted tumours,

* Dublin Hospital Reports, Vol. i. p. 325.
† Transactions of the College of Physicians in Ireland, Vol. i. p. 11.
† Horn's Archiv, Septembre und Octobre 1839.
§ Cases of Sloughing Abscess connected with the Liver, with some remarks on Encysted Tumours of that Organ. By Cæsar Hawkins, Esq. Medico-Chirurgical Transactions, Vol. xviii. p. 98. London, 1833.

Meliceris,[*] *Atheroma,*[†] and *Steatoma,*[‡] were formed in the liver. The instances nevertheless are not well authenticated, and were recorded at periods, when accurate distinctions had not been introduced. Instances of the first and second are believed by the best informed authorities to be degenerated acephalocysts; and those of the last belong mostly to the encephaloid deposit.

B. STRUMA.—Whether struma be always regarded as a heterologous product or not, tubercle is usually considered as such. Struma, however, does not appear, in all instances, in the form of tubercle in the liver. It may take place in that of a sort of infiltration of strumous deposition in the interstitial matter of the gland. Its appearances are then the following. The liver is enlarged, mostly in the transverse direction, with some flattening of the two surfaces. It is also heavier, *i. e.* from five to six or eight pounds. The peritoneum is smooth and tensely stretched. The liver is doughy; generally of a pale yellow or grayish-red colour, sometimes a little variegated, and not vascular. The section is smooth, homogeneous, a little lardaceous looking, but not leaving greasy traces on the knife; and little blood escapes, while a serous muddy liquor oozes from points of the section. The substance is in general friable, flaccid, and lacerable.

Nothing positive or certain is known regarding the anatomico-pathological causes of this change; and, when its physical characters are stated, it is almost all that can be predicated regarding the lesion without committing errors. A new matter is infiltrated into the interstitial tissue of the gland; but what that new matter is, is not known.

This lesion takes place in persons wasted by disease, and with other marks of strumous disposition. It is observed in children and young persons who have enlarged mesenteric glands; and in those who are phthisical. It occasionally proceeds to abdominal dropsy. Yet life may be prolonged for a considerable time with this disorder. Many years ago, I performed several times the operation of paracentesis on a young man labouring under this disease, which had, at the time referred to, been of some duration. In ge-

---

[*] Bianchi, Hist. Hepatica. p. 107.

[†] Columbus, Glisson, and Bianchi, Hist. Hepat. Guettard, Baader.

[‡] Columbus de Re Anatomica. Bianchi, Hist. Hepat. Biumi apud Sandifort, Dissertat. Enaux.

neral, however, it proves fatal, partly by the imperfect digestion from want of proper bile, and partly by the abdominal dropsy.

C. TUBERCLES.—Bodies quite similar to the tubercular masses of the lung have been observed in the liver; and these are then to be viewed as the tubercular form of struma. In other instances strumous abscesses, like those already described, may be regarded as the softening or liquefying stage of the tyromatous deposit. Baillie, however, admits that tubercle is a rare disease of the liver. They appear to have been observed by Portal who, however, has spoken of them as gelatiniform mucous and albuminous formations within the liver. A case in a person of 19 is given by Dr Brämer of Cassel.*

The soft brown tubercles of the liver, mentioned by Baillie as bodies situate at or near the surface of the liver, and consisting of smooth soft brownish-coloured matter, appear to have been either clots of blood, the effects of hemorrhage, or instances of melanosis.

D. SCIRRHUS AND ENKEPHALOMA.—Though instances of scirrhus are represented by many writers to have been found in the liver, yet if we apply the elucidations and distinctions of accurate observation and pathology, scarcely one of these can be recognized as genuine examples of that species of structure. I have already shown that skleroma or simple induration and kirrhosis have been referred to the head of skirrhus of the liver; and I think it not doubtful that any kind of hard structure of unusual characters has been considered as instances of scirrhus. On the whole, genuine skirrhus is a rare formation in the liver; and probably only appears in it by extension from other organs, especially the stomach. From the observations in the next article, however, it must be allowed that if genuine skirrhus be not observed in the liver, it has its representative in the kindred form of morbid structure called *Enkephaloma.*

ENKEPHALOMA must be regarded as the true form in which skirrhus appears in the liver; and in this organ it is extremely common.

It appears in three forms, which are probably only different stages of the same morbid change.

First, there are formed in the liver irregularly rounded nodules, of whitish or whitish-gray matter, varying from the size of a filbert to that of a walnut, or larger. When these bodies are divided, they have a consistence between that of cream cheese and the unboiled potato. The section is quite homogeneous, and totally void of any

* Pabst's Allgemeine medizin. Zeitung, 1838. N. 15-19.

arrangement like vascularity or proofs of organization. Examined very minutely they present the appearance of infinitely minute granules aggregated together. The sections occasionally present an appearance of fibrous radiation very much like that of the radiated zeolite; the fibrous lines diverging and radiating either from one or two points towards the periphery of the tumour, or from a line passing through the middle or centre of the tumour.

In some instances the colour of these tumours internally is of a drab-gray, or fawn, or giraffe tint. But the consistence and physical characters are the same.

In general these moderately sized masses are pretty firm, softer than the unboiled potato, but firmer than lard, something like new cheese of moderate firmness, but less tough and more friable.

In another variety this deposit may appear in the form of irregularly spherical, spheroidal, or ovoidal masses, varying from the size of a filbert to that of a walnut or small egg, yet softer and more elastic than those last described, and presenting at the surface more or less vascularity, and not unfrequently with some vessels ramified through their substance. The aspect of these is in some instances like a smooth strawberry or raspberry.

Tumours of this character proceed early to the formation of fungous growths, which discharge blood freely and often. Some observers deny that this is a softening process.

The consistence of these tumours is generally about that of brain, pulpy, soft, and compressible; and in several parts they may be more pulpy than in others.

Cruveilhier distinguishes this variety into two subspecies according to their less or greater degree of vascularity. For this distinction there may be some foundation; but, if we consider that a degree of vascularity is the general attribute of this form, it seems unnecessarily to multiply subdivision, to derive the characters from differences in degree only.

If a stream of water be directed on tumours of this species, the soft pulpy matter is washed away, and nothing is left but a cellulovascular frame-work.

These reddish rasp-like bodies are found both at the surface and in the substance of the liver. They are in general formed in a short time, like all the varieties of encephaloid disease; but they are peculiar in proceeding rapidly to the formation of bleeding fungi.

These two forms of enkephaloma appear to correspond with the TUBERA CIRCUMSCRIPTA first well described by Dr Farre.

Though I describe these two forms of enkephaloid disease as appearing usually in small masses of definite size, yet it does not follow that they may not be larger. Two or more masses may be growing, and extending, may coalesce, and thus form, instead of twenty or thirty small tuberosities, five or six large irregular-shaped masses. In short, I have strong reason to believe that neither colour nor size are essential and invariable characters; and that the same structure may appear sometimes in small nodules, sometimes in large masses, and that its colour may vary from tallow-white to light fawn.

A third form which the disease assumes is the following.

Large irregularly rounded masses, generally of a whitish colour, are formed in the substance of the liver, projecting from its surface, and rendering that surface irregular and firm. These masses vary in volume from the bulk of a middle-sized potato to that of a large orange. They are never exactly spherical, but only irregularly rounded, oblong, or quite incapable of being referred to any ordinary known figure.

These masses are so large as not only to alter very much the shape of the liver, but to encroach extremely on the original structure of the organ. When the liver is divided, the sections show that the morbid deposition has extended throughout the whole gland.

These masses are whitish, or whitish gray in colour, firm, of a consistence between tallow and cheese; and the section has some resemblance to that of the unboiled potato or yam. The section is not quite so homogeneous and uniform as that of the small tuberosities, and it presents more or fewer minute cavities containing a sero-gelatinous liquid which readily oozes from them. Traces of organic arrangement cannot be distinctly recognized; yet, in some instances, one or two large varicose-like vessels may be seen passing through the mass. In some instances the appearance of radiating fibres, like that of zeolite, may be seen as in the small-sized tuberosities. But this is less frequent than in the latter. The radiating appearance also is greatly less regular, and often appears in the form of irregular lines or fibres.

The shape and outline of these masses is irregularly round, or globular, or spheroidal, and often so irregular that it is impossible to compare them to any known figure. In some instances two or three masses appear to have coalesced into one continuous mass,

3 M

and in this manner to have rendered the figure of the whole still more irregular.

In size, the masses now described are generally large; that is from the size of an apple or orange, to three or four times that magnitude. The masses now described form the *tubera circumscripta*, and the *tubera diffusa* of Dr Farre, who first after Baillie gave, in 1812, a particular account of these growths. Those first described, or the small-sized tumours, are the *tubera circumscripta*; those last described are the *tubera diffusa*. For this distinction the reasons appear not satisfactory. The *tubera circumscripta*, Dr Farre believed to be confined chiefly to the liver, while the *tubera diffusa* might affect not only the liver, but all other organs. We now know that though the former growth appears most commonly in the liver, yet it is not confined to that organ; and we know also that both are mere varieties of the same morbid deposition.

The disease has been regarded and described as the same as the medullary sarkoma or fungus, and the hematoid fungus; and probably it is. But though it bears a close resemblance to this in the great rapidity of its growth, and its mode of invading the substance of organs, it is in some respects different from this. The most probable view is, that the medullary fungus is the advanced stage of the enkephaloid tumour.

The microscopical structure of *enkephaloma* has been examined by Müller and Vogel, under the name of the medullary fungus. According to both, the tumour consists of nucleated cells, round, oval, caudate, varying in magnitude from $\frac{1}{500}$ part of a line to $\frac{1}{50}$. Some contained a nucleolus within a nucleus. By addition of vinegar these cells become pale, and the *nuclei* and *nucleoli* are more distinctly brought into view.[*] Gluge states that enkephaloma consists of clear serum, and very numerous white spherical globules, which show no nucleus, but a ragged undulating surface, or they are colourless and even. These globules are larger than pus-globules.[†] The fluid contains crystals.

From the circumstance of enkephaloid tumours presenting these nucleated cells as other tissues, Müller infers that they are not heterologous growths. But this does not touch the question. The

---

[*] Ueber den feinern Bau und der Formen der Krankhaften Geschwülste von Dr Johannes Müller in Zwei Lieferungen. Erste Lieferung. Berlin, 1838.

Julii Vogel Icones Histologiæ Pathologicæ. Tabula. vi. Histologiam Pathologicam Illustrantes. Lipsiæ, 1843.

[†] Atlas des Pathologischen Anatomie. Erste Lieferung. Jena, 1843.

cells may be the same; yet the structure, that is, the arrangement and contents of the cells, may be totally different. The question is further one which, it is clear, the microscope is not adequate to determine. Careful comparison of the enkephaloid structure shows that it resembles neither cellular tissue, nor fat, nor lard, nor brain, nor gland, nor cartilage, nor bone, but is peculiar in resembling itself alone, and in undergoing peculiar changes.

Enkephaloma appears in the liver in several different modes.

First, It may appear in that gland and in no other tissue ; and the masses may gradually enlarge until they coalesce and occupy the largest portion of the hepatic structure. They may attain a considerable size before the fatal event takes place.

Secondly, Encephaloma may appear in the liver along with or after the development of enkephaloid tumours in one or more of the abdominal viscera, or in the interperitoneal and mesenteric cellular tissue.

Thirdly, A mode not unusual in which it appears is the following. A tumour of suspicious character appears in the breast of a female, and after some time it is removed by the surgeon. The wound is healed ; but in the course of eight, ten, or twelve months, the patient complains of tightness and fulness in the right hypochondriac region, and in the abdomen generally. In the former there is irregular swelling; fluid is effused within the abdomen; and after two or three months more, death ensues. The liver is found quite occupied with large enkephaloid, whitish, or whitish gray masses. The same structure affects the diaphragm, and spreads into the lower lobe of the right lung. This I have seen take place more than once. The tumour removed from the breast is not always quite the same. Sometimes it presents the whitish lard-like structure of enkephaloma; sometimes it presents the characters of pancreatic sarkoma ; and in various instances it has presented those of alveolar or areolar cancer.

Fourthly, Dr Alderson gives several examples of disease of the stomach and liver, in which the former organ presented the areolar and colloid cancer, and the latter presented distinct and unequivocal masses of enkephaloid structure.

If all the facts now adduced be well ascertained and constant, and I can vouch for the truth of the three first, it follows that enkephaloma is allied to other forms of cancerous disease, and that it may be regarded as the form which pancreatic or alveolar cancer of the external organs assumes in the liver. The same morbid action which produces the pancreatic and alveolar deposit in the mamma, and that which produces the colloid structure in the stomach, may produce the encephaloid deposit in the liver.

Fifthly, It occasionally happens that the encephaloid structure appears both in several external parts, for instance in the glands of the neck, those of the female breast, among the muscles of an extremity, or in a bone or joint, and also, either at the same time or soon after, in the liver.

Enkephaloid deposit may affect the liver at any period of life. But it appears most usually between the ages of 30 and 45 or 50. I have seen an instance beyond 60; but this must be regarded as unusual.

Death is produced, not so much by the mere nature of the disease as by its mechanical pressure and pathological irritation on the chylopoietic and assistant chylopoietic viscera. The enlarged liver compresses the stomach, duodenum, and blood-vessels; impedes the function of digestion; and causes intra-abdominal effusion.

Dr Carswell shows that in many if not all instances, the enkephaloid matter is previously found in the blood and blood-vessels; and that from the blood it is conveyed by the vessels to various organs, and especially to the liver. He thinks that in the liver the enkephaloid matter is infiltrated or deposited within the *acini*, or glandular elements; and as the form and size of these bodies is not altered, he infers that this new matter is introduced in the same order and manner as the normal element of nutrition.*

The presence of enkephaloma in the liver is in general recognized during life with little difficulty. A tumour in the site of the right hypochondre and epigastric region, sometimes extending downwards to the space of two or three inches, with an irregular nodulated surface, with the peculiar complexion and expression indicating the presence of heterologous disease, are the marks which it presents.

E. MELANOMA. MELANOSIS.—This, which consists in a deposition of black ink-looking or umber-brown matter, semifluid, solid, like black paste, or liquid, sometimes in points, sometimes in masses contained in cysts, sometimes in layers, is an affection of the liver not very uncommon. Yet it rarely takes place in the liver unless at the same time or previously it has taken place in other tissues. The most usual situation for the melanotic matter to be deposited when it is found in the liver, is in the adipose tissue between the folds of the mesentery, the mesocolon, in that round the rectum, and in the lumbar glands and loins in general. It seems to be not

---

* Illustrations of the Elementary Forms of Disease. By Robert Carsewell, M. D., &c. London, 1838.

doubtful that in these parts it is deposited before it is formed in the liver. The melanotic deposit may, when forming in the liver, have been also previously deposited in organs still more remote, for instance, in the adipose tissue of the eyeball. Melanoma is in short a deposit which is first formed in some of the divisions of the adipose tissue, and then may be formed, to all appearance, in a secondary way, in one or more of the internal organs, most commonly the liver or the lungs.

When melanosis takes place in the liver, it affects one of two forms; first, either the form of black points which are deposited in the *acini*, or black semifluid or consistent masses, which may be tuberiform, and may be or not contained within cysts.

MELANOSIS, viewed as a morbid deposit, consists of a sort of frame-work, and a colouring matter or pigment. The frame-work or tissue is a fibrous structure arranged in the areolar manner, that is, forming areolae or interstices, of a pearly aspect, and which is probably allied to the fundamental structure of areolar cancer, only much softer.

The pigment or colouring matter is of two sorts. It may be either as black as the ink of the cuttle-fish, or it may be of an umber or bistre-brown tint. The former is the most frequent. This Thenard regards as charcoal, and Barruel and Breschet as the colouring matter of the blood. According to the best analyses, those of Barruel, and Clarion, and Lassaigne, this colouring matter consists of albumen 15 per cent., fibrin 6 per cent., carbonaceous matter 31 per cent., oxide of iron 1¾ per cent., and the usual salts of the blood. These facts give a high degree of probability to the opinion promulgated by Breschet, that melanotic matter is blood extravasated and changed, with a large proportion of colouring matter. If this be correct, it seems that it is a mistake to regard melanosis as always a malignant or heterologous growth. The deposit, nevertheless, takes place under circumstances which scarcely permit us to call this in question. It may be that there is a simple or innocuous form of melanosis, and one associated with the carcinomatous structure.

When melanotic matter is deposited in the liver so as to present the solid form, it is usually in the *acini*; and then it gives the gland the aspect of a piece of syenite, or rather black micaceous rock, from the peculiar glistening aspect of the fundamental tissue.

§ 15. d. Dr John Gairdner and Mr Thomas M. Lee described in 1844 a species of hydatid, which, though perhaps noticed by previous observers, had not been accurately distinguished or carefully described. Though the morbid condition connected with the presence of this parasite was not confined to the liver, and affected not merely the right lobe of that organ, but the omentum, part of the pancreas and spleen, part of the intestinal canal, and the surface of the peritoneum in general, yet it may be well to notice shortly the characters of the animal.

In the case given by Dr Gairdner, the hydatids consisted of globular or rounded bodies aggregated in masses or groups, not unlike the egg-bed of the common fowl. Each hydatid consisted of gelatinous matter contained within striæ or fibres; and each had an external membrane provided with *stomata*, or orifices which lead into *tubuli*. Each group consisted of many hydatids attached or covered by one common membrane, which further dipped between them. This membrane presented numerous disks varying in size, and round which the orifices or stomata were arranged. This it has been proposed to denominate, from the circumstance now specified, *Diskostoma acephalocystis.*

In the case which occurred to Mr Lee, the hydatid had a gelatinous body like the last noticed, and membranous investments; but the animal itself, which varied in size from a millet seed to the bulk of an orange. This animal is without aperture or apparent organ of nutrition; and hence it has been proposed to term it *Astoma acephalocystis.*

Those under the size of a filbert were globular. As soon as they advance beyond this size, they assume on the surface a nodulated appearance, which increases with the size of the animal, and which is owing to the simultaneous growth and enlargement of the young cysts contained within it.

The *Astoma acephalocystis* forms a sort of intermediate link between the common acephalocyst (*Acephalocystis simplex*) and the *Diskostoma acephalocystis.**

Some observers have called in question the independent animal existence of these two species of parasite, as others have doubted that of the common acephalocyst. So far as it is possible to form an inference from appearance and characters, they seem entitled to be regarded as animals, though of a low and imperfect type; and it seems most convenient to notice them in this place.

---

* Cases and Observations illustrating the History of two kinds of Hydatids, hitherto undescribed. By John Gairdner, M. D. and Thomas M. Lee. Edin. Medical and Surgical Journal, Vol. lxi. p. 269. Edinburgh, 1844.

The Gall-Bladder and Ducts. The Bile.—§ 1. The gall-bladder, and cystic duct, and common duct are all liable to inflammation, sometimes of a spreading and catarrhal character, or phlegmonous and limited. In either case the process may cause a temporary attack of jaundice.

§ 2. Hydatids have been found in the gall-bladder.*

Parasitical animals, as the *Fasciola hepatica*, it has been already stated, may take place in the biliary ducts.

§ 3. The most usual and important disorder of the biliary excretory system consists in the formation of gall-stones, which may be formed in any part of these ducts, and in the gall-bladder, but most commonly in the latter.

Gall-stones occur of all sizes, from that of a pin-head up to the magnitude of one inch in diameter. When small, they are generally numerous, and may occur to the amount of sixty or seventy in the gall-bladder at one time. Their figure in that case is polyhedral or tetrahedral, with rounded edges and angles, from mutual attrition and polishing. When there are only two or one, then the size may be considerable, that is, from half an inch to three-quarters of an inch, or a whole inch and more in diameter. Their figure is then spherical, oblong spheroidal, or pyriform, more or less regular. In this state they may be contained either within the gall-bladder, or in certain dilated portions of the biliary ducts.

These bodies are lighter than water. Soemmering states he has seen them sink; yet his facts show that they are lighter. They are inflammable, and, when burned, are slowly reduced to charcoal almost pure. Their interior structure presents a resinous glistening fracture, and a yellow or yellowish-brown colour, and, when closely inspected, the broken part exhibits numerous minute brilliant, crystalline scales, which resemble mica or scales of spermaceti. These scales are almost pure cholesterine, which, indeed, constitutes the larger portion of almost all gall-stones. Some gall-stones consist of pure cholesterine; others consist of cholesterine with the colouring matter of the bile; and a very small proportion contain the matter of bile inspissated and altered.

Cruveilhier states, that in most *calculi* of cholesterine, the nucleus consists of concretions of thickened bile. This does not correspond with what is observed in this country. In general, the nucleus or central portion consists of cholesterine in more or less purity, and round this are lamellae or strata, still of cholesterine

* Museum Anatomicum, a Johanne Gottlieb Walter. Berolini, 1805. 4to, p. xix.

in scales, but with colouring matter of bile; and the only part which, in a small proportion of cases, is inspissated bile, is the outer portion of the concretion.*

These facts regarding the chemical composition of biliary calculi show that, previous to their formation, a great and decided change takes place in the bile. Bile does not in the normal state contain cholesterine; but there is no doubt that the cholesterine is formed from the bile. A new arrangement, therefore, of the elements of bile must take place. Cholesterine consists principally of carbon and hydrogen, and the ingredients of the bile must so alter their relations as to form in this manner cholesterine.

The presence of gall-stones in the *tubuli*, the gall-ducts, or in the gall-bladder, gives rise to various effects in these parts. The most common is believed to be jaundice; and certainly in the case of gall-stones of moderate size becoming fixed in either the *tubuli*, the *pori*, the hepatic duct, the cystic duct, or the common duct, more or less jaundice, continuing for a longer or shorter time, usually takes place. On the other hand, numerous instances have been recorded of gall-stones being discharged either by the bowels, or by ulceration through the parietes of the abdomen, in which no jaundice had at any time appeared.

When gall-stones are small, their presence probably gives rise to few or no symptoms. But when they are large, there is strong reason to believe that they induce symptoms of considerable severity. These symptoms may be of two sorts. In one set of cases they are supposed to be those of excruciating pain, and that of a spasmodic character. In another set of cases they induce well-marked symptoms of either peritoneal inflammation, or of intestinal obstruction, or ileus, or of both combined.

When gall-stones are small and numerous, and are contained in the gall-bladder, they cause little uneasiness; and numerous examples show that they may remain in that situation to the end of a long life without giving rise to prominent symptoms.

When, on the other hand, they are large, and either are contained in any of the ducts or get into these canals, they cause very serious evils. Pain in the epigastric region, often of an excruciating character, relieved only by incurvating the trunk, vomiting, jaundice, constipation, are all effects which have been observed to result from the presence of gall-stones in the ducts. These symp-

* An Account of an unusually large Biliary Calculus voided from the Rectum. By James A. Wilson, M. D. Med.-Chirurg. Trans., vol. xxvi. p. 80. London, 1843.

tòms are caused either by the presence of a large distending body in the ducts, or by the efforts made by the ducts and other textures to expel that body.

When gall-stones are unusually large, they may be discharged either by vomiting from the stomach; or by the intestinal canal; the whole of which, as well as the cystic and common ducts, they must traverse; or they procure for themselves a route to the surface of the body by means of ulceration, most commonly through the parietes of the intestinal canal and abdominal muscles. Indeed it is not unlikely that, in various instances, they cause ulceration through the hepatic ducts or gall-bladder, in both the previous cases; and instances are recorded in which ulceration must have been previously effected in the gall-bladder or hepatic and cystic ducts, before the gall-stone could get either into the intestinal canal, or come to the surface.

1. It is not very usual for gall-stones to be expelled from the stomach by vomiting. Schurig, nevertheless, mentions not fewer than eight instances in which gall-stones had been ejected in this manner.* Orteschi records one case in his Diary.† One is given in the Gazette Salutaire; and one is given by Biondi.‡

2. Through the intestinal canal it is greatly more common to observe gall-stones expelled; and while numerous cases are recorded, many must have taken place without being noticed. The following are the best authenticated.

F. Ruysch, Thesaurus Anatomicus Quintus, n. 32.

Dr Musgrave records an instance of an oval gall-stone nearly one inch long, and weighing 59 grains, being voided by a gentleman, after an attack of jaundice, with much pain in the epigastric region.§

Bezold records the case of a woman of 52, who, after much suffering, passed a wedge-shaped hard biliary concretion, weighing, immediately after discharge, one ounce two drachms and half a scruple, which measured in its long circumference from two inches and a half to three inches and a half, and in the middle was about four inches and a half.||

Mr J. Yonge, in a letter to Hooke, informs him that he had lately seen a gentlewoman almost dead in jaundice relieved by the

* Lithologia. † In Diario, p. 283. † Giornale di Medicina, i. p. 282.

§ A Letter from Dr William Musgrave to Dr Hans Sloane concerning Jaundice occasioned by a stone obstructing the *Ductus Communis Biliarius*. Phil. Transact, No. 306, p. 227. London, 1706–1708.

|| Georgii Bezold Dissertatio de Cholelitho. Argentorati, 24th May 1725. Apud Haller, Dissert. Medico-Practicas, Tom. iii. p. 605.

evacuation of a gall-stone as large as a pullet's egg; and another from a man as big as a nutmeg; both followed with a lask (looseness) discharging prodigious quantities of choler.[*] John Baptist Bianchi relates the case of a lady of rank who had been subject to periodical jaundice from twelve to fifteen days at a time; and from whom a gall-stone larger than a walnut was brought away by the operation of a strong purge.[†] Dr James Johnstone records a case in which a corpulent old lady, after suffering for two days severe pain in the epigastric region with vomiting, voided an oblong pyriform biliary concretion, about one inch and a quarter long, and fully one inch in diameter, and weighing 126 grains. She had no jaundice, but seven hours of most excruciating pain.[‡] Lavernet relates a case in which a large biliary concretion weighing three drachms was voided.

Petit mentions the case of a lady who had jaundice with colicky pains. After the use of the warm-bath three times, she discharged with much blood a gall-stone, rough like the skin of the shark, weighing four drachms and two scruples, and measuring two inches and a half long, one inch and a half in diameter, and three inches and a half in circumference.[||]

Walter mentions shortly the case of a female of about 70 years who voided two gall-stones, weighing together two drachms two scruples = 160 grains. The largest was oblong spheroidal, a little more than one inch long, and a little less than one inch in transverse diameter.[¶]

M. Gosse records in a married lady during pregnancy the escape of two concretions of a burnt umber colour, which had been originally one, at an interval of ten hours, weighing together about four drachms (3 gros,) and the first of which was 14 lines long and 23 in circumference. She suffered much previously from colic pains; but had no jaundice.[**]

[*] Philosophical Experiments and Observations of the late Dr Robert Hooke, F. R. S. &c. published by William Derham, F. R. S. London, 1726, p. 79.

[†] Historia Hepatica Joannis B. Bianchi, M. D. Tom. i. p. 189. Genevae, 1725.

[‡] An account of two extraordinary Cases of Gall-stones. By James Johnstone, M. D. of Kidderminster. Phil. Trans. vol. l. p. 543. London, 1758 ; and Medical Essays and Observations, &c. Evesham, 1795, 8vo, p. 200.

§ Journal de Medecine Continué, vol. xv. p. 404.

|| Traité des Maladies Chirurgicales, Tome i. p. 325. Paris, 1774 and 1790.

¶ Henkel's Neuen Medizinische und Chirurgischen Anmerkungen. 1769. And Walter Anatomisches Museum, T. 112, 213. Taf. 2.

** Observation d'un Calcul Biliare expulsé par les selles ; par M. Gosse. Journal de Medecine et Chirurgie, &c. T. xxxiv. p. 45. Paris, 1770.

M. Brillouet gives, in a lady of 68, a case in which, after colic pains, vomiting, and constipation, lasting apparently about a month, there was voided first a gall-stone, five lines long and eighteen in circumference, and weighing forty-three grains ; and fourteen days after a similar concretion, six lines long, and weighing fifty grains ; both fragments of one gall-stone weighing together one drachm thirty-three grains.*

Dr Lettsom records the case of a military gentleman of Jamaica, who had laboured for years under severe pain of the epigastric region, which was ascribed to gout.   As he had intervals of ease for eight or ten days, Dr Lettsom suggested that his complaints depended on the presence of gall-stones.   At length, in one of the fits, he voided an oblong spheroidal concretion $2\frac{1}{4}$ inches long, with a contraction or collar in the middle, weighing 1 ounce 2 drachms and 23 grains.   No jaundice took place in this case.†

F. G. in Meyer Epist. ad Zimmermannum Hannoveræ, 1789, Editio secunda, 1790.

John Gottlieb Walter notices the case of a man of 71 who voided an oblong spheroidal gall-stone, weighing two drachms, two scruples, ten grains = 170 grains, about one inch and a half in the greatest diameter, and nearly one inch in the small diameter.   The patient suffered violent spasmodic pains in the abdomen ; but all ceased on the discharge of the concretion.‡

Heberden mentions a case, in which a female, who had suffered from jaundice for many years, at length voided a concretion, of which the smaller circumference was two inches.§

Mr H. L. Thomas records in a woman of 63 an instance of a globular gall-stone being evacuated, 1.6 inch largest diameter, 1.1 inch small diameter, weighing 228 grains.||

Mr T. Brayne records in a woman of 55 an instance of a gall-stone of the shape of a pigeon's egg being expelled from the bowels, measuring $1\frac{3}{8}$ greatest diameter, $1\frac{1}{4}$ shortest diameter, and

---

* Observation sur un Calcul Biliare expulsé par les selles, par M. Brillouet. Journal de Medecine, T. xxxvi. p. 233.   Paris, 1771.

† Case of a Biliary Calculus. By J. C. Lettsom, M. D. Read 4th September 1786. Memoirs of Medical Society, Vol. i. art. xxx. p. 373.   London, 1787.

‡ Anatomisches Museum Gesammelt von Johann Gottlieb Walter, S. 96, Taf. iv. Berlin, 1796.   4to.

§ Commentarii de Morborum Historia et Curatione. Lond. 1797. 8vo. Cap. 50, p. 209.

|| Case of Obstruction of the Large Intestines occasioned by a Biliary Calculus of extraordinary size. By H. L. Thomas, Esq. Medico-Chirurg. Transactions, vol. vi. p. 99. London, 1815.

weighing 162 grains. Occasional slight jaundice. Symptoms of ileus.*

The same gentleman records, in a female of 65, an instance in which, after much suffering, a flat cubical concretion, with rounded angles and concave depressed sides, weighing 176 grains, and one inch in diameter, was voided ; and another, six days after, hemispherical in shape, and 159 grains, was expelled. ⁚No jaundice.

I met, in March 1824, with a case in an elderly lady, who, after being very ill for eight days with symptoms of obstinate *ileus*, voided a large spherical biliary concretion, weighing, when dried, 160 grains, and measuring one inch two lines in diameter. In this case no yellowness ever was observed.†

Dr Robert Paterson of Leith presented to me, in 1842, the half of a spherical gall-stone, fully one inch in diameter, which had been voided some time previously by a patient of his, after presenting symptoms of obstinate obstruction, without jaundice.

Dr James Arthur Wilson records a case in which a gentleman of 73, after suffering from constipation, with jaundice and hiccup, and vomiting for many days, voided a large biliary concretion, consisting of cholesterine in the centre, and inspissated bile with cholesterine externally.‡

The question has often occurred to my mind since I witnessed the violent and obstinate symptoms both of inflammation and intestinal obstruction, with which the case now referred to was attended, whether these large *calculi* merely distend the ducts before getting into the intestinal canal, or pave to themselves a passage by inflammation and ulceration. It appears to me that though, in some instances, dilatation of the ducts may take place, and be sufficient for the transport of the concretion, yet in several inflammation and ulceration had taken place. Though I distinguish this class of cases from those which are to come next, yet we must remember that nature knows no distinction of this kind. When a gall-stone is fixed either in one part of any of the three ducts, or in the gall-bladder, it may there give rise to inflammation and suppuration of the surrounding textures; and it will depend on several

---

* An Account of two Cases of Biliary Calculi of extraordinary Dimensions. By T. Brayne, Esq. Medico-Chirurg. Transactions, Vol. xii. p. 255. London, 1823.

† History of a case in which the symptoms of Iliac Passion arose from the transit of an unusually large gall-stone, terminating favourably. By David Craigie, M. D. Edinburgh Medical and Surgical Journal, vol. xxii. p. 235. Edinburgh, 1824.

‡ An Account, &c. Medico-Chirurg. Transactions, vol. xxvi. London, 1843.

circumstances what course this inflammation is to take, what textures it will affect, and by what channel the concretion will finally proceed. The suppurative process may then be either confined more or less strictly to the tissues immediately concerned, as the gall-bladder, the cystic duct, the hepatic duct, or common duct, or two of these at once according to the position of the concretion, and the cellular substance of the capsule of Glisson and the duodenum; or it may extend to a larger portion of the intestines, and even by ulceration and adhesion to the *parietes* of the abdomen themselves. The latter result is most likely to happen when the concretion is in the gall-bladder, the *fundus* or base of which is very near the abdominal muscles. Yet there is no assurance that the same course may not be followed when the concretion is in the cystic or common duct, or even in the hepatic duct. In the first case, the concretion is discharged into the cavity of the intestines,—viz. thè *duodenum*, the *ileum*, or the transverse arch of the colon. In the latter, it is almost uniformly expelled by an ulcerated opening through the abdominal parietes.

The reason which induces me to think that these concretions may pass into the intestinal canal by means of ulceration, is found in such cases as that given by Tyson of an abscess in the liver, in which gall-stones were found in the gall-bladder, the *ductus cysticus*, common duct and in the *porus biliarius*, or hepatic duct;* a case mentioned by Walter (at page 126), in which he infers that the gall-bladder must have been inflamed and suppurated, forming around it a pouch or sac, connected with the transverse arch of the colon;† that already mentioned at page 867 of this work; and that given by Dr Scott, in which the patient died during inflammation of the gall-bladder, caused by the presence of a concretion as large as an olive; and which, had life been prolonged, must have found its way by ulceration into the intestines or to the surface of the body.‡

3. The latter appears to be the mode of exit most common in

---

* Anatomical observations of an abscess in the liver, a great number of stones in the gall-bag and bilious vessels, &c., by Edward Tyson, A. M., &c. Oxon. Phil. Trans., No. 142, p. 1035. London, 1678, voL xi.

† Anatomisches Museum Gesammelt von Johan Gottlieb Walter. Berlin, 1796. 4to.

‡ Case of Death from Inflammation of the Gall-bladder, occasioned by the irritation of a Stone. By David Scott, M. D. Edin. Med. and Surg. Journal, Vol. xxiii. p. 297. Edin. 1825.

the case of large concretions; yet it is not confined to them, but serves as the channel for evacuation of moderate-sized gall-stones also. Of this mode of expulsion, many instances are recorded; but I mention only the following in illustration of the circumstance. In the Ephemerides Naturæ Curiosorum cases by many authors. Tolet states that he saw a gall-stone as large as a pigeon's egg discharged by an ulcer at the navel.*

The editor of the Bologna Commentaries gives, from the practice of Tacconi, in 1739, the following case. A married woman of 27 suffered for some time under pain at the epigastric region, squeamishness, occasional vomiting, and at length a suppurating swelling near the site of the right lobe of the liver. Into this an incision was made; when four ounces of matter and seven biliary concretions came away. In the course of fourteen days, other concretions came away, varying in shape, size, and weight, one as large as a nutmeg. After this, recovery took place. No jaundice was observed.†

Cheselden mentions a case in which two gall-stones, six lines in diameter, were discharged through the abdominal integuments.‡

Hoffmann mentions a case in which eighty gall-stones were discharged by an ulcer in the abdomen.§

Wislicen records the case of a man who, after suffering for one year much pain in the abdomen, had a tumour in the right groin, which was opened by caustic, and discharged at length upwards of fifty concretions of the size of beans and peas.||

Petit mentions three instances. The first was that of a lady who had a pointing tumour in the right hypochondre, which, on being opened, discharged at first pure bile; and from which, seven or eight months afterwards, there escaped a gall-stone.¶ The second one, from Lapeyronie, in a woman of 37, in whom a tumour appeared in the epigastric region, which, on being opened, discharged purulent matter with bile, and five or six concretions of the size of

---

* Traité de la Lithotomie. 8vo, 4trieme edition, Utrecht. Chap. iv. p. 24. 1693.

† De Bononiensi Scientiarum et Artium Instituto atque Academia Commentarii, T. 2di, Pars prima. Bononiae, 1745. 4to, p. 212.

‡ Anatomy, Book iii. chap. v. p. 166. 12th edit. London, 1784.

§ Crell Chemische Annalen 1789. viii. St. Seite 128.

|| J. Andreae Wislicen Lapides per Abdomen ulceratione exclusi. Lipsiae, 1742. Apud Haller Dissertationes Medico-Fracticas, T. iii. p. 629.

¶ Traité des Maladies Chirurgicales, Ouvrage Posthume de J. L. Petit. Tome i. p. 313. Mis au jour, par M. Lesne. Paris, 1790.

4

peas.* In a third, a female of 74, he extracted from a fistulous opening in the right hypochondre first one concretion four inches long and three in circumference, and afterwards another smaller concretion.

A case in the *Commercium Norimberg.* 1743, p. 81.

Dr James Johnstone mentions the case of a woman of upwards of 30 labouring, in 1752, under jaundice and excruciating pain, striking from the right hypochondre to the back, with frequent fits of vomiting. At this time, hardness was felt at the pit of the sto-mach. About three months after this time, the tumour suppurated, and discharged with matter several gall-stones. She recovered, and died in 1763.†

M. Marechal and Guerin, in attending a lady of rank, who had a suppurating tumour at the margin of the right hypochondre, opened it by incision, and removed a gall-stone as large as the largest acorn.‡

Haller mentions the instance of a woman in whom, from an ulcer in the epigastric region, several biliary *calculi* were discharged, an-gular, trihedral ; the patient surviving.§

Bloch saw several concretions come away from an ulcer under the false ribs ;‖ and Buttner saw thirty-eight gall-stones discharged from an aperture near the navel.¶

Civadier saw several gall-stones come away from an ulcer in the right groin.**

Acrell published in 1788 at Upsal a dissertation on gall-stones escaping by ulceration through the abdominal parietes; and Sand-torff published at Helmstadt†† a dissertation on the same subject, containing accounts of various cases. Vogler gives an instance of the occurrence ;‡‡ and Bruckmann observed several gall-stones escape successively through an abscess in the abdomen.§§

* Lapeyronie, Memoires de l'Academie de la Chirurgie, T. i. p. 185.   Paris, 1743 ; and Petit, Oeuvres Posthumes, Tome i. p. 320 and 325.   Paris, 1774 and 1790.

† Philosophical Transactions, Vol. l. p. 543, and Essays, p. 207.

‡ Observations par M. Morand, Memoires de l'Academie Royale de Chirurgie, Tome iii. p. 470.   Paris, 1757.

§ Opuscula Pathologica, Lausannae, 1767 et 1768.   Obs. 38, Hist. 8.

‖ Medicinische Bemerkungen.   Berlin, 1774.

¶ Funf Besondere Wahrnehmungen.   Koenigsberg, 1774.

** Nouvelles Economiques et Litteraires, Tom. xx.

†† Dissertatio de Cholelithis ex ulcere abdominis elapsis.   Helmstadii, 1810.

‡‡ Museum der Heilkunde, iv. Band, p. 91.

§§ Horn's Archiv, 1810, p. 231, 144.

Mr George White, formerly a practitioner in this city, informed me, in May 1825, some time after I had published the account of the large gall-stone voided, as already mentioned, from the bowels, of an instance in which first inflammation, and suppuration, and then ulceration of the abdominal parietes took place, and through the aperture thus made a gall-stone of considerable size was discharged, with recovery of the patient.

I may add also, that, in the Museum of Guy's Hospital, there are preserved two biliary concretions, which made their escape through an abscess at the navel in a female patient of Mr T. Calloway, one of the surgeons to that institution.

Dr Macnish gives an interesting case, in which, some months after an attack of acute hepatitis, an abscess was formed below the margin of the ribs, which was at length laid open by incision. About twenty-five days after this, a gall-stone as large as a nutmeg was discharged from the wound; and four days after another concretion and some fragments were discharged. A good deal of bile was afterwards mixed with the discharge. But the patient made a good recovery, the wound having completely cicatrized about twelve months after the date of incision.*

In short, there is no lack of evidence to show, that biliary concretions of all sizes may find their way to the surface of the body by a process of progressive inflammation and suppuration, the parts behind and around being united by the effusion of lymph, so as to prevent the concretion from getting into the peritoneum. It is, indeed, important to observe, that while numerous cases of this mode of exit are recorded, in all of which the movement of the concretion must have been attended with ulceration, and not less numerous cases of their transit into the intestinal canal, in several of which, probably, the same process took place, no instance is recorded of a gall-stone dropping into the cavity of the peritoneum, except in one doubtful instance.†

After the foregoing detail, it is superfluous to say that the gall-bladder and biliary ducts are liable to be affected by inflammation and ulceration. The ducts are liable to become obliterated in the course of the process.

* Case of Tumour in the Region of the Liver, with discharge of Biliary Calculi through the abdominal parietes. By William Macnish, M.D. &c. Edinburgh Medical and Surgical Journal, Vol. xli. p. 169. 1834.

† Andree.

One cause of tumour and eventually abscess has been pointed out by Petit in France, and Amyand in this country. This consists in an accumulation of bile, too thick apparently to flow through the duct, attended probably with some obstruction either in the cystic or common duct, by which the bile is prevented from getting into the duodenum, and consequently distends the gall-bladder, which then is inflamed.

§ 4. The gall-bladder is liable to be involved in the heterologous deposits by which the liver is affected.

§ 5. The gall-bladder has been found altogether wanting by Marcellus Donatus, Schenke, Huber,† Targioni Tozzetti,‡ Sandifort,§ and Wiedemann.‖

§ 6. It is liable to be ruptured, to be wounded or lacerated, and to be ossified.

Section V.
Morbid States of the Kidney.

The kidney is liable to be the seat of inflammation of various sorts, and its effects, especially suppuration within the *calyces ;* to the formation and presence of calculi within the *calyces* and *pelvis ;* to enlargement and dilatation, and hemorrhage ; to granular degeneration (*steatosis*); to the formation of serous cysts ; to atrophy ; to hypertrophy ; and to the heterologous growths.

§ 1. Nephritis. Inflammation and its Effects.—The kidney is, like other glands, liable to inflammation ; but this is more particularly the consequence of certain circumstances residing either in the general system of the individual ; or in the organ itself; or in the relation of the organ to the stomach, and the function of digestion and assimilation. It is said that idiopathic inflammation of the kidney is a rare affection ; and that most commonly the disease is symptomatic, that is, is supposed to indicate the presence and operation of some irritant agent. This may be correct as to acute attacks ; but it is not applicable to chronic affections, which come on and are established either without perceptible cause, or depend on the state of the blood and of the organs of digestion. The idiopathic form is liable to take place in the gouty, as a symptom of the gouty diathesis and internal gout, being one form in

---

* Philosoph. Transact. 492.   † Journal de Medecine, Tome iv. p. 283.
‡ Tabulae Anatomicae, Fasciculus iii.
§ Reil Archiv fur die Physiologie, v. Band, p. 145.

which gout affects the kidney; and it is known by the individual having presented more or fewer of the symptoms of gout, and by the disease terminating in or being associated with a paroxysm of regular gout.

Renal inflammation may ensue on blows or contusions on the loins; falls in which the kidney, with other organs, suffers concussion; carrying heavy loads on the back, or wrenches in consequence of falling in carrying loads; riding on horseback; riding in a carriage over a rough road; the presence of renal concretions or sabulous matter in the infundibula or pelvis, especially if the former be rough, or angular; various irritants taken into the stomach, which either induce acidity, or being absorbed by the blood-vessels, are enabled to irritate the tissue of the kidney, as some of the vegetable acids and fruits, acid wines; the application of cantharides externally, or their use internally; the terebinthinate, resinous, and balsamic substances; cold applied to the lumbar region, especially when overheated; inflammation of the adjoining organs, as the liver, spleen, duodenum, colon, psoas muscle, the dorsal or lumbar vertebræ; and in some instances inflammation of the bladder, extending upwards through the ureters, either resulting from excessive distension of these organs, or without distension.

Of the whole of these circumstances which may be regarded as exciting causes, the operation is very much favoured by the presence of the gouty or calculous diathesis already mentioned.

Inflammation may attack either the pelvic and calycine membrane of the kidney; or the substance of the gland; or the external surface of the gland, with or without its investing membrane.

The most common is inflammation of the calycine membrane, or that part of the mucous epithelial membrane of the kidney, which extends upwards from the pelvis into the *calyces* and *papillæ*. This membrane is then injected into blood, covered by a coating of lymph more or less thick, and the free surface of which is formed into a multitude of minute processes or scales, while purulent matter is eventually deposited within this. The subsequent course of this process shall be noticed presently.

When the substance of the kidney is inflamed, it becomes of a deep red or reddish brown colour, abounds in blood-vessels, much loaded with blood; the whole organ is enlarged in all its dimensions; and its substance is copiously infiltrated with bloody serum. As to consistence, nothing is certain; the inflamed kidney being

3

sometimes softer than natural, sometimes harder. This difference depends probably on the duration of the inflammatory process. Blood may be expressed from the papillæ. In some instances small points and drops of purulent matter, or purulent matter and fluid lymph,.are infiltrated into the substance of the gland.

The terminations vary according to the causes on which the disease depends, the method of treatment, and the nature of the affection.

Idiopathic renal inflammation may terminate in resolution, in an attack of gout, in the deposition of sand or sabulous concretions (*lithiasis*), in suppuration, in suppuration with extenuation of the kidney, in induration or softening of the kidney, and perhaps in granular deposition and transformation, or in death.

Idiopathic *nephritis* may, under the prompt use of remedies, terminate in resolution on the third, fifth, or seventh day. In this case the pain gradually or speedily abates and finally disappears; the vomiting ceases, the heat and thirst are diminished, the patient becomes less restless, and at length falls asleep; and the skin becoming moist, he awakes in general without any feeling of his former sufferings, with the pulse down at 80 or even lower, and begins to discharge without pain or uneasiness a considerable quantity of urine, usually dark-coloured, like brown dirty water or coffee, which deposits on cooling a sediment dark-coloured, and sometimes slightly bloody. In the course of a day or two, if this amendment continue, the urine returns to its natural standard in quantity, quality, and appearance.

In cases of gouty diathesis, the pain of the renal region subsides or disappears, and at the same time pain, redness, and swelling appear on the foot or hand, and pass through their usual course.

If neither of these results take place on or before the fifth or the seventh day, it may be apprehended that the disease is to terminate either fatally, or in suppuration or abscess, or distension and attenuation of the kidney, or one or other of the events already specified.

When the fatal termination takes place, it is generally preceded by complete suppression of the urinary secretion, slow full pulse, stupor proceeding to coma, and a urinous exhalation from the surface of the body.

When *nephritis* terminates neither in resolution nor in death, it may be apprehended that it is to end in suppuration or some similar disorganizing process in the kidney; and though this may take place in the spontaneous or idiopathic form of the disorder, it is much more likely to ensue in cases in which the disease is induced by the mechanical irritation of an urinary concretion.

It is requisite here, therefore, to specify the circumstances under which suppuration is most likely to take place, and the usual forms under which it appears.

§ 2. Though suppuration of the kidney may take place either in its cortical or secreting part, or in its tubular or excreting portion, yet, so far as the evidence of morbid anatomy goes, the most usual mode in which suppuration, or rather the secretion of purulent matter takes place, is the following.

1. An attack of renal inflammation may, if it affect mostly the tubular part of the kidney and the *infundibula*, terminate in the secretion of puriform mucus, plastic lymph and blood from the calycine membrane, that is the delicate mucous surface of these cavities, and the *papillæ*, and from the mucous surface of the *pelvis;* and these morbid secretions may either escape through the ureter into the bladder, and be expelled, or they may remain and produce obstruction of the pelvis, secondary inflammation, and distension of the *pelvis* and *infundibula*.

In the former case, the matter escapes by the ureters into the bladder, partially or entirely, and is discharged in the form of purulent matter, mixed with urine or purulent urine (*pyuria*); but it is liable again to accumulate, unless the inflammatory action is totally subdued. If it do accumulate, it then becomes, in all respects, similar to the latter case, and a peculiar state of the kidney is presented, (NEPHROTASIA; NEPHROPYEMA). The matter retained within the *pelvis* and *infundibula*, or at least not permitted to escape by the ureter, either mixed with urine, or by itself, gradually accumulates and increases in quantity, and causes more or less distension of the pelvis and *infundibula*. If this be moderate, and if death take place, the kidney, when divided, presents as many cavities containing purulent matter as there are *infundibula;* and while the substance of the kidney is rendered much thinner than usual, these cavities are sometimes supposed to be purulent cysts into which the kidney has been converted. This is the true explanation of such cases as that mentioned by Cheston, who states that in a boy of seven, " the substance of the kidneys was so dissolved into matter, that they appeared little more than cysts full of *pus*, the one weighing four ounces and the other three."* I have seen several cases in which observers otherwise able were deceived by his appearance, and were led to imagine that the kidney was converted into purulent cysts. The mistake is rectified by removing the purulent matter cautiously, and washing the cavities in pure water, when it is observed that the fine membrane covering the *papillæ* and lining the *infundibula* (*membrana calycina*) is a little rough and thickened, very generally covered with lymph, but not destroyed or marked by any breach of continuity; that the papillæ may be recognized also entire; and that the only change which has taken place is considerable distension by purulent matter, and consequent attenuation of the tubular and cortical part of the kidney.

The quantity of matter accumulated, however, may be considerable, the distension great, and the consequent attenuation of the renal substance may be carried to a great extreme. The first effect of this increased accumulation is, by the distension, to force two or more *infundibula* into one common and considerable cavity or sac; the next effect is gradually to force several *infundibula* into one considerable sac; and if the accumulation continue and the distension proceed, the *infundibula* and pelvis are converted into one general extensive sac, containing purulent matter. In cases of this description, the cortical and tubular substance of the kidney are so much stretched and attenuated, that not unfrequently they are not thicker than a crown or a half-crown piece; and it might be imagined that these tissues were almost or altogether destroyed by suppuration, and that nothing is left but the external capsule. When, however, a proper section is made, the purulent matter evacuated, and the parts washed with pure water, the calycine membrane and the *papillæ* may be recognized,—the former rough with lymph and thickened mucus, the latter much compressed; the individual tubular cones may be traced, though much stretched and separated; and the cortical structure may be perceived in the form of a thin exterior coating.

The size which the expanded and attenuated kidney may in these circumstances attain, is often very great, and the quantity of matter with or without urine very considerable. The older authors, as Blasius and Ott, have not distinguished the disease with accuracy or precision; and consequently I can make little use of these

* Pathological Inquiries, Chap. ii. p. 9. Gloucester, 1766.

cases. But the kidney has been in this state found to be as large as the head of a child, and to contain almost two pounds or more of purulent, sero-purulent, or urino-purulent fluid; and in one case which was known to me, the left kidney was so much enlarged and distended, that it occupied the whole left side of the abdomen and extended into the pelvis. An excellent case is given by Corvisart in his journal.*

This disease has been described by Frederic Augustus Walter in one stage, under the name of expansion of the kidneys, (*expansio renum*,) and in another under the title of dropsy of the kidneys, (Nierenwasserseuche,) (*hydrops renalis*.)† Neither of these names are appropriate; and the latter is particularly improper, in so far as it conveys a just idea neither of the origin of the disorder, nor its nature, and is liable, in the present state of pathological knowledge, to be confounded with the secondary dropsical effusions which take place in consequence of granular degeneration of the kidney. The expansion is the effect of inflammation, which, by giving rise to morbid products, causes distension of the kidney, and dilatation of its *infundibula* and *pelvis*, much as sero-purulent fluid within the *pleura* separates the lungs from the *pleura costalis* and ribs, and extrudes the walls of the chest. The sero-purulent, purulent, or urino-purulent fluid contained within the expanded *infundibula* and *pelvis* of the kidney, constitutes no resemblance or analogy between the fluid and those of dropsical effusions; and the name should therefore be discarded. If a particular denomination be wished for the disease, the term *Nephropyema* or *Pyonephria* is the proper one, and the term *Nephrotasia* may be used to signify the distension. It may be observed, however, that the latter is a mere effect of the accumulation of purulent fluid.

I think that Mr Howship has been misled by the same circumstance, when, in speaking of this change under the head of distension of the kidneys, he observes, that " by this means a degree of pressure is established, which, as it increases, induces by degrees a total resolution of the whole of the natural structure of the gland, which is ultimately found converted into an assemblage of large and small cysts, or thin membranous capsules."‡

* Journal de Medecine, Tom. vii. p. 387.

† Einige Krankheiten der Nieren und Harnblase. Berlin, 1800. 4to.

‡ A Practical Treatise on the Symptoms, Causes, Discrimination, and Treatment of some of the most important Complaints that affect the Secretion and Excretion of the Urine, &c. By John Howship, Member of the R. C. of Surgeons in London. London, 1823. Section vi. p. 13.

That the great distension which in some cases takes place may be sufficient to separate and detach forcibly from each the individual component cones of the kidney, is a circumstance which I will not deny. But I must say that everything known regarding the effect of suppuration in this part of the kidney shows, that this is not a common result; and that the most frequent consequence by far is that which I have here represented it to be. It is quite impossible to imagine the great changes produced by mere pressure and distension in the human body, without absolute destruction of the organization of parts, were it not the subject of daily observation, aided by accurate inspection of the state of the parts.

In some instances this purulent distension is confined to one or two *infundibula*, which do not readily communicate with the others; and in consequence the purulent matter contained within them does not escape into the other, but, being incessantly increased, causes expansion and enlargement at one part of the gland. In other cases it is confined to the pelvis, and produces on that the same effect which it would elsewhere, but leaving the kidney for some time comparatively uninjured.

The fluid contained may be purulent, sero-purulent, or sero-purulent mixed with urine, that is urino-purulent. In some of the cases described by Walter, the fluid is represented to have been clear and diaphanous.

It is proper, however, to say, that Walter, who had seen several examples of this disorder from obstruction of the ureter by concretions, represents the whole kidney as so changed, that nothing seemed to be left except the exterior membrane or capsule, which was so much extenuated by the pressure of the contained fluid, that the part which was previously a kidney, presented the appearance of an expanded bladder. This distension he ascribes solely to the accumulation of urine, which, not being allowed to pass by the ureter, stagnates in the *pelvis* and *infundibula*, and by compression upon their excreting and secreting parts and vessels, first impedes and then suspends the secretion and excretion of the gland.

In instances of great distension he mentions, that not only is all the perinephral fat absorbed, but the exterior membrane itself may be transformed into an osseous capsule, as was exemplified in various preparations preserved in the collection of his father. The description now mentioned is most applicable to that obstruction which arises from the presence of a concretion in the pelvis or ureter.

§ 3. NEPHROPSAMMIA ; LITHIASIS NEPHRITICA.—An attack of
renal inflammation may terminate in the secretion of a considerable
quantity of sabulous matter, with or without puriform or morbid
mucus and blood; and if this escape not by the ureter into the
bladder, and be thence expelled in the usual manner, the sabulous
matters are aggregated by the viscid mucus and other morbid
secretions into masses moulded in one or more of the *infundibula*
or the pelvis; and there they remain constituting urinary renal
calculi; in which case they may, either with or without inflammation, cause obstruction in the excretion of the urine, and consequent
expansion of the renal *infundibula*.

§ 4. NEPHROPYEMA CALCULOSA.—Though it is well ascertained
that calculi if round do not always give rise to symptoms of uneasiness or pain in the dorso-lumbar region, or to symptoms of
renal inflammation, yet they are very liable to do so during the
operation of any of the ordinary exciting causes of inflammation,
as external violence, exposure to cold, or a long and fatiguing
journey on horseback, or the operation of the particular causes of
renal irritation, as the use of acidulous articles of food or drink,
the absorption or the internal use of cantharides, or the use of the
turpentine, or resinous, or balsamic articles.

Either after or without the operation of one or other of these
causes, the patient is attacked with the symptoms of pain in the
dorso-lumbar region, shivering, squeamishness, numbness of the
thigh, pain or soreness or retraction of the testicle of the same side,
scanty urine or total suppression, or bloody sedimentous urine and
constipation.   In some cases the severity of these symptoms undergoes, either in consequence of remedies or spontaneously, temporary alleviation ; urine tinged brown with blood is expelled; and
shortly after, quantities of sabulous matter or minute concretions
are discharged.

In some instances purulent matter is voided more or less copiously with the urine, and is observed to fall to the bottom of the
vessel, presenting its usual appearance and characters.   Such a
circumstance is generally conceived to indicate suppuration of the
kidney.   In one sense it certainly does denote the presence of this
process, but not in the sense commonly understood.   Though it
be generally said that the kidney then suppurates, yet this is not
necessary either to the termination of the disease, or the appearance
of purulent matter in the urine.   A more common result is puru-

lent or suppurative inflammation of the fine mucous membrane of the *pelvis* and *infundibula,* and consequent distension of the renal tubular cones, but without destruction of their substance. It should never be forgotten, that the presence of a urinary concretion in the pelvis or ureter may cause inflammation and suppuration without that suppuration affecting the proper substance of the kidney; and that suppuration of the kidney may take place without the presence of a concretion in the *pelvis,* or ureter, or any of the *infundibula.* If the stone be by any means expelled and carried into the bladder, the purulent matter may also escape, and after being discharged, the kidney may contract; and the morbid secretion may cease. Hence it is found that discharges of purulent urine may take place for some time, and eventually cease, without preventing the patient from recovering temporarily.

More frequently, however, the reverse is the case. Though the calculus may be discharged, the purulent matter may not be evacuated, or the purulent inflammation continues; and even the stone itself, forming a sort of cyst of the pelvis or ureter, may remain firmly impacted, and prevent the issue either of urine or purulent matter. In either case, the expansion of the kidney (*Nephrotasia*) continues and increases; the tubular cones are distended, compressed, and extruded; the *papillæ* are compressed, flattened, and almost obliterated; the cortical covering is also distended and extenuated; and the exquisite stage of the lesion already described as *Nephropyema* (*Pyonephria*) is fully established. Even ulceration of the parts around the concretion, wherever it happens to be fixed, may take place, and give rise to great and irreparable ravages in the renal tissue, and that of the contiguous organs.

§ 5. It is not uninteresting to trace the subsequent progress of this disorder, and to observe what singular and extraordinary efforts are sometimes made to counteract the mischief in the kidneys, and its effects on the constitution, and to prevent the immediately fatal effects of the disorder.

Eight different terminations may in this state of the disorder be mentioned.

a. The first termination requiring notice is, that the disease may pass into the chronic state, in which the inflammatory process in the *infundibula* and *pelvis* continues, causing the secretion of purulent matter, which is voided with the urine, (*pyuria*), and attended with quick pulse, nocturnal sweatings, wasting, and all the symp-

toms of hectic fever.   It is further requisite to observe, that this
state is liable to alternate with, or terminate in, an acute attack of
the disease, in which the purulent secretion is suddenly suspended
or stopped, pain in the renal region is induced or augmented, with
the other symptoms of renal inflammation, and terminate not unusually, if not checked, in sopor and fatal coma, with urinous exhalation from the surface of the body.

In those instances in which a calculus remains impacted in the
pelvis or ureter, these attacks are several times repeated, until the
kidney is very much enlarged, distended, and attenuated by the
large quantity of purulent or sero-purulent fluid, which never being allowed to escape, is progressively augmented by the addition
of that which is secreted at each new attack.   Death seems then
to be the united result of the repeated inflammatory attacks, and
the lesion inflicted on the structure of the kidney.   Of this mode
of termination instances are given by Tulpius,* and Job a Meek'-
ren,† and a melancholy and remarkable example occurred, in 1821,
in the person of a medical practitioner of this city, in whose body
the left kidney was found dilated so much, as to contain nearly
three pounds of sero-purulent fluid, which had been the product of
several attacks of renal inflammation, occasioned by the presence
of a small mulberry calculus, weighing only 1½ grain, impacted in
the upper end of the ureter.‡

In such circumstances, there is reason to believe that the diseased kidney ceases to secrete urine; since its texture is so much
injured, and its circulation is employed in the maintenance of a
morbid secretion; and that the functions of both are performed by
the sound one.

b. In the second place, ulceration may take place through the
pelvis or ureter, and purulent matter escape into the lumbar and
pelvic adipo-cellular tissue.   Such a termination is necessarily fatal,
as it induces a sloughy mortified state of the lumbar and pelvic
adipose membrane, the effect of which on the system at large is
speedily fatal.   Of this mode of termination a good case is given

* Nicolai Tulpii Observationes Medicæ, 8vo.   Amstelod. 1652 and 1672.   Lib. ii.
cap. 45.
† Jobi A Meek'ren, Chirurgi Amstelodamensis Observationes Medico-Chirurgicæ
Amstelodami 1682, cap. xlv.   The Memoirs of the Royal Society of Medicine (1780–81
Paris, p. 272) ; Fourcroy, Medecine Eclairée par les Sciences Physique, ii. p. 253.
‡ Edinburgh Medical and Surgical Journal, vol. xviii. p. 557 and 561.

by Mr Howship, in case 7, (p. 43), in a person between 60 and 70 years of age, in whom the matter eventually passed by a small round ulcerated aperture of the peritonæum into the general abdominal cavity. A similar case is recorded by Chomel.*

c. In the third place, the matter may pass directly through the *peritonæum* into the cavity of the abdomen, establishing a direct communication between the *infundibula* and *pelvis* of the kidney and the latter cavity. This is mentioned by Chopart; but it seems to be questioned by Chomel, because no cases are specified by the former. It is proper to mention, therefore, that an instance of this mode of suppurative destruction is afforded in the sixth case by Mr Howship, (p. 49,) taking place in the person of a boy of 7, who had laboured under symptoms of urinary disorder from the age of 18 months, and in whom both kidneys, but especially the left, presented marks of suppurative inflammation, and a communication had been established between the surface of the left kidney and the cavity of the peritonæum, and the matter had thereby escaped into the interior of the latter.

d. A fourth mode in which the purulent matter may escape, is into the transverse arch of the colon, especially if it be the left kidney. Of this mode of issue Fantoni records an instance; and in the year 1832, in inspecting the body of a woman destroyed by cholera, I found a state of parts which shows that the same issue must have taken place in that case. In the transverse arch of the colon was a fistulous opening leading into the pelvis of the right kidney, in which and the expanded renal substance was contained a large calculus.

e. In the fifth place, the communication may open, and the matter be evacuated into the sigmoid flexure or rectum. Of this an instance is recorded by Bonnet† in the person of a young woman.

f. A sixth mode in which renal abscess has been observed to procure an outlet for itself is by producing ulcerative destruction of the diaphragm and *pleura*, and evacuating its contents into the lungs and *bronchi*. Of this De Haen gives an instance, in which, in the person of a young man of 15, after symptoms of renal inflammation, purulent matter was first voided with the urine, and,

---

* Archives Gen. xliii. p. 12.

† Journal Hebdomadaire, Tome vii. p. 397. Archives Generales, Tome xxiv. p. 278.

after the interval of three or four years, during which the individual recovered his health so far as to be able to marry, he was attacked with symptoms of intense inflammation of the chest, he expectorated fetid sanious reddish purulent matter, and had most laborious breathing; and eventually he died hectic. It was then found that the left kidney was dilated into a large sac or cyst without any trace of the original gland; the ureter was distended to the size of the small intestine, and was filled with purulent matter; a large aperture was found in the diaphragm, forming a direct communication between the left kidney and the lower lobe of the left lung, which was destroyed, with the lower part of the upper lobe.*

g. A seventh mode in which the renal abscess may procure an issue for its contents is into and through the liver or spleen, the right kidney by the former, the left by the latter, towards the surface. This mode of termination, which is assigned by Peter Frank, is received with doubt by Chomel. It may be observed, however, that Mr Howship gives in his eighth case, (p. 47), the history of an attack of inflammation of the right kidney, in which a large abscess of the right kidney pointed over the region of the liver, and was there opened, and discharged five pints and a half of matter; and though after death, which took place forty-two days after the operation, the substance of the liver was found healthy, its inferior surface was united by adhesion to the superior extremity of the right kidney.

h. In the eighth place, the matter of the renal abscess may open a path for itself posteriorly through the back part of the pelvis or ureter or kidney, and the dorso-lumbar cellular tissue, muscles, and fasciae, so as to point on one or other side of the spine. Of all the modes of proceeding outward, this is the one which has been most frequently observed; and as it has often suggested to surgeons the expediency of making an incision in suspected cases of renal concretion, it is chiefly in the writings of surgeons that accounts of it are given.

Of this mode of issue, instances are recorded by Fantoni, Tulpius,† Job a Meek'ren,‡ Cheselden,§ Petit.‖

The concretion giving rise to ulceration, first of the kidney or its

---

* *Ratio Medendi*, Tom. x. p. 103.
† IV. chap. 27.   ‡ Cap. xliv.   § Anatomy, Book iv. chap. 1.
‖ Oeuvres Posthumes, iii. p. 73, and in the Memoirs of the Academy of Chirurgery, ii. p. 233.

pelvis, or the top of the ureter, causes at the same time suppurative and adhesive inflammation, proceeding gradually to the surface, where it forms a prominent tumour, red, painful, soft, and fluctuating, and, either a spontaneous opening taking place or after an incision, matter is discharged, and not unusually with that one or more urinary calculi, or sabulous matter and urine. The swelling subsides after the first discharge of matter ; but the aperture evinces no disposition to close, and matter continues to be discharged for months or years, while a long sinus or fistula leading to the kidney is maintained. It is then a renal fistula, discharging matter, and sometimes urine and sand, or urinary concretions. If the opening happen to become closed, much pain is produced, and all the former symptoms of nephritis ensue, until fresh suppuration takes place, and the aperture is reopened. Hence Lassus,[*] Monteggia,[†] Boyer,[‡] and other surgeons, recommend that the fistula be kept open by a bougie, a cannula, prepared sponge, or a bit of charpie, in short, by some dilating body.

As in most of the cases now specified, the local disorder of the kidney, if it do not prove immediately fatal, gives rise to more or less hectic fever, with wasting and loss of strength. The condition of the system thus induced was early designated by the name of renal consumption, (*phthisis renalis*)[§]. This name, though retained by Hildenbrand and several moderns, is not proper, because it is liable to lead to confusion ; since the term *phthisis* is no longer general, but has been by most modern nosologists restricted to the particular form of wasting which depends on tubercular destruction of the lungs. A more convenient appellation would be *tabes renalis*.

§ 6. GANGRENE.—The question whether renal inflammation ever terminates in gangrene has been proposed by Chomel. Fabricius Hildanus mentions that in his own son, a boy of 9, he found the kidneys and neighbouring parts inflamed and degenerated into gangrene; and Chopart records the case of a person of 62, who died on the ninth day of symptoms of nephritis, in whose body he found the kidneys bulky, livid, mottled with blackish spots, and easily lacerable. In neither of these cases does the pathologist re-

---

[*] Pathologie Chirurgicale, i. xxvii. p. 163.
[†] Istituzione Chirurgiche.
[‡] Traité des Maladies Chirurgicales, T. viii. p. 505, 508.
[§] Jac. Fabricii, Disputatio de Phthisi Renali. Giessæ, 1699.

cognize positive evidence of gangrene; and Chomel is therefore inclined to doubt the termination; but he allows that, in cases of persons who have died after long continued suppuration of the kidney, some parts of the suppurating surface presenting the dark colour, or grayish, the peculiar odour, the softness, and the absence of apparent organization observed in mortified sloughs.

As an instance of this lesion, Walter records a curious case which took place in the person of a young woman who had laboured for many years under violent pains in the region of the kidneys; and who was at length attacked with inability to void urine, in place of which she had a continual discharge of purulent matter, mixed with blood and fine sand. The belly swelled so much that she was imagined to be pregnant; but she suddenly fell down dead. Upon inspecting the body, Walter found the right kidney enlarged into a great spheroidal swelling, ten inches in the long diameter, six in the transverse, its substance of a brownish-red colour, very soft, and so easily lacerable, that on the slightest touch an opening was made. Internally it was altogether consumed, and its cavity was filled with an astonishing quantity of coagulated blood, purulent matter, and dissolved renal substance. This mixture, which resembled a sort of soup, enclosed two concretions, one weighing two drachms, the other two scruples, which could not be discovered till some of the mixture was emptied. On further investigation, Walter found that some of the large renal vessels had been eroded and laid open, and to this he ascribed the sudden death of the woman, and the quantity of blood found in the kidney.*

This, I think, must be regarded as a pretty unequivocal case of gangrene of the kidney. The termination must, nevertheless, be regarded as rare.

Vogel gives, in a man affected with jaundice, an example of the kidney labouring under gangrene. The chief characters are masses of clotted and decomposed blood disseminated through the parenchyma of the gland.†

Mortification of the perinephral adipose membrane is a common consequence of inflammation of that tissue. But it belongs to another head.

§ 7. *a.* SUPPURATIVE INFLAMMATION OF THE KIDNEY.—Though

---

* Einige Krankheiten der Nieren und Harnblase. 4to. Berlin, 1800. § 11, seite 5.

† Tabula xxiii.

I have represented suppuration of the kidney to commence, in ordinary circumstances, in the interior of the *calyces* and pelvis, and rather to produce a sort of expansion and distension of the gland than an actual purulent destruction, it is, nevertheless, necessary to say, that purulent destruction does take place in the substance of the kidney. Of this I have seen several instances. In these cases, the whole kidney was completely converted into a quantity of thick purulent matter, partly like thin putty, partly more fluid, all of which was contained within the renal capsule, like atheromatous matter in a bag or cyst.

In all the cases of this disorder, excepting one, the patients presented no evident or prominent symptoms which could lead to the suspicion that the kidney was in a state of inflammatory disease. In one case, death took place after an obscure illness of a few days. In the case which I have mentioned as an exception, the patient was hectic, and had uneasiness in the bladder and along the ureters; but, as it was plain that the lungs were tuberculated and presented open *vomicae*, the hectic symptoms were justly ascribed to the presence of the pulmonary disorganization.   If we say that this lesion is of strumous origin, we merely give another answer, without coming more closely to the explanation.   It seems as if the whole renal tissue, cortical and tubular, were liquefied or dissolved in purulent matter.

b. Small patches of purulent matter are occasionally observed in the cortical or in the tubular part of the kidney, without apparent connection with inflammation of the *calyces*.   These, I think, must be admitted to be of strumous origin.   In one instance, in which I witnessed this state of the kidneys, it took place in the body of a sickly strumous boy of fifteen years, who died of lobular *pneumonia*; and it is usually seen in young subjects.

c. In some instances of inflamed vein, purulent matter has been found in the substance of the kidney.   This has been regarded as metastatic; but it is most correct to look on it as transported from the vein inflamed to this in common with other internal organs.

§ 8. *Cartilaginous induration of the Ureters and Pelvis, producing or accompanied with Renal Inflammation.*—It is proper to mention here, that the ureters and pelvis are liable to a particular kind of chronic inflammation, inducing great thickening and induration of the mucous membrane, with roughness of its inner surface.   In the most marked case of the disorder which I have seen, this state extended from the bladder upwards, through the ureters on both sides into the pelvis and calyces of the kidneys. The ureters were rendered thick and firm like cartilage; their size was increased to about five or six times the usual dimensions; their canal was also enlarged; and their firmness prevented them from collapsing, as in the healthy state. The morbid state now mentioned appeared to have originated in the mucous membrane, but eventually to have affected the other tissues. It was difficult to say whether it had commenced in the membrane of the *calyces* or in that of the ureter, and extended to the former; for both were affected in nearly equal degrees.

This change was accompanied with painful and difficult micturition, the urine containing puriform mucus and sand; with quick pulse, much thirst, hot dry skin, alternating with shiverings and sweatings, wasting, loss of strength, a most anxious miserable expression of the countenance, and slight incurvation of the person, as if under the suffering of much pain. The disease had been of long duration, at least several months.

§ 9. *Disease of the Kidneys simulating disease of the Spinal Chord; and inflammation of the Calycine Membrane from injury or disease of the Spinal Chord.*—A singular effect of renal inflammation and suppuration is to induce *paraplegia* and symptoms of diseased spine. It has been long known that injuries and diseases chiefly of an inflammatory character in the spine or spinal cord, are liable to be followed by various morbid states of the urinary secretion, which is generally rendered alkalescent or ammoniacal, sometimes deposits the ammoniaco-magnesian phosphate, sometimes the carbonate of ammonia. Bellingeri had observed, that in animals, after experiments on the spinal chord, inflammation was liable to attack the kidneys and the *peritoneum,* and render the former red and vascular, and cover them with lymph. Mr Stanley has shown, by a judicious selection of cases, that when the spinal chord is supposed to be diseased or injured, either directly or in consequence of disease or injury of the vertebræ, causing pain in the back and *paraplegia,* the symptoms so produced do not originate from disease of either the *vertebræ,* the chord, or the membranes, all of which are sound, but from inflammation or suppuration of the kidneys, in which in general are found collections of purulent matter. From such cases it must be inferred, as Mr Stanley has done, that disease originating in the kidneys simulates, and may give rise to disease in the spinal chord, probably by a reflected influence from the diseased gland through its nerves to those connected with the spinal chord. It may conversely be inferred, that in any morbid state of the spinal chord, the impaired influence of the nerves over the renal action allowing the urine to be secreted in the kidney in an alkaline state, gives rise to a new train of evils, by the irritation necessarily induced in the tubular part of the kidney and in the calycine membrane. The ammoniacal urine then irritates perhaps both the cortical and the tubular part of the glands, and must certainly irritate the calycine membrane, and is the cause of the inflammatory states which it often presents. On this head I refer the reader to the paper of Mr Stanley,* and to what I have in another place said under the section on *Myelitis*.†

The PROGNOSIS in *Nephritis* is in general not favourable. But it is more favourable when the disorder is the result of external violence, than when it is the effect of any internal cause. In gouty and calculous patients, the prognosis is unfavourable, because it generally after one attack recurs several times, until it undermines the strength by renal or vesical calculus, or by the formation of renal abscess, or by total suppression (*Ischuria renalis*), causes speedy death.

Renal abscess or *fistula*, though almost uniformly leading to death, is not necessarily a fatal disorder ; but in whatever of the forms specified it appears, life is always maintained in a most uncomfortable and precarious condition. The least unfavourable is, where none of the unnatural communications or *fistulæ* have taken place, and where the purulent matter has procured an outlet for itself through the ureter into the bladder, and thence been discharged externally. In some instances, recovery has been effected after this event had taken place. Forest mentions (lib. xxiv. obs. 37), the case of a priest, who, after discharging purulent urine for three months, and being reduced to the greatest emaciation, recovered under the use of proper regimen, consisting chiefly of milk. M. Chomel records a case from M. Meniere of the Hotel Dieu, in which a similar recovery must have taken place. The right kidney was shrunk into an irregular mass, about the size of a pigeon's egg, forming a species of membranous sac, consisting of the *calyces*, pelvis, and ureter, containing about half an ounce of clear fluid,

* On Irritation of the Spinal Chord and its Nerves in connection with Disease in the Kidneys. By Edward Stanley, F. R. S., &c. Medico-Chirurgical Transactions, xviii. p. 260. London, 1833.

† Elements of Practice of Medicine, Vol. ii. p. 398.

but totally void of any trace of cortical or tubular portions. This constitutes what some have named Atrophy of the kidney, which, doubtless, is the effect of suppurative destruction, followed by contraction of the remaining parts.

Renal inflammation must be distinguished from the symptoms produced by a calculus in the ureter, from lumbago, from *psoitis* and lumbar abscess, from *peritonitis*, intestinal inflammation, colic, granular disease of the kidneys, and from spinal irritation and inflammation, and disease of the spine generally.

§ 10. GRANULAR DISEASE—STEATOSIS—STEAROSIS of Gluge. This consists in a change in the structure of the kidney, especially its cortical or secreting portion, in which it is penetrated with grayish, whitish, yellowish, or fawn-coloured adipose matter, in the form of minute granules; and in which, at the same time, the density of the urine is diminished, and the urine contains less urea than it ought, and more or less albumen or serum, the presence of which may be shown by the application of heat, or the addition of any of the acids or the metallic salts.

The texture of the kidney, especially its cortical portion, is liable to become changed in various modes, and it presents in the different stages of each different appearances.

It is rare to observe kidneys in the first stage of this disease in any of its forms, as it is not at that period by itself fatal; and it may be doubted whether it has been seen in the incipient stage. The following varieties, however, may be regarded as the most usual.

1. The kidney may be of a very dark-red, or brown colour, much loaded with blood, and its vessels very much enlarged. The tubular is always of a darker colour than the cortical part; but the latter is in this case extremely dark-coloured. When it is divided by a longitudinal incision, the surface of the section is altogether much darker than natural, being a deep chocolate brown, while the cortical portion appears, though darker than natural, yet lighter coloured than the tubular, and presents the aspect of a brownish red mass, surrounding and enclosing dark-brown, or amber-brown coloured tubular cones. The outer surface of the gland, stripped of its tunic, is also very dark-coloured, reddish brown, inclining to chocolate red, is less smooth than natural, and may even be a little rough and irregular, presenting small depressions containing blood-vessels in clusters, and the gland is in general, in this variety and

stage of the disorder, soft and flaccid. The whole gland is large, flabby, and very vascular.

This form of the disorder is seen chiefly in persons who have died from fever or pneumonia, or pleurisy, or in children with symptoms of affection of the brain.

2. In one variety next to be mentioned, the kidneys are large, soft, and flaccid; and when the tunic is stripped, the exterior surface, though less deep in colour, is still more irregular than in the last mentioned variety. The colour, indeed, begins to assume a gray or fawn tint, the brown being less deep, and giving place to chestnut-brown or yellowish-brown. The irregular appearance on the surface is produced by numerous depressions with alternate elevations. In the last case, the depressions are so few in number that they leave between them considerable smooth spaces of the outer surface of the kidney. But in this variety the spaces between the depressions are so small, and the depressions are so numerous, that the whole outer surface appears to consist of manifold alternate pits and elevations. These pits are remarkable for containing little clusters of red vessels. Sometimes, if the surface be attentively inspected by the eye, and always by the aid of the microscope, minute gray-coloured bodies like grains may be recognized deposited in the cortical substance, decidedly differing from the latter in the lighter colour which they present. Upon dividing such a kidney as this by a longitudinal section, the change in structure is still more conspicuous. The cortical portion has throughout become of a lighter colour than natural, and is generally some shade of orange, fawn, or yellow. Thus it may be buff-orange, which is a light stone colour, or reddish orange,—a salmon red tint, or deep reddish orange, or it may vary between these and honey-yellow, sienna-yellow, or ochre-yellow. When inspected carefully, even by a good practised eye, and much more by the aid of a glass of moderate magnifying powers, this change in colour may be traced to innumerable little granular bodies, infiltrated, as it were, or deposited in the cortical substance, varying in size from the point to the head of a pin. These bodies consist of the epithelial cells of the *tubuli* infiltrated with fat, and the *tubuli* themselves infiltrated with albuminous deposit. The cortical or secreting matter of the kidney has then in general lost most of its peculiar striated arrangement; and presents the appearance of reddish orange, or honey yellow, or fawn-coloured matter, enclosing the tubular cones, and

appearing as it were to encroach on their bounds and pass between them. The tubular cones, though retaining their colour, seem then rather smaller than usual, and appear like reddish oval-shaped bodies, enclosed, as it were, in the gray or orange-coloured cortical matter.

The extent to which this transformation proceeds varies in different kidneys and in different portions of the same kidney. In some cases it commences in one of the extremities of the gland, and either extremity is then seen to be more remarkably changed than other parts. In other instances, it commences in the centre of the gland or rather the central part of the cortical matter; and then this part is most completely transformed.

In consequence of the peculiar change in the colour of the surface, the pits in which are of a darker colour than the elevations and intermediate portions, the kidney now described is said to be mottled.

3. Without increase in size or change in consistence, the cortical part of the kidney may be penetrated or infiltrated with granular albuminous matter in various modes and degrees.

a. In one variety which appears to be comparatively in an early, though not an incipient stage, when the gland is stripped of its tunic, the surface is irregular, rough, or as it were sprinkled with fine sand, of a reddish gray colour, with more of the former than the latter; and part of the cortical matter not unusually comes off adhering to the tunic. The surface presents also small hollows or pits, containing blood-vessels as in the last variety; and, indeed, this appearance is one of the most constant. When the surface is closely inspected, numerous minute reddish gray granules may be recognized, not aggregated together, but separately infiltrated into the cortical matter. When the gland is divided by a longitudinal section, part of the striated texture of the cortical part is still recognized in the form of reddish-coloured streaks, extending from the circumference to the tubular cones; but all the rest of the cortical part of the kidney is of reddish gray colour, lighter than usual, and when minutely inspected either by the eye or with the aid of a lens, small cream-coloured or grayish coloured granular bodies are observed dispersed through the cortical matter.

In such a kidney as this, if coloured glue or isinglass be thrown into the blood-vessels, it does not perfectly, as in the healthy state, fill the cortical matter of the gland. The healthy parts only, or those which still retain the striated texture, are reddened by the injected size; while the diseased and gray-coloured portions receive little or none of the injected size.

In general, kidneys in this state are of the natural size, and, instead of being soft and flaccid, are either of normal consistence, or a little firmer than natural.

b. In a variety, which is perhaps in a more advanced stage of progress, the outer surface of the gland, if stripped of its capsule, is still more extensively marked with pits containing clusters of blood-vessels, so that the whole surface is irregular and vascular.   These blood-vessels are star-like or asteroid, branch-like or ramiform, or in the shape of small dots and points, stigmatoid ; and, according to the number, the size, and the aggregation of these clusters, the external surface of the gland is red and vascular or otherwise.   Besides this vascular redness in pits and hollows of the surface, the whole gland is moulded as it were into irregular large hollows and elevations, so as to seem tuberculated or mammillated.   Of the parts not vascular the colour is a sort of stone-gray or light reddish yellow, or fawn-coloured, in considerable masses, so as to render the surface mottled or rather marbled.

A longitudinal section of a kidney in this state often shows a very complete change in the cortical texture.   It presents little or no remains of striated matter ; but the whole cortical portion is one uniform mass of yellowish gray, or buff-orange, or sienna yellow, or cream-yellow.   In this case the new matter is not merely infiltrated, but it is so diffused that the cortical portion is transformed into it.   A few tubular cones still remain more or less complete ; but either they become transformed into the gray-coloured deposit, or the transformed cortical matter has so much encroached on them as to have diminished much their usual dimensions.

The shape of the kidney in this variety sometimes presents a singular deviation from the natural standard.   The gland is tapered at each end, so as to present an apex more or less acuminated, instead of the usual rounded end of the gland.   I am unable to say, whether this change in figure is congenital or the effect of the disease.

The cortical matter of the kidneys, so far transformed as in this variety, is almost altogether incapable of receiving injection.

4. In the next varieties, it may seem doubtful whether they are different from the last, or only the most advanced stages of the transformation and deposition.

The external surface of the kidney is of a slate-gray or leaden-gray colour, and presents, or may be said to consist of, numerous globular granules aggregated together. These globules vary in size from a small pin head to a millet seed, or the grains of sago, and are mostly of the sienna yellow, or cream-yellow, or stone-gray colour, but in some parts they are of leaden-gray. Various patches also of the kidney present this leaden-gray tint, which may be traced partly to the intermediate spaces or lines, partly to the globular granules themselves. None of the striated texture of the cortical matter can be recognized in this variety, in which the cortical matter appears to be completely converted or transformed into the new formation. In the longitudinal section of this all that is seen is the appearance of a uniform mass of sienna-yellow animal matter, without trace of distinct organization, sometimes minute granular bodies, but almost never any striated texture.

The tubular cones retain a colour more or less bright red, and, being enclosed in this buff-coloured morbid texture, present a striking contrast to the state of the healthy kidney. Sometimes they are diminished in size, and sometimes in the section made one or two of them seems either to have disappeared, while in the place which they should have occupied, buff-coloured matter is deposited, or to have been converted into a firm, solid, gray-coloured matter. This variety of change is also unsusceptible of injection.

The kidneys in this state are almost invariably firm and hard, and are sometimes smaller than usual.

5. It is very difficult, if not impracticable, to distinguish all the various forms of this buff-coloured or sienna-yellow transformation of the cortical matter of the kidney. Most of them differ chiefly in the shades of colour which the transformed cortical matter assumes, and the degree in which the striated matter has disappeared, and in which, consequently, the kidney has become incapable of receiving injection. The most usual colour in this stage, which is perhaps the concluding, is some shade of sienna-yellow, sometimes inclining to buff-orange, or to tile-red. In some rare cases the colour of the new deposit is lemon-yellow or gamboge-yellow. In others, it is of a tawny colour. In all these cases the kidney is in general small and firm, sometimes almost cartilaginous.

The kidney is liable to the same kind of change in the dropsy which follows scarlet fever. In some instances, the cortical portion is merely mottled or marbled, and its surface presents superficial hollows containing clusters of blood-vessels, while the section of the gland shows part of it changed in colour, though with remains of the striated texture. The change most usual in this class of cases is buff-orange, or tile-red; but in some instances it is so light as to be of a straw-colour or sienna-yellow.

6. In all the cases now mentioned, the transformation either affects chiefly, or is confined wholly, to the cortical matter of the gland. In a small proportion of cases, however, it either affects first and mostly the tubular portion of the kidney, or it affects that after previously affecting the cortical portion. In either case, it renders the tubular cones so affected very hard, almost cartilaginous, white or gray-white, or sienna-yellow. The nature of this change and its effects on the tubuli are not known. The tubuli are still pervious; but their tissue is probably thickened and indurated. The cortical matter is at the same time of a buff-colour, or tile-red, or sienna-yellow, but differing in shade from the colour of the tubular matter.

In some of these varieties of renal disorganization, the kidney externally is marked by fissures so as to appear lobulated like the fœtal kidney. It is uncertain whether this is the remains of the original fœtal structure, or whether it is to be regarded as a return to the type of the fœtal structure, as the effect of disease.

To complete the morbid anatomy of this disease it is necessary to advert to the state in which other organs are occasionally found.

The subcutaneous cellular membrane is in general more or less infiltrated with serous or sero-albuminous fluid.

The serous membranes often present marks of inflammation, as lymph, soft or firm, purulent fluid, masses of lymph, and adhesions between their free surfaces. In the sub-arachnoid tissue of the brain serous fluid is sometimes effused. But the parts most commonly presenting lymph or purulent fluid are the pleura and peritoneum. In other instances, sero-sanguine fluid alone is found within the cavities of these membranes. In several cases I have met with lymph in the pericardium.

The bronchial membrane is often lined with puriform mucus, or muco-purulent matter streaked with blood; and the other appearances of chronic bronchial inflammation are manifest.

The lungs are in several cases affected with pneumonia; being in a state of red or gray hepatization. In some instances tubercles and vomicæ are found. In some there are the remains of pulmonary apoplexy.

In a certain proportion of cases the heart is found hypertrophied; the mitral and aortic valves are ossified, and the apertures contracted.

The intestinal mucous membrane is in persons who have present-ed diarrhœa during life, rough, villous, and vascular ; the follicles of Peyer are enlarged ; more frequently the isolated follicles are enlarged, prominent or ulcerated ; and in some instances the isolated follicles of the colon are found the seat of ulceration.

In a small proportion of cases the liver is found enlarged and its *acini* of a nutmeg colour. In some it has been found affected with *kirrhosis ;* and in a few with adipescence.

The bladder is generally much shrunk, and contains a small quantity of urine, which when heated furnishes more or less coagulable matter, sometimes in considerable quantity.

The blood generally contains urea.

The period at which the change now described in the structure of the kidney commences varies under different circumstances. I have seen a partial and limited form of it affecting one portion of the cortical matter between the second and third years. One specimen I met with in a complete form affecting the whole cortical matter with the buff-orange transformation, in a boy between six and seven years.

Of its rate of progress almost nothing is known, At first the change was observed mostly in the kidneys of adults ; and in them there were few or no means of ascertaining the exact period at which the disease began. From various circumstances, however, which appear in the course of the symptoms, it may be inferred, that it takes some time before it seriously impairs the functions of the gland, and that years may elapse from the first commencement of the disorder to the time, when the change in structure is so considerable as to impede in a vital degree the function of the kidney.

PATHOLOGICAL DEDUCTIONS.—Regarding the nature of this change, and its origin, various opinions are entertained. Dr Bright, who first directed attention to this change in the structure of the kidney, regards it as a species of degeneration ; but thinks that there is in the kidneys in the early stage a process of slow inflammation, which lays the foundation of their future change in structure.[*] Granular degeneration, as it is usually found after death by long-continued bad health, with or without *anasarca*, Dr Christison regards as essentially a chronic disease ; but allows that, when the kidneys are dark-coloured, flabby, and enlarged, in connection with coagulable urine and eventual suppression, they may have been in the state of ordinary inflammation ; (*nephritis.*[†]) It is

---

[*] Reports of Medical Cases, Vol. i. London, 1827, p. 72.
[†] On Granular Degeneration of the Kidneys, p. 10 and 11.

also to be observed, that while several of the appearances found in the kidneys after death denote unusual congestion of the cortical matter, in the early stage the symptoms of pain and weight in the, region of the loins, dryness of the skin, and thirst, indicate the presence of a febrile or inflammatory state of the system.

M. Martin Solon regards the disease as a hyperemic, that is, a congestive inflammatory state of the kidneys, consequent on irritation of their vessels from the use of stimulating drinks; and to this hyperemic state he ascribes all the early symptoms, and the sero-albuminous state of the urine.* The granular interstitial deposit, and the yellow degeneration, he considers as the effect or remote consequence of the previous hyperemic state, for this reason, that the marks of hyperemia are still found associated with the yellow degeneration.   In some other passages of his work, however, he questions the necessary presence of inflammation in the disease.

M. Rayer, entertaining no doubt of the inflammatory nature of the disease, applies to it the name of *nephritis albuminosa*, and distinguishes it into two varieties, the acute and chronic.   He is indeed the most decided and confident advocate for the inflammatory nature of the disease that has yet appeared; and his views have been espoused, explained, and defended by his pupil, M. Littré.   The chief grounds on which M. Rayer maintains the inflammatory nature of the fawn-coloured degeneration of the kidney are, the vascular redness of the gland in the early stage of the distemper, the enlargement or swelling of the gland, the occasional presence of pain, and the general presence of feverishness; and at a later period the presence of vascular spots and patches, with the grayish or gray-yellow granular deposit.   He is also of opinion, that the red points and spots seen in the substance of the kidney in the early stage of the distemper, (first form of M. Rayer,) in general correspond to the glandules of Malpighi, greatly injected with blood.

Dr Gulliver showed in 1843, that in kidneys affected by this disease, fatty globules and crystalline plates of cholesterine can be seen by the microscope; while Dr Davy obtained from them margarine, cholesterine, and a trace of oleine.†

Gluge maintains, from microscopical examination of kidneys in this state, that the infiltrated matter is in general oil or fat.

In the first form, which is that in which the surface of the kidney is yellowish with red points and millet-seed-like granulations, in-

* De l'Albuminurie, &c. p. 258.
† Edinburgh Medical and Surgical Journal, vol. lx. p. 162.   Edinburgh, 1843.

flammation, with inflammatory globules and purulent matter, is associated with fatty infiltration or *steatosis*. The *tubuli*, especially those of the cortical substance, are filled with fat globules large and small. These distend the tubuli, the convolutions of which form the granulations, and afterwards appear more in the medullary (straight tubular) substance. At length the fat globules are effused between the *tubuli*, and form masses of 10, 15, or more fat-globules, which are occasionally enclosed within a membrane. The Malpighian bodies and the capillary vessels are at first filled with blood; but in the further progress of the disease they are bloodless and pale. The vessels of the medullary substance undergo a like change, though to a smaller degree. Not unfrequently the membrane of the *tubuli* entirely disappears. The fat globules observe in their mode of deposition at first the direction of these *tubuli;* afterwards this is lost, and a confused mass of fat-globules takes their place. In rare instances the fat-globules are deposited not at first in the tubuli, but in the blood-vessels and Malpighian bodies.

In the second form, in which the kidneys are red-brown in their cortical as well as in their medullary substance, and in which, in consequence of a reddish striated arrangement of the medullary, the two portions can scarcely be distinguished. The renal substance is recognized as a reddish, soft, almost soluble, jelly-like matter, in which only the cellular frame-work with wide meshes appears as a separate solid element; no trace of tubules or blood-vessels is to be found either in the cortical or medullary matter; and fat globules, scattered among tubules and empty colourless Malpighian bodies, lie in the residual cellular texture of the glands.

In the third form, in which the outline of the kidneys remains unchanged or diminished, and their outer surface and the section of the cortical substance is occupied with prominent pisiform granulations, giving the glands a rough aspect and hardish appearance ; sometimes inflammatory globules are found with fat-globules ; yet these are always in smaller proportion ; the granulations contain many urinary tubules dilated by a yellowish granular mass and fat-globules, which are also deposited between the tubules.

In short, the fat globules may be deposited within the tubules, without them, and between them, and without or around the Malpighian bodies.*

According to Vogel, the cortical substance in one form of the

* Atlas der Pathologischen Anatomie. Stearose der Niere, Taf. 3.

disease, which is the inflammatory, is thick, white-yellowish, variegated with red dots and lines, and very compact like lard. The
substance contains little blood. The vessels of the Malpighian
bodies are much less distinct than in the normal state. The tubules are indistinct and confused, and between and around them
plastic matter is infiltrated. A similar infiltration is observed
among the medullary tubules.*

The views of Gluge have been confirmed in this country by the
researches of Dr Johnson and Mr Toynbee. The former believing
that the epithelial cells of the healthy kidney contain a minute
quantity of oil in the form of yellowish highly refracting globules,
maintains that granular kidney consists primarily in an exaggera-
tion of the fatty matter which naturally exists in small quantities
in the epithelial cells of the healthy gland. The epithelial cells
of the tubules may be in every degree and stage of distension with
fat-globules, until the cell is so filled that the nucleus is no longer
visible. The Malpighian bodies are the only parts which escape,
a few particles only being scattered over their interior.

The different modes and degrees in which the fatty deposit takes
place give rise to the different external appearances of the kidney.
As the accumulation of fat increases, the kidney becomes granular
or mottled on the surface. The smooth mottled kidneys are those
in which the greatest number of the tubes in the cortical portion
are almost uniformly distended. The granular and atrophied or
small shrunk kidneys are those in which the accumulation of fat
takes place less rapidly and less uniformly. Some convoluted tubes
become distended with fat, forming prominent granulations ; and
these compressing surrounding parts produce obliteration of vessels
and atrophy of tubes ; and thus the entire gland is wasted and contracted.

Dr Johnson further finds that granular disease of the kidney is
often associated with fatty disease of the liver and the steatomatous
degeneration of the arteries, which is also an adipose deposit.
Among 22 cases of granular disease of the kidney examined in the
summer of 1845, in 17 of these there was in a most marked degree
fatty degeneration of the liver. In 4 of the remaining 5 cases
there was a decided increase of fat in the hepatic cells ; and in only
one case was no increase observed. During the same period Dr
J. met with only 4 cases of fatty liver in which there was no attendant disease of the kidney.

* Julii Vogel Icones Pathologicae, Tabula xxvi. p. 107.

GENERAL AND PATHOLOGICAL ANATOMY.

It is also associated with tuberculation of the lungs, though in a much less common degree.*

Similar are the views of Mr Toynbee. In the first stage fat begins to be deposited in the tubules, in the form of soft white spots. In the second stage he represents the Malpighian tufts to be broken up; the *tubuli* to be greatly enlarged; and the parenchymatous cells enlarged, and containing adipose deposits; and in the third stage the tubuli to be filled with oily cells, granular matter, particles of various sizes, and blood-globules.†

What is the cause of this fatty infiltration? Is it an aberration in nutrition, or the effect of a particular form of inflammation. Though in favour of each of these views various plausible arguments may be adduced, the question appears to be one incapable of positive determination. I add the following remarks, not so much with the intention of solving the difficulty, as in illustration of the general question.

It seems scarcely possible to doubt, that, whether inflammation be the cause of the steatomatous transformation of the kidney or not, the process of inflammation is often present as an accompaniment. Two views, indeed, may be taken of the incipient agent or generating cause, and the nature of this disease. The first is, that inflammation of a particular form attacking the cortical portion of the kidney, may be the cause of all the subsequent changes. The second is, that the cortical portion of the kidney may be liable to an aberration of nutrition, in consequence of which its vessels deposit not the usual proper matter of the cortical portion, but a different substance altogether, in the form of albuminous, caseous or steatomatous matter, in the interstices of the cortical tissue.

The first of these opinions, namely, that inflammation of a peculiar kind, most probably chronic, is the main cause of the several changes, is perhaps in a large proportion of cases true. To the correctness of this conclusion it is not necessary that the change should terminate in suppuration. There may be, and we know that there are, different forms of the inflammatory process; and it is possible that the cortical or secreting portion of the kidney may be

---

* On the Minute Anatomy and Pathology of Bright's Diseases of the Kidney, &c. By George Johnson, M. D., Medico-Chirurgical Transactions, Vol. xxix. p. 1. London, 1846.

† On the Intimate Structure of the Kidney, &c. By Joseph Toynbee, F. R. S. Medico-Chirurg. Trans. Vol. xxix. p. 303.

liable to a peculiar form of the inflammatory process, which may neither be sufficiently rapid to proceed speedily to the disorganiza-tion of the kidney, nor sufficiently violent to evince its presence by well-marked symptoms. That the process, whatever it may be, is chronic, may be inferred from two circumstances. The first is the fact, that the disease is often observed to have existed for months or even years without giving rise to any marked external symptom, excepting occasional diarrhœa, and sometimes attacks of rheumatic pain ; and its existence is never suspected until some new symptom renders it requisite to examine the urine, which is then found to contain serous fluid. Rarely, indeed, do patients apply for assist-ance in the commencement of this distemper ; and it is only when a train of long-continued bad health has prevailed for some time, or a smart attack of acute disease has come on, that the case be-comes known in its true characters. The second circumstance, showing the disease to be most commonly chronic, is, that when its true characters have become known by various unequivocal symp-toms, it does not proceed very rapidly to the fatal termination. Some patients remain under the dropsical symptoms even for months, and eventually recover from them, though the primary disease may not be cured.

That the process is of the nature of vascular injection, afflux, and inflammation, seems to be highly probable, from the following cir-cumstances. The appearances in the kidneys are analogous if not similar to those which are found in other glandular organs when the seat of the congestive and inflammatory process. The dark-brown colour, the increased size, and the loaded state of the vas-cular system of the renal cortical matter in the early stage, are suf-ficiently indicative of a congestive state to justify the inference, that the cortical tissue is unduly loaded with blood, which, as in all con-gested and inflamed organs, moves at first slowly, next accumulates, and then stagnates in the vessels. In those stages, which may be placed after the very first, the vascular pits on the surface of the kidney, with the asteroid clusters of vessels, if not to be regarded as indicative of an inflammatory process, show a great derangement in circulation, which is caused either by the new deposit compres-sing certain vessels, or by some similar obstruction. This process, nevertheless, seems to be peculiar in this respect, that it causes ab-sorption, or at least forms hollows in the cortical portion of the gland. The elevations, according to Dr Johnson, consist each of a set of gorged tubules, presenting itself either at the surface of the gland, or in its substance on the surface of a section.

In those stages of the disorder in which yellowish-gray or fawn-coloured granules are infiltrated as it were through the cortical substance, it seems consistent with correct pathology to ascribe this infiltration to the effect of the inflammatory process. One of the most constant effects of that process, if unchecked, is to give rise to morbid products of albuminous, tyromatous, or steatomatous characters; and it seems reasonable to regard this deposit, which is known to be steatomatous, as the effect of the inflammatory process.

In the aggregated slate-gray granular deposit, the same views are applicable. If the isolated granular infiltration be the effect of inflammatory action, à fortiori, the aggregated granular deposition is the effect of the same action. It appears as the termination of that process, of which the others are earlier and immediate effects.

One of the strongest arguments in favour of the disease originating in congestion or inflammation is found in the fact, that it takes place after the operation of various agents which act as remote causes of inflammation. Thus it often ensues as a sequela of scarlet fever, especially if the patient have been exposed to cold. In that disease, and for some time after the disappearance of the eruption, the action of the skin remains feeble and languid; and the blood, which ought to circulate through the cutaneous vessels, is determined in excessive quantity to the kidneys and other internal organs. The quantity of blood thus thrown upon the different internal organs is greater than their vessels can readily transmit; these, consequently, become unduly loaded and distended; and hence inflammation and often discharges of blood take place at this period in convalescents from scarlet fever; and, among other indications of this, the albuminous and occasionally the colouring matter of the blood is forced through the kidneys, and is found in the urine.

The inflammatory character of this disease may be illustrated by considering the influence of another agent in its production. Nothing seems so certainly to be followed by the formation of granular disease of the kidney as the use of mercury in certain constitutions. In some instances, one single course of mercurial medicines has been known to be followed by the development of the disorder; and in all cases in which repeated courses have been given, the dis-

3

ease is sooner or later observed to ensue. Now it is to be observed, that the use of mercury not only induces an inflammatory state of the system, rendering the blood sizy, and the individual liable to attacks of inflammation in various organs, but it also renders the urine serous.* Mercury further acts as an irritant of the glandular organs ; and it is impossible to doubt that a mineral which we know is circulating with the blood, and carried to all the organs, must induce in organs so vascular and complicated a high degree of orgasm and the deposition of new morbid products.

Another agent, which operates in unduly stimulating the kidney and its vessels, is the use of spirituous liquors. It is well ascertained that among the subjects of this disorder a considerable proportion are addicted to the habitual use of these pernicious stimulants ; and as they are often taken for their supposed diuretic properties, the delusion leads patients to continue their use, until the disease attains its confirmed and incurable stage. We know that the habitual use of these stimulants tends to favour the formation of the steatomatous or fatty degeneration in arteries ; and it seems reasonable to infer that their use is equally capable of favouring this deposition in the kidneys.

Exposure to cold acts both as a predisponent and exciting cause ; and in its operation causes that subverted balance in circulation which generally precedes congestion and inflammation in various internal organs.

It is probable that the primary cause, nevertheless, is seated in disorder of the digestive organs. It is observed, that the use of various indigestible articles of food, as pastry, is followed by a serous state of the urine ; and if a single meal of this kind be followed by such a result, it is easy to see that the frequent use of such articles will induce a habitual or constant serous state of the urine. It is manifest, however, that, as this state cannot be induced without more or less disorder in the vascular system of the kidney, the continued irritation may give rise to the change in structure which is eventually observed in the kidneys of persons who have become victims of this disease.

The second opinion, that the glandular deposit is the effect of a peculiar aberration in nutrition, may be true without being incon-

---

* Observations on the Dropsy which succeeds Scarlet Fever, Art. xv. ; and on the Presence of the Red Matter and Serum in the Blood in the Urine of Dropsy after Scarlet Fever, Art. xvii. By Charles Wells, M. D., &c. Transactions of a Society, iii. p. 230. London, 1812.

sistent with the presence of the inflammatory process, either as a cause or as a concomitant. Every aberration in nutrition is preceded and accompanied with a considerable change in the circulation of the part; and whenever the aberration consists in the infiltration or deposition of new matter, the change in circulation is similar to, or the same with inflammation. This is seen in the induration of other organs as the lungs, the brain, the liver, and the prostate gland. When, therefore, the granular disease of the kidney is called degeneration and transformation, it does not follow, that the ideas thus conveyed exclude the presence of the inflammatory process.

The urine and the blood are much changed in granular disease of the kidney.

The urine contains less urea than the normal proportion, and always presents more or less sero-albuminous matter. Its density at the same time is diminished; and may vary from 1008, or 1010, or 1011 to 1115.

The urine may be in colour brown, straw-coloured, or reddish; or it may be pale and nearly colourless. Viewed by refracted light, it has a peculiar pale-blue opalescent tinge.

The serum of the blood is less dense than usual, being about 1013, and rarely above 1022. The solid contents are reduced from 100 or 102 per 1000, to 68, 64, or 61 per 1000. The serum in this state forms when heated a loose coagulum. It contains urea, and not unusually it contains more or less oil; in which case it is milky.

The proportion of fibrin is increased in the early stage. But as the disease advances it is diminished. The hematosin at the same time is diminished in quantity.

When the kidneys are affected with steatosis, it is observed that there is a strong disposition to the production of various inflammatory and irritative disorders in different organs. The most usual are the following.

1. In the brain and its membranes. Epileptic and apoplectic symptoms; death by either, or by stupor. Comatose symptoms terminating in death. The disease named by various authors Nervous and Simple Apoplexy is occasionally observed in persons labouring under steatosis of the kidney.

2. In the chest. Bronchitis. Emphysema of the lungs. Pneumonia and *anasarca pulmonum*; tuberculation and *vomicæ* of the lungs. Pleurisy, terminating sometimes in empyema. Hydrotho-

rax. *Endocarditis*, causing valvular disease ; hypertrophy, simple, excentric, and concentric ; pericarditis.

3. In the abdomen. Spontaneous or irritative vomiting, and various dyspeptic symptoms. Diarrhœa frequently recurring in fits ; and connected with enlargement of the agminated or isolated follicles of the *ileum*. Effusion within the abdomen. Hypertrophy of the liver, fatty degeneration, and kirrhosis.

4. In the extremities. Anasarca. Rheumatic pains and swellings ; especially synovial rheumatism, affecting the knee-joints and other articulations. Erysipelas of the face or extremities.

All these morbid states are more or less dependent on the morbid state of the blood, and especially the presence of urea in it, which acts as an irritant to the different textures and organs.

§ 11. HYDATOMA.—The kidney is liable to the formation of small watery cysts or *vesiculæ*, generally of an ovoidal shape, sometimes roundish, varying in size from tares or vetches up to that of small beans. These bodies appear on the cortical surface of the kidney as soon as the outer tunic is torn off. In some instances, they are few in number, two, three, or four ; but I have seen them so numerous that it was impossible to count them. They penetrate through the whole cortical substance of the gland ; but seldom encroach much on the tubular or medullary part, which, however, may present two or three of them.

On the origin of these serous cysts no correct information has been adduced. Some have thought that they are degenerated Malpighian bodies. But this idea is totally at variance with any thing hitherto known as to these bodies. They may be enlarged and dilated portions of the serpentine tubules. But there are no means of proving this idea. The most probable opinion is, that they are mere serous cysts developed as other serous cysts in the cellular tissue of the kidney. The cortical matter is always removed or absorbed to make room for them ; and a kidney affected by this disease presents the aspect of an immense number of small ovoidal cavities excavated in the cortical portion.

This change is often associated with granular degeneration ; and the urine is usually albuminous.

§ 12. ATROPHY.—This term is applied in the kidney to two forms of disease. First;—In steatosis or granular degeneration, after the adipose matter has been infiltrated into the cells and tubules, the cortical and vascular portion of the kidney becomes shrunk and wasted. The kidney, at least its cortical portion, is, in short, in a state of atrophy.

. Secondly; when *Nephropyema* proceeds to a great extreme, causing distension of the calyces and extenuation of the whole cortical portion of the kidney, it may happen that the greater part of the matter is discharged either through the ureter and bladder, or by a new opening formed into the transverse arch of the colon, through that bowel, or even externally; part is removed by absorption; and the purulent inflammation of the calycine membrane ceases. As these processes advance, the distended and attenuated residue of the kidney contracts; the *calyces* contract, and some may be united by mutual adhesion of their walls and membrane. Eventually the whole residual portion of the kidney is contracted and shrunk into a small, flattened, shapeless body, not larger than a dried fig; and when divided, it is difficult to recognize in the remains the vestiges of the original structure. The ureter alone remains, to prove the fact that this body represents all that was a kidney. The pelvis sometimes is left in a contracted form : and not unusually the pelvis and ureter are obstructed and converted into a solid chord. Some small traces of one or two calyces remain; but in general the tubular portion of the kidney is gone, and the cortical is either very much shrunk, or so changed, that its characteristic structure can no longer be recognized. This is atrophy of the kidney after *Nephropyema.*

The lesion is not common; for the disease of which it is the sequela is usually fatal. I have nevertheless seen three examples of it; the preparation of one of which is preserved in the collection of the University.* Job A. Meek'ren records three instances of it, in one of which the right kidney was so destroyed, that it is stated to have been wanting.† I have already shortly noticed a case which occurred to Chomel.‡

§ 13. HYPERTROPHY.—The kidney may be enlarged in all its dimensions without serious change in its intimate structure. In the most usual case, that of atrophy of one kidney after *Nephropyema,* or any similar form of destruction, the opposite kidney is always

---

* Notice of a case of Cyanosis or the Blue Disease, with mutual adhesion of the semilunar valves of the Pulmonary Artery. By David Craigie, M. D.   Edin. Med. and Surg. Journal, Vol. lx. Case I. p. 268.   Edinburgh, 1843.

† Jobi A. Meekren, Observationes Medico-Chirurgicæ. Amstelodami, 1682. Cap. 39, 40, and 44.

‡ P. 945.

much enlarged both in its cortical and tubular portion ; its vessels are large and numerous ; and little doubt can be entertained that it performs the functions of both glands. Such I found to be the state of the residual kidneys in the instances of atrophy already mentioned.

§ 14. HETEROLOGOUS PRODUCTS.—The kidneys are liable to be affected by these, chiefly by *enkephaloma*, and sometimes by *carcinoma*. But most usually they are involved in the growth extending from other organs. In other circumstances, these growths in the kidney present nothing peculiar.

SECTION VI.

DISEASED STATES OF THE FEMALE BREAST.

THESE are inflammation and its effects ; suppurative induration ; chronic inflammation ; lacteal tumour ; simple chronic tumour ; strumous enlargement ; the hydatomatous tumour ; irritable or neuralgic tumour ; adipose tumour ; atrophy ; hypertrophy ; scirrhus ; pancreatic sarcoma, and enkephaloma.

§ 1. Inflammation is seen sometimes spontaneously, more frequently as the effect of the irritation from the first attempt at the secretion of milk. It usually proceeds to abscess, which, however, is seated most in the cellular tissue of the gland.

§ 2. Induration is a common effect of inflammation, and depends on the infiltration of lymph which undergoes coagulation, and on the presence of blood in the vessels, from which the lymph is separated.

§ 3. Strumous enlargement is common in young females. Tubercular matter or a liquid containing fat and caseous matter is infiltered within the tubes and around them. In certain cases, after this has subsisted some time, it undergoes an imperfect suppuration ; and causes a peculiar copious secretion of matter and abscesses of the perimastoid cellular tissue.

§ 4. HYDATOMA. CYSTOSARKOMA SIMPLEX and CYSTOSARKOMA PROLIFERUM of Müller—In the hydatomatous tumour, a number of serous cysts is formed in the breast, which is generally consolidated by adhesive inflammation. The cysts may be only one or two, but are generally more numerous. In certain cases they appear to be true hydatids or Acephalocysts ; and in others, the serous cyst (*hydatoma*). In the latter case they are either a cyst composed of numerous lamellae, like the crystalline humour, or they are a bag containing serous fluid.*

The *cystosarkoma* is in short a tumour or growth, consisting of a fibrous or fibro-vascular frame-work or stroma, containing cysts more or less complete, of various sizes, and more or less numerous. Dr Hodgkin describes a tumour consisting of hydatid cysts as incident both to the female breast and testis of the male.†

§ 5. The irritable or neuralgic tumour consists in painful hardness with or without swelling of one or two lobes of the mamma. The pain is disproportionate to the hardness or enlargement. The surface is tender, and does not bear handling. This is more a dynamic affection than a disease of the mamma; and its presence is connected with the state of the uterus and ovaries. It occurs in young females between 15 and 30.

§ 6. The adipose tumour is sometimes an increased deposit of the natural adipose tissue; or fat may be deposited in one or more cysts. Fatty matter is also liable to be infiltrated within the lacteal tubules when the period of menstruation ceases, causing a sort of steatosis of the gland.

§ 7. ATROPHY.—The breasts undergo a species of shrinking or atrophy in all females after menstruation ceases and the period of child-bearing is past. In some instances, apparently in connection with some morbid state of the ovaries, one or both breasts are liable to become shrunk in this manner previous to the normal time for the cessation of menstruation. In other instances fat is deposited and the glandular structure diminishes or disappears.

§ 8. HYPERTROPHY.—In some females, particularly about the age of 18, 20, or between that and 25, a peculiar enlargement of the breast is observed. The gland becomes enlarged and heavy; the skin over it is likewise enlarged. If the enlargement continue, the breast is so bulky and pendulous that the tension of the skin is no longer adequate to support it; but it hangs down loose, bulky, and pendulous. The nipple is flattened; the areola expanded. So far as can be judged, this is a true hypertrophy of the glandular structure.

§ 9. Cartilaginous and ossific transformation has been observed

---

* Illustrations of the Diseases of the Breast. By Sir Astley Cooper, Bart. London, 1829. 4to.

† On the Anatomical Characters of some Adventitious Structures. By Thomas Hodgkin, M. D. Medico-Chirurg. Transactions, Vol. xv. London, 1829.

in the breast. The change is most likely confined to the galacto-
phorous tubes.

§ 10. SKIRRHUS.—In no organ has skirrhous structure been more
frequently studied than in the mamma. Yet information is not
very precise and presents several discordant points.

a. It seems certain that different forms even of morbid structure
belonging to skirrhus may affect the breast. In one set of cases,
the gland is affected with hardness in lumps or masses, to which
the skin is drawn down in a shrivelled corrugated manner, and adheres over various points of the surface. Internally, white, firm,
fibrous lines are seen intersecting each other through the gland;
and within these is deposited a softer gray-coloured matter, which
presents numerous minute irregular cells and granules, from the
surface of which oozes a serous fluid. The nipple is retracted
and introverted.

In one of these tumours of the breast Vogel found the two elements now mentioned united in the following manner. In the
centre or middle of the tumour were longitudinal bands apparently
cylindrical, thick at middle, but pointed at each end, not straight,
but slightly contorted. These were crowded very closely in the
centre; but at the margin where their pointed extremities terminated, they were more apart. In the interstices between these firm
longitudinal chords were deposited granules spherical, spheroidal,
or pyriform, which were cellular, and had *nuclei* and *nucleoli*. Besides these, were very minute granules, which seemed to be fat.*

b. In another set of cases the same matter is deposited in a tubercular form, and assuming the appearance of irregular masses of
reddish-gray coloured hardish tubercles aggregated together, giving
the whole the aspect of the pancreas.

According to Müller, the gray structure of simple scirrhus of
the breast bears only a remote resemblance to cartilage. Whitish
chords are not regularly observed. Skirrhus of the mamma presents sometimes at various points fibres, in which may be recognized
a canal, containing a colourless, or whitish, or yellowish content.
These white fibres may be formed from the thickened walls of the
milk-tubes and lymphatic vessels. In skirrhus of parts not glandu-

---

* Julii Vogel Icones Histologiæ Pathologicæ. Tabula xxv. Lipsiæ, 1843.

The above description was written from personal examination of a number of skirrhous mammæ long before the engravings of J. Vogel were published. The only point
deserving notice is, that they correspond as accurately as can be expected. I refer to
the engraving of Vogel because it illustrates the subject well.

lar, these hollow white lines are not observed. The mass of the skirrhus consists of a fibrous and granular gray substance. The fibrous mass is rarely manifest on section; but it is distinguished by scraping the gray mass, for which the fibrous seems the frame-work. When the gray globular mass is removed by scraping or maceration, the fibrous framework appears to be a very irregular network of solid fibrous bundles. The gray matter, which is easily removed from this framework by scraping, consists entirely of microscopical globules, which have little mutual connection. They are transparent, hollow cells or *vesiculae*, varying from $\frac{45}{100.000}$ to $\frac{100}{100.000}$, and $\frac{120}{100.000}$ of a Paris inch in diameter. They are insoluble in vinegar and water cold and boiling. In many of these cells are seen only some *punctula* or dots like small granules; in others may be recognized a larger corpuscle like a nucleus, or like a smaller *vesicula* contained within a cell-globule. After examining many scirrhous mammae, Müller could not satisfy himself of the existence of small or young cellules in the formation-globules; yet these he saw evidently in some.[*]

c. A form of cancer more common than simple scirrhus in the breast, is, according to Müller, that which he denominates reticular carcinoma. This attains in a shorter time than simple skirrhus a large size, and it differs from the latter in its tendency to the lobular arrangement. In consistence it sometimes approaches skirrhus, and sometimes is softer, approaching that of enkephaloma.

Reticular carcinoma consists of a gray globular frame-work, imbedded in a reticular texture of fibrous bundles, which is recognized when the gray granular mass is scraped or macerated. The gray mass consists of transparent formation-globules or cell-globules, similar to those observed in simple scirrhus. These contain often one, two, or more small *vesiculæ* with colourless nuclei. In other instances the smaller germinal cells cannot be recognized within the larger formation-globules. On the other hand, in the interior of the transparent cell-globules, appear very many granules. Similar small granules are also observed sometimes in large quantity, free between the vesiculæ,—the smallest with molecular action. The colourless cell-globules have a diameter of from $\frac{21}{100.000}$ to $\frac{36}{100.000}$ and $\frac{40}{100.000}$ of one Paris inch. The diameter of the enclosed granules is only from one-fifth to one-fourth of the diameter of the cells.

[*] Ueber den Feinern Bau und die Formen der Krankhaften Geschwülste. von Dr Johannes Müller. Erste Lieferung. Berlin, 1838. Seite 14.

3

This form of cancer is distinguished by the peculiarity of the constant white or whitish-yellow reticulated figures being more or less manifest. These figures are irregularly net-like, sometimes branched or spotted. There are no dilated vessels with thickened walls as are sometimes seen in simple carcinoma, but characteristic formation. The reticulated figures arise from the deposition of white granules in the gray mass. These granules appear not cellular, but resemble most a conglomeration of opaque granules with roundish or elongated corpuscles.

Cavities are sometimes formed in this structure; and in these is enclosed a coagulable albuminous matter; while the walls are occupied by whitish bodies.

Though this sort of cancer is very common in the female breast, it is not peculiar to that organ, being found also in other parts. This shows that its presence and formation are not necessarily connected with the structure of the lacteal glands.*

d. The female mamma is further liable to be attacked by enkephaloma, which appears with its usual characters. It forms, however, a softer and more compressible tumour; and it appears more lobulated; and some of these lobules seen to be cysts containing fluid. It appears also in younger subjects; and is more a disease of early life than scirrhus.

This disease, however, when it appears in the mamma, is rarely confined to this gland. The same structure is usually developed in the liver, or more or fewer of the internal organs.

e. The nipple is liable to various morbid changes. The most common is excessive development or growth in its *nucleus*, which is attended with pain and some swelling. Usually it ceases of its own accord. But if it do not, it is liable to form a small tumour, which is said often to pass into the malignant state. This I believe is very doubtful, if the subjacent gland remain sound. Other morbid conditions are atrophy, hypertrophy, or excessive nutrition, tubercular skirrhus, and enkephaloma.

SECTION VII.

MORBID STATES OF THE TESTIS.

THE diseased state incident to the *testis* are inflammation and its effects; hydrocele; suppuration within the *testis*; strumous dis-

---

* Ueber den Feinern Bau und die Formen den Krankhaften Geschwülste.

ease; atrophy; hæmatocele; hydatoma or cystic disease of. the testis; cystosarcoma; fibrous disease; skirrhus; *enkephaloma ;* and *kolloma.*

§ 1. ORCHITIS.—Inflammation is acute or chronic. In acute inflammation the anatomical characters are more or less swelling and enlargement; sero-albuminous matter effused within the *tunica vaginalis ;* lymph lining the tunic; the gland redder and more vascnlar than natural, though not much enlarged; bloody serum infiltrated into its parenchyma; and effusion of a brownish coloured fluid into the cellular tissue of the epididymis and that connecting it to the testis,—causing enlargement and induration of that body.

Inflammation affects more frequently the right *testis* than the left. Among 138 cases of *orchitis,* in 78 the right testis was affected; in 49 the left; and in 11 cases both glands.

The most usual causes are the poison of gonorrhœa; a blow or other violence on the gland; urethral irritation; the previous existence of mumps; and probably rheumatism.

This process may leave the testis a little enlarged and indurated; the epididymis much enlarged and indurated; or effusion of fluid within the vaginal coat forming hydrocele.

§ 2. ABSCESS IN THE CENTRE OF THE TESTIS.—Suppuration is not a common result; but it may after some time ensue; and then it generally appears in the form of a collection of matter within the centre of the testis. This is not easily distinguished from chronic disease, as there is constant pain, some induration and some enlargement. The disease is liable to be mistaken for malignant; and the *testis* may accordingly be removed. But there is found only a quantity of greenish-yellow opaque purulent matter in a cavity or cyst in the centre of the gland, the walls of which are lined with lymph. This I have seen many years ago; and I find that the same had been met with by Sir A. Cooper.

§ 3. OBSTRUCTION OF THE TUBULI.—One of the effects of inflammation, if obstinate and long continued, is the effusion of sero-albuminous matter within and around the *tubuli.* The serous part disappears; the albuminous or plastic matter remains, filling and obliterating the tubules, causing enlargement and induration, and afterwards if extensive, atrophy of the testis. When this effusion affects only a portion of the tubules it obliterates them so completely that they no longer perform their functions of secreting canals; and the lymph outside causing them all to adhere, the part

4

so affected is hard, of a reddish gray colour, sometimes with white fibrous lines, the remains of the tubules. This portion afterwards shrinks, and is in the state of partial atrophy.

§ 4. STRUMOUS DISEASE. TYROMA.—Chronic inflammation in the strumous is an affection of the testis not unusual. It gives rise to effusion of tyromatous sero-albumen within and around the tubules, filling and obstructing their cavity with tyromatous matter, and uniting the whole in a mass of tubercular matter. The testis is more enlarged than in common inflammation; and it is more or less irregular and nodulated on the surface according to the irregularity of the agglutinated masses of tubules composing the gland.

Of this disease there are two forms; one mild, another more severe. In the former, the matter deposited is a peculiar yellow homogeneous substance, which when first formed is fluid or semifluid and afterwards acquires consistence and firmness. It adheres closely to the *tubuli*, and involves them so completely as to convert them into one mass. In this state it may remain a long time, forming merely a much enlarged testis, or rather a tumour involving the *testis*.

In this form, however, it is liable to undergo ulterior changes. Portions of the mass, which are always of a low degree of vitality, may undergo inflammation. Some of these become dead; or portions are perhaps struck with death previously, and excite the vital parts to reaction. Sloughing and suppuration proceed, until considerable portions of the new mass are ejected; and if the patient's general strength is adequate to endure all this process, the parts eventually heal after the separation of the greater part or the whole of the new growth, which generally involves the original tubular structure of the testis.

In another form of this disease, the matter deposited contains a large proportion or consists wholly of tubercular matter. This tubercular matter possesses a degree of vitality still lower than the last, and more readily passes into disorganizing processes. Strumous abscesses are formed at the surface, or in the substance of the new growth; and terminate in fistulae and sinuses. Some parts become dead, and these slough away as in the former case. The process, however, is more enfeebling, whether from its natural violence or the weakness of the constitutions of those in whom it takes place. Many patients die under the process.

The main cause of the sloughing in this form of disease appears to be the dense and unyielding nature of the *tunica albuginea* and its processes, and the tension with which it encloses the testicular tubes, in consequence of the constriction by which, when new matter is infiltrated into the tubular structure, as no adequate expansion takes place, the enclosed parts are, as it were, strangulated and deprived of vitality by the compression of their blood-vessels by the *tunica albuginea*.

§ 5. ATROPHY.—Under this head are comprehended arrest of development and wasting.

a. *Arrest.* Most commonly the testis has not descended from the abdomen; and when it has, one or both are smaller than usual, shrunk, and manifestly not adequately nourished. The tubular portion is imperfectly developed.

b. *Wasting.* When the testis has been fully developed, it may be attacked by wasting. Either after a blow, contusion, or other violence, or sometimes, as was observed in the soldiers of the French army in Egypt, after sexual excesses, the testis becomes at first a little larger, then softer than natural, then small and shrunk. In this form of atrophy, the tubules undergo a species of chronic inflammation, causing obliteration from infiltration of lymph, and sometimes of oily matter. The secreting structure is thus disorganized. The blood-vessels shrink, and less blood than usual is conveyed to the gland.

In a testicle affected by wasting, the testis feel soft; and its texture is pale and with few blood-vessels. The fluid expressed from the *tubuli* is void of spermatozoa. Mr Gulliver found fatty matter in the glandular substance.

§ 6. HAEMATOCELE; or effusion of blood takes place most usually within the *tunica vaginalis*, constituting the affection called *Haematorchis*, already noticed.

§ 7. FIBROUS TRANSFORMATION. DESMOSIS.—In some instances, not very common, the testis has been found converted into a species of fibrous mass; while its proper secreting structure has disappeared. This change I regard as depending on increased development of the *tunica albuginea* and its processes, all of which become thick, dense, and increased in size; and by compressing the tubular structure cause its absorption. . The lesion is not very common; but in the instances in which I have seen it, this view appeared to be directly suggested by the phenomena and characters of the change.

§ 8. OSSIFICATION is probably always to be traced to the *tunica albuginea.* Patches of bone appear in this and in its processes.

§ 9. HYDATOMA. CYSTO-SARKOMA.—The testis resembles the female mamma in the frequency with which this growth is formed in its substance. Cysts, similar to hydatids, one, two, or several in number, sometimes many, are formed in the parenchyma of the gland. These may be so numerous as to occupy the whole body of the *testis,* the natural structure of which is displaced and disappears. The nature and origin of this disease is imperfectly known. Sir Astley Cooper was inclined to regard it as formed from enlarged and obstructed seminiferous tubes, because they are not distinct bags, but send out solid processes by which they are connected with other bags. Dr Hodgkin regards them as serous cysts formed in the substance of the gland. It must be allowed that the cysts are rarely so large as in the breast; and it is quite possible that this lesion of the *testis* may be different from the *hydatoma* of the breast.

It merely remains to be observed, that cysts of the kind now described seem common to the kidney, the *mamma,* and the testis.

§ 10. Of the HETEROLOGOUS GROWTHS, both skirrhus and enkephaloma are observed in the *testis.* It is difficult to say which of these two is the most common. Skirrhus occurs, as in other organs, rather at a late period of life. *Enkephaloma* may take place at any age, but shows a preference for the early period, that is, before 40. A character of distinction more important is that, when *enkephaloma* appears in the testis, the same structure is generally found in the abdomen.

The anatomical characters of both are similar to those in other organs.

§ 11. COLLOID or GELATINIFORM cancer takes place in the *testis;* but much more rarely than the other two lesions now mentioned, and infinitely more seldom in the testis than in the stomach and some other organs.

§ 12. MELANOMA also occurs, but not very frequently, unless at the same time at which it appears in the abdomen.

SECTION VIII.

DISEASED STATES OF THE PROSTATE GLAND.

The principal morbid states of the prostate gland are suppuration within the ducts; chronic enlargement or hypertrophy of the gland and its effects; and enlargement of the middle lobe.

§ 1. PROSTATOPYEMA.—Suppuration within the ducts, or suppuration of the mucous membrane of the ducts, is a disease of strumous character. The whole mucous membrane, from their outlets into the urethra upwards to their remote extremities, is inflamed, secretes lymph, and a foul imperfectly formed purulent matter, which does not easily escape, but remaining, as it is increased by fresh secreted matter, distends and enlarges the ducts into small or middle-sized cavities, with narrow outlets. A prostate gland in this state is large, bulging, and elastic-compressible, as if containing fluid, and lobulated on the surface; and when divided by incision, it appears, as if it consisted of several distinct encysted abscesses. These apparent abscesses are formed by the ducts of the gland distended and enlarged by purulent matter and lymph. When the matter is removed, the epithelial membrane of the ducts is observed lined with lymph, yet not in a state of ulceration. The surface is indeed unbroken.

This disease may take place at any period of life, but is most common in strumous subjects between the ages of 20 and 30.

It causes great disorder of the general health, occasionally hectic, and peculiar depression of spirits.

§ 2. CHRONIC ENLARGEMENT AND HYPERTROPHY.—This may affect either one lobe, or both, or part of both. The substance of the gland is enlarged, firm, and greatly more crowded with veins and arteries than usual. The veins are distended, enlarged, and varicose. Blood and lymph is infiltrated into the substance of the gland; and eventually, if the process be not arrested or stop spontaneously, either one or two abscesses are formed; or the prostatic substance becomes extremely hard, dark-coloured, and almost cartilaginous; while its original structure can no longer be recognized. The substance of the gland shows whitish specks and lines, which are manifestly lymph effused.

When the prostate gland is in this state it is liable to two morbid actions. One is a secretion of ropy viscid, almost puriform mucus from the ducts of the gland, and occasionally the purulent collections within these ducts noticed under the last head. The other is a discharge of blood from the vessels of the gland more or less copious. The latter is caused by the previous distended state of the vessels, and the pressure exerted on them by the enlarged and condensed parenchyma of the gland.

Similar enlargement may affect the third lobe of the prostate gland.

BOOK VI.

THE LUNGS AND HEART.

CHAPTER I.

The Lungs.

Section I.

The Minute Structure of the Sound Lung.

THE lungs may be regarded as the ramifications and terminal ends of the bronchial tubes, pulmonary artery, and pulmonary veins, all united by filamentous-cellular tissue and enclosed within the *pleura*.

The filamentous-cellular tissue now mentioned forms with these enclosed textures the pulmonic substance, tissue, or parenchyma.

The main point, however, which it is important to know, in order to understand either the structure of the lungs, as explanatory of their morbid condition, or the functions of these organs during health, is the mode in which the bronchial tubes are distributed and terminate.

This point has been partly considered already, when speaking of the ultimate termination of the bronchial mucous membrane. A few points I have here to add, in consequence of the question of these terminations having been again made the subject of research.

Malpighi, who first studied the structure of the lungs with attention, maintained that the *bronchi* terminate in closed ends, slightly expanded into the form of spherical or globular *vesiculae* (*vesiculae orbiculares*), which he in one passage compares to the cells of bee-hives.* This shows that he believed that these *vesiculae* communicate with each other. He thought it also probable that these *vesiculae* are continuations or processes from the inner membrane of the windpipe,—in other words, from the bronchial membrane.

Duverney maintained, in 1699, that these vesicles or cells communicate with each other; and Stephen Hales, who examined them in the calf by the microscope, represents them as little cubes or hexaedral figures, not spherical, and estimates their diameter at $\frac{1}{100}$ part of one inch.†

* De Pulmonibus, Epistola I. J. Alphonso Borelli. Marcelli Malpighi, Opera Omnia. Londini, 1686. Folio. Tomus Secundus, p. 133 and 134.

† Statical Essays Vol. i. pp. 239 and 241. London, 1731.

Senac next maintained that the lungs consist of lobules; that each lobule consists of *vesiculae*, in each of which ends a bronchial tube; and that each *vesicula* consists of small polyedral cells, not more than the sixth part of one line in diameter.

This idea of vesicles or small cells was adopted by James Keill, Cheselden,* Winslow,† and various systematic authors; and the idea of Duverney that they communicate, appears at the same time to have been added.

Helvetius on the other hand was of opinion, from various examinations and experiments, that the representation of round *vesiculæ* or cells was entirely a fiction; that what Malpighi describes as air vesicles are the cells of the cellular tissue; and that the closed ends of the bronchial tubes are the last recipients of the atmospheric air.‡

Haller, though inclined to the doctrine of Helvetius, inferred nevertheless, that considering all the circumstances and the phenomena of experiments and dissections in living or recently dead adult animals, each bronchial tube does not terminate in an individual cavity, but that there is in the human as in the reptile lung, a cellular arrangement, the imperfect chambers of which communicate freely with each other, until the investment of each lobule delays the passage of the air and prevents it from proceeding from lobule to lobule.

All these observers speak in a manner rather confused and sometimes contradictory; and, though it seems singular, that any one accustomed to inquiries of this kind could confound the terminations of the bronchial tubes, whether forming cells or not, with the cells of the pulmonic cellular tissue, there is reason to believe that this was done by Dr Hales.

The doctrine of communicating air-cells was accordingly very generally taught by anatomists, and is distinctly presented by Soemmering, who may be taken as the representative of anatomical

---

* " They are each composed of very small cells, which are the extremities of the *aspera arteria* or *bronchos*. The figure of these cells is irregular, yet they are fitted to each other so as to have common sides and leave no void space."—Anatomy, Book iv. Chap. vii. p. 173. Lond. 1784.

† Exposition Anatomique de la Structure du Corps Humain. Par Jacques-Benigne Winslow, de l'Academie R. des Sciénces, &c. Paris, 1732. 4to. N. 104 et 136.

‡ Memoires de l'Academie des Sciences, 1718, p. 24—28.

§ Elementa Physiologiæ, Lib. viii Sectio ii. § xxix. § xxx. Tom. iii. p. 179. Lausannæ, 1766.

doctrine at the close of the 18th century, and for the first fifth of the 19th. According to Soemmering the substance of the lung consists of small air-cells or *vesiculæ*. Several of these *vesiculæ* form a cluster, (*acervulus*); several clusters compose small lobules; these unite into large lobules; and these by their union form the lobes of the lungs.

These cells appear to be round, polygonal and irregular. When inflated they are about the eighth or the tenth part of one line in diameter; and they communicate with each other through the wind-pipe, in such manner that air blown into one cell easily passes from this into the bronchia, and by these penetrates into all the other cells of the lungs. The cells of neighbouring lobules, however, do not communicate with each other; and it is only the cells belonging to each cluster and lobule that thus communicate.*

If this description be understood literally, it implies that the alleged cells of the lungs do not communicate with each other by themselves, but only by the arrangement of the bronchial tubes terminating in them. From this it follows, that these air-cells are mere shut ends of the bronchial tubes.

In 1808 Reisseissen examined in various modes the terminal ends of the bronchial tubes, and arrived at the conclusion, that the lung possesses no arrangement like that described as air-cells, and that closed ends of the bronchial tubes, not communicating with each other however, but which retaining the peculiar structure to their extremities, present the appearance of air-cells or air-vesicles.†

The essay of Reisseissen was not published till 1822; and it was only subsequent to that time that his statements became known or their correctness ascertained.

Magendie examined in 1821 the minute structure of the lungs by inflating and drying small portions; and concluded that there is a cellular or vesicular arrangement at the extremities of the bronchial tubes communicating with these tubes, and in which these tubes finally terminate; that these cells present no regular form, and appear to be void of membranous walls; that they are formed by the last divisions of the pulmonary artery, the *radiculæ* or roots of the pulmonary veins, and the numerous anastomoses of these vessels; that all the cells of one lobule communicate with each

---

* De Fabrica Corporis Humani. Tomus sextus, § xxi.

† Franz Daniel Reisseissen über den Bau der Lungen. Berlin, 1822. Folio; and Edinburgh Medical and Surgical Journal, Vol. xxi. p. 444. Edinburgh, 1824.

other, but not with those of contiguous lobules; and that these
cells vary in size at different ages.*

Reynaud, who examined the bronchial tubes with the view of
ascertaining the accuracy of the representations of Reisseissen,
arrives at the following conclusions.

Any given bronchial tube when traced through the lung is found
to divide before and behind, and on each side into small branches;
which again traced still further are found to be subdivided into
branches still smaller than these.   These divisions become shorter
and shorter, and of smaller calibre, end in becoming rounded, as
if they had formed at their side a number of small shut ends or depressions, and at length they terminate in an extremity shut and
scarcely enlarged.   This is shown by mercury poured into them
and urged forward by pressure, when the mercury demonstrates, as
it were, the last divisions of the diminutive bronchial tree,—and also
by insufflation and dissection.;   These small tubes all terminate
at right angles to the *pleura*, which allows the observer to recognize only the assemblage of their terminal sacs, and not the bronchial tubes from which they proceed.

He mentions, however, the following disposition also.   A greater
or smaller number of bronchial tubes larger than others do not
end thus at the *pleura;* but having come near it, instead of terminating more or less rectangularly at the pleura, proceed beneath
this membrane parallel to it, and terminate at the distance of two,
three, four, or five lines from their point of emergence.   The air
which filled these tubes appeared like the mercury, in the instance
above mentioned, to represent these small trees with perfect regularity, and to demonstrate their arborescent disposition to that
point, when pressure more or less forcible was inadequate to urge
the air onward, and where it was evident it had reached its last
limits.

These ends of bronchial tubes are about two lines from the
pleura, or even less; and to demonstrate them fully, it is often
requisite to open them the whole length, and urge a bristle through
them, so as to perforate that membrane, or to make a small counter
opening.   In this manner the end of the bronchial tube is displayed,
showing the membrane continuous from the upper part of the tube

† Memoire sur la structure du poumon de l'homme ; sur les modifications qu'
eprouve cette structure dans les divers ages ; et sur la premiere origine de la phthisie
pulmonaire ; par M. Magendie. Journal de Physiologie, Tome i. p. 78. Paris, 1821.

throughout. The only other circumstance is, that at. two lines from the termination, it looks as if perforated by many small depressions, which it had not previously presented. Small apertures leading into small ultimate branches are likewise seen more and more near to each other.*

The general correctness of this description is strongly confirmed . by the phenomena of obliteration of the bronchial tubes.

Bourgèry made known to the Academy first in 1836, and afterwards in 1842, the results of researches on the minute structure of the lungs, of which the following is a summary. To every minute lobule of the lung is sent one central bronchial tube, which proceeds to the peripheral basis of the lobule, and is distributed with progressive ramification to the terminal ends of the same. During this course, the central stem sends within the lobule alternately, radiating in all directions, subordinate shoots, which are to be considered as terminal branches of the proper air-tube tree, and which Bourgery denominates *ramified bronchial canals*. Beyond these commences, according to M. Bourgery, the capillary air-sucking system. Each ramified bronchial canal ends in a small, irregular, winding, elongated dilatation, which is sometimes two-lobuled or three-lobuled. These are bounded, in their course and in their dilatations, by walls perforated in a sieve-like fashion by small orifices, by which the branched and ramified bronchial tree, as an inferent and efferent apparatus, is connected with those parts of the lungs which are to be viewed as the proper functional substance. This part forms a labyrinth of tubes expanded in three directions, which are distributed in a tortuous course along the windings of the vessels, observe a. proportional diameter, and at their ends also, as in the lateral walls, communicate with each other by many orifices.†

Dr Thomas Addison maintains the existence of a collection of cells in which a filiform bronchial tube terminates.

Mr William Addison gave in 1842 an account of the results of various researches which he had made by the aid of the microscope, on the distribution of the ends of the bronchial tubes, and arrived at the conclusion that these tubes do not end in closed sacs ; and that after dividing into numerous minute branches, which take their

* Memoire sur l'Obliteration des Bronches ; par A. G. Reynaud, D. M. &c. Memoires de l'Academie Royale de Medecine, T. iv. p. 115. Paris, 1835. 4to.

† Extrait d'un Memoire sur la Structure intime des Poumons dans l'homme et les Mammiferes, (lu a l'Academie des Sciences, 11 Juillet 1842,) by J. M. Bourgery. Gazette Medicale, 1842, Tom. x. N. 20.

course in the cellular interstices of the lobules, they terminate in their interior in branched air passages, and freely communicating air-cells.

It is proper to premise, that to each lobule of the lung belongs one bronchial tube of some size ; that the divisions or branches of this bronchial tube are confined to the lobule to which it belongs, which indeed it forms, and do not communicate with the branches of adjoining lobules ; and that each lobule is enclosed in cellular or filamentous tissue, firmer than that within the lobule, and which thus separates that lobule from the surrounding ones. The small bronchial divisions within each lobule are *intralobular ramifications.*

In the fœtal lung, these intralobular bronchial divisions pursue a regular branched arrangement, subdividing in all directions, and terminating at the boundary of the lobule in closed extremities. Many also terminate in the interior of the lobule. These intralobular branches do not anastomose.

In the fœtal lung, there are no air-cells properly speaking. But when an animal breathes, the air entering by its pressure into the windpipe and bronchial tubes proceeds to the intralobular branches ; and in this manner distends each lobule speedily to as great extent as these intralobular branches allow. After this they are found to form a series of communicating cells, which are permanently occupied by air ; and in this all the trace of the original branched arrangement is lost or obscured. These cells are pentagonal or hexagonal in shape.

This may be regarded as the statement of the fact as given by Mr Addison. The cause of this cellular formation is twofold ; first, the forcible pressure of the air which enters by the windpipe, and is perpetually impelled to the ultimate extremities of the tubes and their intralobular ramifications ; and the delicate and yielding membrane of these ramifications, which, by presenting an unequal resistance, is thus distended into cells.

The air-cells do not, however, communicate with each other in the interior of a lobule in an indiscriminate and general manner. As the intralobular bronchial ramifications do not anastomose, the air-cells formed along one branch do not communicate with those formed along another ; and so on through the whole lobule.

The lobules nevertheless present in their interior branched passages forming a communication between the cells. But these passages are stated to be neither tubular nor cylindrical. They are denominated lobular passages.

3

When a thin section of inflated and dried lung is placed under the microscope, a number of large well-defined oval FORAMINA, with a sharp delicate edge, is seen thickly distributed among the cells. These FORAMINA are portions of lobular passages. They are smaller near the pleura and surface of the lung than in the interior of the organ.

When mercury is poured into the lungs of a rabbit which have been macerated, so as to expel the air, it gets into the air-tubes, and appears at the surface of some in the form of globules, at that of others as beaded and nodulated branches, which, according to Mr Addison, combine the character of cells and passages.

The membrane of these air-cells, when examined by the microscope, does not form round or even rounded cells, but flat membranous plates, circumscribing polyhedral spaces. They present ovate bodies as part of their structure. They possess an epithelium in the form of large, round, nucleated scales, in each of which from one to fifteen or more nuclei may be counted.

Mr Addison found, like Magendie, the cells in early life small, and in old age large. At the age of 45, they vary from $\frac{1}{200}$ to $\frac{1}{500}$ part of one inch in diameter.[*]

The correctness of these statements has on the whole been confirmed by the researches of Mr George Rainey.

Mr Rainey finds that when the bronchial tubes have arrived at about one-eighth of one inch from the surface of the lung, the membrane terminates abruptly; that the passages conveying the

* On the Ultimate Distribution of the Air-Passages and the Air-Cells of the Lungs. By William Addison, Esq. F. L. S., &c. Read 7th April 1842. Philosophical Transactions, London, 1842.

On the use of the term vesicle, Mr Addison pronounces a criticism which partakes more of boldness than wisdom or knowledge. " Anatomical writers," says Mr Addison, " generally use the terms air-vesicles and air-cells synonymously, so that they are convertible terms ; but, strictly speaking, an air-vesicle is an air-bubble, and may exist either in or out of a pulmonary air-cell."—Phil. Trans. vol. for 1843, p. 158.

It is rather the term vesicles than air-vesicles, that anatomical writers use as synonymous with that of air-cells. By what means Mr Addison has arrived at the inference that vesicle means air-bubble, I know not. But, with deference to Mr Addison, he will find that all the anatomical writers who have spoken of these bodies—Malpighi, Senac, Winslow, Haller, and Soemmering—employ the term in its original acceptation, that is, a small *vesica*, or bladder, or small membranous bag or cell. The words of Soemmering are ; " *Pulmonum substantia* parvis *cellulis, vesiculis*, vel *sacculis* aere plenis conflatur.—Plures ejusmodi vesiculæ in acervulos congeruntur." Tomus sextus, § xxi.—The idea that the word *vesicula* is ever used to signify an air-bubble is a modern invention, not sanctioned by classical use. *Bulla* is the word used.

air, which he terms *intercellular,* continue in the same direction as the tubes of which they are continuations, but without perceptible membranous lining ; that the diameter of the ultimate bronchial tubes is from $\frac{1}{50}$ to $\frac{1}{80}$ of one inch ; that they communicate with but few cells ; that the intercellular passages, the intralobular of Mr Addison, are at first of a circular form, communicating also with few cells ; but as they approach the surface of a lobule, their number increases, and at length these communicating openings are so numerous and so close, that the intercellular passage loses its circular figure, and forms an irregular-shaped passage running between air-cells, and communicating with them in all directions, and having arrived at the surface of a lobule, it terminates in an air-cell, which is not dilated, but is in truth of the same size as the passage.

The air-cells are small, irregularly-shaped, yet most frequently four-sided cavities, varying in size in different parts of the same lung. Those are smallest, as well as most vascular, which are situate nearest the centre ; while their size increases, and their vascularity diminishes, as they extend into remote parts. The air-cells situate close to the bronchial tubes, or intercellular passages, open into them by large circular apertures ; while those placed further from these passages, communicate with them through the medium of other cells.

Besides these intervening air-cells, there are others which fill the angle formed by the bifurcation of the intercellular passage, and which thus appear to form a communication between them.

Mr Rainey controverts the statement made by Mr Addison, that in the lungs of the fœtus, the air-cells are not developed. He injected the lungs of various fœtal animals which had never breathed, and found, on examining them with the microscope, that the air-cells were developed proportionally with other parts of the lungs.

He adds, however, that in the very young fœtus, the *septa,* or partitions between the air-cells, consist almost entirely of minute cellules or granules, and a small quantity of fibrous tissue, with scarcely any blood-vessels ; and that, as the age of the fœtus advances, this granular matter diminishes, while the capillaries increase, so that at birth the same arrangement of the air-cells and the other parts of the lungs is observed as in after life.

. . The capillaries of the lungs are situate, or contained within, a fold of membrane. Traced from the peripheral to the central parts, this membrane lines first the air-cells which are next the surface of a lobule, whether next the pleura or adjoining lobules; then the cells enclosing the capillary vessels; and thence extending from cell to cell, it arrives at the intercellular passages, and at the termination of the bronchial tubes becomes identified with the bronchial membrane.*

In several points these statements agree; in others they greatly differ. On two points all agree. The first is, that within each lobule there is a separate or proper system of minute bronchial ramifications, with terminal ends, between which there are communications within the lobule only. The second is, that these bronchial divisions and terminations, whether named air-cells or not, do not communicate with those of the contiguous lobules. The air which enters the interior of one lobule never can find its way into the interior of the contiguous lobules.

SECTION II.

MORBID STATES OF THE LUNGS.

THE morbid states of the lungs are, inflammation and its effects; hepatization of various kinds; suppuration; hæmorrhagic peripneumony; gangrene; dilatation of the air-cells; emphysema; hemorhage; tuberculation and vomicæ; parasitical animals, and various heterologous growths.

§ 1. PNEUMONIA.—The anatomical characters and morbid effects of inflamed lung may be stated in the following manner. 1st, On opening the chest and admitting the air, though there are no adhesions, the lung does not collapse at all, or does so very slightly. 2d, The pulmonic substance, when inflamed, becomes harder and denser than natural, and does not float completely in water. If the induration is considerable or extensive, it sinks entirely. 3d, It loses its elasticity and compressibility, or cannot be inflated, and no longer crepitates as in the healthy state, but resembles a piece of solid flesh. 4th, When divided by the knife, a portion of inflamed lung is more or less firm; its spongy or vesicular structure appears much redder than usual, the colour being chiefly florid but partly of a darker hue; a white or yellowish fluid, somewhat frothy, flows from the cut bronchial tubes; the substance of the lung is dark red or brown-red, and very much loaded with

---

* On the Minute Structure of the Lungs, and on the Formation of Pulmonary Tubercle. By George Rainey, Esq. M. R. C. S. Medico-Chirurgical Transactions, vol. xxviii. p. 581. London, 1845.

blood within vessels and out of them; while bloody serum escapes copiously from the proper pulmonic cellular tissue.

These may be regarded as the general characters of inflamed lung. These characters nevertheless vary according to the progress of the disease; and it is observed, that a lung in a state of inflammation presents different characters, as that inflammation is in its commencement, is established, is completed, or is subsiding.

Laennec describes three different degrees of pneumonic inflammation, and distinguishes them; 1*st*, according as the lung is red or violet, but crepitates and discharges, when cut, a frothy blood-coloured fluid; the stage of obstruction; 2*d*, as the portion of lung is destitute of crepitation, and is red and granulated interiorly, without discharge of fluid when cut, unless squeezed; the stage of hepatization or carnification; 3*d*, as it is consistent and granular, its section a pale yellow, a straw or stone-gray colour, and as it discharges a considerable quantity of opaque, yellowish, viscid fluid, from many points of its cut surface;—the stage of gray hepatization or purulent infiltration. ʹIn this state the substance of the lung is friable and lacerable, and easily gives way.

I think four different stages may be recognized, exclusive of effects.

In the first, the lung is dark red, or reddish-brown, or violet-coloured, and does not collapse when the chest is opened. It feels also slightly more firm and resisting, but not so much as in the next stage. When cut, it is observed to be loaded with blood, which is very abundant in the filamento-cellular tissue; much blood and bloody serum escapes; frothy serous fluid also is observed to issue from divided bronchial tubes. The lung still crepitates, but is slightly œdematous, or at least receives the impression of the finger.

When a lung in this state is examined by the microscope, no morbid product is seen in the filamento-cellular tissue. The vessels, that is, the capillaries, are injected and loaded with fluid blood, generally dark coloured, and with serum. The air-cells, or at least the small divisions of the bronchial tubes, are filled with serum mixed with air. This is the stage of injection or bloody congestion, and it affects the capillary vessels, the filamento-cellular tissue, and the air-cells of the lungs. It is therefore *pneumonia* with vesicular *bronchitis*.

This state of lung may affect one or both lungs. When it affects both, it often proves fatal, from the great extent, not the intensity of the lesion. In cases in which it affects only one lung, or part of one, or part of both, recovery is more easily effected.

In the second stage, the lung is a little firmer and more resistent, and may project beyond the ribs when the chest is opened. It is more thoroughly loaded with blood; and blood begins to be separated into blood-*plasma* (*liquor sanguinis*), and serum, in being effused into the filamento-cellular tissue. The blood is sometimes found infiltrated extensively into the lower part of the lung, and is not separated decidedly into lymph or clot and serum. Its presence, however, renders the lung dark-red or brown, massy, and consistent; yet it crepitates in various parts; and in others it is œdematous, not unfrequently receiving the impression of the ribs. In this state it commonly affects most the lower and middle lobes.

A lung in this state shows, when examined, that its tissue is rather closer than usual, and contains a large quantity of blood in its vessels and filamento-cellular tissue; and blood is beginning to be effused into the air-cells. This is the state called obstruction by Laennec. It is the close of the state of congestion or injection.

In the third stage, a new series of phenomena is observed. The blood, which had been previously in vessels mostly, and was fluid or at most only beginning to become fixed, is now observed to be extravasated into the interstices of the filamento-cellular tissue. The part or parts of the lung thus affected are not only dark-red or violet-coloured, but solid, firm, do not crepitate, and when cut and washed, though they effuse blood and bloody serum, the section shows patches of a rough granular aspect, as if they consisted of small granules aggregated together, and which are solid, not compressible, and manifestly totally different from the contiguous portions of lung. At first these patches or portions with soft intervals are small. Afterwards they are large; and in some instances a large portion of lung at once passes into this red, solid, rough, granular condition.

The appearance now described is produced by blood effused into the filamento-cellular tissue; and the effusion thus taking place closes and obliterates the small bronchial tubes and air-cells. Blood may be effused into these parts also, and commonly is effused.

This is the stage of red solidification, consolidation, or hepatization. Its colour is various shades of red, according to the state of the effusion and the duration of the disease. In some instances it is brown, and in some violet or purple. The lung so affected loses tenacity and becomes friable.

In some instances this change is of a chronic character, and it appears to occupy weeks or even months in its progress to completion.

In other instances it seems to proceed a certain length and then to stop, leaving considerable portions of the middle and lower lobes in a state of red hepatization. These patches are easily distinguished by being dark-coloured, while the adjoining lung is more or less red; by being solid and incompressible, and void of crepitation, while the other parts are soft, compressible, and crepitating, by being quite insusceptible of inflation; and by sinking in water. Sections of such portions of lung show the close granular appearance and compact structure of the pulmonic tissue already mentioned. In these circumstances the *pleura* is in general healthy, and it is not uncommon to find that membrane in its usual state over considerable portions of lung that have been long in a state of red or brown solidification.

As a fourth stage of *pneumonia* has been generally enumerated the change denominated gray hepatization. It appears to me not certain that this view is correct. Gray hepatization appears to be often a change not succeeding to red or brown consolidation, but one which follows a certain stage of the disease in a particular form and in certain constitutions. Its anatomical characters are the following.

The whole lung is firm, solid, inelastic, and more or less incompressible. It fills the chest completely, and usually projects a little when the sternum is removed. The pleura is very generally covered with patches of lymph, and sometimes it adheres extensively and more or less firmly. The lung itself is most solid at the middle and lower lobes, and the upper lobe alone is soft and a little compressible. Sections of the lung show the substance to be of gray-red, or dirty yellow colour; sometimes with portions of bluish-gray, green, orange, and in short variegated. The substance is solid, compact, but friable and very easily rent; in short, it comes away under the fingers. Much serous fluid, more or less turbid, with some blood-coloured purulent matter, oozes from the surface of the sections. When examined by the microscope, pus globules are seen both in the interstitial matter and oozing from the cut surface. Granules of lymph and blood are also observed infiltrated into the interstices of the filamento-cellular tissue. When the part has been macerated or well washed, the section presents a granular compact aspect like the section of the lung in red consolidation. But it is more varied; the substance of the lung is more thoroughly destroyed or disguised, and the lung is softer and more lacerable. In some instances the portions of lung present a sort of tubercular induration, that is, hardened masses, bluish-gray or gray in colour, and of irregular form, interspersed among whitish-gray softened portions. In other instances, gray portions, firm, yet lacerable, are interspersed among reddish portions.

It is impossible to doubt, that these changes depend partly on blood infiltrated and changed, and in a greater degree on lymph, and purulent matter infiltrated into the filamento-cellular tissue. Various products also, as blood, *liquor sanguinis,* and lymph, are poured into the air-cells and obliterate them. It is supposed by some that this causes the appearance of whitish granules in the lung affected by gray hepatization. It may do so; but the infiltration of this matter takes place also into the filamento-cellular tissue; and while the presence of one set of granules may depend on the former cause, that of another, it appears to me, depends on the latter.

In short, there are effused blood-corpuscles; *liquor sanguinis* or plasma, afterwards formed into granules; and pus-globules all at the same time and in the same tissue. The blood-corpuscles after some time undergo changes in colour, and hence arise the bluish-gray, greenish, and reddish brown or orange colours of the parts affected.

The changes now specified may come on rather gradually and insidiously, without very great disorder in the breathing, until the greater part of one or both lungs is destroyed by consolidation. The disease, if it do not begin in, certainly affects mostly the substance of the lung, that is the filamento-cellular parenchyma; and along with this it involves the pulmonic air-cells, which are filled with blood and obliterated. From the substance, it affects eventually the *pleura* which is covered with lymph recent and soft, or firm. In several instances which have come under my own observation, the patients did not complain of uneasiness or disorder until the *pleura* began to be inflamed. In general death was then not remote, and took place in the course of a few days.

Inflammation usually commences in the lower part of the lung, and generally attains there its greatest intensity. Thus, the whole of the lower lobe may be in a state of extensive induration and he_ patization, while the middle lobe is only reddened and infiltrated with serum, sero-sanguine fluid, or blood, and the upper lobe is comparatively healthy. The centre of the lung also, especially opposite to the lower angle of the scapula, is often the seat of inflammation. Inflammation may take place in one lung or in both; and in the same manner it begins first, and attains its greatest intensity in the lower lobes of both. In the former case, it is said to be simple; in the latter, it is double pneumonia. It is not easy to estimate the comparative prevalence of pneumonia in either lung, or in both; but from the attempts made, it appears that pneumonia of the right lung is more common than in the left, in the ratio of more than two to one, and that single pneumonia is more common than double pneumonia in the ratio of six to one.*

It must not be imagined, however, that inflammation is always seated in the lower part of the lung. Morgagni, Frank, and Broussais often found the upper part of the lung inflamed. In the summer of 1837, I found, in the body of a woman who had died rather suddenly, the upper part of both lungs in a most complete state of gray hepatization; and in several cases since that time, I have found the upper parts of the lungs affected with pneumonia in various degrees, while the lower was in comparative soundness. The same occurrence is admitted by Andral, who allows that it is not uncommon, and by Chomel, whose experience leads him to regard it as frequent.

Pneumonic inflammation may terminate in resolution; effusion of blood or simple hepatization; effusion of blood and lymph or granular hepatization; and suppuration; or it may become chronic, and terminate in mixed hepatization; or it may terminate in gangrene.

It is very important to observe with regard to gray hepatization, that persons labouring under it die apparently very unexpectedly, if not suddenly. These persons have perhaps been only in a sort of general ill-health, when all of a sudden they are attacked with great difficulty in breathing and extreme weakness, and in this state die, or even without this preliminary difficult breathing, they suddenly fall down and are found dead.

Though this shows that the disease is chronic in progress, yet

* Of 210 cases of pneumonia, 121 were in the right lung, 58 in the left, 25 double and 6 not ascertained. Among 75 cases given by M. Jules Pelletan, in 58 inflammation was in one lung, in 17 in both at once; in the right the disease occurred 42 times; in the left 16 times; in the base of the lung 24 times; in the apex 7 times; all over 24 times. Memoire Statistique in Memoires de l'Academie, Tome viiiieme Paris, 1840.

other points regarding chronic forms of the disease shall be immediately considered.

Pneumonia has been distinguished by practical authors and nosologists into several varieties, according to certain modifying circumstances. The following list comprehends the most important, 1. Hemorrhagic peripneumony; 2. The spurious or bastard Peripneumony (*Peripneumony Notha*); 3. The chronic, slow, or latent (*Pneumonia Chronica*); 4. The gastric or bilious (*Pneumonia gastrica vel Pneumonia biliosa*); 5. The nervous or Typhoid Pneumonia (*Pneumonia Nervosa et Typhodes*); and 6. The malignant, pestilential, or gangrenous (*Pneumonia septica vel Pneumonia maligna*) *gangraena pulmonum*.

Hæmorrhagic peripneumony (*Pneumonia Hæmorrhagica.*) Cullen observed, that pneumonia had a termination peculiar to itself, namely, the effusion of a quantity of blood into the cellular texture, (*i. e.* the filamentous or parenchymatous tissue) of the lungs, which soon interrupting the circulation of the blood through these organs produces fatal suffocation. In some instances, however, this extravasation of blood does not produce immediate suffocation. These appear to be principally when the effusion takes place in limited and isolated points, for instance, forming small amorphous masses about the size of a filbert or walnut in the lower lobes of one or both lungs. The portions of lung thus the seat of bloody extravasation become firm, resisting, uncrepitating, dark-coloured and granular in structure. The boundaries are generally distinctly circumscribed, and the difference between them and the surrounding portion of lung is distinctly marked. When near the surface of the lung they are both felt and seen through the *pleura* by the deeper brown colour over them, by their firmness and solidity, by not collapsing while the rest of the lung collapses, and by breaking down instead of collapsing when they are compressed. In these dark-brown, hard, granular masses, the blood-vessels and the bronchial tubes and vesicles are completely obliterated, and their canals closed, and the membrane of the contiguous bronchial tubes is dark brown, thick, and friable.

The change, indicated by the presence of these masses in the lung, which had originally been described by Baillie under the name of the brown tubercle of the lungs, was afterwards made the subject of particular attention by Laennec, under the denomination of pulmonary apoplexy. The chief objection to the term is that it converts into a disease, that which in correct pathology is the effect of morbid action; and that its author represents this lesion as the pathological cause of hæmoptysis. Had he said that hæmoptysis or hemorrhage from the lungs, and this dark-brown circumscribed induration of the lung were effects of the same cause, the representation would have been more just. Both these phenomena are the effects of the previous congestion and injection of the lungs which terminates in this extravasation; and, providing the extravasated fluid get into the bronchial tubes, it may be coughed up in the form of blood more or less pure. In general, even when blood is coughed up in this manner, a quantity, more or less considerable, is at the same time effused into the interstices of the pulmonic filamentous tissue, where it stagnates, and at length coagulating gives rise to the granular dark-coloured solid indurated masses found on dissection, disseminated through the lung. These masses are not the cause, but the effect of the hemorrhage, which is itself the effect of previous congestion.

The change now mentioned is often found in the lungs as an effect of disease of the heart, especially degeneration, ossification, and arctation of the mitral valve. But I have observed it take place independent of this; and I have met with a remarkable instance of it in the lungs of an infant of twelve or thirteen months.

These and other circumstances lead me to regard this change as one of the effects of pneumonic inflammation, and I therefore refer it to the present head under the name of hemorrhagic peripneumony, (*pneumonia hæmorrhagica.*)

Of the other varieties, the second is rather a species of vesicular bronchitis, and as such has been already described under its proper head.

The third, viz. the chronic or latent peripneumony, occurs under two forms, chronic inflammation of the pulmonic tissue, and inflammation of the lobules.

§ 2. CHRONIC PNEUMONIA.—In the first it presents the same anatomical characters as the acute disease, but comes on in a more insidions and gradual manner. Andral, indeed, represents the anatomical character of chronic pneumonia to be hardening of the pulmonic tissue, with a yellow, gray, blue, black, or brown tint, with impermeability to air. This, however, is the ultimate result of a series of changes, in which the portion of lung has been previously the seat of red coloration and congestion, infiltration of blood, and at length infiltration of blood and lymph. In this mode it most frequently steals on imperceptibly, with cough aggravated in the winter season and on exposure to cold, slight dyspnœa which increases gradually, very slight febrile symptoms aggravated during the night, gradual wasting and eventually death, either by bastard peripneumony, a sudden and unexpected attack of the acute disorder, or the establishment of pleuritic inflammation.

In less frequent cases the same change is sometimes left as a residue of the acute form of the disorder.

§ 3. LOBULAR PNEUMONIA.—In the second form of chronic pneumonia the inflammatory disorder comes on in a different manner. Either at the same time, or successively inflammatory congestion, indicated by redness, induration, and at length the effusion of blood and lymph, takes place in several, sometimes many points, of one or both lungs. This goes on for weeks or months, until the whole of both lungs present a multitude of roundish or irregular formed nodules about the size of small nuts, diffused through their substance. When these are divided by the knife they present an exterior of reddish, firm vascular substance, inclosing in general small grains of grayish-coloured matter, sometimes like coagulated lymph, sometimes like purulent matter. They are manifestly confined to the minute divisions or lobules of the lungs, and as the inflammatory action has thus originated in, and been chiefly confined to these lobules, the disorder has not improperly been denominated *lobular pneumonia*, (*pneumonia lobulorum*.) The lungs at the same time are infiltrated with serum; the bronchial tubes contain puriform mucus; the *pleura* is invariably more or less inflamed and covered with patches of albuminous exudation, especially opposite to those inflamed lobules which approach nearest to the *pleura pulmonalis*; the pulmonic and costal *pleuræ* are often united by soft recent adhesions; the upper part of the apex of the lung generally adheres extensively; and sero-albuminous or puriform fluid is found in the cavity of the *pleura*.

The symptoms of this disorder are imperfectly known. In the few cases which have fallen closely under my observation, the existence of disease of the lungs was not even suspected; and in one case which I had occasion to inspect, the patient, a boy of fifteen, was supposed to have died of continued fever. Febrile symptoms, indeed, he presented for about eight or nine days previous to the fatal event, and at the same time the breathing was rapid, he complained of headach, and afterwards a little delirium and coma ensued. I learned from his relatives that he had habitual difficult breathing, but I could not ascertain that he had cough or expectoration.

Besides the morbid state of the lungs in this form of disorder, it is usual to find inflammatory redness and enlargement of the muciparous follicles of the colon, the cæcum, and sometimes of the ileum, and these may be affected with ulceration.

The *meninges* also are generally injected, and fluid is formed in the subarachnoid tissue, within the ventricles, and within the spinal theca.

This form of pneumonic inflammation is most usually found in children and young persons. Its causes are imperfectly known. But, from the circumstance of its being often associated with the disorders of the joints, bones, and similar tissues usually imputed to the influence of the strumous diathesis, its development may be inferred to be dependent on the presence of this diathesis, and created by exposure to cold or some similar exciting causes. From the peculiar form which it assumes, and from its association with ulceration of the intestinal follicles, as well as the circumstances in diathesis already mentioned, I regard it as the early stage of tubercular consumption. The only reason that it is not so frequently met with as the other ordinary forms of pneumonia, is, that it seldom proves fatal in the early stage, or before it has not only occupied the whole of both lungs with the morbid deposit, but produced more or less excavation.

Marks of chronic diffused pneumonia are always found, in every case of tubercular infiltration and destruction of the lung.

The gastric or bilious *pneumonia* has been rendered a subject of great importance by Lepecq de la Cloture,* Stoll,† Romain,‡ Ackermann,§ Jansen,‖ Guidetti,¶ Borsieri, Goeden, Hauff, and various other foreign physicians. Its existence as a form of peripneumony is almost denied by Andral, and I confess that in this country it is seen so rarely, as to justly give rise to doubts of its

* Lepecq de la Cloture Observat. sur les Maladies Epidemiques.   Paris, 1776.
† Ratio Medendi, Vol. iii. iv. and v. Part II. v. vii. p. 112, 117, 346.
‡ Romain Essai sur la Maniere de Traites les Peripneumonies Bilieuses. Metz, 1779.
§ Ackermann Pleuritidis Biliosæ brevis adumbratio. Kiliae, 1785.
‖ Dissert. de Peripneumonia Biliosa.   Goett. 1787.
¶ Guidetti, Dissert. de Pleuritide Biliosa.   Heidelberg, 1790.

individual and independent reality. Pneumonia doubtless takes place in persons in whom the alimentary functions are disordered, and sometimes the hepatic secretions perverted or deranged; and it sometimes happens that symptoms of gastric and hepatic disorder simulate symptoms of pneumonic inflammation. The first must be regarded as a mere complication, such as is very frequently met with in practice. The second must be viewed as a distemper totally different, and requiring different treatment.

The class of persons in whom pneumonia and bronchitis is observed to assume the bilious or gastric disorder in this country most frequently are the intemperate, especially spirit and wine-bibbers, the gouty, and those labouring under mental anxiety and distress.

§ 4. The term nervous or typhoid *pneumonia* has been applied to pneumonia taking place, as it often does, along with typhoid fever, or giving rise to symptoms of typhoid fever. Of this variety two forms may be specified.

1*st*, Either a person attacked with continued fever presents in the course of it symptoms of bronchial inflammation or even pneumonia, not very well marked, but still sufficiently so to be recognized by the skilful observer. Sometimes, not always, there is cough; for in certain cases the patient is so feeble that he is unable to cough or expectorate. In general the respiration is laborious, limited, and irregular; the face, cheeks, and lips are livid; the hands and feet livid and cold; and the pulse small, soft, and sometimes irregular or intermitting. Upon employing auscultation the presence of pneumonia in the posterior and inferior region of one or both lungs is recognized. In this form of the disorder it is said to be typhoid fever with pneumonia.

2*d*, In a person attacked with pneumonic inflammation, the symptomatic fever does not assume the open and distinct symptoms usually presented, but observes a slow, latent, and insidious form, in which the symptoms of great feebleness (*adynamia*) and nervous irritation (*neurasthenia*) are predominant. Of these the most prominent are great oppression at the breast, intolerable anxiety, and jactitation; a sense of internal heat; great difficulty in breathing and coughing; total cessation of pain if previously felt; a deceitful calm or listlessness; delirium in the night especially, or *typhomania;* dryness and tremulousness of the tongue, unquenchable thirst, meteorismus of the belly, dry burning skin, faintings, subsultus tendinum, feebleness of the voice or aphonia, extreme debility of the voluntary motions, great softness and weakness of the pulse, which is also sometimes quick, sometimes natural. In some cases vomiting or hiccup, or both ensue. The surface of the skin presents dark-coloured petechial spots or a miliary eruption, especially on the anterior part of the trunk. Hemorrhages from the nostrils, throat, lungs, stomach, and intestinal tube are liable to take place; the urine is sometimes dark-coloured and bloody; and discharges of blood from the *uterus* in females are not unusual. The blood, if drawn from a vein, presents in general a loose, soft coagulum, with a small proportion of serum. In a few rare cases the clot is firm.

As the symptoms proceed, the delirium or typhomania passes into lethargic sopor; the breathing becomes stertorous, and is attended with general tracheo-bronchial rattling; the pulse becomes small, and can scarcely be felt; convulsions occasionally ensue; the head, neck, and chest are covered with cold fetid sweats; the extremities become cold, and death follows.

Morbid anatomy shows, that this distemper is of the kind denominated pleuropneumony, with vesicular bronchitis. Gluge and Vogel however both represent the substance of the lungs to be consolidated with infiltration of dark-coloured blood in patches. The lungs are found gorged with blood, dark-coloured and dense towards the posterior part, not indurated or consolidated, but rather œdematous and doughy. The surface of the lung presents dark livid patches. The pleurae contain sero-sanguine or sero-purulent fluid, with shreds of lymph. Sometimes even the pericardium and the peritoneum present fluids of the same kind, with flocks of lymph. The chambers of the heart also and the large vessels contain large, loose, soft coagula of blood. In some epidemics the intestinal tube contains *lumbrici*.

A state of the lungs very similar to this is observed to take place in persons labouring under sea-scurvy.[*]

§ 5. PNEUMONIA SEPTICA. GANGRÆNA PULMONUM.—It may be doubted whether pneumonia ever legitimately terminates in mortification or gangrene of the lung; and there is some reason to think, that, when mortification does take place in these organs, it

---

[*] *Vide* Huxham, chapter ii. p. 186, and Henderson, Edinburgh Medical and Surgical Journal, vol. iii. p. 10.

is the result not of ordinary inflammation, but of a peculiar kind of inflammation, the tendency of which is to gangrene.

Gangrene of the lungs takes place either as a part and conco-mitant of continued fever with typhoid symptoms and pestilential fevers in general, or it may occur, so far as it is possible to judge, as a primary species of inflammatory disorder of the lungs.

α. In the first case, a person with the usual symptoms of aggra-vated and rather intense typhoid fever, and commonly with marks of imperfect general circulation and perverted and imperfect pul-monary circulation, as lividity of the face, nose, cheeks, lips, and extremities, coldness of the extremities, hiccup, and small pulse, presents obscure symptoms of disorder of the lungs, laborious and irregular respiration, sometimes hurried, sometimes slower than natural, slight cough, at first dry, afterwards moist with sputa, very viscid, glutinous, orange-coloured, streaked with blood, and very fetid offensive breath. The sound upon percussion is more or less dull; and upon auscultation, either the crepitant rattle, sometimes with large bells, is heard, or this is heard with inaudi-bility of the vesicular sound most usually in the subscapular and inferior convex region of one or both lungs. With these symp-toms are usually associated great feebleness, delirium or typho-mania, intermittent, irregular small pulse, a tendency to gangrene of the extremities and sacrum, hiccup, subsultus tendinum, diar-hœa; and at length with increasing difficulty of breathing, fetor of the breath, and tracheo-bronchial rattling, death ensues. Some-times hemorrhage takes place from the lungs, and contributes, with the other marks of feebleness, to accelerate the approach of the fatal event.

β. In the second case, the distemper appears to come on at first in general as an affection of the lungs. Either the patient has an attack of pneumonic inflammation, or bronchial disease, or spitting of blood, (*hæmoptysis*), with more or less dull pain in some part of the side or chest, most commonly in the mammary or submammary region before, and the subscapular region behind, and sometimes as if passing between these two points. Cough continues and in-creases, with *sputa* in general reddish, brown, or bloody, and sometimes with pure blood, and very offensive fetid breath. The countenance is anxious and livid; the complexion dingy, wan, and leaden coloured; the cheeks occasionally tinged with a reddish or pink-coloured flush; the eye heavy and pale, sometimes wild,

3 R

glaring, and slightly suffused, in other instances hollow and ghastly. In the other symptoms considerable variety takes place. Thus in one case, no complaint or symptoms appear which indicate a serious disorder of the lungs. The patient is merely feeble, with dingy wan complexion, irregular breathing, cough, and a little expectoration. In other cases, pains, more or less acute, are felt in the chest, and the labour of respiration, with debility, is considerable. The most characteristic symptom of the distemper, the fœtid offensive breath, is not an early symptom. It does not take place till the disease has subsisted for some time, two weeks, or even a longer period; and indeed it appears only to take place after a communication between the seat of disorder and the bronchial tubes and the air inspired and expired has been established. When it takes place it is impossible to entertain any doubt of the presence of the distemper; but gangrene of the lungs may, on the other hand, exist, and have proceeded to a considerable extent, yet with-out giving rise to fœtor of the breath and expectoration.

As the disease advances, expectoration becomes more abundant, with sputa reddish, brown, blood-coloured, or consisting of blood more or less pure, and the characteristic fetid odour. Respiration becomes very irregular and laborious, being at one time slow, at another quick and panting. In general, immediately before the fetid odour of the breath and sputa is manifest, more or less stupor and much anxiety come on, with small, feeble, irregular pulse.

In general, after the fœtor of the breath and sputa is established, the distemper tends rapidly to the fatal termination. In one case which fell under my own observation, the distemper continued thirty days before the fœtid odour of the breath was evinced. The breath and *sputa* were fœtid on the thirtieth day of the disorder, and death took place the second day afterwards. In one of the cases by M. Schrœder, death took place nine days after the first occurrence of fœtor. In another case attended by myself, the offensive fœtor of the breath and *sputa* was recognized on the 23d of February, and death took place on the 6th of March, eleven days after. This, I believe, may be regarded as nearly as may be, the latest period that life is likely to be prolonged, after the occurrence of well-marked fœtor of the breath and *sputa*.

The duration of this disease varies from four weeks to two months. It is rare that physicians witness its commencement; for it is only when the patient can no longer move about, or pursue his ordinary occupations, that he applies for assistance ; and in general the disease has been proceeding for eight days or two weeks when he is **first seen.**

The appearances found after death are of two kinds. One is indicative of what is named diffusive gangrene of the lungs, the other is circumscribed. In the first case, a mass of lung, about two inches and a half or three inches wide, but irregular in figure and outline, is converted into a soft, pulpy, dark ash-coloured substance, which, when it is handled or pressed by the finger, falls down into a loose moist mass—emitting a fœtid offensive odour, without trace of the usual structure of the lungs, except a few bronchial tubes, and blood-vessels and filaments and shreds of filamentous tissue. This mass is in general bounded by, but it does not terminate abruptly in, healthy lung. It is soft, dingy, and infiltrated with a dark, ash-coloured, dirty serous liquor. Occasionally the surrounding portion of lung is hepatized or infiltrated with blood, or blood-coloured serum ; the bronchial tubes always contain much blood-coloured viscid mucus ; and sometimes the *pleura* is reddened, covered with lymph or adhesions, and contains fluid in its cavity.

The part of the lung most usually thus mortified is either in the lower lobe, the upper part of the lower and lower part of the middle or upper lobe on the left side, or the middle lobe alone on the right side ; that is, the central part of the lungs, but verging toward the lower part.

In the second form, or that which is circumscribed, a portion of the lung generally towards the surface, presents a dark-coloured hard patch, varying in size from a shilling to a half-crown piece or more, often pretty exactly circular, bounded all round by healthy lung, and not unusually a distinct reddened circle of vessels, or vessels with lymph. This circular hard patch, which resembles closely an eschar produced by caustic potass, or any of the cauteries, may either adhere or be detached. In the latter case, it generally leaves disclosed a cup-like cavity, a little larger than the detached eschar, not loose or filamentous, or shreddy-like as in diffuse gangrene, but firm, granular, with the blood-vessels and bronchial tubes closed, and with the surrounding lung more softened, but generally presenting marks of pleurisy, *pneumonia*, and *bronchitis*, all united. Sometimes albuminous exudation over the *pleura* and within its cavity is found to have taken place,—a circumstance which is to be ascribed to secondary pleurisy caused by the inflammation induced to detach the dead eschar.

Though these forms of gangrene of the lung are sometimes distinct, they occasionally take place at the same time in the same lung. Thus in the case of one of the patients who was treated by myself, a man of fifty-six, diffuse gangrene was observed towards the internal and anterior surface of the left lung, and circumscribed gangrene in the form of a cup-like cavity at the outer surface of the same lung.

Laennec represents this disease as occasionally terminating favourably. Of this I have never seen an instance, either in my own practice, or in that of any of my colleagues at the Royal Infirmary. It is, indeed, a disease almost necessarily fatal, whether from the kinds of constitution in which it occurs, or its deleterious effects on the lungs and their functions.

The causes of gangrene of the lungs are little known. The disease occurs either along with typhoid fever, or gives rise to typhoid symptoms. It is more common in persons beyond the ages of forty-five or fifty, and especially in those who have lived intemperately. It also occurs in persons much younger, or between twenty and thirty-six. But very often in persons at this age, it is found to have taken place either during a mercurial course, or shortly after its completion.

Some authorities regard it, especially when circumscribed, as the effect of pulmonary apoplexy.

I have, when treating of the transporting power of the veins, adverted to the fact, that when gangrene affects the lungs, suppuration, or a purulent deposit, is liable to take place in the brain. From the cases in which this has been observed, not many indeed, I think that it is impossible to doubt, that however it may be explained, under certain circumstances purulent deposit, either within the veins and sinuses of the brain, or within the substance of the brain, takes place after gangrene of the lungs has been established. Yet the necessity of the gangrenous affection to the production of the effect is not obvious. On the other hand, mere suppuration of the lung may be adequate.

Gangrene is liable to attack certain forms of tubercular excavation and vomicæ of the lungs. To this attention shall be directed afterwards.

In certain circumstances, this disease appears to prevail epidemically, whether it be the effect of a typhoid or pestilential fever which gives rise to it, or it depends on the prevalence of some peculiar telluric or atmospheric miasma. In the year 1348, a febrile disorder, with intense pneumonic symptoms, often terminating fatally by profuse or continued hemorrhage from the lungs, appeared in Italy, and spread between that year and 1350 over many parts of Europe, destroying much of the population of different countries in an incredibly short space of time. This disorder, which was emphatically denominated by the populace the black death, appears to have possessed the character of fever with gangrenous pneumonia. In many pestilential epidemics, however, as in that of Marseilles, Transylvania, and other countries, carbuncular and glandular plague appears to have been attended with symptoms of pulmonary mortification.

Pneumonic inflammation, very often with vesicular *bronchitis*, occurs secondarily in ague, remittent fever, typhoid fever, smallpox, measles, pulmonary consumption, rheumatism, and rheumatic gout, and disease of the kidney. I have also observed the disease take place in a latent or insidious manner in the insane from chronic meningeal inflammation.

§ 6. VOMICA OR ABSCESS OF THE LUNGS.—To complete the history of pneumonic inflammation, I add a few remarks on abscess of the lungs, and a form of suppurative inflammation to which they are liable.

The formation of a distinct abscess of the lungs as a consequence of inflammation, was at one time generally admitted among pathologists. Laennec, however, who describes suppuration of the lungs under his third degree of pulmonary induration, maintains that it .is exceedingly rare, and gives it as the result of his observation, that small abscesses are found in the pulmonic tissue not above four or five times, and an extensive one not above once, in many hundred cases. Gray hepatization is in one sense suppuration of the lungs; for pus-globules are found in the interstices of the filamento-cellular tissue, and are observed oozing from it. This however is infiltration of purulent matter, not an abscess or deposit in a particular cavity. Many of the reported cases of pulmonary abscess, or suppuration of lung, as a consequence of inflammation, may be regarded as excavations or *vomicæ* formed by the softening of extensive tubercular masses. Several also, I am satisfied, are instances of chronic pleurisy terminating in *empyema* and condensed lung. It is possible that suppuration, as a consequence of inflammation of the lungs, may be rare, for two reasons; *1st,* Because the disease may prove fatal by suffocation, before it has attained the complete suppurative stage; 2d, Because under the influence of remedies, it may be so much modified as to prevent the formation of purulent matter in a distinct sac or cavity. But it must not be regarded as so rare as M. Laennec represents it. Instances are recorded by Morgagni, in which a considerable portion of the pulmonic tissue was converted into a purulent abscess, with the contiguous structure apparently healthy, or indurated as a consequence of previous inflammation. Dr Baillie expresses himself with some uncertainty; for his language may be interpreted so as to apply either to tubercular vomicæ, or to pulmonary abscesses; though it is evident, and more especially from what he says in his engravings, that he believed in its ordinary occurrence.

On this subject evidence is defective; and several good cases, with the appearances after death are required, in order to ascertain the frequency or the general occurrence of abscess as a consequence of pneumonic inflammation.

It is impossible to doubt, nevertheless, that suppuration of the lungs, that is, the proper pulmonic filamentous tissue, does take place as an effect of inflammation of that tissue. In this instance, purulent matter of a gray dirty aspect is formed beneath the pleura or the subserous cellular tissue, and extends in this direction between the lobes. An excellent example of this lesion occurred to me in the course of July 1843. A man in an extreme state of feebleness presented himself for admission to the hospital. It was manifest that he was in the last stage of some serious disease of the lungs; and death took place in the course of a few hours. Inspection disclosed the following state of the lungs. The *pleuræ* of both lungs, but especially of the right, were detached from the subjacent substance of the lung by a quantity of dirty ash-coloured purulent matter. In the right lung, this detachment with the corresponding purulent matter extended into the division of the lobes and lobules, which were thus separated from each other. The filamento-cellular tissue appeared as if it had been dissolved and carried away in the purulent collection; for it was no longer cognizable in its wonted characters. When the matter was washed away, bronchial tubes and blood-vessels were all that was left; and these did not adhere as they are wont to do. In short the cohesion of the whole of the lower and middle lobe of the right lung was entirely destroyed.

Another example of the same lesion is recorded by Dr Stokes in the third volume of the Dublin Medical Journal. This gentleman found in the body of a young man who died after labouring for fifteen days under symptoms of pneumonic inflammation, a considerable collection of purulent matter beneath the pulmonic *pleura* of the lower lobe of the left lung, and between it and the bronchial tubes and vesicles of the lung—dissecting away as it were the *pleura*, from the lung, destroying, or at least converting into purulent matter, the pulmonic filamentous tissue, and leaving the pulmonic vesicles and bronchial tubes comparatively untouched. This must be regarded as not only an example of suppuration of the lung, but as proving clearly, that the seat of this form of *pneumonia* is in the pulmonic parenchyma or filamentous tissue, as already inculcated.[*]

§ 7. PULMONARY PHLEBITIS. COLLECTIONS OF MATTER IN THE VEINS OF THE LUNGS.—I have met with two or three examples, in which, without expecting any morbid appearance, I found the pleura sound, the lungs interspersed at considerable distances with numerous minute abscesses, but the intermediate tissue quite healthy. As it occurred that these were softened tubercles, the whole organ was carefully examined, yet without finding anything but minute spherical abscesses of various sizes, and with the surrounding texture natural. The peculiarity, therefore, of this species of suppuration, is its not being preceded by tubercles, the surrounding pulmonic tissue being neither inflamed nor indurated, and the simultaneous formation of many purulent points.

Dr Baillie, by whom this species of suppuration had been seen, thought it probable that the abscesses were produced by a number of scattered tubercles taking on the process of suppuration. When however these purulent collections are carefully examined, they are found to take place within the veins of the lungs. Of this I am satisfied from having observed these deposits ensue after inflammation of the veins of the arm, consequent on blood-letting. They take place also after amputation of the extremities, in which the medullary membrane and veins of the bones have been inflamed and suppurate, and occasionally after other injuries which proceed to suppuration.[†]

[*] Dublin Journal of Medical Sciences, vol. iii. Contributions to Thoracic Pathology, by Dr Stokes, p. 51.

[†] Observations on Depositions of Pus and Lymph occurring in the Lungs and other viscera after injuries of different parts of the Body. By Thomas Rose, Esq. &c. Medico-Chirurgical Transactions, Vol. xiv. p. 251. London, 1828.

This has been mentioned by Gluge as taking place after glanders and metastatic inflammation ; and he considers the purulent matter as deposited in the pulmonic filamento-cellular tissue.* It appears to me that though this may take place occasionally, yet these collections are very generally in the veins of the lungs.

In one case of inflammation of the uterine veins, with matter in them and the common iliac veins and *cava*, Dr Lee found, with hepatization of the lower lobe of the left lung, matter in the pulmonary veins and lymph in the pulmonary trunk.†

§ 8. DEPOSITS OF BLOOD IN THE PULMONARY ARTERIES AFTER PHLEBITIS.—Another effect of inflammation of the veins consists in deposits of blood, or lymph, or both, in the pulmonary artery and its branches. While the last mentioned deposit of purulent matter succeeds purulent *phlebitis,* this, there is every reason to believe, follows lymphy or plasmatic *phlebitis,* in which either clots of blood or lymph are formed in the inflamed vein. The following is the ordinary mode in which I have seen this take place.

Symptoms of inflammation appear in a vein of the extremities ; most usually in the common femoral or external iliac vein, which is painful, and in the site of which a hard firm swelling is felt, with general swelling and pain of the veins of the extremity. This proceeds for days and weeks, until the interior channel of the vein is more or less, sometimes completely obstructed.

Other symptoms indicative of more or less disorder in the organs of respiration take place. In some instances purulent effusion within the pleura follows. In others there are indications of derangement in the action of the heart, as palpitation, forcible pulsation in the cardiac region, irregular or intermittent pulsation and dropsical effusion. At length, after weeks or months, death ensues, when the following facts are observed.

A bloody or lymphy clot more or less firm, sometimes completely solid, in the external iliac and common femoral artery ; the coats of the vein thickened and not collapsing, and their inner membrane rough and reddened for a considerable space.

In some cases a clot of blood or lymph adheres most firmly to the *laciniæ* of the tricuspid valve, or to the walls of the right ventricle. When the pulmonary artery is examined, one or two of its branches is filled more or less completely with a brownish firm clot

---

* Atlas Der Pathologischen Anatomie. Sechste Lieferung. Seite 5.

† Case of Pulmonary Phlebitis. By Robert Lee, M. D. &c. Medico-Chirurgical Transactions, Vol. xix. p. 45. London, 1835.

of blood, and dispersed through the lungs are similar clots, brownish-coloured, all of which may be traced to divisions of the pulmonary artery.

- This disease is sometimes chronic in its course, and may take ten or twelve months before it renders the lungs unable to perform their functions. But in one case it terminated in about seven or eight weeks.

The occurrence of these clots of blood within the branches of the pulmonary artery has been noticed by Cruveilhier,* M. Baron,† Mr James Paget,‡ and Dr Dubini.§ It does not appear that in all the cases recorded by these observers, there was proof that the circumstance was preceded by inflammation in any veins of the extremities, or the formation of clots within their channels. In several of the cases, the obstruction came on to all appearance spontaneously, and without indications of previous disease. In the case given by Cruveilhier, the obstruction was connected with uterine *phlebitis*. But Mr Paget thinks that there is between these cases and those which he records a great difference. The cases mentioned he thinks, connected either with pulmonary apoplexy, especially if dependent on disease of the heart, or with pneumonia, or with the presence of enkephaloid matter in the blood, or with that of urea in the blood, as in the case of granular disease of the kidney, in which he finds these deposits to be frequent. It appears, therefore, that the formation of these deposits depends on several different causes, all however agreeing in some morbid state of the blood or the veins.

§ 9. PNEUMONORRHAGIA. HEMORRHAGE FROM THE LUNGS.— Discharge of blood by coughing occurs under two forms. One is that of bronchial hemorrhage, sometimes copious, but often in small quantity. The other is that of pulmonary hemorrhage, which may be small in quantity, but is generally very copious. Of the former sufficient notice has already been taken under the head of diseases of the bronchial membrane. The latter is to be considered in this place.

· * Anatomie Pathologique, Livraison xi.

† Recherches et Observations sur la Coagulation du Sang, Dans l'Artere Pulmonaire et ses effets. By M. C. Baron, Archives Generales de Medecine, T. xlvii. p. 5. Paris, 1838.

‡ On Obstructions of the Branches of the Pulmonary Arteries. By James Paget, F. R. C. S. and Medico-Chirurgical Transactions, Vol. xxvii. p. 162. London, 1844. Additional Observations on Obstructions of the Pulmonary Arteries. By James Paget, F. R. C. S. Medico-Chirurgical Transactions, Vol. xxviii. p. 352. London, 1845.

§ Annali Universali di Medicina di Febraio. 1845.

On the exact source and pathological causes of spitting of blood, physicians entertained either erroneous or indistinct ideas. The ancients ascribed it to rupture of some of the pulmonary vessels; and this opinion was adopted by many practitioners, and is still entertained by the vulgar, to whom this disease has been long known by the name of *rupture of a blood-vessel.* This opinion, however, is manifestly contradicted by anatomy and by observation. In modern times this opinion regarding the pathology of pulmonary hemorrhage is found to be correct in two cases only; first, when an aneurismal tumour or a diseased artery bursts into the air tubes (*bronchia,*) or the windpipe; and secondly, when an arterial branch passing through a tubercular excavation has given way during the progress of ulceration. Neither of these cases, it is obvious, are necessarily connected with true pulmonary hemorrhage. Both are followed by immediate or very speedy destruction. But the process of hæmoptysis may recur from time to time during months or years in the same individual, or even the whole of a long life; yet without being the direct cause of death.

In modern times, the opinions on the nature of pulmonary hemorrhage may be referred to two heads. According to one of these views, hæmoptysis is the result of an actual wound or breach in the bronchial or mucous membrane of the lungs. This was the opinion of Barry, Grant, Gilchrist, and even of Cullen, if we understand him aright. According to the other view, which is more recent, hæmoptysis is believed to depend on some disorder of the bronchial membrane, and its exhalant vessels; in consequence of which they discharge blood instead of mucus. This opinion was that of Bichat, who has been followed by all the physicians of the Parisian school, and by many in this country. This opinion is, as I have already shown, well-founded within certain limits only. There are cases of hæmoptysis in which the bronchial membrane and its capillaries only or principally are affected; and then the blood which is occasionally coughed up is the result of exhalation, or of destillation, as it used to be named by the older pathologists. Such are the discharges of blood which take place in slight cases of hæmoptysis or pulmonary catarrh, about the termination of peripneumony, about the commencement of consumption, and in young females after the suppression or retention of the menstrual discharge.

There are, however, many instances of bleeding from the lungs in a violent and extreme degree, for which it is impossible to account by capillary exhalation only.

Dr William Stark was the first who described accurately the state of the lungs in these instances of hæmoptysis. The air vesicles in some parts of the lungs he found filled with blood or bloody serum. These parts did not collapse on opening the chest, but were firm, very dark or light-red in colour, and could neither be compressed nor distended by the usual inflation. When cut into, thick blood or bloody matter issued from the cut surfaces; and portions of the diseased parts, after being for some time macerated in water, still sank as before maceration. He further showed by blowing air into the blood-vessels and air-tubes of the sound and diseased portions respectively, that in the latter, air passed from the branches of the pulmonary artery and veins into the bronchial tubes,—in other words, that the minute arteries and veins or capillary vessels of the lungs communicated freely with the bronchial tubes and air-cells.*

This description is extremely accurate, but appears to have been altogether overlooked. Its accuracy has been confirmed by various subsequent observers, and especially by the researches of Laennec. The facts ascertained in this manner show that a considerable change takes place in hæmoptysis in the pulmonary substance, or the proper tissue of the lungs. A portion of the organ becomes uniformly hard, of a dark-red colour, and impermeable to the air. The indurated spot is always partial, from one to four cubic inches in extent, pretty exactly circumscribed, with healthy or pale-coloured lung, and looks not unlike a clot of venous blood; circumstances by which it is to be distinguished from pneumonic induration, which terminates more or less gradually in sound lung. These changes consist in effusion of blood into the parenchyma of the lungs, and into the bronchial tubes; and as they are analogous to those which take place in the brain in apoplexy, Laennec applies to them the name of pulmonary apoplexy. These are confined chiefly, however, to the severer forms of pulmonary hemorrhage.

Not even is this description, however, sufficient to explain all the phenomena of pulmonary hemorrhage. The changes of the pulmonic tissue described by Laennec, are rather the effects of a previous morbid state of the capillary circulation of the lungs, than the actual state of the morbid process, which gives rise to effusion of red blood from the bronchial membrane. When the lung is in the

* The Works of the late William Stark, M. D., &c. London, 1788, p. 34.

state described by this pathologist, the blood has been already discharged from the vessels, or extravasated not only into the cells of the pulmonic tissue, but into the minute extremities of the bronchial tubes, which are thus filled and obstructed within, while they are compressed and obliterated without. But it is the agent that causes this effect, which it is the object of the pathologist to know ; it is the state of the capillary circulation which terminates in this effusion, which it is necessary to explain in unfolding the pathology of pulmonary hemorrhage. This it will be found consists in more or less injection and distension of the capillaries or minute arteries and veins which are distributed through the pulmonic tissue, to wind round, and ramify in the minute or extreme bronchial tubes, in consequence of some derangement or impediment in the circulation.

The truth is, that in all the instances of the lesion described as hemorrhage into the substance of the lungs, whether recent, or in the form of pulmonary dark-brown induration, it is preceded either by disease of the heart, or disease in the substance of the lungs.

1. Bichat, and particularly Corvisart, observed that, in certain forms of disease of the heart, especially the active aneurism of the latter, or what is at present termed hypertrophy, expectoration of blood was a symptom of the second and third stages of the disease. The same circumstance was also noticed by Mr Allan Burns, who, however, has hypothetically connected this symptom with dilatation of the right side of the heart. All the best marked cases of pulmonary hemorrhage with hemorrhagic induration which I have seen, have been connected with ossification of the mitral valve, and arctation of its aperture, or hypertrophy of the left ventricle. The operation of the former it is easy to understand. The blood does not pass with its wonted facility through the mitral valve into the left ventricle ; the left auricle is consequently kept in a constant state of over-distension ; this distension is propagated along the pulmonary veins to the pulmonary capillaries, which are thus perfectly filled and distended with blood, which is not allowed to be moved into their trunks in the usual manner, and with the wonted regularity. As this distension is every hour and day increasing, with the persistence and increase of the obstruction in the left auriculo-ventricular aperture, it is not wonderful that the blood is extravasated into the pulmonic filamentous tissue, and through the bronchial membrane, causing in the former the dark brown-coloured circumscribed masses which are found after death, and in the latter the bloody expectoration which takes place during life.

It is remarkable, nevertheless, that this extravasation and its effects are greatest and most conspicuous in young persons. A degree of degeneration of the mitral valve and arctation of its aperture, which produces little inconvenience at or beyond the age of sixty years, causes between the ages of twenty and thirty extreme *dyspnœa* and *orthopnœa*, cough, hæmoptysis, and all the aecompanying symptoms, with serous infiltration into the different cavities and the subcutaneous cellular tissue.

Much the same phenomena may take place in consequence of dilatation or hypertrophy, general or partial, of the left ventricle. Often, indeed, the dilatation or excentric hypertrophy and the concentric hypertrophy are the result of disease of the semilunar valves at the origin of the aorta; but, in several instances, they take place independently of this. When they do ensue, they give rise to a similar state of imperfect transmission of the blood out of the ventriele into the aorta; the left ventricle, auricle, and pulmonary veins become unduly distended; and eventually the pulmonary capillaries are constantly distended with an unusual load of blood, which at length is extravasated, and causes the same state of the lung, and the same expectoration of blood, which takes place at an earlier period in the degeneration of the mitral valve.

In either of these cases now specified, but especially in disease of the mitral valve and arctation of the auriculo-ventricular aperture, in hypertrophy, and in that rare disease called partial aneurism of the heart, hemorrhage of the lungs may take place in one or other of the following modes.

After a fit of great difficulty of breathing, generally with orthopnœa, a quantity of blood varying from one to six ounces is brought up forcibly by coughing. In one instance I saw nearly two pounds coughed up in the course of about thirty hours. In such cases the large fluid rattling and gurgling, is heard all over the chest, generally on both sides. From this state recovery is sometimes but rarely effected. Death usually takes place in the course of a few days, not so much from loss of blood, which rather relieves the patient than otherwise, as from the extreme difficulty in breathing. The state of the lungs is then the following. They are completely gorged with blood; of a dark-red or very livid colour; and in several points brown masses not firm are formed, which are blood effused into the filamento-cellular tissue. When the case is recent, these masses are few and small, sometimes on the margins of the lungs, sometimes deep in their substance. They are also soft, and the blood is imperfectly coagulated. A curious appearance in lungs of this kind is that of red-spotting or maculation all over the surface and into their substance. When the *pleura* is removed by dissection, these spots are observed to lie beneath it on the substance of the lungs, and are found to depend on blood poured into the bronchial tubes and extending to their ultimate terminations.

Sprinkling or maculation with blood in the lungs from its presence in the bronchial tubes and air-vesicles, I have in like manner observed in the lungs of persons who had committed suicide by cutting the throat, and in sheep slaughtered in the same manner.

The lungs in this state are heavy, compact, and partially condensed; and though they crepitate and contain air in certain points, yet they generally sink in water.

In another set of cases, the patient is attacked with a fit of extreme breathlessness, amounting to orthopnœa, in which the lips, nose, and cheeks are blue or violet-coloured, and by coughing he brings up at length frothy mucus, at first streaked, then mixed with blood. This may continue for two, three, or eight days, when the urgent symptoms subside, and the bloody expectoration disappears. This is repeated several times at intervals more or less remote. The fits however are less violent, though longer continued. At length the individual has fewer and less distinct intervals of relief. Breathlessness is either constant, or very nearly so. Cough continues, with expectoration of bloody mucus, and blood, sometimes in considerable quantity. When death ensues, the following is the state of the lungs.

Masses of variable size, but sometimes very considerable, that is, as large as a walnut or small pippin, dark-brown, firm and solid, are found dispersed through the lungs. These masses are solid, granular, and friable, and, though firm, may be broken between the fingers. These also sink in water. When examined carefully, it is easy to see that they are blood extravasated into the filamento-cellular tissue of the lungs. The vessels are closed; the bronchial tubes obliterated, at least not permeable to air. Little of the lungs, indeed, is left in their elastic compressible crepitating condition.

The heart is found either in a state of great hypertrophy, or with the mitral valve ossified, and its aperture greatly contracted. In some instances, though less numerous, the same state is found when the aortic valves are ossified, and the aortic aperture is closed,

The same state of lungs takes place in partial aneurism of the heart.*

These facts may be regarded as established. But another question remains for solution. What is the cause of this distension or injection of vessels, when it cannot be traced to disease of the heart? What is the nature of that condition of the pulmonary capillaries which allows them to be so unusually distended? What change in properties do they undergo in living persons in that particular portion of lung, in consequence of which they become distended with blood, which stagnates in them, and at length is forced from them by extravasation? And lastly, why does this state not give rise to inflammation and its consequences? To these questions no satisfactory answer has hitherto been given.

2. Profuse hemorrhage from the lungs takes place in consequence of tubercular deposition and infiltration. In various persons the deposition of tubercular matter, either in the lungs or at the extremity of the bronchial tubes and vessels, induces the same disorder in the motion of the blood through the pulmonary capillaries which takes place in diseases of the heart. As the presence of these bodies encroaches both upon the lungs and the blood-vessels, the different vessels of the lung become distended with blood, which is not allowed to move through them with the natural facility and rapidity; accumulation consequently ensues; and afterwards extravasation, and sometimes even vessels have been found ruptured.

When the tubercular deposition is extensive, and beginning to cause vascular congestion, serous extravasation, and softening, it also happens not unfrequently that the vessels become much enlarged and distended; their tunics at the same time are involved in the morbid changes, become thickened and covered with morbid products, and are thereby rendered brittle and lacerable; and in this condition they often give way and cause profuse hemorrhage.

3. Lastly, it has been observed, in inspecting the lungs of persons who have died during the breaking down of tubercular masses, and after these masses have been excavated, that, though in general some provision is made against the ulcerative destruction of the blood-vessels by coagula being formed in them, and by their cavities being obliterated, yet in some instances a vessel has been found passing near or across a tubercular cavity, and, having been opened, has

* Observations and Cases illustrating the Nature of False consecutive Aneurism of the Heart. By David Craigie, M. D. &c. Edinburgh Medical and Surgical Journal, Vol. lix. p. 356. Edinburgh, 1843.

poured forth much blood, which has been partly brought up by coughing, and partly filled the cavity with bloody clots, as was ascertained by inspection after death.

The causes of hæmoptysis may be understood from the account already given of the different circumstances under which hemorrhage may take place. They may be shortly enumerated in the following manner : *First*, inflammatory action and induration ; *secondly*, hemorrhagic induration, with or without disease of the heart ; *thirdly*, disease of the arteries ; *fourthly*, tubercular deposition ; *fifthly*, tubercular destruction and excavation ; and *sixth*, bronchial hemorrhage.

§ 10. TUBERCULATIO. TYROMATOSIS. TUBERCULOSIS. STATE OF THE LUNGS IN PULMONARY CONSUMPTION.—In the bodies of those who have died after suffering from the usual symptoms of pulmonary consumption, as already specified, the lungs are always more or less changed in structure and more or less destroyed. In those who have been long ill, and who have been much wasted, the upper regions of one or both lungs are much indurated, and occupied by one or more irregular-shaped cavities or caverns, containing either air, or air and a little viscid puriform dirty-looking matter adhering to their walls.

Very generally the apex of one or both lungs is firmly attached to the inner part of the chest, by the pulmonary *pleura* adhering closely to the costal pleura by means of false membrane, which is usually thick, firm, and cartilaginous. The extent of this adhesion may be such, as, while it surrounds the whole lung, not to descend below the third or the fourth rib ; beneath which the pleura may be free from inflammatory exudation or adhesion ; it then forms a sort of cartilaginous cap or covering of the apex of the lung. But in some instances, while the pleura investing the upper lobe adheres firmly to the costal pleura, that covering the lower lobes and the middle lobe on the right side is covered by a layer more or less thick of albuminous exudation, while a quantity of sero-purulent fluid is found in the posterior part of the thoracic cavity. Almost invariably the lobes adhere by interlobular false membrane.

Sometimes the greater part of one upper lobe is hollowed into one large irregular cavity ; more frequently the upper lobe presents two or three caverns, either isolated or communicating ; and in some instances the upper lobe is occupied by a number of cavities of moderate size, some containing air, others puriform dirty-look-ing mucus. The largest cavities are most commonly formed in the apex or upper region of the upper lobe; but occasionally a con-siderable cavity is found near the middle, or tending towards the base of the upper lobe, and corresponding with the pectoral and axillary regions externally. Cavities filled entirely or partially with matter have been named *Vomicæ*, sometimes abscesses rather im-properly, and with greater propriety softened tubercular masses. When wholly or partially emptied, they are usually named tuber-cular cavities, or cavities, tubercular excavations, or simply excava-tions.

Lower down, for instance in the lower part of the upper lobes, the cavities are few, small, or none; in the middle lobe of the right side, also cavities are rarely observed; and the lower lobes of both sides are in general entirely free from cavities. The whole of these parts, however, are more or less indurated by the presence of hard, solid, irregular-shaped masses, variable in size, but in general larger and more numerous in the upper and middle region of the united lungs than in the lower region.

When the caverns (*vomicæ*,) above noticed, are examined, they are observed to vary, not only in size, but in shape. They vary from the size of a large pea or small bean to that of a walnut, a pigeon's egg, or even a small pippin. Though their shape is more or less ovoidal, they are always irregular, and sometimes consist of one large or considerable cavern with two or three small append-ages. The interior is always irregular, and more or less traversed by cylindrical bands or chords, (*septa*,) (*trabeculæ*,) about the twelfth, the tenth, or the eighth of an inch in diameter, passing in various directions, but generally observing that of the longitudinal diameter of the lung, or observing a slight degree of obliquity.

These bands or chords (*trabeculæ*,) are formed in various modes. Laennec believed them to be formed of the natural tissue of the lungs, condensed as it were, and charged with tubercular matter, and maintains that he in no case found them to present traces of having contained blood-vessels. Schroeder, on the other hand, who frequently injected tuberculated and excavated lungs, represents them to be formed chiefly by the gradual and progressive oblitera-tion of small blood-vessels by means of inflammation, the large ones receiving nutriment after the small ones have ceased to do so.*

* Observationes Anatomico-Pathologici et Practici Argumenti, Auctore J. C. L. Schroeder Van der Kolk, Med. et Art. Obstet. Doct. Fasciculus I. Amstelodami, 1826, 8vo, p. 77 and 78.

It is not improbable that they consist partly of inflamed and con-densed cellular, that is, filamentous tissue, especially that investing the lobules, and partly of obliterated blood-vessels.

The inner surface of a cavity, chiefly or altogether emptied, though irregular, rugged, and hollowed into several subordinate depressions and eminences, presents, nevertheless, a smooth firm surface, which is observed to be owing to the presence of a newly formed membrane. When, indeed, the fluid and granular matter is removed by washing it repeatedly in water, it appears, though hard and somewhat cartilaginous, to be almost like an imperfect mucous membrane, or rather the villous surface of a fistula or sinus. This Laennec regards as a false membrane, or newly formed product; and certainly it presents several of the characters of false or morbid mucous membrane. Thus it is thin, smooth, whitish, or gray, semitransparent, soft, friable, and easily removable by the scalpel. In some instances subjacent to this thin semitransparent membrane, are one, or portions of one a little firmer, rather more opaque, and more closely adherent to the walls of the cavity.

When the texture surrounding the cavity, and forming its walls, is examined, it is found to be solid, firm, incompressible, almost cartilaginous, entirely void of elasticity, more or less dark-red or brown, and serous fluid oozing abundantly from the divided sur-faces. The bronchial tubes passing through such parts, and open-ing into the cavity or cavities, are often enlarged, and their mem-brane is invariably of a deep or bright-red colour, rough and villous, and lined with viscid mucus. In general these bronchial tubes are cut transversely across, or truncated at the point of junction with the cavity. In some rare cases, one bronchial tube is found passing through a cavity or a vomica, showing that it has escaped, or resisted the destroying process which commonly cuts it through. This fact, noticed by Schroeder, I have also seen. But in general such bronchial tubes are at length destroyed, if the life of the patient be sufficiently prolonged. Neither Laennec nor Louis ap-pear to have met with bronchial tubes within cavities; and perhaps the occurrence is rare.

The solidity and firmness of the surrounding texture is caused by two circumstances; the first, the presence of tubercular deposi-tion in the lungs; and the second, inflammatory induration.

The tubercular deposit appears in the form of hard masses, which are amorphous or void of regular shape, and variable in size. When divided, these masses are solid, firm, sometimes almost cartilaginous, of a bluish or dirty gray colour, and when closely.inspected, consist of granular bodies, various in size, from a millet-seed to a small pea, closely aggregated together, and mutually pressing each other. In various points are observed portions of whitish or grayish coloured viscid semifluid matter, which when removed are observed to be contained in small cavities. Such masses cannot be said to be homogeneous. Though invariably much more firm and incompressible than the surrounding lung, and than healthy lung, they consist of portions of different degrees of consistence, and of different colour. To the masses and their component parts, the name of tubercles is indiscriminately applied. It would be more correct if the denomination of tubercle were confined to one or the other, especially to the smaller component portions ; in which case the large masses might be denominated tubercular.

The tubercular masses, as thus described, may occupy the superior and middle parts of the lungs, leaving very little of the sound lung intermediate between them. Lower down, and especially in the lower lobe, they are less extensively diffused, and smaller in size, so that portions of the lung are unoccupied by them. In general, also, they are more abundant at the posterior than at the anterior part of the lungs.

Tubercular masses vary in size, and may be distinguished in this respect into small, middle-sized, and large. · The small masses are those about the size of garden peas, or small beans ; the middle-sized are those about the size of a filbert, or small gooseberry, and all those above this may be designated as large. In general, when they have attained the latter dimensions, they have either become partially softened, or they have begun to soften.

Though the tubercular masses vary in size, their component parts, viz. the minute tubercles, are generally about the same magnitude. These are commonly about the size of a millet-seed or a little larger ; but in general the whole of the interior of a tubercular mass presents in the advanced stage such a confused mass of morbid texture, that it is impossible then to recognize the individual tubercles, or distinguish them from each other and the whole mass. It is only by examining ttuberculated lungs in the early stage, and before the disease has proceeded far, that it is possible to form an accurate notion of the characters of a tuberculated mass.

The tubercular masses receive not injection, and hence cannot be said to receive vessels from the large vessels of the lungs. Attempts to inject tuberculated lungs were made by Dr William Stark; and he always found that the injection reached neither the vomicæ nor the tubercular masses. He found that blood-vessels which were of considerable size, at a little distance from a tubercular mass or masses, speedily became contracted, so that a large vessel, which at its origin measured nearly half an inch in circumference, could not be cut open further than an inch; and that when cut open, such vessels presented a very small canal, which was filled by fibrous substance, evidently albumen or coagulated blood. The same fact he also proved by blowing air into the vessels, or injecting them with wax. When air is blown into the vessels of a tuberculated lung, the air either does not pass along the vessels at all, or does so in a very imperfect manner, nor does air in this manner reach the vomicæ. If coloured wax or isinglass be thrown into the pulmonary artery and vein, the parts least affected by disease, and which before injection are soft and elastic, become afterwards the hardest and firmest; and the parts most occupied by tubercular masses, and which before injection are hardest, become after it much softer than the others. When a lung so injected is divided by incision, numerous minute branches filled with injected matter are seen in the sound parts; but in the diseased parts, few or no injected branches; and the matter is observed never or seldom to enter the tuberculated masses or their vomicæ.

These and similar experiments were performed by Schroeder, who found that no vessels pass through the centre of a vomica, but are closed, and as it were truncated at the margin of the vomica; that in cases in which numerous vessels pass transversely across a vomica or ulcer, though many of them are filled with wax, when injected, yet the small or capillary branches adhere to the trunks externally like filaments, or in the form of slender cellular tissue, but are obstructed and impervious, so that they do not admit the injected matter; whereas the trunks penetrating the vomica are surrounded by no pulmonary parenchyma, excepting the filaments described as the remains of the capillary vessels.

From these facts M. Schroeder concludes that the obliteration begins in the small vessels and proceeds to the large trunks; that this obliteration is the effect of inflammation of the *vasa vasorum*,

by which lymph is effused into the canal of the vessel which unites
its walls and renders its trunk impervious; that the *vasa vasorum*
may not be so much affected by this inflammation, as to interrupt
their circulation, and may continue, consequently, to nourish the
obliterated trunk, which then forms the *septum* of Laennec, and
the *trabecula* of Schroeder; but that in those instances in which
these nutrient vessels have become involved in the inflammation
and obstructed, the trunk becomes black, dies, and is dissolved in
the general suppurative destruction of the tubercular mass.

The state of the lymphatic vessels it is extremely difficult to distinguish in the lungs; and though M. Schroeder injected with
mercury in lungs affected with *vomicæ*, some lymphatic vessels of
the pulmonic *pleura*, yet he never found any one of them penetrating the substance of the lung. Subsequently, however, in the
sound lung, he succeeded not only in injecting with mercury the
lymphatics of the whole surface of the lung (the pulmonic *pleura*
I presume), but traced several branches into the pulmonic *parenchyma* so distinctly, that he was satisfied that the lymphatics en-
compassed the lobules like meshes of net-work; and further traced
to a small black tubercle in the surface of the lung, not far from
the windpipe several lymphatic vessels, which partly penetrated the
tubercle, and partly poured mercury into it. From this circumstance, and from the analogous one, that tubercles in this situation
often contain calcareous matter, M. Schroeder thinks it not un-
unlikely, that the calcareous tubercles are the result of degeneration of the lymphatic vessels or glands.

It appears that the nervous filaments terminate with the vessels
at the margin of the *vomica*, so that they appear to have been converted into a species of cartilage or tough cellular tissue. In one
case described by this author, the nervous branches were reddened
and thickened, numerous vessels being brought into view upon
them by means of injection. Like Mr Swan, M. Schroeder saw
in phthisical persons the pneumogastric nerve reddened and thickened; but in other cases he admits that he found it quite unchanged, so that he is averse to make any positive conclusion.

Before proceeding to describe the state of the other respiratory
and circulating organs, and that of the intestinal canal, it is proper to consider here the mode in which these tubercular masses are
formed, their nature, their progress and progressive changes, and
their termination.

The question of the original formation of tubercles requires the previous consideration of three points; in which texture of the lungs are the tubercular bodies first deposited; in what form, fluid or solid, are they first deposited; and what is the cause of the deposition.

1. Dr Stark represents tubercles as formations in the filamento-cellular substance of the lungs; and Baillie inferred from dissection, that tubercles were deposited in the cellular, that is the filamentons tissue of the lungs. This opinion, which has been very generally received without much question or inquiry, and is espoused by Laennec, derives verisimilitude from the appearances presented on dissection of the lungs of phthisical persons, in which in general it is impossible to distinguish anything but the tubercular masses, imbedded as it were, in the parenchyma of the lungs. We shall see, that, in order to obtain just views on this point, it is requisite to examine lungs in which the diseased deposit is just beginning, or not very far advanced, or very generally diffused through the lungs.

2. Another opinion, originating in the idea that consumption is a strumous distemper, and that strumous distempers are seated in the lymphatic system, is that tubercles are morbid formations or a degeneration of the lymphatic glands of the bronchi and lungs. This opinion has been more or less strongly maintained by Portal, Heberden, Broussais, and Nasse. "Upon dissecting the bodies of consumptive persons," says Heberden, "I have seen the lung crowded with swelled glands, some of which are inflamed, and some suppurated or even burst."* " After the most attentive examination," says Portal, " I think that the tubercles constituting primary consumption are formed both by enlargement of the lymphatic glands distributed in almost all the parts of the lungs, or remote from the *bronchi*, and also by lymphatic swellings of the cellular tissue of the lungs, which, after becoming more or less indurated, frequently end in bad suppuration."†

The same doctrine has been not less explicity and forcibly taught by Broussais in several of his writings; and more recently by Nasse.‡

* Commentarii. London, 1782.

† Observations sur la Nature et le Traitement de la Phthisie Pulmonaire, Tome ii. p. 309.

‡ Horn's Archiv. 1824, Juli, Aug. p. 106, et *apud* Rust Handbuch der Chirurgie, B. xvi. *Tuberculosis*, p. 439.

The great objection under which this doctrine labours, is its being at variance with anatomical facts.   The lymphatic bronchial glands are situate chiefly round the ramifications of the *bronchi;* and though these glands are sometimes enlarged, and sometimes infiltrated with tyromatous matter in young subjects, this change is not uniformly or even often observed in pulmonary consumption. The bronchial glands, further, may be affected by tyromatous deposition, when the lungs are themselves either healthy, or at least not affected by tubercular deposit.   Lastly, in those instances in which the bronchial glands are enlarged, indurated, infiltrated with tyromatous matter, or softened into suppuration, along with tubercular deposit, and tubercular excavations of the lungs, the former can always be readily distinguished from the latter, by the peculiar site which they occupy, and still more by their appearance, figure, and other physical characters.   It is chiefly in children that this tyromatous enlargement, and transformation of the bronchial glands is observed; and in those cases in which the enlargement is associated with tubercular disease of the lungs, dissection at once shows the difference between the two lesions.   The sections of the bronchial glands are large, homogeneous, circular, or elliptical, whitish, or grayish coloured, or grayish-blue surfaces round the large bronchial tubes.   The sections of the tubercular masses are irregular, variable in consistence; hard points and spots being mixed with softer portions, and the colour gray-blue, or bluish-red, situate in the substance of the pulmonic lobes and lobules.

As the affection of the lymphatic glands, therefore, is not adequate to account for the morbid appearances presented by phthisical lungs, Portal admitted that tubercles might be seated in other two textures.   The first of these was in the lymphatic glands of the lungs, properly so called, which are smaller than the bronchial glands, more regularly rounded, and harder; and these he conceived became the seat of tubercular infiltration in certain forms of consumption, in which the disease began by plethoric or inflammatory symptoms.

The other texture in which he admitted that tubercles might be formed, is the cellular or filamentous tissue around the lymphatic glands, that is, the parenchyma of the lungs, agreeing in this respect with Stark and Baillie.   This takes place, however, only under particular circumstances.   After adverting to the induration of the lungs of phthisical persons, and their increased weight above the average, he states that this is owing to the extravasation of glutinous matter (albuminous matter,) which, after filling the lymphatic glands and the lymphatic vessels terminating in them, is further extravasated into the tissue of the lungs, and forms these tubercles sometimes in infinite numbers.

Part of this doctrine seems to be well founded, and part of it is perhaps open to objection. When it is admitted that tubercles may arise from extravasation of albuminous matter into the substance of the lung, the exclusive deposition of these bodies in the bronchial or lymphatic glands is virtually abandoned. The only question is, whether this effusion is the effect of the preliminary abundance of fluid in the glands and lymphatic vessels; and whether this alleged extravasation, which forms tubercles in the filamentons tissue of the lungs, may not take place without affection of the glands, and does not take place, as Broussais seems to think, previously to that affection of the glands. It is proper to add, that M. Andral admits that this mode of the formation of tubercles in the lungs, viz. by tubercular matter being deposited in the lymphatic ganglions of the interior of the lung, is not improbable.[*]

3. An opinion, which appears to be most consonant to the facts, is that which was brought forward in 1821 by Magendie, and in 1826 by M. Schroeder, who fix the seat of tubercular deposition in the extremities of the bronchial tubes, or in what are named the pulmonic vesicles, in which the tubercles are deposited from the fine mucous membrane in a state of inflammation.

According to Magendie, the first indications of tubercular phthisis consist in the deposit of a certain quantity of grayish-yellow matter, in one or more cells of the lung. The yellow matter sometimes fills completely and distends the cells; but it is easy to perceive the small blood-vessels which circumscribe the matter deposited. In other instances the yellow matter is movable within the cells, and may probably be expelled from them.

In some instances only one or two cells contain yellow matter; but most frequently it fills all the cells, forming a lobule. In this case the matter adheres to the small vessels; and these soon disappear; on which the whole lobule seems formed by yellow or tubercular matter.

After opening numerous bodies, M. Magendie never saw in the

---

[*] Clinique Medicale, Partie iii. sect. iii.

cells the small pearly granules which, according to certain authors, are the first germs of phthisis. On the contrary, the matter first seen is that named tubercular matter, which is presented as if secreted by the walls of the small pulmonary blood-vessels.*

These views on the first origin of tubercular deposition, were afterwards elaborated and illustrated by M. Schroeder and Dr Carsewell; and they seem from various facts to be most probable.

In order to form a clear conception of the origin of the process of tubercular deposition in the lungs, it is necessary to examine these organs in the bodies of persons cut off by other diseases, and in the earlier stages of consumption, when the disease has made little progress. At this stage of the disease it is still uncomplicated with marks of general inflammation of the lung, or its component tissues; and at the worst there is merely topical change.

If in this state tubercles be divided and inspected by the aid of the microscope, it then appears that the air-cells of the lungs are filled with some opaque material, which renders them less pellucid, the nearer the eye is directed to the edge of the tubercles. The cells filled with pellucid coagulable lymph are harder than the neighbouring sound cells, and do not admit the air, as easily appears by slight pressure in water. This lymph contained in the cells is sometimes so limpid, that the tubercle can scarcely be distinguished by the eye from the sound structure of the lung, and requires the aid of touch.

In other spots, however, the centre of the tubercle is already white, and losing its transparency, has become opaque; so that by the aid of the microscope, in the centre of the cell little or nothing can be distinguished, and their *parietes* appear united with the matter of the tubercle, while the adjoining cells still contain transparent matter. From this fact the author infers, in opposition to the representation of Laennec and Lorinzer, that in certain air-cells, or in a lobule of the lung, local inflammation may be developed, and produce effusion of lymph which obstructs the air-cells.

As this exudation proceeds, the walls of the cells are at length compressed on all sides, and not only unite with the contained lymph; but, as the effusion hardens and becomes opaque princi-

* Memoire sur la structure du poumon de l'homme, &c. &c., et sur la premiere origine de la phthisie pulmonaire ; par M. Magendie. Journal de Physiologie, Tome I. p. 78. Paris, 1821.

pally from the centre to the circumference, a mass of lung thus occupied becomes solid and granular in the centre, and softer at its margins.

The shape of the tubercular mass thus formed depends on the structure of the lung,—a circumstance on which authors have not bestowed sufficient attention. The lobes of the lungs consist of lobules united by cellular tissue; and each lobule receives a separate bronchial tube, which terminates in many air-cells, all pervious to air,—and a peculiar artery and vein, each subdivided into many minute vessels, all penetrable by injected fluids in the sound state. It hence results that the beginning of tubercular deposition is confined at first to one lobule only, without affecting the contiguous lobules, and is recognized only by the greater opacity and firmness of that lobule than of the healthy ones. It is also found, by injecting the arteries and veins of the lung, that some lobules are less penetrated with this tubercular deposition than others, the vessels of the former being more susceptible of injection, while those of the latter are few in number and less penetrable by injection, and diminish in this manner in number and susceptibility of injection, till in the truly and perfectly tuberculated lobule the small vessels are completely shut and obliterated, and the large one only remains pervions. In such lobules the structure of the lung can no longer be traced; the shape of the air-cells is destroyed; and in the centre of these tuberculated lobules, which is hollow, suppuration has commenced. Such tuberculated lobules are whiter than the adjoining ones, and are surrounded by thick cellular tissue separating them from the adjoining lobules, which may at this stage of the disease be less affected. Very soon, however, the air-cells of these lobules become penetrated by the same deposition, which in like manner becomes opaque and firm, and agglutinates the cells into a similar firm, inelastic mass, also surrounded by indurated filamentous tissue. When at length several lobules have in this manner become penetrated and occupied by tubercular deposition, with the suppurative destruction proceeding in their respective centres, the coalescence into a single undistinguishable mass is followed by the union of their respective minute cavities into one or more larger ones. In the course of this process, the cellular, or rather what I term the filamentous, tissue of the lung being placed outside the penetrated cells, naturally resists longest the suppurative process, and may even become thickened and indurated. At length, however, this also may give way, and be destroyed partially or entirely; and hence appears the reason why some anatomists maintain that the tubercle or small *vomica* is surrounded by a membrane, while by others this is denied.

From this account of the progressive formation of tubercles, it results that not only the air-cells are filled, and then obliterated by the exudation of coagulable lymph, but that the areas of the blood-vessels are so contracted, that they no longer admit the wax of injection, and become obliterated, and incapable of receiving and conveying blood to the ultimate terminations; and hence the centre of the tubercle wastes, and is consumed and degenerated; and that the vessels, still pervious, assuming the inflammatory action, secrete purulent matter, which dissolves the tubercle already softened and macerated. M. Schroeder van der Kolk further regards this deposition as coagulable lymph, because by immersion in spirit it is coagulated and rendered opaque; and he therefore contends that it is impossible to adopt the view of Laennec and Lorinzer, or Nasse, that tubercles are formed without previous inflammation. The argument also adduced by the latter author, that tubercular deposition takes place generally in the upper lobe of the lung, whereas peripneumony occurs more frequently in the lower one, he thinks of no moment. He admits the fact, but maintains that it merely shows that tubercular deposition and the consequent *vomicæ* differ from peripneumony, and that chronic inflammation differs from the acute form of the disease.

The question regarding the origin of tubercles from degenerated bronchial glands, he allows to be more difficult of decision,—from the fact, that frequently degeneration and inflammation of the glands of the neck, or some other part, precede the appearance of consumption, and that strumous persons are very liable to the disease. He observes, however, that in examining carefully the bodies of the strumous, when the vessels were filled with fine injection, he found very minute tubercles occupied in different points by concretions, and in general calcareous rather than tubercular matter deposited. In examining such lungs microscopically, he found the minute branches of the bronchial tubes, at least to one-fourth of a line in diameter, everywhere reddened within by injected vessels, and a beautiful net-work expanded on the internal mucous membrane; in some of the minute branches, he saw the smaller glands thick and somewhat whiter; the miliary tubercles were surrounded by a net-work of vessels, in which he could distinguish the air-cells still open. These tubercles generally adhered externally to the branches of the bronchial tubes, or to the pulmonary arteries and veins; in some cases a small bronchial tube seemed to end in a tubercle. Externally the pulmonic *pleura* was marked by black round lines like rings, which appeared to be lymphatic vessels. Where the degeneration was a little greater, the cells were obliterated, and the tubercles, the vessels of which were impervious, appeared to have coalesced into a whitish mass.

- This author doubts, nevertheless, whether these bodies, which he denominates *miliary tubercles*, were not obliterated vessels, which, when cut across, presented the appearance, but had not the reality of tubercles, the more so, that these tubercles could be traced through the lungs in the direction of ramification. He further expresses the opinion, that these tubercles are first formed by thickening, and inflammatory degeneration of lymphatic glands, and that this is the reason why they present a different appearance from that of the ordinary tubercles of the air-cells already described,—since they seem to adhere most to the small bronchial tubes.

As to the origin of the calcareous matter, he does not admit that these concretions can be formed by the inhalation of dust or sand, since their structure is too complex, and the opinion is sufficiently refuted by analysis; but he thinks, that the surrounding membrane, whether that of a gland, or an air-cell, had so degenerated by inflammation as to assume the fibrous character, and the faculty of osseous or calcareous secretion.·

He infers, therefore, that the lungs present two kinds of tubercles; one produced by chronic inflammation of the air-cells, by which .their membrane ˙is made to secrete lymph, which fills and unites them into a mass; the other more calcareous, produced apparently by degeneration of the minute glands; but both agreeing in inducing inflammation of the adjoining air-cells, and *vomicæ*. The suppuration which produces the latter change, and which commences most frequently in the centre, though sometimes in the side of the .tubercle, presents this peculiar difference from common suppuration, or that which takes place in wounds, that whereas in the latter granulations are formed by which the cavity is filled, in the former no granulations take place, because no new vessels are formed; and as the vessels are obstructed and convey· no new matter, the tubercular mass is softened by a species of partial death. When this suppurative destruction begins, it proceeds in general till the tubercular mass is broken down and excavated; and it is much less common to find a tubercle partly dissolved than entire, or a small *vomica*, after the tubercle has been destroyed by suppuration. In this state the *vomica* is lined by a thin vascular membrane, sometimes by a thick yellowish one; and if small, it is rarely traversed by any vessel; but this is not unusual in large *vomicæ*. The author also observes, that these tubercular masses afford, in the process of softening, an illustration of the general principle formerly laid down, that every inflamed part and ulcer presents at the same time different degrees of inflammation. The centre of the tubercle may be dead or expelled after the process of solution; its crust may be in a state of suppurative softening; the circumference may be inflamed; and this process diminishes in the parts of the lung farthest removed from the margin of the air-cells.

In the manner now mentioned, the cavity of a *vomica* is progressively enlarged, until in desperate cases of consumption the patient sinks under the disease. The extent to which the lung is destroyed before this event takes place, varies according to the age of the parties.

Similar views of the mode in which tubercles are originally deposited in the lungs have been taken by M. Andral, Dr Carsewell, M. Ravin,* and other pathologists. The bronchial tubes terminate in shut sacs, lined by a fine mucous membrane, and enclosed by the submucous or filamentous tissue. This fine mucous membrane is liable to various forms of inflammation, in which it secretes a fluid or semifluid matter which contains much albumen, and consequently is liable to undergo spontaneous coagulation. This has been sometimes named strumous matter, glutinous matter, (Portal,) plastic lymph, (Schroeder,) coagulable lymph, purulent matter of particular nature, (Lerminier and Andral,) and tubercular matter. None of these denominations convey a just notion of the object; and the latter is objectionable, because it is applied indiscriminately to several kinds of morbid texture, different both in nature and in form. But it is sufficient to know that the mucous membrane of these bronchial terminations or vesicles is liable to a kind or form of inflammation, which is perhaps peculiar, and that in this state it secretes matter, which, though at first fluid, afterwards be-

* Memoire sur les Tubercules, pour repondre a la question proposée par l'Academie Royale de Medecine dans 28 Aout 1827. Par F. P. Ravin, D. M., &c. Memoires de l'Academie Royale de Medecine, Tome IV. Paris 1835, p. 324.

comes solid, filling up and obstructing the terminations of the tubes. As the matters effused become solid, they naturally assume the rounded or oblong-rounded form of the pulmonic vesicles; and in this state, as they are small, firm, rounded bodies, harder than the neighbouring parts, and giving them a knotty appearance, they are tubercles (*tubercula*), or little tuberosities.

That this is one and perhaps the most usual mode in which tubercles are formed, must be regarded as established by the accurate and beautiful delineations of Dr Carsewell, who has represented the tubercular matter, as he terms it, when deposited on the free surface of the bronchial mucous membrane, at the extremities of the bronchial tubes. Andral manifestly takes the same view of one of the modes in which pulmonary tubercles may be formed.

Frederic Peter Ludovic Cerutti, who published in 1839 a short but learned dissertation on the subject, states, that after repeated observations, he had not been able to satisfy himself of the facts adduced by Schroeder; but allows it to be proved that the cells of the lung in those parts becoming occupied by tubercular matter, and which differ from healthy cells, in presenting a different colour, contain no air, because not only individual portions of lung sink in water, but also a whole lobe, which still fresh, on being immersed in water, sunk more than one-half, immediately after being inflated by air, rose to the surface.

From this fact, he is convinced that tubercles in their origin consist of a fluid exudation, which moistens the walls of the pulmonic cells, which, he argues, are mutually compressed by the increased weight caused by this humidity, to such a degree only, that though the inspired air is unable to enter them, they may nevertheless be expanded by artificial inflation.*

In the first commencement of this distemper, the colour of the affected portion of the lung only is changed; and as yet the secreted matter is probably soft and semifluid, or at least not very firm. But after some time, when the effused matter has acquired consistence, and become a little firm, the part is felt between the fingers as if it contained several hard knots. These are granular or graniform bodies within the air cells, filling, distending, and preventing them

---

* Collectanea quaedam de Phthisi Pulmonum tuberculosa scripsit et in Universitate Lipsiae in die xviii. Junii A. C. 1839, publice defendet, Dr Frid. Petrus Ludovicus Cerutti, Pathologiæ et Therapiae Specialis, P. P. O. Des. Lipsiae, 1839. 4to, p. 22.

from collapsing. The size of these bodies in this stage is about that of a pin-head, rising to a millet-seed or a grain of mustard-seed. These bodies, now described, have been, in this state, regarded as the miliary tubercles of Bayle and Laennec, the disseminated tubercles of Gendrin, and the simple tubercles of Dr Lombard and Dr Home. But this does not appear to be established with unquestionable certainty. One variety, at least, of the miliary tubercle, I am inclined to think, is formed in the filamentous tissue of the lungs; and certainly differs widely from the arrangement and appearance of the bodies now mentioned.

A good method of demonstrating the origin of the most usual forms of pulmonary tubercles, is by observing what takes place in lobular pneumonia. In this disease inflammation attacks the lung in individual lobules, perhaps beginning first like vesicular *bronchitis*, that is, affecting the terminations of the bronchial tubes, and the air cells, and perhaps in a slight degree the submucous filamentous tissue, or the parenchyma of the lung in which these vesicles are imbedded. The result of this inflammation is effusion within the vesicles of a species of soft semifluid matter, intermediate between albumen and gelatine, but which undergoes coagulation, and thereby fills the vesicles with an equal number of small roundish bodies, of moderate consistence, but which eventually become firm, and at length hard, while their mutual proximity aggregates them together into small hard masses, isolated, and limited to each pulmonary lobule, or part only of a lobule. As the disease proceeds, it affects the whole lobule, and its investing tissue or capsule, giving it the appearance of a hard knotty mass, irregular in shape and figure, and surrounded by natural pulmonic tissue. This disease may either affect one or two, or many lobules simultaneously and successively; and in proportion to the extent over which it is diffused, the lung is occupied by bodies having all the characters of tubercles, and which eventually constitute pulmonary tubercles.

In this state, these masses, when divided, are firm, of a bluish-gray colour, and consist of minute portions aggregated together, in a confused manner, so as to form a mass not quite homogeneous, but firmer than the surrounding lung. In this state, before these masses have become softened, they constitute what has been named by Laennec crude or yellowish tubercles (*tubercula cruda*), agglomerated tubercle by Gendrin, multiple tubercle by Lombard, and aggregated tubercle by Dr Home. These masses vary in size, from that of a garden pea or a cherry-stone, to that of a walnut or even larger. Though the surrounding lung may be sound, yet the portions of lung which previously were in the place of these tubercular masses are completely solidified; and hence neither bronchial tubes nor blood-vessels are traced into them.

Another lesion, which has been believed to form a certain stage of this process of the conversion of isolated or simple tubercles into aggregated tubercles, is that which has been named gray, semitransparent granulations, and which, indeed, are the miliary or cartilaginous tubercles of Bayle. It is certain, both from the researches of Dr Carsewell, Andral, and Cerutti, that they may exist in the lungs without giving rise to the peculiar structure already described as tubercular. They are generally isolated, very seldom aggregated, disseminated or dispersed through the lungs almost indiscriminately; and it is very doubtful whether, if they be formed in the air-cells, they are always formed in them.

Andral regards these gray granulations as indurated and hypertrophied air cells. I have several times observed them in the filamentous tissue of the lung, in such circumstances that I thought it scarcely possible for them to be formed in the cells. In some instances they appear like transformation of certain portions of the lymphatic vessels or glands of the lungs. They are occasionally observed in the lungs of quarry-men, stone-cutters, and hewing-masons.

In certain cases, however, of this sort of lesion, it has been ascertained that these gray, semitransparent, hard tubercles are deposited originally in the pulmonic vesicles. Thus, Dr Home mentions that a specimen of this kind of tubercle, occurring in a hewing-mason, was presented in 1838 to the Anatomical Society, in which it was found that in the centre of each tubercle was contained a grain of sand or earthy matter, ascertained to consist of silica and carbonate of lime, and which had no doubt been inhaled, and gave rise, by mechanical irritation, to chronic inflammation in the ends of the bronchial tubes.

A third lesion, which has been sometimes rather vaguely called tubercular, is what may be termed gray hepatization, occurring in definite masses, or circumscribed gray hepatization, or, what might be less objectionable, circumscribed tyromatous deposition.

In this state, a portion of lung, more or less extensive, becomes the seat of considerable induration and solidification; and when a portion thus affected is divided, it is observed to consist of various minute, gray-coloured, firm bodies or grains aggregated together, and which give the section a gray or light-yellow colour, and a granular aspect. There is no doubt that this change in the consistence and appearance of the lung is the effect of inflammation, acute, subacute, or chronic; but it is not quite certain that the presence of this state is a necessary step in the formation of tubercles. This change may probably take place in any part of the lung; but the situations in which I have most usually seen it are the upper lobe near its apex, and sometimes the middle lobe of the right side. This has been observed by Baillie, and is described by Laennec, under the name of tubercular infiltration, and by Dr Home under the name of diffuse tubercle.

In this form of the disorder, the morbid deposition does not begin in the air-cells exclusively, as in the first described, but affects all the elementary tissues of the lung by lobules, at once in one uniform disorder; and it gives rise to extravasation of albuminous or tyromatous matter, over the whole space which it affects, but effused into the cells and filamentous tissue, and compressing and thereby obliterating the air vesicles, the tubes, and the blood-vessels all at once. Often also the surrounding tissue of the lobule is converted into a sort of membrane or capsule, so that the tyromatous deposit appears as it were encysted. The size which these masses acquire, varies from that of a small gooseberry to a large one or more. When divided, besides the yellow or gray colour already mentioned, they present a much more uniform or homogeneous aspect than the other forms of tubercular deposit.

The state of the surrounding lung, though often congested or reddened, varies much both in these different forms of deposition and also in different stages of its progress. In the early stage, or that of crudity, the substance of the lung around may be crepitating, elastic, and compressible; and even in the advanced stage, some observers have found the lung interposed and surrounding, free from induration or much redness. Thus Baillie and Soemmering found the substance of the lung surrounding considerable tubercular masses healthy; and Laennec and Louis appear to have observed the same fact. Much more frequently, however, there are more or less reddening, vascular congestion, and infiltration of serum into the substance of the lung; and in a considerable number of cases I have observed pneumonic inflammation either in its first or in its second stage.

3 T

In the case of the isolated tubercular infiltration, chronic pneumonia is very common. At least in the cases of that form which have fallen under my own observation, I have observed, that symptoms altogether like those of pneumonia or peripneumony took place during life, and, upon inspection after death, the usual appearances left by inflammation of the substance of the lung were found.* These tubercles, indeed, do not appear readily to undergo the process of softening, and most usually prove fatal either by being complicated with or inducing pneumonic inflammation.

It may be here mentioned, that, both in simple red or brown and gray consolidation, and when these changes are accompanied by the presence of tubercles, fat-globules and adipose particles may be recognized.

The manner in which tubercular masses are softened or broken down and discharged, or what may be termed the mechanism of tubercular softening and excavation, has attracted some notice, and deserves consideration. At one time, it was imagined to be either identical with, or analogous to, suppuration in other tissues; and it was supposed that tubercular *vomicæ* were merely abscesses of the lungs. But the process, though perhaps analogous to, is not the same with suppuration. It seems to be more complicated, and not so uniform in its progress. It seems to be difficult to ascertain at what part softening commences. In one case it may begin in the centre, and proceed to the circumference; in another it may begin at the circumference, and go round the whole mass, detaching it from the surrounding lung; in a third case it may begin at once at the centre, and at the margins; and, in other cases, it has been observed to commence at the same time in several parts of the substance of the tubercular mass. The latter is the course, especially in the case of large tubercular masses. Cerutti,† who entertains this opinion, states that, in the section of a tubercular mass in this state, the portion or spots about to be softened appear to lose firmness and to become friable, and, if examined by the microscope, they present numerous minute holes, as if punctured by a needle. This condition extends over the whole mass, until its parts are detached from each other; and minute grains are found amidst a semifluid or fluid opaque mass. While this is proceeding,

* Two Cases of Tubercular Deposition, &c. By D. Craigie, M.D. Edin. Med. and Surg. Journal, Vol. xliii. p. 273.

† Collectanea quædam de Phthisi Pulmonum tuberculosa scripsit et in Universitate Lipsiae in die xviii. Junii A. C. 1839, publice defendet, Dr Frid. Petrus Ludovicus Cerutti, Pathologiae et Therapiae Specialis, P. P. O. Des. Lipsiae, 1839, 4to, p. 22.

a communication is established with one or more bronchial tubes, the small end of which are destroyed or dissolved in the softening process, and the semifluid matter reaching them irritates them, causing secondary catarrh, and excites coughing, by which it is expelled. The transition of this semifluid matter through the bronchial tubes is the cause of the redness and villous appearance of the mucous membrane of the bronchial tubes, so generally observed in the lungs of those destroyed by this distemper.

On the means by which this softening is effected, different opinions have been entertained. An opinion very generally received is, that the tubercular masses, acting in some manner as foreign bodies, give rise to irritation and vascular action in their vicinity, and thereby induce a sort of congestive and inflammatory afflux of fluids, in which they are dissolved in imperfect suppuration. This opinion is supported by those facts which show that tubercles begin to soften near the circumference of the masses.

Many tubercular masses, nevertheless, seem to possess an internal and innate tendency to destruction. Their texture is imperfect;* and in some instances the internal substance begins to soften, apparently whether any irritation of the surrounding lung has taken place or not. There is no doubt that, in a considerable proportion of cases, the presence of the irritation of severe *bronchitis* or peripneumony appears to have pushed the tubercular masses into speedy liquefaction; and the frequency with which the symptoms of pneumonic inflammation are succeeded by those of consumption, shows that in the formation of softening at least, if not in the development of tubercular deposits, inflammatory congestion has great influence.

As softening proceeds, whether it has been attended with pneumonic inflammation or not, it is speedily followed by that, and by bronchial inflammation, the latter being chiefly induced and maintained by the incessant irritation kept up by the transition over the membrane of the contents of the tubercular softening. If the tubercular mass be large, or if the degree of pneumonic inflammation be considerable, it affects a third membrane, viz. the pleura. In all cases, indeed, in proportion to the size of tubercular mass, and the consequent excavation to be formed, and as that advances from the substance to the surface of the lungs, pleurisy takes place. The

* See p. 1012.

great use of this inflammation, or what may be termed its final cause, in the softening and expulsion of tubercular masses, is, by the effusion of lymph and the formation of adhesions between the pulmonic and costal pleura, to prevent perforation of the lung, the escape of air and tubercular matter into the cavity of the *pleura* (*pneumothorax*, and *empyema*), and the consequent formation of pleurisy complicated with pneumothorax,—a lesion generally fatal. By the slow and gradually advancing inflammation of the pleura, and the consequent albuminous exudation and adhesion, this accident is prevented. This is so common, that in one case only among 112 were the lungs free of adhesions.

It, nevertheless, sometimes happens that this accident takes place. The apex of the lung, I have already said, is very generally covered all round with a thick, cartilaginous coat of false membrane, uniting it to the interior of the thoracic walls; and any cavity formed in this region is thus prevented from opening into the pleura, and the general cavity. But if in the lower region of the lower lobe, any large tubercular mass is softened and expelled, and leaves a considerable cavity, verging towards the pectoral and axillary regions, it occasionally happens that adhesion has not taken place there, and that the walls of the cavity, already extenuated to an extreme degree, give way, or are perforated, especially during a fit of coughing, air and once tubercular matter escape into the pleural cavity, and there produce first collapse of the lung, and then pleuritic inflammation. Among 112 cases observed by Louis, perforation was known to take place in eight cases, and in seven of these it took place on the left side. Among 100 cases recorded in the Royal Infirmary Report, perforation took place in six, in three on the right side, and in three on the left. Since the publication of that report, I have met with two cases of perforation, among eighteen cases inspected under my own care; and in one case, perforation took place in the left side, in the lower part of the superior lobe, and another in the middle lobe of the right side.

MORBID ANATOMY OF THE APPENDAGES OF THE LUNGS AND THE OTHER ORGANS.—Besides the state of the lungs above described, the trachea, larynx, and epiglottis are liable to present various lesions. The membrane of the epiglottis is always reddened, and sometimes softened; and the whole laryngeal and tracheal membrane is reddened and softened, or rendered flaccid. Ulcers also, various in size and shape, may be formed in these parts.

Among 102 cases examined by Louis, ulcers of the epiglottis were found in eighteen cases (one-sixth), ulcers of the larynx in twenty-two cases (one-fifth), and ulcers of the trachea in thirty-one cases (one-third).

Most of the ulcers of the epiglottis are confined to the lower or laryngeal surface of that cartilage. The ulcers are generally small, one, two, or three lines in diameter. They are more common in males than in females.

The most frequent seat of ulcers of the larynx is the junction of the vocal chords; then the vocal chords themselves, especially their posterior part; and lastly, the base of the arytenoid cartilages; the upper part of the larynx, and the interior of the ventricles. In some rare cases one or more of the vocal chords are denuded or destroyed, and the base of the arytenoid cartilages exposed.

Ulcers of the trachea, sometimes very large, are found chiefly in the posterior or fleshy part of the canal, and are attended with a red colour, more or less deep, of the contiguous mucous membrane, and some softening and thickening. In rare cases, the ulceration spreads so much as to denude or destroy more or less completely several of the cartilaginous rings; and in that case the ulcerated ends of the rings give the margins of the ulcer a peculiar, irregular, and denticulated appearance.

The only general result that can be established regarding the heart is, that it is rendered smaller and softer than usual, or is atrophied.

Mr Abernethy found that, in severe cases of pulmonary consumption, in which the lungs were much occupied by tubercular masses, by injecting the arteries and veins of the heart, the injection readily flowed into the chambers of the organ, and that the left ventricle was first and most completely filled. He found that the channels of this injection were the *foramina Thebesii*, which, though in the natural state few and small, becomes numerous and large in disease of the lungs, especially tubercular induration, which impedes the circulation of the pulmonary artery, and thereby distends and gorges the right chambers of the heart. Mr Abernethy also found the *foramen ovale* more or less open in the hearts of persons destroyed by pulmonary consumption.*

In about from one-tenth to one-fifth of cases of consumption, the

* Observations on the *Foramina Thebesii* of the Heart. By John Abernethy, F.R.S. Phil. Trans. 1798. Part I. p. 10.

stomach is enlarged or distended to two or three times its usual bulk. The mucous membrane of the organ is very generally in an unhealthy state, either wholly or partially. It may be in the splenic end softer and thinner than natural, with a bluish-white or yellowish colour. This takes place in one-fifth.

The same part may be reddened or softened. In about one-fifth the mucous membrane of the anterior coat is red, thickened, and softened,—generally in connection with enlargement of the liver. Ulcers, prominences, and granulations, are found in a smaller proportion of cases. Most of these lesions are to be viewed as the effect of some form of inflammation; and it is established that, in the phthisical, irritation or inflammation of the gastric mucous membrane is very readily induced.

By far the most constant lesion in the alimentary canal of the phthisical, consists in some change in the mucous membrane of the ileum or of the colon.

The most common lesion in the former is the presence of ulcers, which are observed in five-sixths of the cases. In one-sixth they occupy the whole tract of the intestine; and in the other two-ninths they are found only at the lower part of the *ileum.* These ulcers always correspond to the aggregated glands of Peyer, in which they begin; but as the disease proceeds, if life be protracted, they extend to the mucous membrane in general, and thus are found to occupy the greater part or the whole circumference of the bowel. Their shape is elliptical, annular, or linear. In general, at the commencement, they appear in one or two points, that is, in one or two follicles of one of the aggregated glands. In the advanced stage of the disease, several of these coalescing may form a large and extensive ulcer. The latter is mostly seen at the lower end of the ileum, where that bowel enters the colon. In some instances, these ulcers may commence in the isolated follicles; but this is not common.

A lesion less frequent is the presence of granulations, semicartilaginous or tubercular, in the ileum. These lesions, which appear to be seated in the isolated follicles of the bowel, and which consist in tubercular degeneration of the follicles, take place in three-eighths of the cases.

Much in the same manner, and at the same rate, is the mucous membrane of the colon liable to be diseased. It is reddened either continuously or in patches. The most common lesion is the presence of ulcers, which are formed in from eight-elevenths to seven-ninths, or about nine-twelfths. They may be large, middle-sized, or small. The most common situations are the cæcum, the ascending colon, the transverse arch, and the rectum, in the order now specified. When the cæcum is affected, the ulceration is often extensive, being associated with ulcers or ulceration of the lower end of the *ileum*, the ileo-cæcal valve, which is often stripped of its mucous membrane, or altogether destroyed, and over the whole inner surface of the cæcum. In the ascending colon and transverse arch, the ulcers present the appearance of broad flattish patches, the largest diameter being across the intestine, the converse of what is observed in the ileum. These ulcers may commence in the mucous follicles of the colon; but they eventually pass to the mucous membrane in general.

Tubercular granulations are found in the colon in a smaller proportion of cases.

Of these ulcers or ulcerated patches it is a pretty general result, that, as they destroy the mucous membrane, and advance through the subjacent coats to the peritoneum, they cause in the latter inflammation in minute isolated points or spots, followed by effusion of albuminous fluid, which coagulates and adheres in an equal number of minute points, opaque, elevated, and generally isolated, but touching each other, so as to form a rough patch, circular or oval in shape. In this state, these small whitish opaque bodies present the appearance of tubercular specks, and are hence called by many authors tubercles of the peritonæum. Whatever be the name applied to them, they are formed in the mode now mentioned.

The final cause of this peritoneal inflammation is to counteract ulcerative perforation, and to thicken and strengthen the bowel. In some rare cases, however, this object is defeated, and the ulceration destroys all the textures, and the *peritoneum* suddenly gives way, allowing the escape of air and the intestinal contents into the abdomen, and causing sudden fatal *peritonitis*. This accident is, however, not very common. One example only have I met with among nearly one hundred instances of fatal consumption.

In other instances, effusion of sero-purulent or purulent fluid is found in the peritoneum, and soft coagulable lymph between the intestinal folds, showing that it must have been inflamed during life.

In the bodies of the phthisical the liver is very generally in a morbid state. The most frequent change in this country is that of *kirrhosis*, with more or less enlargement and induration, in which sections of the gland show it to have a peculiar yellow colour, with a darker hue of the *acini*. This takes place in rather more than one-third of the cases. The most common change in France ap·pears to be the adipescent transformation of the organ which occurs in one-third of the cases. In this the organ is pale, fawn-coloured, more or less tender and friable, chequered with red outside as well as within. The bulk of the organ is always increased, some-times to the amount of twice its usual dimensions. In this coun-try, this change does not take place in so many as one·sixth of the cases. The former lesion is most common among males; the lat-ter among females.

The brain is very generally slightly softer than natural. The membranes are injected; and fluid is effused beneath the arachnoid membrane and within the ventricles.

Tubercular deposits or tyromatous matter, fluid or semifluid, or solid, are found in various other organs besides the lungs. Thus the ileum and the colon are said to become the seat of this deposit; but perhaps it is rather the albuminous effusion in the granular shape, than real tyromatous matter, which has received this cha-racter. The deposit, however, is found in the mesenteric glands, the cervical lymphatic glands, the lumbar glands, the prostate, the spleen, ovaries, kidneys, womb, brain, and *cerebellum*, in the order now mentioned.

The usual termination of the lesions of the lungs above described is in death. As the contents of the tubercular masses are softened and expelled into the bronchial tubes, they cause in these and in the windpipe and lungs most violent irritation and inflammation, with consequent copious secretion of puriform mucus, which is mingled and spit up with the proper tubercular matter. As this process advances with several tubercular masses simultaneously and successively, very general bronchitic and tracheal inflammation is induced; and at the same time with them symptoms of peripneu-mony and pleurisy may be combined from the causes already spe-cified. In this state of matters, the function of respiration is gradually confined in its extent and effect, until it is nearly anni-hilated, when perhaps not more than one-fourth, or, in some cases, one·sixth, or one-tenth of the lungs is left permeable to air and blood. Death then ensues, partly as the effect of the exhaustion from constant tracheo-bronchial irritation, partly as the effect of exhaustion from annihilated respiration.

Notwithstanding the frequency of this as the usual termination of the process of tubercular destruction, softening, and excavation, there is reason to believe that, in an extremely small proportion of cases, recoveries from very ominous states take place after all the usual signs of consumption have existed for a sufficient time to render the conclusion probable that these symptoms were caused by tubercular softening and excavation. As the evidence of this fact is at once doubtful and important, it is best to state it, as it most usually is observed.

1. It occasionally happens, that, in inspecting the bodies of persons destroyed by several different diseases, there is observed in the upper lobe of the lungs a peculiar morbid state. The *pleura* is puckered and shrivelled into small, firm, irregular portions, in which there is distinctly felt a sort of leathery firmness, and beneath that a spot or body or round globular, pretty firm and resisting. When this is divided, the pleura is found to be shrivelled and a little indurated, contracted downwards and inwards upon the hard body, and the substance of the lung hardened and shrinking, enclosing the hard body, which is then found either like a portion of soft putty, or more consistent like chalk, slightly moistened with water. This is regarded as a cicatrized or contracted vomica. The putty-like or chalky contents are the thicker part of the softened matter of the tubercle after the thinner have been expectorated or removed by absorption. In cases of this kind, in which such chalk-like masses usually encysted, are contained in the apex or upper regions of the upper lobes, the rest of the lungs are in general either free from tubercular masses, or are little occupied by them, or present some miliary tubercles disseminated through their substance.

In some instances, these solid bodies are perfectly firm and almost stony, grating against the knife.

Changes of this kind, however, M. Louis thinks, do not depend on any determinate lesion. From the soundness of the rest of the lung, and the small space which such bodies occupy, it is possible that these putty-like bodies may be tyromatous masses in the early stage degenerated, and the calcareous concretions, phlebolites, or concretions in parts of the lungs previously inflamed.

2. In other instances, however, appearances of a less equivocal nature are recognized. In examining the bodies of persons who

have previously suffered from cough, breathlessness, expectoration, and wasting, there are found in the upper lobe of the lungs, irregular cavities lined by a semicartilaginous membrane, similar to that formerly described, but firmer and smoother, containing particles of whitish chalky-like matter, or even putty-like matter adhering.   In other instances, cavities irregular in shape, but marked by septa or partitions, are found lined by a firm smooth false membrane, empty, that is containing only air; while in the same lung may be found tubercular masses partially or wholly softened, and in some instances, crude tubercular masses.

At the near extremity of such cavities the bronchial tubes, which are truncated, are in general also dilated or enlarged in diameter; while those at the further extremity are shrunk and contracted, or altogether impermeable.   These cavities also themselves show a tendency to contraction by the lung, and even the thoracic parietes pressing them mutually together.   When this contraction or shrinking of the cavities takes place, the extremities of the nearer bronchial tubes also are contracted, from participating in the centripetal pressure; and, in some instances, they are impermeable and obliterated.   This lesion has been well represented by Reynaud in his fourth plate, fig. 1, who has detailed several cases, showing the frequency of obliteration of the tubes, in cases both of fatal phthisis, and in those in which partial recovery appeared to take place.

Lastly, In some instances in the apex of the lungs are found simply masses, fibrous and cellulo-fibrous, with firm cartilaginous intersections without cavity, and without permeable bronchial tubes.

From these several facts it is inferred, 1*st*, that the cavities now mentioned are tubercular cavities emptied and partially or wholly cicatrized; and 2*d*, that the solid firm portions are cavities in which great or complete contraction had taken place.

§ 11. KIRRHOSIS.—This name Dr Corrigan applies to the following condition of the lung.   The substance of the lung is firm and solid to touch, and void of crepitation; it is of grayish-red colour and tough; when divided, it is traversed, in all directions, by thick white bands of fibro-cellular tissue.   The bronchial tubes, instead of growing smaller in diameter as they proceed to their terminations, increase in size and capacity, until they terminate in oval or rounded cavities, in some of which are seen crowded together the openings of the small *bronchia*, giving them an appearance similar to that of the *bronchia* of the tortoise.   The lining membrane of the large dilated bronchia is red and thickened. The small bronchia are not permeable beyond their orifices. The tubes are generally filled with viscid puriform mucus. The lung itself is generally smaller than natural or contracted. No tubercles are observed. But it is common to find the pleura covered with lymph, or adhering to the costal pleura.

These changes Dr Corrigan ascribes to the previous existence of chronic inflammation in the filamento-cellular tissue of the lung, converting it into a fibro-cellular structure, which contracts toward the centre of the organ, and in its contraction draws along with it the elastic substance of the lung, in the same manner as the cellular tissue of the liver is supposed to contract that organ.*

This explanation is hypothetical. The lesion has been described and represented by Andral, Reynaud, and Dr Carsewell as hypertrophy and dilatation of the bronchial tubes. These are manifestly both dilated and their walls are thickened and hypertrophied, while their cellular or vesicular terminations are obliterated. These are facts. All the rest are opinions. All that can be said of this change is, that it seems to be the result of an inflammatory condition of the bronchial tubes, with obliteration of their extremities, sometimes with pleuritic exudation.

It seems impossible to establish any analogy between this morbid state of the lung and kirrhosis of the liver. In the latter disease, the acini or granular elements are hypertrophied, and they contain bile or the matter of bile, (taurine), and colouring matter, and crystalline fatty matter. Nothing analogous to this is seen in the lung with hypertrophied bronchial tubes.

§ 12. CONCRETIONS.—Hard gritty or stony bodies are very frequently found in the substance of the lungs.† The most usual situation for these bodies is at the apex of one or both lungs, or somewhere in the upper part of the upper lobe. In some cases the *pleura* adheres to the costal *pleura* over the site of these bodies, so that they are not recognized until the lung is removed from the chest. If the pleura do not adhere, it is observed that a shrivelled contracted appearance of the spot with some depression has taken place, as if it were the mark of a cicatrix or healed scar of the lung, while the

---

* On Cirrhosis of the Lung. By D. J. Corrigan, M. D. &c. Dublin Journal of the Medical Sciences, Vol. xiii. p. 206. Dublin, 1838.

† A Case of Obstructed Deglutition from a preternatural dilatation of, and bag formed in, the Pharynx. By Mr Ludlow, Surgeon, Bristol. Medical Observations and Inquiries, Vol. iii. London, 1769, p. 98.

substance of the lung, to the extent of one-third or half of a cubical inch is indurated. When this is divided, the centre of the mass is found to consist of a whitish-gray or bluish matter, very hard, and distinctly gritty, or with gritty particles disseminated through the mass. These bodies have been regarded by Laennec as the remains or vestiges of cicatrized *vomicæ*. It is possible that this may be the case. But it is to be observed that these concretions occur in lungs in which there are no tubercles and no *vomicæ* or traces of these cavities elsewhere.

Hard stony bodies may occur also in other parts of the lungs. These are variable in size, from the bulk of a millet seed to that of a bean. They are traced to blood-vessels, and are vein stones; (*phlebolitha*).   •

§ 13. PARASITICAL ANIMALS.—a. HYDATIDS.—The acephalocyst has been found in the lungs by many observers ; and in several instances, acephalocysts have been discharged by coughing.   They are formed either in the filamento-cellular tissue, or in the *pleura ;* from either of which they may find their way into the *bronchi* by suppuration, and hence be discharged by coughing.   Instances of this kind are not uncommon.*

On the origin and pathological relation of these bodies, a new, and, in several respects, peculiar view has been given by M. C. Baron, who, from the phenomena of various cases, traces an intimate connection between hemorrhagic effusions, and the presence of acephalocysts.   This author thinks, that when blood is effused into the pulmonic substance, the mass undergoes various changes, the central continuing red, the peripheral yellow.   The central portion may be expelled through orifices formed in the peripheral; or it is partly absorbed by the peripheral portion; which is thus progressively transformed into a cyst, which after some time may become a hydatid.†

This method of explanation seems more applicable to the origin

* Case of Hydatids discharged by Coughing.   Related in a Letter from John Collett, M.D., Newbury, Berkshire. Transactions of College of Physicians, Vol. ii. p. 486.   Lond. 1772.   135 acephalocysts coughed up in the course of 116 days.

Case of Hydatids coughed up from the Lungs.   By Dr Doubleday of Hexham. Medical Observations and Inquiries, Vol. v. p 143.   Lond. 1776.

Hydatids in the Air Tubes of the Lungs.   In a Letter from a Physician in London (Dr Pearson). Edinburgh Med. and Surg. Journal, Vol. vii. p. 490.   Edin. 1811.

Case of Hydatids discharged from the Lungs.   Guy's Hospital Reports, Vol. i. p. 507.   Lond. 1836.

† De la Nature et du Developpement des Produits Accidentels.   Par M. Le Doc. teur Ch. Baron.   Memoires de l'Academie, Tome xi. p. 381.   Paris, 1845.

of serous cysts than that of acephalocysts. The author nevertheless maintains its validity, because hydatids are found in the
blood, and their ova may therefore be effused with it. To this it
may be answered, that, admitting that hydatids or their germs
exist in the blood, it must be easy for them to find their way into
the lungs without the effusion of blood.

Hydatids, when existing in the lungs, either cause suppuration
and then expulsion with more or less disorder, general and local;
or they may die; the cysts contract and become opake; and they
then form a sort of lamellated tumour, the presence of which does
not appear to be detrimental.

b. WORMS.—Instances are recorded by several authors, among
others Schenke, of worms having been discharged from the lungs.
It has been generally believed—that these cases were the result of
the credulity of the recorders; and so perhaps some of them may.
The same objection, however, can scarcely be urged against a case
recorded by Dr Thomas Percival, who mentions that a patient,
aged 49, after cough and oppression at the breast, expelled
by coughing, in February 1774, two masses, the largest the
size of a nutmeg, of a chocolate colour, upon dividing which it
was found to contain a number of worms like maggots. The cough
and expectoration diminished in severity; but the result as to final
recovery is not stated.*

§ 14. HETEROLOGOUS GROWTHS.—Both skirrhus and enkephaloma have been represented to be found in the lungs. As to the
latter there is no doubt. The occurrence of the former is more questionable.

Bayle was the first who in 1810 directed attention to the precise
character of cancer in the lungs. He gives three cases; in the first
of which the cancerous masses were hard, and presented the white
shining appearance of fresh bacon or lard. In the other two the
tumours bore the characters of brain or genuine enkephaloma.
These were instances of enkephaloid disease affecting the lungs.

Laennec was decidedly of opinion that the structure named
Skirrhus does not take place in the lung, and that the only species
of Cancer found in these organs is the medullary sarkoma, or
enkephaloid deposit; and if careful attention be given to the cases
which were published both before and since his time, we shall see
reason to admit, that this inference is well founded.

* Philosophical, Medical, and Experimental Essays. By Thomas Percival, M. D.
Vol. iii. Lond. 1778.

.. The cases of enkephaloid disease published in 1817 and 1818 by Mr Langstaff showed, so far as negative evidence goes, that skirrhus does not affect internal organs; and that enkephaloma is the usual form in which malignant disease attacks the lungs. With the exception of one case referred to the head of tuberculated sarkoma, all presented the usual characters of enkephaloma; and probably this was enkephaloid deposit in the tuberculated form.*

These facts and considerations deducible from them, have led Mr Travers to consider skirrhus and enkephaloma as dependent on the same generating cause, and that this, whatever it be, produces in one order of organs, mostly external, the skirrhus deposit, and in another order, mostly internal, the enkephaloid formation.† · It is not easy to say whether this view be the correct one or not; but the facts which support it, show the truth of the doctrine which has been several times stated in the course of this volume, that enkephaloma is the most common malignant deposit that affects internal organs.

It seems indeed doubtful whether genuine skirrhus has been found in the lungs; for all the authentic cases hitherto recorded present the characters of the enkephaloid deposit.‡ It has been observed to pass from the *mamma* to the pleura, and thence to the lungs. This, however, is not the primary affection of the lungs by skirrhus.

ENKEPHALOMA is greatly more common, and, according to the most authentic evidence hitherto adduced, must be regarded as the principal form in which cancer affects the lungs. It may appear in four different modes.

In the first place, the enkephaloid matter is deposited in the bronchial glands, and causes the gradual enlargement of these bodies and their encroachment on the bronchial tubes, and the substance of the lungs. As this enlargement proceeds, the breathing is increased in difficulty, and fluid is effused within the *pleuræ*. The masses

---

* Cases of Fungus Haematodes with Observations, &c.   By George Langstaff, Esq., &c.   Medico-Chirurgical Transactions, Vol. viii. p. 272, &c.   London, 1817.

Cases of Fungus Haematodes, Cancer, and Tuberculated Sarkoma, &c.   By George Langstaff, Esq.   Medico-Chirurgical Transactions, Vol. ix. p. 297.   London, 1818.

† Observations on Local Diseases termed Malignant.   By Benjamin Travers, F.R.S., &c. Parts I. and II.   Medico-Chirurgical Transactions, vol. xv. p. 195 and 228.   Lond. 1829.   Part III. Vol. xvii. p. 300.   London, 1832.

‡ Case of Extensive Carcinoma of the Lungs.   By George Burrows, M. D., &c.   Medico-Chirurgical Transactions, Vol. xxvii. p. 118.   Lond. 1844.

Cases of Malignant Disease of the Lungs.   By H. Marshall Hughes, M. D.   Guy's Hospital Reports, Vol. vi. p. 330.   Lond. 1842.

vary in size according to the duration of the disease, from the bulk of a gooseberry or a filbert to that of small pippins. Most commonly several masses are found united in one irregular tumour; or they form a chain of tumours extending through the posterior mediastinum along the bronchial tubes. They are gray or gray-white, moderately firm, and present the usual characters of enkephaloma.

The presence of these bodies produces a peculiar form of breathlessness with *orthopnoea*; at first recurring in fits, afterwards constant, and causing a hissing, wheezing, roaring noise over the site of the bronchial tubes, with crowing inspiration.

In the second form, the disease affects the lungs in the chest, commencing either in the pleura, or in the substance of the lungs. The enkephaloid deposit may appear either in the encysted or the unencysted form. But in whichever way it appears, it rapidly occupies the whole interior of the chest, pushing the lung away from the ribs towards the mediastinum. After some time it occupies the whole of the interior of the chest with one continuous, yet lobulated mass of enkephaloid deposit. The presence of this may be known during life by the complete dulness emitted by the chest on percussion, and the total absence of respiratory murmur, with great breathlessness and debility.

After death, which follows quickly, the *demithorax* is found occupied with this enkephaloid mass, and the lung compressed into a very small space at the upper part of the thorax and the mediastinum, is scarcely to be recognized. The tumour presents the usual characters of enkephaloma. Some parts are soft, pulpy, and semifluid, like brain, or the brain of the fœtus; others are firm and consistent like cream-cheese; others are a mixture of soft gray-coloured cerebriform matter with blood and blood-vessels.

In the third mode of approach, the enkephaloid matter appears first in the liver, and after occupying the greater part of that gland, it proceeds to affect the diaphragmatic peritoneum, the diaphragm itself, the *pleura*, and the lower lobe of the right lung. Through this the enkephaloid deposit extends gradually until it occupies the middle lobe and the lower part of the upper lobe. In this case it is not easy to say whether the tumour displaces the lung, or the enkephaloid matter is infiltrated into the pulmonary substance, as it is in that of the liver. In the instances in which I have observed this mode of occupation, the new growth seemed to advance by successive steps from one texture to another, and the lungs appeared to be occupied from their proximity the organs first attacked.

In this mode of approach, the new growth passes to the left side of the diaphragm, the tendinous centre, the *pericardium*, heart, and part of the left lung. The extent to which the growth proceeds in this direction is a mere question of time. If life be sufficiently prolonged, the growth is found affecting a considerable portion of the left lung. If the patient be destroyed early, then less of that lung is involved.

It must further be allowed that enkephaloma appears to be deposited in the form of tuberous masses in the lungs, much in the same manner in which they are deposited in the liver. Such was the mode of deposition in the cases given by Mr Langstaff and Mr Lawrence. The tuberosities are further stated to have been enclosed within very delicate cysts. Some of these were very vascular. In one case given by Mr Langstaff, the deposit had affected the uterus and lungs, but not the liver or other abdominal viscera. These masses vary in size from the bulk of peas to that of small apples.[*]

When the disease appears in the left *demithorax*, it by its increasing size, not only displaces the lung to the mediastinum and upper part of the chest, but it thrusts the heart over towards the right side of the chest.[†]

Dr Warren records the case of a man of 25 in whom colloid cancer affected the subcutaneous cellular tissue, the absorbent glands, the skull, the muscles, the heart, the lungs, the liver, pancreas, and kidneys.[‡] Other instances, however, would be required to confirm the inference that colloid cancer affects the lungs.

§ 15. MELANOSIS.—Of this deposit two forms are observed to take place in the lungs; one true melanosis; the other consisting of a deposition or formation of carbonaceous matter from smoke and small dust inhaled, and which has been distinguished by the name spurious melanosis. Between these affections, however, though similar, there is no natural alliance.

In true melanosis the deposit takes place in two modes. In one it affects first the bronchial glands, infiltrating them with a dark-blue-coloured matter, most commonly solid, sometimes slightly fluid, semi-fluid, or pasty. The glands are at the same time enlarged, and. usually increase in size as the deposit proceeds; and

---

[*] Cases of Fungus Haematodes, &c. By George Langstaff, Esq. Medico-Chirurg· Transactions, Vol. viii. and ix.

[†] On Malignant Tumours connected with the Heart and Lungs. By John Sims, M. D., &c. Medico-Chirurgical Transactions, Vol. xviii. p. 281. London, 1833.

[‡] Peculiar Case of Gelatiniform Cancer, &c. with the Appearances on Dissection. By John C. Warren, M. D. Med.-Chirurg. Trans. Vol. xxvii. p. 385. London, 1844.

thus encroach on the lung. In the other mode, the melanotic matter is either infiltrated into the substance of the pulmonic filamentocellular tissue, or it is deposited in cysts contained or formed within the same. Of this, instances are given by various authors, among others, by Mr Langstaff.

The melanotic deposit is liable to occur in conjunction with the enkephaloid. In the first variety of the second case, the melanotic matter appears in the form of black or blue specks, patches, or lines and streaks disseminated through the pulmonic parenchyma. In this instance, they are probably in the interlobular filamentocellular tissue.

In spurious melanosis, the black matter is diffused pretty regularly through the whole lung. The expectoration is always more or less black; and the bronchial tubes are filled with black or darkblue puriform mucus. The bronchial membrane is tinged of a dark colour; and the substance of the lung is more or less extensively black; while it is often occupied with blue or black indurated patches and masses, and not unusually with tubercular masses and *vomicae*. From a lung in this state, a large quantity of black-coloured fluid may be expressed.

The cause of the blackening in spurious melanosis or the coal-miners' lung is various. In one set of cases, the black matter has been found to be coal in a state of very minute division, most probably mechanical. In another set of cases, it has been represented to be carbonaceous matter inhaled from the smoke of the lamps and candles used by the miners. In a third set, again, it has been maintained, that it is the carbonaceous matter inhaled after explosions of the adjoining strata by means of gunpowder. For farther information on all these points, I refer to the papers by Dr James Gregory,* Mr Graham,† Dr William Thomson,‡ Dr Hamilton, and Dr Stratton;§ and a memoir by M. Natalis Guillot.‖

* Case of peculiar Black Infiltration of the whole Lungs resembling Melanosis. By James C. Gregory, M. D. Edin. Med. & Surg. Journ. Vol. xxxvi. p. 389. Edin. 1831.

† On the Existence of Charcoal in the Lungs. By Thomas Graham, F. R. S. E., &c. Edinburgh Medical and Surgical Journal, Vol. xlii. p. 323. Edinburgh, 1834. Cases by G. Hamilton, M. D. &c. Case 2d. Edinburgh Medical and Surgical Journal, Vol. xlii. p. 297. Edinburgh, 1834.

‡ On Black Expectoration and the Deposition of Black Matter in the Lungs, particularly as occurring in Coal-miners, &c. By William Thomson, M. D. Med.-Chir. Trans. Part I. Vol. xx. p. 230. Lond. 1837; and Part II. Vol. xxi. p. 340. Lond. 1838.

§ Case of Anthracosis or Black Infiltration of the whole Lungs. By Thomas Stratton, M. D. Edin. Med. and Surg. Journal, Vol. xlix. p. 490. Edinburgh, 1838.

‖ Archives Generales, T. lxvii. p. 1. Paris, 1845.

· I merely observe that the general conclusion, which results from the history of all the cases recorded and their phenomena, as also from those which have fallen under my own observation, is, that, though black infiltration observed in coal-miners may exist without disease, or with little disease of the lungs, yet most commonly it is associated with very considerable disease both of the bronchial membrane and lungs. The former is almost constantly in a state of chronic inflammation. In the latter there are often tubercles, *vomicae*, or indurated portions, sometimes stony concretions. The lungs are also emphysematous. The pleura is often adherent over the apex, sometimes all over. The coal dust is inhaled by all coal-miners, and is stated to be freely spit up daily and from time to time without inconvenience or injury. When, however, the bronchial membrane becomes inflamed, either from exposure to cold or the inhalation of stony particles, or in working at stony strata, then the evil becomes urgent. The lungs are often occupied by tubercles; and the diseased state of these and the bronchial membrane aggravates into most deleterious effects the inhalation of carbonaceous matter, which seems not to be of itself very detrimental, unless it has been continued for a long time.

CHAPTER II.

THE HEART.

SECTION I.

STRUCTURE OF THE HEART.

THE heart is a complex organ consisting of muscular fibres, arranged so as to form its different chambers, covered externally by *pericardium*, and lined internally by a very delicate transparent membrane to which the name *endocardium* is given. The latter is the only element requiring notice here.

The endocardium is a very thin transparent membrane, which resembles much the inner membrane of the arteries, and which is composed, according to Henle, of four separate tunics. Its free surface is perfectly smooth, and is formed by a sort of epithelium, which is in immediate continuation with the epithelium of the vessels; that of the right chambers with the venous epithelium; that of the left with the pulmonary-venous and aortic epithelium. Next to this free or epithelial membrane is a layer of delicate and greatly

contorted fibres, similar to those which form the striated membrane
of the vessels.   Then is a layer of elastic fibres, which may be regarded as an elastic tissue.   Lastly, is a tissue which is called by
Henle ligamentous, but which is manifestly the filamentous tissue
that unites it to the muscular fibres of the heart.

Of these four tunics, the three first only are proper to the endocardium.   The fourth is common to it and the muscular fibres of the
heart.

This description applies most to the *endocardium* of the auricles.

Within the ventricles, the *endocardium* is altogether more delicate than in the auricles; the striated tunic is thinner; and the
strong elastic fibres are entirely wanting.

The tricuspid and mitral valves are formed by duplications of
this membrane; and in them the elastic tissue is abundant.

Section II.

Morbid States of the Heart.

The heart is liable to manifold lesions, which it would require a
considerable space to describe with the requisite detail and accuracy.
Several of these have already received consideration, for instance
inflammation and various lesions of the substance of the heart, under the head of diseases of the muscular system, and *pericarditis*
under that of diseases of the serous membranes.   The most important which deserve consideration here are inflammation of the
lining membrane, (*endocarditis*), and its effects, induration or ossification of the valves; hypertrophy, partial or general; atrophy; and
passive aneurism.

§ 1. Abscess of the heart.—This has been already considered
at some length.   Besides the cases there mentioned, I may notice
the following as not less conclusive.   Dr Chambers of Colchester
records an example of the lesion in a boy of fourteen.   An
abscess, containing two ounces of purulent matter, was found
deeply seated in the substance of the heart, and extending from
auricle to auricle round the apex of the organ.   In an instance of
partial inflammation of the substance of the heart, described by M.
Gintrac, matter was formed in the parietes of the left ventricle and
burst into the pericardium.

Mr Stallard of Leicester records an instance in a man of 60

* Case of Suppuration of the Heart. By Richard Chambers, M. D.   Lancet,
1844. July 27th. P. 557.

years, who was attacked suddenly, while at work, with coma, cyanosis, and great feebleness. On the third day death followed. The heart was fat, flabby, and rather larger than usual, and the pericardium contained about one ounce of dirty serum. The right auricle and ventricle were of normal size, and the valves were healthy. The lining membrane was of a deep violet or wine-coloured red. The left ventricle being opened, an abscess was observed situate near the apex, of an irregular shape, being· most pointed towards the apex, from which it was separated by two or three lines of sound structure. Above it projected into the cavity of the ventricle, with which it communicated by a small fissure. The interposed space was one line thick, and appeared to consist of thickened *endocardium.* The cavity of the abscess contained bloody purulent-looking fluid. Its lining membrane was of a light red colour, and was granular in appearance. The surrounding muscular tissue was darker than usual, and fibrinous clots were infiltrated. The coronary arteries were much ossified.*

In a female of 35, who had been suffering for some time under rheumatism of the right knee, I found, with the cribriform state of the aortic valves, in the walls of the auricles near the origin of the aorta, a cavity containing purulent matter, and extending into the attached margin of the semilunar valves. This was caused by inflammation of the muscular part of the auricles.

These cases merely confirm the truth of the general conclusions formerly established regarding this lesion.

· § 2. ENDOCARDITIS ET ENDOCARDOSTIA VALVULARUM. INDURATIO ET IN OS CONVERSIO. ARCTATIO VALVULARUM.—The lining membrane of the heart (*Endocardium*) is liable to inflammation, sometimes idiopathically, sometimes in consequence of rheumatism. The effect of this is, to render the folds, especially which form the mitral valve and sometimes those of the semilunar valves, thick, irregularly tuberculated with small hard eminences, inflexible, shrivelled, and contracted. At first albumen appears to be deposited in the interstices of the membranous folds; then the folds are shrivelled and thickened and indurated; the tendinous chords at the same time are shrivelled, thickened, and indurated; and, gradually, the three valvular folds, by the inflammatory action continuing both at their apices and their base, produce disorgani-

---

* Observations on the Pathology of Abscess of the Heart, with a Case. By J. H. Stallard, Esq. &c.   Provincial Transactions, Vol. xv.   London, 1847.

zation of the former, and a considerable degree of contraction in the latter.

As this process advances, it progressively renders the valve more stiff, hard, and unyielding, until it is converted into a sort of irregular ring of cartilage or bone, or cartilaginous matter, with patches of bone intermixed. The valve is then said to be ossified. The auriculo-ventricular aperture at the same time is so much contracted, that the blood no longer flows from the auricle into the ventricle with its wonted facility; and a small quantity only passes into the ventricle, while the auricle is kept in a constant state of distension, and is dilated, and sometimes its walls are thickened. In this state the auricle is said to be affected with hypertrophy.

In some instances the valve is occupied at its apices with warty tumours or growths, which have the same effect in rendering it stiff and immovable.

: The tendinous chords have been known to give way during great efforts, or long-continued running; and the rupture lays the foundation of disease of the tendinous chords and the valve. .

The change now described may take place at any period of life.; and it has been observed in persons aged 18, 22, and at all ages under 30. But it is more frequent beyond 40 than previous to that age.

It seems very often to be the effect of inflammation of the lining membrane of the heart, affecting chiefly the valve, taking place along with or after rheumatism; and even when it appears to take place slowly in the course of a long series of years, it is the effect of chronic inflammation of the membrane forming the valves.

The semilunar valves, at the origin of the aorta, are liable to be affected with the same stiffness and induration, and to be penetrated by steatomatous matter, cartilaginous matter, or portions of calcareous matter. In the beginning, and the slightest form of this kind of change, the semilunar valves lose their pliancy, and can no longer be made to fold completely into the axis of the artery. This is easily known in the dead body, by pouring a stream of water into the aorta, which, falling on the valves in their healthy state, detaches them from the sides of the artery, and makes them meet in the centre, so that the column of water is sustained by them. When they become rigid, cartilaginous, shrivelled, and lose their pliancy, they cannot be detached in this manner from the the sides of the vessel, but remain more or less fixed, so that the water passes from the artery into the ventricle. The valves are

thus inadequate to perform their function of preventing the blood
from flowing backwards into the ventricle, when propelled from that
chamber. In more advanced stages of this disorder, the valves are
more rigid, more firm, and more penetrated by calcareous matter;
their margins become rough, irregular and tuberculated or warty;
their substance thickened and firm, but very much shrivelled, so
that they no longer retain either their membranous character or
their semilunar figure; they gradually are transformed into a ring
of firm cartilaginous or calcareous matter; and, at the same time,
the orifice of the aorta is considerably contracted. In some instances, they remain in the horizontal position, as to the axis of the
artery, projecting from its walls in the form of hard firm growths,
and impeding much the issue of blood from the left ventricle.

Cartilaginous or osseous degenerations of the semilunar aortic
valves are not uncommon lesions. They may take place at any
period of life, after the fortieth year; but are found earlier; and
are most common in advanced life.

With or without the changes now mentioned in the aortic semilunar valves may be observed steatomatous and calcareous deposits
at the commencement of the aorta, and extending into the coronary
arteries. In the aorta, these deposits may be in the shape of flat
patches, or warty prominences and elevations, and sometimes the
inner membrane is detached, and it is observed that the blood has
been flowing over a hollow sac with a rough continuous surface,
like a small and imperfect aneurism. In some instances, these
patches are of the nature of bony spiculæ, and a considerable
space of the aorta is converted into a rigid calcareous tube.

The coronary arteries are occasionally affected with the same
deposit; and then become rigid, firm, and unyielding, deranging
the circulation through the heart, causing atrophy of the organ,
and rendering it feeble and unable to contract with due force on
the blood. Such a change has been supposed to give rise to the
symptoms of *Angina pectoris;* but it has been observed to take
place without inducing any symptoms, yet causing sudden death
either by syncope or paralysis of the heart.

These steatomatous deposits consist of fat in a crystalline state or
cholesterine.

Cartilaginous or calcareous transformation of the tricuspid and
semilunar pulmonary valves is much more rare; a fact noticed by
Bichat, and repeated since his time by most pathological writers,
as distinctive of the difference between the internal membrane of

6

the arterial system and that of the venous. The lesion, however, is not unknown. Instances of its occurrence are given by Vieussens, Hunald, Morgagni, Bertin, the elder Horn, Cruwel, Corvisart, Burns, and Mr Bransby Cooper. In a slight degree, that is, in the state of cartilaginous induration, it is occasionally observed in the tricuspid valve, and less frequently in the semilunar pulmonary valves. It is a remarkable circumstance, that the cartilaginous or ossified state of the valves of the right chambers of the heart is found chiefly in the persons of those who present a preternatural communication between the right and left chambers of the organ; and from this, Laennec infers that the action of the arterial blood has considerable influence in the production of these calcareous deposits.

Small granular bodies loosely adhering to each other are liable to grow on the valves, especially in the left chambers of the heart, and sometimes from the walls of the heart itself. These loose granular bodies, which have been usually denominated warty growths, (verrucæ), and vegetations, have been ascribed by Kreysig, Bertin, and Bouillaud to the influence and effects of inflammation. The justice of this opinion Laennec questions, though he admits that a false membrane, produced by inflammation, might form in some rare cases the nucleus or rudiment, as it were, of the concretion. Laennec further ascribes these productions to partial coagulation of the blood. It seems to me doubtful, nevertheless, whether Laennec has not in this view adopted too limited notions on the nature of inflammation. Though these substances are so loose and soft that it is difficult, if not impossible, to preserve them, yet it appears to me that they may be the result of chronic inflammation of the lining membrane of the heart; and it is some argument in favour of this idea, that these productions are often associated with other changes, which are known to be the result of inflammatory action; for instance, cartilaginous and steatomatous transformation and calcareous deposition. By Scarpa and Corvisart they are ascribed to the influence of the syphilitic poison. It is a well ascertained fact that they are frequent in the bodies of those who have been subjected to the full and repeated influence of mercury.

The lesions now described may exist for some time alone. But the most usual course is, that they either give rise to, or are complicated with, certain changes in the dimensions and capacity of the chambers of the heart, and various changes in the muscular walls of the organ.

Thus when the mitral valve is rendered firm or calcareous, and the auriculo-ventricular aperture is contracted, the left auricle be-comes dilated and sometimes hypertrophied, that is, its walls become thick and firm.

The most common changes of this kind are dilatation of the ven-tricles, dilatation of the right chambers, and hypertrophy of the ventricles.

§ 3. ATROPHY OF THE VALVES.—PERFORATING OR CRIBRIFORM ATROPHY.—The valves of the aorta and the folds of the mitral' valve are liable in certain circumstances to become extremely thin, and at length to be perforated by small irregular holes. In this state they are unable to perform their functions as sustaining and resisting membranous folds, against the weight of the blood; and not only does the lesion cause regurgitation, but the valves may give way and be ruptured.

This cribriform state is most common in the aortic valves; next to these in the mitral valve. It is occasionally seen in the triens-pid valve, and sometimes, though rarely, in the pulmonary semi-lunar valves. It appears to be a species of wearing, the effect of previous brittleness and attenuation, and these again the result of chronic inflammation.

§ 4. CONTRACTION AND ABRIDGMENT.—Under the operations of chronic inflammation and aberration in nutrition, the valves are liable to be not only indurated and thickened as already de-scribed, but to be shortened. Thus the semilunar valves at the origin of the aorta are liable to be in this manner drawn together, and shortened. In some instances two valves appear to be united, or to have coalesced into one; or one is unusually short and con-tracted; or the whole three may be drawn together at their margins. In the same manner he *laciniæ* of the mitral valve are liable to become very much shortened, thickened, and drawn together.

It may be doubted whether this last mentioned change is justly de-signated as atrophy. It is evidently one of the contracting effects or remote consequences of the shrivelling ensuing in certain forms of the inflammatory process in certain tissues. It appears to be the result of inflammatory action in the elastic fibrous tissue of the middle valvular tunic.

These changes are most frequently observed in the mitral and aortic semilunar valves; less usually in the tricuspid and pulmo-nary semilunar valves.

§ 5. The latter are liable to a lesion of a very important nature from its connection with various malformations of the heart.

The orifice of the pulmonary artery is liable to three forms of lesion. The first is an unusually contracted or narrow state of the cylinder of the artery, the capacity of which may be not half its normal size, or at most between that and three-fourths. A second is narrowing, sometimes obstruction even to obliteration of the channel of the artery. This is usually accompanied with, if not caused by, more or less thickening of the arterial walls, and may be accompanied with some effusion of lymph or blood in the interior of the vessel at the part. In some instances it is like false membrane uniting the opposite sides of the artery.

The third is more or less occlusion of its interior by coalescence and mutual adhesion of the valves. The most usual form of this is for the three semilunar valves to be united by their margins, leaving at their *apices* only a very moderate sized aperture. Of this there are various degrees, regulated mostly by the size of the central aperture. In some cases it is large enough to admit the tip of the little finger. In others it is so contracted that it allows only a catheter of middle size to pass. And in others, the aperture is so small that it admits only a common probe. Several instances of this lesion I have published ;* and others are given in the work of Kreysig on Diseases of the Heart, and in that of Gintrac on *Cyanosis.* The latter author mentions that the pulmonary artery was thus contracted in 16 among 53 cases of cyanosis, and in five more the orifice was obliterated.

The semilunar valves are in general thickened, and sometimes they are indurated. They form in short a septum or diaphragm, perforated in the centre, stretched across the orifice of the pulmonary artery.

The cause of this lesion is not known. In several cases it is manifestly congenital, and must have originated in the fœtus. It is possible that at that period when the artery and its valves were small, slight inflammation may have taken place at the origin of the pulmonary artery, and thus produced there mutual adhesion and coalescence. If this were the case, then it is easy to see, that this lesion would keep the pulmonary artery almost if not wholly in its fœtal state, so that enlargement and expansion with the other organs of the body could not advance. This might be in different

* Notice of a Case of Cyanosis or the Blue Disease connected with mutual adhesion of the Semilunar Valves of the Pulmonary Artery. By David Craigie, M.D., &c. Edinburgh Medical and Surgical Journal, Vol. lx. p. 265. Edin. 1843.

degrees; but in all the effect would be to keep the orifice of the artery more or less obstructed.

Such I believe to be the cause of the coalesced state of the semilunar valves in cases of this class.

This coalition of the valves is very constantly connected with more or less malformation of the heart, by which the two sides of that organ communicate. Thus it is observed in open *foramen ovale*, in perforation or deficiency of the septum, and in cases in which the aorta arises from the right ventricle, or from both ventricles at once. I have elsewhere attempted to show that, taking into consideration all the circumstances of this lesion, it is probably the cause of these communications, or bears to them such a relation that the arctation of the pulmonary artery renders these communications between the right and left chambers requisite.

In some rare cases only two semilunar valves are found at the orifice of the pulmonary artery; and Dr Theophilus Thomson records a case of· unusually large pulmonary artery in which it was provided with four valves.*

§6. DILATATION OF THE VENTRICLES, (*Ampliatio,*) PASSIVE ANEURISM of Corvisart, consists in enlargement of the chambers of the heart, with thinning of their walls. The muscular substance is at the same time unusually soft and flaccid, sometimes of a violet colour, in other instances pale and almost yellowish. In such instances the substance of the heart must be regarded as in a state of atrophy, hypotrophy, or imperfect nutrition. The substance is at the same time lacerable. The extenuation may be so extreme that the thickest part of the ventricle does not exceed two lines, and the apex is scarcely half a line; or the muscular substance may be so stretched, attenuated, and absorbed, that nothing but a little fat covered by pericardium retains the blood. Laceration, in such circumstances, as ·Burns imagined, seems not impossible; yet neither Corvisart nor Laennec met with any instance of this accident in consequence of dilatation of the left ventricle; and in none of the recorded instances of rupture does the accident appear to have been the result of extenuation, so much as friability or ulceration.

This disease M. Bertin ascribes to the operation of obstacles or impediments to the circulation; for instance, ossification of the valves, and arctation of their apertures, congenital straitness of the pulmonary artery or the aorta, professions requiring painful efforts,

---

* Account of a Case of Irregular Formation of the Heart, &c. By Theophilus Thomson, M. D. Medico-Chirurgical Transactions, vol. xxv. p. 247. London, 1842.

and certain diseases of the lungs, as consolidation and tubercular induration. Though the influence of these causes is considerable, the most general and the most powerful is original conformation ; that is, an unusually narrow pulmonary artery as to the right ventricle, and a narrow aortic orifice as to the left ventricle. Several instances of passive dilatation of the left ventricle, I have seen associated with ossification of the aortic semilunar valves, and consequent arctation of the orifice. When the right ventricle is dilated, the lesion is usually connected with more or less disease of the lungs ; and the right auricle becomes at length affected in the same manner.

§ 7. HYPERTROPHY or excessive nutrition of the heart may be said to consist in increased thickness of the muscular substance of the organ, which is at the same time, in general, firmer and more dense than natural. It may exist in one ventricle only, or extend to both ; and it may be general or partial. When the left ventricle is affected, it may exceed one inch, or be even eighteen lines in thickness at the base, which is fully double or three times thicker than in the natural state. When the ventricle is generally affected, it is thickest at the base, and diminishes gradually to the apex ; but the apex sometimes participates to the extent of from two to four lines. If the apex is affected, the disease is generally local. In other instances, partial thickening appears most commonly in the neighbourhood of the valves. In the case of the right ventricle, the increased thickness is more uniform, extending over the whole, and rendering it so firm as not to collapse when cut open. The preternatural change, however, is always most distinct in the neighbourhood of the tricuspid valve, and in that part of the ventricle which gives origin to the pulmonary artery. The bulk of the fleshy pillars (*columnae carneae*), is always much increased ; and this condition, which is more conspicuous than in the left, with the great firmness of the muscular substance, forms a striking feature in the anatomical characters of hypertrophy of the right ventricle.

Hypertrophy has been distinguished by M. Bertin into three forms, according to the effect it exerts on the capacity of the chambers of the heart, or according to the mode in which the increased deposit of material is applied ;—1*st*, simple hypertrophy; 2*d*, excentric hypertrophy; and 3*d*, concentric hypertrophy.

In the first form, the walls of one or more of the chambers of the heart are thickened, while the chambers are neither enlarged nor diminished in capacity. This is *simple hypertrophy*, in which the increase of matter may be regarded as applied from the inner surface outwards.

In the second form, the walls of the chambers are thickened, while the capacity of these cavities is enlarged. This is *excentric hypertrophy*, in which, with the increase of matter from within outwards, there is exerted in the same direction a dilating or distending force. This corresponds with the *active aneurism* of Corvisart.

In the third form of the disorder, the thickening of the walls of the heart is combined with diminution in the capacity of the ventricles, as if the new matter had been added chiefly to the interior of the ventricle, or had been deposited, at least, from the exterior to the interior surface. This is, therefore, named *concentric hypertrophy*.

No doubt has ever been entertained as to the existence of the two first forms; for instances of simple hypertrophy have been observed by Morgagni, Corvisart, and others, though they have not been carefully distinguished; and excentric hypertrophy is by far the most common lesion to which the heart is liable. It is different with concentric hypertrophy, the existence of which has been called in question by Cruveilhier in France, and Dr Budd in this country, both of whom ascribe to the mode and circumstances in which death takes place, the appearance deemed characteristic of that lesion.

Cruveilhier has observed in the bodies of those who had suffered death by decapitation and those cut off by violent death, the two phenomena of great contraction or even obliteration of the ventricle, and proportional thickness of the walls of the heart, and he infers, therefore, that these phenomena are the effect of this species of death, and regards the concentrically hypertrophied hearts of M. Bertin and Bouillaud as hearts more or less hypertrophied in persons overtaken by death in the full energy of contraction. He further argues, that, as it is always possible to open and dilate these hearts apparently without cavity, by introducing several fingers, these circumstances indicate more forcibly that the state of the heart is the effect of the last vital contractions.*

Dr Budd, finding that in such hearts the ventricle becomes re-

* Dictionnaire de Medecine, Art. Hypertrophie.

laxed to its usual capacity after the heart had been macerated a few days, and that during life there was no intermittence or irregularity of pulse, no dilatation of the right cavities, and no symptoms of impediment to the circulation, arrives at the same conclusion.*

It cannot be denied, that, in various instances of sudden death, as death by hemorrhage, and also in many instances of death by cholera, the left ventricle is found in this greatly contracted state, hard, firm, with thick walls, and almost no cavity, the internal surfaces of the ventricle being closely applied to each other, and the ventricle being entirely empty. It is also to be observed, that this state of the heart is found in persons, in whom none of the usual symptoms of disease of the heart were observed to take place during life, and consequently in whom the existence of such a lesion was not suspected. It may be admitted, then, that, in a certain number of cases, especially where this state of the heart is found after violent death, sudden death by hemorrhage, or sudden death from other causes, it is not positively indicative of a peculiar morbid state of the heart during life.

It seems, nevertheless, a conclusion too violent to infer, that, of all cases in which this state of the heart is found, none is to be regarded as the effect of morbid thickening of the ventricle with contraction of its chambers. M. Bouillaud, accordingly, who maintains the correctness of the views of M. Bertin, records in his work on Diseases of the Heart, eight cases of concentric hypertrophy of the right ventricle, and five of concentric hypertrophy of the left ventricle.

I have met with a few cases of this state of the heart, independent of those which I observed in the bodies of persons destroyed by cholera; and in the Clinical Report for 1832-1833, are mentioned three cases, in two of which I think no doubt could be entertained of the existence of this lesion. In the one case, in which death was caused by granular disease of the kidney, the cavity of the left ventricle was almost obliterated by the close mutual application of the walls, which were very thick, firm, and hard. In the other case, in which death was caused by an attack of erysipelas, the cavity of the ventricle was equally contracted, and its walls were nearly as thick and firm as in the former; and the patient had presented during life symptoms of *angina pectoris*.†

* Medico-Chirurg. Transact. Vol. xxi. London, 1838.
† Clinical Report for 1832-1833, Edinburgh Med. and Surg. Journal.

Excentric or aneurismal hypertrophy is, nevertheless, by far the most common lesion; and the extent to which the heart may be enlarged by it is very great. The circumference of the base of the heart may amount to from 12 to 16 inches; its transverse dia. meter, 6 or 9; and the longitudinal diameter, from base to apex, from 5 to 7 inches.

The increase in weight is the most conspicuous change. The minimum weight of the adult heart is about 6 ounces 2 drachms; the average weight about 8 ounces. In the state of hypertrophy, however, the weight is increased to 12 or 13 ounces at least, and may be so great as 22, 26, or 28 ounces. The average of seventeen cases recorded by Bouillaud amounts to 16 ounces. The thickness of the walls of the left ventricle varies from 7 to 14 lines. The thickness of those of the right ventricle varies from 3 to 5 lines.

This lesion gives rise to, or is connected with, others very important to be known. It is often associated with a bloody or hemorrhagic consolidation of the lungs and hæmoptysis; and, in a considerable proportion of cases, it gives rise to softening or hemorrhage in the brain.

Excentric hypertrophy is often associated with cartilaginous or calcareous degeneration of the semilunar aortic valves, and sometimes with that of the mitral valve.

Excentric hypertrophy is, in a large proportion of instances, the result of rheumatism affecting the heart, and giving rise to *endocarditis*. This can in general be known by the fact, that the individual has suffered rheumatic pains in the wrists and ankles, or in the elbows and knees, previous to the appearance of the symptoms of hypertrophy. In some cases, hypertrophy, adhesion of the pericardium to the heart, and valvular disease, are united in the same individual.

§ 8. PARTIAL ANEURISM, OR CONSECUTIVE FALSE ANEURISM.— This consists in a portion of the muscular fibres of the heart giving way, so as to form in the muscular walls of the organ a cavity, sac, or pouch, communicating by an opening with the cavity of the chamber, in the walls of which the pouch has been formed.

This change may take place in any part of the muscular substance of the heart; but it is most usually seen in the left ventricle, near or towards the apex. In various affections of the heart, but especially in dilatation, with more or less disease of the aortic semilunar valves, it is not uncommon to observe, formed near the apex of the left ventricle, small cavities or pouches, while the muscular walls at that part are rendered extremely thin. These cavities, which contain blood in the shape of adherent clots, are formed by a gradual separation of the muscular fibres and some degree of dilatation; but no laceration or breach of continuity is in general to be perceived.

It is different with partial aneurism. The muscular fibres undergo an interruption or solution of continuity in the transverse direction quite perceptible; and by their retraction and separation, a cavity or pouch, variable in size and shape, but generally round or ovoidal, is formed in the walls of the heart. In some instances the fibres are completely destroyed, and the outer wall of the pouch is formed by the pericardium alone. This appears to have taken place in a case by M. Dance, and in the case of the actor Talma.

The interior of these pouches or cavities in the walls of the heart may be filled with coagulated blood, adherent to the walls, and, in some instances, arranged in the form of *laminæ*, as in aneurism of arteries. In some instances they are empty, or contain only a little clotted blood or blood plasma adhering to the walls of the pouch.

This lesion generally takes place in the anterior or lateral part of the walls of the left ventricle, or near the apex in the anterior and left side. In ten cases among seventeen well-marked instances of the disease collected by myself, the tumour was situate near or formed in the apex. In a few cases it is found in the *septum cordis*. In one case which was under my own care, the pouch or sac was formed in the base of the septum;* and it formed a large round prominence in the right ventricle. In an instance given by Dr Pereira, the cavity was formed in the substance of the *septum*, and consisted of four subordinate pouches, one of which had burst into the right ventricle.† Mr Thurnam mentions three instances, also in the *septum*,‡ and Bouillaud gives one.§ In a case given by Zannini, the origin of the aneurismal tumour was

* Observations and Cases illustrating the Nature of False Consecutive Aneurism of the Heart. By David Craigie, M. D. Edinburgh Medical and Surgical Journal, Vol. lix. p. 356. Edinburgh, 1843.

† Case of Partial Aneurism of the Left Ventricle of the Heart. By Jonathan Pereira. Medical Gazette, October 1845, and Edinburgh Med. and Surg. Journal, Vol. lxvi. p. 503. Edinburgh, 1846.

‡ On Aneurisms of the Heart, with Cases. By John Thurnam. Medico-Chirurgical Transactions, Vol. xxi. p. 187. London. 1838.

§ Traité Clinique des Maladies du Cœur. Par J. Bouillaud. Paris, 1835. 2ième Edition. Tome i. p. 594. Paris, 1841.

situate in the lower end of the septum, and extended into the apex
formed by the walls of the heart.*

. In size these aneurismal pouches vary. Some are small, not
larger than a gooseberry; others are much larger, and make a
large projecting tumour externally, altering much the usual figure
of the heart.

. The disease has been observed in general in persons above 25;
and several of the cases have occurred in persons advanced in life.
In only one case among 58 was the patient under 20 years. In the
case given by Dr Pereira, the disease took place in a girl of 15
years, which is the earliest period yet recorded at which it has been
observed.

. Partial aneurism of the heart is generally associated with other
lesions of that organ and its valves. Thus the aortic valves are
very generally rigid, steatomatous, or penetrated with specks and
patches of bone. In some instances they are cribriform or perforated by holes. In a few cases, the mitral valve is rigid and slightly
ossified. In most cases, the lining membrane is more or less thickened, and not unfrequently white opaque spots in it are visible.
Round the pouch itself there is usually observed a layer of fibres,
rough, firm, and rigid, not unlike horse-hair. The ventricle,
either right or left, is usually in a state of hypertrophy. In the
case examined by myself, the heart weighed with the aorta 32
ounces; and if for the latter one ounce and a half or two ounces
be deducted, it makes the heart 30 ounces, which is about three
times more than the average weight of the adult heart in a state of
health.

Upon the mode in which these pouches are formed, it is not easy
to give a decided opinion. It seems certain that, in most instances,
the muscular fibres of the heart are lacerated transversely, and separated in their longitudinal direction. When the pouches are
carefully examined, one portion of the sac is always more or less
distinctly formed, by what we know must be the ends of the contorted muscular fibres of the heart. These, it is true, are lined
or covered by lymph and blood; but when this is removed, and
even sometimes without, it is possible to trace the fibres ending
abruptly.

On the mode in which the laceration takes place, or the causes
by which it may be produced, much difference of opinion prevails

* Observations and Cases, &c.. By Dr Craigie. Case 9.

among writers on pathology. M. Breschet, regarding it as false consecutive aneurism of the heart, and, therefore, analogous to the false consecutive aneurism of the arteries, studies to illustrate its nature and origin by appealing to the history of the cases of rupture or laceration of the heart. Many instances of this lesion have been recorded, and the successive observations of Harvey, Lancisi, Verbruggen, Morgagni, Senac, Lieutaud, Morand, Portal, Corvisart, and recently of Ferrus, Laennec, Rostan, Blaud, Bayle, and the two MM. Rochoux, have furnished so much information on the circumstances, in which rupture is most likely to take place, that we cannot expect to know much more on that subject. It is known that these accidents, though they may occur in any part of the organ, are, nevertheless, by far the most common in the left ventricle, and especially at the apex. This circumstance is probably to be ascribed at once to the greater thinness and weakness of the parietes at the apex, and to the strength and energy with which the left ventricle contracts. It is almost clear to demonstration, that, of any muscular organ, of which the greater part is thick and strong in structure, and forcible in action, while one part is a little thinner, the latter is most likely to give way during any action of the organ unusually forcible or violent. This will, of course, be much more likely to happen where either unusual resistance is presented, as in disease of the aortic valves, or where the action is morbidly increased from morbid though partial increase in the thickness of the parietes of the heart.

M. Breschet seems to think that the position of these lacerations may be employed to explain the origin of the false consecutive aneurism of the heart, and he directs attention to the important fact, that, in the ten cases which he records, and most of which are abridged in the memoir referred to, in most the lesion was situate at or near the apex of the left ventricle. The right ventricle, he observes, presents nothing of this nature, nor did his researches bring him acquainted with any instance of its occurrence in the right ventricle. He allows, however, that we are not entitled, from so small a number of cases, to deduce any very positive conclusions.

M. Breschet, nevertheless, very properly refers to three conditions which have been believed to be, almost necessarily implied in the sort of lesion now described. These are; 1st, softening of the tissue of the heart, that is, of its muscular fibres; 2d, ulceration of the inner membrane; and 3d, rupture of the muscular fibres; and while he questions the effective operation of the two former, be advocates somewhat strongly the influence of the third cause. I must refer my readers to the original paper for the arguments by which he maintains the justice of his cause.

In point of fact, while Mr Thurnam has shown that this species of aneurismal dilatation or rupture may occur not only in the left ventricle, but in the right, and also in the auricles, the 22d case which is recorded in the memoir by the author, and the instances of the lesion taking place in the *septum cordis*, prové that the lesion may take place not merely at the apex of the heart, but at the base of the septum. It must be allowed, therefore, that, though the lesion is most liable to take place at or near the apex of the left ventricle, it may be found in other parts of the heart, and consequently that the circumstances concerned in its production must be applicable not to the apex only, but to other parts.

By M. Bouillaud an idea somewhat different has been advanced, viz. that the false consecutive aneurism of the heart is one of the effects or terminations of inflammation in the muscular substance of the heart. This author informs us, " that the formation of an aneurismal cyst consecutive to ulceration of the internal and middle membranes of the heart, is accomplished by the same mechanism as that of an aneurismal cyst of the arteries. The lamellar disposition of the coagulum is exactly the same in the false consecutive aneurism of the heart, as in the false consecutive aneurism of the arteries. I need not, therefore, dwell at length here on the anatomical description of this accident of the ulcerations of the heart. The tumour formed by the blood infiltrated and coagulated is very different in quantity. Thus it may in some instances not be equal to the size of a walnut or filbert, while in other cases it exceeds the bulk of an egg, and may even be greater than that of the two ventricles together."

It cannot be denied that this mode of explaining the origin of the aneurismal cysts of the heart is to a certain extent plausible. Several of these cysts present appearances of ulceration ; and if it could be proved that the ulceration always precedes the formation of the cysts, and is always the effect of previous inflammation, the question would be decided. This is, however, very far from being the fact, or the constant result in all cases. Not only do instances of aneurismal cysts in the substance of the heart take place without any indications of previous inflammation or ulceration ; but in several of the cases, indeed the majority, the lesion exists for a long time without presenting any of the symptoms of the inflammatory or ulcerative process. Thus, in the well-known case of Talma, there was no indication of previous inflammation or ulceration, and after it had taken place, and lasted for at least three years, it did not indicate its presence by any very marked symptom of any kind, and assuredly by none indicating the presence of inflammatory action, either acute or chronic. In almost all the other cases also no conspicuous or urgent symptoms took place to denote the exact date of the commencement of the lesion, which has, in most instances, been discovered unexpectedly in examining the heart after death.

It must be allowed, nevertheless, that the inflammatory process, without proceeding to ulceration, as Bouillaud requires, may have a tendency to produce this lesion, by the change which it effects on the tissues, in which it is seated. It is one of the most constant, perhaps, of the properties of this process, to impair or destroy the tenacity, elasticity, cohesion, and resisting power of the animal tissues, and in none more decidedly than in the muscular. All textures after inflammation are rendered more fragile and more lacerable. This is particularly the case with the arterial tunics, with tendons, with cartilages, and with the bones, and above all, with the muscular tissue, which becomes less distensible, less contractile, and more rigid than before. It is possible that some new deposit may have been formed in it. But even this does not seem necessary; and the simple pre-existence of the inflammatory congestion appears to be all that is requisite to induce this sort of lacerability.

It is not improbable that these facts and considerations appeared so conclusive to M. Cruveilhier, that, in proposing another circumstance as a preliminary or predisposing cause of false consecutive aneurism, he found it difficult, if not impracticable, to exclude the influence of the inflammatory process. From various phenomena presented by the tumours and cysts in this lesion, but especially from the phenomena presented by the preparation described in Case 17 in the memoir by myself, he infers that, in every instance of false consecutive or partial aneurism of the heart, one of two processes is in operation ; one the inflammatory action, and the other the fibrous transformation of the muscular tissue of the heart. To the latter, however, which he believes to be often primary or idiopathic, and not accompanied by inflammation, he assigns the principal place. Numerous facts, he informs us, lead him to conclude that the idiopathic fibrous transformation of the muscular fibres of the heart performs a greater part in the formation of partial aneurism than inflammation ; and if the apex of the heart be often the seat of the lesion, the reason is, that it is the weakest part of the left ventricle, and therefore the most frequent seat of the fibrous transformation, so common a consequence of distension of the muscular tissue.

The reason why the right ventricle, he adds, is less frequently affected by partial dilatation is, that its walls are less thick, and its structure more areolar than that of the left ventricle. The vigour and force with which the left ventricle contracts is the anatomico-physiological cause of its predisposition to this disease.

When the fibrous transformation has commenced in one point of the walls of the heart, he infers that the distension which takes place at each contraction becomes an incessant cause of irritation ; and there are formed in this non-contractile sac clots which may serve as a barrier to oppose the enlargement of the tumour. He adds that he has seen cases, in which the shape of the heart was not sensibly altered externally, though its apex presented the commencement of this fibrous sac or recess, and the presence of such a state had been denoted by no symptom during life. The correctness of this observation I can confirm from personal knowledge ; and of this the case of the young man, No. 21, which occurred in my own practice, is an excellent example.

When, however, the part thus transformed into fibrous tissue is dilated into a sac superadded to the ventricle, or pushed beyond the level of its internal surface, yet communicating with its cavity by a narrow orifice, it constitutes the partial aneurism described by authors.

M. Cruveilhier, however, does not apply to all these tumours the name of false consecutive aneurism ; and he makes a distinction between this and partial aneurism of the heart. By partial aneurism of the heart, M. Cruveilhier understands dilatation of one portion of the heart into a cyst, in consequence of the fibrous transformation of the tissue of the organ. These parts, however, may become eroded, and hence may be lacerated ; and while the cardiac pericardium prevents complete rupture, either alone or by its having contracted adhesion with the capsular pericardium, the partial aneurism of the heart would then be converted into false consecutive aneurism.*

* Cruveilhier Anatomie Pathologique, Livraison xxi.

He maintains also that the partial aneurism of the heart commences always by dilatation, and ought, therefore, to be regarded as a true aneurism.

Throwing aside this distinction in the meantime, it must be admitted, that the point for which M. Cruveilhier contends, as the main predisposing cause of aneurism of the heart, namely the previous fibrous transformation of the muscular tissue, is one which derives considerable force from the appearance of many of the examples of the lesion. In the majority of these, the aneurismal sac or cyst has presented, as in the 17th case of the essay, more or less of the fibrous structure. In the case which occurred in my own practice, this fibrous transformation was remarkably distinct, both on the side of the left ventricle, and also on that of the right, most so certainly in the latter, where it formed a firm strong prominent mass, convex in shape towards the right ventricle. This fibrous structure was also distinctly visible and very strong at the margin of the opening of the sac into the left ventricle. In all the cases detailed in my own memoir, the fibrous structure is remarked at the margin of the orifice of the cyst, which is described as firm, elevated, and generally whitish.

The only question for consideration would appear to be, whether has this fibrous transformation taken place before the aneurismal dilatation or after its occurrence? I am not sure that any of the facts which I have recorded, or which have come to my knowledge, are capable of determining this point.

With regard to the other point maintained by M. Cruveilhier, viz. the distinction between *true or partial aneurism* of the heart and *false consecutive aneurism* of the heart, it appears to me that, in the present state of knowledge, it must be considered as a distinction rather in the degree and stage than in the nature and kind of the lesion. Several of these aneurismal cysts appear to commence at first by slight laceration, and then to be enlarged by dilatation. Several, on the other hand, especially those near the apex of the heart, appear to commence first by dilatation, and then to be enlarged by some degree of laceration. In many the two processes are conjoined; and it seems difficult to say which of them is the first. It is admitted even by M. Cruveilhier himself, that the form of the disease which he denominates *partial aneurism* is earlier and less advanced than that named *false consecutive aneurism*, and in which the fibrous transformation, not yet effected in the former, is far advanced or completed.

One word only have I to add on the probable mechanism of such cases of aneurismal cyst as that which occurred to myself. The septum at its base becomes very thin ; and if it be carefully dissected or boiled, it is found that, at the base, its muscular fibres, gradually attenuated, are stopped by cellular tissue, and that on the base, as it were, is fixed that part of the heart containing the two auricles and the commencement of the pulmonary artery and aorta. If, therefore, by any morbid action, the base of the septum were rendered fragile or brittle, or its cohesion with the auricular part of the heart were weakened or destroyed, it is not difficult to understand that it might be thus detached, and gradually made to give way and form an aneurismal sac at its base.

Though it is doubtful whether abscess is the cause of this lesion, I think various facts show that chronic inflammation is the main predisposing cause of its origin. In the first place, the disease takes place in persons rheumatic or gouty, or who have had rheumatism ; and in whom often the *endocardium* is or has been inflamed. In the second place, the effect of inflammation, it has been shown, on the muscular tissue is to destroy its elasticity, to render it brittle and easily lacerable, and sometimes to soften it. If therefore inflammation were attacking either the *endocardium* and spreading to the muscular fibres, or were attacking the latter from the first, it is easy to see that it might cause in an organ so liable to distension and in action so incessant, laceration. In the third place, we find the lesion preceded or accompanied by various changes in different textures of the heart, which are generally regarded as effects of chronic inflammation.

§ 9. ATROPHY. STEATOSIS.—The muscular fibres are pale, or yellow-coloured, soft, flaccid, and lacerable. The organ is small and shrunk, and collapses. Fat-globules and cholesterine are infiltrated into the cylinders of the muscular fibres.

§ 10. MALFORMATIONS.—These must be mentioned very shortly. The most important are those which cause the communication of the right and left chambers, or the venous and arterial sides of the heart ; with various degrees of that blue or violet colour of the skin, called *Kyanosis*.

These are the following. 1*st*, The *foramen ovale* or aperture of Botallus, more or less open, sometimes forming a large and direct communication between the auricles. 2*d*, The *septum cordis* being deficient, or open, or perforated, congenital, or acquired ; or the two last mentioned united ; as in the case by Landoury.* 3*d*, The aorta arising in such a manner that its orifice corresponds to a congenital aperture in the *septum*, most commonly at the base of that partition. 4*th*, The aorta arising at once from the right and left ventricle, as in the case recorded by Sandifort, that by Dr Nevin, and in the 47th case given by Gintrac, the case of M. Olivry, in the case recorded by Dr George Gregory, in one given by Chassinat,† and in one given by Casper.‡ 5*th*, The pulmonary artery arising from the left ventricle, while the aorta arises from the right, as in the case recorded by Baillie, one by Hildebrand,§ and one by Dr Walshe.‖ 6*th*, The aorta and pulmonary artery arising from the left ventricle, as in the case recorded by M. Marechale. 7*th*, Only one auricle and one ventricle, the latter giving rise to one trunk, which afterwards divides into the aorta and pulmonary artery. 8*thly*, One auricle and one ventricle, giving rise to a separate aorta on the right, and a pulmonary artery on the left, as in the two cases given by M. Thore.¶

These errors in formation may be traced to one of two causes ; arrest or interruption in the process of development ; and misadaptation of constituent parts. All of them, however, are further connected with some form and degree of that obstruction or arctation in the orifice of the pulmonary artery already noticed. My limits and the nature of this work do not allow me to enter into detail on the consideration of this subject ; and all that I can here

---

* Observation de Communication Anormale entre les cavités du Coeur, &c. Par H. Landoury. Archives Generales, T. xlviii. p. 436. Paris, 1838.

† Observations d'Anomalies Anatomiques remarkables de l'appareil circulatoire, &c. Par M. le Docteur Raoul Chassinat. Archives Generales T. xli. p. 80. Paris, 1836.

‡ Wochenschrift fur die Gesammte Heilkunde. Herausgegeben von den D. D. Casper, Romberg und v. Stosch. Jahrgang, 1841. No. 13.

§ Merkwurdige Missbildung des Herzens und der Grossen Gefüsse. Von Dr Hildebrand. Graefe und Walthers' Journal der Chirurgie und Augenheilkunde, Bd. xxix. Heft 3, Seite 490.

‖ Case of Cyanosis depending on Transposition of the Aorta and Pulmonary Artery. By W. H. Walshe, M. D. Medico-Chirurgical Transactions, Vol. xxv. p. 1. Lond. 1842.

¶ Memoire sur le Vice de Conformation du Coeur, consistant seulement en une Oreillette et un Ventricule. Par M. Thore. Archives Generales, T. lx. 316. Paris, 1842.

Note sur une Anomalie du Coeur chez un Enfant nouveau-né. Par M. Thore. Transposition of the Aorta which is on the right ; the pulmonary artery and auricular appendages on left ; one Ventricle. Archives Generales, T. lxi. p. 199. Paris 1843.

say is, that the facts carefully examined render it highly probable, that this obstruction and impediment in the orifice of the pulmonary artery is the incipient phenomenon in the series of changes, in short, must be regarded as the main cause of those imperfections, to which the name of malformations is applied.   While this impediment is in any manner formed at an early period of fœtal existence, the other changes with *kyanosis* follow as matter of course.

The first two defects, open *foramen ovale*, and imperfect septum, are the most usual.   These are the immediate consequences of arrest of development in the formation of the heart.

In the early period of fœtal existence, it is known, that the heart consists of two chambers only, that is, one auricle and one ventricle.   The auricle, in the natural progress of formation, begins about the end of the second or the beginning of the third month to be divided into two portions,—a right and left,—by one thin membrane proceeding from its posterior surface forwards, and another thin membrane advancing backwards from its anterior surface. These have crescentic margins, which in the natural course meet and pass, overlying or imbricating each other, so as at the period of birth, or soon after, generally to complete the partition.   When however, from obstruction or impediment in the orifice of the pulmonary artery, the blood which enters the right ventricle cannot obtain by that vessel and the *ductus arteriosus*, a ready outlet, its copious passage from the right to the left division of the auricle continues uninterrupted and undiminished, and the membranous folds are not only prevented from meeting and overlapping each other, but their increase is suddenly stopped, and the *foramen ovale* remains unclosed.

The *septum* of the ventricles is a growth partly from the posterior wall of the common single ventricle, partly from the anterior wall, beginning at the apex and proceeding in growth towards the base.   In the early period of fœtal existence, the blood which enters the right ventricle, and which is supposed to be chiefly that which comes from the head, neck, and superior extremities, enters also the left, and there partly proceeds to the aorta without, it is believed, entering the pulmonary artery.   There is at least nothing to prevent this, as the right ventricle communicates directly with the left at the base till the seventh week, when the opening is still large.   As intra-uterine life advances, however, provision is made for stopping this by the gradual growth of the *septum* towards the base ; and at the end of the second month the *septum* is usually completed, and the orifice is closed. This growth, however, may be interrupted at any stage of its progress, early or late; and the interruption is most likely to take place, when the orifice of the pulmonary artery is small and more or less obstructed. If the interruption take place early, the *septum* is very imperfect, perhaps perforated in the middle. If it take place late, it is still imperfect, though less so, and is deficient only at the base of the heart, so as to allow blood easily to enter the aorta. Hence it results that the septum is imperfect or perforated, and that often with that is necessarily conjoined either the aorta communicating with the right ventricle, that is, its orifice corresponding with an aperture in the septum, or arising from that chamber and the left at once.

The rare example of the heart consisting of only one auricle and one ventricle is merely the extreme degree of this form of arrest of development.

The case of the pulmonary artery arising from the left ventricle, while the aorta issues from the right, takes place in a different manner. A degree of mal-apposition in the vessels and the ventricle must have taken place at an early period of fœtal existence. This we know takes place with other organs, with bones for instance, and with certain portions of the abdominal and thoracic viscera.

All these lesions now mentioned are in different degrees incompatible with the continuance of life. Their incompatibility is very nearly in the order in which they are arranged. But to this must be added, that their incompatibility and fatality are regulated, to a certain extent, by the degree in which the orifice of the pulmonary artery is contracted and obstructed. If the contraction be not very great, life may be continued for years; and the individual, though feeble, and evidently imperfectly nourished, may attain the adult age or beyond that. If the contraction be greater, and so considerable that the blood does not readily enter the orifice of the artery, though he attain the age of puberty, life is rarely prolonged beyond that period. *Kyanosis* is considerable and almost constant. If the aperture be still smaller, the individual dies in infancy, or may be cut off a few days after birth. And when the artery is entirely obstructed, death takes place shortly after birth.

§ 11. HETEROLOGOUS GROWTHS.—The heart is observed to be involved in enkephaloma when that structure appears in the lungs and in the liver; and it is also affected by the melanotic deposit. In the first case the enkephaloid matter forms a species of investing mass encroaching on the whole substance of the heart. In the latter case, the melanotic deposit may either appear in this manner, or it may be infiltrated into the substance of the organ.

§ 12. EKTOPIA. DISPLACEMENT.—The heart is pushed to the right side in cases of empyema of the left pleura, with copious effusion. This, however, is the mere effect of the effusion; and disappears when that is absorbed. This is not *ektopia*.

This term is applied to those displacements of the heart, in which, from some deficiency in the formation of the enclosing parts, as the sternum, the ribs, the diaphragm, the heart is found in a situation different from its natural. The common point or character is, that the heart is out of the cardiac region; and it may be either in that of the head, that of the chest, or that of the abdomen. The first is rare. The second and third, which are more common, have been distinguished by Fleischmann and Weese under the names of *Ektopia Pectoralis* and *Ektopia Ventralis*.

Under the head of *Ectopia Pectoralis* are comprehended all those instances of displacement, in which the heart protrudes on the surface of the chest, either with deficiency of the sternum and ribs, or these remaining entire, at either extremity of the sternum.

Under the head of *Ektopia Ventralis* are comprehended those instances in which, from deficiency of the diaphragm, the heart is protruded among the abdominal viscera.

In the first case it is rare to find the heart protruded without deficiency of the sternum and ribs. It has been observed, however, by Weese in the sheep. More commonly the sternum is wanting, or it is divided by a fissure. With this other malformations are usually associated; for instance the *foramen ovale* open, the *septum* perforated, and the aorta connected with both ventricles. The *pericardium* is sometimes wanting; and in some instances the mediastinum is deficient.

Ektopia Ventralis may be attended either with integrity or more or less deficiency of the sternum and ribs. The prolapsed heart is sometimes surrounded by a membrane like that of a hernial sac.

To these forms of *Ektopia* Breschet has added that in the region of the head, *Ektopia Cephalica*.

For details I refer to the Commentary of Weese,* and the Memoir of Breschet.†

* De Cordis Ectopia Commentatio Anatomico-Pathalogica. Auctore Carolo Weese, M. et Ch. D. Accedunt Tabulae Aeneae vi. Berolini, 1819. 4to.

† Memoire sur l'Ectopie de l'Appareil de la Circulation, et particulierement sur celle du Coeur. Par G. Breschet, D. M. &c. Repertoire Generale, T, ii. p. 1. Paris, 1826.

INDEX.

Cæcum, inflammation of   Page 632
Calcareous and osseous deposits in
  brain   .   .   .   347
———— concretions in lungs, on
  their origin and indication 1033, 1035
Capillary vessels, system of, characters 131
———————— morbid processes
  taking place in   .   .   136
Cartilage, its structure and forms   490
———— its morbid states   .   492
———— adventitious deposits of, in
  serous membranes   .   .   740
Cartilaginous union of ribs and other
  bones   .   .   .   478
Cauliflower excrescence of the uterus 680
Cerebellum, morbid states of   .   300
Cheloid tumour   .   .   541
Chest, malformation in bones of 478, 481
Chondroma, character of in brain   344
———— of serous membranes   740
Chondrosis of ureters   ●   . 943
Choroid plexus, inflammation in   724
Cirsoid aneurism, its characters   100
Coal miners' lung, on its nature   1041
Colloid cancer in mucous membranes 676
Conarion or pineal gland, morbid
  states of   .   .   . 349
Concretions, lacrymal   .   827
———————— salivary   .   .   829
———————— in pancreas   .   848
———————— in hepatic ducts   .   903
———————— in gall bladder and ducts 919
Congestion, on its characters   .   139
Consolidation of lungs, on its nature
  and causes   .   .   . 983
Contraction, morbid, of hand and fingers   .   .   .   421
Corpuscula of bone described   432
Croup, its nature and seat   .   577
Cystidia, chronic inflammation of
  bladder   .   .   :   657
Cystirrhœa, suppurative catarrh of
  bladder   .   .   .   655
Cystosarkoma of mamma   .   963
———————— in testis   .   971
Cysts in cellular tissue   .   48
—— in kidney   .   .   961
—— in liver   .   .   909
—— in mamma   .   .   963
—— in testis   .   .   971
Delirium taking place in the phthisical 722
Demodex Folliculorum, the follicular
  worm, its characters   .   530
Desmodia, inflammation of ligament
  and fascia   .   .   417
Desmosis of testis   .   .   970
Diastasis or separation of epiphyses   447
Diffuse inflammation, its pathological
  characters   .   .   37
Dilatation of bronchi   .   . 605
———————————— the effect of
  aneurismal tumours   .   606

Dilatation of the heart   Page 1050
Disjunctive inflammation, its seat and
  characters   .   .   58, 67
Displacements of mucous membranes 680
Diverticula   .   .   . 682
Dropsies, causes of   .   . 191, 709
Duodenum, morbid states affecting   620
Dura mater, thickening of   .   743
Dysentery, its seat and characters 639, 640
Ear, disease of, giving rise to abscess
  of brain   .   .   .   286
Echinococcus in the liver   .   908
Ekthyma, characters and seat   .   525
Ektopia of heart   .   .   1066
Elephantiasis, its nature   .   194
Emphysema, superficial, pneumatosis 46
———————————— of lungs   594
Empyema, its causes and nature   713
Enkephalia, its nature   .   .   277
Enkephalaemia or apoplexy, state of
  brain and vessels in   .   .   291
Enkephalelleipsis, deficiency of brain
  or its parts, its causes   .   355
Enkephaloma in bones   .   .   488
———————— in brain   .   .   352
———————— in joints   .   .   756
———————— in kidneys   .   963
———————— in liver   .   .   911
———————— in lungs   .   . 1036
———————— in mamma   .   967
———————— in pancreas   .   851
———————— in serous membranes   742
———————— in testis   .   .   971
Entozoa in brain   .   .   904
———— in liver   .   .   917
———— in lungs   .   .   1036
Enteria (enteritis mucosa)   .   620
Epiphora, its seat   .   .   568
Erectile system, its anatomical characters   .   .   .   169
———————————— its morbid states   176
Exanthemata, their seat   .   506
Exfoliation of bones, different sorts of 450
Exhalant vessels, their characters   187
———————————— morbid states in
  them   .   .   .   190
Exostosis, different sorts of   451, 474
———————— medullary exostosis   474
Fascia, palmar, chronic inflammation
  and contraction of   .   .   421
Fat-globules in the renal tubules in
  granular disease   .   .   953
———————————— in arteries   1046
———————————— in liver   .   901
———————————— in heart   .   1062
Fever, on the state of the vessels in   156
—— on the state of the blood in   163
—— state of the brain in   .   316
Fibrous, white, system, its structure
  and distribution   .   .   414
———————————— diseases tak-
  ing place in   .   .   .   417

EDINBURGH : PRINTED BY STARK AND COMPANY,
OLD ASSEMBLY CLOSE.